YOUR GUIDE TO

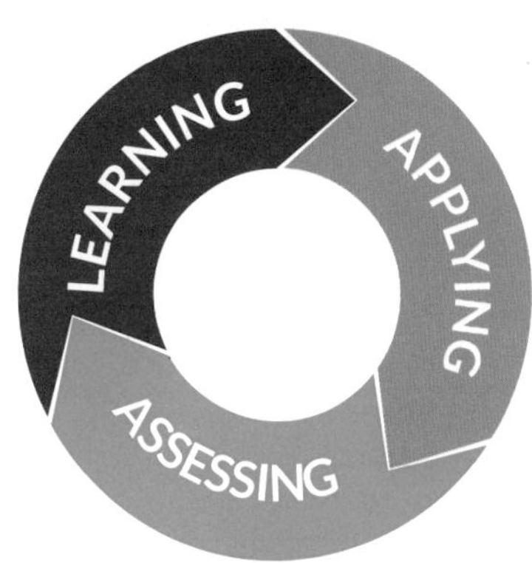

Pediatric Nursing

The Critical Components of Nursing Care

Everything you need to succeed...
in class, in clinical, on exams, and on the NCLEX®

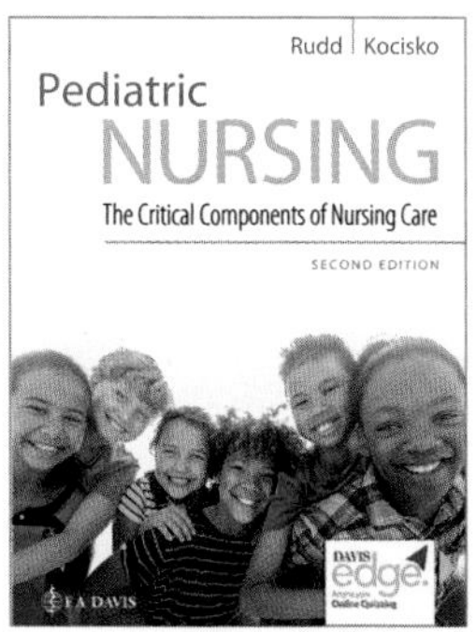

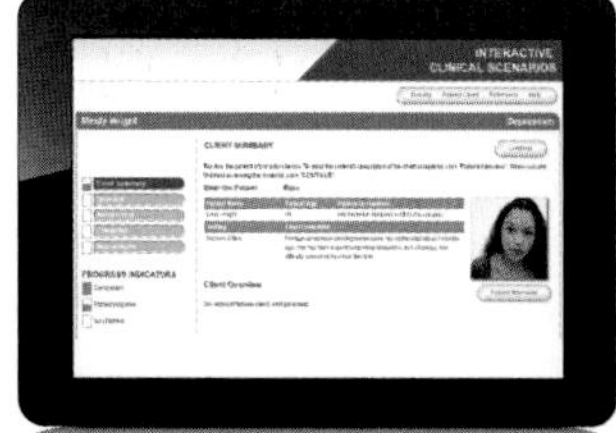

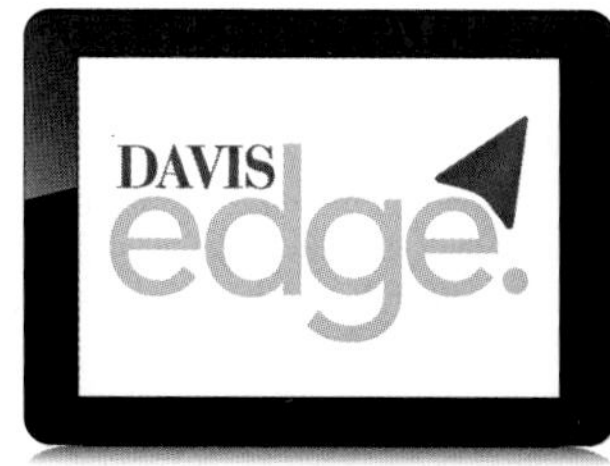

LEARNING

Your text provides the foundational knowledge you need to know.

APPLYING

Interactive Clinical Scenarios show you how theory applies to practice.

ASSESSING

Davis Edge is the online Q&A review platform that evaluates your mastery of the material and builds your test-taking skills.

Your journey to success

BEGINS HERE!

Your text works together with Interactive Clinical Scenarios and Davis Edge to make this often-intimidating, but must-know content easier to master.

Don't miss everything that's waiting online to make learning less stressful... and save you time. Follow the instructions on the inside front cover to use the access code to unlock your resources today.

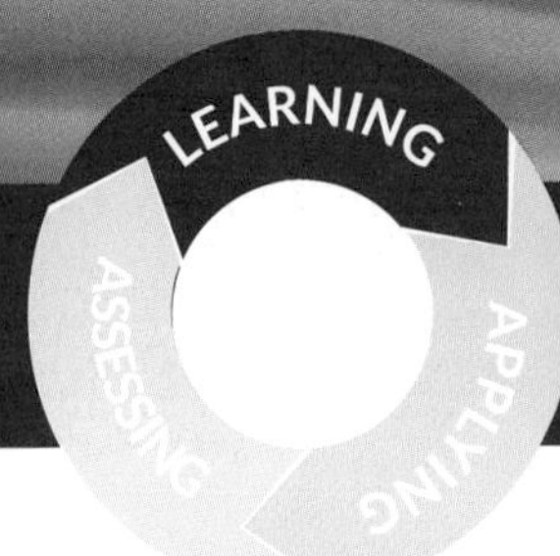

LEARNING

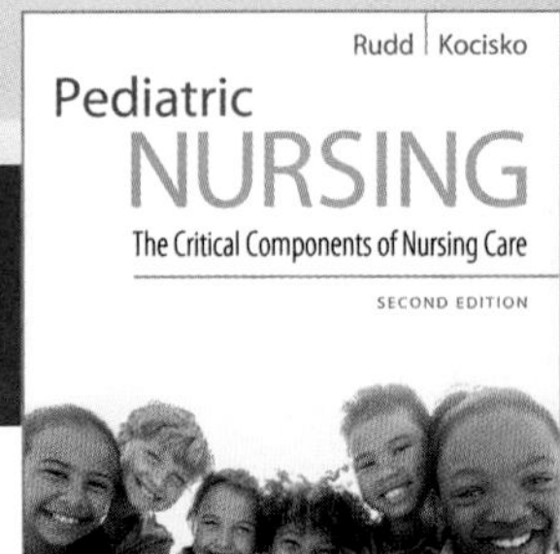

STEP #1

Build a solid foundation.

Critical Component Boxes highlight essential information in each chapter.

CRITICAL COMPONENT

Object Permanence

Object permanence is one of the most important developments in the sensorimotor stage. The child now knows that an object exists even when it cannot be seen or heard. This is a wonderful time to introduce the game peekaboo; by the end of this stage the child will understand that you did not disappear just because your hands are over your face.

SAFE AND EFFECTIVE NURSING CARE: Clinical Pearl

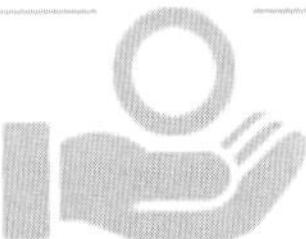

Separation Anxiety

Nurses need to take into account growth and developmental stages when a child is hospitalized or ill. Ages 6 to 9 months often go through separation anxiety. They will often find more comfort in familiar people than strangers. Being in the hospital can trigger separation anxiety for toddlers (2–3 years). Preschoolers can fear body mutilations, the dark, being left alone, and ghosts (Beckett & Taylor, 2016).

Safe and Effective Nursing Care Boxes summarize important safety concepts, such as understanding medications and patient education.

Evidence-Based Practice Boxes focus on current research-based and practice guidelines related to nursing care.

Evidence-Based Practice: Adult Literacy and Readability of Health-Care Education

Healthy People. (2017). Health communication and health information technology. Retrieved from https://www.healthypeople.gov/2020/topics-objectives/topic/health-communication-and-health-information-technology

Healthy People 2020 identified health literacy as one of its core objectives. In 2017, the Centers for Disease Control and Prevention (CDC) estimates that 90 million adults have low health literacy (CDC, 2017). In 2011, 64.1% of people aged 18 years and older reported that instructions from health-care providers were easy to understand (Healthy People, 2017).

Objectives of *Healthy People 2020* include:

- Improving the health literacy of the population
- Increasing the proportion of patients who indicate that communication with health-care providers was satisfactory
- Increasing the proportion of patients who use electronic health management tools
- Increasing individual internet access
- Increasing the number of quality health-related websites
- Increased social marketing in health promotion and disease prevention
- Increased crisis and emergency risk messages to protect the public health (CDC, 2017)

Background

Multiple studies have demonstrated a correlation between low literacy and poor health-care behaviors and outcomes, such as frequent emergency care visits and hospital admissions, decreased compliance with medications, improper use of metered-dose inhalers, incorrect installation of infant car seats, failure to seek screening and later diagnosis of cancer, and poorer glycemic control, to name just a few examples (CDC, 2017).

According to the Centers for Disease control health literacy is "the degree to which individuals have the capacity to obtain, process, and understand basic health information and services needed to make appropriate health decisions" (CDC, 2016, para. 1)

Recommendations

- Health education materials intended for *adults* should be created at a reading level no higher than eighth grade, although most are written at a more difficult level.
- Try the SMOG (Simple Measure of Gobbledygook) approach to assess and adjust readability. Details on this method and a SMOG calculator are available through a website belonging to its originator, Harry McLaughlin (see the later "Additional Resources" section for the link.)

Case Study

Emily is a manager in a technology company who is currently on maternity leave following the birth of her second child. While she is on leave, she attends the community center sporadically with her two daughters. Audrey has just turned 4 years old and will be attending kindergarten soon. Kathryn is 4 months old. Emily usually does not interact much with staff at the community center, but today she asks questions about Kathryn's sleep patterns. Kathryn still wakes up two to three times per night and Emily is exhausted. Her wife is a company executive and travels a lot. Emily admits that her wife thinks she must be doing something wrong with Kathryn, because Audrey was a better sleeper. She can't stand Kathryn's crying in the evening and her frequent waking at night. Emily has been reading some books and thinks she should be able to get Kathryn into a routine that includes sleeping for 8 hours at night. She is very frustrated. While you are talking with Emily, Kathryn is playing with a toy and is watching other children playing nearby. She coos and makes sounds. As soon as she makes a noise Emily puts a pacifier in her mouth. Audrey is playing with some of the other children. A little boy takes the toy she has been playing with, and she tries to take it back. When that doesn't work, she throws herself on the floor and screams. Emily quickly offers her treats from her purse. Emily states Audrey has frequent outbursts at home and she does not know how to deal with them.

1. What stage of development are Audrey and Kathryn in according to Erikson?
2. What factors can have an impact on Audrey's development?
3. What strengths and weaknesses does the family have?
4. What strategies based on Kathryn's development can the nurse suggest?
5. What concerns can you identify regarding Emily's parenting of the girls?

Case Studies at the end of the chapter let you test your understanding and apply your knowledge in a clinical context.

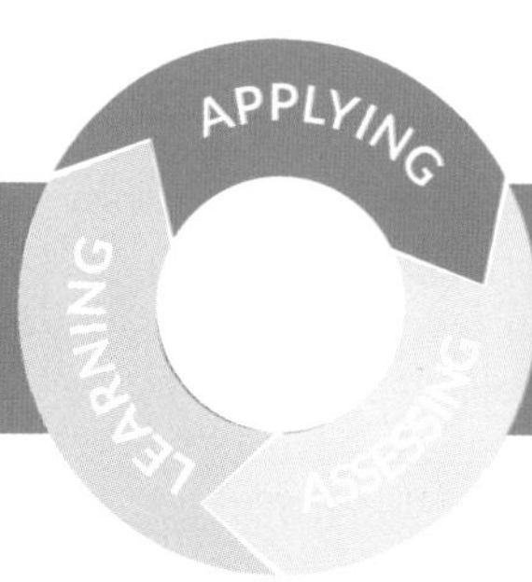

APPLYING

STEP #2

Practice in a safe environment.

- Ethics
- Failure to Thrive
- Growth & Development
- Teen Sexuality
- Tetralogy of Fallot
- Child with Gastroesophageal Reflux
- Cupping
- Trauma
- ADHD
- Respiratory Syncytial Virus
- Child with Type 1 Diabetes Mellitus
- Anorexia Nervosa

Interactive Clinical Scenarios walk you through the nursing process with client summaries, multiple-choice questions with rationales, drag- and drop activities, and so much more.

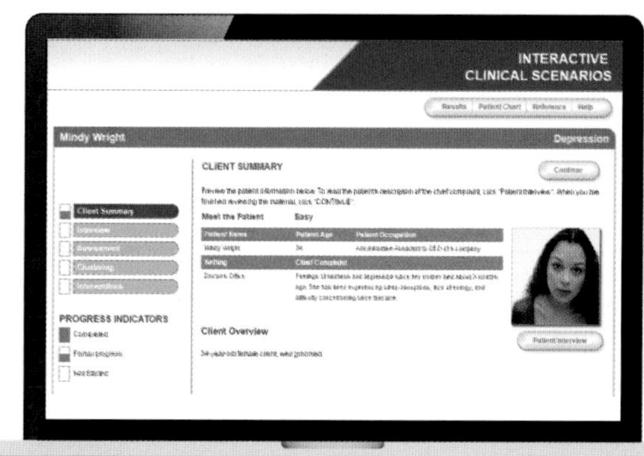

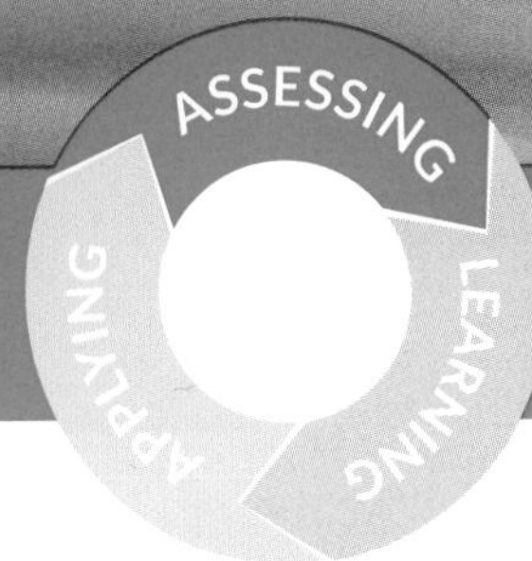

ASSESSING

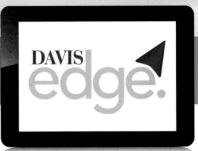

STEP #3

Study smarter, not harder.

Davis Edge is the interactive, online Q&A review platform that provides the practice you need to master course content and to improve your scores on classroom exams. Access it from a laptop, tablet, or mobile device for review and study on the go.

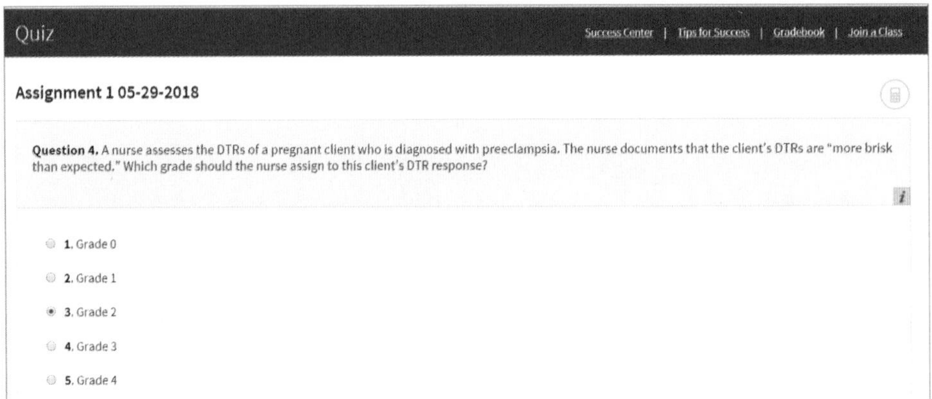

Assignments are made by your instructor. Or, create your own practice quizzes to review before an exam.

Comprehensive rationales explain why your responses are correct or incorrect. Page-specific references direct you to the relevant content in *Pediatric Nursing.*

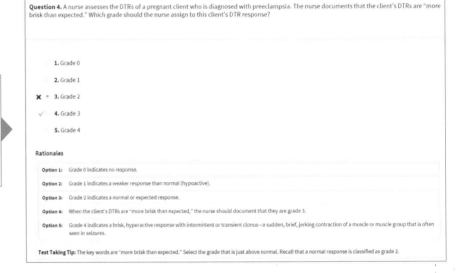

Test-taking tips help you understand how to tackle difficult questions.

The Success Center offers a snapshot of your progress and identifies your strengths and weaknesses.

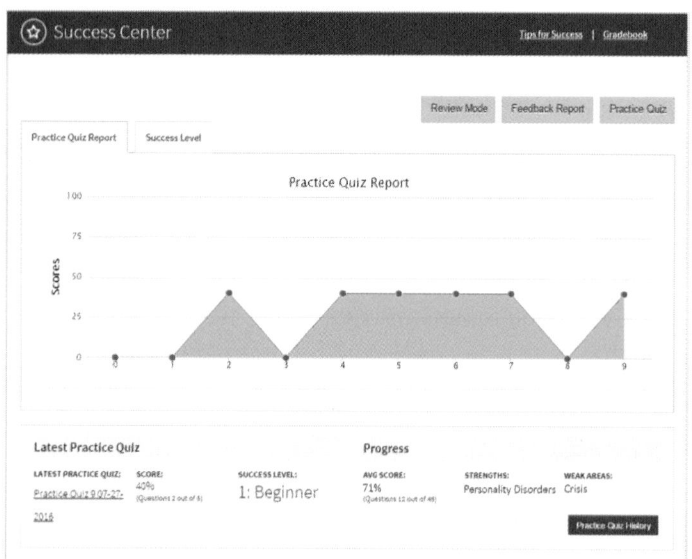

Feedback Report

Success Center | Tips for Success | Gradebook

Feedback Report

Create Practice Quiz On Weak Areas | Course Topic

Strengths and Weaknesses will appear for a specific course topic or concept once you have answered a minimum of 10 questions in that area. Select to view by Course Topic or Concept from the drop down box above. Choose 'Create quiz on weak areas' above to begin creating a new quiz based on all weak areas.

Course Topic	Strength / Weakness	Number of Questions Answered	Success Level	Create Quiz
Anxiety, Obsessive-Compulsive and Related Disorders	● Needs More Practice	10	1: Beginner	Create Practice Quiz
Bereaved Individual, Mental Health Nursing of	● Needs More Practice	25	1: Beginner	Create Practice Quiz
Biological Implications	Strengths and Weaknesses will appear for a specific course topic or concept once you have answered a minimum of 10 questions in that area	6	1: Beginner	Create Practice Quiz

The Feedback Report drills down to show your performance in individual content areas. It's easy to create new practice quizzes that focus on your areas of weakness or to select the topics or concepts you want to study.

★★★★★

"Davis Edge is the reason why I passed my course."

– Sakina Anderson, Student at La Grange College

95% of students surveyed received a B or higher in their class using Davis Edge.

SECOND EDITION

Pediatric NURSING

The Critical Components of Nursing Care

Kathryn Rudd, DNP, RN, C-NIC, C-NPT
Clinical and Didactic Educator
Cuyahoga Community College
Notre Dame College
Capella University
Cleveland, Ohio

Diane M. Kocisko, MSN, RN, CPN
Director, Nursing Education & Professional Practice
The MetroHealth System Department of Nursing
Cleveland, Ohio

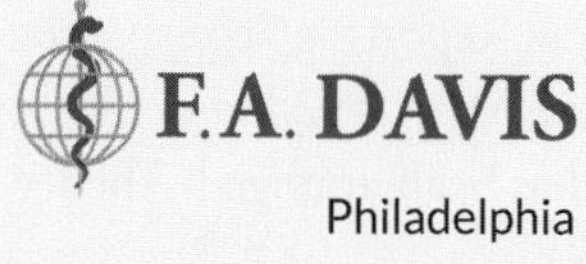

Philadelphia

1915 Arch Street
Philadelphia, PA 19103
www.fadavis.com

Printed in the United States of America

Last digit indicates print number: 10 9 8 7 6 5 4 3

Acquisitions Editor: Jacalyn Sharp
Developmental Editor: Andrea Miller
Manager of Project and eProject Management: Catherine Carroll
Content Project Manager: Amanda Minutola
Design & Illustration Manager: Carolyn O'Brien

Library of Congress Cataloging-in-Publication Data

Names: Rudd, Kathryn, editor. | Kocisko, Diane M., editor.
Title: Pediatric nursing : the critical components of nursing care / [edited by] Kathryn Rudd, Diane M. Kocisko.
Other titles: Pediatric nursing (Rudd)
Description: Second edition. | Philadelphia : F.A. Davis Company, [2019] | Includes bibliographical references and index.
Identifiers: LCCN 2018024560 (print) | LCCN 2018025032 (ebook) | ISBN 9780803694002 | ISBN 9780803666535 (pbk.)
Subjects: | MESH: Pediatric Nursing—methods | Nursing Care—methods | Child | Infant | Adolescent
Classification: LCC RJ245 (ebook) | LCC RJ245 (print) | NLM WY 159 | DDC 618.92/00231—dc23
LC record available at https://lccn.loc.gov/2018024560

To my husband, Daniel Rudd,
and
my mother, Joan Antesberger, for their love and support.
Kathryn Rudd

To my mother, Kathleen Kocisko, for her love,
encouragement, and affirmation.
Diane M. Kocisko

Preface

FOCUS

Pediatric Nursing: The Critical Components of Nursing Care is a pediatric nursing textbook that emphasizes fundamental pediatric nursing content focusing on evidence-based practice. This textbook with its accompanying ancillaries presents pediatric concepts that may be useful for programs designed to present the subject of pediatrics in an abbreviated or condensed manner. It was designed to address the contemporary changes in nursing education and to assist today's student who must juggle work and family responsibilities by providing clear and concise content while maintaining the integrity of the content. Developing knowledge in pediatric nursing is essential to all nurses, regardless of whether they ultimately become pediatric nurses. Our focus is not to have the student memorize terms and data. We want students to learn how to apply the information to the clinical setting. We encourage the use of electronic devices during the learning process. We believe that learning is not memorizing information for a test. Learning is the ability to apply new information to the clinical situation. For this reason, we have included features within each chapter to facilitate the application of information.

Most pediatric texts contain detailed information about every aspect of pediatric care. As pediatric nurses, we have found that this information can quickly become outdated. We revised this textbook based on the recommendations of those who have used it—faculty from across the United States, students in all types of programs, and through our own experiences. Today's technology provides the nurse with the opportunity to look up information within minutes. We included multiple web links to encourage the reader to quickly validate and reference information. We recognize that student nurses must synthesize data from texts and life, laboratory, and clinical experiences to care for children. This text is organized to first present foundational information followed by complex information. Our concise format facilitates teaching pediatric nursing at all licensure levels and within varying time frames. We have updated content to keep current in standards of practice, including new guidelines for blood pressure monitoring, obesity, cultural diversity, growth and development, common childhood illnesses, common medications and treatments for children, safety, preventative care, and end-of-life issues. Professional standards of care for pediatric nursing are also discussed that are based on current practice guidelines and research.

CRITICAL COMPONENTS

Our text is titled *Pediatric Nursing: The Critical Components of Nursing Care* because our aim is to provide the most crucial information in pediatric nursing. This text, although not all-inclusive, does provide the critical components and major areas of knowledge essential for a basic understanding of pediatric nursing that is crucial for students and new pediatric nurses to know. The text is intended for prelicensure students and may be used for pediatric certification preparation. The critical components were derived from the authors' combined 50 years of teaching pediatric nursing in both traditional and accelerated programs, and years of laboratory and clinical practice in a variety of pediatric settings. Current guidelines and standards are integrated and summarized to present not just what is "normal," but to anticipate deviations from the norm. Early detection, especially in children, will lead to early interventions and improved outcomes.

ORGANIZATION

This text uses theory and evidence-based clinical knowledge of pediatric nursing according to systems, but can be easily used in concept-based curriculums. Professional practice, ethical principles, family theories, and cultural aspects of pediatric family-centered nursing are strong features of this edition. The text includes many online references to allow students to get up-to-date information in the rapidly changing landscape of health care. *Pediatric Nursing: The Critical Components of Nursing Care* reflects current knowledge, standards, and trends in pediatric nursing, including census data trends, projected population, and racial changes.

FEATURES

This textbook presents the critical components of pediatrics in a pragmatic, condensed format by using the following features:

- *Bulleted format:* For easy-to-read content
- *Figures, tables, and boxes:* Summarizes information in a visual way
- *Learning Outcomes:* Identifies what the reader will know and be able to do by the end of the chapter
- *Critical Components:* Highlights critical information in pediatric nursing
- *Evidenced-Based Practice:* Highlights current research and practice guidelines related to nursing care
- *Case Studies:* Ties it all together by applying critical components in clinical context
- *Safe and Effective Nursing Care (SENC):* Highlights safe and effective nursing care concepts as they apply to the chapter content
  - *Cultural Competence:* Stresses the importance of cultural factors in nursing care
  - *Understanding Medication:* Highlights commonly administered medications during childhood

- *Promoting Safety:* Focuses on important safety concepts
- *Clinical Pearl:* Provides tips on applying critical thinking in a clinical setting

APPENDICES

The appendices include:

- Asthma Action Plan
- 2018 Recommended Immunization Schedule
- Car Seat Safety
- Growth Charts

RESOURCES AVAILABLE

Student

Use the unique code from the inside front cover to access the following student resources:

- *Interactive Clinical Scenarios:* Experience real-world challenges while working through each step in the nursing process
- *Davis Edge + e-book:* An online Q&A review platform with integrated interactive e-book that seamlessly blends into the classroom to give students the additional practice questions they need to perform well on course and board examinations

Instructor

Instructors will have access to:

- *Active Classroom Instructor's Guide:* Maps resources and activities for an active classroom approach
- *PowerPoints:* Fully customizable slides summarizing key concepts from each chapter
- *Test Bank:* NCLEX®-style questions with rationales for correct and incorrect answers in ExamView Pro
- *Davis Edge + e-book:* Create assignments, track your students' progress, and access the complete text with our online Q&A review platform
- *Image Bank:* Includes all images from the text

Contributors

Kelly J. Betts, EdD, RN, CNE
Assistant Professor
University of Arkansas for Medical Sciences (UAMS)
College of Nursing
Little Rock, Arkansas

Ludy Caballero, MSN, APRN, FNP-C, EMT-P
Family Medicine/Express Care Nurse
The MetroHealth System
Cleveland, Ohio

Margarita Diaz, BSN, RN
Manager of Health Equity
The MetroHealth System
Cleveland, Ohio

Irene Cihon Dietz, MD, FAAP
Assistant Professor of Pediatrics
Case Western Reserve University
The MetroHealth System
Cleveland, Ohio

Suzanne M. Fortuna, DNP, APRN-BC, CNS-BC, FNP-BC
CNP Pediatrics Complex Care Coordinator
University Hospitals Case Medical Center/Rainbow Babies and Children's Hospital
Cleveland, Ohio

Tina Goodpasture, MSN, RN, NP-C
Family Nurse Practitioner
Cone Health Child Neurology
Greensboro, North Carolina

Mary Grady, DNP, RN, CNE, CHSE
Associate Professor
Lorain County Community College
Elyria, Ohio

Bonnie Kitchen, MNSc, APRN, PPCNP-BC
Acute Care APRN, Hospitalist Medicine
University of Arkansas Medical Science
Arkansas Children's Hospital
Little Rock, Arkansas

Lillian M. Kohler, MSN, RN
Clinical Nurse & Quality Improvement Facilitator, Labor & Delivery
The MetroHealth System
Cleveland, Ohio

Courtney A. Kwapinski, MSN, RN
Quality Specialist
The MetroHealth System
Cleveland, Ohio

Rebecca Loth Luetke, PhD, MSN, BS, BA, RN, SANE-P
Professor of Nursing
Colorado Mountain College, Spring Valley
Glenwood Spring, Colorado

Jill Reiter Matthes, RN, DNP, CHSE
Assistant Professor
College of Nursing
Ashland University
Mansfield, Ohio

Judith D. McLeod, DNP, RN, CPNP
Dean, School of Nursing
California Southern University
Costa Mesa, California

Jill Morinec, RN, BSN, CCRN
RU-ICU Resource
The MetroHealth System
Cleveland, Ohio

Daniel C. Rausch, BSN, RN
Sr. Clinical Application Analyst, MLM Knowledge Engineer
University Hospitals—Cleveland
Pediatric Clinical Instructor
School of Nursing
Cleveland State University
Shaker Heights, Ohio

Andrea Warner Stidham, PhD, RN
Assistant Professor
Kent State University
College of Nursing
Kent, Ohio

Sheryl D. Stuck, MSN, APRN-CNS, CDP
Professor
School of Nursing
University of Akron
Akron, Ohio

Teresa Whited, DNP, APRN, CPNP-PC
Director of MNSc Program
Specialty Coordinator of PNP Program
College of Nursing
University of Arkansas for Medical Sciences (UAMS)
Little Rock, Arkansas

Reviewers

Sharon Anderson, DNP, NNP-BC, APNG
Assistant Professor
Rutgers School of Nursing
Newark, New Jersey

Pamela F. Ashcraft, PhD, RN
Associate Professor
University of Central Arkansas
Conway, Arkansas

Sue Anne Bell, PhD, FNP-BC
Clinical Associate Professor
School of Nursing
University of Michigan
Ann Arbor, Michigan

Susan N. Benner, MSN, RN
Instructor
Ball State University
Muncie, Indiana

Janice Bidwell, RN, MN, CNS
Lecturer Pediatric Nursing, RN to BSN Program Coordinator
School of Nursing
San Diego State University
San Diego, California

Ann M. Bowling, PhD, RN, CPNP-PC, CNE
Assistant Professor
Wright State University
Dayton, Ohio

Jacqueline Brandwein, RN, MA, CPNP
Assistant Clinical Professor
Adelphi University
Garden City, New York

Jutta Braun, RN, MS, CNE
Assistant Professor of Nursing
County College of Morris
Randolph, New Jersey

Denise Brehmer, MSN, NP-c
Assistant Professor
Indiana Wesleyan University
Marion, Indiana

Kathleen M. Cahill, MS, RN, CNE
Professor Pediatrics
Saint Anselm College
Manchester, New Hampshire

Corine K. Carlson, MS, MSN, RN
Associate Professor
Luther College
Decorah, Iowa

Sheri Carson, MSN, RN, CPN, CPNP
Clinical Instructor
University of Arizona
Pediatric Nurse Practitioner
Asthma & Airway Disease Research Center
Tucson, Arizona

Beth Desaretz Chiatti, PhD, RN, CTN, CSN
Assistant Professor
Drexel University
Philadelphia, Pennsylvania

Joyce Clay, RN, MS
Professor of Nursing
Richland Community College
Decatur, Illinois

Georgina Colalillo, MS, RN, CNE
Professor
Queensborough Community College/CUNY
New York City, New York

Elizabeth Conoley, MSNEd, RN, CPN
Assistant Professor
Brenau University
Gainesville, Georgia

Suzy Cook, MN, RN, CNE, CHSE
Professor, Nursing
Olympic College
Bremerton, Washington

Claire M. Creamer, PhD, RN, CPNP-PC
Assistant Professor, Nursing
Rhode Island College
Providence, Rhode Island

Lana K. Davies, MSN, RN, CPNP
Assistant Professor
Research College of Nursing
Kansas City, Missouri

Lynette DeBellis, MA, RN
Chairperson and Assistant Professor of Nursing
Westchester Community College
Valhalla, New York

M. Kathleen Dwinnells, MSN, CNS, CNE
Associate Lecturer/Nursing Coordinator
Kent State University at Trumbull
Warren, Ohio

Karen Ferguson, PhD, RNC, FNE
Division Chair
Martin Methodist College
Pulaski, Tennessee

Jeffrey S. Fouche-Camargo, DNP, APRN, WHNP-BC, RNC-OB, C-EFM
Assistant Professor of Nursing
Georgia Gwinnett College
Lawrenceville, Georgia

Sue Gabriel, EdD, MSN, MFS, RN, SANE-A, CFN, CFC
Associate Professor of Nursing
Nebraska Wesleyan University
Lincoln, Nebraska

Kim Green, MSN, RN, PNP, CNE
Associate Professor of Nursing
School of Nursing
Western Kentucky University
Bowling Green, Kentucky

Anna Gryczman, DNP, RN, AHN-BC, CNE
Nursing Faculty
Century College
White Bear Lake, Minnesota

Jennifer Harwell, MSN, RN
Assistant Professor
The University of West Alabama
Livingston, Alabama

Iris Hobson, DHEd, MSN, RN, FNP-BC
Professor
Dallas Nursing Institute
Dallas, Texas

Teresa Jodway, MSN, CPNP
Assistant Professor of Nursing
Bethel College
Mishawaka, Indiana

Carol Johnson, MS, RN
Upper Division Nursing Director/Faculty
Arizona College
Mesa, Arizona

Gwendolyn Jordan, RN, MSN
Faculty
Carolina College of Health Sciences
Charlotte, North Carolina

Laura M. Karges, MSN, RN, CPN
Associate Professor
Union College
Lincoln, Nebraska

Amber Kool, MSN, RN
Faculty
Arizona College
Mesa, Arizona

Barbara Lane, MSN, RN-BC
Program Coordinator, Department of Nursing and Allied Health
Lincoln University
Ft. Leonard Wood, Missouri

Ann M. Laughlin, PhD, RN
Associate Professor of Nursing
College of Nursing
Creighton University
Omaha, Nebraska

Resa Lord, RN, MSN, CPNP
Chairperson, Health Sciences
Chattahoochee Valley Community College
Phenix City, Alabama

Tabatha Mauldin, RN, MSN, CPN
Instructor
Winston-Salem State University
Winston-Salem, North Carolina

Sandra McChristy, RN, MSN, FNP-C
Instructor
Pittsburg State University
Pittsburg, Kansas

Barbara McClaskey, PhD, APRN CNS-BC, RNC
University Professor
School of Nursing
Pittsburg State University
Pittsburg, Kansas

Amy J. McClune, PhD, RN
Associate Professor, Nursing
Edinboro University
Edinboro, Pennsylvania

Florence T. McCutchen, RN, MSN
Associate of Science in Nursing Instructor
Southern Regional Technical College
Family Nurse Practitioner
Thomasville, Georgia

Bernita Missal, PhD, RN
Professor
Bethel University
St. Paul, Minnesota

Carol M. Moore, MSN, CRNP
Assistant Professor of Nursing
Bloomsburg University
Bloomsburg, Pennsylvania

Joann M. Oliver, MNEd, RN, CNE, CBIS
Professor, Nursing and Health Care Initiatives
Anne Arundel Community College
Arnold, Maryland

Helen Papas-Kavalis, RNC, BSN, MA
Professor of Nursing
Bronx Community College/CUNY
New York City, New York

Jane C. Parish, BBA, PhD, RN, CPN, CNE
Professor of Nursing
Walters State Community College
Morristown, Tennessee

Rhonda Phillips, MSN, CNS, RN
Associate Dean, Nursing
City Colleges of Chicago
Chicago, Illinois

Colleen M. Quinn, EdD, MSN, RN
Professor
Broward College
Pembroke Pines, Florida

Denice Reese, RN, DNP, CPNP
Associate Professor of Nursing
Davis & Elkins College
Elkins, West Virginia

Candice Rome, DNP, RN
Chair, Prelicensure Programs; Associate Professor
Gardner-Webb University
Boiling Springs, North Carolina

Alice Rosanski, RN, MSN, CPN
Assistant Professor of Nursing
Alderson Broaddus University
Philippi, West Virginia

Donna Sandretto, MS, RN, CNE
Assistant Professor
Niagara County Community College
Sanborn, New York

Elizabeth M. Scarano, MSN, RN
Associate Professor of Nursing
Lewis-Clark State College
Lewiston, Idaho

Cynthia Scaringe, RN, MSN
Department Chair of Nursing; Nursing Instructor
Nursing Program
Skagit Valley College
Mount Vernon, Washington

Robin G. Seal-Whitlock, RN, PhD, MSN
Professor of Nursing
Chesapeake College/MGW Nursing Program
Wye Mills, Maryland

Diana Shenefield, PhD, MSN, RN
Director of Nursing
Huntington University
Huntington, Indiana

Jennifer Storer, MSN, RN
Associate Professor of Nursing
Kirkwood Community College
Cedar Rapids, Iowa

Linda A. Strong, MSN, RN, CPNP, CNE
Associate Professor, Pediatric Nursing
Cuyahoga Community College
Cleveland, Ohio

Zelda Suzan EdD, RN, CNE
Associate Professor, Course Coordinator
Phillips School of Nursing
Mount Sinai Beth Israel
New York, New York

Allison Swenson, MSN, RN
Assistant Professor
Utah Valley University
Orem, Utah

Maureen P. Tippen, RN, C, MS
Clinical Associate Professor
University of Michigan, Flint
Flint, Michigan

Theresa Turick-Gibson, MA, PNP-BC, RN-C
Professor
Hartwick College
Oneonta, New York

Geri M. Tyrell, DNP, RN, CNE
Director, Associate Professor of Nursing
Bethel College
North Newton, Kansas

Susan Warmuskerken, MSN
Professor of Nursing
West Shore Community College
Scottville, Michigan

Beverly B. West, PhD(c), MSN, RN
Clinical Associate Professor
University of Memphis, Loewenberg College of Nursing
Memphis, Tennessee

Becky White, MNSc, RN
ADN Faculty
National Park College
Hot Springs, Arkansas

Acknowledgments

I am grateful to my husband, Daniel Rudd, and my children, Ashley, David, Matthew, and Mary Kathryn, for their continued love and support throughout this long project.

Thanks to my colleagues for their suggestions and support. I would like to thank the expert contributors for their hard work on this project and the reviewers on this project.

Thanks to my teachers and mentors Alice DeWitt, RN, and Rosemary Bolls, RN, at St. Alexis School of Nursing, who instilled in me a love of nursing and education.

Kathryn Rudd

I am thankful for my mother, Kathleen Kocisko, for her ongoing encouragement, prayers, and support.

Thanks to my teachers and mentors Maureen Mitchell, EdD, RN, and Marylin Weitzel, PhD, RN, for their encouragement, instilling in me the love of nursing education, pediatrics, and developing students.

I would like to thank my colleagues at Cleveland State University and The MetroHealth System for their ongoing support of this project.

Diane Kocisko

Thanks to our F.A. Davis team—Jacalyn Sharp, Andrea Miller, Amanda Minutola—for their guidance.

Thanks to our contributors for sharing their expertise and taking on the task of writing these chapters despite their continued workload.

Contents in Brief

Table of Contents

UNIT

1

Pediatric Nursing: An Overview

1 Issues and Trends in Pediatric Nursing

Diane M. Kocisko, MSN, RN, CPN
Lillian Kohler, MSN, RN

LEARNING OUTCOMES

Upon completion of this chapter, the student will be able to:

1. Define *pediatric nursing*.
2. Describe the differences between nursing care of infants, children, and adolescents and care of the adult population.
3. Describe the history of pediatric nursing.
4. Describe the projected racial population changes in the United States.
5. Identify models of care applied to pediatric nursing.
6. Describe the roles of the pediatric nurse.
7. Identify the different fields of pediatric nursing and the education required for each.
8. Identify current issues and trends in pediatric nursing practice, education, and research.
9. Identify evidence-based resources that are available for pediatric nurses.

INTRODUCTION TO PEDIATRIC NURSING

The nursing care of children from birth through adolescence includes health promotion, disease prevention, illness management, and health restoration (Fig. 1–1).

Nursing Care for Children Versus Care for Adults

Pediatric nursing care requires the nurse to use assessment and evaluation tools that are unique to infants, children, and adolescent populations.

- Pediatric nurses must assess attainment of developmental milestones (see Chapter 6).
- Pediatric nurses monitor growth and development, including:
  - Physical maturation
    - Development and mastery of gross and fine motor skills
    - Height, weight, and head circumference, tracked via growth charts that are adapted as needed for specific populations (e.g., Down syndrome)
    - Physical maturation of each body system (see Chapters 8–10)
    - Onset of puberty using the Tanner scale
    - Required immunizations
  - Cognitive maturation (see Chapter 6)
    - Erikson's stages of psychosocial development
    - Piaget's stages of cognitive development
    - Freud's psychosexual stages of development
    - Kohlberg's stages of moral development
    - Language development
    - Presence of learning and developmental disabilities where indicated

CRITICAL COMPONENT

Role of Development

In pediatric nursing, the unit of care is the child and the caregiver(s). Caring for children is not just caring for "little adults." The needs of children will vary by developmental level.

HISTORY OF PEDIATRIC NURSING

Before pediatrics became a specialty, newborns were delivered by midwives and cared for in the home (Fig. 1–2). The first pediatric hospital in the United States was the Children's Hospital of Pennsylvania, founded in 1855. As early hospitals became more industrialized, the following were common practices in infant and child care:

- Nursing care focused on preventing the spread of infectious disease and was often cold and rigid.
- Parents were unable to visit or stay at the bedside of their children, relinquishing all care responsibility to the staff.
- Including the family in the plan of care was believed to be detrimental to patient outcomes.
- The emotional and psychological needs of children were not considered in care planning.

In the late 19th and early 20th centuries, nurses became involved in many public and private health-promotion initiatives, including the care of children (Fig. 1–3). As the field of pediatric nursing progressed, efforts were made to improve nursing education. In 1917, the *Standard Curriculum for Schools of Nursing (Standard Curriculum)* suggested that special educational preparation should occur when training nurses to care for children. The curriculum included content on diseases of infants and children, nutrition and cookery, therapeutics, orthopedics, gynecology, psychology, and ethics, to name a few (Committee on Education of the National League of Nursing Education, 1917). The content covered is similar to the diverse nursing courses that are taught in today's schools of nursing.

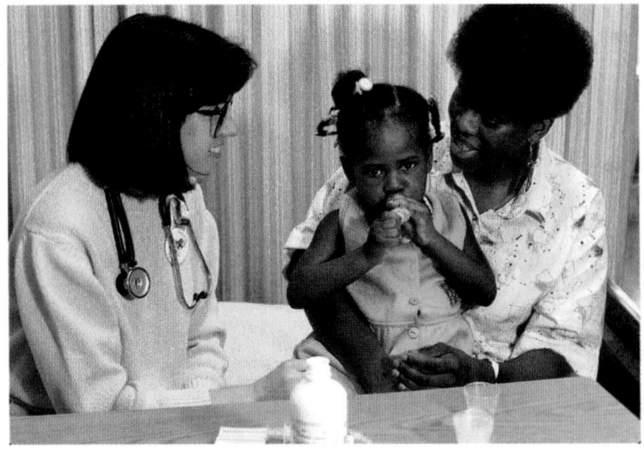

FIGURE 1–1 Nurse engaged with a child who requires health care.

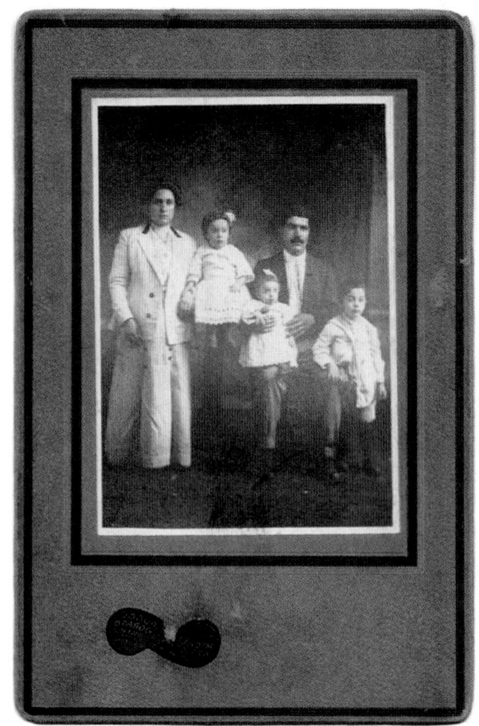

FIGURE 1–2 Family in early 1900s. *(Courtesy of D.M. Kocisko)*

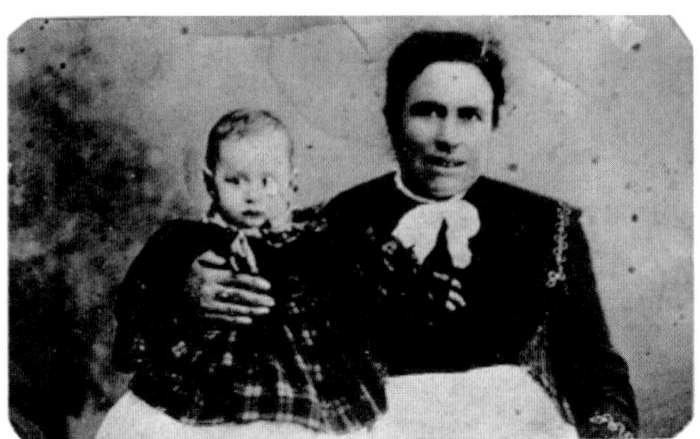

FIGURE 1–3 Child from the late 19th century. *(Courtesy of D.M. Kocisko)*

Research conducted in the mid-20th century indicated the negative effects of separating parent from child, resulting in a push toward more family-centered care. The early field of pediatric nursing influenced the later development of advanced practice roles (e.g., neonatal nurse practitioner, pediatric nurse practitioner). Pediatric nurse practitioners were the first nurse practitioners. In the latter half of the 20th century, the nursing profession continued to define itself through:

- Development and publication of professional standards of practice
- Availability of certification programs
- Formation of professional organizations
- Continued nursing research
- Continued educational opportunities

RACIAL MAKEUP OF AMERICAN CHILDREN

The racial population of the United States continues to evolve, which in turn changes the demographics of the pediatric population. It is important for the nurse to identify the illnesses and chronic diseases the child is at risk for acquiring based on his or her cultural and ethnic background. These are the projected demographics for the U.S. pediatric population in 2020 (Federal Interagency Forum on Child and Family Statistics, 2016):

- Less than half of children aged 0 to 17 years will be white non-Hispanic. This is the first time in history that non-Hispanic whites do not account for 50% or more of the population.
- Hispanic children will represent 26% of the pediatric population. This is an increase from 25% in 2015.
- Black, non-Hispanic children will represent 14% of the pediatric population. No change from 2015.
- Asian, non-Hispanic children will represent 5% of the pediatric population. No change from 2015.
- Non-Hispanic children who represent two or more races will reflect 5% of children. This is an increase from 4% in 2015.
- American Indian and Alaska Native, non-Hispanic children will reflect 0.8% of the pediatric population. This is a decrease from 0.9% in 2015.
- Percentage of Native Hawaiian and other Pacific Islander, non-Hispanic children will remain unchanged from 2015 at 0.2%.

MODELS OF CARE IN PEDIATRIC NURSING

Family-centered care, relationship-based care, and pediatric medical home are three models of care for providing nursing care to children. In all models, the importance of the family to the child is emphasized.

- Core concepts of family-centered care include the following:
  - Dignity and respect for the child and family
  - Information sharing with the family
  - Family participation in care, including collaboration in care planning and provision
- Core concepts of relationship-based care include the following:
  - The child and family remain the focal point in the plan of care.
  - The nurse strives to develop a relationship with the child's family members and engages in one-to-one conversations with the child and family on each shift.
  - Care is individualized to meet the specific needs of the child based on issues that arise in these one-to-one conversations with the child and family.
  - All staff members strive to respect, understand, and address the child's and family's concerns.
  - Children and families are actively engaged in all aspects of care, including decision making.
  - Open communication must occur between child, family, and staff.
  - The child's well-being and dignity must be safeguarded in all aspects of communication and care.

Pediatric Medical Home

Health-care reform has driven development of initiatives to improve population health. Pediatric medical homes provide children with better health outcomes and a better patient experience. This is especially important for children with socioeconomic, racial, and ethnic health disparities.

Core concepts of pediatric medical home-care coordination include:

- Proactive outreach to ensure timely well-child care
- Comprehensive care during vulnerable patient care transitions
- Care coordination, including hospital discharge to primary care
- Referral from primary care to community services for additional nonmedical needs
- Care coordination to enrollment in available home visiting programs (Brown, Perkins, Blust, & Kahn, 2015).

ROLE OF THE PEDIATRIC NURSE

When caring for children and their families, the pediatric nurse must assume several critical roles. He or she:

- Incorporates knowledge of human growth and development when providing care to children
- Recognizes the physiological differences between children and adults
- Provides care in a developmentally appropriate manner to promote the optimal physical, psychological, and social well-being
- Recognizes the integral role of family in a child's health and incorporates the family in the plan of care
- Provides culturally sensitive care by integrating knowledge of cultural and religious practices into the plan of care
- Implements models of care that are specifically applicable to infants, children, and adolescents

Where Pediatric Nurses Work

Pediatric registered nurses with undergraduate preparation work in many settings and capacities. Some of the most common include:

- Acute care—bedside nurse
- Hospital nurse manager (BSN or MSN required for some positions)
- Hospice and palliative care
- Surgical care

- Ambulatory care
- Outpatient care
- Home care
- School nurse
- Camp nurse
- Travel nurse
- Day-care consultant
- Community educator
- Public health nurse
- Research trial coordinator
- School-based health centers

Pediatric nurses with master's degree preparation are often employed in the following settings and capacities:

- Pediatric nurse practitioner (inpatient/outpatient)
- Family nurse practitioner (inpatient/outpatient)
- Neonatal nurse practitioner (inpatient/outpatient)
- Clinical nurse specialist (inpatient)
- Nurse educator (hospital/college or school of nursing)

Pediatric nurses with doctoral preparation may be employed in leadership roles. They develop and implement research programs for hospitals, colleges, or schools of nursing. The focus is more global and directs the paths of evidence-based practice. Many doctoral nurses work in colleges and universities. Many academic settings that teach nursing require instructors to have a nursing doctorate or be actively working to obtain a doctorate degree.

Additional Training and Certification

Pediatric nurses at all levels who wish to further specialize their careers can obtain additional certification in many practice areas. Available programs include:

- Neonatal Resuscitation Program (NRP)
- Pediatric Advanced Life Support (PALS)
- End of Life Nursing Education Consortium—PEDS (see Chapter 5 for more information on death and dying)
- Pediatric nursing certification:
  - Certified Pediatric Emergency Nurse (CPEN)
  - Certified Pediatric Nurse Practitioner (CPNP; acute and primary care)
- Pediatric Primary Care Mental Health Specialists (PMHS through the Pediatric Nursing Certification Board, Inc.)
- Certified Pediatric Oncology Nurse (CPON)
- Neonatal/pediatric and critical care nurse certification (CCRN)
- Maternal Child Nursing RN-BC (American Nurses Credentialing Center)
- S.T.A.B.L.E. Program (post-resuscitation and pretransport stabilization care of sick infants)
- National Certified School Nurse (NCSN through the National Board of Certification of School Nurses)
- Sexual Assault Nurse Examiner (SANE-P through the Forensic Nurse Certification Board)

Additional certifications for advanced practice nurses include:

- Certified Pediatric Nurse Practitioner (CPNP; acute and primary care)
- Certified Neonatal Nurse Practitioner (NNP-BC)
- Certified Clinical Nurse Specialist (CCNS; neonatal or pediatrics)
- Certified Clinical Nurse Specialist (PCNS-BC; pediatrics)

ISSUES IN PEDIATRIC NURSING

Nurses considering a career in pediatrics must become familiar with common issues in this area of health care. In general, there is an expected nursing shortage in the United States due to an aging population and many nurses near the age of retirement (American Association of Colleges of Nursing, 2017). The shortage will impact all areas of nursing, including the subspecialty areas. As a result, many children who need ongoing medical care must remain in a hospital setting longer than necessary while a pediatric home-care nurse is located and trained.

There may also be a lack of nurses who are equipped to carry out research projects in the pediatric population. Ethical considerations in pediatric nursing research impact clinical practice. Children aged 7 years and older can assent (agree) or dissent (disagree) to be in a clinical trial. This means that even if the caregivers want the child in the study and signs the consent, the child can refuse and the researcher will not include the child in the study. Caregivers of infants and children younger than 7 years may be hesitant to participate in a drug study because of the potential risks of injury to the child's vital organs. The caregiver may be more inclined to want the child to receive medications that have been tested in children.

In addition, the lack of research studies using ethnically and culturally diverse participants means that the indications of research results from studies with participants of one ethnic/cultural group are often applied to infants, children, and adolescents of another ethnic/cultural group in clinical practice.

Additional issues in pediatric nursing include the following:

- As the number of chronically ill children continues to increase because of medical advances, continuity of care between hospital, home, and school must improve. Children are now exceeding previous life expectancies for chronic illnesses, but still require ongoing medical management.
- Maintaining communication with families and caregivers has become more challenging with the increased number of divorced parents, blended or reconstituted families, and grandparents as primary caregivers.
- Pediatric nurses must also consider the special issues in working with foster parents, extended families, single-parent families, lesbian/gay/bisexual/transgendered (LGBT) families, cohabitating families, and families with adopted children.

- Ensuring adequate health education and follow-up services for children and families is a primary nursing responsibility that becomes more challenging when working with those with limited health literacy and/or for whom English is a second language.
- As health-care costs continue to increase, families' adherence to recommended therapy and treatments may be negatively affected by having little or no health insurance. Uninsured and underinsured families may be unable to afford follow-up care.

TRENDS IN PEDIATRIC NURSING PRACTICE

Pediatric nurses should be aware of existing trends in this area of practice and consider how these factors impact their roles and responsibilities. These include:

- Increased numbers of children who require mental health services
- Increased numbers of children becoming ill because of antibiotic-resistant organisms
- Increased usage of blood conservation techniques for hospitalized children
- Increased emphasis on provision of safety education (e.g., internet safety, dealing with bullying)
- Increased admissions based on environmental risk factors, such as dangerous living environments, unstable households, and risky behaviors
- Increased admissions based on deficient knowledge base of caregivers, such as not following or understanding the treatment regimen
- Increased admissions based on lack of primary care access
- Earlier onset of puberty and its ramifications for adolescent sexual health
- Shift in the focus of medical/nursing care from disease treatment to health promotion and disease prevention
- Provision of health education in the school system
- Increased incorporation of families in the overall care of children
- Increased numbers of children who require home care
- Increased prevalence of autism spectrum disorders and childhood depression, requiring more education and research in these areas
- Increased childhood incidence of:
  - Obesity
  - Hypertension
  - Diabetes
  - Asthma
- Increase in children and adolescents who identify as transgender

Obesity

The prevalence of obesity among adolescents has doubled since the 1990s, increasing from approximately 10% (in 1990) to 20% in 2014 (Federal Interagency Forum on Child and Family Statistics, 2016). Childhood obesity can be difficult to overcome in adulthood. Obese children are at increased risk for poor health outcomes, including diabetes, stroke, heart disease, arthritis, and certain cancers. Hypertension, early puberty, and asthma often result from adolescent obesity. The psychosocial impact can also be significant and include issues such as impaired body image, decreased self-esteem, and eating disorders (see Chapter 14). Pediatric caregivers have an opportunity and responsibility to promote health and wellness in the obese population by:

- Promoting the intake of healthy foods and avoidance of unhealthy foods
- Promoting physical activity and reducing sedentary behaviors in individuals and families
- Providing guidance and support for healthy diet, sleep, and physical activity
- Promoting healthy school environments, health and nutrition literacy, and physical activity in school-aged children and adolescents
- Providing family-based, multicomponent weight-management services for obese and overweight children (Pizzi, 2016).

Lesbian, Gay, Bisexual, and Transgender Youth

Although individuals are born with a biological sex, this is separate from gender identity—the awareness and sense of oneself as male or female that develops in early childhood. Transgender is a term used to describe individuals whose gender identity differs from their biological sex.

Pediatric caregivers have an opportunity and responsibility to promote health and wellness in individuals with gender discrepancy by:

- Protecting the health, well-being, and civil rights of transgender children and adolescents in society
- Providing nondiscriminatory care with equal treatment
- Providing inclusive care that prevents feelings of isolation
- Assessing risk factors for depression, suicidal thoughts and behaviors, and substance abuse
- Assessing, educating, and supporting youth who are at risk for or experiencing bullying, violence, victimization, or discrimination
- Supporting and educating children and families on gender identity and transgender youth (National Association of Pediatric Nurse Practitioners, n.d.)
- Providing anticipatory guidance to specialized care
- Supporting healthy emotional development
- Providing comprehensive, inclusive sexual education, including HIV prevention and treatment options
- Providing gender-affirming care to transgender youth
- Following evidence-based best practice guidelines for LGBT youth
- Considering interpersonal and structural stigma that may impact equity in health-care resources, training, and competencies (Adelson, Dowshen, Makadon, & Garofalo, 2016).

Nonheterosexual orientations and nonconformity in gender expression are not new concepts, but they are more visible in society than ever before. Competence in caring for LGBT youth and their families' unique needs must be a core skill provided by pediatric caregivers.

TRENDS IN PEDIATRIC NURSING EDUCATION

As pediatric nursing practice and patient population evolves, education programs for aspiring nurses in this realm must keep pace with new initiatives. Some of these include:

- Inclusion of multicultural care topics and family theory in nursing programs
- Incorporation of growth and development concepts into nursing curricula
- Clinical experience in a range of settings, including acute care, community, school, and well care
- Increased focus on health promotion and disease prevention in nursing programs (e.g., screenings and preventive education)
- Increased focus on community-based nursing education through events such as health fairs and public screenings
- Clinical education supplemented with simulation as fewer pediatric clinical sites are available for nursing students (Fig. 1–4)

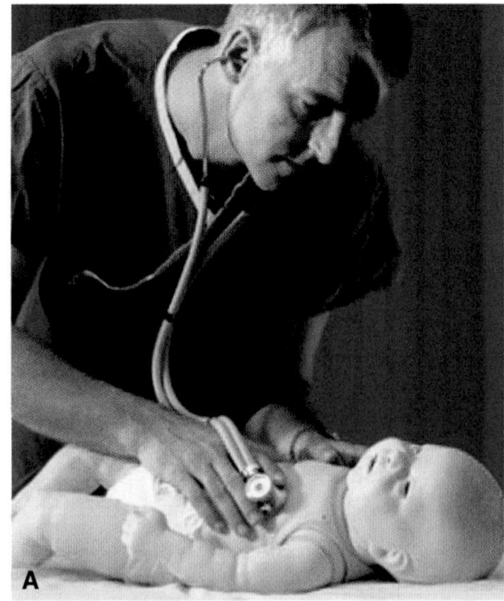

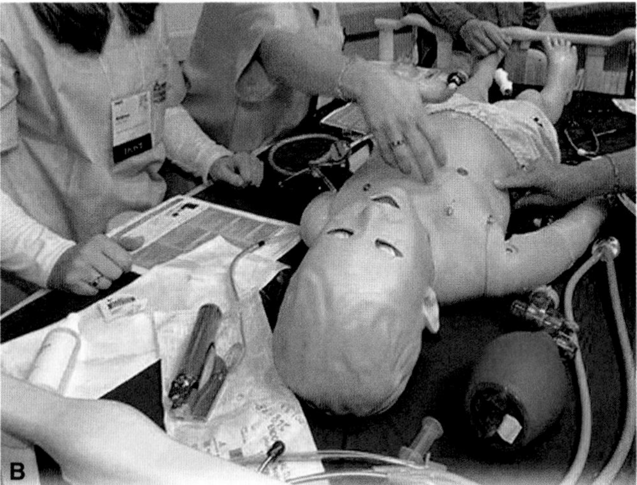

FIGURE 1–4 **A,** Infant and **B,** child patient simulators.

TRENDS IN PEDIATRIC NURSING RESEARCH

Research initiatives have the potential to improve health outcomes for children worldwide and have a significant impact on pediatric nursing practice. In 2007, the U.S. Congress reauthorized the Best Pharmaceuticals for Children Act, the Pediatric Research Equity Act, and the Pediatric Medical Device Safety and Improvement Act. These laws require that medications, medical devices, and interventions be tested on children if they are intended for use in children. This represents a new direction for research, as children were rarely used as research subjects before the passage of these laws. Because research studies now more frequently involve child participants, interventions will be safer for children because they are no longer based on data from adult response to treatment. For example, more medications are being researched for off-label use. Recently, tiotropium bromide and lurasidone hydrochloride have been approved for pediatric patients by the U.S. Food and Drug Administration (U.S. Department of Health & Human Resources, 2017).

RESOURCES FOR PEDIATRIC HEALTH DATA

The following reliable resources contain valuable pediatric health data for nurses:

- Child Stats
- CDC Wonder
- Data Resource Center for Child and Adolescent Health
- National Database of Nursing Quality Indicators
- National Children's Study
  - The study is intended to determine how environmental factors influence health and development.
  - Participants in the study will be tracked from birth until age 21 years.

RESOURCES FOR EVIDENCE-BASED PEDIATRIC NURSING PRACTICE

- Pediatric nursing journals:
  - *Journal for Specialists in Pediatric Nursing (Journal of the Society of Pediatric Nurses)*
  - *Journal of Child Health*
  - *Journal of Pediatric Nursing*
  - *Pediatric Nursing*
  - *Journal of Child and Adolescent Psychiatric Nursing*
  - *American Journal of Maternal/Child Nursing* (MCN)

- Online resources for pediatric nursing:
  - American Academy of Pediatrics (AAP). (2008). *Bright Futures: Guidelines for Health Supervision of Infants, Children, and Adolescents* (3rd ed.)
  - Agency for Healthcare Research and Quality (AHRQ) resources:
    - Innovations Exchange, a review of innovations and quality tools
    - Research updates
  - Child Health Care Quality Toolbox
  - U.S. Food and Drug Administration (FDA), information on pediatric pharmaceuticals
  - National Institute of Child Health and Human Development (NICHD)
  - National Institute of Nursing Research
  - Immunization Action Coalition
- Pediatric professional organizations:
  - American Academy of Pediatrics (AAP)
  - Academy of Neonatal Nursing
  - Association of Camp Nurses
  - Association of Child Neurology Nurses
  - Association of Pediatric Hematology/Oncology Nurses
  - National Association of Neonatal Nurses
  - National Association of Pediatric Nurse Practitioners
  - National Association of School Nurses
  - Society of Pediatric Nurses

REFERENCES

Adelson, S. L., Dowshen, N. L., Makadon, H. J., & Garofalo, R. (2016). Introduction to lesbian, gay, bisexual, and transgender youth health. *Pediatric Clinics, 63*(6), xvii–xxi. Retrieved from http://dx.doi.org/10.1016/j.pcl.2016.09.002.

American Association of Colleges of Nursing. (2017). Nursing shortage. Retrieved from http://www.aacnnursing.org/News-Information/Fact-Sheets/Nursing-Shortage

Brown, C., Perkins, J., Blust, A., & Kahn, R. (2015). A neighborhood-based approach to population health in the pediatric medical home. *Journal of Community Health, 40*(1), 1–11. doi: 10.1007/s10900-014-9885-z

Committee on Education of the National League of Nursing Education. (1917). *Standard curriculum for schools of nursing (standard curriculum).* Baltimore, MD: The Waverly Press.

Federal Interagency Forum on Child and Family Statistics. (2016). America's children in brief: Key national indicators of well-being, 2016. Merrifield, VA: Health Resources and Services Administration Information Center. Retrieved from https://www.childstats.gov/pdf/ac2016/ac_16.pdf

National Association of Pediatric Nurse Practitioners. (n.d.). Supporting and educating children and families on gender identity and transgender youth. Retrieved from https://www.napnap.org/supporting-and-educating-children-and-families-gender-identity-and-transgender-youth

Pizzi, M. A. (2016). Guest editorial. Promoting health, well-being, and quality of life for children who are overweight or obese and their families. *American Journal of Occupational Therapy, 70*(5), 7005170010p1–7005170010p. doi: 10.5014/ajot.2016.705001

U.S. Department of Health & Human Resources. (2017). New pediatric labeling information data base. Retrieved from https://www.accessdata.fda.gov/scripts/sda/sdNavigation.cfm?sd=labelingdatabase

Standards of Practice and Ethical Considerations

2

Kathryn Rudd, RN, DNP, c-NIC, c-NPT

LEARNING OUTCOMES

Upon completion of this chapter, the student will be able to:

1. Identify and describe sources of standards of practice relevant to the day-to-day practice of pediatric nurses.
2. Identify and elaborate on the key themes related to pediatric nursing standards of practice.
3. List the six standards of practice and 11 standards of professional performance highlighted in *Pediatric Nursing: Scope and Standards of Practice* (American Nurses Association [ANA], 2015e), and discuss associated measurement criteria.
4. Describe the value and functions of the *Code of Ethics for Nurses* (ANA, 2015c).
5. Identify the nine provisions of the *Code of Ethics for Nurses* and relate them to practical situations encountered in the day-to-day practice of pediatric nursing.
6. Identify ethics controversies commonly encountered in the practice of pediatric nursing, and discuss relevant principles, duties, rights, and virtues.
7. Differentiate consent, permission, and assent, and discuss how promoting the best interests of children in the issue of consent differs from obtaining informed consent from a competent adult.

INTRODUCTION

The care of children and their families requires the application of the nursing process in accordance with accepted standards of practice, professional performance, and ethics. Quality pediatric care is developmentally appropriate, family centered, culturally sensitive, and evidence based. Compassion, advocacy, care coordination, continuity of care, and a holistic approach are additional hallmarks of quality care, and together provide the context for standards that direct the practice of pediatric nurses.

ETHICS IN NURSING PRACTICE

Codes of ethics and standards of practice and professional performance serve as benchmarks of quality and accountability, providing protection for the public and guidance for professionals. Although *Code of Ethics for Nurses With Interpretive Statements* (American Nurses Association [ANA], 2015c) and *Pediatric Nursing: Scope and Standards of Practice* (ANA, 2015e) must be considered primary, the sources of standards relevant to the practice of pediatric nursing are actually many and varied. Table 2–1 provides a representative listing of just a few of these sources.

Familiarity with codes of ethics and standards of practice fosters decisiveness, consistency, empowerment, and accuracy in the practice setting. Pediatric nurses must also develop an understanding of basic principles of ethics and consider the types of ethical dilemmas they will likely encounter in nursing practice, have a process for resolving ethical issues, and know the resources to consult when ethical issues arise.

ANA *Code of Ethics for Nurses*

The *Code of Ethics for Nurses With Interpretive Statements* (ANA, 2015c) outlines and elaborates on the values and moral standards

CRITICAL COMPONENT

Public Perception of Nursing

Nursing is a highly trusted profession. As of December 2016, nursing was ranked in first place for the last 13 of 14 years in the annual Gallup survey of professional honesty and ethics. The only time the profession was ranked in second place was following the terrorist attacks of 9/11 in 2001 (see the later "Additional Resources" section for a link to this study). This is largely a testament to the relationships nurses develop with patients and their families, as well as the principles, values, and standards by which they aspire to conduct themselves (Norman, 2016).

that should guide nurses in practice. It is a formal and public declaration of the principles of good conduct expected of members of the profession. The ANA *Code of Ethics for Nurses* can be characterized as:

- A foundation for all we do, serving as a source of guidance for and empowerment of individual nurses and for the profession as a whole
- A covenant between the profession and the patients who nurses serve
- A reflection of key ethics philosophies, principles, rights, duties, and virtues as they apply to interactions with patients, their families, and the broader community, as well as colleagues and other stakeholders in the promotion and facilitation of quality health care
- An evolutionary document that responds to and anticipates a constantly changing health-care delivery environment, emergent scientific knowledge and technological capabilities, the demands of increasingly better-educated and outcome- and quality-focused health-care consumers, and the realities of resource availability

The *Code of Ethics for Nurses* has a relatively short history, and yet has changed significantly over time (Box 2–1). The "legacy and vision" (Ellenchild Pinch & Haddad, 2008) of the Code are instructive, motivating, and deserving of exploration in greater detail than possible here. The Nightingale Pledge (1893), based largely on the Hippocratic Oath, was an early predecessor of today's Code and was often unofficially referred to as the code of ethics for the profession. The first formally sanctioned version of the Code, which included 17 provisions, appeared in 1950. Today, the

TABLE 2–1 Sources of Standards That Inform Pediatric Practice

TYPES AND SOURCES OF STANDARDS		SELECT EXAMPLES
Laws Rules of law Policies Codes of ethics Position statements Professional standards Practice standards Clinical standards Administrative standards	International federal legislation and regulatory agencies	• UN Convention on the Rights of the Child • Department of Health and Human Services (DHHS): *Healthy People 2020* • Food and Drug Administration (FDA) • Centers for Disease Control and Prevention (CDC) • Health Insurance Portability and Accountability Act (HIPAA) • Patient Self-Determination Act (PSDA)
	State and local legislation and regulatory agencies	• Nurse practice acts • State boards of nursing • State pharmacy boards • State chapters of the American Hospital Association (AHA)
	Nongovernmental organizations/ not-for-profits and public advocacy groups	• The Joint Commission (formerly Joint Commission on the Accreditation of Hospitals) • National Association for Children's Hospitals and Related Institutions (NACHRI) • National Association for Children's Hospitals (NACH; NACHRI policy affiliate) • National Institute for Children's Healthcare Quality (NICHQ) • 5 Million Lives Campaign: Institute of Healthcare Improvement (IHI) • Institute for Safe Medication Practices (ISMP) • The Leapfrog Group
	Professional associations	• American Nurses Association (ANA) • Society of Pediatric Nurses (SPN) • National Association of Pediatric Nurse Practitioners (NAPNAP) • National Association of Neonatal Nurses (NANN) • National Association of Neonatal Nurse Practitioners (NANNP) • National Association of School Nurses (NASN) • American Professional Society on the Abuse of Children (APSAC) • American Academy of Pediatrics (AAP)
	Hospitals and other health-care settings	• Institutional review boards that approve and monitor research • Institution-specific policies (clinical and administrative)

CRITICAL COMPONENT

The Code of Ethics: A Source of Nursing Character and Strength

The ANA *Code of Ethics for Nurses* is so fundamental to our practice and so richly developed that every nurse should own and periodically reread a copy. The Code takes on new meaning as the nurse gains professional experience, so each rereading has the potential to reveal nuances that further enlighten personal practice. The *Code of Ethics for Nurses* serves as a source of both inspiration and professional pride (ANA, 2015c; used with permission).

Code's provisions have been reduced from 17 to 9, and modified in terms of content, emphasis, language, and format.

PEDIATRIC NURSING SCOPE AND STANDARDS OF PRACTICE

Standards are statements that carry varying degrees of authority, impose responsibilities, outline correct processes, identify target outcomes, specify acceptable levels of performance, and/or define desirable professional attributes and qualifications. Other notes about standards include the following:

- A distinction can be made between "standards" and "guidelines," but for the purposes of this chapter, the terms will be used interchangeably.
- Standards may be labeled as such or may be embedded in laws, rules, policies, position statements, and codes of ethics, among other documents (see Table 2–1).
- Many standards of practice and professional performance are derived from and/or reflect principles embodied in codes of ethics. In some instances, to separate discussions of standards from discussions of ethics is to draw an artificial distinction.

Primary Source of Standards

Although far from the only source of standards of practice for nurses who care for children and their families, the ANA publication *Pediatric Nursing: Scope and Standards of Practice*, 3rd ed. (2015d) is a definitive and primary source. This compilation of standards results from a collaborative effort between the National Association of Pediatric Nurse Practitioners, the Society of Pediatric Nursing, and the ANA to modify and unify previously distinct documents. The revised version specifies 6 standards of practice and 11 standards of professional performance (Box 2–2), elaborating on both with meaningful measurement criteria. It reflects key themes and trends that impact all pediatric health-care settings, and provides the framework for specific standards to emerge.

The scope and standards of pediatric practice are relevant to both nurse generalists and advanced practice nurses, and should be used in conjunction with *Nursing: Scope and Standards of Practice*, 3rd ed. (ANA, 2015e), *Nursing's Social Policy Statement: The Essence of the Profession* (ANA, 2010), and Population-Focused Nurse Practitioner Competencies (Nurse Practitioner Core Competencies Content, 2013).

BOX 2–1 | The Nine Provisions of the ANA *Code of Ethics for Nurses*

"The Code of Ethics for Nurses was developed as a guide for carrying out nursing responsibilities in a manner consistent with quality in nursing care and the ethical obligations of the profession" (ANA, 2015b, para. 1). This code is nonnegotiable.

1. The nurse, in all professional relationships, practices with compassion and respect for the inherent dignity, worth, and uniqueness of every individual, unrestricted by considerations of social or economic status, personal attributes, or the nature of health problems.
2. The nurse's primary commitment is to the patient, whether an individual, family, group, or community.
3. The nurse promotes, advocates for, and strives to protect the health, safety, and rights of the patient.
4. The patient's right to self-determination must be upheld. Limitations to self-determination must always be seen as a deviation from the standard of care, justified only when there are no least restrictive means to preserve the rights of others, justified by law, and maintain public safety.
5. The nurse owes the same duties to self as to others, including the responsibility to preserve integrity and safety, to maintain competence, and to continue personal and professional growth.
6. The nurse participates in establishing, maintaining, and improving health-care environments and conditions of employment conducive to the provision of quality health care and consistent with the values of the profession through individual and collective action.
7. The nurse participates in the advancement of the profession through contributions to practice, education, administration, and knowledge development.
8. The nurse collaborates with other health professionals and the public in promoting community, national, and international efforts to meet health needs.
9. The profession of nursing, as represented by associations and their members, is responsible for articulating nursing values, for maintaining the integrity of the profession and its practice, and for shaping social policy.

BOX 2–2 | Pediatric Nursing Standards of Practice and Professional Performance

"The six Standards of Practice describe competent levels of nursing care, as demonstrated by the nursing process, including assessment, diagnosis, outcome identification, planning, implementation, and evaluation" (ANA, 2015e, p. 6). The 11 Standards of Professional Performance describe competent behavior in a professional role that relates to "quality of practice, outcome measurement, education, communication, ethics, collaboration, research and clinical scholarship, resource utilization, leadership, accountability, and advocacy" (ANA, 2015e, p. 7).

Practice

#1 Assessment: The pediatric nurse collects comprehensive data pertinent to the patient's health or the situation.

#2 Diagnosis: The pediatric nurse analyzes the assessment data to determine the diagnoses or health-care issues.

#3 Outcomes identification: The pediatric nurse identifies expected outcomes for a plan of care individualized to the child, family, and the situation.

#4 Planning: The pediatric nurse develops a plan of care that prescribes strategies and alternatives to attain expected outcomes.

#5 Implementation: The pediatric nurse implements the identified plan of care.

- **5a** Coordination of care and case management: The pediatric nurse coordinates care delivery.
- **5b** Health teaching and health promotion, restoration, and maintenance: The pediatric nurse employs strategies to promote health and a safe environment.
- **5c** Consultation: The pediatric nurse provides consultation to health-care providers and others to influence the identified plan of care for children, to enhance the abilities of others to provide health care, and to effect change in the health-care system.
- **5d** Prescriptive authority and treatment: The advanced practice pediatric nurse utilizes prescriptive authority, procedures, referrals, treatments, and therapies in providing care.
- **5e** Referral: The advanced practice pediatric nurse identifies the need for additional care and makes referrals as indicated.

#6 Evaluation: The pediatric nurse evaluates progress toward attainment of outcomes.

Professional Performance

#7 Ethics: The pediatric nurse integrates ethical considerations and processes in all areas of practice.

#8 Education: The pediatric nurse attains knowledge and competency that reflects current nursing practice.

#9 Research, evidence-based practice, and clinical scholarship: The pediatric nurse integrates research findings into practice and, where appropriate, participates in the generation of new knowledge.

#10 Quality of practice: The pediatric nurse systematically enhances the quality and effectiveness of nursing practice.

#11 Communication: The pediatric registered nurse communicates effectively in a variety of formats in all areas of practice.

#12 Leadership: The pediatric nurse provides leadership in the professional practice setting and the profession.

#13 Collaboration: The pediatric nurse collaborates with the child, family, and others in the conduct of nursing practice.

#14 Professional practice evaluation: The pediatric nurse evaluates one's own nursing practice in relation to professional practice standards and guidelines, relevant statutes, rules and regulations.

#15 Resource utilization: The pediatric nurse considers factors related to safety, effectiveness, cost and impact on practice in planning and delivering patient care.

#16 Environmental health: The pediatric registered nurse practices in an environmentally safe and healthy manner.

#17 Advocacy: The pediatric nurse is an advocate for the pediatric client and family.

Reprinted with permission from the National Association of Pediatric Nurse Practitioners, Society of Pediatric Nurses, and American Nurses Association, *Pediatric Nursing Standards of Practice and Professional Performance*, ©2015.

Role of Therapeutic Relationships

In pediatrics, as in other nursing specialties, the relationship formed between the nurse and the patient/family provides the framework for care delivery. Professional boundaries must be respected but can at times be difficult to define. Therapeutic relationships are respectful, caring relationships between the patient, family, and the child's nurse that are bound by ethical and professional boundaries. These relationships are guided by the six Cs: care, compassion, competence, communication, courage, and commitment (Roberts, Fenton, & Barnard, 2015). (see Chapter 3 for details). Therapeutic communication should be mutually positive and acceptable to all stakeholders, and recognize the individualism and uniqueness of the child, family, and health-care situation. Therapeutic relationships include these characteristics:

- Goal-directed
- Mutual respect and trust
- Empathy
- Advocacy
- Avoidance of the extremes of the relationship continuum (i.e., enmeshment and disengagement)
- Resultant empowerment of the patient/family (McAliley, Lambert, Ashenberg, & Dull, 1996)

Enmeshment occurs when the nurse becomes personally involved with the patient and/or the family unit without regard for professional boundaries. Disengagement is a protective measure used by nurses to protect themselves from difficult situations that may result in patient neglect. Disengagement can also be a professional measure to end the nurse–patient relationship at the conclusion of care.

Therapeutic Relationship Challenges in Pediatric Care Settings

Infants and children are innately vulnerable, and this vulnerability increases when parents or guardians are not present and/or unable to participate in the child's care. This inherent vulnerability may lead the nurse to either distancing or overinvolvement, especially in cases that involve children who are:

- Abused and neglected
- Terminally ill
- Addicted to drugs
- Chronically ill with a condition such as cystic fibrosis, cancer, or sickle cell anemia that leads to repeated hospital admissions
- Tough, street-wise adolescents who challenge everything and everyone
- Children or families who are perceived as noncompliant or nonadherent
- Children of parents diagnosed with borderline personality disorder or other types of mental illness

As in any field of nursing, the cultural background, life experiences, and values of the nurse can result in biases and blind spots—especially when they differ from those of the patient or family. The Safe and Effective Nursing Care: Clinical Pearl box describes potential pitfalls for the pediatric nurse and strategies he or she can use to develop a truly therapeutic patient/family relationship.

Professional Boundaries and Personal Authenticity

Provision 2.4 of the ANA *Code of Ethics for Nurses* acknowledges the challenge of maintaining appropriate professional and personal boundaries while supporting positive outcomes for the patient (ANA, 2015c). Discovering and respecting professional boundaries and the keys to a therapeutic relationship are lifetime pursuits, but very few studies about boundaries provide specifics as to where the boundaries should be drawn.

Policies and rules governing professional boundaries sometimes conflict, making it necessary for the pediatric nurse to use professional judgment and collaborative decision making. It is prudent to articulate a shared concept of what constitutes a therapeutic relationship and to identify explicit guidelines for interactions with patients, families, and colleagues in the workplace. Individuals should commit to holding themselves and their colleagues accountable for maintaining boundaries and revisit agreements as problems arise or staff turnover occurs.

The Roots of Challenging Patient and Family Behaviors

Because of the fiduciary nature of the connection between nurse and client, the nurse bears greater responsibility than the family for promoting and sustaining a therapeutic relationship; however, this does not imply that the patient and family have no responsibility, or that the nurse has total control over the outcome. Nurses should avoid the use of labeling and instead use assessment skills to determine the roots of a problematic relationship, which will:

- Reduce the impulse to personalize the patient/family behavior.
- Help the provider maintain compassion.
- Avert a defensive or adversarial response.
- Facilitate identifying and addressing personal contributions to the situation.
- Provide insights regarding appropriate intervention.

Once contributing factors have been identified, the nurse must use judgment with respect to whether the primary focus should be on addressing the underlying factors, more directly addressing the disruptive behaviors, or taking a combined approach (Box 2–3).

SAFE AND EFFECTIVE NURSING CARE: Clinical Pearl

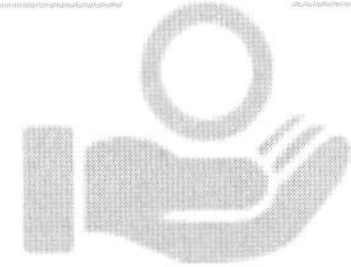

Therapeutic Relations, Family-Centered Care, and Relationship-Based Nursing: A Cautionary Note

The elements of family-centered care and relationship-based nursing are key to quality care, but they are also associated with potential hazards, the avoidance of which requires thoughtful analysis and application of self as the nurse develops a therapeutic alliance. Common issues include the following:

- Some nurses may believe that an interaction or intervention that feels "warm and fuzzy" and makes patients and families happy must be therapeutic and laudable, when in fact, these moments can actually result in boundary violations and staff splitting, create unrealistic expectations of staff on the part of the family, and interfere with achievement of key outcome goals
- Lack of distinction between being a friend and being a friendly professional
- Lack of distinction between being a parent substitute and being a caring, nurturing professional
- Lack of distinction between using good nursing judgment and being prejudiced or judgmental

Recognizing these distinctions and acting accordingly is where some of the "art" of nursing comes into play. This can be particularly challenging in the pediatric setting because of patient vulnerability.

FAMILY-CENTERED CARE

Family-centered care recognizes that families are central to the well-being of children and, subsequently, the impact a child's illness may have on the family. This type of care promotes a partnership between patients, families, and health-care professionals to the benefit

SAFE AND EFFECTIVE NURSING CARE: Clinical Pearl

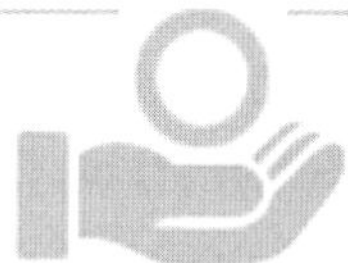

Therapeutic Relations: Sorting Out Boundaries

Nurses must consider boundaries and guidelines regarding:

- Sharing/disclosure of personal information with patients/families
- Accepting gifts from and giving gifts to patients/families
- Loaning money to patients/families
- Offering rides to family members
- Babysitting for or socializing with patients/families outside the workplace
- Assignments and patient contact when a patient or family member is a relative, friend, or acquaintance
- Visiting the patient when he or she is admitted or transferred to another clinical location
- Funeral attendance when patients die

Criteria for Analysis

- What objectives do these actions meet, and whose needs do they serve?
- What are the potential impacts on others?
- How do these actions impact outcome goals?
- How do these activities relate to workplace mission and policies?
- What safeguards must be put in place?
- Would you do the same with or for every patient/family in your care under similar circumstances?
- When nursing judgment suggests the usual standard may or should be ignored, what issues should be considered and who else (if anyone) needs to be involved in the decision?

(ANA, 2015c; McAliley et al., 1996)

of all. The presence and involvement of the family can be as important to the child in some respects as any medication or treatment.

Family may be defined in a variety of ways. Nurses should be prepared to accommodate single-parent families, adoptive families, foster families, blended families, second-generation (grandparenting) families, same-sex partners or marriages, families involving mixed cultures or religions, and other family configurations (see Chapter 3).

Overview of Family-Centered and Family-Focused Strategies

When caring for patients and families, the pediatric nurse should keep in mind family-centered strategies to improve outcomes and build a therapeutic relationship. For example:

- Involve parents in medical rounds, nursing change-of-shift reports, and the child's plan of care.

BOX 2–3 | Potential Contributing Factors to Challenging Family Behaviors

As the nurse cares for children and their families, many factors influence how these children or families respond or cope. Some external factors cannot be controlled by the nurse but affect the health-care environment.

- Anxiety regarding the child's condition/prognosis, unexpected changes in condition, the risks and burdens of treatment, transfers to a new environment
- Guilt over child's condition
- Family is in possession of inadequate information or misinformation
- Fear of loss of control (common among people with professional/leadership backgrounds)
- Unmet expectations (realistic or otherwise)
- Competing work/family/financial worries/concerns
- Altered thought process (mental health, substance abuse)
- Previous bad hospital experience or fears inspired by national focus on hospital errors and hospital-acquired infections
- Conflicting communications from professionals involved in the child's care
- Delays in availability of care/equipment
- Failures/errors of health-care team
- Environmental issues (dirty, lack of parental accommodations and privacy, noisy)
- Staff rude, impatient, slow to respond to need for assistance
- Unreasonably inflexible hospital/unit rules that fail to permit individualized care

- Adapt schedules as possible to suit the patient/family's routines and preferences.
- Implement noise-reduction efforts, including quiet hours and placing cellphones and other devices on vibrate mode.
- Decrease lighting during evening hours.
- Plan periods of "quiet time" when diagnostic and therapeutic intrusions are limited.
- Implement programs that provide free or reduced-cost food for breastfeeding mothers.
- Provide access to refrigerators and the means to prepare and heat food brought from home.
- Provide dedicated family space in patient rooms, and laundry and lounge facilities for rooming-in parents.
- Place signs on doors reminding providers to knock.
- Consider whether family-centered initiatives of other organizations and similar programs could be adopted in your workplace. For example, for more than 35 years Ronald McDonald House Charities has sponsored "Ronald McDonald Family Rooms" that provide free access to a living room environment and host/hostess services. Many hospitals offer their own version of a hospitality center.

- Create staffed "Family Resource Centers" with library and computer services to facilitate access to medical educational information, health-care support groups, and special services.
- Create staffed "Family Learning Centers," where families can learn common procedures such as blood glucose testing and administration of insulin injections. The center should include:
  - Dedicated instructors
  - Formal teaching modules and videos
  - Simulated, hands-on practice with anatomically correct dolls
  - Consistent educational practices
  - Opportunities to develop confidence and competence to perform required care procedures in a low-pressure setting
- Create "Family and Patient Advisory Councils" that permit input into policies, programming, building renovation or design, food services, or other areas.
- Create "Foster Grandparent" or "Special Visitor" programs that provide visitors for children who do not have family members rooming-in or visiting with frequency.

Rewards of Family-Centered Care

The benefits of family-centered care are:

- Enhanced patient and family learning of new information and skills
- Decreased levels of patient and family stress
- Increased likelihood of adherence to plans of care
- Reduced likelihood of medical error
- Improved patient/family sleep and nutrition
- Decreased disruption of normal patient/family routines and responsibilities
- Increased patient and family satisfaction

For additional information about family-centered care, visit the websites of the Institute for Patient- and Family-Centered Care and the Family Voices (see the later "Additional Resources" section for links).

Role of Child Life Specialists

Like nurses, child life specialists are key proponents of family-centered care, and their presence in inpatient settings, clinics, emergency departments, intensive care units, rehabilitation settings, procedural planning, and other areas is of incalculable value. Child life specialists possess expertise in the field of child development, including a 4-year degree in child psychology or a related field. After 480 hours of field experience, they are eligible to take an examination to achieve Child Life Specialist Certification from the Child Life Council. They promote effective coping, ongoing development, and normalization for children and families by:

- Preparing children and families for and supporting them through procedures
- Providing therapeutic play and self-expression opportunities
- Helping design and maintain child- and family-friendly environments
- Working closely with art and music therapists, and acting as liaisons with hospital- and community-based teachers

DEVELOPMENTALLY APPROPRIATE CARE

Children are not simply mini-adults. They are in the process of developing in the physiological, motor, cognitive, psychosocial, psychosexual, moral, and spiritual realms. In addition to facility with child development, the pediatric nurse must also recognize that families go through stages of development. (See Chapters 3 and 6 for overviews of family and child development theories.) A complex interplay of genetic, experiential, and environmental factors influences the developmental course and outcomes of a given child and family. Familiarity with developmental theories, principles, and milestones enables:

- Effective communication and support that maximizes cooperation and minimizes anxiety
- Developmentally appropriate and effective assessments, goals, plan of care, and education
- Safely structured environments, routines, and procedures
- Facilitation or minimal disruption of ongoing development

Child Development and Pain Management

Prompt and effective pain management is an absolute moral imperative, and there are definite developmental implications for the assessment and management of discomfort in children. Children differ from adults in physiological responses to pain; ability to describe, localize, and quantify pain; and tolerance of and response to medications.

Many tested tools are available for assessing the need for and response to pain management interventions in children of different ages or stages of development (see Table 2–2). Assessment tools can be classified as behavioral observation scales (infants) or self-report rating scales (young child through adult).

Infant behavioral scales rely on specifically defined indicators, such as vital signs, need for oxygen, breathing patterns, facial expressions, presence and nature of crying, and movement of extremities (Hamil, Lyndon, Liley, & Hill, 2014). Use of infant behavior observation tools requires staff training and achievement of interobserver reliability, which means similar results are obtained by different observers.

Self-report rating scales necessitate preliminary teaching with the child and family, and assessment of the child's readiness to use a specific tool. These scales may require a child to:

- Point to drawings or photos of facial expressions reflecting varying degrees of pain.
- Pick up a number of poker chips that correlates with the amount of pain.
- Point to a spot on a visual scale that is associated with a number (usually 0 to 10) and/or words that describe pain feelings.

Success in using the self-report rating scales necessitates preliminary teaching with the child and family, and assessment of the

TABLE 2–2 Overview of Select Pain Assessment Scales

BEHAVIORAL AND PHYSICAL INDICATOR SCALES			
PIPP: Premature Infant Pain Profile (Stevens, Johnston, Taddio, Gibbins, & Yamada, 2010)	**NIPS:** Neonatal Infant Pain Scale (Srouji, Ratnapalan, & Schneeweiss, 2010)	**CRIES** (Krechel & Bildner, 1995)	**FLACC** (Voepel-Lewis, Zanotti, Dommeyer, & Merkel, 2010)
Neonates (28–40 weeks of gestation)	Preterm and full-term neonates	Preterm and full-term neonates	2 months to 7 years of age
0–3 points each for gestational age, behavioral state, heart rate, O_2 saturation, brow bulge, eye squeeze, nasolabial furrow	0–1 (2 for cry) points each for facial expression, cry, breathing patterns, arm movements, leg movements, state of arousal	0–2 points each for **c**ry, **r**equires O_2, **i**ncreased vital signs, **e**xpression, **s**leeplessness	1–3 points each for **f**ace, **l**egs, **a**ctivity, **c**ry, **c**onsolability
SELF-REPORT SCALES			
FACES (Witt, Coynor, Edwards, & Bradshaw, 2016)	**Oucher** (Beyer, 2009)	**VAS: Visual Analogue Scales (variety of scales and descriptors)**	**Adolescent Pediatric Pain Tool** (multidimensional) (Savedra & Crandall, 2005)
3 years through adolescence	3 years and older	6 years and older	8–17 years
Six line drawings of faces with expressions from happy to neutral to crying, each associated with a number from 1 to 6	Series of photographs of facial expressions from neutral to crying (Caucasian, Hispanic, African American, First Nation, Asian) associated with ratings of 0 to 10	Horizontal or vertical line with linguistic pain descriptors and equidistant markings associated with numbers (usually 0–10)	Body outline (draw location of pain); word-graphic scale (mark on a line closest to the intensity descriptor); word list (circle the sensory, affective, and evaluative words that apply)

child's readiness to use a specific tool. Growth and developmental status also influence choice of pharmacological and/or nonpharmacological pain management techniques:

- In the first few months of life, nonnutritive sucking and/or the administration of small amounts of 24% sucrose solution have been demonstrated to effectively reduce physiological and behavioral responses to pain and hasten the recovery from simple procedural pain.
- Distraction (e.g., toys, television, video games) can work to some extent with children of almost all ages who are experiencing pain at the lower end of the pain scales.
- Hypnotherapy, biofeedback, and other complementary and alternative treatment approaches may be suitable for children able to follow instructions and use their imaginations.

Medication dosages are calculated based on weight or body surface area, and formulations of oral medications depend on the child's ability to swallow pills versus liquid. Most children's pain medications are flavored to increase acceptance, but some may need to be disguised further (American Academy of Pediatrics, Committee on Fetus and Newborn, 2006; Butchelor & Marriott, 2013; Ivanovska, Rademaker, vanDijk, & Mantel-Teeuwisse, 2014; Lopez, Ernest, Tuleu, & Gul, 2015).

Patient and Family Education

The nurse provides children and their families with learning opportunities related to health maintenance and promotion, illness and injury management, and decision making and coping. In the role of patient educator, the nurse is responsible for:

- Assessing learning preference styles with guidance from parents when possible
- Assessing learning readiness (interest and motivation; freedom from pain, anxiety, distractions)
- Provision of accurate, useful information that is developmentally appropriate and culturally sensitive, as well as tailored to individual needs
- Assessment of information understanding and retention, as well as the need for reinforcement and/or additional education
- Documentation of the above

Children are active learners and should be provided with developmentally appropriate and culturally sensitive health-care education materials such as videos, comic books, drawings, reader-friendly diagrams, computer-assisted learning, and hands-on experience with anatomically correct dolls and actual materials and equipment.

Evidence-Based Practice: Adult Literacy and Readability of Health-Care Education

Healthy People. (2017). Health communication and health information technology. Retrieved from https://www.healthypeople.gov/2020/topics-objectives/topic/health-communication-and-health-information-technology

Healthy People 2020 identified health literacy as one of its core objectives. In 2017, the Centers for Disease Control and Prevention (CDC) estimated that 90 million adults have low health literacy (CDC, 2017). In 2011, 64.1% of people aged 18 years and older reported that instructions from health-care providers were easy to understand (Healthy People, 2017).

Objectives of *Healthy People 2020* include:

- Improving the health literacy of the population
- Increasing the proportion of patients who indicate that communication with health-care providers was satisfactory
- Increasing the proportion of patients who use electronic health management tools
- Increasing individual internet access
- Increasing the number of quality health-related websites
- Increased social marketing in health promotion and disease prevention
- Increased crisis and emergency risk messages to protect the public health (CDC, 2017)

Background

Multiple studies have demonstrated a correlation between low literacy and poor health-care behaviors and outcomes, such as frequent emergency care visits and hospital admissions, decreased compliance with medications, improper use of metered-dose inhalers, incorrect installation of infant car seats, failure to seek screening and later diagnosis of cancer, and poorer glycemic control, to name just a few examples (CDC, 2017).

According to the CDC, health literacy is "the degree to which individuals have the capacity to obtain, process, and understand basic health information and services needed to make appropriate health decisions" (CDC, 2016, para. 1)

Recommendations

- Health education materials intended for *adults* should be created at a reading level no higher than eighth grade, although most are written at a more difficult level.
- Try the SMOG (Simple Measure of Gobbledygook) approach to assess and adjust readability. Details on this method and a SMOG calculator are available through a website belonging to its originator, Harry McLaughlin (see the later "Additional Resources" section for the link.)

Child Development, Privacy, and Confidentiality

Privacy and confidentiality are related but distinct concepts that must be addressed from a developmental perspective, because both give rise to challenges of an ethical nature in the pediatric setting. Standards require increasing respect for the needs for privacy and confidentiality as children get older. With maturity, minors become increasingly more involved in providing their own medical history and begin to approach health-care professionals with their own agendas.

Older children cannot be expected to provide reliable information or request education or services with respect to sensitive subjects if not provided with privacy and some assurance of confidentiality. Such sensitive subjects include:

- Family violence
- Substance use/abuse
- Depression and suicidal thoughts
- Struggles with weight or eating disorders
- Gender identity issues and sexual activity

Privacy measures must also be taken with respect to the physical examination, and the older child or adolescent may request confidentiality of some clinical findings and even diagnoses.

Conflicting Duties to Child and Parents

Respecting the privacy and confidentiality of pediatric patients may create some tension for nurses when they experience a sense of conflict with between duties owed to the child and those owed to the parent. Parents must instill values and provide for the health and safety of the child, which can be difficult to do if they have limited information. The pediatric nurse must educate parents and older children and adolescents about privacy and confidentiality. Education in this area supports the child in developing identity and autonomy through the protection of that child's privacy.

It is also important to specify practical limitations and legal exceptions. Although pediatric nurses should encourage frank and open discussion about sensitive matters between adolescents and their parents, they must also be aware that sometimes such discussions will not happen, and, in select cases, that honest discussion could be dangerous for the child. When unable to convince the child to disclose to parents or provide consent to do so on his or her behalf, confidentiality will be maintained to the degree that is practical and legal. Even though information may sometimes be withheld from parents, the professional should not lie on behalf of the child.

Practical Limitations and Legal Exceptions Regarding Confidentiality

Practical considerations may preclude confidentiality. These include:

- Parental right to access medical records: Although some confidential information may be omitted by the nurse when documenting histories and examinations, other sensitive information must be documented to justify care given, direct the care of others, record responses to treatment, or as required by law or professional standard.
- Parental financial responsibility: Parents are not obligated to pay for nonemergency care for which they did not provide consent. This is a major practical barrier to confidentiality for minors without access to a free clinic or funds to pay for treatment. When insurance is used, parents may receive billing information that discloses the nature of the visit/condition.

- Mandatory pregnancy testing: Some important diagnostic procedures and treatments or medications require pregnancy testing and may have to be withheld or significantly modified if the test results are positive. Adolescents and their parents must be informed of the need for the pregnancy testing and told what will be done with the results before the test is performed.

In certain circumstances, the health-care provider is required by law to break confidentiality. Professionals have legal and moral obligations to disclose "reasonable concerns" that a child may intentionally harm himself or herself or another person, as well as suspicions that the child may be the victim of any form of abuse. The child should be given the option to participate in telling his or her parents if that is the professional's intended course of action. Health-care providers should anticipate, prepare the child for, and help mitigate potential fallout from disclosure to family.

In the case of suspected abuse, a report must be made to a child protective services agency and/or to law enforcement (depending on local requirements). There is no need to have proof when reporting suspicions, and the individual who is making the report is immune from liability regardless of the investigation's outcome if it can be shown that the report was made in good faith and not frivolously or maliciously. If it is workplace policy that such reports are filed by a social worker, the nurse must confirm that the patient's record contains documentation of the report, thus fulfilling his or her obligation as a mandated reporter.

SAFE AND EFFECTIVE NURSING CARE: Clinical Pearl

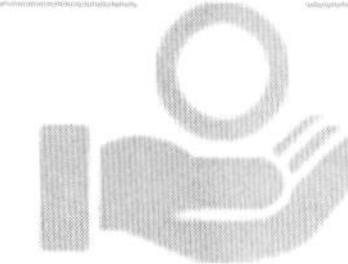

Source of Information Regarding State Parental Consent Requirements

The Alan Guttmacher Institute is a research, policy analysis, and public education organization with the stated aim of advancing sexual and reproductive health on a worldwide basis. Regularly updated state-by-state summaries of adolescent consent regulations are available through its website, along with fact sheets, research articles, policy updates, media kits, slide shows, and other educational aids. Materials for and about adolescents are available. (See the later "Additional Resources" section for link.)

Use of Chaperones

Although their presence can be viewed as a barrier to privacy and confidentiality, an offer of a medical chaperone is highly advisable under potentially sensitive circumstances such as the following:

- Any examination or procedure involving exposure and/or touching of breasts or anal-genital areas
- Examinations involving children/parents known to be anxious, suspicious, seductive, mentally or cognitively impaired, and/or litigious
- A medical history that requires detailed questions of a sensitive nature that could be misinterpreted as inappropriate by the patient (e.g., a history specific to sexual abuse)

Chaperones are an equally wise precaution for nurses as for physicians because they afford protection for both the patient and the professional regardless of whether they are of the same sex or opposite sex. Parents make effective chaperones in most cases with infants and young children, but are often not acceptable to older children and adolescents for privacy reasons. Chaperones must be aware of the responsibility to witness safe and appropriate care delivery, and to maintain privacy and confidentiality. The presence and identity of the chaperone should be documented in the medical record. The patient/family and chaperone should receive a full explanation of the nature and purpose of the examination or procedure so that surprises, misperceptions, and charges of impropriety are less likely. They should also be informed that the same confidentiality safeguards apply to the chaperone as to the examining physician/nurse.

If the offer of a chaperone is declined, the professional should use judgment as to whether the examination/procedure should take place without one or be canceled or deferred to someone else. When possible, the wishes of the patient/family should be honored. The offer and the refusal should be documented.

SAFE AND EFFECTIVE NURSING CARE: Clinical Pearl

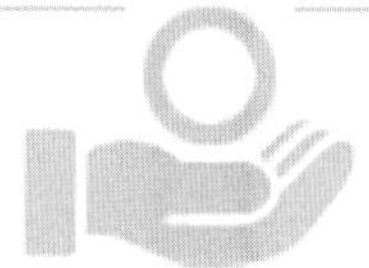

Child Development and Health-Care Decision Making

The extent and manner to which children of various ages can be involved in their own medical decision making is the source of abundant ethical controversies in clinical settings. The concepts, principles, and legalities involved in these issues deserve serious attention. Nurse familiarity with bioethics basics is valuable.

Confidentiality and the Health Insurance Portability and Accountability Act of 1996

Among other provisions, the Health Insurance Portability and Accountability Act of 1996 (HIPAA) requires standards for electronic health-care transactions and mandates the security and privacy of personal health information.

HIPAA imposes obligations with respect to how we dispose of personal health information, shield information on computer screens from the view of others, and afford privacy when registering a patient at a desk in a public lobby or when obtaining a medical history; what we talk about in hospital elevators and hospital cafeterias; and how and where we give change-of-shift nursing reports and make patient rounds.

HIPAA has implications for policies about what we can do and say in front of grandparents who are visiting, how we respond to a telephone caller claiming to be a parent, what we do when a patient asks for an update regarding another patient with whom he or she is friendly and shares information, and how we protect parts of the record the patient wishes to remain confidential.

SAFE AND EFFECTIVE NURSING CARE: Clinical Pearl

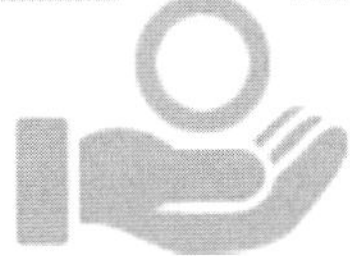

Privacy Passwords

Privacy passwords may be used in the case of custody issues or suspected child abuse, where health information privacy needs to be protected from unauthorized individuals. At admission, have parents select a personalized password. Instruct them to share this password only with persons with whom they permit staff to share the patient's personal information. Remind them they will need to remember the password when calling from outside the hospital. Record this password in an easily retrievable section of the medical record and in a protected area at workstations.

PEDIATRIC DECISION MAKING

Pediatric health-care providers are often confronted with situations in which the parents disagree with each other, the parents disagree with the child (children should be given an increasingly stronger role in decision making as they mature), and/or the parents disagree with the child and/or with the health-care team. The best-interest standard, in which decisions are made based on the child's best interest, sounds good in principle but in practice presents substantial challenges for health-care providers. Figure 2–1 provides a generic template for decision making in such circumstances.

Best Interest: Who Gets to Decide?

When the patient is a minor, the parent or legal guardian makes the decisions, although this default position is not without limits. Parental decision-making rights should never be revoked casually, and the burden of proof should rest with those challenging those rights. The following are examples of circumstances that may warrant revocation:

- The parents are making decisions based on the interests of someone other than the child or have an apparent conflict of interest. For example, a profoundly brain-injured child with no prospect of recovery or a meaningful interactive life was the victim of parental abuse. Removal of life support would result in the parent being charged with murder instead of child endangerment and other lesser crimes, so the parent refuses to give permission for withdrawal of life-sustaining interventions.
- The parents are insisting on unduly burdensome interventions with very little hope of benefit and that would result in a quality of life that the average person would find intolerable. Individuals may sometimes be misguided in attempts to thwart nature, thus prolonging death rather than preserving life.
- To the clear detriment of the child, the parents are refusing interventions that have a high likelihood of success and benefit, are associated with limited burden, and would be favored by the average person.

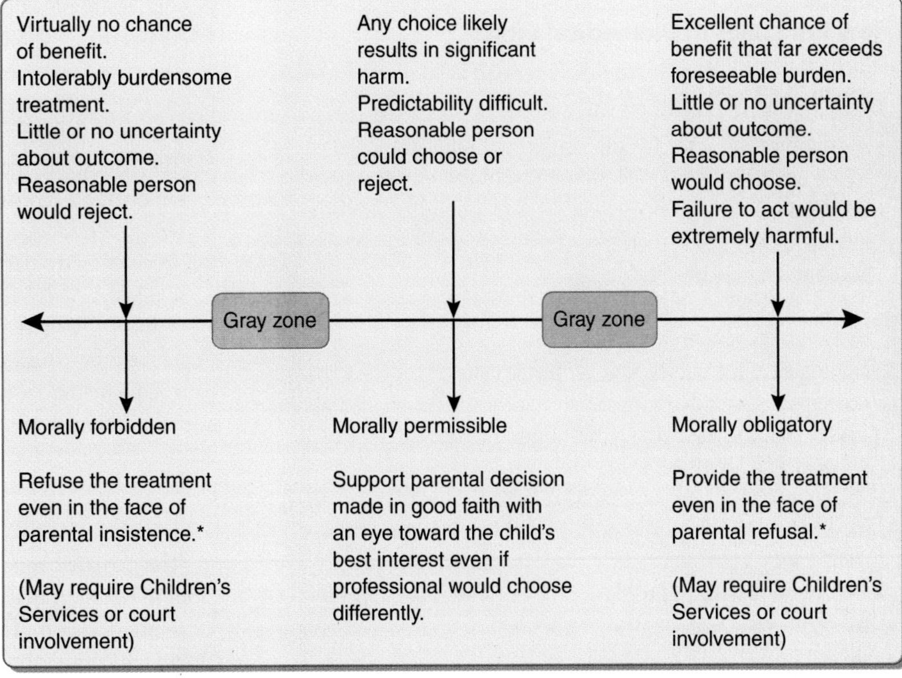

FIGURE 2–1 The best interests of the child: a generic paradigm.

- The parents do not demonstrate the capacity to understand the factors involved in or the implications of the decision they are being asked to make.

It is critical to note that overruling parental or patient preferences (regardless of whether child protective agencies or the courts are involved) should not equate to total disregard for those preferences. The health-care team should:

- Make authentic attempts to understand the family's wishes and the priorities and values behind them.
- Make any partial accommodations or compromises that are possible.
- Continue to update the parents about the child's condition and give them the opportunity to be involved in ongoing planning and care of the child.

The wishes of the child matter, and for some decisions, the child's wishes may be a determining factor. For example:

- A 15-year-old with acute appendicitis who is fearful of and actively resisting the surgery will generally be taken to the operating room even against his wishes. However, a 15-year-old who is fearful of scoliosis surgery and unwilling to deal with the recovery process need not be taken for the procedure against his wishes, because there is time to work with him so that he might come to understand the benefits of the procedure.
- An 8-year-old refusing blood because of religious beliefs will generally be given the transfusion anyway if all else fails, but a 16-year-old's informed, passionate, and insistent refusal of the same on religious grounds may be persuasive, given what we understand of the stages of spiritual development.

CRITICAL COMPONENT

Key Principles of Biomedical Ethics

The following principles are commonly viewed as primary to the analysis and resolution of bioethics dilemmas.

- Autonomy: The right for the competent adult to accept or refuse any medical treatment based on his or her own values, priorities and preferences regardless of potential outcome, including death. Basis for privacy, confidentiality, and informed consent & refusal policies.
- Beneficence*: The duty of health-care providers to do things that are beneficial or good.
- Nonmaleficence*: The duty of health-care providers to do no harm.
- Justice: Fair access to and distribution of resources—treat patients with like needs in like ways.
- Veracity: This may be seen as the duty to tell the truth or may merely be viewed as the duty not to lie. The distinction is significant.
- Fidelity: Duty to keep promises (some promises are implied in the context of a nurse–patient relationship rather than expressly stated).
- Sanctity of life: Do not kill.

*It is often not possible to benefit patients without causing harm (for example, if the patient has bone cancer, it may not be possible to cure the cancer without exposing the child to amputation and toxic chemotherapy and radiation). Beneficence and nonmaleficence are therefore often combined and treated as one principle—that of "utility": do things that provide proportionately greater good than harm and avoid doing things that are disproportionately burdensome. The focus is on consequences or outcomes and brings quality-of-life considerations into play. Outcomes can be difficult to predict with confidence and quality of life can be very subjective.

(Veatch, R.M. 2011); (Fox & Demarco, 2008); (Beauchamp & Childress, 2001).

CRITICAL COMPONENT

Standards of Ethical Decision Making & Relationship to Child Development/Capacity

- Gold standard—autonomy—competent individual makes informed choice based on personal priorities and values and free of coercion. Applies to most adults.
- Primarily a negative right: The right to be left alone.
- No right to care that is futile or exceedingly and disproportionately burdensome or fails to meet recognized standards of practice and care.
- Silver standard—substituted judgment—a surrogate stands in for a previously competent individual who is currently unable to express personal preferences.
- The surrogate chooses what he has good reason to believe (based on prior written instructions or past conversations or observations of the way the patient lived his life and made other relevant choices) the patient himself would have chosen.
- Applies to previously competent adults who may now suffer dementia or who may be comatose or intubated and sedated or under the influence of mind altering drugs, etc.
- Bronze standard—best interest—a surrogate makes the decision on behalf of an individual who is not and never was competent (or who may have been competent in the past but for whom there is no friend or relative or document that can tell us what his preferences might have been).
- Decisions are based on what is judged to be in the patient's best interest.
- Applies to infants, young children, and most adolescents most of the time as well as to significantly cognitively impaired and/or mentally ill adults.

(Veatch, 2011); (Beauchamp & Childress, 2001).

The pediatric nurse and health-care team should involve children in decision making even when they will not be making the ultimate decision. This should include developmentally appropriate education about his or her condition, treatment options, and rationale for choices, as well as solicitation of the child's preferences and associated reasons for these preferences.

SAFE AND EFFECTIVE NURSING CARE: Cultural Competence

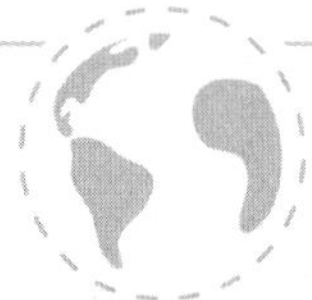

Strategies for Achieving Concordance Between the Family and the Health-Care Team

Before overruling parental decisions, the following strategies should be used, assuming the child's condition permits the time required:

- Tincture of time/repeated discussions that are goal and outcome focused: For example, this strategy may be effective when repeated instructions to the parents are not implemented, resulting in a detriment to the child's condition.
- Family should be encouraged to spend substantial time bedside, so the reality of the child's situation and experience is apparent.
- Goal and outcome-focused care conferences should be conducted with all involved specialists, family members, and key family support persons.
- Ethics consultation with Ethics Committee involvement may be required in some circumstances.

CRITICAL COMPONENT

Consent, Assent, and Permission

Informed consent: An individual with presumed (or demonstrated) adult decision-making capacity agrees to (or refuses) diagnostic or treatment interventions for himself or may accept or reject participation in a clinical research trial.

- In the United States, the age of consent for most medical decision making is 18 years.
  - "Emancipated Minor" status and "Mature Minor Doctrine" provide for exceptions to the 18-year age requirement (see below).
- In parts of Canada, the age of consent for medical decision making is 14 years.
- In parts of the United States, teenage parents may make medical decisions for their babies that they are not in the same legal position to make for themselves and this can be the source of confusion and frustration for those adolescents, for health-care providers, and for the grandparents of the babies.

Informed assent: A child or other individual thought not to have full capacity to make freely chosen and informed decisions is asked his thoughts about treatment or participating in a research trial (if parent or guardian has provided prior approval).

- Basic information about the child's condition and proposed treatment is provided at the level of the child's ability to comprehend it and his support is sought.
- If the child refuses:
  - Treatment may be modified until it is acceptable to the child,
  - Treatment may not be provided at all,
  - Treatment may be delayed to permit further discussion until the child is in agreement, or
  - Treatment proceeds and child is given developmentally appropriate explanations why the plan is going ahead despite his expressed rejection.
- Research assent is requested as young as 7 years of age.
  - Standards are stricter for child participation in research as the child is generally being exposed to risks with little or no hope of benefit for himself or, as in the cases of some cancer treatment protocols, there is the hope of benefit but the risks are significant and the outcomes are very uncertain.

Informed parental permission: A parent or guardian makes an informed and freely chosen decision to permit (or refuse to permit) the treatment or research participation the professional has recommended for the child. If we are to be precise in our use of terminology, individuals provide "consent" to their own care but surrogates provide "permission" for the care of others.

Best Interest: What Criteria Count?

How do we decide what factors should be taken into consideration and how much weight should be assigned to any given factor? Common metrics include:

- Reasonable person standard: This refers to what the "average person," "most people," or the "reasonable person" would choose. In any group of 10 people debating a true bioethical dilemma, there will likely be a diversity of opinion, and yet it is just as likely that all 10 individuals believe his or her choice represents what "reasonable people" would choose.
- Consensus or majority standard: This means taking a vote. However, the group must determine whether the decision will be made based on 100% agreement, a clear and convincing majority, or just a majority of one. It is important to note that major support alone is not sufficient to prove a course of action is "right."
- Basing the decision strictly on medical criteria: However, this metric disregards the important elements of religion, finances, resource distribution and utilization, impact on marriage and family, and other key factors.

Role of Parental Religion in Best-Interest Determinations

With few limitations, parents have the right to raise their children according to the tenets of their religion and in keeping with the practices of their culture. Health-care professionals must make an authentic attempt to understand the religious and cultural beliefs of the child and family, respect the right for individuals to have and express those beliefs, and attempt to honor them to the extent that is feasible and safe.

Paraphrasing a famous legal quote from the Supreme Court decision in the case of *Prince v. Commonwealth of Massachusetts* (1944), parents are free to martyr themselves based on their own religious beliefs but may not make martyrs of their children, who do not yet have the capacity to make the same decisions in an informed and freely chosen manner. Parental religious beliefs and cultural practices that expose children to significant, reasonably imminent, and avoidable harm, suffering, or death should not be honored.

Partnering With Children in Decision Making

As children grow up and their capacity for decision making develops and matures, they can and should become more actively involved in promoting their own health care. In specific circumstances, some adolescents are accorded autonomy by law for their health-care choices. Nurses and parents can help prepare the minor to transition from pediatric to adult health care by gradually increasing his or her responsibility for:

- Providing his or her own medical history
- Making appointments independently
- Making sure prescriptions do not run out
- Contributing to the development of the plan of care

Patient Self-Determination Act and Advance Directives

Young adults with chronic childhood conditions may continue to receive care in pediatric inpatient and ambulatory care settings, so pediatric nurses must be familiar with policies and their role regarding the Patient Self-Determination Act (PSDA) and advance directives. The PSDA is an amendment to the Federal Omnibus Budget Reconciliation Act of 1990 that, strictly speaking, applies to those who are 18 years of age or older, but it has implications with respect to participation of adolescents in decision making regarding end-of-life care. (See the later "Additional Resources" section for an online link that provides government accountability office review of implementation of the PSDA.) The PDSA requires Medicare and Medicaid facilities and health-care providers to inform competent adults of their right to accept or refuse treatment and to express their preferences through advance directives such as a living will or durable power of attorney for health care. Other important factors related to the PDSA include the following:

- Although minors are not qualified to draw up formalized advance directives that have guaranteed legal standing, discussions concerning these documents should be held from time to time with older children and adolescents who have chronic or life-threatening conditions. These conversations are of clinical, ethical, and legal importance even without *automatic* legal standing. They can carry significant weight with parents, health-care professionals, and, if necessary, with courts in times of crisis and/or conflict. Delaying these discussions until times of crisis or conflict adds to the stress experienced by all involved, potentially creating a barrier to thoughtful decision making.
- Ethics consultants recommend documenting any conversations of this nature; not only does doing so create an opportunity to influence the family, but it also allows the health-care team to influence the guardian *ad litem* or court if necessary.

An advance directive is more than a legal document; it's a reflection of a process over time between health-care professionals, their patients, and the families and loved ones. Even though discussions surrounding advance directives can be quite emotional, they also build and strengthen bonds among the patient and members of his or her support system. The pediatric nurse should encourage children and their parents to have these discussions together and provide them with guidance and support; even when another member of the child's medical team sees these discussions as his or her prerogative or has had the task formally assigned, children and families may seek out the nurse as the person who spends the most time at the bedside. (See Chapter 5 for further discussion.)

SAFE AND EFFECTIVE NURSING CARE: Clinical Pearl

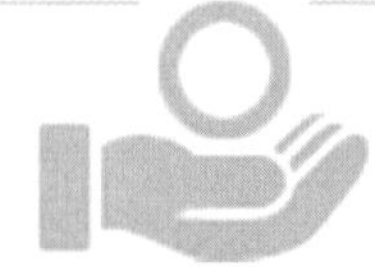

Approaching Children About Advance Directives

Discussions with children about advance directives do not have to be formal, lengthy, or directed toward specific end-of-life issues. They generally are not conducted in a single setting but take place over time. The discussions may be planned and initiated by the health-care provider, or they may be impromptu and initiated by the patient or the provider. Questions that may help determine the patient's values, priorities, and preferences include:

- What things are most enjoyable and most important to you in life?
- What do you hope to accomplish during your life?
- What, if anything, would make life seem intolerable to you?
- What things worry you?
- What things do you believe worry your parents?

The health-care provider can capitalize on situations the child or adolescent has seen other patients encounter or has seen in the news, and ask questions such as:

- Is that something you've ever thought about or worried about?
- If you were in that situation, what do you think you would want?
- What do you think your parents would want for you?
- Have you ever discussed this with them? If yes: How did they react, and how do you feel about the discussion you had? If no: What keeps you from having this discussion, and what do you think would happen if you brought it up?
- We've helped other children like you talk with their parents—would you like some help from someone here to have this kind of discussion with your family?

If discussions are based on the direct experiences of the patient, questions similar to the following are appropriate:

- You were in the intensive care unit last month and you were supported with a ventilator for several days. What was that like for you?
- If you were to require the support of a ventilator again, what would you think about that?
- What would you want if it was determined that you could not be successfully weaned from the ventilator but would need it for the remainder of your life?

CRITICAL COMPONENT

Documenting Advance Directive Discussions

When discussing advance directions with a patient, make sure to document the following:

- Context, including who raised the topic and how
- Specific topics and scenarios discussed
- Specific options introduced and preferences expressed
- Underlying values and priorities the patient might reveal

The last element can be difficult to elicit from children, but it is helpful information to seek, because one cannot anticipate all possible scenarios and options (McAliley, Hudson, Gunning, & Rowbottom, 2000).

SAFETY IN THE PEDIATRIC SETTING

Health-care safety concerns are monitored both within the health-care industry and by educated consumers and watchdog agencies. These concerns have spawned a multitude of studies and standards that strive to protect patients from:

- Medication errors
- Hospital-acquired infections
- Wrong-surgery/wrong-site incidents
- Falls
- Skin breakdown in bedridden patients or those with limited mobility
- Abduction (in pediatric facilities)

National Patient Safety Goals

National Patient Safety Goals (NPSGs) are issued by The Joint Commission (formerly known as the Joint Commission on Accreditation of Healthcare Organizations) and updated annually. The Joint Commission is a private nonprofit organization that accredits hospitals and other health-care organizations. Accreditation is a voluntary process that promotes health-care safety and quality based on hundreds of benchmark standards, including NPSGs identified each year for nationwide priority attention. NPSGs that are especially critical or that need constant reinforcement may be carried over from year to year. As with other standards, some of the NSPGs require adaptation in the pediatric setting. (See the later "Additional Resources" section for an online link to the current year's NPSGs.)

Two NPSGs that were focuses of previous years and require pediatric adaptation or considerations are:

- Requirement for the use of two patient identifiers
- Requirement for implementation of a program aimed at the reduction of patient falls

Two Patient Identifiers

Two patient identifiers must be checked every time a patient is admitted, transported, transferred, or discharged; every time a medication or blood product is administered; every time a laboratory specimen is obtained; and every time a procedure is performed, no matter how long the patient has been known to the nurse or admitted to the facility.

In most inpatient settings, the identifiers are the patient's first and last name and the patient's medical record number, manually read from a patient ID band and scanned with a bar code wand. The room or bed number may not be one of the identifiers. In ambulatory care settings where patients may not wear an ID, the most common identifiers are name and birth date.

There are challenges associated with checking two identifiers in a pediatric setting:

- Premature infants are so tiny that bands often do not fit, and their fragile skin may be easily irritated.
- Older infants and toddlers often find ingenious ways to remove ID bands that adults have a hard time removing.
- Teens may not like being identified as patients and remove the IDs when their friends are visiting.
- Children in outpatient settings who may be old enough to tell their names may still not be able to provide their birth dates.
- When parents are not present and an ID has been removed from a child or infant who cannot provide his or her own ID, there must be a standard in place for verifying the child's identity before applying a new ID.

Child identification is not the only challenge; parent identification is also a safety issue. This can be especially true when a child is the subject of a custody dispute. Many children's hospitals lock all entrances and exits from patient care units and require all visitors to wear photo ID. In some settings, children are tagged with ID equipment that sets off alarms if the children are removed from the setting in an unauthorized manner. The manner in which these safety precautions are presented to patients and families is important. Parents may become insulted or frustrated by insistence that the ID be worn at all times and checked every time a treatment or medication is administered, even though the staff members know the child and family well. Everyone on the care team must be held accountable for following ID safety standards all of the time to preserve parental trust in the staff and prevent children from receiving the wrong care or being removed by noncustodians.

Patient Falls Reduction Standards

Health-care facilities are required to implement programs to reduce the number of patient falls and evaluate the effectiveness of those programs; identify patients at risk for falls and notify everyone on the care team; develop standardized strategies for addressing risk and document their application; and educate staff and families on these protocols. Children present special challenges for fall reduction:

- Older infants and toddlers who are learning to walk frequently fall (although not very far and usually without sustaining any injuries).
- Preschool children run as much as they walk and are not particularly safety conscious.

- Cribs, infant seats, beds, examination tables, wheelchairs, and high chairs present their own safety challenges if children are not secured or monitored appropriately, or equipment is not maintained properly.

Until recently, most of the data and literature addressing falls risk factors and reduction strategies were specific to adult patients and adult-care settings. Statistics are now being compiled and risks evaluated in pediatric health-care settings. Notably, Miami Children's Hospital developed a pediatric falls reduction program that has widespread implementation, use, and evaluation in other settings across the country.

SAFE AND EFFECTIVE NURSING CARE: Promoting Safety

Humpty Dumpty Falls Prevention Program

Miami Children's Hospital developed a pediatric falls reduction program that is available for use by other facilities and includes:

- Risk assessment scale
- Prevention protocol
- Educational materials for staff and for patients and families
- Room signage and patient ID stickers
- Access to onsite or teleconference training sessions

The program is customizable and provides both tools for promoting safety and a basis for quality monitoring. Additional details and ordering information are available through the online link provided in the "Additional Resources" section at the end of the chapter.

Understanding Medications

Medication safety standards that emanate from The Joint Commission and other sources are usually generic and apply to adults as well as children, so it is often up to the pediatric health-care facility to tailor them to reflect the special vulnerability and needs of children. Important considerations include the following:

- Children's medication dosages are largely based on formulas that involve the child's weight and/or body surface calculations. This adds opportunities for error in dosing, such as wrong weight or height, wrong formula, and math errors.
- Children's medications come in a variety of formulations and strengths, presenting additional opportunities for error in preparation and dispensing.
- Infants and young children will not recognize that the wrong medication is being given, and some older children who suspect something is wrong may not feel they can challenge adults by questioning why the pill is a different color or why there are three pills instead of two.
- Most medications given to children have never been researched using child subjects. Furthermore, children may be unable to communicate symptoms of adverse reactions, so they must be monitored closely for more objective signs.

Medication Safety Precautions

Pediatric nurses can help ensure medication safety with the following measures:

- Reconciliation of medications given at home with those given in the hospital, as well as reconciliation of medications given in different areas of the hospital when the child is transferred
- Computer order entry to ensure use of standardized formulas, to reduce human calculation errors, and to prevent mistakes caused by difficulty reading handwriting
- Special labeling and storage of look-alike and sound-alike medications
- The banning of medication order abbreviations and careful attention to guidelines for placement of decimal points
- Special labeling and two-person verification of high-risk or "high-alert" medications (see the later "Additional Resources" section for link)
- Labeling of all medications and medication containers (including medicine cups and syringes) as they are drawn up/poured
- Use of unit-dose dispensing
- Use of pumps with built-in, customizable software to prevent errors in infusion of IV fluids and medications
- Careful labeling of all patient lines so that medications are not administered via the wrong route or mixed in solutions with which they are incompatible

STANDARDS OF PRACTICE AND CULTURALLY SENSITIVE CARE

Living and working in a society with a broad mix of ethnic and cultural diversity is both enriching and challenging. Culture is a multidimensional term that may refer to:

- Culture of origin, usually referring to ethnicity
- Culture of poverty
- Religious culture
- Culture associated with gender and with sexual preferences
- Culture associated with age
- Culture associated with workplaces, professional organizations, hobby and special interest groups, and other interests

The nurse is obligated by standards of practice and ethics to make an authentic attempt to understand the cultural beliefs and practices of patients and their families, and accommodate them to the extent feasible, safe, and in keeping with standards of practice and care. Cultural sensitivity may require considerations such as:

- Dietary accommodations: For example, patients may keep Kosher or prefer a vegetarian diet.

- Interpreters for those who speak little or no English or who are hearing impaired and use sign language: Children and family members should not be asked to serve in this role because this introduces issues of privacy and confidentiality, capacity to understand medical matters, and willingness and ability to accurately and fully translate.
- Scheduling accommodations: This includes awareness of prayer times for Muslim patients and Sabbath restrictions such as the use of electricity and phones for orthodox Jewish families.
- Treatment accommodations: For example, Jehovah's Witness adults may refuse lifesaving blood for themselves, but not for their children. Health-care providers can take measures to avoid giving these children blood while still providing effective care and having a comprehensive blood conservation program or knowing of a program that can be consulted if appropriate.
- Gender accommodations based on culture: For example, Muslim women are not supposed to be alone with or seen by men who are not their husbands. Attempts should be made to provide female caretakers, but care should be taken not to make such a promise if staffing will not permit it.
- Home-care accommodations: For example, an Amish client who is going home with a family member will probably not have electricity or a phone and may need arrangements made for a generator and installation of a phone or use of a neighbor's phone.
- Knowledge of and tolerance for complementary and alternative medicine (CAM) approaches such as Reiki, acupuncture, hypnotherapy and biofeedback, homeopathy, and the use of herbs and supplements: Although CAM treatments may be helpful, some may be ineffective but harmless, and still others may be harmful themselves or interact in harmful ways with elements of traditional or Western medicine. When taking a patient history, nurses should routinely ask about CAM treatments in a nonjudgmental manner.
- Cultural practices: Some cultural practices (such as coining, spooning, and cupping, and perhaps even some carefully applied forms of moxibustion) that are minimally painful and cause temporary damage may be acceptable, whereas others, such as female genital circumcision, would be considered painful and harmful to the extent of being classified as abuse. Even though some scarring and tattooing rituals have cultural significance, these may be used abusively as well.
- Families may be encouraged and supported in praying for their child's recovery from pneumococcal meningitis, acute appendicitis, or leukemia, but health-care providers are obligated to advocate on behalf of the children when the antibiotics, appendectomy, or chemotherapy is being rejected in favor of simply putting faith in God. It can be helpful to invite (with the family's permission) respected pastors or elders from the religious or ethnic community to participate in decision-making discussions.

Geographic medicine departments of medical schools or large medical centers that serve international clientele may have experts available to consult with health-care professionals in local practices. (For further discussion of cultural issues, see Chapter 4.)

TRUTH-TELLING STANDARDS AND PEDIATRIC NURSING

Veracity is a principle that implies a duty to tell the truth or at least not to tell a lie. Truth-telling contexts in the clinical setting include, but are not limited to:

- Disclosing diagnosis and/or prognosis
- Withholding some or disclosing all treatment options
- Adequately informed and noncoerced consent
- Conflicts arising from confidentiality requests
- Consideration of the use of placebos in treatment or research
- Disclosures regarding medical errors
- Misrepresenting the qualifications of patients who otherwise would not receive health-care or social welfare services

In general, children prefer the truth and may develop distrust for health-care providers when just one health-care provider deceives them. They usually do understand the subtle moral distinctions adults must sometimes make between lying and withholding information, sharing partial truths, and using euphemisms. Good intentions may not matter. For these reasons, when children ask questions, health-care providers must discern exactly what they want to know before anguishing over how to reply and how much detail to provide. The traditional example is the 4-year-old who comes home and asks where babies come from. He is probably not asking about sperm and ova and intercourse—he may just want to know which hospital.

When parents or patients prefer to trust the recommendations of the team and avoid disclosing details, this desire can sometimes be respected as an "informed choice," although it depends on the nature of the decision and the risks and burdens involved. For example, if the recovery process will be arduous and burdensome, and require ongoing motivation and cooperation on the part of the patient and family to realize a successful outcome, the patient and family must have that information.

Culture may play a role with respect to truth telling. Some individuals with traditional Navajo beliefs, for example, do not want to hear potential risks because hearing them spoken out loud is synonymous with inviting them to occur (Andrews & Boyle, 2012; Joint Commission, 2016). However, the nurse cannot assume that anyone of a particular culture subscribes to all of its traditionally held beliefs and should be prepared to explore all possibilities.

Medical Errors

In the event of a medical error, prompt disclosure and transparency along with sincere apologies and attempts to repair damages may help maintain client trust in health-care professionals and lessen the likelihood of a lawsuit. It can also be prudent and therapeutic to inform patients and families about changes put in place as a result of the error to prevent the same thing from happening to other patients. Most health-care facilities have policies that outline who must be informed of medical errors, the nature of the investigation that will take place, who should disclose to the family and in what manner, and what contact, if any, the person(s) most directly involved in the error should continue to have with the patient/family.

ADVOCACY

Advocacy entails speaking up on behalf of those who cannot speak for themselves and helping to further empower those who do have a voice. For nurses, advocacy involves the championing of care as much as it does the actual provision of care. Children are vulnerable to varying extents from developmental and political perspectives, and are particularly in need of surrogate voices. Nurses advocate for safe and quality care on behalf of patients and families within the practice setting. They may also engage in advocacy efforts on a broader scale on behalf of the rights and health of all children on a local, national, or international level. Advocacy may require risk taking, organizational sensitivity, political savvy, and activism. Good communication skills are essential.

Advocacy is not an option; it is an obligation that is reflected in the ANA *Code of Ethics for Nurses* and in *Pediatric Nursing: Scope and Standards of Practice*. The UN Convention on the Rights of the Child and versions of Pediatric Patient Bill of Rights and Responsibilities that can be found in most children's health-care settings (Box 2–4) highlight the rights that direct many pediatric nursing advocacy efforts.

Advocacy and Child Maltreatment

Prevention, detection, and treatment of child maltreatment are a major advocacy focus. Pediatric nurses must be familiar with risk factors (Box 2–5), possible medical and behavioral indicators of maltreatment (Box 2–6), effective interventions, and the availability of resources for various types of maltreatment, including:

- Physical abuse: An injury is inflicted that results in or poses the risk for significant physical harm or death. Even if intent was not to harm, if the damage was reasonably predictable and avoidable, due care and protection were not afforded the child.
- Sexual abuse: "The engaging of a child in sexual activities that the child cannot comprehend, for which the child is developmentally unprepared and cannot give informed consent and/or that violate the social and legal taboos of society" (Campbell & Hibbard, 2014).
- Emotional abuse: "Systematic, psychologically destructive behavior that attacks a child's development of self and social competence" (Children's Bureau, 2016).
- Medical abuse (also referred to as "pediatric condition falsification"): The child is needlessly exposed to diagnostic and

BOX 2–4 | Pediatric Patient and Family Bill of Rights

Many versions of the Pediatric Patient and Family Bills of Rights are available. The now-defunct Association for the Care of Children's Health is generally credited with a national push to document and respect pediatric patient and family rights. Each hospital, clinic, or professional organization modifies the document to capture its mission, vision, and values and to appeal to its constituents. Commonly expressed rights include:

- Respectful interactions with the health-care team
- Quality, individualized, professional care that meets or exceeds national standards
- Prompt and ongoing assessment and management of pain and other discomforts
- Confidentiality
- Understandable, comprehensive, accurate information regarding condition, prognosis, and diagnostic and treatment options
- Participation in the development of the plan of care
- Parent/guardian or surrogate rooming-in
- Identity of all persons involved in care delivery
- Safe environment
- Second opinions/specialty consultations
- Respect for religious and cultural beliefs and practices, and provision of interpreters or signers as needed for communication purposes
- Informed participation in medical research as appropriate and available
- Knowledge of hospital services, mission, vision, values, and rules
- Prompt attention and response to concerns
- Knowledge of hospital charges and access to financial counseling

Commonly expressed responsibilities of patients/families include the responsibilities to:

- Interact respectfully with the health-care team.
- Provide comprehensive and accurate information regarding health status, medical history, and response to treatment.
- Collaborate in the development of the plan of care, including the requirement for parents to be readily available in person or via phone when decisions need to be made.
- Comply with plan of care or discuss difficulties and renegotiate.
- Keep appointments and be on time or provide prompt notification when appointment must be canceled.
- Respect hospital rules and safety measures.
- Report complaints and/or compliments to the appropriate individuals.
- Make good-faith arrangements to meet financial responsibilities.

BOX 2-5 | Child Maltreatment Risk Factors and At-Risk Populations

Research has indicated the risk factors associated with maltreatment (Children's Bureau, 2016). "A combination of individual, relational, community, and societal factors contribute to the risk of child abuse and neglect" (CDC, 2016, para. 1). Some of the more common risk factors are:

- Young, immature parents with unrealistic expectations
- Parents with unmet emotional needs
- Economic crises
- Domestic violence
- Lack of parenting knowledge
- Parental depression or other mental health problems
- Substance abuse
- Families with premature and/or chronically ill children
- Families with children with attention deficit-hyperactivity disorder or mental health disorders such as oppositional defiant disorder
- Families with the presence of a nonbiological father or maternal boyfriend (sexual abuse)

Sources: Giardino & Alexander (2005), Reece & Christian (2008), and Roesler & Jenny (2008).

BOX 2-6 | Potential Medical and Behavioral Indicators of Child Maltreatment

The presence of one or two isolated indicators does not necessarily portend child maltreatment, and developmental factors must always be taken into consideration.

Nonspecific Indicators

These are general indicators of stress or distress that might be observed in a variety of circumstances that include, but are not restricted to, child maltreatment. They could be a reflection of a move to a new neighborhood, a parent out of work, financial woes, new baby in the family, parent in jail, parental discord, substance use or abuse within the household, bullying, death in the family, and other factors. When reflections of maltreatment, they could be indicative of physical abuse, sexual abuse, emotional abuse, or neglect. Nonspecific indicators include:

- Sudden personality changes
- Mood swings (emotionality, aggression)
- Depression, including being disinterested, withdrawn
- Change in appetite
- Change in eating habits
- Sleep disturbances
- Problems with concentration
- Sudden change in school performance or behavior
- Excessive absences from school
- Regressive behavior
- Stuttering
- Run-away behavior or threats
- Cruelty to animals
- Self-injury
- Suicide threats or attempts
- Low self-esteem
- Too eager to please
- Fear of going home
- Destruction of homework, books, learning aids, or favorite toys

Physical Abuse

- Frequent injuries ("accident prone")
- Injuries inconsistent with explanation or explanation changes over time
- Placing blame for infant's injuries on siblings—too young to speak up for themselves
- Delays in seeking medical attention for significant injuries
- Injuries to sites that are not commonly injured accidentally (e.g., neck, back of shoulders and upper arms, lower back, buttocks, back of thighs)
- Patterned injuries, such as from a belt, brush, cigarette lighter, cords, heating grates, curling irons, or irons
- Parents are rejecting, ignoring, belittling
- Child is hypervigilant; startles easily; shrinks from adults (or from males or females)

Sexual Abuse

- Genital pain, itching, swelling, discharge, or lesions; diagnosed with sexually transmitted infections
- Difficulty walking or sitting comfortably
- Frequent, painful, or bloody urination; painful or bloody bowel movements
- Stained or bloody underclothing
- Seductive, sexualized behaviors, including touching other people; humping behavior with other people or with objects; tongue kissing; making sexual sounds (moaning, sighing, heavy breathing)
- Excessive or public masturbation; inserting of fingers or objects in anal or genital area
- Excessive or age-inappropriate curiosity about sex; drawing of sexually explicit pictures
- Seems concerned about homosexuality

Neglect

- Poor hygiene; bad body odor
- Inadequately dressed for weather; tattered, improperly sized, or unclean clothing

continued

BOX 2-6 | Potential Medical and Behavioral Indicators of Child Maltreatment—cont'd

- Poor growth pattern
- Developmental lags
- Constant hunger; stealing or hoarding of food; rooting through garbage for food
- Constant fatigue
- Destruction of homework, books, learning aids, or toys
- Unattended medical needs, such as lack of immunizations, gross dental problems, needs glasses or hearing aids, untreated illnesses or injuries
- Frequently left unsupervised for long periods (may come to school early and hang around late or always wants to go home with another child)
- Infants/toddlers: Bald spots, listlessness, self-stimulation behaviors, rocking, head banging, lack of interest/curiosity

Medical Abuse/Pediatric Condition Falsification

- Unexplained, persistent, or recurrent condition, or one that is unusually unresponsive to therapy
- Symptoms and signs for which the onset has not been witnessed by anyone other than the parent or caregiver, or that do not occur when the parent or caregiver has no access to the child
- Caretaker observations that are not in keeping with health-care provider observations
- The patient reportedly does not tolerate the treatment regimen
- Finding of unexpected drug in blood, urine, or stool, or finding of blood that is not of the same type as the child in emesis, urine, or stool
- Polymicrobial infections or infections with organisms not commonly associated with site
- Alternate diagnoses included in the differential are very uncommon, even in the experience of a specialist
- Frequent change in medical providers and expensive or extensive evaluations in more than one medical center
- Repeated parental requests for invasive or risky diagnostic tests or treatments
- Feeding tubes and central lines that provide easy means to introduce infection or toxins

Sources: Giardino & Alexander (2005), Reece & Christian (2008), and Roesler & Jenny (2008).

therapeutic interventions for symptoms or conditions that have been exaggerated, totally fabricated, or purposefully induced. The person lying about or inducing the symptoms can be the patient, but in pediatrics, it is most commonly a caretaker (usually, although not always, the mother or mother figure) (Campbell & Hibbard, 2014).

- Neglect: Failure to provide for basic needs to the extent that the child is harmed or put at significant risk for harm. Deficits might be in the areas of food, shelter, clothing, education, health care, and/or safe supervision.

Health-care providers are mandatory reporters of child maltreatment and cannot be held liable for good-faith reports, but could suffer legal penalties for failing to report to law enforcement or the appropriate children's service agency.

Ethical Issues and Child Maltreatment

Issues of ethics emerge in dealing with cases of possible child maltreatment:

- Professionals may not have a high enough index of suspicion regarding abuse among families that seem "nice" or "respectable" and may be disproportionately suspicious of those who are poor or are members of minority groups.
- It can also be difficult to decide how much of a concern warrants a formal report to the authorities in the absence of clear proof. Even if a family is cleared following the medical or social services investigation, the fact that a report was made remains on the books, so reporting is a serious step that should not be undertaken lightly.
- Health-care providers may wonder if the family should be informed about the report before it is made. Honesty and advance notice are usually the best choices. A report should only be made without the family's knowledge in the rare circumstance when there is good reason to believe the child or staff will be in danger.

Child Advocacy Strategies and Skills

Although advocacy usually begins with the efforts of one lone player, it is most effective as a team sport. For those who are interested in advocacy beyond the boundaries of the practice setting, a multitude of opportunities and avenues exist:

- Membership in professional organizations can include involvement in the development of position statements and participation on legislative affairs councils. Even without time for active participation, paying dues to these organizations facilitates their advocacy efforts.
- Letters to legislators and participation in campaign efforts for those supportive of children's health and welfare, and on behalf of ballot issues that impact children.
- Participation in local initiatives to improve health of children in the community: Some examples include working on programs to get smoke detectors in every home, supply families with car seats, supply children with bike helmets and cycling safety education, and improve immunization rates.
- Community education regarding child health and welfare issues, hospital newsletters and websites that highlight hot topics, speaking engagements, and other platforms.

SAFE AND EFFECTIVE NURSING CARE: Clinical Pearl

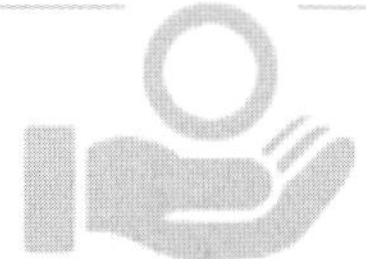

The Power of Child Advocates

"Never doubt that a small group of thoughtful, committed citizens can change the world. Indeed, it is the only thing that ever has."
—Margaret Mead

Case Study

Family-Centered Care Scenario

Baby Williams is a 26 weeks' gestation premature infant in the neonatal intensive care unit. His mother is a 17-year-old single mother with a 1- and 2-year-old at home. She has dropped out of school and is working part time. The father, also age 17, remains in school and works part time. He helps when he can but does not live with his children.

- What can be done to keep in touch with parents and support their involvement in decision making if they cannot often visit the neonatal intensive care unit?
- What practical steps might be taken to support a relationship between a premature infant in the neonatal intensive care unit and his toddler brothers, who are not permitted to visit during respiratory virus season?
- How can daily medical rounds and nursing change-of-shift reports be structured to include the Williams family when they are present, without becoming prohibitively time-consuming?
- How can we accommodate unmarried minor parents who want to room-in and need to learn the details of the complex care their child needs, but also must keep up with school attendance and homework?
- Because peers are critical in the life of adolescents and are, in a sense, part of their "family," how can we keep them "in touch" with normal teen life during hospitalizations? What can we do for teens who miss out on important school events, such as the high school senior who will miss her prom or the injured basketball player who will miss out on the championship game?

REFERENCES

American Academy of Pediatrics, Committee on Fetus and Newborn. (2006). Prevention and management of pain in the neonate: An update. *Pediatrics, 118*, 2231–2241. doi: 10.1542/peds.2006-2277

American Nurses Association (ANA). (2010). *Nursing's social policy statement: The essence of the profession* (3rd ed.). Silver Spring, MD: American Nurses Association. Retrieved from http://Nursingworld.org

American Nurses Association (ANA). (2015a). About code of ethics. Retrieved from http://www.nursingworld.org/codeofethics

American Nurses Association (ANA). (2015b). *Code of ethics for nurses.* Spring Hill.

American Nurses Association (ANA). (2015c). *Code of ethics for nurses with interpretive statements* (2nd ed.) Silver Spring, MD: American Nurses Association. Retrieved from http://Nursingworld.org

American Nurses Association (ANA). (2015d). *Nursing: Scope and standards of practice* (3rd ed.) Silver Spring, MD: American Nurses Association. Retrieved from http//Nursingworld.org

American Nurses Association (ANA). (2015e). *Pediatric nursing: Scope and standards of practice* (2nd ed.) Silver Spring, MD: American Nurses Association. Retrieved from http://www.Nursingworld.org

Andrews, M., & Boyle, J. (2012). *Transcultural concepts in nursing care* (6th ed.). Philadelphia: Lippincott Williams & Wilkins.

Beauchamp, T., & Childress, J. F. (2009). *Principles of biomedical ethics* (6th ed.). New York: Oxford University Press.

Beyer, J. (2009). The Oucher: A summary. Retrieved from http://www.oucher.org/the_scales.html

Beyer, J. E., Villarruel, A. M., & Denyes, M. J. (2009). The Oucher: User's manual & technical report. Retrieved from http://www.oucher.org/downloads/2009_Users_Manual.pdf

Butchelor, H. K., & Marriott, J. F. (2013). Formulation for children: Problems and solutions. *British Journal of Clinical Pharmacology, 79*(3), 405–418.

Campbell, A. M., & Hibbard, R. (2014). More than words: The emotional maltreatment of children. *Pediatric Clinics of North America, 61,* 959–970. doi: 10.1016/j.pcl.2014.06.004

Centers for Disease Control and Prevention (CDC). (2016). What is health literacy? Retrieved from https://www.cdc.gov/healthliteracy/learn/index.html

Centers for Disease Control and Prevention (CDC). (2017). Health literacy in the United States. Retrieved from https://www.cdc.gov/healthliteracy/training/page669.html

Children's Bureau. (2016). Definitions of child abuse and neglect. Retrieved from https://www.childwelfare.gov/pubPDFs/define.pdf

Ellenchild Pinch, W. J., & Haddad, A. M. (2008). *Nursing and health care ethics: A legacy and a vision.* Silver Spring, MD: nursesbooks.org

Fox, R. M., & DeMarco, J. P. (2008). *Moral reasoning.* Mason, OH: Cengage Learning.

Giardino, A. P., & Alexander, R. (2005). *Child maltreatment.* St. Louis, MO: G. W. Medical Publisher.

Hamil, J. K., Lyndon, M., Liley, & Hill, A. G. (2014). Where it hurts: A systematic review of pain-location tools for children. *Pain, 155*(5), 851–858.

Healthy People. (2017). Health communication and health information technology. Retrieved from https://www.healthypeople.gov/2020/topics-objectives/topic/health-communication-and-health-information-technology

Ivanovska, V., Rademaker, C. M. A., vanDijk, L., & Mantel-Teeuwisse, A. K. (2014). Pediatric drug formulations: A review of challenges and progress. *Pediatrics, 134*(2), 361–372.

Joint Commission. (2016). The facts about patient-centered communications. Retrieved from http://www.jointcomission.org/facts_about_patient-centered_communications

Krechel, S. W., & Bildner, J. (1995). CRIES: A new neonatal postoperative pain measurement score. Initial testing of validity and reliability. *Pediatric Anesthesia, 5*(1), 53–61.

Lopez, F. L., Ernest, T. B., Tuleu, C., & Gul, M.O. (2015). Formulation approaches to pediatric oral drug delivery: Benefits and limitations of current platforms. *Expert Opinion Drug Delivery, 12*(11), 1727–1740.

McAliley, L., Hudson, D., Gunning, R., & Rowbottom, L. (2000). The use of advance directives with adolescents. *Pediatric Nursing, 26,* 471–480.

McAliley, L. G., Lambert, S., Ashenberg, M. D., & Dull, S. M. (1996). Therapeutic relations decision making: The rainbow framework. *Pediatric Nursing, 22,* 199–203.

Norman, J. (2016). Americans rate healthcare providers high on honesty, ethics. Retrieved from http://www.gallup.com/poll/200057/americans-rate-healthcare-providers-high-honesty-ethics.aspx

Nurse Practitioner Core Competencies Content. (2013). Population-focused nurse practitioner competencies. Retrieved from http://www.mc.vanderbilt.edu/documents/CAPNAH/files/Scope%20of%20Practice/PopulationFocusNPComps2013-Intro.pdf

Prince v. Commonwealth of Massachusetts, 321 U. S. 158 (1944).

Reece, R. M., & Christian, C. W. (Eds.). (2008). *Child abuse: Medical diagnosis and management.* Elk Grove Village, IL: American Academy of Pediatrics.

Reid v. Covert 354 U. S. 701 (1955). Retrieved from https://www.law.cornell.edu/supremecourt/text/354/1

Roberts, J., Fenton, G., & Barnard, M. (2015). Developing effective therapeutic relationships with children, young people and their families. *Nursing Children & Young People, 27*(4), 30–35.

Roesler, T. A., & Jenny, C. (2008). *Medical child abuse: Beyond Munchausen syndrome by proxy.* Elk Grove Village, IL: American Academy of Pediatrics Press.

Savedra, M., & Crandall, M. (2005). Multidimensional assessment using the adolescent pediatric pain tool: A case report. *Journal for Specialists in Pediatric Nursing, 10,* 115–123. doi: 10.1111/j.1744-6155.2005.00023x

Srouji, R., Ratnapalan, S., & Schneeweiss, S. (2010). Pain in children. Assessment and nonpharmacological management. *International Journal of Pediatrics, 110,* 474838. doi: 10.1155/2010/474838

Stevens, B., Johnston, C., Taddio, A., Gibbins, S., & Yamada, J. (2010). The premature infant pain profile: Evaluation 13 years after development. *Clinical Journal of Pain, 26*(9), 8813–830.

Veatch, R. M. (2011). *The basics of bioethics* (3rd ed.). Upper Saddle River, NJ: Prentice Hall.

Voepel-Lewis, T., Zanotti, J., Dommeyer, J. A., & Merkel, S. (2010). Reliability and validity of the face, legs, activity, cry, consolability behavioral tool in assessing acute pain in critically ill patients. *American Journal of Critical Care, 19*(1), 55–61.

Witt, N., Coynor, S., Edwards, C., & Bradshaw, J. (2016). A guide to pain assessment and management in the neonate. *Current Emergency Hospital and Medicine Reports, 4,* 1–10. doi: 10.1007/s40138-016-0089-y

ADDITIONAL RESOURCES

Institute for Patient- and Family-Centered Care (http://www.familycenteredcare.org)

Family Voices Organization (http://www.familyvoices.org)

SMOG website (http://www.readabilityformulas.com/smog-readability-formula.php)

Guttmacher Institute (https://www.guttmacher.org)

GAO review of implementation of Patient Self-Determination Act (http://www.legistorm.com/showFile/L2xzX3Njb3JlL2dhby9wZGYvMTk5NS84/ful25813.pdf)

Current year's NPSGs (http://www.jointcommission.org; Click on "Patient Safety" and then click on "National Patient Safety Goals")

Humpty Dumpty Falls Protection Program (http://www.mch.com/content.aspx?PageID=2257)

Institute for Safe Medication Practice (http://www.ismp.org)

ISMP High-Alert Medications Tool (http://www.ismp.org/Tools/highalertmedications.pdf)

National Association for the Care of Children in Hospitals & Related Institutions (NACHRI) (http://www.childrenshospitals.net)

Institute for Health Improvement (http://www.ihi.org/ihi)

National Institute for Children's Healthcare Quality (http://www.nichq.org)

UNIT 2

Psycho-Social-Cultural Assessment of the Child and the Family

Family Dynamics and Communicating With Children and Families

3

Kathryn Rudd, DNP, RN, c-NIC, c-NPT
Diane M. Kocisko, MSN, RN, CPN

LEARNING OUTCOMES

Upon completion of this chapter, the student will be able to:

1. Describe the process of normal communication.
2. Describe the patterns of family communication.
3. Describe family dynamics.
4. Describe family theories.
5. Identify family function roles.
6. Describe family structures and the approaches to communication within each structure.
7. Identify age-specific approaches for communicating with parents, families, toddlers, school-age children, and adolescents.
8. Explain various influences in communication, including body language, tone, pitch, and environment.
9. Describe strategies for incorporating communication into assessment.
10. Describe communication with families during periods of emergency care.
11. Identify the role of family-centered care in caring for the hospitalized child.

COMMUNICATION AND FAMILIES

Communication is a two-way process by which information is exchanged between individuals with a common use of language, mannerisms, behaviors, or symbols.

Principles of Communication in Families

The manner of communication used by families provides information about the family style and the structure and function of family relationships. Functional communication influences the decision-making process and is based on mutual trust; dysfunctional communication inhibits nurturing and results in a decrease in self-esteem and self-worth in communication partners.

Communication is influenced by culture, so the nurse must have cultural awareness to facilitate effective communication with clients (see Chapter 4). In addition, it is important to note that ill and hospitalized children may regress to a lower level of communication than is typical of their communication pattern.

Process of Communication in Families

The communication process in families possesses these characteristics:

- Bidirectional process: needs both sender and receiver
- Constantly in motion
- Transactional
- Irreversible
- Learned through culture and society

- Denotation: the dictionary meaning of a word
- Connotation: the meanings and feelings associated with a word based on an individual's past experiences

Patterns of Family Communication

While working with families, the pediatric nurse will observe a range of communication patterns (Fig. 3–1). These most commonly include:

- Clear and direct, the most productive form of communication, is a clear message directed to the appropriate family member. For example, "Daughter, I'm irritated that you didn't put the dishes in the dishwasher away as I asked you."
- Clear and indirect is a clear message directed to the wrong family member. The mother tells the father: "I can't stand it when people don't put the dishes away when asked."
- Masked and direct means an unclear message is delivered to the appropriate family member: "Daughter, it's really annoying to us when our children do not work as hard as they should in this family."
- Masked and indirect communication is the least productive, characterized by an unclear message not directed to a specific family member: "Kids are all lazy" (Oster, 2017).

Components of the Communication Process

The importance of establishing good communication cannot be overstated because it affects all aspects of a child's care.

- Verbal:
  - Spoken words: Choose clear, concise language; avoid distancing language such as assigning gender; and do not use avoidance language, such as euphemisms (e.g., "passed on" instead of "died").
  - Written words: Written communication can be in the form of using storybooks that highlight certain information or encouraging journaling for adolescents; do not write directions above the reading level of the child or family, and do not use complex wording or medical jargon.
- Nonverbal:
  - Body language: An open stance is welcoming; crossed arms indicate coldness or displeasure.

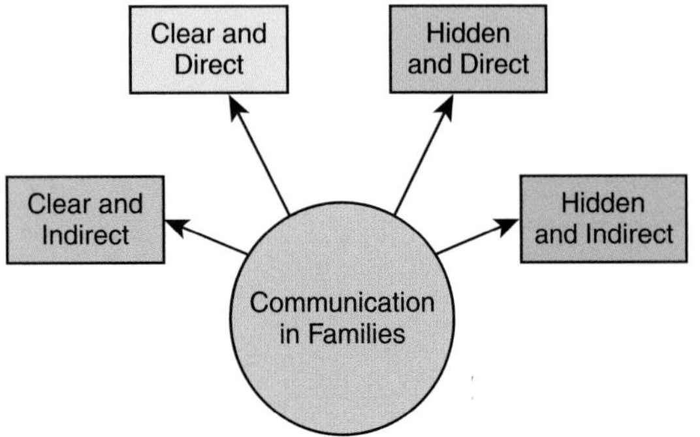

FIGURE 3–1 Concept map of patterns of family communication.

- Gestures:
  - Confirming behaviors such as nodding of your head, restating what you hear
  - Nonconfirming behaviors such as tapping your foot, standing in the doorway, being in one's personal space, or looking at your watch
- Paralanguage: Pitch, volume, and pausing

Children are very aware of anxiety and fear in their caregivers, which can be conveyed through both nonverbal and verbal behaviors. Speak slowly and be mindful of long pauses and the tone or manner in which you speak to the child. Nurses should practice effective listening; this key to successful communication requires active involvement in the communication process.

Empathy enhances the communication process. Empathy is an understanding of a person's feelings—not sympathy, which is not therapeutic. Responding positively to an individual helps develop communication skills, language, self-esteem, and trust.

Typically, children communicate in a manner consistent with their developmental level (see Chapter 6 for growth and development information).

Health and Communication Issues Within Families

Although children learn health habits from their families, this does not occur in a vacuum; lifestyle is also influenced by their community and environment. The National Coalition on Healthcare (2016) provides a framework for community health education through schools. This includes eight initiatives focused on health education, health promotion and literacy, reducing health risks, and addressing health behaviors influenced by family, peers, media, or the culture (U.S. Department of Health & Human Services, 2014). In addition, decision-making and goal-related skills are included to help enhance the community, the family, and the individual. Another resource, National Health Education Standards (NHES), provides a framework for teachers, administrators, and policymakers to design or select curricula, allocate resources, and assess progress in education (Centers for Disease Control and Prevention, 2016).

Access to health care varies among U.S. families. In 2015, 29 million Americans did not have health insurance despite the Affordable Care Act (Kaiser Family Foundation, 2016). The term *underinsured*, which describes individuals or families who have insurance coverage considered inadequate, applied to 31 million Americans in 2014, an increase of 6 million from the last reporting in 2010 (The Commonwealth Fund, 2015). The insurance status of uninsured or underinsured families affects their health-care practices. They may:

- Forgo treatment until a condition worsens
- Use emergency rooms for primary care in the absence of a relationship with or access to a primary care physician
- Miss follow-up appointments because of transportation, employment, inadequate knowledge, and other barriers
- Lack resources to obtain needed medication to treat acute or chronic conditions

Communicating With Families: Nurse's Role

When communicating with children and their families, the pediatric nurse should:

- Identify his or her role.
- Provide appropriate introductions for the nurse, caregivers, and family members. Identify the stakeholders and the caregivers, including the child in the process.
- Record all telephone calls during office hours and after, and log all incoming and outgoing calls, advice given, and questions answered. Include date, time, and who was involved in the communication process (Bell & Condren, 2016; Institute for Healthcare Communication, 2017).
- Establish an appropriate setting to communicate information.
- Ensure privacy.
- Provide anticipatory guidance, a critical communication strategy that improves care and supports competence in caregiving by offering information, guidance, and education for family caregivers.

SAFE AND EFFECTIVE NURSING CARE: Clinical Pearl

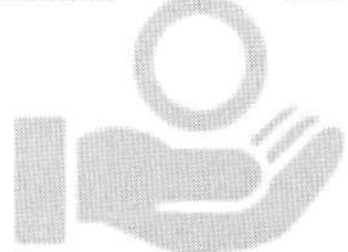

Health Insurance Portability and Accountability Act

In 1996, the Health Insurance Portability and Accountability Act (HIPAA) was enacted to protect the privacy of patients' health records and information. The law protects "individually identifiable health information" (U.S. Department of Health & Human Services, 2017). It also limits access to health information in any format (e.g., written, oral, facsimile, social media) to authorized individuals who have a "right to know." "Right to know" includes disclosure of a person's health information to individuals who have a direct need to know on a specific date in which that health-care provider is caring for the client. For example, if a coworker has had a baby in your institution and as a nurse you are caring for newborns on that particular floor but not this patient, it is unlawful for that nurse to look up his or her coworker's baby information. Deviations from this federal law have resulted in imprisonment and fines for the offending individuals or institutions. Recent updates to HIPAA are related to increases in transmission security, cybersecurity, auditing, workforce screening, and the encouragement of reports of abuse (U.S. Department of Health & Human Services, 2017).

Communication With Family Members During Emergencies

When families are under stress during emergencies, communication can be challenging. Nurses can help ensure their message is received in trying times with these strategies:

- Provide a quiet environment for conversation.
- Communicate slowly.
- Avoid medical jargon.
- Sit down and face caregivers at eye level.
- Allow plenty of time for questions.
- Avoid giving false hope.
- Allow for repetition of what caregivers have heard to ensure understanding.
- Be empathetic and sincere (Lederman, 2016; Porter, Cooper, & Taylor, 2014).

CRITICAL COMPONENT

Emergencies

Critical components and interventions during emergencies include:

- Provide clear and concise information.
- Do not make promises.
- Inform family members that the physician will speak with them as soon as possible.
- If possible, give them a private environment.
- Call clergy, child life specialists, and social workers if available to offer support.

Barriers to Effective Communication

The pediatric nurse can facilitate effective communication by identifying potential barriers to client/family communication and removing them when possible. Barriers to effective communication may include:

- Physical abnormalities such as cleft lip or cleft palate
- Physiological alterations such as hearing or visual impairment (Fig. 3–2)
- Cognitive barriers may affect perceptions, expression, concrete or abstract thinking; for example, this may include the use of jargon, sarcasm, or irony
- Avoidance or distancing language, for example, acting out, denial, projection, rationalization, or trivializing (Vertino, 2014)

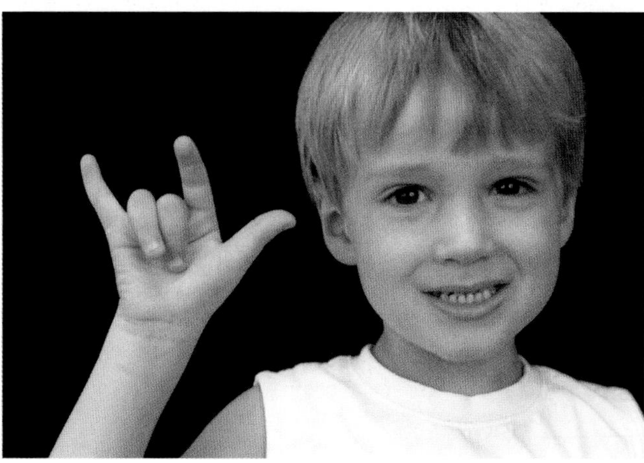

FIGURE 3–2 Child using American Sign Language for the word *love*.

- Environmental noise
- Cultural differences, particularly when the message sender does not focus on the beliefs, values, goals, and outcomes of the child and family (see Chapter 4 for further cultural factors).
- Language barriers, hearing or speech difficulties
- Psychological alterations: children with disabilities have communication rights that must be met by the health-care practitioner (Brady et al., 2016; Limiñana-Gras, Sánchez-López, Calvo-Llena, & Corbalán, 2015)
- Sender and receiver biases
- Closed-ended, yes-or-no questions: use only when the nurse needs focused information
- Ignoring family and psychosocial issues (U.S. Department of Health & Human Services, 2014)

Additional barriers are described in Table 3–1.

SAFE AND EFFECTIVE NURSING CARE: Clinical Pearl

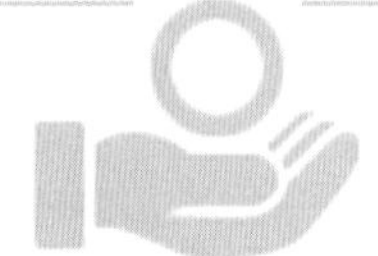

Protection for Individuals With Hearing Disabilities

"Title III of the Americans with Disabilities Act (ADA) prohibits discrimination against individuals with disabilities by places of public accommodation" (42 U.S.C. §§ 12181–12189). Private health-care providers are considered places of public accommodation. As noted by the National Association of the Deaf (2017), "the U.S. Department of Justice issued regulations under Title III of the ADA at 28 C.F.R. Part 36. Health care providers have a duty to provide appropriate auxiliary aids and services when necessary to ensure that communication with people who are deaf or hard of hearing is as effective as communication with others. 28 C.F.R. § 36.303(c)."

SAFE AND EFFECTIVE NURSING CARE: Clinical Pearl

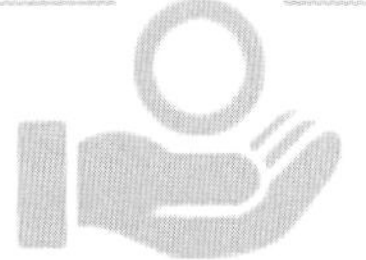

Hearing Screenings

Hearing screenings are performed before discharge on all infants born in the hospital. This evaluation detects deviations in hearing that may prevent the child from reaching developmental milestones such as turning the head toward a sound, being soothed by the voice of a caregiver, mimicking sounds heard, and learning to talk. These primary skills of communication must be obtained before the development of the communication process. Infections passed from the mother and the antibiotics used to treat such infections may cause ototoxicity and alter hearing. In addition, chronic ear infections or infections transmitted in utero can cause limitations in hearing.

SAFE AND EFFECTIVE NURSING CARE: Cultural Competence

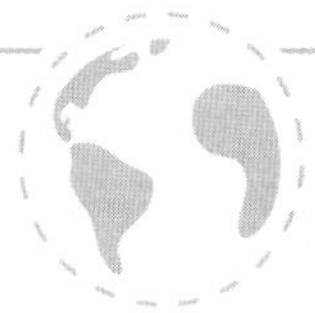

Communication

To facilitate communication with children and families from other cultures, the nurse should:

- Include family members in interactions.
- Be an active listener.
- Observe verbal and nonverbal cues.
- Understand that family responses to wellness and illness strongly influence behaviors.
- Learn culturally appropriate interactions, such as whether to use eye contact and whether shaking hands is welcomed in the client's culture. Be mindful of pauses and personal space.
- Repeat important information more than once, and speak slowly.
- Avoid medical jargon, instead using terms family members can understand.
- Allow time for questions.
- Give information in the family's native language, with the use of certified interpreters as necessary.
- Address intergenerational needs.

SAFE AND EFFECTIVE NURSING CARE: Cultural Competence

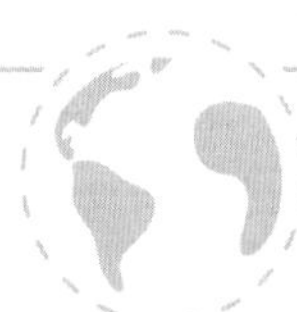

Legal Requirements for Interpretation

The 1964 Civil Rights Act states that no person should be denied the benefits of or experience discrimination in any program receiving federal assistance based on his or her race, color, gender, or natural origin. The Supreme Court determined that discrimination based on language amounts to discrimination based on natural origin. This legally requires health-care institutions to provide language accessibility for their patients. Many states, such as California, New Jersey, and Washington, have enacted health-care interpreter certification as directed by the National Council on Interpreting in Healthcare, which advocates for the development and implementation of national standards of practice for interpreters in health care (Chen, Youdelman, & Brooks, 2007; Friedman, 2014; National Conference of State Legislators, 2016). Facilities not covered by federal funds may still be subject to individual state laws (National Conference of State Legislators, 2016). The lack of trained medical interpreters in a health-care setting puts children and families at risk and is a form of discrimination.

TABLE 3–1 Barriers To Communication

BARRIERS TO COMMUNICATION WITH CHILDREN AND FAMILIES INCLUDE:

1. Closed-ended questions with yes-or-no answers
2. Prejudiced or preconceived messages based on race, age, ethnicity, culture, gender, lifestyle, wealth, appearance, or status
3. Preconceived messages based on the practitioner's beliefs of what constitutes *correct* family structure, function, or roles
4. Unaddressed fears of the child or the caregiver
5. Child, family, or caregiver not being treated with respect
6. Insufficient information
7. Not answering minor questions, such as those related to diet
8. Failure to include parents in the care plan
9. Parents not being treated as partners in their child's care
10. Failure of nurses to understand parent–child relationships
11. Failure to meet the developmental needs of the child
12. Failure to consider cultural aspects or speaking in nuanced language that is specifically culturally based

DEFINITION OF A FAMILY

A family consists of two or more members who interact and are dependent on one another socially, financially, and emotionally. Until the early 1960s, nuclear families consisting of a husband, wife, and children were the norm in the United States (Fig. 3–3). The exception was during the Great Depression, when multiple generations living together as extended families became more common because of economic necessity (Fig. 3–4). Nuclear families were portrayed by the media in television by *The Adventures of Ozzie and Harriet* and *Leave It to Beaver*. Single widowed parents were also shown with television shows such as *The Andy Griffith Show*.

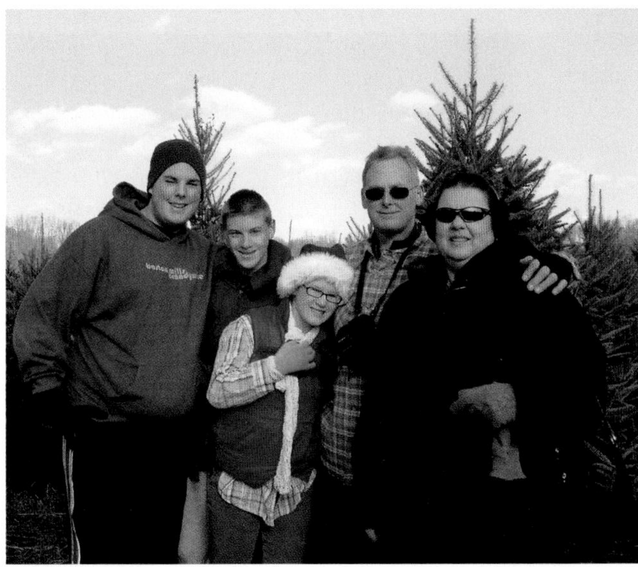

FIGURE 3–3 A nuclear family (mother, father, child, or children).

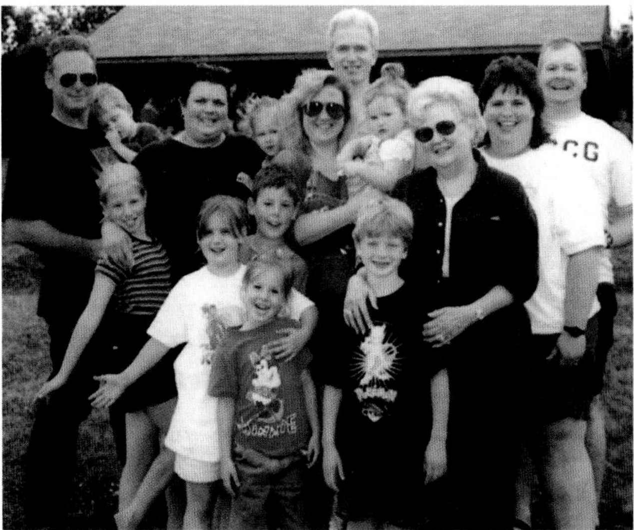

FIGURE 3–4 An extended family may have three generations of a family living together.

The 1960s saw tremendous turmoil caused by political, social, and cultural changes resulting from the Vietnam War and the emergence of civil rights for women and minorities. Social attitudes began to shift during this time and were reflected in television and movies. Single parenthood, women's changing roles, birth control, and divorce were now shown in the media (Angier, 2013). Blended families, those consisting of remarried parents and the children of their former marriages, first appeared in the media during the 1960s; that included single-parent and same-sex-partner families. Over the decades, sitcoms like *Roseanne* and *Modern Family* reflected the nation's changing demographics.

Although divorce rates have essentially remained unchanged since the 1990s, changes in family structure continue to occur. Children are more likely to live in a single-parent family or a cohabitating family (consisting of unmarried adults and the children of one or both adults) at some time in their lives. According to the Pew Research Center (2015), two-parent families represented 69% of all families, compared with 73% in 2000 and 87% in 1960. Fifteen percent of children live with parents who are remarried, 7% of children live with a parent who is cohabitating with a partner (Pew Research Center, 2015). In 2015, one-parent families constituted 26% of all families, compared with 22% in 2000 and 9% in 1960 (Pew Research Center, 2015). The Pew Research Center (2015) notes that 78% of the children in white households, two-thirds of Hispanic children, and 84% of Asian children lived in a two-parent household. Conversely, 54% of black children lived with a single parent, with 38% living in a two-parent household. Children in households with a college-educated parent were more likely to be living in a two-parent household (Pew Research Center, 2015).

Regardless of family structure, the available resources such as goods, services, information, and influences impact a child's health, development, and ability to adapt to disease and illness. Race, ethnicity, and immigrant status also affect families and children through cultural influences (see Chapter 4 for details). Nurses must be aware of these influences and assist in strengthening the family structure to maintain and support the parenting and family process. Referring the family unit to social service within the institution will assist in helping to identify resources.

SAFE AND EFFECTIVE NURSING CARE: Clinical Pearl

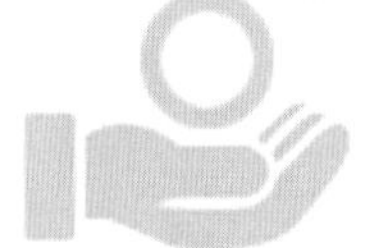

Diversity of Families

Family is also defined as the structure or the relationship between individuals that provides the financial and emotional support needed for social functioning (Friedemann, 1989). Nurses should not be judgmental when caring for children and families. We must remember that every family acts as a unique unit.

SAFE AND EFFECTIVE NURSING CARE: Cultural Competence

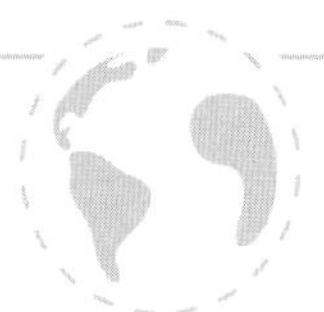

Types of Family Units

The family unit of today varies. Family members do not have to be related by blood to be considered a unit. Families of today can be nuclear, extended, single-parent, blended, foster, and adoptive. Parents can be of different sexes or the same sex. One family unit is not better than another. The most important thing is for children to be in a positive, supportive environment so that they can grow and develop to their highest potential.

Family Types and Functions

Family structures commonly seen in the United States include:

- Family of origin—family that raises the child
- Family of choice—family formed through marriage or cohabitation
- Nuclear family—male and female parents and their children living separately from grandparents
- Extended family (multigenerational family)—three or more generations of family members living within the same house, with children influenced by and interacting with all adults living in the home
- Married—family consists of married parents and their biological or adoptive children
- Single-parent family—family headed by a divorced, widowed, or unmarried biological or adoptive parent
- Grandparents functioning in the role of parents
- Same-sex-partner family—family headed by lesbian or gay partners (Fig. 3–5)
- Adoptive family—family includes a nonbiological adopted member; can be a subset of other family types (Fig. 3–6)
- Blended family—family consisting of members of two or more prior families; can be a result of death or divorce, as well as other factors
- Cohabitating family—family in which the parents are unmarried
- Solely extended family or no-parent family—a family in which children are cared for by other relatives, such as grandparents or aunts and uncles, rather than parents
- Dyad family—A couple living together without children
- Communal families
- Foster families (legal implications)

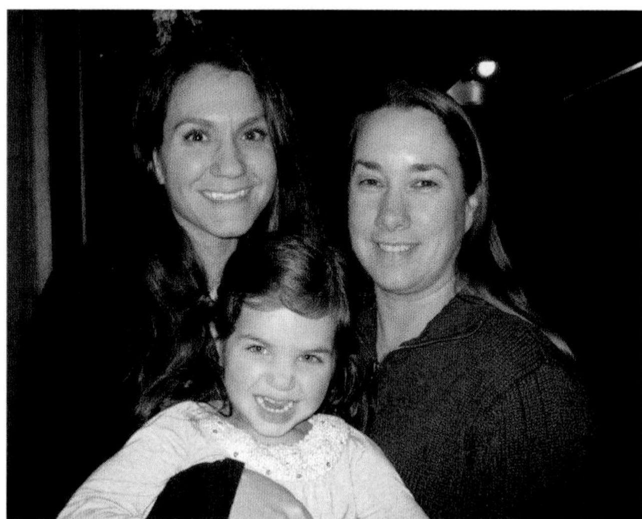

FIGURE 3–5 This nontraditional family represents the diversity in family types.

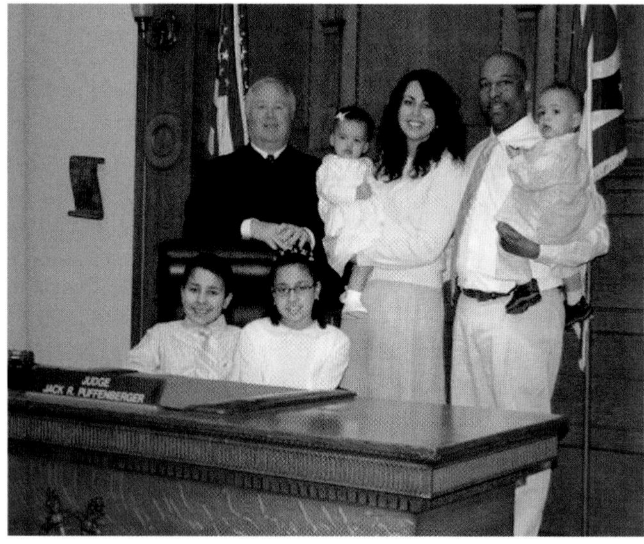

FIGURE 3–6 Adoptive family.

Roles and Developmental Tasks of the Family

Families provide for a child's physical needs, such as shelter, food and water, and clothing, as well as economic needs. Beyond these basics, families also provide nurturing, a sense of love and belonging, financial organization, and boundary management. Coping strategies help families deal with stresses of life and provide a nurturing environment. Role strain and time constraints because of dual-career demands present problems for families. Communication may need to be expanded to meet the emotional and behavioral needs of the child. Socialization of the family is necessary to meet the demands of society and facilitate the assumption of values, morals, and socially acceptable behavior (Duvall, 1985).

Family Dynamics

Nurses should be aware of family dynamics that may affect communication. For example:

- Family members interact and participate in activities with one another.
- A single adult may function as the disciplinarian.
- Children in the home interact and learn skills from each other.
- Sibling rivalry may occur (Fig. 3–7).
- The birth order of children, their ordinal place, influences communication, personality, relationships, and careers. First-born and only children are exposed more to adults, so they tend to be motivated perfectionists who are more direct in their communication (Miscioscia, Blavier, Pagone, & Simonelli, 2017). Middle children develop as conflict avoiders, mediators, or balanced with avoidance communication patterns (Miscioscia et al., 2017). The youngest are more immature and tend to have self-centered communication patterns (Miscioscia et al., 2017). If there are more than three children, then these roles tend to overlap.
- A same-sex parent and child or opposite-sex parent and child may interact with stronger alliances with the same sex, resulting in improved family interactions and communication (Miscioscia et al., 2017).

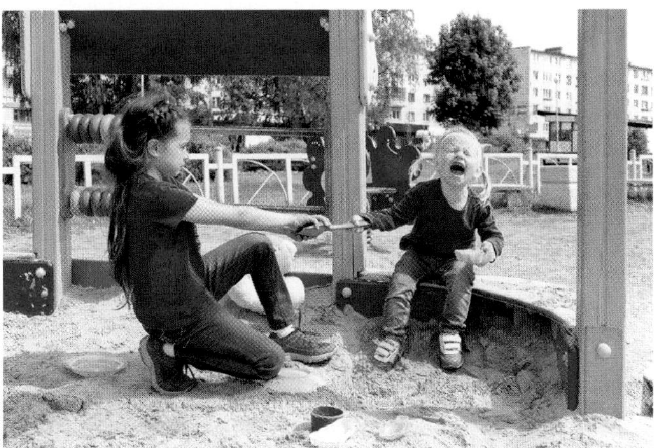

FIGURE 3–7 Sibling rivalry.

Stressors on Families

Families can become stressed by many environmental factors, such as:

- Overwhelming concern for the child
- Feelings of neglect of other children and family structure
- Loss of income
- Impact on social status
- Employment constraints like unemployment or underemployment
- Insurance issues, including being underinsured or uninsured
- Poverty
- Homelessness
- Mental illness, chronic physical illness, or catastrophic illness or injury in the family unit
- Addition of family members placing a strain on finances
- Lack of support systems
- Cultural and religious constraints
- Inadequate coping skills
- Societal pressures, HIV, suicide
- Inadequate public education
- Time at work necessitating the use of day care and nonfamily care providers

Family Reaction to a Child's Illness

Families have a range of emotional reactions to learning their child has an acute or chronic illness. These may include:

- Disbelief
- Frustration
- Worry
- Anger
- Denial
- Anxiety
- Depression
- Fear
- Guilt

Specifically, siblings of the child who is ill may experience:

- Isolation
- Fear
- Feelings of being responsible because they had bad feelings about the sibling (magical thinking)
- Disruption in family roles and routines
- Problems in school
- Acting-out behaviors
- Sibling rivalry or jealousy
- Ambiguity

Nursing Interventions to Assist Families

When a child is admitted to a hospital, all family members are affected. Central themes related to increased family stress include parents experiencing a lack of control, changing roles, loss of family togetherness, demands on family coping skills, and a loss of financial support. Nurses can support the families of children they are caring for by:

- Communicating openly with the parents, which may just mean listening to the parent speak about his or her situation, child, or fears.
- Encouraging the parents to care for the child.
- Supporting the parental role and providing positive feedback on their care and role fulfillment.
- Developing a trusting relationship with parents, by providing honest communication and strong clinical skills; these attributes may help the parent feel comfortable leaving the child when they cannot be present at the hospital.
- Beginning discharge instructions as soon as the child is admitted, especially if the child has a long-term condition.
- Encouraging siblings to visit and bring familiar objects to the hospital; preparing siblings for what they can expect to hear, see, and smell; child life specialists are an excellent resource in this regard.

SAFE AND EFFECTIVE NURSING CARE: Clinical Pearl

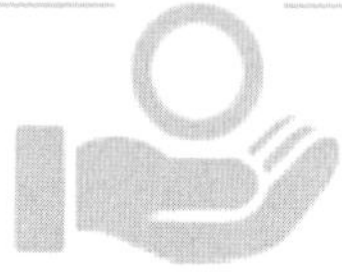

Legal Custody/Legal Power of Attorney

With the increase of nontraditional family types, nurses must be aware of who has legal custody and who has legal power of attorney. These questions must be asked on admission to the hospital.

COMMUNICATION THEORY

Communication theory was identified by Schudder in the early 1900s and first published in 1980. This theory states that all living beings communicate, although the manner of communication is different (Boyer, Campbell, & Ling, 2015). Staying connected is a social norm and provides social connectedness that is essential in family life (Boyer et al., 2015). When evaluating family dynamics, the nurse should consider the following questions:

- How does the family exchange information, values, and emotional connections?
- Are messages supporting or attacking?
- Does nonverbal communication stifle verbal communication?
- Are love and support withheld when differences of opinion occur?

Healthy Families

Families characterized as having healthy communication and dynamics:

- Give clear, congruent, and consistent verbal and nonverbal cues.
- Help children move forward in the decision-making process.
- Foster the child's attainment of autonomy through support and guidance (Bindman, Pomerantz, & Roisman, 2015).
- Encourage interactions and consistently interact in a positive manner.
- Derive pleasure, companionship, kinship, and love from one another (Fig. 3–8).

Evidence-Based Practice

Bindman, S. W., Pomerantz, E. M., & Roisman, G. I. (2015). Do children's executive function account for associations between early autonomy supporting parenting and achievement through high school? *Journal of Educational Psychology, 107*(3), 756–770.

This study demonstrated a correlation between a mother's autonomy support (providing instruction to identify, nurture, and develop the child's inner thoughts, feelings, or actions) during the first 3 years of a child's life, including warmth and cognitive stimulation, with subsequent achievement not only in kindergarten but also throughout middle and high school.

Unhealthy Families

Families with unhealthy communication and dynamics:

- Give inconsistent, noncongruent verbal and nonverbal messages.
- Humiliate, intimidate, or control communication.
- Do not promote decision making through communication.
- Neglect interactions because of lack of knowledge, time, or interest in the child, as well as other barriers.

FAMILY THEORY

When a group of individuals comes together as a family unit, they go through a series of developmental stages as described by

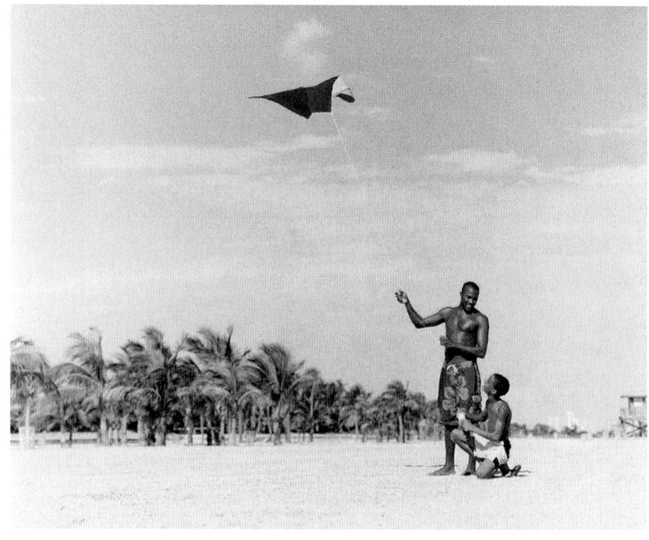

FIGURE 3–8 Family members sharing activities together form healthy bonds.

Tuckman in 1966. Group theory as applied to the family unit is as follows:

- Forming stage—marriage or cohabitation, birth or adoption of children
- Storming stage—two or more personalities realize their differences, such as emotional clashes with teenagers
- Norming stage—adjustment to individual members and rules; parental rules are imposed; children agree to obey rules
- Performing stage—family or group accomplishes goals and produces results
- Adjourning stage—death, divorce, or children leave to form their own families

Family Systems Theory

Family systems theory is focused on the family as an emotional unit. This theory describes how triangulation occurs when a third individual is introduced to a relationship that began with two individuals. The relationship created by this triangulation requires de-triangulation, in which the third individual begins to differentiate himself or herself (Bowen Center, 2017).

- Changes that occur in aspects of one family member's life affect the entire family.
- The family shares a unique identity.
- The family is characterized by the concepts of wholeness and the interdependence of its parts (Fig. 3–9).
- The family is dynamic.
- Interactions with work, church, school, and friends are encouraged, but family boundaries remain intact.
- Subsystems within a family may form, such as alliances between siblings or with one parent.
- Families strive to maintain balance during a crisis.

Resiliency Model of Family Stress, Adjustment, and Adaptation

The resiliency model assesses a family's ability to adjust during times of stress and crisis, function effectively, and adapt to stressful hospitalizations and disease processes. This model also determines a family's ability to adjust to members who are physically or mentally disabled and focuses on family strengths and capabilities (Bindman et al., 2015; McCubbin, Thompson, & McCubbin, 1996; Phillips & Prezio, 2017). This model also describes how family stress, adjustment, and adaptation affect all members of the family.

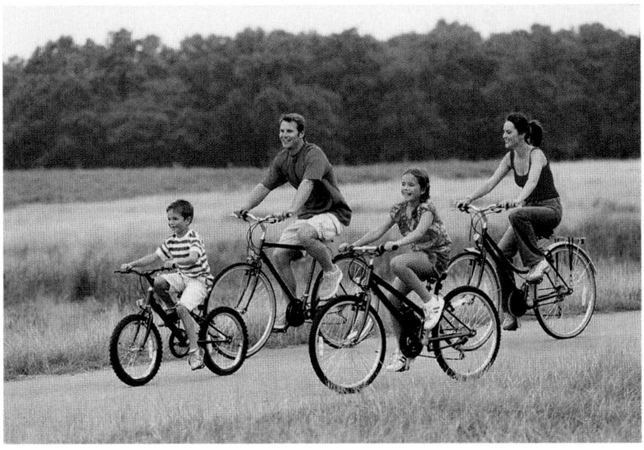

FIGURE 3–9 Biking together as a family helps to develop a sense of belonging.

Murray Bowen and Family System Theory

Psychiatrist Murray Bowen developed the family system theory based on human behavior. According to Bowen, the family is a unit in which members are emotionally connected and interdependent; thus, a change in one member's role or functioning will impact the functioning and roles of the other members. This interdependence assists in promoting cohesiveness and cooperation of the family members (Bowen Center, 2017). The theory helps to identify family problems that result from failure to communicate and allows parents to teach values that are important to the family. Bowen's theory includes eight interrelated concepts:

1. Triangles—a three-person relationship is the smallest stable relationship
2. Differentiation of self—whether good or bad, feelings of self will influence family relationships
3. Nuclear family emotional system
4. Marital conflict
5. Dysfunction in one spouse
6. Impairment of one or more children
7. Emotional distance (Bowen Center, 2017)
8. Multigenerational transmission process—small differences between parent and sibling transfers over generations; individuals choose mates with concepts of self similar to their own (Bowen Center, 2017)

Virginia Satir and Family Therapy

Satir's theory of family therapy states that the goal of family therapy is to deal with family pain that is manifested in one family member but affects other family members in one way or another (Family Therapy, 2015). The family is seen as an interactive unit. For example, a dysfunctional marital relationship results in dysfunctional parenting patterns. Family dysfunction is then tied to dysfunctional parenting (Family Therapy and the Theories of Virginia Satir, 2015). Satir was key in the development of family therapy. She believed that:

- A healthy family was one that was open and reciprocal in sharing love, support, and ideas.
- Love and nurturance are key concepts of family healing and health (Evans, Turner, & Trotter, 2012; Leslie, 2016).

Duvall and Family Development Theory

Duvall's theory involves eight stages that are based on Erickson's theory of psychosocial development. The oldest child in the family marks the transition of the family into the next stage. The family unit changes over time, with members moving through developmental stages. Duvall describes the family as a small, semiclosed system that interacts with a larger social system. As this occurs, the role of the health-care practitioner caring for family members must also adapt as follows:

- Beginning family: Practitioner aids in identifying a common goal, choosing career paths, and planning for children. In this stage the task of couples is to establish themselves as a family unit of two.
- Childbearing stage: The couple prepare for the introduction into the family unit of a child. All members of the family then must adjust to new roles as parents and/or grandparents.
- Preschool stage: As the oldest child transitions to early childhood, the family begins to learn to socialize and prepare the child for entry into school. Practitioner notes evolving parenting skills and is alert for signs of abuse or neglect.
- School-age stages: As the oldest child transitions to this stage, the family unit must assist the child in developing social connections that are outside of the family unit. Practitioner aids in health promotion, including providing information on drugs and sex.
- Adolescent stage: As the oldest child transitions into this stage, independence and launching of the child is a major focus. The parents can now refocus on their marriage.
- Launching, middle-age, and retirement stages: Family comes full circle to return to the self and couple building, refocusing on extended family relationships. Practitioner roles vary (Duvall, 1985).

The family's life-cycle stages are based on changes in the structure, function, and roles within the unit. Understanding a family's current stage of development can assist the nurse in identifying areas where education and anticipatory guidance may be needed.

Neuman's System Theory

Neuman's system model views the client as an open system that responds to stresses in the environment. Stresses may be intrapersonal, interpersonal, or extrapersonal, and result from internal, external, and created environments (Khatiban, Oshvandi, Borzou, & Moayed, 2016). Nursing interventions are related to three primary areas of prevention:

- Primary prevention occurs before the stress affects the client in alleviating possible risk factors.
- Secondary prevention occurs after the stress affects the client and addresses symptomology.
- Tertiary prevention occurs when the nurse assists in maintenance factors to bring the individual back to the primary state (Khatiban et al., 2016).

In Neuman's system theory the family is viewed as a target that should be assessed and to which nursing interventions should then be applied. Variables within the child's internal and external environments comprise the whole system. All members of the family express themselves differently, and this influences the group as a whole. The goal in this theory is to keep the family structure stable in its environment through the three areas of prevention (Khatiban et al., 2016).

Family-Focused Care

The philosophy of family-focused care is based on the belief that a child receives the best quality care when health-care providers work with the parents and family. In family-centered care, family members and health-care professionals work as a team to promote quality care for the child. Families assist children in meeting their psychosocial and developmental needs. Other tenets of this care philosophy include:

- Acknowledgment of diversity, differences in family backgrounds, and support systems
- In acute-care settings, stress is placed on family communication patterns
- Focusing on family relationships, values, coping strategies, and perceptions
- Enabling family caregivers by encouraging them to room-in with the child
- Nurses empowering and assisting families to make informed choices
- Provision of a place for families to spend quality time with the child in care settings
- When appropriate, allowing the family to spend time talking and playing with the child in the absence of medical staff
- Encouraging and supporting the family to make decisions and implement care
- Recognition of caregivers as experts in caring for their child
- Recognition that the illness or injury of a child affects the entire family (Institute for Family-Centered Care, 2017)
- Assessment of support and education needs for all family members
- Encouragement of visitation and providing age-appropriate information for siblings

SAFE AND EFFECTIVE NURSING CARE: Clinical Pearl

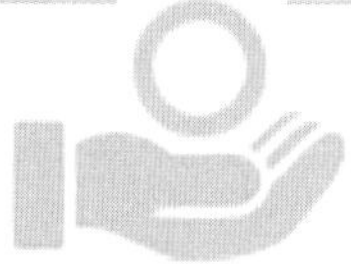

Benefits of Family-Focused Care

Family-focused care benefits the child and the family. For the child, these benefits include decreased anxiety, reduced need for pain medication, and improved coping during hospitalization (Institute for Family-Centered Care, 2017). As for the family, members who participate in care conferences and in the child's care feel empowered by being included in the decision-making process, which allows them to develop the skills needed to care for and support the child. It also decreases feelings of stress and dependency on others. The nurse's role is to support the family and provide members with the knowledge needed for self-care.

SAFE AND EFFECTIVE NURSING CARE: Clinical Pearl

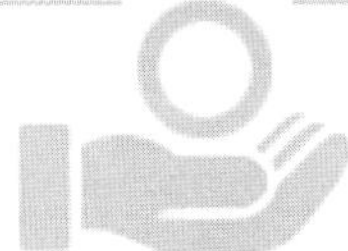

Separation Anxiety

Nurses should be aware that separation anxiety occurs during the toddler years (1–3 years of age), but can begin as early as 6 months of age (see Chapters 7 and 8 for further details). Separation from caregivers is stressful for toddlers and can be even more stressful if the child is hospitalized. Care should be given to include the parents in necessary procedures for the child when possible.

Structural-Functional Theory

Structural-functional theory sees the family as a social institution that is essential for the continuation of a strong society. Each family must successfully perform four main functions to be considered functional. These functions include sex, procreation, economic function, and socialization (Altman, Dumas, Odden, Velez, & Weinhold, 2013). If a family does not perform these functions, it is considered dysfunctional (Altman et al., 2013). This theory focuses on the promotion of family function and is strongly tied to the traditional nuclear family (Altman et al., 2013). Familial roles include:

- Provider
- Housekeeper
- Child caregiver
- Socializer and recreational organizer
- Sexual partner
- Therapist
- Kinship (Harper, 2011)

King's Theory of Goal Attainment

Imogene King's theory of goal attainment looks at the recognition of interactions that occur in the family unit. It addresses three interrelated systems—personal, interpersonal, and social (King, 2017)—with goal achievement attained through all three. The family is an interpersonal social system. The nurse, child, and family communicate information, set goals together, and then apply interventions to achieve these goals. Nurses use the nursing process to assist the child and the family in achieving their goals through action, reaction, and interaction (King, 2017).

Roy Adaptation Model

This model, formulated by nurse theorist Sister Calista Roy, holds that God and humans have a relationship with the environment, and humans are an adaptive system that strives to maintain balance with either healthy or unhealthy adaptations. People are viewed as individuals, but they can also be viewed as existing within groups, families, or populations. In Roy's theory, the nurse's role is to promote adaptation for groups, families, or populations (Connell School of Nursing, 2014).

This model has four components:

- Psychological mode: Behavior in this mode is related to the physiological activity of cells and includes oxygenation, nutrition, elimination, activity and rest, and relaxation (Connell School of Nursing, 2014).
- Self-concept mode: This mode looks at the personal side of how one sees his or her own physical being and the psychological side that looks at his or her qualities, values, and worth (Connell School of Nursing, 2014). The basic need is psychic integrity (Connell School of Nursing, 2014).
- Role function mode: This mode looks at the position and functioning capacity of one's role in society. The basic need is self-identity (Connell School of Nursing, 2014).
- Interdependence mode: This mode is associated with relationships and interactions with others. Basic needs are nurturance and affection (Connell School of Nursing, 2014).

FAMILY ASSESSMENT

Family resources and processes are primary influences on the child's health and development, so family assessment provides the nurse with critical information that will impact the provision of quality care.

Family Size and Shape

Family structure, socioeconomic status, resources, physical and mental health, and identity are influential factors. Average family size has decreased compared with a generation ago and is culturally dependent. Family structure is very diverse, and family members are not necessarily blood-related. Families may be defined differently by the child and the parent (Ward & Hisley, 2014a).

Parenting Styles

Parenting style influences a child's developmental outcomes. Children view their parents as powerful protectors and problem-solvers who have access to resources. Common parenting styles include:

- Authoritarian-dictatorial parenting
  - Absolute rules, strict expectations
  - Children have little decision-making power
  - Punishment by withdrawal of approval
  - Children may become shy, sensitive, loyal, and honest
- Permissive (laissez-faire) parenting
  - Children control their environment and make their own decisions
  - Few rules to follow
  - Children may have difficulty following rules that are expected in the public environment
  - Children may grow up to be irresponsible, disrespectful, and aggressive

- Authoritative or democratic parenting
  - Combination of authoritarian and permissive styles, drawing on the positive aspects of each
  - Firm rules that allow some freedom (rules with discussion)
  - Children are taught the correlation between actions and the consequences of those actions
  - Children may become self-reliant, assertive, and display high self-esteem (Ward & Hisley, 2014a)

Roles and Relationships

Nurses can gain information about family roles and relationships by observing:

- Delegation of tasks, including household chores
  - How is good and bad work rewarded/punished?
  - Are traditional sex (gender) roles observed?
- Clothing and personal hygiene
  - Is personal hygiene congruent between the caregiver and the child?
- The condition of the home
  - Who makes the decisions? Who has the control?
  - How are problems solved?

Tools for Assessment

Assessment tools are designed to evaluate the strengths and protective components of the family unit (Ward & Hisley, 2014a). Conduct the assessment in a comfortable environment after a relationship has been established with the child and the family.

Genogram

A genogram goes beyond the traditional family tree and includes family relationships and medical history. In family health, genograms can be used to illuminate family dynamics through psychological factors. It does not go as far as a pedigree, which involves investigating genetic code information to assist genetic counselors (see Chapter 18 for further details on genetics). A genogram comprises the following elements:

- Pictorial representation of the family unit (Fig. 3–10)
- Diagrams of health concerns and behavioral patterns

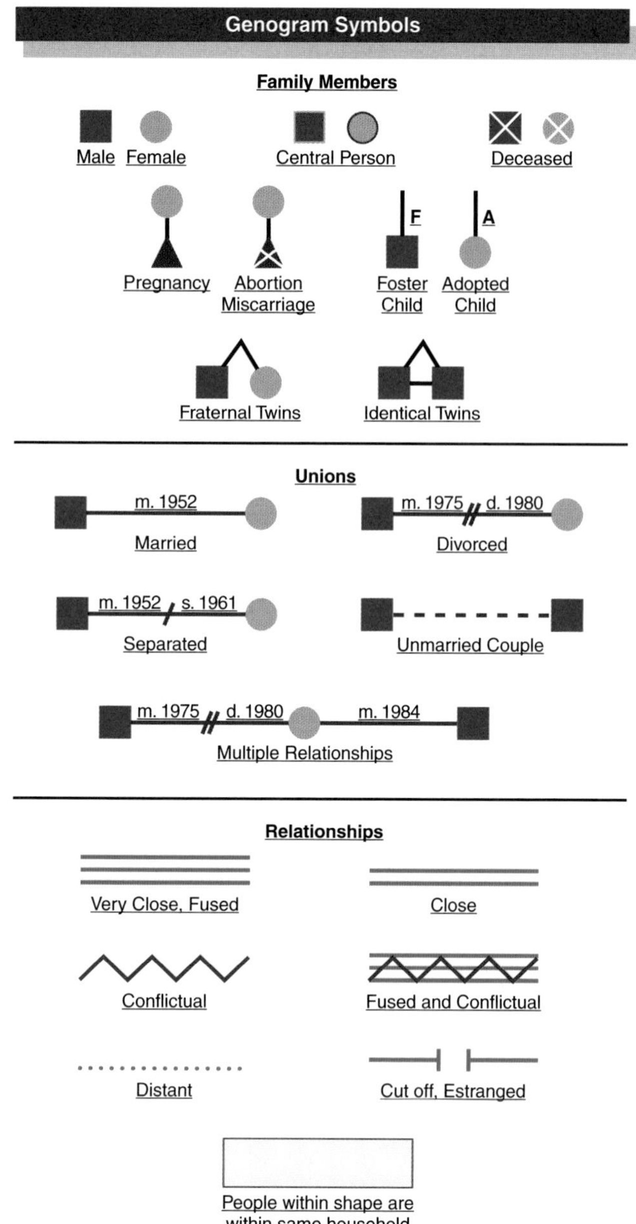

FIGURE 3–10 Example of a genogram template.

Kinetic Family Drawing

With kinetic family drawing, the child draws a picture of the family unit (Fig. 3–11). This drawing depicts the child's view of the family and can reflect the family's health and areas of distress.

Structural Family Assessment

The structural family assessment uses interviews and questionnaires to determine:

- Who lives in the home?
- What is the social, economic, cultural, and religious makeup?
- What is the family composition?
- What are the occupations and education levels of family members? (Gehart, 2016)

A structural family assessment may include the following elements: family developmental stage, family rituals, and triangulation.

Family Developmental Stage

The family can exist in a variety of stages, such as having a preschooler and sending a child off to college. Children go through the stages of development noted by Erik Erikson (1959), with tasks that must be met at each stage to proceed to the next. The success in meeting the tasks of the various stages of development will influence the communication demonstrated by the child. Family developmental stage is assessed by interview, observation, tools, and surveys.

Family Rituals

Family rituals consist of the routines or activities taught by the family to maintain stability. The nurse assesses, through observation

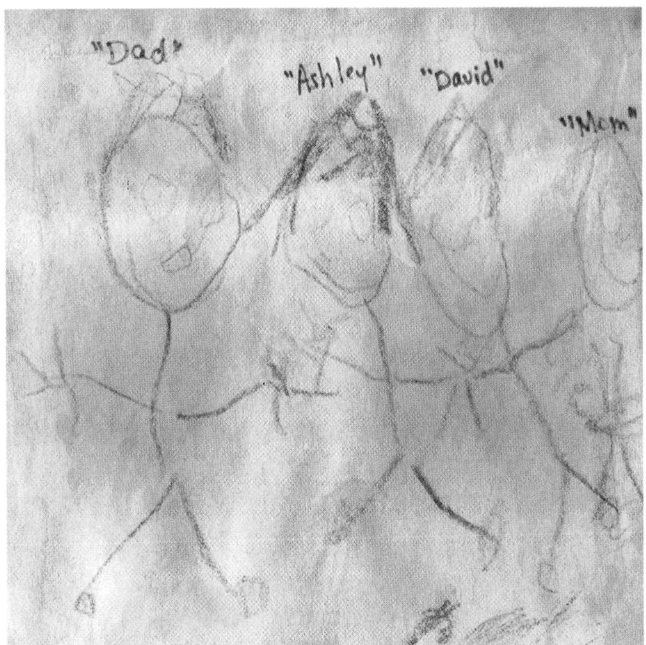

FIGURE 3-11 A kinetic drawing illustrates the family unit.

or surveys, the importance of these rituals. The nurse must allow these rituals to be maintained as much as possible for the continuity and stability of the family unit.

- When possible, permit families to share meals together.
- When possible, maintain regular nap times and nighttime rituals.
- When appropriate, permit families to maintain involvement in the child's routine care.

Triangulation

Triangulation occurs when two or more family members team up against a third family member. It can also occur when one family member will not speak to another family member but communicates through a third family member. This places the third family member in a triangular relationship. A dyad is the formation of a two-person bond or subsystem within the family unit, such as a husband-and-wife dyad or a twin-to-twin dyad.

Functional Family Assessment

With this assessment, the nurse interviews members of the family and records his or her observations, such as:

- Who has the power or makes decisions in the family?
- What characterizes family interactions and roles?
- What communication methods are used, and are they successful?

This type of assessment allows the nurse to develop cultural sensitivity in recognizing cultural factors that shape family perceptions, as well as cultural competence as a nursing assessment tool (see Chapter 4). Sub-roles of the nurse conducting this assessment include:

- Stranger
- Resource person
- Teacher
- Leader
- Surrogate
- Counselor (Child Welfare Group, n.d.)

Family APGAR Five-Item Questionnaire

The APGAR questionnaire is used to determine family members' satisfaction with the functional status of the family (Box 3–1). It is usually completed in an outpatient or home environment and consists of the following five items:

- A—Adaptation: the ability to use resources for problem solving in a crisis
- P—Partnership: the ability to share responsibilities and nurturing roles in a crisis
- G—Growth: the ability to achieve physical or emotional growth
- A—Affection: the ability to demonstrate love and attention to family members
- R—Resolve: the ability to devote time to other family members in the nurturing process

Results are scored numerically from 0 to 20 and categorized as highly functional, moderately dysfunctional, or highly

BOX 3-1 | Examples of Family Nursing Diagnoses

Any North American Nursing Diagnosis Association (NANDA) diagnosis may be appropriate for describing an individual family member's health status. A family diagnosis is intended to describe the health status of the family as a whole. Examples of family diagnoses include the following:

- Caregiver role strain (actual and risk for)
- Dysfunctional family processes: Alcoholism
- Family coping: Compromised
- Family coping: Disabled
- Impaired parenting (actual and risk for)
- Ineffective family therapeutic regimen management
- Readiness for enhanced family copying
- Readiness for enhanced parenting
- Risk for parent–infant–child attachment
- Social isolation
- Spiritual distress

Nursing Outcomes Classification (NOC) designations specifically for families as units are included in the NOC domain "Family Health." This category includes the following classes: family caregiver status, family member health status, and family well-being and parenting. Outcomes from other domains may also apply. Nursing Intervention Classification (NIC) designations for families as units are included in the NIC domain "Family." This category includes the following classes: childbearing care, childrearing care, and life-span care.

Wilkinson, J.M, et al (2015) Fundamentals of Nursing (3rd ed.) Philadelphia: F.A. Davis.

dysfunctional. Higher scores indicate higher family satisfaction (Smilkstein, 1978; Takenaka & Bon, 2016).

COMMUNICATING WITH THE FAMILY

Pediatric nurses should use the following strategies for effective communication:

- Encourage parents to talk openly regarding their concerns.
- Use open-ended questions.
- Use careful, nonjudgmental statements.
- Men may prefer a focus on cognitive, problem-solving talk (Reiss, 2016).
- Women may prefer a focus on the process rather than the outcome (Reiss, 2016).
- Be aware and considerate of generational, cultural, and other differences.
- Incorporate active listening skills.
- Use silence, empathy, respect, genuineness, and trust as nursing interventions.
- Follow the established policies and procedures the hospital has in place for communication with nontraditional and noncustodial parents.
- Remember to observe and record nonverbal communication factors, such as tone of voice, body language, and facial expression. Be aware of your own nonverbal communication factors, and make sure you are not communicating unintended messages.
- Allow family members to voice their understanding of the current situation.
- Clarify or provide teaching points to decrease misunderstandings.

Communicating With Children

Even though most communication will take place between health-care practitioners and parents, the child cannot and should not be excluded. Child health decision making is a result of family health-care decision making (Cherry, 2015). A decision should be made by collaborating with the parents, the health-care practitioner, and the nurse as to who will speak to the child about the health-care issue at hand—the practitioner, the caregiver, or a combination of the two. When communicating with the pediatric client:

- Incorporate active communication strategies.
- Incorporate an understanding of growth and development.
- Observe body language, facial expressions, and other nonverbal gestures.
- Incorporate play into nursing assessments and interactions where appropriate (Fig. 3–12).
- Use special toys or games to assist with assessments/education (Fig. 3–13).
- Be aware of both verbal communication, including words, speech patterns, crying, and other cues, and non-verbal communication, including gestures, body language, posture, and eye contact (see Chapter 7).

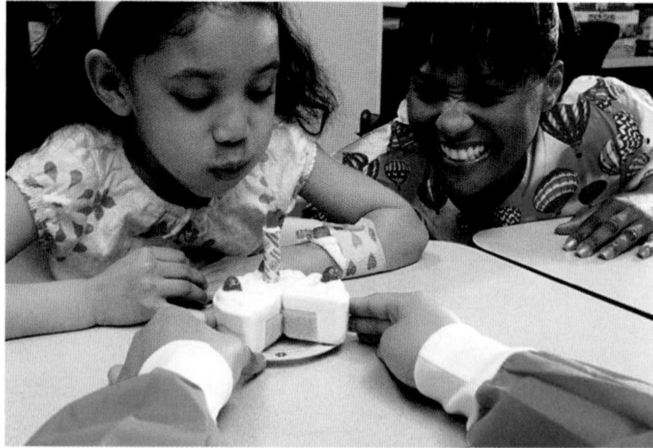

FIGURE 3–12 Incorporate play into family assessments.

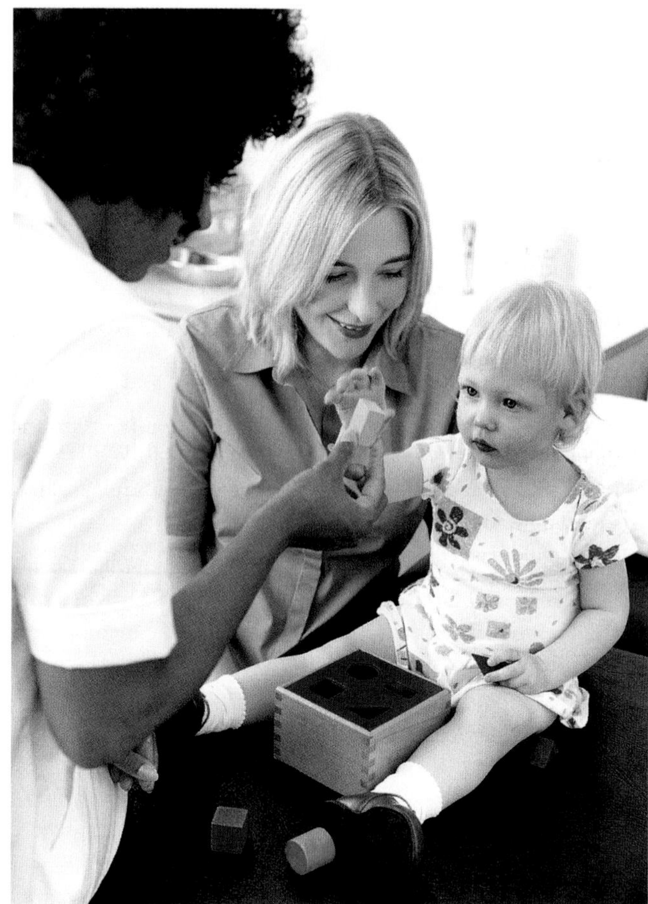

FIGURE 3–13 Use special toys or games to assist with assessments.

- Use visual forms of communication, including signs, photos, and illustrations, as appropriate.
- Incorporate play, which allows children to express feelings and concerns nonverbally (Fig. 3–14).

Communicating With Infants

The infant period, from birth to 12 months, is a time of rapid physical and developmental growth. The body systems are maturing, and skill development is taking place. Social development

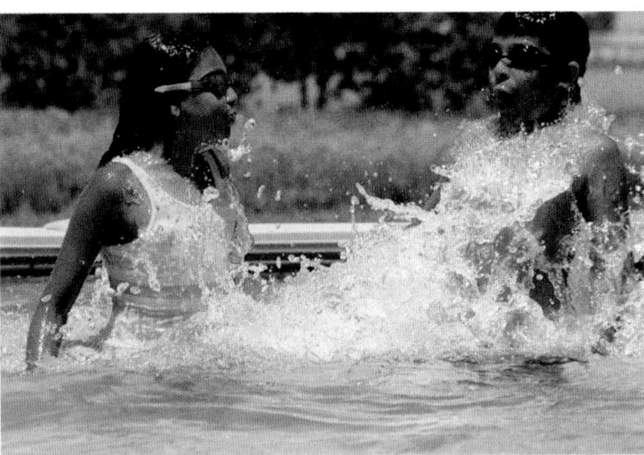

FIGURE 3–14 Play allows children to express feelings and concerns in a nonverbal manner.

is influenced by the infant's environment and the attachment developed with his or her parents and caregivers. When caring for an infant, the pediatric nurse should be aware of the following communication characteristics of this age group:

- Infants are unable to verbalize needs, concerns, and discomforts.
- Nonverbal behaviors, such as smiling, promote socialization.
- Infants cry when they are hungry, when their diapers need to be changed, when feeling pain or discomfort, and when feeling lonely or wanting to be held.
- Infants coo when they are content or happy.
- Infants are often quiet, observing the environment around them.
- Infants respond to the nonverbal behaviors of adults: touch, sound, and tone of voice.
- If the child has attained understanding of object permanence, he or she will know when a parent is missing (see Chapter 6).
- Observing parent and caregiver interactions with the infant can provide information about:
  - Separation anxiety
  - Fear of strangers
  - Temperament and disposition

Nursing Interventions for Infants

- Communicate primarily with parents and/or caregivers.
- Learn the infant's routines—feeding, changing, sleeping schedule—and incorporate them into nursing care.
- Use gentle touch when handling the infant to provide a sense of security and comfort.
- Allow the infant to suck on the pacifier to promote stress relief and relaxation.
- Talk to the infant when providing care to console him or her.
- Use music and sounds to assist in soothing the infant.
- Quickly respond to the infant's crying by feeding, diapering, or picking up the infant, all the while talking to the child about what you think he or she is communicating (Fig. 3–15).
- Use sing-song approaches to communication—singing and music can quickly gain the infant's attention, as does wide-eyed, high-pitched communication (Traub, 2016).

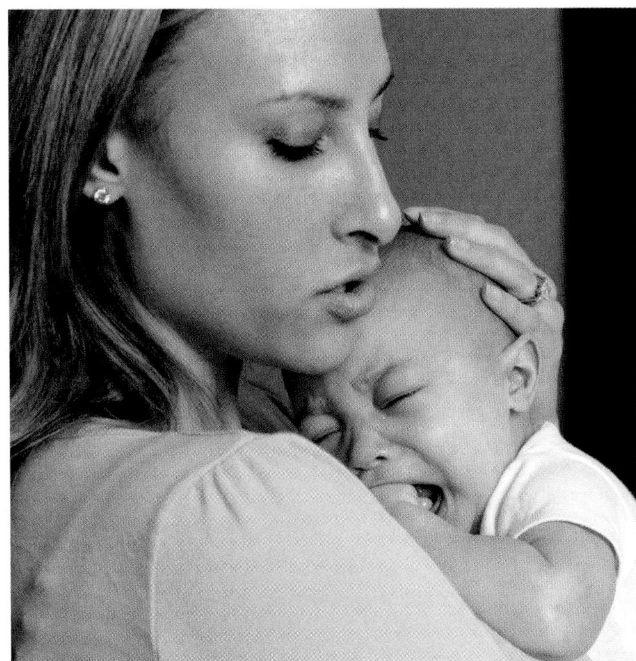

FIGURE 3–15 Quickly respond to the infant's crying by feeding, diapering, or picking up the infant.

- Incorporate visual, auditory, tactile, and kinesthetic stimulation into nursing care and activities.
- If the hospital uses child-care specialists who come and provide interaction, include such specialists in the provision of the child's care.
- Incorporate continuance of care so that the same nurses are providing care as much as possible. The infant will become familiar with the nursing staff.
- Incorporate consistency in nursing care and contact to allow the infant to develop trust.
- Consistent nursing staff will allow the nurse to better interpret the nonverbal communication patterns of the infant.
- To decrease problems with temperament and disposition, incorporate as much of the infant's normal routine as possible in care provision.

Communicating With Toddlers and Preschoolers

The period between ages 1 and 5 is a time of intense exploration of the child's environment. The speech of a 5-year-old should be understood by anyone listening. The young child learns more about the environment while also exhibiting some negative behaviors, including tantrums. Children of this age are typically egocentric, or unable to think from another person's point of view. Although this time can be overwhelming and challenging for parents and caregivers, substantial cognitive, social, psychosocial, and biological growth and development are occurring. When communicating with a child in this age group, the nurse should be aware of the following:

- Use statements such as "good job" praise, instead of "good boy/girl."

- The child is unable to separate his or her actions from the origin of pain experienced.
- Exploring objects through touch helps children gain knowledge of and experiment with unknown environments (Fig. 3–16).
- Medical play may be useful in demonstrating how a procedure will take place.
  - The child may practice or pretend that a doll is having a procedure done.
  - If appropriate, allow the child to handle a stethoscope, pulse oximeter, and blood pressure cuff, and explore these items in a nonthreatening environment.
- Children of this age are very concrete and literal, and are often unable to conceptualize that one word may have more than one meaning.
  - "IV" means "intravenous" to the nurse, but may be translated as "ivy," a known plant, by the young child (Fig. 3–17).
  - "Stick" or "poke" refers to a needle insertion for the nurse, but the young child views a stick as a small piece of wood found in the yard.
- Bleeding may be perceived as a child's "insides leaking out." Young children are often comforted by an adhesive bandage used to cover an open area.
- When having an x-ray procedure, the child may smile when getting his or her "picture" taken.
- Children assume that inanimate objects feel and act as humans do. For example, they might think that something inanimate could bite them.
- The child may call an instrument "bad" if it has caused pain or discomfort to them.
- They are fearful of unfamiliar objects and environments.
- When possible, allow the child to tour a facility or treatment room before the actual treatment.
- Preschoolers begin to develop skills in fantasy and pretend play.
- This is a period of social, language, and behavioral development.
- Children of toddlers are developing a sense of autonomy (Fig. 3–18; see also Chapter 6).

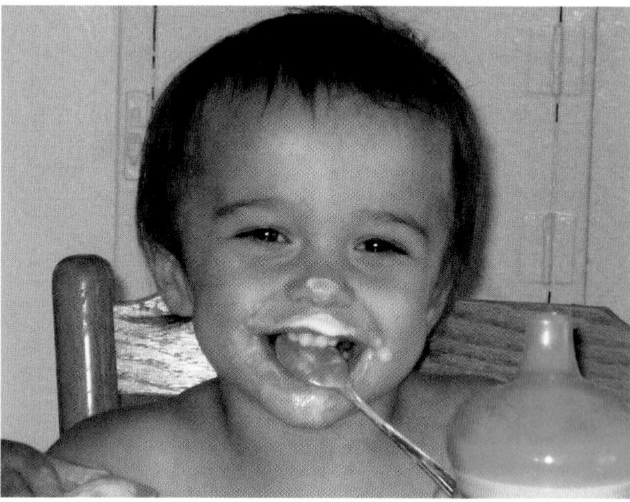

FIGURE 3–16 Infants need to feel and touch the environment around them.

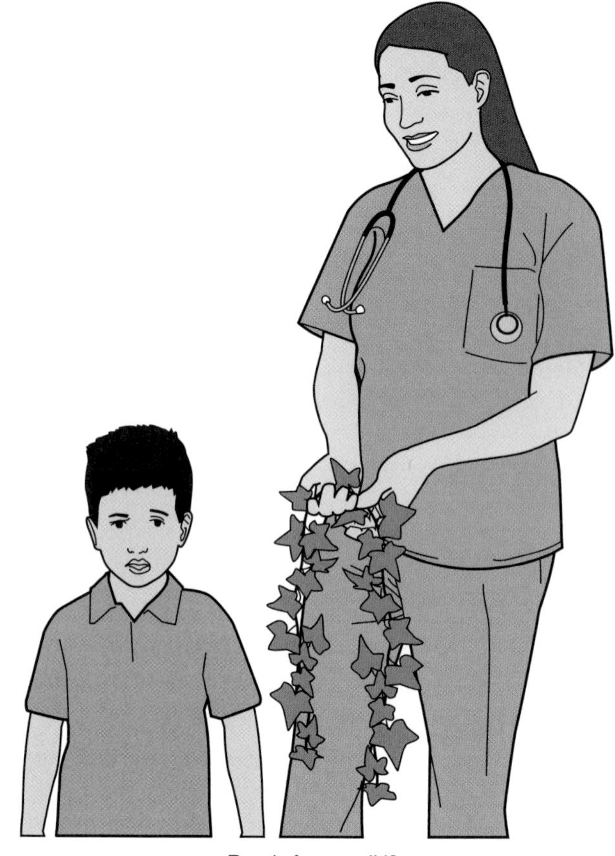

FIGURE 3–17 Toddlers are very concrete and literal, and are unable to conceptualize that one word may have more than one meaning.

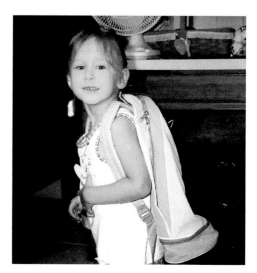

FIGURE 3–18 Developing a sense of autonomy.

Nursing Interventions for Communicating With Toddlers and Preschoolers

- Use simple terminology. Young children are unable to understand certain concepts. Those concepts should be discussed in concrete terms that the child can understand.

- Do not use euphemistic or idiomatic phrases such as "a small stick in the arm," which may be misunderstood.
- Assume the same position as the child. If the child is sitting in a small chair, sit in a chair at his or her eye level.
- Keep unused equipment out of the room until it is needed.
- Use the treatment room for painful procedures so that the assigned child's room is a haven.
- Label the child's emotions to validate feelings of fear and anxiety.
- Have toys available during procedures. Allow the child to perform the procedures on a doll or stuffed animal so he or she can better understand what will occur. Supporting pretend and fantasy play with the child provides opportunities to express fears and anxieties.
- Use the parents and caregivers to assist with providing care and communication.
- Support preschoolers who self-talk (internal speaking that helps to identify information about emotions, attitudes, and beliefs). This practice encourages the alignment of thought patterns (Traub, 2016).
- When appropriate, offer the child choices so that control can be maintained (e.g., do you want water or juice after you swallow your medicine?)
- Prepare the child for the procedure just before the procedure, not days in advance.

Communicating With School-Age Children

The period of physical and psychosocial development from ages 6 to 12 years includes many milestones, such as entering school, communicating independently, and beginning to conceptualize the environment. Direct communication with children of this age is equally important as communicating with their parents. School-age children are energetic and want answers to their questions. They develop connections between new information and existing knowledge. Other communication characteristics of the school-age child include:

- Curiosity
  - Used to asking questions in school when they cannot understand
  - Want to know why or how things happen
- Knowledge gained by hands-on experience
  - Enjoy having a job or task to complete
  - Eager to please and want to complete a task independently
  - Work well with positive feedback
  - May bargain to postpone an intervention
- Concreteness
  - Unable to think abstractly
  - Learns well when given physical examples
  - May overreact if feeling threatened
  - Able to verbalize thoughts, feelings, or concerns

Nursing Interventions for Communicating With School-Age Children

- Tell the child that he or she is part of the medical team that will help to get him or her well.
- Assign daily jobs, such as an exercise or a task, so that the child can assist with care.
- When appropriate, offer the child choices so that control can be maintained (e.g., do you want water or juice after you swallow your medicine?).
- Explain the why and how in simple, nondescript, and nonfearful terms.
- Remember that abstract thinking has not yet been accomplished at this age.
- Allow the child to participate in procedures safely, such as taking off an adhesive bandage or depressing a blood pressure cuff.
- Allow the child to voice his or her concerns.
- Encourage children to ask questions and answer honestly and simply, in concrete verbiage.
- Allow the child to have time to play, explore questions, and have fun.
- Older children may wish to journal their experiences.
- Other children may serve as a support group.
- Facilitate playtime, which allows the child to communicate thoughts or feelings in a nonthreatening environment.

Communicating With Adolescent Children

Adolescence, from ages 13 to 18 years, is a time of developing independence and maturity. The adolescent child typically focuses on social networks and friends and may seek counsel and feedback from sources other than parents and caregivers. Sexual development, including menstruation and emission, has already occurred. Behavior may fluctuate between adult and childlike. Adolescents are independent with activities of daily living, but still require adult supervision and input (Fig. 3–19). Trust is extremely important in their relationships and influences the extent of communication. Adolescents tend to develop their own language and culture, which may be different from those of parents and caregivers. Medical decisions may be influenced by the adolescent's peer group.

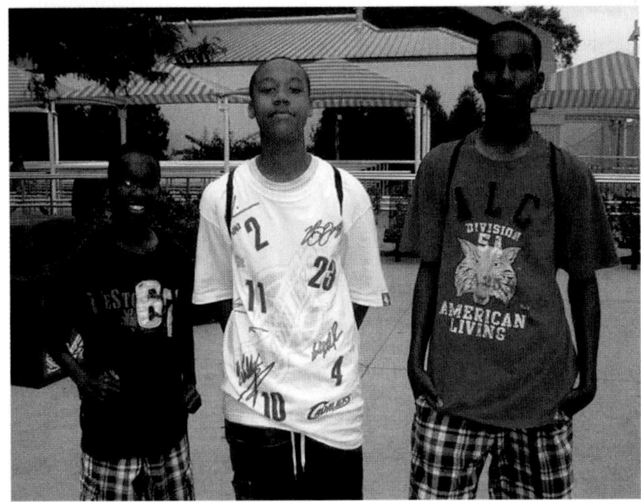

FIGURE 3-19 Adolescents are becoming more independent, but still require adult supervision and input.

Nursing Interventions for Communicating with Adolescents

- Use open-ended questions.
- Encourage the child to express his or her feelings and concerns.
- Provide privacy, as many adolescents will not be honest if interviewed in the presence of parents or caregivers.
- Explain the limits of confidentiality.
- Clarify differing opinions and/or reports from parents and child.
- Incorporate genuineness, trust, active listening, respect, and rapport skills into nursing care.
- Do not confuse the adolescent's mature body with emotional maturity.

COMMUNICATING WITH THE ALTERED FAMILY UNIT

Families may be affected by situational crises such as hurricanes, tornados, floods, loss of job, or loss of a family member, as well as developmental crises such as those experienced by adolescents. Common crises that families experiences are described in the following subsections.

Substance Abuse

- Negatively affects the family
- Abuser often enabled because of denial, pride, or embarrassment
- Roles shift to enable the abuser to continue to abuse substances:
  - Responsible or enabler member role: This is usually the nonusing caregiver. In this role, this caregiver does everything he or she can to maintain the family unit while making excuses for the abuser in the family (Low, 2015).
  - Hero member role: This is the family member who takes on responsibilities far beyond his or her role or developmental stage in the family unit. This would include a child caring for younger children, making dinner, or dressing his or her siblings. This child then strives for perfection in himself or herself as he or she takes on more and more responsibility (Low, 2015).
  - Scapegoat role: This is the child who acts out in school or in public to deflect from the dysfunctional home environment (Low, 2015).
  - Lost child role: This is the child who is withdrawn and isolated, and may use fantasy play as a means of escape (Low, 2015).
  - Mascot role: This is the child who uses comedy as a form of relief from the dysfunctional family environment (Low, 2015).
- The family unit is codependent.
- There may be an inability to communicate with outsiders—secret keepers.

Coercive Family Processes

- Members are critical and punitive.
- Punishment is used inconsistently.
- Child's behavior is ignored by the family.
- Rewards are coerced.

Physical, Emotional, or Sexual Abuse

- Secrets are kept within the family unit, preventing a resolution.
- The nonabuser parent may ignore or cover up the abuse, or may take up the role of a sexual, emotional, or physical competitor against the abused.
- Usually one member of the family is singled out for abuse.
- Nurses are legally bound to report suspected abuse in any form.

Chronic Physical or Mental Illness

- Nurses need to educate families on the physical and emotional care needed by members who experience chronic illnesses.
- Educate the child and the family unit on the need to follow the prescribed treatment regimen, schedule of follow-up appointments, and administration of medications.
- Empower the affected member and family unit by discussing options and alternatives.
- Refer the family unit to other specialists or departments, for example, social work, as questions arise related to financial resources, such as Social Security, Medicaid, or other resources related to paying for medications.
- Educate the family unit concerning techniques to assess for deficits, strategies for interventions, and when to call for help (Ward & Hisley, 2014a).
- Provide suggestions, options, and resources available for respite care when caregiver issues arise.

Hospitalization

- Hospitalization of a family member often triggers a crisis.
- Adaptation of the family unit depends on past experiences, coping skills, and resources available.
- Nurses may need to coordinate resources in the community or the home to facilitate the transition from the hospital to the home.

Death of a Family Member

- The developmental levels of family members affect their responses to death.
- Stages of grief vary from family member to family member and from family unit to family unit (Table 3–2; see Chapter 5 for further discussion).
- Responses to death change in children over time as the child's understanding of the concept of death becomes more concrete (Table 3–2; see Chapter 5 for further discussion).

TABLE 3–2 The Grieving Process As Described By Various Theorists

KÜBLER-ROSS'S STAGES OF GRIEVING	RODENBAUGH'S STAGES OF GRIEVING	HARVEY'S PHASES OF GRIEVING	EPPERSON'S PHASES OF GRIEVING	RANDO'S REACTIONS OF BEREAVED PARENTS
Denial (shock and disbelief)	Reeling (stunned disbelief)	Shock, outcry, and denial (external response to loss)	High anxiety (physical response to emotional upheaval)	Avoidance (confusion and dazed state, avoidance of reality of loss)
Anger (toward God, relatives, the health-care system)	Feelings (emotionally experiencing the loss)	Intrusion of thoughts, distractions, and obsessive reviewing of the loss (internal response, isolation)	Denial (protective psychological reaction)	Confrontation (intense emotions, anger, sadness, feeling the loss)
Bargaining (trying to attain more time, delaying acceptance of the loss)	Dealing (taking care of the details, taking care of others)	Confiding in others to emote and cognitively restructure (integration of internal thoughts and external actions to move on)	Anger (directed inwardly, toward another family member, or toward others)	Reestablishment (intensity declines, and the parents resume their lives)
Acceptance (readiness to move forward with newfound meaning or purpose in one's own life)	Healing (recovering and reentering life)		Remorse (feelings of guilt and sorrow)	
			Grief (overwhelming sadness)	
			Reconciliation (adaptation to existing circumstances)	

Source: Ward, S. L., & Hisley, S. M. (2014). *Maternal-child nursing care: The critical components of nursing care* (2nd ed.). Philadelphia: F. A. Davis.

Case Study

Family Conflict and Communication

The Riveras are a blended family in which the father brings two sons and the mother brings one son and one daughter. The children range in age from 3 to 15 years old. Mr. Rivera has recently become disabled and is unable to work. Mrs. Rivera works outside of the home five evenings per week as a waitress. Mr. Rivera is an autocratic disciplinarian, and Mrs. Rivera's style is more democratic. The children have not bonded as a family, despite being blended for 3 years. Mr. Rivera's physical situation does not allow him to do much around the home, except for driving the children to their many after-school activities. Family conflicts are the result of many different personalities, financial concerns, differences in values, and differences in child-rearing.

1. Identify the conflicts in this family that have fostered poor communication.
2. What are the parent–child power struggles in play in this scenario?
3. What factors are hindering the discussion of family values, issues, and other important topics?
4. What are the potential parental conflicts within this scenario?

REFERENCES

Altman, K., Dumas, M. S., Odden, S., Velez, L., & Weinhold, S. (2013). Structural-function theory in family nursing. *Prezi.* Retrieved from https://prezi.com/h9jaz-uhfhrf/structural-functional-theory-in-family-nursing/

Angier, N. (2013, November 25). The changing American family. *The New York Times.* Retrieved from http://www.nytimes.com/2013/11/26/health/families.html?pagewanted=all&_r=0

Bell, J., & Condren, M. (2016). Communication strategies for empowering and protecting children. *Journal of Pediatric Pharmacology and Therapeutics, 21*(2), 176–184.

Bindman, S. W., Pomerantz, E. M., & Roisman, G. I. (2015). Do children's executive function account for associations between early autonomy supporting parenting and achievement through high school? *Journal of Educational Psychology, 107*(3), 756–770.

Bowen Center. (2017). *Bowen theory.* Retrieved from https://www.thebowencenter.org/theory/

Boyer, J. B., Campbell, S. W., & Ling, R. (2015). Connection cues: Activating the norms and habits of social connectedness. *Communication Theory, 26*(2), 128–149.

Brady, N. C., Bruce, S., Goldman, A., Erickson, K., Mineo, B., Ogletree, B. T., & Wilkinson, K. (2016). Communication services and supports for individuals with severe disabilities: Guidance for assessment and intervention. *American Journal on Intellectual and Developmental Disabilities, 121*(2), 121–138.

Carpenito-Moyet, L. J. (2006). *Handbook of nursing diagnosis* (11th ed.). Philadelphia, PA: Lippincott Williams & Wilkins.

Centers for Disease Control and Prevention. (2016). *National Health Education Standards.* Retrieved from https://www.cdc.gov/healthyschools/sher/standards/index.htm

Chen, A. H., Youdelman, M. K., & Brooks, J. (2007). The legal framework for language access in healthcare settings: Title VI and beyond. *Journal of Internal Medicine, 22,* 362–365.

Cherry, M. J. (2015). Re-thinking the role of the family in medical decision-making. *Journal of Medicine & Philosophy, 40*(4), 451–472.

Child Welfare Group. (n.d.). *The functional family assessment process.* Retrieved from http://www.childwelfaregroup.org/documents/FunctionalAssessmentProcess.pdf

Connell School of Nursing. (2014). Sr. Callista Roy, Ph.D. FAAN. William F. Connell School of Nursing. Retrieved from http://www.bc.edu/schools/son/faculty/featured/theorist.html

Duvall, E. (1985). *Marriage and family development.* New York: Harper & Row.

Erikson, E. H. Paul, I. H., & Gardner, R. W. (1959). *Psychological Issues.* International University Press.

Evans, P., Turner, S., & Trotter, C. (2012). *The effectiveness of family and relationship therapy: A review of the literature.* Melbourne, Australia: PACFA.

Family Therapy and the Theories of Virginia Satir. (2015). *Awaken.* Retrieved from http://www.awaken.com/2015/12/family-therapy-and-the-theories-of-virginia-satir/

Friedemann, M.-L. (1989). The concept of family nursing. *Journal of Advanced Nursing, 14,* 211–216.

Friedman, E. (2014). U.S. Hospitals and the Civil Rights Act of 1964. *Hospitals and Health Networks.* Retrieved from http://www.hhnmag.com/articles/4179-u-s-hospitals-and-the-civil-rights-act-of-1964

Gehart, D. (2016). *Theory and treatment planning in family therapy: A competency-based approach.* Boston, MA: Delmar Cengage Learning.

Harper, D. W. (2011). Structural-functionalism: Grand theory or methodology? Leicester, UK: School of Management, University of Leicester. Retrieved from http://www.academia.edu/1973019/STRUCTURAL_FUNCTIONALISM_GRAND_THEORY_OR_METHODOLOGY

Institute for Family-Centered Care. (2017). An excerpt from *partnering with patients and families to design a patient- and family-centered health care system: Recommendations and promising practices.* Retrieved from http://www.http://www.ipfcc.org/resources/downloads-tools.html

Institute for Healthcare Communication. (2017). Communication skills for child health care professionals. Retrieved from http://healthcarecomm.org/training/continuing-education-workshops/communication-skills-for-child-health-care-professionals/

Kaiser Family Foundation. (2016). Key facts about the uninsured population. Retrieved from https://www.kff.org/uninsured/fact-sheet/key-facts-about-the-uninsured-population/

Khatiban, M., Oshvandi, K., Borzou, S. R., & Moayed, M. S. (2016). Outcomes of applying Neuman system theory in intensive care units: A systematic review. *Critical Care Nursing Journal, 9*(4), e8886.

King, I. (2017). King's theory of goal attainment. *Nursing Science Quarterly, 5*(1), 19–26.

Lederman, Z. (2016). Family presence during cardiopulmonary resuscitation: Evidence-based guidelines? *Resuscitation, 105,* e5–e6.

Leslie, M. E. (2016). Widening our lens, deepening our practice: An exploration of energy within the teachings of Virginia Satir. *Satir International Journal, 4*(1), 5–20.

Limiñana-Gras, R. M., Sánchez-López, M. P., Calvo-Llena, M. T., & Corbalán, F. J. (2015). Personality styles, psychological adjustment and gender differences in parents of children congenital disabilities. *Health, 7,* 1492–1505.

Low, M. (2015). Substance abuse and the impact on the family system. *ProTalk.* Retrieved from http://www.rehabs.com/pro-talk-articles/substance-abuse-and-the-impact-on-the-family-system/

McCubbin, H. I., Thompson, A. I., & McCubbin, M. A. (1996). *Family assessment: Resiliency, coping and adaptation: Inventories for research and practice.* Madison, WI: University of Wisconsin Publishers.

Miscioscia, M., Blavier, A., Pagone, P. R., & Simonelli, A. (2017). The desire of parenthood: Intuitive co-parental behaviors and quality of couple relationship among Italian and Belgian same-sex and opposite-sex couples. *Frontiers in Psychology, 8,* 110.

National Association of the Deaf. (2017). Americans with Disability Act. Retrieved from https://www.nad.org/resources/civil-rights-laws/americans-with-disabilities-act

National Coalition on Healthcare. (2016). Coalition for healthcare communication. Retrieved from http://www.cohealthcom.org

National Conference of State Legislators. (2016). State laws and actions challenging certain health reforms. Retrieved from http://www.ncsl.org/research/health/state-laws-and-actions-challenging-ppaca.aspx

Oster, A. (2017). Our everyday life: Family communication styles. Retrieved from http://oureverydaylife.com/family-communication-styles-6196.html

Pew Research Center. (2015). The American family today. Retrieved from http://www.pewsocialtrends.org/2015/12/17/1-the-american-family-today/

Phillips, F., & Prezio, E. A. (2017). Wonders & worries: Evaluation of a child centered psychosocial intervention for families who have a parent/primary caregiver with cancer. *Psycho-Oncology,* 26(7), 1006–1012.

Porter, J. E., Cooper, S. J., & Taylor, B. (2014). Emergency resuscitation team roles: What constitutes a team and who's looking after the family? *Journal of Nursing Education Practice, 4*(3), 124–132.

Reiss, A. (2016). Study finds differences in male, female brain activity when it comes to cooperation. *Stanford Medicine News Center.* Retrieved from https://med.stanford.edu/news/all-news/2016/06/brain-activity-during-cooperation-differs-by-sex.html

Smilkstein, G. (1978). The family APGAR: A proposal for a family function test and its use by physicians. *Journal of Family Practice, 6,* 1231–1239.

Takenaka, H., & Bon, N. (2016). The most important question in family approach: The potential of the resolve item of the family APGAR in family medicine. *Asia Pacific Family Medicine, 15,* 3.

The Commonwealth Fund. (2015). 31 million people were underinsured in 2014; many skipped needed healthcare and depleted savings to pay medical bills. Retrieved from http://www.commonwealthfund.org/publications/press-releases/2015/may/underinsurance-brief-release

Traub, S. (2016). GH6123 Communicating effectively with children. *University of Missouri Extension.* Retrieved from http://extension.missouri.edu/p/GH6123

Tuckman, B. (1966). Developmental sequence in small groups. *Psychological Bulletin,* 63.

U.S. Department of Health & Human Services. (2003). OCR privacy brief. Summary of the HIPPA privacy rule. Retrieved from https://www.hhs.gov/hipaa/for-professionals/privacy/index.html

U.S. Department of Health & Human Services. (2014). The SHARE approach: Overcoming barriers with your patients: A reference guide for health care providers. Workshop curriculum: Tool 3. Retrieved from https://www.ahrq.gov/sites/default/files/wysiwyg/professionals/education/curriculum-tools/shareddecisionmaking/tools/tool-3/share-tool3.pdf

U.S. Department of Health & Human Services. (2017). HIPPA news releases & bulletins. Retrieved from https://www.hhs.gov/hipaa/newsroom/index.html

Vertino, K. (2014). Effective interpersonal communication: A practical guide to improve your life. *The Online Journal of Issues in Nursing, 19*(3), 1. doi: 10.39121OJIN.Vol19No03Man01

Ward, S. L., & Hisley, S. M. (2014a). *Maternal-child nurse care: Optimizing outcomes for mothers, children and families* (2nd ed.). Philadelphia: F. A. Davis.

Ward, S. L., & Hisley, S. M. (2014b). *Maternal-child nursing care: The critical components of nursing care* (2nd ed.). Philadelphia: F. A. Davis.

Cultural, Spiritual, and Environmental Influences on the Child

4

Diane M. Kocisko, MSN, RN, CPN
Margarita Diaz, BSN, RN

LEARNING OUTCOMES

Upon completion of this chapter, the student will be able to:

1. Identify individual cultural bias.
2. Discuss Leininger's theory and how it can be used to plan patient care.
3. Identify effective cross-cultural communication, body language, nurse–patient relationships, and multidisciplinary relationships between the caregiver, family, and the pediatric patient.
4. Identify strategies for overcoming language barriers and describe the importance of doing so.
5. Identify and describe the characteristics that are determined by culture.
6. Describe the components involved in a cultural assessment.
7. Discuss how spiritual beliefs influence the care of a child and family.
8. Identify environmental and societal considerations when caring for the pediatric patient and family.

CULTURALLY COMPETENT CARE

Culturally competent care must consider the client's culture, spiritual beliefs, values, traditions, behaviors, and environment and how these factors impact care to provide optimal outcomes. To provide care that is culturally competent, nurses must be aware of their own belief systems and identify the belief systems of clients and caregivers. Respect for cultures is fundamental to cultural competence. Although each culture has characteristics that are commonly shared among members, nurses must avoid stereotyping. Each family and individual is unique, and family members of the same culture may apply and interpret their culture in different ways. Culture may change with time or be interpreted differently among generations of the same culture. A person's culture will affect both verbal and nonverbal communication styles, and a closed family structure may not allow open communication from individuals outside of the culture. The nurse should be aware of a family's structure and function when caring for the pediatric patient. For example, assessment of function may reveal that the family has a spokesperson or person of authority who will make the medical decisions for the patient. In these cases, input from others will not be accepted or encouraged.

Culture also serves as a template for evaluating the patient's and family's psychosocial needs. When these needs are met, the client is better able to participate in care and focus attention on individualized health education. Children learn about their culture from parents or caregivers who serve as role models and teachers in demonstrating how culture is applied to everyday living, as well as how illness is perceived (Fig. 4–1). They also may dictate the child's cultural needs. The child's age and stage of development will influence his or her ability to recognize and articulate these needs.

Cultural bias may occur when the nurse places his or her own values before the values of a different culture. Nurses must examine how their own belief system may influence the care that is provided to prevent bias from occurring. Although it is not necessary for the nurse to agree with a client's cultural and spiritual beliefs, the health-care team must respect the beliefs of others.

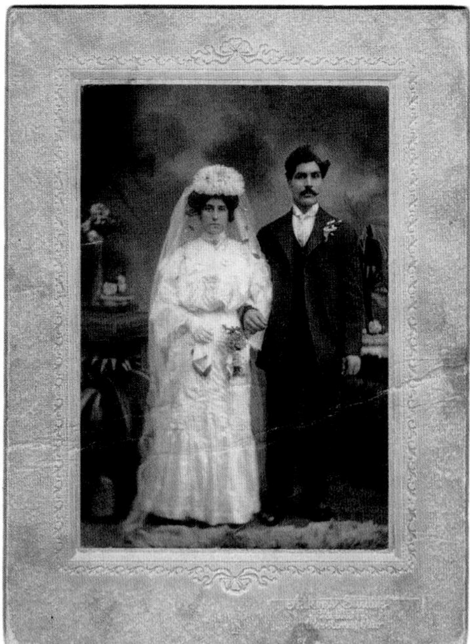

FIGURE 4–1 Parents are role models and teachers of culture. *(Courtesy of D.M. Kocisko)*

Clients may be subject to disparities in provision of or access to health care based on where they live and with whom they live. Awareness of these disparities can allow the health-care provider to tailor care accordingly and help remove barriers to care (Centers for Disease Control and Prevention, 2015) (Fig. 4–2).

SAFE AND EFFECTIVE NURSING CARE: Cultural Competence

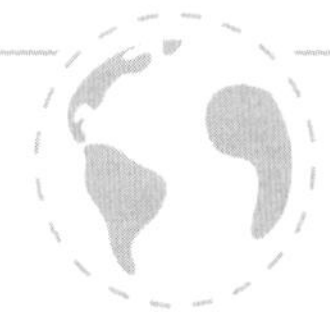

Self-Awareness

To identify one's own belief system and potential cultural bias, nurses should ask themselves the following introspective questions:

- What do I believe in?
- Am I familiar with the patterns of care for children within different cultures?
- What have been my experiences with those of different cultures? Have the experiences been positive or negative?
- Am I treating all caregivers and patients in a way that shows respect for and inclusion of their cultural values and beliefs?
- Have I asked the caregivers for input to help me understand their beliefs?
- How do I view cultures that are different from my own?
- Are there conflicting values between the patient/family and myself?
- In what way am I biased?
- Am I aware of any bias?
- How do I resolve my bias?

CRITICAL COMPONENT

Cultural Care Theory

Transcultural nursing occurs when the nurse incorporates the patient's culture into the care he or she provides (Leininger, 2009). Cross-cultural nursing is delivering care in a manner proven appropriate to the patient's culture. Madeleine Leininger's Cultural Care Theory considers the complexity and interrelatedness of an individual within an environment and the community to which he or she belongs. Dr. Leininger has been termed the founder of cultural care nursing (Leininger, 2009). Dr. Leininger's theory has been able to capture and articulate how culture affects health. Her theory helps to explain how practices handed down from generations can impact an individual's health today. According to this theory, the nurse should include a cultural assessment of the individual when evaluating the support and needs from a cultural and spiritual perspective. This assessment should then be incorporated into the patient's care plan. Dr. Leininger's Web site (http://www.madeleine-leininger.com) provides samples of her work and educational materials helpful to both instructors and students.

Environmental Considerations

A client's home environment has a substantial impact on his or her outcomes. It influences how care is delivered, the types of food available, how medication is stored, whether the patient has privacy at home, and countless other aspects of well-being. When caring for a pediatric client, the nurse should be especially aware of how his or her home environment influences care. For example, witnessed communication between individuals in the home may influence an adolescent's communication style and coping skills. The number of children living in the home may influence the time and amount of attention given to each member. Unstable living arrangements and those within close quarters can have

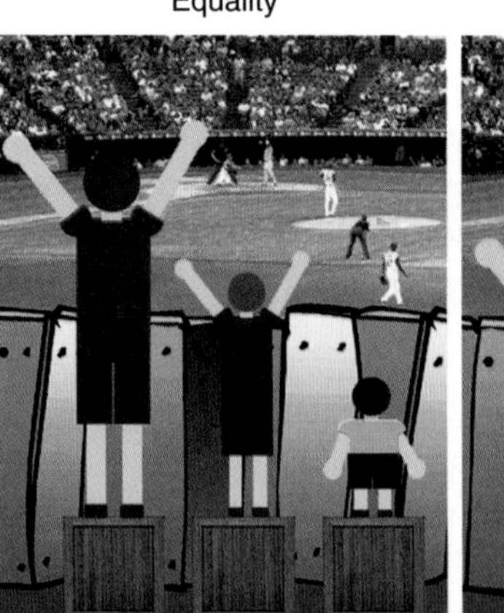

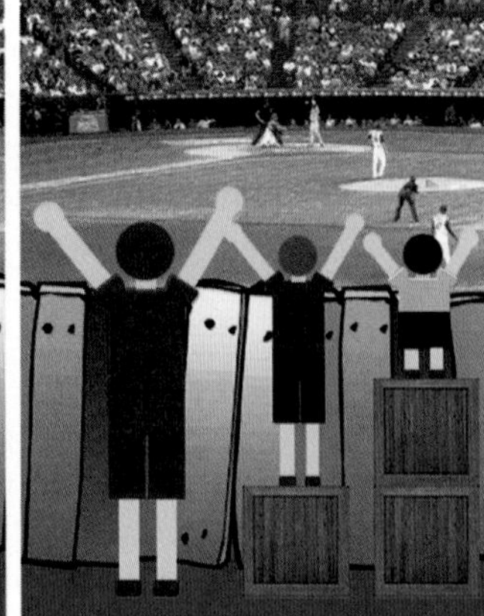

FIGURE 4–2 Equity illustration.

a detrimental effect on a child's development and health outcomes. The pediatric nurse should assess:

- Family composition
- Socioeconomic status
- Employment status of parents
- Safe areas for outdoor play
- The presence of lead-based paint and other environmental hazards
- Lack of safe drinking water
- Inadequate medical help during emergency situations
- Inadequate police coverage to protect neighborhood
- Gas and chemicals released from local industries
- Lack of availability to a Level 1 trauma center to care for the critically ill or injured pediatric patient

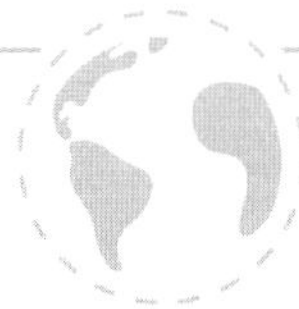

SAFE AND EFFECTIVE NURSING CARE: Cultural Competence

Racial Changes in America

The races of individuals living in the United States are changing. In 2020, less than half of children living in the United States will be classified as white or non-Hispanic white according to the 2020 Projected Ethnicity Breakdown (Table 4–1). These racial changes may also bring health disparities.

Health Disparities

To create a culture of comparable access and equitable care for all patients, it is important to recognize the disparities and inequalities first. Health disparities include social and economic status that adversely affect groups of people who have systematically experienced greater obstacles to health based on:

- Racial or ethnic group
- Religion
- Socioeconomic status
- Sex
- Age
- Mental health
- Cognitive, sensory, or physical disability
- Sexual orientation or gender identity
- Geographic location

Social determinants of health are "the structural determinants and conditions in which people are born, grow, live, work and age" (World Health Organization, 2017). They include factors such as socioeconomic status, education, the physical environment, employment, and social support networks, as well as access to health care. Social determinants of health factor 40% of what creates "health" according to the World Health Commission on Social Determinants of Health (Marmot and Allen, 2014).

For example, hunger and limited access to healthy food are predominant in populations who are in low socioeconomic communities. Food deserts are neighborhoods that lack a full grocer that supplies fresh fruit and vegetables and healthy food options. Families who live in a food desert may not have access to nutritious foods nor the ability to pay for nutritious food. Because children depend on caregivers to provide healthy meals and snacks, food deserts not only result in a lack of nutrition for growing children, but also a lack of role modeling of healthy eating habits by caregivers.

Health equity is not necessarily equality. Equality is giving everyone the same. Equity is giving everyone what they need to be successful. Strategies used for fairness that address inequities should be evidence based and result in best practices. Agency policy, family-centered care, and addressing dietary needs are the most common strategies used. However, challenges to best practice may arise out of agency policy.

TABLE 4–1 2020 Projected Ethnicity Breakdown

White, non-Hispanic	<50%
Hispanic	26%
Black, non-Hispanic	14%
Asian, non-Hispanic	5%
Non-Hispanic children who represent two or more races	5%
American Indian and Alaska Native, non-Hispanic	0.8%
Native Hawaiian and Other Pacific Islander, non-Hispanic	0.2%

Projection for America's children in 2020. Data are from America's Children in Brief: Key National Indicators of Well-Being, 2016 (Federal Interagency Forum on Child and Family Statistics, 2016).

Agency Policy

An agency's policies steer a client's overall care, including visitation and diet. However, these components of care may not be in accordance with the nurse's own beliefs, both cultural and spiritual. The nurse should investigate policies concerning these practices before applying for a job at the facility. If these policies cause cultural or spiritual distress to the nurse, then culturally competent patient care will be difficult to implement. Consider the following best practices:

- Visitation
- Unrestricted parent, caregiver, and grandparent visitation
- Other visitors allowed during the child's waking hours
- Visitors free of communicable diseases and disease-prevention strategies maintained
- Opportunity for the client to get appropriate rest
- Good hand-hygiene practices for all visitors
- Family privacy allowed during visitation

- Patient held and cared for by family members
- Proper seating and space for socialization provided
- Family allowed to take patient out of the room when possible
- Play items and items used for diversion techniques are available

Family-Centered Care Components

- Patient provided some level of normalcy
- Opportunities to play with other children and siblings
- Caregivers may room-in with the patient
- Caregivers have a place to maintain hygiene and eat meals
- Unlimited caregiver access to the patient
- Whenever possible, caregivers given the opportunity to provide care
- Caregivers encouraged to provide input into the plan of care
- Health-care team listens to caregiver suggestions

Dietary Needs

- Caregivers are encouraged to bring familiar cultural foods from home. (Check for any medical dietary restriction.)
- Food preparation and options are adequate and appealing.
- Vegetarian, vegan, kosher, and halal meal options are available.
- Patients and caregivers may select from a variety of foods.
- Nutritious food selections are available and encouraged.
- Patient's restricted food items are documented, and diet restrictions are enforced per the patient's and family's wishes.
- Cultural and spiritual food restrictions are documented and enforced.

Staff Education

The agency's policy and procedures will drive the type of information provided to the nursing staff. Each individual nurse has the professional responsibility to appraise the cultural differences and concerns of the patient. It should be the goal of every health-care professional to tailor care to meet the holistic health needs of the patient. Best practices include:

- Staff is expected to strive for cultural competency and effectiveness in interactions with individuals of different cultures
- Annual education to maintain current knowledge and understand new and evolving practices in culturally competent care
- Identification of cultural groups predominant in the organization's practice, and examination of the beliefs and values of these cultures that may affect care
- Provision of theory and tools necessary to perform culturally competent care for all children and their caregivers
- Encouragement to seek information on unfamiliar cultures

CROSS-CULTURAL COMMUNICATION

Effective cross-cultural communication requires the health-care team to communicate with each patient/family in a manner that is well received within their culture. Communication, a term that encompasses words, tone, body language, and rate of speech, is influenced by the relationship of the individuals in question, the culture of origin, and the individual interpretation of the receiver. Communication involves a sender and a receiver. Even with the best intentions, there can be miscommunication. See Chapter 3 for more information on communication.

SAFE AND EFFECTIVE NURSING CARE: Clinical Pearl

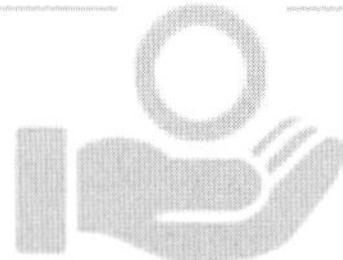

Health Assessments

Health assessments in the United States are typically made in a private setting and contain direct questions that anticipate direct answers. This process may not be effective in eliciting information from other cultures. Cultural awareness can assist the communication process so that health-care providers can obtain accurate health information. Respect for the patient's and family's beliefs is required for all interactions.

Best Practices for Effective Communication

To develop effective communication with clients and families of all cultures, nurses should:

- Learn about interacting with diverse cultures.
- Know who is responsible for making health decisions for the patient.
- Identify the patient's and caregiver's perceptions of the cause of the illness or health alteration.
- Determine whether the gender of the care provider *can* affect the patient's care.
- Communicate in a language understood by the person receiving the information.
- Use a certified interpreter when needed.
- Ensure written communication is legible and in the language that the receiver can most easily understand.
- Determine the literacy level of the individual who is receiving information and making health-care decisions, and explain information at an understandable, appropriate level.
- Do not interrupt when conversing with a client; allow the patient or caregiver time to articulate descriptions of or feelings about care.
- Speak in a tone that is appropriate for the situation.
- Provide undivided attention to the patient and caregiver.
- Be aware that silence, eye contact, and personal space can mean different things in different cultures.

Establishing a Nurse–Patient Relationship

A therapeutic relationship with the client and family is based on mutual respect and trust. Pediatric nurses should take these best practices into account:

- Information is kept confidential.
- The relationship is developed on mutual respect.

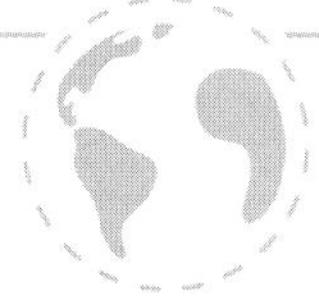

SAFE AND EFFECTIVE NURSING CARE: Cultural Competence

Body Language and Touch Awareness

When caring for a patient of another culture, be aware of the types of body language and touch acceptable in that individual culture. Consider elements that may be interpreted differently by those of other cultures, such as:

- Eye contact (direct or indirect)
- Nodding of the head
- Touching the top of the head
- Shaking hands, particularly with a member of the opposite sex
- Hand and arm gestures

- Recognize that you are developing a new relationship within a different culture.
- Recognize appropriate boundaries and maintain those boundaries.
- By law, all nurses must report suspicion of and actual child abuse or neglect. These "secrets" cannot be kept.
- Patients are treated as unique individuals.
- All patients are treated equally.
- Relationships are kept within the boundaries of the care setting.
- When appropriate, provide the patient with opportunities to make choices.

Multidisciplinary Relationships

- Health-care providers work as a team and share information as appropriate.
- Individuals have different perspectives and different experiences.
- Respect differences of opinion.
- Respect does not equate with agreement.
- Support each other.
- The patient's best interest is kept in mind by all care providers.
- Ethics consultations should take place when differences are identified between care providers or families and care providers.

CRITICAL COMPONENT

Understanding Nurse Discomfort

Developing a new relationship with a patient from a different culture may feel uncomfortable. This discomfort is likely due to your own uncertainty and the mental strain involved in interpreting and understanding the culture in a manner that is organized or makes sense for you.

Language Barriers

Language barriers include any circumstances in which the sender of communication and/or his or her message is not accurately understood by the intended receiver of communication.

- Both sender and receiver may become frustrated.
- Feelings of frustration may lead to anger.
- Remain calm and contact an interpreter.
- Patients and families with language barriers are to receive the same information, education, and support as those without language barriers.

Working With Interpreters

- Avoid using "charades" to communicate; wait for the interpreter.
- Pictures can be used to communicate ideas when an immediate interpreter is not available.
- Family members may serve as an interpreter, but take caution that interpretation is accurate to the message that is being conveyed by the care providers. Always best to use an interpreter.
- Document the name and certification number of the interpreter used.
- Interpreter services are available free of charge to the patient.
- An interpreter should be used for teaching or need for consent.
- Always speak directly to the patient/family and not the interpreter.
- Interpreter services, including for the deaf, should be readily available to clients.
- The internet can sometimes aid in interpretation; ensure that you are only using sites that have been approved by your facility.

SAFE AND EFFECTIVE NURSING CARE: Clinical Pearl

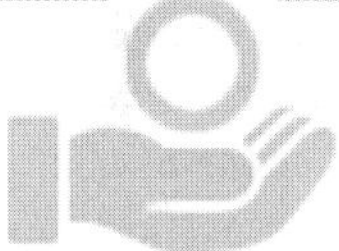

Tips for Communicating With Individuals With Language Barriers

1. Remain calm and provide appropriate support via body language as appropriate to culture.
2. Contact an interpreter.
3. Hand gestures mean different things in different cultures, so avoid their use if possible.
4. When appropriate, allow parents to remain with their child.
5. When appropriate, use touch and facial expressions to communicate concern.
6. Use pictures that may be able to accurately depict concepts.
7. Pictures are only a temporary intervention and should be used when an interpreter is not available.
8. You and the patient/caregiver may point at pictures to communicate if immediate interventions are needed.
9. Use the internet for basic interpretation of words and phrases.
10. Do not provide elective procedures without the consent of the caregiver.

When an interpreter is not available at your organization:

- Use a language listing that enables the patient or family to point to the language that is spoken.
- Phone services should be available that allow the medical provider to contact an interpreter and have a three-way conversation between the caregiver, translator, and patient or family (Fig. 4–3).
- Video services should be available for those who are hearing impaired.
- Become familiar with the resources that your organization uses for interpretation.

Characteristics and Behaviors Determined by Culture

- Individuals will act and respond as they have been taught to act and respond.
- Children may "pretend" by responding in the way that their caregivers would respond, or by responding in an "acceptable" way rather than one that accurately communicates their feelings.
- Social skills are acquired through an individual's normal interactions.
- Full patient disclosure is needed for safe care in the following areas:
    - Individual medical history
    - Family history
    - Description of symptom
    - Length of symptom occurrence
    - Potential embarrassment and disgrace of having the disease/condition

Personal Space

The nurse's interpretation of personal space may be different from that of individuals from other cultures. Know what physical space between communicators is expected, and respect that space in personal discussions.

Eye Contact

Know the etiquette of eye contact among different cultures—some may prefer direct eye contact, whereas others may not. Provide eye contact if unsure whether it is appropriate.

Diet

- Most children do not have control over what food is stored in the home.
- Processed foods are cheaper than fresh foods.
- Fresh fruits and vegetables can be costly.
- Most nutritious foods cost more than nonnutritious foods.
- Children will more likely eat foods they have often.

LanguageLine Solutions® Interpreting Services Available

English Translation: Point to your language. An interpreter will be called. The interpreter is provided at no cost to you.

American Sign Language Point to your language. An interpreter will be called. The interpreter is provided at no cost to you.	**Korean** 한국어 귀하께서 사용하는 언어를 지정하시면 해당 언어 통역 서비스를 무료로 제공해 드립니다.
Arabic عربي أشر إلى لغتك. وسيتم الاتصال بمترجم فوري. كما سيتم إحضار المترجم الفوري مجانًا.	**Mandarin** 國語 請指認您的語言， 以便為您提供免費的口譯服務。
Bengali বাংলা আপনার ভাষার দিকে নির্দেশ করুন। একজন দোভাষীকে ডাকা হবে।দোভাষী আপনি নিখরচায় পাবেন।	**Nepali** नेपाली आफ्नो भाषातर्फ औंल्याउनुहोस्। एक दोभाषेलाई बोलाइनेछ। तपाईंको विना कुनै खर्चको, एकजना दोभाषे उपलब्ध गराइनेछ।
Burmese မြန်မာ သင့်ဘာသာစကားကို ညွှန်ပြပါ။ စကားပြန် ခေါ်ပေးပါမယ်။ သင့်အတွက် စကားပြန် အခမဲ့ ပေးပါမယ်။	**Polish** Polski Proszę wskazać swój język i wezwiemy tłumacza. Usługa ta zapewniana jest bezpłatnie.
Cantonese 廣東話 請指認您的語言， 以便為您提供免費的口譯服務。	**Portuguese** Português Indique o seu idioma. Um intérprete será chamado. A interpretação é fornecida sem qualquer custo para você.
Farsi فارسي زبان مورد نظر خود را مشخص کنید. یک مترجم برای شما درخواست خواهد شد. مترجم بصورت رایگان در اختیار شما قرار می گیرد.	**Punjabi** ਪੰਜਾਬੀ ਆਪਣੀ ਭਾਸ਼ਾ ਵੱਲ ਇਸ਼ਾਰਾ ਕਰੋ। ਜਿਸ ਮੁਤਾਬਕ ਇਕ ਦੁਭਾਸ਼ੀਆ ਬੁਲਾਇਆ ਜਾਵੇਗਾ। ਤੁਹਾਡੇ ਲਈ ਦੁਭਾਸ਼ੀਆ ਦੀ ਮੁਫਤ ਇੰਤਜ਼ਾਮ ਕੀਤਾ ਜਾਂਦਾ ਹੈ।
French Français Indiquez votre langue et nous appellerons un interprète. Le service est gratuit.	**Romanian** Română Indicaţi limba pe care o vorbiţi. Vi se va face legătura cu un interpret caare vă este asigurat gratuit.
Haitian Creole Kreyòl Lonje dwèt ou sou lang ou pale a epi n ap rele yon entèprèt pou ou. Nou ba ou sèvis entèprèt la gratis.	**Russian** Русский Укажите язык, на котором вы говорите. Вам вызовут переводчика. Услуги переводчика предоставляются бесплатно.
Hindi हिंदी अपनी भाषा को इंगित करें। जिसके अनुसार आपके लिए दुभाषिया बुलाया जाएगा। आपके लिए दुभाषिया की निशुल्क व्यवस्था की जाती है।	**Somali** Af-Soomaali Farta ku fiiqluqadaada... Waxa laguugu yeeri doonaa turjubaan. Turjubaanka wax lacagi kaaga bixi mayso.
Hmong Hmoob Taw rau koj hom lus. Yuav hu rau ib tug neeg txhais lus. Yuav muaj neeg txhais lus yam uas koj tsis tau them dab tsi.	**Spanish** Español Señale su idioma y llamaremos a un intérprete. El servicio es gratuito.
Italian Italiano Indicare la propia lingua. Un interprete sarà chiamato. Il servizio è gratuito.	**Tagalog** Tagalog Ituro po ang inyong wika. Isang tagasalin ang ipagkakaloob nang libre sa inyo.
Japanese 日本語 あなたの話す言語を指してください。 無料で通訳サービスを提供します。	**Vietnamese** Tiếng Việt Hãy chỉ vào ngôn ngữ của quý vị. Một thông dịch viên sẽ được gọi đến, quý vị sẽ không phải trả tiền cho thông dịch viên.

© 2016 LanguageLine Solutions www.LanguageLine.com

A

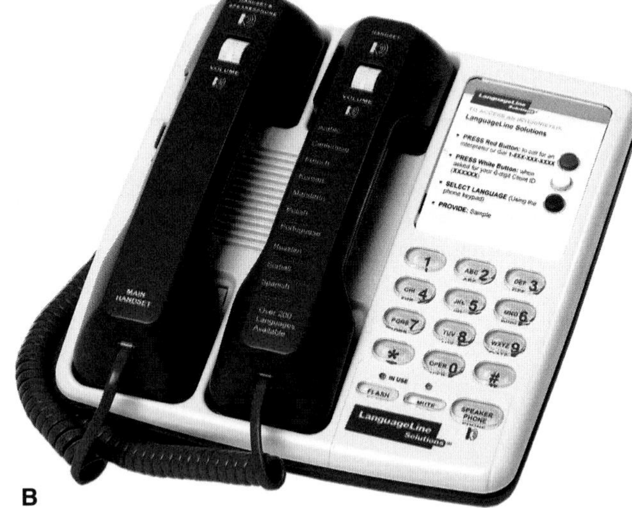

B

FIGURE 4–3 **A,** Language ID desktop display and **B,** language line phone.

- Home eating times should be maintained as much as possible during the hospital stay.
- Encourage parents to eat meals with their child to promote normalcy and socialization.
- Food storage practices may require two separate refrigerators.

Time

- Perceptions of time may be different among individuals of varying cultures.
- Personal time may be required for prayer.
- Preferred times for visitation may not be consistent with visiting hours, presenting difficulties.

Touch

- Touch with communication may be offensive to patients and caregivers.
- It can be interpreted differently and may be dependent on the care environment.
- Touch also may be interpreted differently between genders.

Family Use of Alternative Medicine

- Herbs may have drug interactions.
- Treatments or remedies may be called "old wives' tales."
- A family leader may dictate how to treat symptoms.
- Treatments should be accepted if they will not harm the patient.
- Alternative treatments and medicines, proposed or being used, should be discussed with the multidisciplinary team.

CULTURAL ASSESSMENTS

In the health-care setting, the cultural assessment is a mechanism through which the nurse gathers subjective data to identify beliefs and values associated with the patient's culture. Undergoing this process:

- Assures the patient that the care provider is interested in the patient's values
- Allows the care provider to individualize care and incorporate cultural beliefs and values
- Provides data to incorporate subjective and objective information into holistic assessment

The cultural aspect of a patient assessment usually comes last and is often inaccurately perceived as having less importance than other assessment data. A cultural assessment should evaluate the following areas that impact health care and may differ by culture:

- Religious beliefs
- Client and family perception of current health status
- Food preferences
- Typical daily schedule

Nurses must also consider these questions:

- Will an interpreter be required to communicate?
- What is the patient's or caregiver's preferred language?
- Who is responsible for making the health decisions for the client?
- Will health-care interventions interrupt or interfere with any cultural or spiritual beliefs?
- Does the patient or caregiver need you to contact a spiritual leader for assistance in care?
- What are the patient's and caregiver's perceptions of the cause of the disease?

SAFE AND EFFECTIVE NURSING CARE: Clinical Pearl

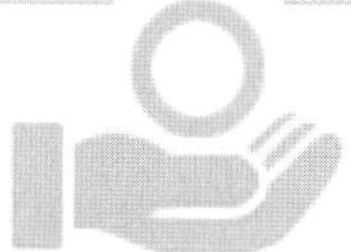

Questions to Ask or Consider During the Cultural Assessment

- What culture do you consider yourself belonging to?
- Are your cultural beliefs important to you?
- How long have you been in this country?
- Are you having difficulty meeting your health-care needs?
- Do you have a social support system within your cultural community?

Giger and Davidhizar Transcultural Assessment Model

Giger and Davidhizar (2002) note that individuals are unique, and they provide a transcultural assessment model that consists of evaluating the following six aspects:

- Communication and how thoughts and feelings are expressed
- Personal space between the individuals who are communicating
- Biological variations, such as appropriate weight and development
- Time, both the perception of time in general (e.g., fast-paced, time-centered lifestyle versus more leisurely lifestyle) and when daily events should occur (e.g., mealtimes)
- The degree to which individuals feel they can influence or control their environment or experiences
- Social organizations that the patient and family are part of (e.g., family, religious affiliation, social groups)

SAFE AND EFFECTIVE NURSING CARE: Clinical Pearl

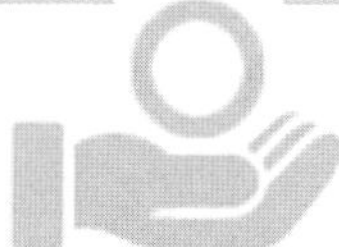

What Defines a Family?

A family is defined by who the child and caregiver say is the family. Families are not necessarily blood or legally related. Many times, a child may have a sitter or care provider who spends an extended amount of time with that child. The child may be more familiar and comfortable with the non-blood-related care provider than an actual family member. A parent or grandparent figure may also play an important role in the child's life. Even though family is defined in many ways, only the legal guardian can sign consent or discharge forms.

Spirituality

Spirituality describes a person's belief in a greater being that affects his or her daily and world events. This belief typically encompasses the person's concept of where and how humanity began, as well as views of the afterlife. For many individuals, spirituality takes the form of a religious affiliation: a group or formal community of individuals with shared spiritual beliefs. Health-care providers must be aware of a client's religious beliefs and alter care as appropriate. However, it is important to note that all individuals within a religious group are unique, and each may accept some but not all of a specific religion's beliefs. Also, a person may be spiritual without belonging to a specific religious group.

SAFE AND EFFECTIVE NURSING CARE: Cultural Competence

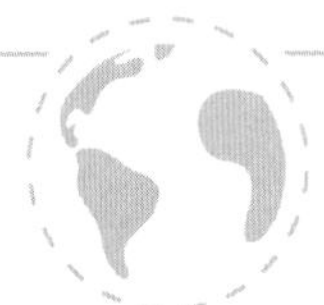

Respecting Religion

Nurses should become familiar with the religious beliefs of the patient and caregiver. Information about a particular religious affiliation can be obtained from the patient, caregiver, books, or caregiver-suggested internet sites. Patient and caregiver beliefs should be respected, regardless of the beliefs of the care provider.

FICA Assessment Tool

The FICA tool can be used by the nurse to identify the patient's spiritual and religious history (Box 4–1; Puchalski, 2006; Puchalski & Romer, 2000). FICA stands for Faith, Importance, Community, and Address, the four components of the tool, which provide the nurse with baseline patient data that can be used to individualize care. It also offers an opportunity for the nurse to identify spiritual distress and collaborate with other disciplines as needed. Most importantly, the FICA tool allows patients and families to describe their spiritual beliefs and concerns in their own words and to participate in the creation of their plan of care. The nurse will also better understand the patient's viewpoint when providing care.

SAFE AND EFFECTIVE NURSING CARE: Cultural Competence

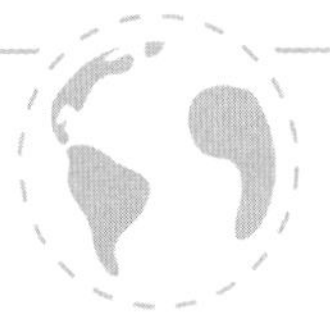

Pediatric Spiritual and Cultural Assessments

Health-care providers are challenged by time constraints, financial constraints, and knowledge deficits regarding the cultural and spiritual needs of a child. Professional nurses need specific knowledge about the major groups of culturally diverse individuals, families, and communities they serve, including but not limited to specific cultural practices regarding health, definitions of and beliefs about health and illness, biological variations, cross-cultural worldviews, acculturation, and life experiences such as immigration and refugee status, which may include history of violence, oppression, and trauma. Cultural competency skills are essential to facilitate communication and ask culturally sensitive questions about beliefs and practices. The more knowledge a nurse has about a specific culture, the more accurate and complete the cultural assessment. For example, patients of some Hispanic cultures may use traditional healers; if nurses are not aware of this, they will not ask the appropriate questions about the individual's use of alternative practitioners and alternate therapies.

Evidence-Based Practice

Bull, A., & Gillies, M. (2007). Spiritual needs of children with complex healthcare needs in hospital. *Pediatric Nursing, 19*, 34–38.

Bull and Gillies (2007) identified that minimal research has been done to study the spiritual needs of children with conditions that require complex medical care. The only three research studies identified by these authors took place in the United States. The small number of available articles on studies of this subject demonstrates that little research attention has been directed toward children and spirituality.

The study by Bull and Gillies (2007) was performed in the United Kingdom with five children aged 8 through 11 years, and used pictures to prompt storytelling. Only five children were involved in this study; therefore, generalizations cannot be drawn. However, four main themes were identified: relationships, hospital environment, coping with invasive procedures, and belief (Bull & Gillies, 2007). The researchers concluded that health-care providers must evaluate and meet the spiritual needs of children when providing care.

BOX 4–1 | FICA Spiritual Assessment Tool

F—Faith and Belief

"Do you consider yourself spiritual or religious?" or "Do you have spiritual beliefs that help you cope with stress?" If the patient responds no, then the health-care provider might ask, "What gives your life meaning?" Sometimes patients respond with answers such as family, career, or nature.

I—Importance

"What importance does your faith or belief have in your life? Have your beliefs influenced how you take care of yourself in this illness? What role do your beliefs play in regaining your health?"

C—Community

"Are you part of a spiritual or religious community? Is this of support to you? If so, how? Is there a group of people you really love or who are important to you?" Communities such as churches, temples, and mosques, or a group of like-minded friends, can serve as strong support systems for some patients.

A—Address in Care

"How would you like me, your health-care provider, to address these issues in your health care?"

As with any other part of the patient interview, the spiritual histories should be patient centered. Thus, the tool is meant to

BOX 4–1 | FICA Spiritual Assessment Tool—cont'd

create an environment of trust by indicating to the patient that the physician or other health-care professional is open to listening to the patient about his or her spiritual issues, if the patient wants to talk about those issues. There are ethical guidelines to which the physician or health-care provider should adhere when taking a spiritual history. Health-care professionals are encouraged not to use the FICA tool as a checklist, but rather to rely on it as a guide to aid in open discussion of spiritual issues.

Sources: Puchalski & Romer (2000); George Washington Institute for Spirituality & Health (2009).

Case Study

You are assigned to care for a child who belongs to a culture that is different from your own. Kathleen is a 10-year-old child who often asks for her mother. Many other visitors come throughout the day and night. Yesterday, visitors came in at 1 a.m. They identified themselves as close family friends and insisted on waking the child up to visit. The nurse used the phone translation service to communicate with the visitors. At the end of the conversation, the visitor agreed that it was not appropriate to wake up the child. The mother of this patient comes in to visit at various times during the day and night and insists that the child eat dinner with her while she visits. The dinner trays on the unit arrive at 5 p.m., and the child consistently states that she would rather eat when her mother comes to visit. Unfortunately, the mother does not visit daily. It has become challenging to have the child eat when there is uncertainty around the mother's visitation. It has been noted that the family does not comply with the visitation policy of the unit. Parents can come anytime, 24 hours a day. Extended family may visit from 8 a.m. to 8 p.m. This is Kathleen's fourth day in the hospital and once again visitors arrive at midnight.

1. How will you address this issue with the family?
2. Identify some of the obstacles to providing culturally competent care.
3. How will you resolve the visitation issue with the family and caregivers?

REFERENCES

Bull, A., & Gillies, M. (2007). Spiritual needs of children with complex health-care needs in hospital. *Pediatric Nursing, 19*, 34–38.

Centers for Disease Control and Prevention. (2015). *Adolescent and school health.* Retrieved from https://www.cdc.gov/healthyyouth/disparities/

Federal Interagency Forum on Child and Family Statistics. (2016). *America's children in brief: Key national indicators of well-being, 2016.* Retrieved from https://www.childstats.gov/pdf/ac2016/ac_16.pdf

George Washington Institute for Spirituality & Health. (2009). *FICA for self-assessment.* Retrieved from http://smhs.gwu.edu/gwish/clinical/fica/spiritual-history-tool

Giger, J. N., & Davidhizar, R. (2002). The Giger and Davidhizar transcultural assessment model. *Journal of Transcultural Nursing, 13*, 185–188.

Leininger, M. (2009). *Madeleine-Leininger.com FAQ.* Retrieved from http://www.madeleine-leininger.com/en/faq-1.shtml

Marmot, M., & Allen, J. J. (2014). Social determinants of health equity. *Journal of Public Health, 104*, S517–S519.

Puchalski, C. (2006). Spiritual assessment in clinical practice. *Psychiatric Annals, 36*, 150–155.

Puchalski, C., & Romer, A. L. (2000). Taking a spiritual history allows clinicians to understand patients more fully. *Journal of Palliative Medicine, 3*, 129–137. Retrieved from http://www.liebertpub.com/products/product.aspx?pid=41

World Health Organization. (2017). *Social determinants of health.* Retrieved from http://www.who.int/social_determinants/sdh_definition/en/

5

End-of-Life Care

Rebecca Loth Luetke, PhD, RN

LEARNING OUTCOMES

Upon completion of this chapter, the student will be able to:

1. Understand causes of infant and pediatric death.
2. Understand and describe appropriate communication with the patient and family in end-of-life care.
3. Understand and describe appropriate communication within the multidisciplinary care team in end-of-life care.
4. Define the roles of family-centered care and culturally competent care in end-of-life care.
5. Define and describe hospice care, including the roles of the nurse and multidisciplinary team.
6. Discuss assessment and treatment of pain in the hospice care of an infant or pediatric patient.
7. Understand and explain the role spiritual and cultural care have within end-of-life care.
8. Define and compare the stages of grief.
9. Understand and describe the role of nursing education in end-of-life care.
10. Define and understand withdrawal of care in infant and pediatric end-of-life care.
11. Define and describe the role of the nurse in infant and pediatric end-of-life care.
12. Understand and describe organ donation and procurement.
13. Define and describe legal aspects of infant and pediatric end-of life-care.

INTRODUCTION

Death is defined as the end of sustainable life; for infants and pediatric patients, death is the end of a short life caused by a terminal diagnosis or disease. A terminal diagnosis results from either trauma or physiological causes. Categorizations include:

- Trauma, caused by outside forces
  - Accidental, such as a car accident or drowning
  - Nonaccidental, such as intentional self-injury or abuse
- Physiological, caused by forces within the body
  - Disease such as cancer
  - Congenital defect, such as Edward's syndrome

Routine nursing care in pediatrics differs from end-of-life care in pediatrics, based on the hospice needs of the patient's family rather than treatment of a diagnosis or disease. The goal is a peaceful death rather than continuation of a healthy life.

COMMUNICATION IN CARE OF THE DYING PATIENT

Communication with the patient and family is an essential nurse role in end-of-life pediatric care. When communicating with the family, nurse assessments should be conducted to:

- Determine how the family unit functions.
- Understand the level of information the family desires.
- Determine the cognitive level of family members to provide appropriate education.

SAFE AND EFFECTIVE NURSING CARE: Promoting Safety

Accidents or unintentional injuries are the leading cause of death in pediatrics (National Institutes of Health, 2015). The primary cause of sudden unexpected infant death is sudden infant death syndrome or SIDS, one of the leading causes of death for infants 1 month to 1 year of age (Box 5–1). The peak time for SIDS deaths is 2 to 4 months of age (American Academy of Pediatrics, n.d.). Parents of newborns and infants up to 1 year should be educated on strategies to prevent SIDS, such as the "safe to sleep" campaign that encourages parents to place infants on their backs to sleep (Fig. 5–1). This can reduce the incidence rate of SIDS by 50% (National Institutes of Health, 2015). One emerging SIDS prevention method is providing new parents with a baby box that contains supplies to help the parents care for the newborn. Once the supplies are removed it becomes a safe, portable sleeping area for the newborn with a firm mattress with a fitted sheet (Southern New Jersey Perinatal Cooperative, n.d.) (Fig. 5–2).

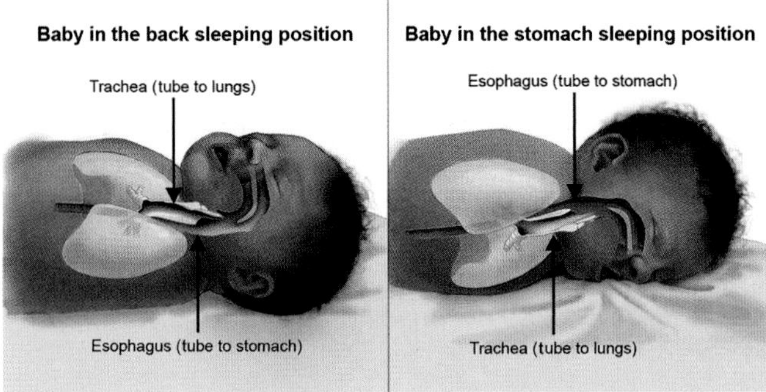

FIGURE 5–1 Always educate parents to put their infants on their backs to sleep to help prevent sudden infant death syndrome by keeping the airway fully open.

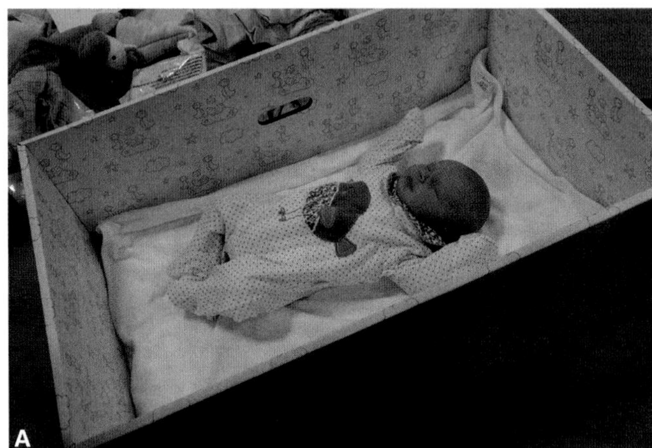

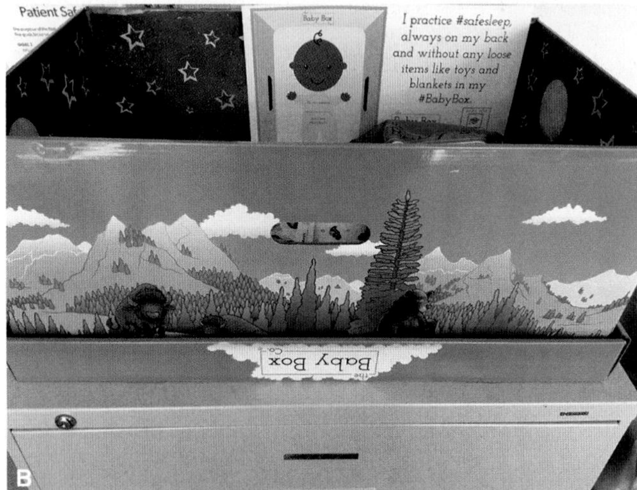

FIGURE 5–2 A, B The box provides a safe sleep zone for the newborn to help prevent sudden infant death syndrome.

BOX 5–1 | Causes of Pediatric Death

Causes of pediatric death in the United States in 2015 varied by age range, as noted in the following list (Centers for Disease Control and Prevention, 2015):

1–4 Years of Age

- Number of deaths: 3,830
- Deaths per 100,000 population: 24
- Leading causes of death
  - Accidents (unintentional injuries)
  - Congenital malformations, deformations, and chromosomal abnormalities
  - Assault (homicide)

5–14 Years of Age

- Number of deaths: 5,250
- Deaths per 100,000 population: 12.7
- Leading causes of death
  - Accidents (unintentional injuries)
  - Cancer
  - Intentional self-harm (suicide)

15–19 Years of Age

- Number of deaths: 9,586
- Deaths per 100,000 population: 45.5
- Leading causes of death
  - Accidents (unintentional injuries)
  - Suicide
  - Homicide

- Determine the family's overall understanding of the patient's diagnosis and potential outcomes.
- Establish who can legally receive information about the patient.

More information about family communication is available in Chapter 6.

Family-Centered Care in End of Life

Family-centered care is the basis for all interactions with the family of a patient who is receiving end-of-life care. Communication with the family should be compassionate, cognitively appropriate, and based on the health-care provider's assessment. Communication with the patient should be both compassionate and developmentally appropriate. Family-centered care at end of life requires communication that is:

- Culturally appropriate: considers culture of patient and family in all communications
- Developmentally appropriate: considers developmental level of siblings when communicating with them and in their presence
- Compassionate: treats patient and family with kindness
- Informative: includes details regarding the diagnosis and the death and dying process as appropriate and desired
- Honest: discusses the outcome of death with the patient and family without giving false hope

In addition to patient communication, communication within a multidisciplinary care team takes place during rounds or through charting. Nurses have an important communication role in end-of-life care; within the multidisciplinary care team, the nurse has the most contact with the patient and family, and acts as an advocate and voice for their care. Nurse communication with each member of the care team on an individual basis ensures optimum care of the patient and family. The nurse must communicate to all staff that end-of-life care is occurring so there is an understanding of the process and the patient's and family's needs by the entire unit. Communication within the hospice care team can be different from communication within the routine multidisciplinary care team; nurses must understand the role of hospice care to provide professional education (Fig. 5–3).

HOSPICE CARE

Hospice care for pediatric patients is provided at end of life to promote patient comfort and family involvement. It promotes a graceful, natural death rather than attempting to prevent death with treatment. The patient with a terminal diagnosis receives compassionate care focused on his or her comfort with as few invasive devices and procedures as possible. Hospice care can occur in any unit of the hospital or at home with visiting nurses and care aides.

Multidisciplinary, Family-Centered Approach

Initiation of hospice care is generally done by the physician with input from the multidisciplinary care team. A multidisciplinary approach is essential for successful hospice care. Team roles and responsibilities are as follows:

- Nurses serve as patient and family advocate and bedside patient care provider.

CRITICAL COMPONENT

End-of-Life Nursing Education Consortium

End-of-Life Nursing Education Consortium is dedicated to excellence in hospice care (American Association of Colleges of Nursing, 2016). The goal of the project is to ensure that all nurses are educated on hospice care, ensuring patients receive the highest quality care during end of life. The education provides nurses the knowledge and skills to positively impact the lives of patients and their families while they are experiencing the impending death of the patient.

- Pharmacy provides medications to increase comfort in appropriate administration route for patient.
- Nutrition provides desired diet and food choices for the patient as needed.
- Social work ensures that the family's nonmedical needs, such as housing and employer notification, are met.
- Chaplain or pastoral care focuses on the spiritual and religious needs of the patient and family.
- The child life specialist provides age- and developmentally-appropriate toys and environment for patient and siblings.
- The physician leads care and orders medications and interventions while providing the patient and family with education regarding the diagnosis.

Family communication with staff, including sibling care, must be an important aspect of all daily care. Sibling care can include playtime or activities for siblings allowing for some normal childhood activates. Sibling care should also include respect for what the siblings are experiencing and acknowledgment of their feelings. Outcomes of using family-centered care include a more cohesive family unit during the death of a child and possibly promoting healing after death.

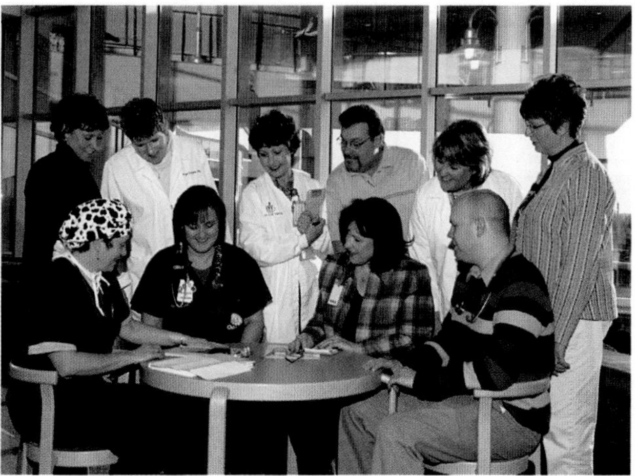

FIGURE 5–3 The multidisciplinary health-care team provides communication, support, and guidance during the death of an infant or child.

SAFE AND EFFECTIVE NURSING CARE: Clinical Pearl

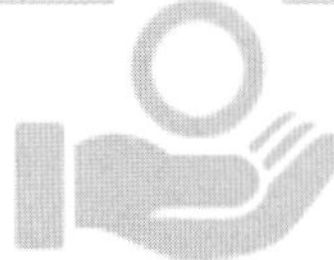

Child life therapists are specially trained therapists who are experts in how children play, socialize, and develop (Fig. 5–4). Children's hospitals generally have a child life department dedicated to the proper development of hospitalized children. The child life therapist focuses on the individual patient and his or her siblings, and works with the family during the hospitalization. For end-of-life patients, the child life therapist will help the patient and siblings understand the process and develop coping skills for the inevitable.

Pediatric Pain Control

Pain control is an important aspect of the definition of hospice care and is the job of the nurse, physician, and pharmacist. In end-of-life pediatric care, pain is defined as any uncomfortable feeling that prevents patient relaxation or rest. Pediatric pain can manifest very differently than adult pain, with symptoms that are very different from adult pain symptoms. Pediatric pain assessment techniques include using vital signs, positioning, and parent/caregiver input. Pain interventions include pain medication and other therapies to increase comfort and decrease anxiety, promoting relaxation.

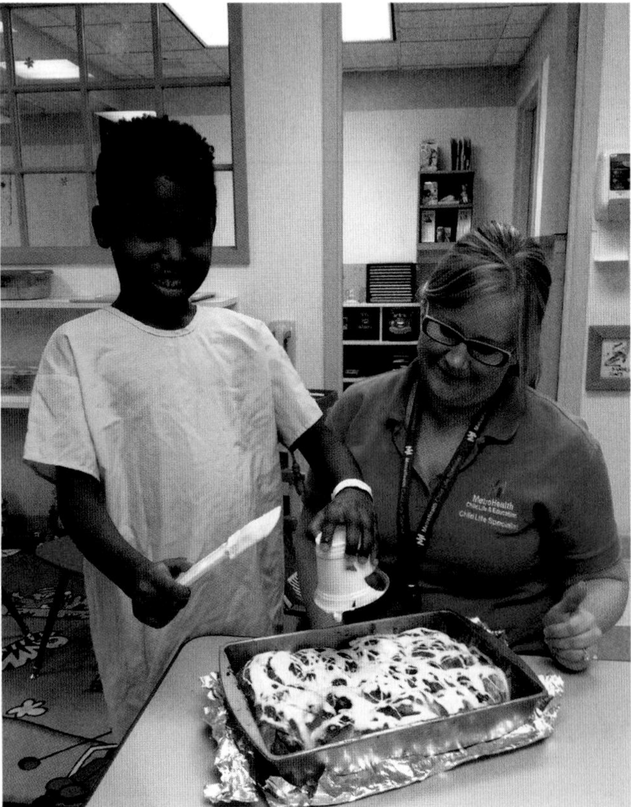

FIGURE 5–4 A child life therapist provides developmentally appropriate interventions for patients and siblings.

The multidisciplinary care team members involved in pain control include the physician, nurse, pharmacist, and child life specialist. Involvement of family in determination of pain is an important aspect of pediatric pain control; parents/caregivers can be excellent judges of their child's comfort level. Involvement of family in alternative pain treatments includes discussing and suggesting options such as the following:

- Massage therapy provides relaxation for the patient and potentially decreases pain.
- Relaxation therapy helps the child relax using techniques such as music, holding, and positioning. Some facilities offer complementary or alternative therapies such as healing touch or aromatherapy.
- Play therapy distracts the patient from the pain with calm, developmentally appropriate activities such as puzzles and coloring.

Pain must be properly assessed using the appropriate pain assessment tool. The following tools are commonly used in pediatric pain assessment:

- NIPS: Neonatal and Infant Pain Scale for newborns. This assesses the newborn's cry, facial expression, respiratory pattern, the position and flexion of the arms and legs, and the level of alertness (Srouji, Ratnapalan, & Schneeweiss, 2010).
- FLACC: Faces, Legs, Activity, Cry, Consolability Scale for newborn to 7 years. This assesses the patient's facial expression, leg positioning and flexion, activity level, crying level, and consolability (Srouji et al., 2010).
- Faces Scale: The Faces Scale is only for patients aged 3 years and older; the child must be developmentally able to read and recognize faces drawn with various levels of painful expressions. This pain scale asks the child to choose the face that best represents his or her pain level (Srouji et al., 2010).
- Visual Analog Scale (VAS): The VAS is for children aged 7 years and older who have the developmental ability to use the traditional pain scale based on numbers 0 to 10 for pain rating (Srouji et al., 2010).

SAFE AND EFFECTIVE NURSING CARE: Clinical Pearl

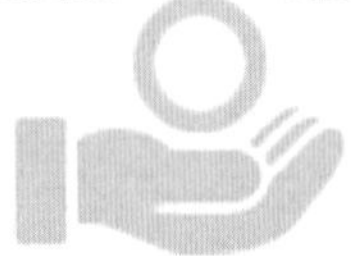

Role of the Pain Team

Many pediatric hospitals offer a pain team as part of the multidisciplinary care team. The pain team is generally headed by an anesthesiologist, and its primary purpose is to assess and alleviate a patient's pain. The pain team is responsible for writing and ensuring follow-through on all pain-related medical orders and interventions.

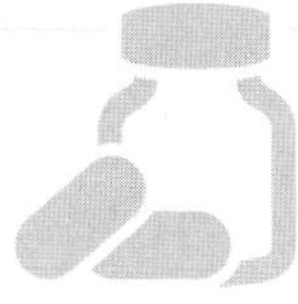

SAFE AND EFFECTIVE NURSING CARE: Understanding Medication

Administration

When administering end-of-life pain medication, the least invasive administration route should be chosen. Various routes are available, including topical, oral, intravenous, inhaled, and rectal. The various routes of administration allow the child to be free of most invasive devices at the time of death. An example is morphine sulfate, a pain medication often given intravenously. If a patient does not have an IV line, the medication can be given orally as a liquid placed in the buccal cavity for absorption; if the patient cannot swallow the medication, it can be given as a topical patch or via nebulizer in an inhaled form.

Cultural and Religious Care During End of Life

Cultural considerations for pediatric end of life include respecting the cultural beliefs of the family and patient. Providing culturally competent care requires the nurse to incorporate the cultural beliefs of the family and patient into daily care. The spiritual needs of family and patient require the nurse to incorporate the spiritual beliefs of the family and patient into daily care (Fig. 5–5). Family-centered care encourages the nurse to consider the cultural and spiritual needs of the family while providing care. See Chapter 4 for further details.

CHILD DEVELOPMENT

An understanding of overall child development and how it relates to a child's view of death is necessary to provide competent care. (See discussions of development in Chapters 7–10.) Nursing interactions with children at the end of life should be based on the child's developmental level and cultural needs. A child's view of life is based on his or her developmental level and created from his or her experiences and perception. If a child is dying from a congenital condition or disease, his or her developmental level may be lower than expected for his or her age; delays must be considered in the developmental assessment. A child's view of death is based on developmental stage and life experiences, so expect varied behavior and opinions related to death (Table 5–1). In providing family-centered care, the nurse must incorporate care of the siblings at the appropriate developmental level. Child behavior at end of life may be developmentally abnormal based on the stress and confusion of death and dying. Parent and family education related to the child's developmental stage is important to convey how the dying child and any siblings understand death.

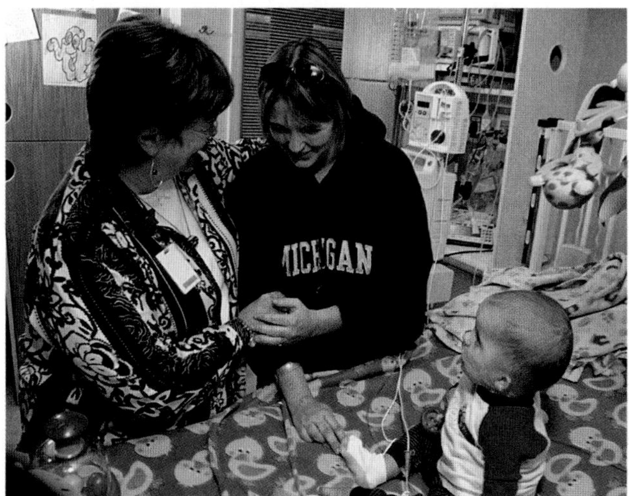

FIGURE 5–5 The hospital chaplain or spiritual care staff can provide support to the patient and family.

GRIEF

There are many theories on grief, or bereavement, including those of Kübler-Ross, Bowlby, Engle, and Worden. Most theories indicate that individuals progress through their grief on an individual timeline but through similar stages. Kübler-Ross (2009) is a respected grief theorist who defined the common stages of grief (Table 5–2). These include:

- Anticipatory grief occurs before the stages of grief and is common in infant and pediatric death, when the family of a patient with a terminal diagnosis prepares for death before the dying process (Kübler-Ross, 2009).
- Denial: Following anticipatory grief is denial, which is a refusal to believe that an infant or child is dead or dying (Kübler-Ross, 2009).
- Anger: Anger concerning death results in feelings of wrath or indignation; it will often manifest as anger toward the disease, the cause of death of the infant or child, or even the medical staff and caregivers of the child (Kübler-Ross, 2009).
- Bargaining or negotiations: These are an attempt to create a change in the situation through an agreement for services exchanged (Kübler-Ross, 2009).
- Depression or depressed mood: This stage of grief often manifests as loss of interest in life and normal activities, along with feelings of guilt or low self-worth (Kübler-Ross, 2009).
- Acceptance: Acceptance is to receive or agree with what is offered. In pediatric grief, it is when the parents or family come to terms with the event and the associated loss.

Family members may grieve at different stages; everyone will not grieve in the same manner at the same time. The family should be educated that this may occur and is normal. Staff feelings of grief over the loss of a patient are common and should be expected and addressed as a normal reaction to the loss of a pediatric patient.

TABLE 5–1 Child's View of Death Based on Developmental Stage and Life Experiences

AGE GROUP	EMOTIONAL DEVELOPMENT	CONCEPTUAL VIEW OF DEATH
Infants and toddlers (birth to 35 months) Preschoolers (3–5 years)	Fear and anxiety over separation Magical thinking, formation of peer relationships, gender identification	No or little understanding of death (Brown & Warr, 2007) Death is something that happens to others Death is not a permanent state; death is reversible Curious about dead animals and flowers (Brown & Warr, 2007)
Early childhood (6–12 years)	Enthusiasm for learning and work Developing strong interpersonal relationships Building self-esteem	Death is final Death is universal Death is only in the distant future (Brown & Warr, 2007)
Adolescents	Identity formation Development of complex cognitive skills	Understand death in a logical manner similar to adult understanding Death is permanent (Brown & Warr, 2007)

TABLE 5–2 Kübler-Ross Stages of Grief

COMMON STAGES OF GRIEF	EXPECTED BEHAVIORS FROM FAMILY MEMBERS
Denial	Unwillingness to accept diagnosis, lack of trust in medical staff (Kübler-Ross, 2009)
Anger	Anger or aggression toward staff or family members; verbal arguments and confrontations are common (Kübler-Ross, 2009)
Bargaining	Reliance on a higher power to prevent death, belief that promises of future behavior will prevent death of the child (Kübler-Ross, 2009)
Depression	Crying, withdrawal from family and friends, loss of appetite (Kübler-Ross, 2009)
Acceptance	Statements of understanding of the loss, positive outlook, discussion of the future (Kübler-Ross, 2009)

NURSING EDUCATION IN END-OF-LIFE CARE

Education for the patient (when appropriate for age and development) should include:

- Explanation of cause for terminal diagnosis and how the disease will cause death.
- Explanation of current medical interventions needed and what the patient should expect.
- Explanation of the dying process, with appropriate explanation of what to expect.

Parent/caregiver education should include information about:

- How the disease process will affect the child
- Current medical treatments available for patient diagnosis, including all possible information about available options
- Potential disease outcomes, with discussion of time frame when possible
- What to expect during the dying process, in terms appropriate for the child, siblings, parents, and family members. Every child's death experience will be unique based on his or her underlying diagnosis. Ensure that parents and family members are educated on the decline that will occur, including physical changes such as cool and mottled skin, swelling, altered verbalization, swallowing, and breathing pattern, and altered state of consciousness.
- What to expect at the time of death, such as how the child will look, the involvement of the staff, and whom the family wants in the room
- What to expect after death, such as care and disposition of the body and funeral arrangements

WITHDRAWAL OF CARE

Withdrawal of care occurs when the family decides to stop all lifesaving measures and allow the infant or child to die naturally with the family at the bedside, rather than an end-of-life attempted resuscitation with the child surrounded by medical staff. Parental rights in withdrawal of care allow them to consent to end interventions and determine when the interventions will be stopped; they also have the right to change their minds and continue care. Parent and family education regarding withdrawal of care—how it is done and what to expect in the child's response—is important to prevent misunderstandings. When appropriate, the siblings and patient should also be educated on withdrawal of care and what to expect.

Initiation of withdrawal of care is determined by the condition of the patient, the physician's opinion, and parent/caregiver desires. Nursing interventions in withdrawal of care include turning off the monitor, disconnecting all invasive lines, and creating a comfortable, undisturbed, peaceful, and private environment for the family.

FAMILY PRESENCE IN CODE SITUATIONS

Family presence in pediatric code situations is handled differently in all hospitals, so knowledge of hospital-specific guidelines is paramount. Considerations include the following:

- Family involvement in pediatric code situations provides family-centered care in a very stressful situation.
- The desired outcome of family-centered care in pediatric code situations is to create greater communication and decrease confusion for the family.
- This can be positive because the family knows everything possible was done to save the patient.
- A negative aspect is that the family sees the child in the worst situation possible.
- The family may attempt to be at the bedside, which can be inappropriate with specific interventions.

SAFE AND EFFECTIVE NURSING CARE: Promoting Safety

Resuscitation

It is common procedure to invite families to remain with the pediatric patient during resuscitation (Emergency Nurses Association, 2009; Smith McAlvin & Carew-Lyons, 2014). Research has demonstrated that presence during resuscitation was beneficial for the family members, and they often felt that being present was both a right and an obligation (Emergency Nurses Association, 2009; Smith McAlvin & Carew-Lyons, 2014). Most facilities have policies to guide family presence during resuscitation.

During a pediatric code situation, it is critical to provide for the safety of the patient's family. Nurses should:

- Ensure that a staff member is assigned to be with the family during the entire code event.
- Ensure that family members are not touching the bed or medical equipment during cardiac shock delivery.
- Ensure that family members are not in the way of medical staff.
- Ensure that family members are not in the way of medical equipment.
- If family members are unsteady on their feet, ensure that they are given a place to sit.

NURSING ROLE IN CARE OF THE DYING CHILD

Family involvement in the daily nursing care of the dying child will be different for all families, but when appropriate and desired, the family should be involved in all aspects of care. Bathing and dressing of the infant or child will depend on the parents' wishes. When appropriate, have the parents choose clothing for the child and assist with bathing and dressing. Accommodating visitors despite unit visitation rules is the role of the nurse and should be done in an appropriate way while respecting the needs of the other patients on the unit. Accommodations for religious or spiritual ceremonies must be included in the bedside care of the dying patient. When appropriate, assist hospital pastoral care in meeting the spiritual needs of the family and patient. Allow the family time to say goodbye to the child and spend time alone with him or her. When possible and desired, allow family to hold the child or lay in the bed next to the child. Creation of mementos and keepsakes for the family of dying pediatric patients provides them with a tangible memory of their child (Fig. 5–6). This can include:

- Handprints and footprints created using molds or ink
- A lock of hair cut and placed in a secure envelope or bag to prevent loss
- Pictures are very common for the family who has lost an infant or child; some hospitals provide a camera for the staff to take digital photographs, and some professional photographers take end-of-life pictures as a gift for the family

When the child dies, follow hospital protocol for declaration of death and disposition of the body, which will vary based on facility policy. Depending on the cause of death, the body will go to the coroner or funeral home; be sure to properly label the body and respect the body at all times. Follow state regulations and hospital protocol for autopsy. Some patients will require an autopsy, and it is generally at the discrimination of the local

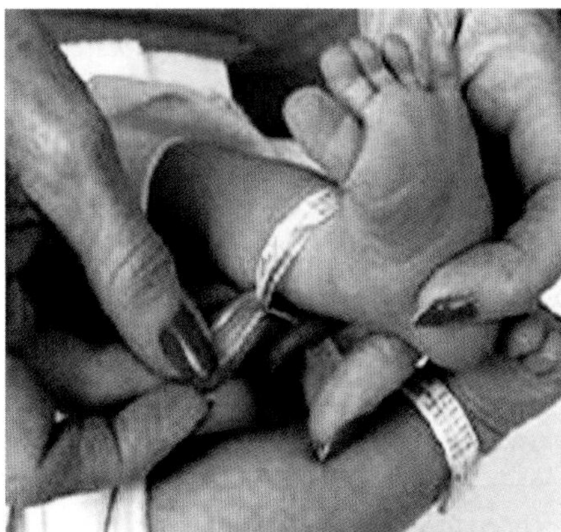

FIGURE 5–6 A patient's name band is often kept as a keepsake by the family.

coroner. Follow facility protocol related to patient death and contacting the coroner. Proper documentation at time of death is the responsibility of the nurse. Ensure that all care, nursing interventions, and patient outcomes are documented thoroughly in the child's medical record.

ORGAN DONATION

Organ donation is the giving of viable organs from a dying patient to patients in need of specific organs. Pediatric organs can be transplanted into adult and pediatric patients. A patient is considered a viable donor when the organs are not damaged by disease, trauma, or medication. These protocols for organ donation must be followed:

- When a child is considered a viable candidate for organ donation, the family is approached by an organ donation approach team. This multidisciplinary team of health-care providers and ancillary staff is specially trained in approaching families to request that they donate the patient's organs.
- Consent is needed from the legal guardians for organ donation.
- Once consent is given, blood is drawn from the patient to determine the patients on the transplant list who are the best match for the organs available.
- Procurement of organs is commonly done by the transplanting surgical team. The team travels to the site of the organ donor, and the patient is taken to the operating room to remove the organs.
- Parents and family members should say goodbye to the patient before transfer to the operating room; the patient will die in the operating room.

Family education regarding organ donation is critical and should include:

- Information about how the patient will be kept alive via medical intervention until the procurement surgeon arrives
- Details of how the infant or child will pass away in the operating room, and the fact that the family cannot be in the operating room
- The benefits of organ donation to the recipient

A national government-funded organ donor branch of the federal government oversees and acts as a watchdog for organ donation, which currently works in conjunction with the United Network for Organ Sharing.

- The Organ Procurement and Transplantation Network (OPTN) is the unified transplant network established by the U.S. Congress under the National Organ Transplant Act in 1984 (U.S. Department of Health and Human Services, 2017).
- The OPTN oversees the federal laws related to organ donation and procurement, and ensures that organs are distributed fairly and given to patients based on diagnosis, stage in life, and matching percentage (U.S. Department of Health and Human Services, 2017).
- The OPTN facilitates organ matching and placement through a computer system and fully staffed organ center operating 24 hours a day that works in conjunction with individual state organ donation networks (U.S. Department of Health and Human Services, 2017).
- Organ donation is generally a closed process; the donating family will not know who has received their child's organs (U.S. Department of Health and Human Services, 2017).

SAFE AND EFFECTIVE NURSING CARE: Cultural Competence

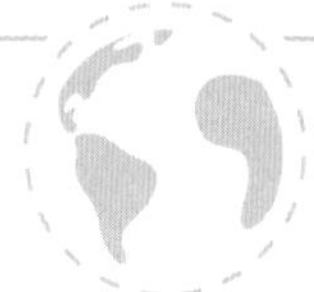

Organ Donation

Not all children who die are candidates for organ donation. Ability to donate is determined on an individual patient basis, and consent of the family must be provided. Some cultures do not approve of organ donation; be sure to understand the family's cultural beliefs before notifying the approach team for organ donation.

LEGAL ASPECTS OF PEDIATRIC END OF LIFE

It is the responsibility of the nurse to understand and adhere to the nursing scope of practice. When caring for a dying child, the nurse must include any legal considerations in the plan of care, including:

- Determination of legal guardians
- Obtaining consent
- Withdrawal of care

See Chapter 2 for more about legal and ethical considerations.

CRITICAL COMPONENT

State Nursing Practice Acts

The nursing practice act of each individual state guides nursing practice; these acts vary from state to state. The nurse practice acts for each state can be found by contacting the specific State Board of Nursing.

Autopsies

Autopsies can be requested by the family, the physician, and/or the coroner; note that autopsy policies and procedures differ by state and facility. Families may request an autopsy if they wish to know the exact cause of the death of their child; if the coroner does not agree that an autopsy needs to be performed, the family may be responsible for the cost of the autopsy. The physician may request an autopsy if the patient's cause of death is not known; if the coroner does not agree with the need for an autopsy, the family may need to give consent. The coroner has the legal right to request an autopsy in any suspicious or unexpected death and does not need consent of the family if it is considered legally necessary.

Do Not Resuscitate Orders

Some terminal children will have a do not resuscitate (DNR) order, and just as in adult medicine, this order must be respected. Nurses should be aware of the following:

- All facilities have specific policies relating to DNR orders; be sure to follow facility policies when caring for a patient with a DNR order.
- Only the legal guardians can determine a minor patient's DNR status.
- A DNR order can be reversed at any time by the legal guardians.
- DNR orders can range from provision of no life-sustaining interventions to provision of partial or limited life-sustaining interventions.
- Parents or legal guardians need to be fully educated on all aspects of a DNR order.
- If you are the nurse caring for a terminal child, it is your responsibility to know if the child has a DNR and the limitations within the specific DNR.
- When a patient has a legal DNR order, it is the responsibility of the health-care team to follow the DNR order.

In the death of a child from suspected abuse or intentional injury, the legal aspects are very important and must be considered. Understand the facility policies and state laws when caring for a child who is the suspected victim of abuse. Nurses must ensure they only release information following the protocols and laws outlined in the Health Insurance Portability and Accessibility Act. All aspects of nursing care require proper documentation and charting, and this includes the death of a child. If you were involved in the care of an infant or child in which the infant or child's death included resuscitation attempts, ensure that everything is documented in the proper form according to hospital policy.

Determination of Legal Guardian

The person who is legally able to give consent for the child needs to be determined on admission based on facility policies and state laws. Many types of family units exist within U.S. society, and people in the patient's life who function as a family unit are not always legally seen as a family unit. Some pediatric patients are able to give self-consent depending on the laws of the state or individual legal rulings making the minor independent. Every state has individual laws that determine the age of consent, or the age at which a child is considered legally an adult and able to sign for his or her own medical care.

When caring for any infant or pediatric patient, nursing must ensure that the people giving consent for treatment are the legal guardians. In cases of abuse or patients who are wards of the state, it is essential that the consent for any and all procedures is only obtained from the legal guardian(s). Always employ social work or case management staff for any unclear family units to ensure the legal guardian is giving consent. As with all nursing care, ensure proper documentation of the determination of legal guardianship and who is able to sign consents for the patient.

Case Study

You are working in a pediatric unit and are assigned to care for an 8-year-old child who has been diagnosed with stage 4 inoperable glioblastoma. Before the diagnosis the child was developmentally appropriate for his age and doing well in school. Since the diagnosis the child has difficulty with his gait and balance, slurs some words, and has significant short-term memory issues, but his long-term memory is currently intact. The child's diagnosis is terminal with days to weeks to live. The child has been at home with his family and was brought in to the hospital today via ambulance and admitted to the floor. The child has been admitted for pain control.

1. What is the most appropriate pain scale to use on this child?

   The child has his large family in the room with him including his parents, his younger sister and older brothers, his grandparents, and several aunts and uncles and cousins. You need to contact the child life therapist.
2. Who are you going to ask the child life therapist to visit and work with?

   As you are interacting with the parents you realize that their primary language is not English, and one of the patient's siblings state that they speak Mandarin Chinese. The patient and siblings are fluent in Mandarin Chinese and English.
3. How do you best communicate with the parents? Is it okay to use the patient or siblings to translate for you?

   Once you have secured appropriate translation services you have a long discussion with the parents. The mother is asking about the patient's schoolwork and how long he will be in the hospital so she can ensure he does not fall behind in school, and the father is asking about when the patient's balance will come back so he can go back to playing soccer.
4. What Kübler-Ross defined stage of grief are the parents in?

   You assess the patient and he is in moderate pain but states he does not want any pain medication because it makes him so sleepy.
5. What alternatives therapies could be provided to help the patient improve his comfort level?

   The patient's aunt approaches you in the hallway and asks if she can bring in home-made food and call their spiritual leader to come visit the patient in the hospital.
6. What is your best response to this question?

REFERENCES

American Academy of Pediatrics. (n.d.). *SIDS handout.* Retrieved from http://www.healthychildcare.org/Doc/SIDSexercise1.doc

American Association of Colleges of Nursing. (2016). *End of Life Nursing Education Consortium.* Retrieved from http://www.aacn.nche.edu/elnec/about/fact-sheet

Brown, E., & Warr, B. (2007). *Supporting the child and the family in pediatric hospice care.* Philadelphia: Jessica Kingsley Publishers.

Centers for Disease Control and Prevention. (2015). *Child health, data for the United States health status.* Retrieved from https://www.cdc.gov/nchs/fastats/child-health.htm

Emergency Nurses Association. (2009). *Clinical practice guideline: Family presence during invasive procedures and resuscitation.* Retrieved from https://www.ena.org/docs/default-source/resource-library/practice-resources/cpg/familypresencesynopsis3bdad0aaaeeb4370856e849f26e553a3.pdf?sfvrsn=21ca66b_16

Kübler-Ross, E. (2009). *On death and dying: What the dying have to teach doctors, nurses, clergy and their own families* (40th anniversary ed.). New York: Routledge.

National Institutes of Health. (2015). Back to sleep education campaign. Retrieved from http://www.nichd.nih.gov/sids/

Smith McAlvin, S., & Carew-Lyons, A. (2014). Family presence during resuscitation and invasive procedures in pediatric critical care: A systematic review. *American Journal of Critical Care 23*(6), 477-485.

Southern New Jersey Perinatal Cooperative. (n.d.). *New Jersey Baby Box Initiative.* Retrieved from https://heartsj.org/what-we-do/family-resources/family-health-wellness.html

Srouji, R., Ratnapalan, S., & Schneeweiss, S. (2010). Pain in children: Assessment and nonpharmacological management. *International Journal of Pediatrics, 2010*, 474838.

U.S. Department of Health and Human Services. (2017). *Organ procurement and transplantation network.* Retrieved from http://optn.transplant.hrsa.gov

UNIT 3

Growth and Development of the Child

Growth and Development

6

Mary Grady, DNP, RN CNE, CHSE
Jill Matthes, DNP, RN CHSE

LEARNING OUTCOMES

Upon completion of this chapter, the student will be able to:

1. Describe general principles of growth and development.
2. Discuss cognitive growth and development according to Jean Piaget.
3. Discuss psychosocial growth and development according to Eric Erikson.
4. Discuss psychosexual growth and development according to Sigmund Freud.
5. Discuss social-moral growth and development according to Lawrence Kohlberg.
6. Discuss the theory of nature versus nurture.
7. Apply principles of family-focused care in approaches toward the child.
8. Analyze factors that affect growth and development.
9. Understand nursing applications of growth and development theories.

GENERAL PRINCIPLES OF GROWTH AND DEVELOPMENT

Growth and development are closely interrelated and interdependent processes that are unique for each individual and influenced by factors such as genetics, environment, and nutrition. Growth, the increase in height and weight, and development, the acquisition of skills and abilities, begin at conception and continue until the end of life. Although highly individualized, growth and development follow an orderly pattern characterized by periods of rapid growth and plateaus (spurts and lulls):

- Cephalocaudal—starts at the head and moves downward
  - Example: The child can control his or her head and neck before it can control his or her arms and legs.
- Proximodistal—starts in the center and processes to the periphery
  - Example: Movement and control of the trunk section of the body occurs before movement and control of the arms.
- Differentiation—simple to complex progression of achievement of developmental milestones
  - Example: The child learns to crawl before learning to walk.

Variation at different ages is based on specific body structure and organ growth.

Developmental tasks are the sets of skills and competencies that are unique to each developmental stage. Certain tasks must be mastered for the child to progress to the next level. Developmental tasks for each stage are detailed in Table 6–1.

Childhood is divided into the following five stages:

- Infant—birth to 1 year
- Toddler—1 to 3 years
- Preschool—3 to 6 years
- School-age—6 to 12 years
- Adolescence—12 to 18 years

See Table 6–2 for an overview of growth and development by age.

SAFE AND EFFECTIVE NURSING CARE: Clinical Pearl

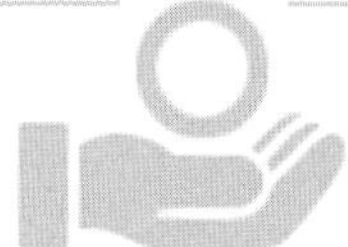

Failure to Thrive

Failure to grow and develop at an expected rate can mean that a child is failing to thrive. The diagnosis of failure to thrive (FTT) is given to children who fall below the 5th percentile ranges on height and weight charts. For infants, it usually presents first with an absence of weight gain or weight loss (Price & Gwin, 2012). Then a drop in height is followed by a drop in head circumference. FTT be caused by organic or nonorganic causes, which can contribute to developmental delays in the child.

SAFE AND EFFECTIVE NURSING CARE: Promoting Safety

Childproofing

Caregivers must be aware of growth and developmental milestones so that they can prevent injury at the different stages. In early childhood, much care and consideration should be given to prevent falls, choking, and aspiration of food or objects. Childproofing the home to prevent injuries is important.

CRITICAL COMPONENT

Reflexes

Nurses need to know normal infant reflexes and recognize when they are not present. Reflexes that remain can be a sign of growth and developmental issues and delays (Beckett & Taylor, 2016). A few of the most common reflexes to watch for are:

- Tonic neck/fencing reflex—disappears around 4–6 months
- Moro/startle reflex—disappears around 4–6 months
- Babinski's—disappears by 1 year of age

SAFE AND EFFECTIVE NURSING CARE: Clinical Pearl

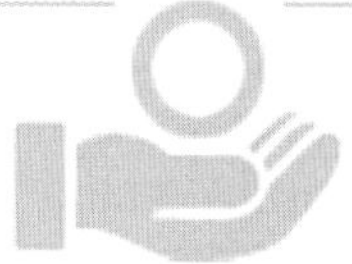

Family-Centered Care

As part of family-centered care, nurses need to adapt their care and nursing interventions to the child's stage of growth and development. They will need to explain what is happening to a child in language and on a developmental level the family can understand. A child's caretaker should always be included in the child's care and interventions. Nurses need to remember that we are not caring for just a child, but for the entire family unit (Institute for Patient- and Family-Centered Care, 2014).

TABLE 6–1 Developmental Milestones

AGE	FINE MOTOR	GROSS MOTOR
2–3 months	Grasps toys, can open and close hands Eyes follow object to midline Blows bubbles	Raises head and chest when lying on stomach Supports upper body with arms when lying on stomach Stretches legs out and kicks when lying on stomach or back
6–8 months	Bangs objects on table Can transfer objects from hand to hand Start of pincer grasp	Can roll from side to side Can sit unsupported by 7 or 8 months Supports whole weight on legs
1 year	Can hold crayon, may mark on paper Begins to use objects correctly	Pulls self up to stand Walks holding on to furniture May walk two or three steps independently
2–3 years	Learning to dress self Can draw simple shapes (e.g., a circle)	Jumps Kicks ball Learning to pedal tricycle
4–5 years	Dresses independently Uses scissors Learning to tie shoes Brushes teeth	Goes up and down stairs independently Throws a ball overhand Hops on one foot

Source: Centers for Disease Control and Prevention (2016).

PSYCHOINTELLECTUAL DEVELOPMENT

The key theorist within cognitive development is Jean Piaget, a Swiss child psychologist who lived from 1896 to 1980. Piaget identified the following characteristics of cognitive development:

- Development is a sequential and orderly process, moving from stages that are relatively simple to more complex (Table 6–3).
- Cognitive acts occur as the child adapts to the surrounding environment.
- The child's experience with the environment naturally encourages growth and maturation.

TABLE 6–2 Overview of Growth and Development by Age

AGE	GROWTH FACTS
Infant: age birth to 1 year	**Weight:** • Doubles by 5–6 months • Triples by 1 year **Height:** • Increase of 1 foot by 1 year of age **Teeth:** • Erupt by 6 months • Has six to eight deciduous teeth by 1 year of age
Toddler: age 1–3 years	**Weight:** • Gains 8 oz or more a month from 1–2 years • Gains 3–5 lb a year from 2–3 years of age **Height:** • From 1 to 2 years of age, grows 3–5 inches • From 2 to 3 years of age, grows 2–2.5 inches per year **Teeth:** • By 3 years of age, has 20 deciduous teeth
Preschool: age 3–6 years	**Weight:** • Gains 3–5 lb a year **Height:** • Grows 1.5–2.5 inches a year
School-age: age 6–12 years	**Weight:** • Gains 3–5 lb a year **Height:** • Grows 1.5–2.5 inches a year
Adolescence: age 12–18 years (Puberty usually will last somewhere around 2–5 years.)	**Variations** **Weight:** The gain that occurs during puberty years • Girls: Gain 15–55 pounds • Boys: Gain 15–65 pounds **Height:** The growth that occurs during puberty years • Girls: 2–8 inches Growth occurs during puberty. Girls usually stop growing taller 2 years after the start of their menstrual periods. • Boys: 4.5–12 inches

- The child must accommodate to new or complex problems by drawing on past experiences.
- There can be overlap between the child's age and stage of development. Each stage does not start and end at exactly the same age for each child.

Key Stages of Piaget's Theory

Piaget's theory of cognitive development defines developmental stages as follows:

- Sensorimotor—birth to 2 years: The child learns through motor and reflex actions, and begins to understand that he or she is separate from the environment and from others.
  - Stage 1: Reflexes—birth to 2 months
    - The child understands the environment purely through inborn reflexes such as sucking.
  - Stage 2: Primary circular reactions—1 to 4 months
    - The child begins to coordinate reflexes and sensations. For example, he or she may find the thumb by accident, find pleasure in sucking it, then later repeat sucking it for pleasure.
  - Stage 3: Secondary circular reactions—4 to 8 months
    - The child focuses on his or her environment and begins to repeat actions that will trigger a response. For example, the child puts a toy rattle in his or her mouth.
  - Stage 4: Coordination of secondary schemata—8 to 12 months
    - To achieve a desired effect, the child will repeat the action, such as repeatedly shaking a rattle to make the sound.
  - Stage 5: Tertiary circular reactions—12 to 18 months
    - The child begins trial-and-error approaches: for example, making a sound to see whether it will get attention from the caregiver.
  - Stage 6: Inventions of new means/mental combinations—18 to 24 months
    - The child learns that objects and symbols represent events, such as that the appearance of a bowl and spoon means dinner is coming.

CRITICAL COMPONENT

Object Permanence

Object permanence is one of the most important developments in the sensorimotor stage. The child now knows that an object exists even when it cannot be seen or heard. This is a wonderful time to introduce the game peekaboo; by the end of this stage the child will understand that you did not disappear just because your hands are over your face.

- Preoperational—2 to 7 years
  - Application of language
  - Use of symbols to represent objects
  - Ability to think about things and events that are not immediately present
  - Oriented to the present; difficulty conceptualizing time
  - Thinking influenced by fantasy
  - Teaching must account for the child's vivid fantasies and undeveloped sense of time

SAFE AND EFFECTIVE NURSING CARE: Clinical Pearl

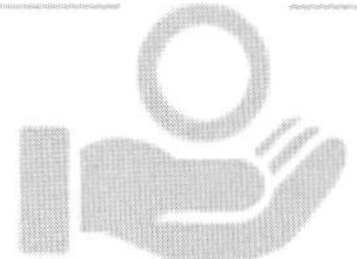

The Procedure From the Child's Perspective

In this stage the child is egocentric, or unable to take the view of others. While the child is hospitalized, the nurse should introduce role-playing and medical play therapy. The child needs to understand the procedure from his or her own perspective, such as by touching and playing with the equipment before its use. In addition, language is not fully developed; therefore, teaching through discussion will not be effective.

- Concrete operational—7 to 11 years
  - Shows increase in accommodation skills
  - Develops an ability to think abstractly and to make rational judgments about concrete or observable phenomena
  - In teaching, give the opportunity to ask questions and explain things back to the nurse. This allows the child to mentally manipulate information.
- Formal operational—11 years to adulthood
  - This stage brings cognition to its final form.
  - The individual no longer requires concrete objects to make rational judgments.
  - Individuals are capable of hypothetical and deductive reasoning.
  - Teaching for adolescents may be wide ranging because they can consider many possibilities from several perspectives.

TABLE 6–3 Piaget's Five Stages of Cognitive Development

	SENSORIMOTOR STAGE	PREOPERATIONAL STAGE*	INTUITIVE THOUGHT PHASE	CONCRETE OPERATION STAGE	FORMAL OPERATIONAL STAGE
Age	Birth to 2 years **Stage 1:** Reflexes Birth to 2 months **Stage 2:** Primary circular reactions 1–4 months **Stage 3:** Secondary circular reactions 4–8 months **Stage 4:** Coordination of secondary schemata 8–12 months **Stage 5:** Tertiary circular reactions 12–18 months **Stage 6:** Inventions of new means 18–24 months	2–4 years	4–7 years	7–11 years	11 years to adulthood
Characteristics	During this stage the child progresses from reflex activity to simple repetitive behaviors. The end result is behaviors that are imitative. By the end of the stage the following concepts should be mastered: • Object permanence • Understanding of cause and effect • Understanding of spatial relationships • Uses make-believe and pretend play	• Egocentric • Magical thinking • Increase in language development • Associates words with objects/symbols	• Less egocentric • Thinks of others • Can think of one idea at a time • Words used to express thoughts	• Continues to become less self-centered • Thought process is more coherent and logical • Solves concrete problems • Still unable to think abstractly	• Adaptable and flexible • Use of rational thinking • Thinks abstractly • Reasoning is deductive

**The preoperational stage often includes ages 2 to 7 years.*

SAFE AND EFFECTIVE NURSING CARE: Clinical Pearl

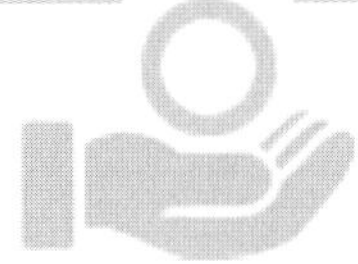

Formal Operational

The child in this stage begins to consider that his or her actions will result in possible consequences. It is important to remember when caring for a patient in this stage that you should explain reasons for the hospitalization, the disease process, and possible outcomes, especially those related to the patient's behavior.

PSYCHOSEXUAL DEVELOPMENT

Freud, a physician from Vienna, Austria, who lived from 1856 to 1939, proposed a theory of psychosexual development and an approach called psychoanalysis to explore the unconscious mind. His psychosexual theory is based on the belief that experiences from our early childhood form the unconscious motivation for the things we do later in life as adults. The theory proposes that sexual energy is stronger in certain parts of the body at specific ages. Sexual feelings are present in different forms depending on age. Fixation of development can occur at a specific stage if needs are not met or conflicts are not resolved. Freud's theory views the personality as consisting of three parts: the id, the ego, and the superego (Beckett & Taylor, 2016) (Table 6–4).

- Id—the basic sexual energy that is present at birth and drives the seeking of pleasure
- Ego—the realistic part of a person, which develops during infancy and searches for acceptable methods to meet impulses
- Superego—the moral and ethical system that develops in childhood and contains values as well as conscious thoughts

According to Freud, human nature has two sides:

- Rational intellect—being able to think about others, and do what is right. Example: delayed gratification
- Irrational desires—following the unconscious mind, which is driven by uncontrollable instincts that are irrational and pleasure seeking. Example: getting what you want when you want it even if the timing is not right or others are affected negatively

TABLE 6–4 Freud's Definition of Personality

THREE COMPONENTS OF PERSONALITY		
Id	**Ego**	**Superego**
Primitive rational • Requires immediate gratification • Inward-seeking behavior • Instincts	Conscious and ideas Acts as a censor to the id Reality	The person's conscience Morality

Source: McLeod, 2016

Key Stages of Freud's Psychosexual Theory

- Oral—birth to 1 year
  - Children at this stage are preoccupied with activities associated with the mouth.
  - Sexual urges are gratified with oral behaviors: sucking, biting, chewing, and eating.
  - Children who do not have their oral needs met may become thumb suckers or nail biters.
  - In adulthood, they may become compulsive eaters or smokers.
  - Normal development requires not depriving oral gratification, such as weaning too soon or a rigid feeding schedule.
- Anal—1 to 3 years of age
  - Preoccupied with the ability to eliminate
  - Sexual urges gratified by learning to voluntarily defecate
  - Sphincter muscles maturing (Beckett & Taylor, 2016)

CRITICAL COMPONENT

Toilet Training

Nurses should explain to caregivers the basic biological characteristics that allow a child to be toilet trained. Freud believed that how a child is toilet trained can have lasting effects on personality. If toilet training is too rigid or scheduled, the child can develop behaviors that are hypercritical or meticulous later in life (Potts & Mandleco, 2013).

- Phallic stage—3 to 6 years
  - Preoccupation with the genitals
  - Curious about childbirth, masturbation, and anatomic differences
  - Girls experience penis envy and wish they had one; boys suffer from castration anxiety, the fear of losing the penis
  - Children develop strong incestuous desire for caregiver of the opposite gender
    - Oedipal complex—attachment of boy to his mother
    - Electra complex—attachment of girl to her father
  - Children need to identify with caregiver of same gender to form male or female identity
- Latency stage—6 to 11 years of age
  - Sexual drives submerged
  - Energy focus on socialization and increasing problem-solving abilities
  - Appropriate gender roles adopted
  - Oedipal or Electra conflicts resolved
  - Identifies with same-gender peers and same-gender caregiver
  - Superego developed to a point where it keeps id under control

- Genital stage—begins at around 12 years of age and lasts to adulthood
  - Struggle with sexuality
  - Sexual desires return and are related to physiological changes and fluctuating hormones
  - Changing social relationships
  - Dealing with struggle of dependence and independence issues with parents
  - Learning to form loving, appropriate relationships
  - Must manage sexual urges in socially accepted ways

See Table 6–5 for more about Freud's stages of development.

SAFE AND EFFECTIVE NURSING CARE: Clinical Pearl

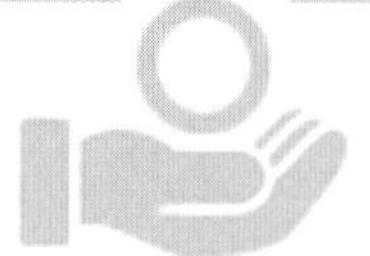

Recognition of Cognitive and Emotional Differences

Children are different than adults. They grow in particular patterns, and their behavior develops in particular stages. Nurses need to recognize the cognitive and emotional features of children of varying ages, based on developmental principles (Berk, 2013).

TABLE 6–5 Freud's Five Stages of Psychosocial Development

AGE	STAGE
Infancy (birth to 1 year)	**Oral stage** Comforted through the mouth
Toddler (1–3 years)	**Anal stage** Derives gratification from control of bodily excretions
Preschool (3–6 years)	**Phallic stage** Becomes aware of self as sexual being Identifies with the parent of the opposite sex, but by the end of stage will identify with same-sex parent Oedipal complex: attachment of a boy to his mother Electra complex: attachment of a girl to her father
School age (6–12 years)	**Latency stage** Focuses on peer relationships Emphasis on privacy and understanding the body
Adolescent (12–18 years)	**Genital stage** Focus on genital function and relationships

PSYCHOSOCIAL DEVELOPMENT

The primary theory of psychosocial development was established in 1959 by Erik Erikson, who lived from 1902 to 1994 and studied under Freud's daughter, Anna. Erikson's psychosocial development theory consists of eight different stages that address development over the life span. Each stage has a crisis that exists; healthy personality development occurs as each crisis, a challenge between the ego and social and biological processes, is resolved (Table 6–6). A person must master these psychosocial crises to grow and progress to the next stage of development. An individual either meets the healthy needs or does not, and this will influence future social relationships.

Key Stages of Erikson's Psychosocial Development Theory

- Trust versus mistrust (birth to 1 year) (Fig. 6–1)
  - An infant requires that basic needs are met—food, clothing, touch, and comfort.
  - If these needs are not met, the infant will develop a mistrust of others.
  - If a sense of trust is developed, the infant will see the world as a safe place.
  - Play is usually considered a psychosocial activity. During this stage play is referred to as solitary (Beckett & Taylor, 2016).
- Autonomy versus shame and doubt (1–3 years) (Fig. 6–2)
  - The child is learning to control bodily functions.
  - Independence starts to emerge; for example, toddlers control their worlds by deciding when and where elimination will occur.
  - They vocalize by saying no to something and direct their motor activity.
  - Children who are consistently criticized for showing independence and autonomy will develop shame and doubt in their abilities.
  - Toddlers also need to recognize the feelings and needs of others; excessive autonomy could lead to disregard for and an inability to play with others (Beckett & Taylor, 2016).
  - Play during this stage is known as parallel (Beckett & Taylor, 2016).

SAFE AND EFFECTIVE NURSING CARE: Clinical Pearl

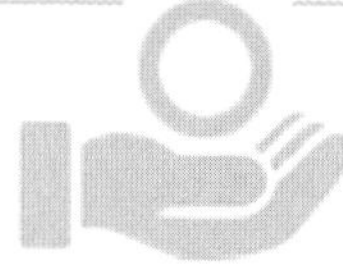

Age-Appropriate Toys

Toys that are age-appropriate for toddlers and account for their growth and development include stuffed animals, building blocks, books, play dough, tricycles, small cars and trains, and pretend toys to play housekeeping, such as pots, pans, spoons, and cups.

TABLE 6–6 Erikson's Five Stages of Psychosocial Development in Children

AGE	STAGE	COMMENTS
Infancy: birth to age 1 year	Trust versus mistrust	The child learns to trust as needs are met by the caregiver
Toddler: age 1–3 years	Autonomy versus shame and doubt	The child becomes more independent Frame of mind: "I am a big kid now." The child starts to have some control over body functions
Preschool: age 3–6 years	Initiative versus guilt	Development of a conscience Learning right from wrong
School age: age 6–12 years	Industry versus inferiority	Rule-following behavior Forming social relationships is seen as important
Adolescent: age 12–19 years	Identity versus role confusion	Changes in the body are great Preoccupied with appearance and what others think of them Peers are very important Working on establishing own identity

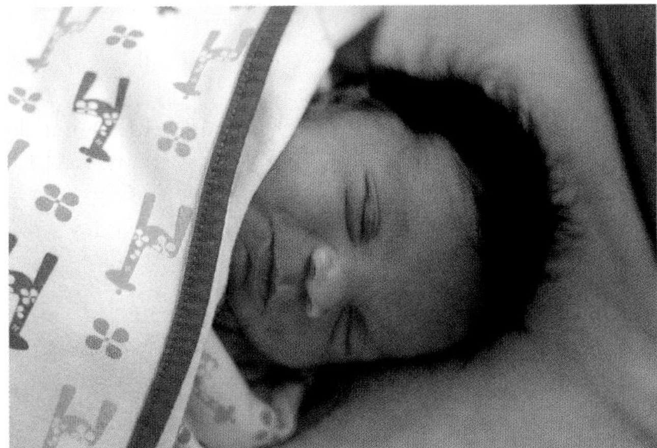

FIGURE 6–1 A newborn infant requires that basic needs are met—food, clothing, touch, and comfort.

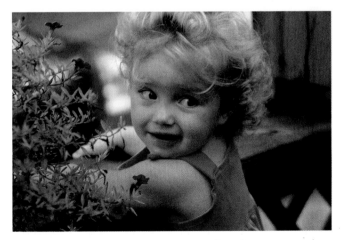

FIGURE 6–2 Toddlers experience the conflict of autonomy versus shame and doubt.

- Initiative versus guilt (3–6 years) (Fig. 6–3)
  - The preschool child is exposed to new people and new activities; the child becomes involved and very busy.
  - The child learns about the environment through play.
  - The child learns new responsibilities and can act based on established principles.
  - The child develops a conscience.
  - If the child is constantly criticized for his or her actions, this can lead to guilt and a lack of purpose.
  - Play at this stage is known as associative play (Beckett & Taylor, 2016).
- Industry versus inferiority (6–12 years) (Fig. 6–4)
  - The child develops interests and takes pride in accomplishments.
  - The child enjoys working in groups and forming social relationships.
  - Projects are enjoyable.
  - The child follows rules and order.
  - Developing a sense of industry provides the child with purpose and confidence in being successful.
  - If a child is unable to be successful, this can result in a sense of inferiority.
  - A child must learn balance, an understanding that he or she cannot succeed at everything and that there is always more to learn.
  - Play during this stage is known as cooperative play (Beckett & Taylor, 2016).
- Identity versus role confusion (12–18 years) (Fig. 6–5)
  - Children of this age are preoccupied with how they are seen in the eyes of others.
  - They are working to establish their own identity.
  - They are trying out new roles to see what best fits for them.
  - If they are unable to provide a meaningful definition of self, they are at risk for role confusion in one or more roles throughout life.
  - Some confusion is good and will result in self-reflection and self-examination.

SAFE AND EFFECTIVE NURSING CARE: Cultural Competence

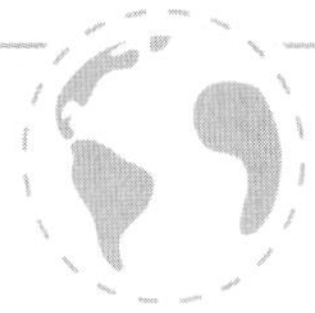

Compared with heterosexual youth, LGBTQ (lesbian, gay, bisexual, transgender, or questioning) teens are more likely to experience:

- Bullying
- Physical violence
- Rejection
- Suicidal thoughts
- High-risk behavior such as sexual and substance abuse

Source: Centers for Disease Control and Prevention (2013).

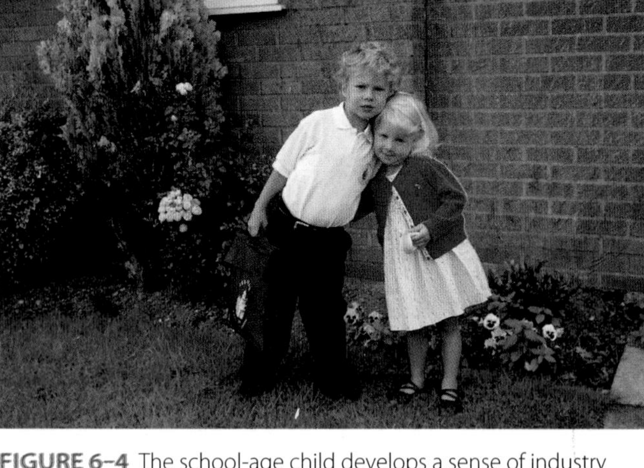

FIGURE 6–4 The school-age child develops a sense of industry that provides the child with purpose and confidence in being successful.

SAFE AND EFFECTIVE NURSING CARE: Promoting Safety

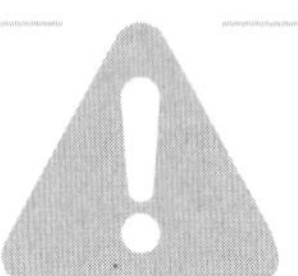

Adolescents feel that nothing bad will happen to them, and because of this they engage in risky behaviors. They are risk takers. Care should be given to educate this age group on safe practices, such as wearing a seat belt when driving, avoiding alcohol and drug use, safe sex practice, and suicide prevention. Noncompliance with a needed medical regimen may occur, and hospitalization may be the outcome. For example, the adolescent with asthma who chooses not to use his or her inhaler during activity may end up in respiratory distress that can result in a trip to the emergency department.

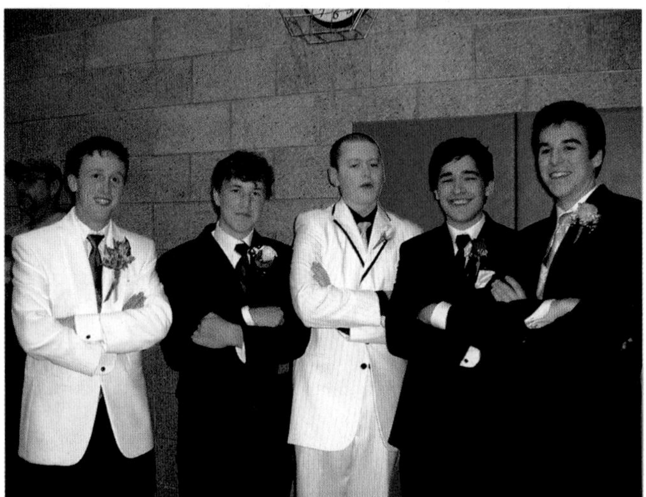

FIGURE 6–5 Teenagers are preoccupied with how they are seen in the eyes of others.

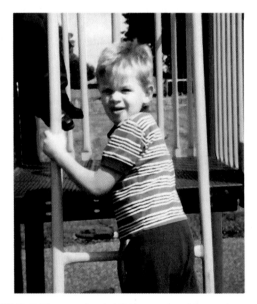

FIGURE 6–3 The preschool child learns about the environment through play.

SOCIAL-MORAL DEVELOPMENT

Based on the cognitive-developmental theory of Piaget, Lawrence Kohlberg theorized that children acquire moral reasoning in a specific developmental sequence. In 1958, Kohlberg developed a stage-based theory established on the premise that at birth, we are void of morals or ethics; thus, moral development occurs through social interaction with the environment around us. Kohlberg analyzed children in Germany, Kenya, Taiwan, and Mexico based on the motives of people when faced with making decisions. Moral development, which according to Kohlberg includes three major levels, can be advanced and promoted through formal education (Beckett & Taylor, 2016). Kohlberg has been criticized for insensitivity to cultural differences, sexual biases, and lack of consideration for family moral development. See Table 6–7 for Kohlberg's theory of moral development.

TABLE 6–7 Kohlberg's Three Stages of Moral Development

LEVEL	PRECONVENTIONAL LEVEL	CONVENTIONAL LEVEL	POSTCONVENTIONAL AUTONOMOUS LEVEL
Stages	1: Obedience and punishment orientation 2: Individualism and exchange	3: Good interpersonal relationships 4: Maintaining the social order	5: Social contract and individual rights 6: Universal principles
Age	2–7 years	7–12 years	12 years and older
Characteristics	• Follows rules that are set by those in authority • Adjusts behavior according to good/bad and right/wrong thinking	• Seeks conformity and loyalty • Follows rules • Maintains social order	• Constructs a personal and functional value system independent of authority figures and peers

NATURE VERSUS NURTURE

To what extent do hereditary factors and environmental influences shape the various personal traits and characteristics of a child? This has been a debated topic in growth and development, also referred to as *heredity versus environment* or *maturation versus learning.* Both nature and nurture play a part in shaping us to be who we are, although the extent of influence of each is debated.

Nature refers to the traits, capacities, and limitations that a person inherits from parents at conception.

- Examples: hair and eye color, body type, and inherited diseases
- Possible examples: athletic or musical ability

Nurture refers to the environmental influences that occur after conception, including the mother's health before birth and the child's environment thereafter. Nurture takes what nature gives us and molds us as we grow and mature. The interaction between the two is a critical influence in our development.

SAFE AND EFFECTIVE NURSING CARE: Clinical Pearl

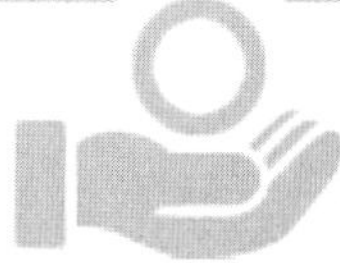

Definition of *Family*

Family is defined as the structure or the relationship between individuals that provides the financial and emotional support needed for social functioning (Friedemann, 1995). Nurses should not be judgmental when caring for patients and their families. We must remember that every family acts as a unique unit.

FAMILY

The nuclear family is composed of a mother, a father, and a biological or adopted child or children. The term nonnuclear family describes family forms other than traditional, such as single-parent homes, grandparents functioning in the role of parents, same-sex parents with a child or children, and blended families, in which families from divorce are joined together by remarriage. This can also occur when a spouse has died and the remaining spouse remarries. (See Chapter 3 for further details on the family.)

BEHAVIORIST AND SOCIAL LEARNING THEORY

Developed as a response to psychoanalytical theories, behaviorist and social learning theories describe the importance of the environment and nurturing of a child. Behaviorist theory was the dominant view from the 1920s through 1960s, with John B. Watson, Ivan Pavlov, and B. F. Skinner as some of the most noted theorists. Behaviorist theories are based on observable behaviors that arise from either classical or operant conditioning.

- Classical conditioning is "a learning process that occurs through associations between an environmental stimulus and a naturally occurring stimulus" (Cherry, 2016).
- Operant conditioning is a change in behavior based on rewards, reinforcement, and punishment (Cherry, 2016).

SAFE AND EFFECTIVE NURSING CARE: Clinical Pearl

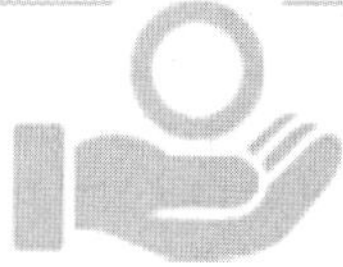

Growth Based on Experiences

Behaviorists believe that children are born with a "blank slate," and as they grow and develop they are changed based on their experiences. Nursing and child life specialists can use stickers, rewards, and praise to let children know they did a great job after a procedure such as an IV insertion or a blood pressure reading.

Social Learning Theory: Albert Bandura

Albert Bandura was born in 1925 and is still alive today. He completed the famous Bobo doll experiment that demonstrated the power of observation. When children observed violent acts, they mimicked them; when an adult was praised for those acts, the children were more likely to repeat them (Bandura, 2006). Bandura's theory posits that children learn through observing others in their environment, as well as from rewards and punishments. Intrinsic reinforcements such as satisfaction and accomplishment lead to learning. Through observing the actions of other people, children develop new skills and acquire new information.

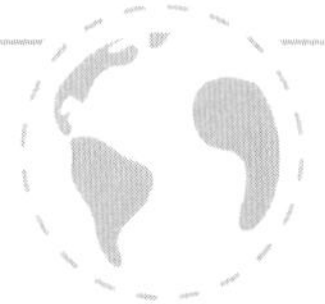

SAFE AND EFFECTIVE NURSING CARE: Cultural Competence

Environment and Culture

A child's ability to master tasks and grow and develop in the proper way is affected by numerous factors. The environment and culture are two areas that should always be assessed. A child needs an appropriate environment and proper stimuli, or development may be delayed.

FACTORS THAT AFFECT GROWTH AND DEVELOPMENT

Although growth and development follow predictable patterns, these patterns are influenced by a number of factors.

Intrauterine Factors

The mother's health and nutritional status while pregnant affect the fetus.

- Poor nutrition in the mother can lead to low-birth-weight babies, as well as slow development, compromised neurological performance, and impaired immune status (Ward & Hisley, 2015).
- Low iron levels in the mother can result in anemia in the infant (National Institutes of Health, 2016).
- Maternal smoking can result in infants with low birth weight and/or congenital anomalies such as cleft lip and cleft palate.
- Ingestion of alcohol during pregnancy may lead to delays and fetal alcohol syndrome.
- Substance and drug abuse prenatally may result in neonatal addiction, convulsions, hyperirritability, poor social responsiveness, neurological disturbances, and changes in the cognitive functioning of the child (Ward & Hisley, 2015).
- Prescription and nonprescription drugs may affect the unborn child.
- Certain maternal illnesses can harm the fetus, such as rubella.
- Exposure of the mother to environmental factors, such as chemicals or radiation, can harm the fetus.

Birth Events (Prematurity, Birth Trauma)

Premature infants can experience delayed growth and development, and are thus expected to reach developmental milestones at the same age they would have reached them if born at normal gestational age. Age is adjusted for assessments: subtract the weeks/months that the infant was born prematurely from the current chronological age. The child should be reaching the adjusted age milestones. Most premature children have caught up with all the milestones/developmental tasks by age 2 years (Beckett & Taylor, 2016).

Chronic Illness and Hospitalization

Illness and hospitalization are stressful events for a child and family. A child's physical state of well-being can affect developmental levels, because illness may interfere with normal progression by causing the child delays in acquiring the skills needed to progress to the next level. When a child is hospitalized, the family routine is disrupted, and the child and family are not able to do what they normally do. The possible separation of family members because of the child's illness adds stress.

CRITICAL COMPONENT

Play as a Stress Reducer

Play is what children do and should not be overlooked when a child is in the hospital. Play can be a diversional activity and a stress reducer, and provides the hospitalized child with an opportunity to act out fears and anxieties. Many children's hospitals provide the ill child with a playroom and the services of a child life specialist who can assist the child in fostering growth and developmental needs through play. The child life specialist has a strong background in growth and development, and can use this training to assist the medical team in preparing a child for hospitalization and procedures.

SAFE AND EFFECTIVE NURSING CARE: Clinical Pearl

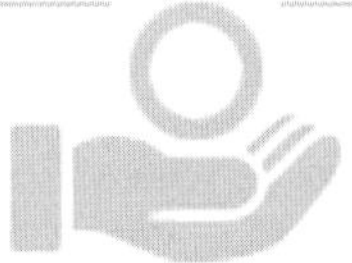

Separation Anxiety

Nurses need to take into account growth and developmental stages when a child is hospitalized or ill. Ages 6 to 9 months often go through separation anxiety. They will often find more comfort in familiar people than strangers. Being in the hospital can trigger separation anxiety for toddlers (2–3 years). Preschoolers can fear body mutilations, the dark, being left alone, and ghosts (Beckett & Taylor, 2016).

Environmental Factors

Children who are abused or neglected experience problems in numerous areas of growth and development; examples of common problem areas are sleeping and feeding disorders. The child may also experience delays in learning to trust others and disorders of attachment.

Abuse can be physical, including beatings, burns, or other physical injuries; emotional, including constantly yelling at, ridiculing, or putting a child down; or sexual, including any sexual activity with a child younger than 18 years and commanding a child to perform sexual acts with another adult or child. Areas that are considered neglect include:

- Medical
  - Not providing common medical care
  - Not allowing a child who is ill to consult a health-care provider
  - Death of a child from an illness that is considered treatable by Western health care
- Emotional
  - Not attending to the child's emotional needs
  - Ignoring the child
  - Leaving the child alone for significant amounts of time
- Educational
  - Not providing education for the child in any manner
  - Not providing the child needed aids to encourage education (hearing aids, speech therapy, etc.)
- Abandonment
  - Leaving a child to care for himself or herself
  - Not providing adequate adult supervision

CRITICAL COMPONENT

Nursing is one of the professions required by law to report any suspected child abuse or neglect. Circumstances, protocols, and paperwork may vary from state to state, but reporting to the authorities when you suspect or have reason to believe a child is in harm is necessary and mandated for the health-care professional. More information about mandatory reporting for the health-care professional can be found at the Child Welfare Information Gateway website.

SAFE AND EFFECTIVE NURSING CARE: Promoting Safety

Physical Home Environment

A safe and healthy home environment is needed for normal growth and development. The quality of housing and access to basic services—such as clean water, sanitation and waste disposal, fuel for cooking and heating, and ventilation—need to be addressed with the family. Exposure to lead paint, radon, and electromagnetic sources should also be assessed, because these can affect normal growth and development (Sly et al., 2009).

BASIC NEEDS

Basic needs at each level of someone's life must be met before they can progress to the next level of growth and development. These are outlined by Maslow's hierarchy of needs:

- Level one: Physiological needs must be met first: food, rest, air, water.
- Level two: The child has the need to be protected from harm and feel safe.
- Level three: Feeling loved and part of a group.
- Level four: Esteem needs to develop—the need to respect yourself and be respected by others.
- Level five: Self-actualization, or becoming a complete person and reaching your greatest potential (Price & Gwin, 2012).

SAFE AND EFFECTIVE NURSING CARE: Clinical Pearls

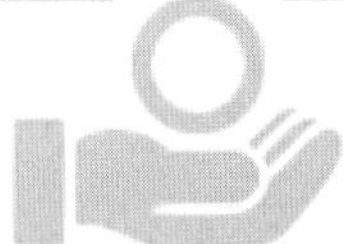

Sleep Deprivation

Children need more sleep than adults. Sleep deprivation can impact the growth and development of a child and cause delays. Preschoolers, for example, need 12 hours of sleep a day (Price & Gwin, 2012).

CRITICAL COMPONENT

Early Parent–Child Relationships

Early parent–child relationships have been shown to play a major role in a child's social-emotional development. This relationship also influences and is linked to cognitive development and learning patterns. Feeling loved and cared for can enhance development in these areas (Ward & Hisley, 2015).

Socioeconomic Factors

Lack of income can affect a child's health and development; families who are struggling to make ends meet may be unable to afford healthy food and lack transportation to health-care facilities. When both parents work, they may have little time to devote to meeting their children's emotional needs.

Cultural Background

Cultural background influences how children are socialized and how they experience the world around them. Beliefs, customs, and values are learned from cultural surroundings. (See Chapter 4 for further discussion of cultural factors.) Everyone is a product of their cultural background. Culture does more than shape our preferences; it is the foundation of our worldviews. The cultural identity of a child and the family is always relevant and must be considered in the care that we give (Price & Gwin, 2012).

SAFE AND EFFECTIVE NURSING CARE: Cultural Competence

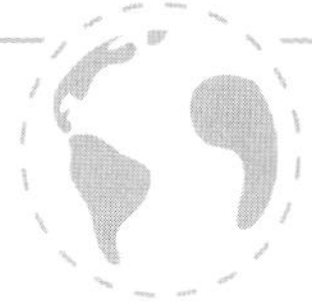

Cultural Factors

Nurses must consider a child's cultural background when doing developmental testing. Children may not be familiar with specific games or activities used in the test. There could be possible language barriers that interfere with reliable testing. Another part of culture, religion, may be meaningful to the family. The need for spiritual clergy can be important to both the child and the family.

Case Study

Emily is a manager in a technology company who is currently on maternity leave following the birth of her second child. While she is on leave, she attends the community center sporadically with her two daughters. Audrey has just turned 4 years old and will be attending kindergarten soon. Kathryn is 4 months old. Emily usually does not interact much with staff at the community center, but today she asks questions about Kathryn's sleep patterns. Kathryn still wakes up two to three times per night and Emily is exhausted. Her wife is a company executive and travels a lot. Emily admits that her wife thinks she must be doing something wrong with Kathryn, because Audrey was a better sleeper. She can't stand Kathryn's crying in the evening and her frequent waking at night. Emily has been reading some books and thinks she should be able to get Kathryn into a routine that includes sleeping for 8 hours at night. She is very frustrated. While you are talking with Emily, Kathryn is playing with a toy and is watching other children playing nearby. She coos and makes sounds. As soon as she makes a noise Emily puts a pacifier in her mouth. Audrey is playing with some of the other children. A little boy takes the toy she has been playing with, and she tries to take it back. When that doesn't work, she throws herself on the floor and screams. Emily quickly offers her treats from her purse. Emily states Audrey has frequent outbursts at home and she does not know how to deal with them.

1. What stage of development are Audrey and Kathryn in according to Erikson?
2. What factors can have an impact on Audrey's development?
3. What strengths and weaknesses does the family have?
4. What strategies based on Kathryn's development can the nurse suggest?
5. What concerns can you identify regarding Emily's parenting of the girls?

REFERENCES

Bandura, A. (2006). Autobiography. In M. G. Lindzey & W. M. Runyan (Eds.), *A history of psychology in autobiography* (Vol. IX). Washington, DC: American Psychological Association.

Beckett, C., & Taylor, H. (2016). *Human growth and development* (3rd ed.). London: Sage-Publications, Inc.

Berk, L. E. (2013). *Development through the lifespan* (6th ed.). Boston, MA: Allyn and Bacon.

Centers for Disease Control and Prevention. (2013). Lesbian, gay, bisexual, and transgender health. Retrieved from https://www.cdc.gov/lgbthealth/links.htm

Centers for Disease Control and Prevention. (2016). *Learn the signs. Act early.* Retrieved from http://www.cdc.gov/ncbddd/actearly/milestones/index.html

Cherry, K. (2016). *Psychology theories.* Retrieved from https://www.verywell.com/behavioral-psychology-4013681

Friedemann, M. L. (1995). *The framework of systemic organization: A conceptual approach to families and nursing.* Thousand Oakes, CA: Sage.

Institute for Patient- and Family-Centered Care. (2014). *Strategies for changing policies.* Retrieved from http://www.ipfcc.org

McLeod, S. A. (2016). Id, ego and superego. Retrieved from https://www.simplypsychology.org/psyche.html

National Institutes of Health. (2016). *Iron dietary supplement fact sheet.* Retrieved from https://ods.od.nih.gov/factsheets/Iron-HealthProfessional/

Potts, N. L., & Mandleco, B. L. (2013). *Pediatric nursing: Caring for children and their families* (3rd ed.). Clifton Park, NY: Thomson and Delmar Learning.

Price, D. L., & Gwin, J. F. (2012). *Thompson's pediatric nursing* (11th ed.). St. Louis, MO: Elsevier Saunders.

Sly, P. D., Eskenazi, B., Pronczuk, J., Sram, R., Diaz-Barriga, F., Machin, D. G., & Meslin, E. M. (2009). Ethical issues in measuring biomarkers in children's environmental health. *Environmental Health Perspectives, 111*, 1185–1190.

Ward, S., & Hisley, S. M. (2015). *Maternal-child nursing care with the women's health companion: Optimizing outcomes for mothers, children and families* (2nd ed.) Philadelphia: F.A. Davis.

7 Newborns and Infants

Kathryn Rudd, DNP, RNC-NIC, c-NPT

LEARNING OUTCOMES

Upon completion of this chapter, the student will be able to:

1. Describe the perinatal factors that affect the newborn during the transition process.
2. Describe the growth and development that occur during the newborn and infancy period.
3. Describe the physical assessment approaches for the newborn and infant.
4. Discuss the variations in nursing procedures related to the care of the newborn and infant.
5. Describe approaches to medication administration in the newborn and infant.
6. Describe the health promotion functions necessary in an infant and newborn's family structure.
7. Discuss the emergency care of the newborn and infant.
8. Describe the specific characteristics of care of the hospitalized newborn and infant.
9. Describe the specific characteristics of a pediatric medical home during the newborn and infancy period.
10. Discuss chronic care of the newborn and infant.
11. Describe the importance and function of play in the newborn and infant's life.
12. Describe the safety measures needed to care for a newborn and infant in the home.
13. Discuss alternative/complementary therapies for the family of the newborn and infant.
14. Describe child abuse considerations in the newborn and infant populations.

CARE OF THE NEONATE

A child younger than 28 days old is a newborn or neonate. The term *newborn* refers to any preterm, term, or post mature child. The infancy period comprises ages 1 month to 1 year.

- Gestation is the duration of pregnancy, measured in weeks.
  - The average full-term baby is born between the first day of the 38th week and the first day of the 42nd week of pregnancy.
  - A preterm infant is born before the end of the 37th week of pregnancy.
- Viability is a term used to determine the rate of survival.
  - Less than 22 weeks' gestation is considered not viable.
  - At 23 weeks' gestation, 17% survive.
  - At 24 weeks' gestation, 39% survive.
  - At 25 weeks' gestation, 50% survive.
  - At 26 weeks' gestation, 80% survive.
  - At 27 weeks' gestation, 90% survive.
  - At 28 to 31 weeks' gestation, 90% to 95% survive.
  - At 32 to 33 weeks' gestation, 95% survive.
  - At 34+ weeks' gestation, survival is similar to that of a full-term infant (Ehrenkranz & Mercurio, 2017).
  - Post mature infant: Refers to infant born after 42 weeks of pregnancy.
- Care associated with most full-term infants at 38 weeks' gestation primarily protects and supports the neonate during its physiological transition to extrauterine life. This includes:
  - Delivery room and transitional care
  - Maintenance of thermoregulation
  - Newborn assessment with a review of the maternal history and a complete physical examination
  - Prophylaxis care to prevent disorders specifically related to respiratory function and decreasing risk for infections

- Family education and discharge preparation related to caring for and feeding the newborn

Pertaining to the immediate needs of the newborn, the predominant role of the nurse is to assess the newborn in the transition period, protect his or her physical well-being, and promote a family-centered environment. Priorities include the following:

- Clear the airway. Wipe mouth and nose with the delivery of the head. If suctioning, suction mouth first, then nose to remove mucus and blood with bulb syringe. Depress bulb first and then insert into the orifice to remove secretions. Infant should be positioned on his or her back with the neck slightly extended or in a "sniffing position." Hyperextension of the neck is contraindicated because it will occlude the airway.

SAFE AND EFFECTIVE NURSING CARE: Clinical Pearl

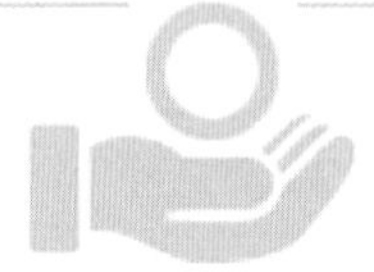

Inserting the Syringe for Suctioning

When inserting the bulb syringe, insert it in the corner of the mouth, not the center. Always suction the mouth first and then the nose. Suctioning the nose first may cause the infant to gasp and thereby force mucus deeper into the respiratory tract (see Fig. 7–1).

Hint for Students: M for mouth comes before N for nose in the alphabet.

- Dry and stimulate the infant.
- Maintain thermoregulation with immediate drying and removal of wet linens. Chilling increases oxygen consumption and metabolism through the process of evaporation.
- Assign the Apgar score, based on the system developed in 1952 by Dr. Virginia Apgar (Table 7–1).
  - The Apgar scoring system evaluates a neonate's ability to adapt to the birthing process.

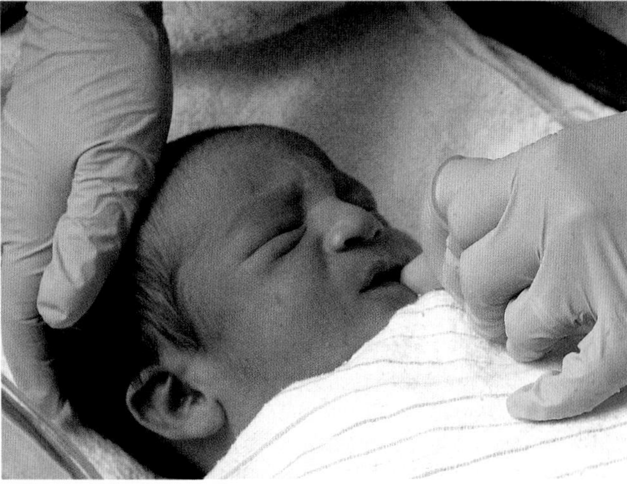

FIGURE 7–1 Bulb suctioning.

  - It determines the need for resuscitation, the effectiveness of the resuscitation, and the neonate's morbidity and mortality risks.
  - The Apgar system measures respiratory rate, heart rate, muscle tone, color, and reflex irritability, assigning an overall score from 0 to 10. The neonate is rated with a zero, a number one, or a number two for each category.
    - Total score of 0 to 2 = severely depressed
    - Total score of 3 to 6 = moderately depressed
    - Total score of 7 to 10 = good condition
  - Number scores are assigned at 1 and 5 minutes. A higher score indicates adequate adaptation.
  - The Apgar score at 1 minute indicates the neonate's ability to transition to extrauterine life, factors occurring during the birthing process, and whether resuscitation is needed.
  - The Apgar score at 5 minutes indicates the neonate's status and/or the effectiveness of resuscitative efforts, as well as neurological deficits and long-term morbidity and mortality.
- Band infant with on-demand or barcode on arm and leg, with corresponding bands applied to the mother and significant other if present in the delivery room.

SAFE AND EFFECTIVE NURSING CARE: Promoting Safety

Security Bands

Alert staff to similar or identical last names on labor, delivery, and postpartum units. All caregivers must check the bands against the correct information, such as infant's name, mother's name, sex, medical record number, and date of birth. Many institutions use umbilical cord clamp bands and electronic tags that if removed from the infant's body will lock and shut down elevators and doors. All infants should also have their own baby bands with their own unique identifiers of name, sex, date of birth, and medical record number. Limited human-readable data are present with on-demand and barcode information. Careful attention should be paid to the identification of multiples. Some institutions use footprints or photos of infants for additional identification.

- Administer baby prophylactic medications (Table 7–2).
  - Phytonadione (vitamin K_1): Newborns are born with a sterile intestinal tract and do not have the bacteria necessary to synthesize vitamin K. Therefore, newborns have decreased levels of vitamin K, the nutrient responsible for clotting and preventing hemorrhages.
  - Erythromycin eye ointment prevents serious eye infections such as gonorrhea and chlamydia eye infections, and should not be washed away.
  - Hepatitis B immunization is given to prevent hepatitis B. Mothers with unknown hepatitis B status are also administered human hepatitis B immunoglobulin G (IgG).

TABLE 7–1 Neonatal Apgar Scoring

Sign	SCORE 0	1	2
Respiratory effort	Absent	Slow, irregular	Good cry
Heart rate	Absent	Slow, below 100 bpm	Above 100 bpm
Muscle tone	Flaccid	Some flexion of extremities	Active motion
Reflex activity	None	Grimace	Vigorous cry
Color	Pale, blue	Body pink, blue extremities	Completely pink

Source: Durham, R., & Chapman, L. (2014). Maternal-newborn nursing: Critical components of nursing care *(2nd ed.). Philadelphia: F.A. Davis.*

- Protect the physical well-being of the newborn.
  - Prevent the spread of infection through strict hand hygiene, limited traffic in the labor and delivery room suite, the use of scrub clothing by personnel to minimize infection exposure, and prohibitions against artificial nails and nail polish.
  - Provide baby cord care, circumcision care, and infant bathing.
- Foster parent–infant bonding; promote family-centered care.

MATERNAL HISTORY

During newborn care, a maternal history should be taken that includes:

- Review of prenatal history, including past pregnancies, complications, genetic factors for both mother and father, and previous pregnancies
- Infections—prenatal as well as past exposures

TABLE 7–2 Prophylactic Medications for Newborns and Infants

BABY MEDICATION	AQUAMEPHYTON, PHYTONADIONE, VITAMIN K	ERYTHROMYCIN, TETRACYCLINE, EYE OINTMENT, SILVER NITRATE	HEPATITIS B, ENERIX-B, RECOMBIVAX HB
Uses	Prevent hemorrhagic disease of the newborn by enhancing the liver's synthesis of clotting factors II, VII, IX, and X	Prevent transmission of infections of gonorrhea and chlamydial ophthalmia during passage through the birth canal	Prevent hepatitis B, a liver disease caused by the hepatitis B virus that can cause serious chronic liver disease and cancer of the liver
Side effects	Pain at the injection site	Silver nitrate can cause eye irritation, goopy discharge of the eyes, or slight redness of the eyes	Pain at the injection site
Administration	Single dose of 0.5 (for preterm) to 1.0 mg (for full term) IM within 1 hour of birth Injection site is vastus lateralis muscle—lies lateral to the midline of the thigh	1-cm thin ribbon administered from inner canthus to outer canthus on lower eyelid	Vaccinate all newborns with monovalent vaccine before discharge—0.5 mL IM for first dose Given within 12 hours with hepatitis B immune globulin if mother is hepatitis B positive or status is unknown; given at discharge if mother's status is known to be negative Massage area for dispersion of the drug Injection site is vastus lateralis muscle
Special considerations	Protect from light Mandated by state laws	Do not delay administration beyond 1 hour following delivery Mandated by state laws	Follow immunization schedule for administration; some parents defer to first pediatrician appointment Series of three doses, given in vastus lateralis

Source: Vallerand, A. H., Sanoski, C. A., (2017). Davis's drug guide for nurses *(16th ed.). Philadelphia: F.A. Davis.*

- Screening tests and risk factors
- Labor and delivery problems or risk factors
- Perinatal substance abuse exposure

Perinatal Substance Abuse

Substance abuse can affect the developing fetus through exposure to nicotine, selective serotonin-reuptake inhibitors, benzodiazepines, alcohol, opiates, or other substances. The incidence of neonatal abstinence syndrome has quadrupled within the last decade and continues to increase (Patrick et al., 2015). Neonatal abstinence occurs secondary to opioid exposure, resulting in central nervous system irritability, autonomic nervous system dysfunction, and gastrointestinal and respiratory dysfunction (Jones & Fielder, 2015).

Biological neonatal specimens are obtained from meconium, hair, cord blood, and urine for testing. The Finnegan Neonatal Abstinence Scoring Tool is the most widely used tool to assign numbers to neonatal symptoms of exposure, including central nervous system disturbances, gastrointestinal disturbances, and metabolic, vasomotor, and respiratory disturbances (McQueen & Murphy-Oikonen, 2016). Scoring should occur every 3 hours before feedings.

Nonpharmacological interventions include swaddling, comfort, and feeding. Pharmacological interventions are with morphine sulfate or methadone adjusted based on scores greater than 8. Doses are then weaned if scores are less than or equal to 8 for 48 hours or more (McQueen & Murphy-Oikonen, 2016). The American Academy of Pediatrics (AAP) recommends opioid replacement therapy for infants who do not respond to nonpharmacological management to alleviate the signs and symptoms of neonatal abstinence syndrome and to prevent seizures, weight loss, and other long-term complications (Boucher, 2017).

TRANSITION TO EXTRAUTERINE LIFE

The transition to extrauterine life begins in utero as the fetus prepares for this transition. Intrauterine changes are dependent on gestational age, maternal health factors, condition of the placenta, and/or defects and congenital abnormalities. In utero, the lungs are filled with amniotic fluid, and the placenta is the organ of respiration and waste removal.

Respiratory System Transition

Transition occurs when the umbilical cord is clamped and the infant takes his or her first breath. All body systems of the neonate transition to extrauterine life, but most significant are the respiratory and circulatory system transitions. When the cord is cut, the placenta is no longer the organ of respiration. Several factors influence the first breath, including:

- Internal stimuli such as chemical changes due to hypoxia and increasing carbon dioxide levels

CRITICAL COMPONENT

Family-Centered Care

The following tenets are central concepts of patient- and family-centered care:

- Dignity and respect: Health-care practitioners listen to and honor patient and family perspectives and choices. Patient and family knowledge, values, beliefs, and cultural backgrounds are incorporated into the planning and delivery of care.
- Information sharing: Health-care practitioners communicate and share complete and unbiased information with patients and families in affirming and useful ways. Patients and families receive timely, complete, and accurate information to effectively participate in care and decision making.
- Participation: Patients and families are encouraged to participate in care and decision making at the level they choose.
- Collaboration: Patients, families, health-care practitioners, and hospital leaders collaborate in policy and program development, implementation, and evaluation; in health-care facility design; and in professional education, as well as in the delivery of care.

Source: Institute for Patient- and Family-Centered Care (2017).

SAFE AND EFFECTIVE NURSING CARE: Clinical Pearl

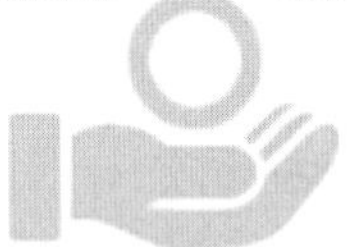

Recognizing Normal Vital Signs

Temperature:

Normal range: 36.5°C–37.0°C (97.7°F–99.4°F)

Pulse:

- 120–160 bpm (count apical pulse rate for 1 full minute)
- Rate increases to 180 bpm if crying and 100 bpm if sleeping

Respirations:

- 30–60 breaths per minute (count respiratory rate for 1 full minute)
- Irregular, diaphragmatic, and abdominal breathing are normal.
- Rate increases when crying and decreases when sleeping.
- Apneic (absence of breathing) is significant if it lasts longer than 15–20 seconds.
- Hold oral feedings if respiratory rate is greater than 60 breaths per minute.

Blood pressure is not a routine part of neonatal vital sign assessments. If requested to perform, blood pressure should be obtained on the arm or leg.

- Systolic 50–75 mm Hg
- Diastolic 30–45 mm Hg

Adapted from Ward & Hisley (2015) and Durham & Chapman (2014).

- External stimuli such as thermal changes, sensory changes, or mechanical changes due to the delivery process (Figure 7–2; Ward & Hisley, 2015)
  - The first breath begins to clear amniotic fluid and fill the lungs with oxygen. This increases alveoli oxygen tension (PaO_2), which dilates the pulmonary artery, decreases pulmonary vascular resistance, increases pulmonary blood flow, and increases O_2 and CO_2 exchange (see Chapter 12).
  - The fetus produces surfactant at 34 weeks' gestation. This phospholipid created in the alveoli of the lungs decreases surface tension, allowing the alveoli sacs to remain partially open on expiration. This decreases the amount of pressure and energy required for the fetus to take the next breath as he or she practices breathing in utero. Alterations in this system's transition result from insufficient production of surfactant because of prematurity, hypoxia, and acidosis, all of which increase pulmonary vascular resistance.
  - Retained alveolar fluid can result in transient tachypnea of the newborn. Insufficient surfactant production can result in collapsed alveoli and the development of respiratory distress syndrome (RDS), a disease that results in poor lung compliance, loss of residual capacity, and chronic lung changes. RDS is prominent in premature infants. Failure of the normal drop in pulmonary vascular pressure can result in persistent pulmonary hypertension of the newborn. These alterations require specialized medical care in neonatal intensive care units that support the neonate's respiratory system.

Newborn Respiratory Assessment and Development

When assessing the respiratory system of a newborn, nurses should be aware of the following:

- Assess the nose for patency. Newborns are obligate nose breathers, but after several months they become nose-and-mouth breathers.
- Chest wall symmetry/asymmetry can be a result of pneumothorax.
- Respiratory pattern is normally very irregular, sporadic, shallow, and diaphragmatic.
- Average rate at birth is 30 to 60 breaths per minute; count for a full minute (McKee-Garrett, Weisman, & Duryea, 2017).
- Respiratory rate decreases with age.
- Acrocyanosis (bluish color of hands and feet) is normal in the term infant in the first 24 to 48 hours. After 24 to 48 hours of life, this may be an indication of cardiac disease (see Chapter 12).
- In dark-skinned infants, cyanosis is better assessed through the mucous membranes.
- Older infants become diaphragmatic breathers.

CRITICAL COMPONENT

Signs and Symptoms of Alterations in Respiratory Transitioning

Newborns who are experiencing alterations in respiratory transitioning may display:

- Cyanosis
- Apnea: a cessation of breathing longer than 15 to 20 seconds; may or may not be associated with change in color or heart rate
- Gasping: deep, slow, irregular terminal breaths (McKee-Garrett et al., 2017)
- Flaring: outward flaring movements of the nostrils on inspiration due to forced airflow
- Excessive mucus or drooling
- Tachypnea: respiratory rate greater than 60 breaths per minute when quiet
- Tachycardia: heart rate more than 160 bpm when quiet
- Chest wall asymmetry
- Grunting: audible expiratory groaning heard on expiration due to a partial closing of the glottis (McKee-Garrett et al., 2017)
- Retractions are backward movements of the sternum or intercostal spaces of the ribs due to increased negative pressure; retractions may be suprasternal, supraclavicular, intercostal, subcostal, and/or substernal
- Congenital abnormalities (see Chapter 11)

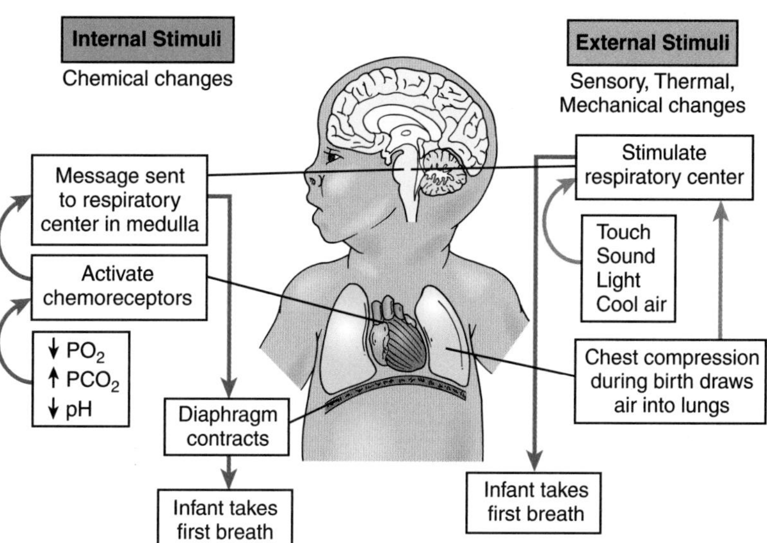

FIGURE 7–2 Stimuli that influence respirations.

Circulatory System Transition and Assessment

Circulatory system transition occurs with the clamping of the cord and the first breath (Figure 7–3). The successful transition is directly influenced by the changes that occur in the respiratory and thermoregulation systems. Three fetal structures maintain fetal circulation:

- The ductus arteriosus, between the pulmonary artery and the aorta
- The foramen ovale is the connection between the right and left atria
- The ductus venosus in the hepatic system (Figure 7–4)

As pulmonary vascular resistance decreases, placental secretion of prostaglandins (PGE_1) decreases, the fetal ducts close, and the transition occurs (see Chapter 12). Nurses conducting an assessment of a newborn's circulatory system should be aware of the following:

- Three vessels should be present in the umbilical cord: two arteries and one vein. The presence of only two vessel cords may indicate renal agenesis or lack of development.
- Cord blood may be obtained from an Rh-negative mom or O blood group. Blood gases may be obtained if O_2 levels are decreased or Apgar scores are depressed at 5 minutes of age.
- Newborn heart rate (apical) averages 120 to 160 bpm at rest but can increase with crying and decrease with sleeping. Count for a full minute. Heart rate decreases as the infant ages.
- All peripheral pulses should be palpable and normal in intensity.
- Blood pressure increases with age (see Chapter 12).

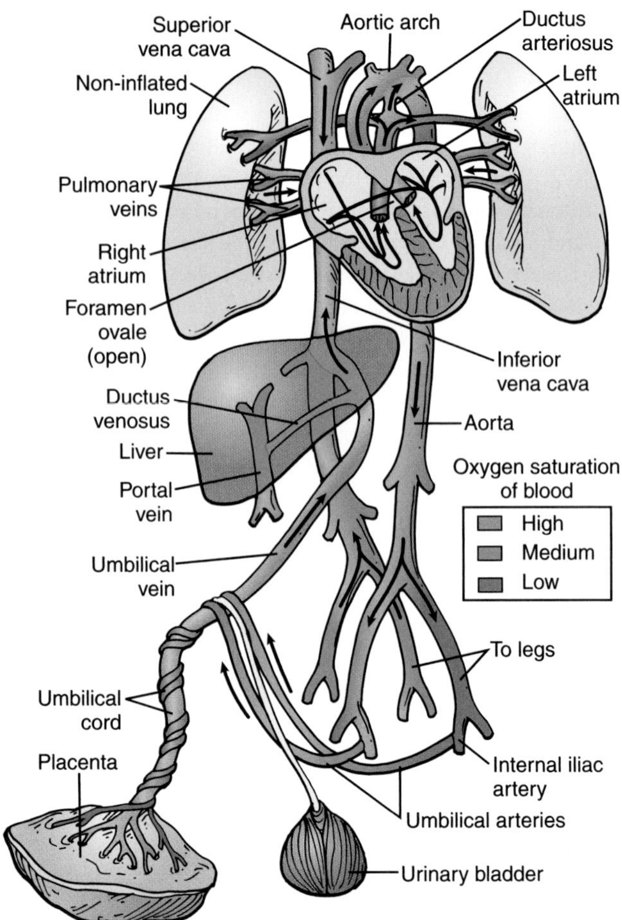

FIGURE 7–4 Fetal circulation.

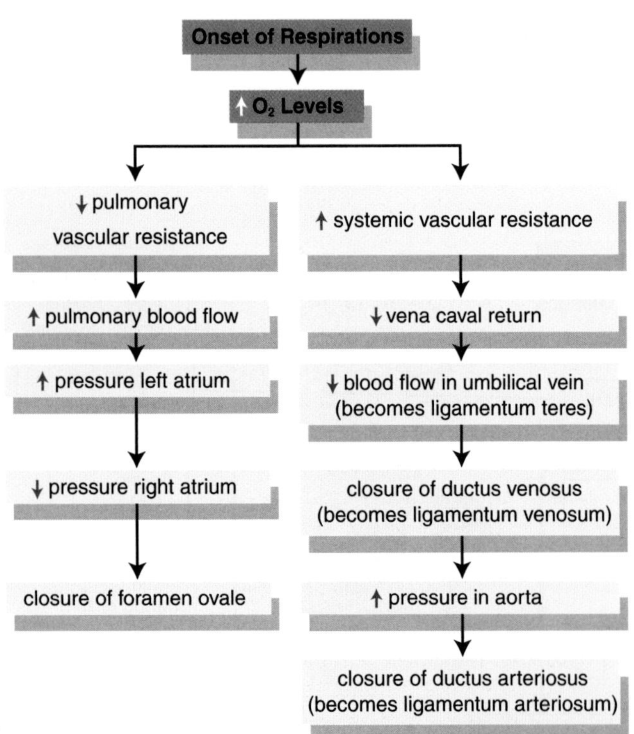

FIGURE 7–3 Transition from fetal to neonatal circulation.

- Four extremity blood pressures are indicated with heart murmur (see Chapter 12), turbulent blood flow heard by a stethoscope as swooshing or whooshing. Murmurs may be present at birth and can be completely normal (see Chapter 12).
- Brisk capillary refill should be less than 3 seconds; abnormal is longer than 4 seconds.
- Congenital abnormalities are related to failure of the fetal structures to close, structural abnormalities, or blood outflow problems (see Chapter 12).

Thermoregulatory System Transition and Assessment

The thermoregulatory system is necessary for sustaining homeostasis and is dependent on external and internal factors. Neutral thermal environment is the temperature the infant requires to minimize metabolic and oxygen needs, prevent metabolic acidosis, and arrest brown fat depletion.

- Normal neonatal temperature is 36.5°C to 37.0°C through axillary method (under the armpit) (see Figure 7–5).
- Normal rectal temperatures range from 36.5°C to 37.5°C; in many institutions, these must be ordered and are performed with great care to avoid rectal injury. A rectal temperature may be done initially to assess for anal patency. This is per hospital policy.

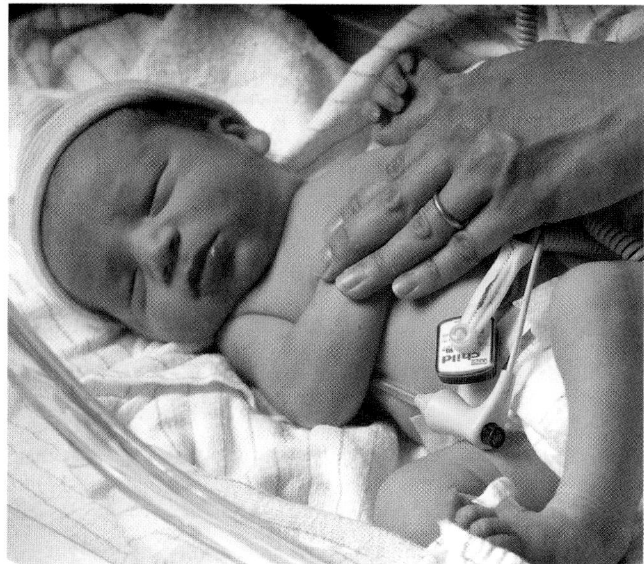

FIGURE 7–5 Taking an infant's temperature.

- Gestational-age term infants have stores of brown fat (brown adipose tissue [BAT]) in the neck, intrascapular region, axillae, groin, and around the kidney area (Figure 7–6). Brown fat is used and burned for heat metabolism. Weight and prematurity affect the infant's ability to regulate body temperature because of decreased brown and subcutaneous fat stores.
- Full-term infants have increased body surface area compared with total body mass.
- Neonates have a higher metabolic rate. Term infants can lose heat even in the first few minutes and hours after birth. Exposure to cold in a newborn sets off alterations in physiological and metabolic processes to generate heat. An infant's response to cold includes the following:
    - Peripheral vasoconstriction and chemical thermogenesis take place.
    - Newborns do not shiver.
    - The sympathetic nervous system responds by decreasing the temperature and stimulation of skin receptors, many in the face, to increase peripheral vasoconstriction.
    - Brown fat utilization breaks down fat into glycerol and fatty acids to produce heat. Rapid utilization of brown fat can result in metabolic acidosis, jaundice, infection, and poor weight gain because of thermogenesis, which increases oxygen demands and caloric consumption.

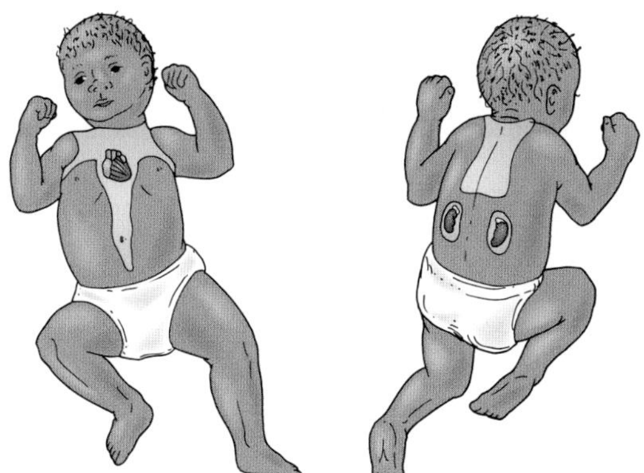

FIGURE 7–6 Sites of "brown fat" (brown adipose tissue stores) in the newborn.

CRITICAL COMPONENT

Signs and Symptoms of Cold Stress

Cold stress occurs when the newborn's body temperature decreases, which results in an increase in oxygen consumption, glucose utilization, and energy. This then increases the burning of BAT, depletion of glycogen stores, a decrease in surfactant, respiratory distress, and metabolic acidosis. Cold stress can result in significant morbidity and mortality in the newborn infant (see Figure 7–7).

Cold stress is characterized by:

- Jitteriness
- Tachypnea
- Grunting
- Hypoglycemia
- Hypotonia (can exacerbate heat loss)
- Pallor
- Lethargy
- Poor sucking reflex

SAFE AND EFFECTIVE NURSING CARE: Clinical Pearl

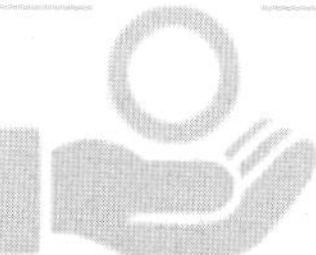

Heat Loss in the Newborn

The newborn can lose heat in a variety of different ways. Heat loss can result in peripheral vasoconstriction, a buildup of lactic acid, and metabolic acidosis. The nurse is responsible for minimizing heat loss through a variety of mechanisms that include the following:

- Radiation heat loss occurs through transfer of heat to the cooler air surrounding the neonate. This can occur when an infant is placed near a window or the cold walls of a single-walled isolette. The nurse should make sure that if a newborn is placed in an isolette that it is a double-walled isolette.
- Conduction—transfer of heat directly from the infant to a cooler surface or equipment. Place the infant on a warm surface, remove wet linens, and cover the infant's head. Cover cold surfaces with a warmed blanket.
- Convection—transfer of heat through drafts passing over the infant, such as from fans, air drafts, blowing oxygen, if the sides of the radiant warmer are down, or air conditioners.
- Evaporation—transfer of heat when water on the surface of the infant's skin is converted to water vapor. The nurse should make sure that the infant is dried after delivery and after a bath.

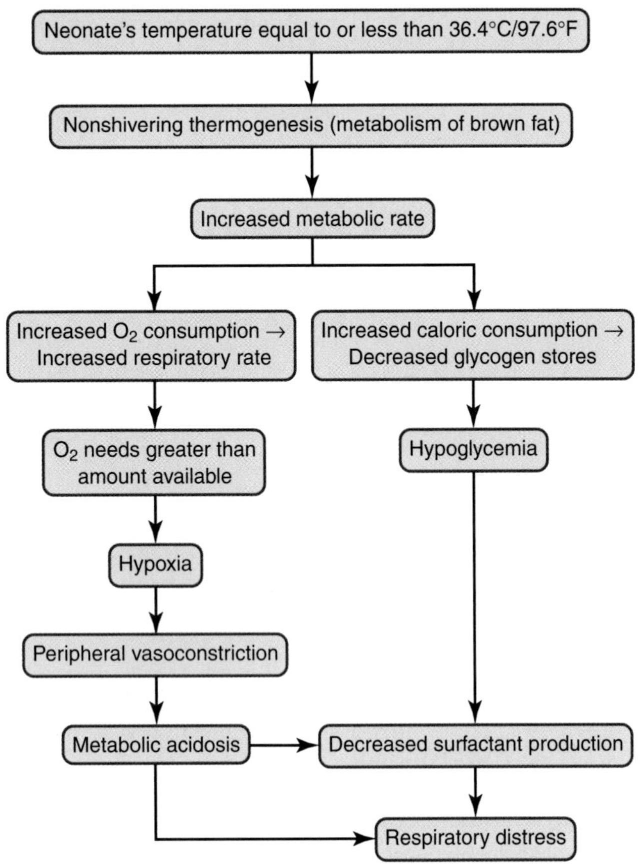

FIGURE 7–7 Cold stress.

Nursing Interventions to Prevent Hypothermia

- Place infant skin to skin (preferably kangaroo care) with mom or on a radiant warmer to rewarm.
- Remove wet linens, which cause heat loss through radiation and conduction.
- Maintain dry, warmed linen as the most effective means of rewarming an infant.
- Delay the first bath until the infant has regulated and stabilized core body temperature. The first bath should be completed in the presence of the mother to support infant bonding and completed with kangaroo care.
- Keep the infant's head (largest surface area) covered with a stocking cap to prevent heat loss due to radiation and conduction, except if the infant is placed in a sleep sack.
- Wrap the infant in t-shirt, pajamas, and two blankets to decrease heat loss from convection and radiation.
- If these measures are not effective, place the naked infant on a radiant warmer, place the servo-control probe on the infant's abdomen (avoiding bony prominences, liver, and brown fat areas), and set the temperature at least to 36.5°C.
- A radiant warmer only heats the outer surfaces, so do not clothe or cover the infant.
- Do not artificially heat an IV bag or K pad device and apply to rewarm the baby's skin. Burns may result from overheating or uneven heat dispersion.
- Closely monitor temperature fluctuations when using a radiant warmer, which may mask the signs and symptoms of temperature instability in the neonate, an indication of sepsis.
- Monitor fluid status to determine insensible water losses if using a radiant warmer.
- Closely monitor the neonate's temperature, respiratory rate, and glucose levels per institution guidelines.
- Recognize that alterations in temperature are directly proportional to gestational age and may indicate the need for physician intervention and notification.

CRITICAL COMPONENT

Kangaroo Care

Kangaroo care (or skin-to-skin contact) has been used in developing countries throughout the world since the 1970s as an alternative to conventional methods of neonatal care, with the aim to improve the health and survival of low-birth-weight infants and stabilize thermoregulation in newborns (Association of Women's Health, Obstetric, and Neonatal Nurses [AWHONN], 2016). The neonatal mortality rate of high-risk babies is significant, with more than 30% of babies dying before stabilization. Evidence to date suggests that the outcomes for these babies improve if kangaroo mother care is started early to allow for earlier stabilization (AWHONN, 2016). Health personnel must be present for the first 2 hours after the initiation of kangaroo care to maintain safety (AWHONN, 2016).

Infant Benefits

- Stabilization of heart rate
- Stabilization of breathing patterns
- Improved oxygenation
- More rapid weight gain
- Decreased crying
- Improved breastfeeding episodes
- Earlier discharge (Ludington-Hoe, 2013)

Mother Benefits

- Increased milk supply
- Increased sense of parental control
- Increased confidence in the care of their child
- Increased bonding (Ludington-Hoe, 2013)

Metabolic System Transition and Assessment

Glucose is the main source of energy for the brain (Chandran, Rajadurai, Alim, & Hussain, 2015), and the newborn brain depends on glucose metabolism for 90% of its needs. In the last 2 months of fetal life, glucose is stored as glycogen in the liver and is used after birth for:

- Coping with the stress of birth
- Breathing
- Heat production
- Muscular activity

Gluconeogenesis is the breakdown of glycogen into glucose. Glucose levels at birth are 80% of maternal blood glucose levels.

Clamping of the cord results in a decrease in the level of circulating glucose, which in turn increases epinephrine, norepinephrine, and glucagon, and decreases insulin levels (Chandran et al., 2015).

Hypoglycemia occurs with levels less than 40 mg/dL and is the most frequent problem experienced by neonates within the first 48 hours after birth (Adamkin & Polin, 2016; Rozance & Hay, 2016). Increased glucose utilization demands can be caused by hypothermia, hypoxia, or sepsis. Prematurity, small for gestational age (SGA), intrauterine growth restriction, and inborn errors of metabolism can result from a decrease in glycogen stores. A decrease in glucose post-maturity can be caused by deterioration of the placenta, which provides nutrition. Decreases can also result from maternal intake of certain medications, such as terbutaline.

Large for gestational age (LGA) babies, infants of mothers with diabetes, erythroblastosis fetalis, and Beckwith–Wiedemann syndrome can result from overproduction of insulin in the neonate because of high intrauterine glucose levels. Infants of mothers with diabetes have high levels of insulin caused by high levels of circulating maternal glucose. After birth, the circulating glucose from the mother is removed, but the neonate's insulin levels remain elevated, resulting in hypoglycemia. A hyperglycemic state in mothers with diabetes results in beta cell hypertrophy, increased fetal oxygen consumption, and inhibited surfactant and insulin production in the neonate (Adamkin & Polin, 2016).

Alterations in glucose levels can predispose an infant to the development of metabolic acidosis. The nurse must monitor glucose levels especially closely with evidence of risk factors, congenital metabolic conditions, birth defects, stress, jitteriness, or neonatal depression. Normal glucose levels vary from institution to institution. Ranges for plasma glucose levels should ideally be between 70 and 100 mg/dL, and heel-stick glucose levels need to be greater than 40 mg/dL (Durham & Chapman, 2014).

CRITICAL COMPONENT

Glucose Levels

Critical glucose levels less than 40 mg/dL obtained with point-of-care devices such as glucometers must be confirmed by serum levels sent STAT to the laboratory. At-risk infants should be fed at 1 hour of age and glucose levels checked 30 minutes after feedings. In infants who are poor feeders, tube feedings should be considered (Rozance & Hay, 2016). The Pediatric Endocrine Society has set a goal of greater than 50 mg/dL for the first 48 hours of life and greater than 60 mg/dL after 48 hours of life (Thornton et al., 2015).

Nursing Interventions

When caring for a neonate, the nurse should perform the following interventions:

- Monitor for signs and symptoms of hypoglycemia.
- Recognize risk factors for hypoglycemia.
- Assess blood glucose with glucometer, i-STAT.

SAFE AND EFFECTIVE NURSING CARE: Clinical Pearl

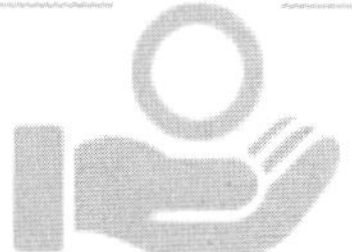

Recognizing Hypoglycemia in the Neonate

Signs of hypoglycemia in the neonate include:

- Irritability
- Jitteriness
- Hypotonia
- Temperature instability
- Apnea
- Poor feeding
- Lethargy
- Seizures

Lack of symptoms does not always indicate absence of alteration.

- Feed the infant when glucose levels are less than 40 mg/dL or as directed by institutional guidelines, generally 5 mL/kg (Durham & Chapman, 2014).
- Assist with breastfeeding.
- Infants of mothers with diabetes should receive 3 to 5 mg/kg/min glucose to prevent overstimulation of insulin secretions (Rozance & Hay, 2016).
- Intrauterine growth-restricted infants should receive 6 to 8 mg/kg/min of glucose if symptomatic (Rozance & Hay, 2016).
- Term or near-term infants should receive 4 to 7 mg/kg/min glucose if symptomatic (Rozance & Hay, 2016).
- Begin intravenous glucose maintenance and rigorously follow guidelines on repeat blood serum glucose levels.
- Maintain neutral thermal environment to prevent cold stress, which increases utilization of glucose.

Newborn Screening

- Every year in the United States, 4.1 million newborns are screened for metabolic disorders at birth, 4,000 of whom are diagnosed and another 1,000 infants in whom these disorders are undetected (AAP, 2017e). The National Newborn Screening and Genetics Resource Center lists the tests each state requires.
- Metabolic disorders occur when absence or abnormality of an enzyme or cofactor leads to excessive accumulation or deficiency of a specific metabolite (Bodamer, 2015). Disorders of amino acids, organic acids, carbohydrates, and the urea cycle, as well as of mitochondrial, fatty acid, peroxisomal, lysosomal, purine, pyrimidine, and metal metabolism, are some of those tested for in the newborn period. Tests can detect up to 100 different inborn errors of metabolism or deviations. Each state has its own regulations for newborn screening depending on family history or diagnosis of a symptomatic infant. Some states require written parental consent.
- Most tests are performed within the first 24 to 48 hours after birth or at follow-up newborn wellness checks. Tests use

capillary blood drawn by nursing or laboratory personnel and placed on filter paper cards (Figure 7–8). In some states, all babies are screened a second time about 2 weeks after birth because of postnatal changes that can alter the inborn errors of metabolism screenings (AAP, 2017e).

Phenylketonuria

Phenylketonuria is an autosomal recessive deficiency of the enzyme phenylalanine and is the most common inborn error of metabolism. Deficiency prevents the conversion of the essential amino acid phenylalanine to tyrosine. The elevated levels of phenylalanine can result in mental cognitive impairment caused by defective myelination and degeneration of the white and gray matter of the brain. This is characterized by developmental delays, poor feeding, irritability, and vomiting (Bodamer, 2015).

- This metabolic disorder is tested for in all 50 states and the District of Columbia.
- Affected infants must be on feedings for 3 full days so that the liver enzyme that converts phenylalanine to tyrosine will be secreted.
- Guthrie blood test is performed.
- A low-phenylalanine, low-protein diet must be implemented for the rest of the child's life.

Congenital Hypothyroidism

- Congenital hypothyroidism, caused by an underactive or absent thyroid gland, can lead to mental retardation and is tested for in all 50 states and the District of Columbia (Wassner & Brown, 2013).
- Symptoms include hypotonia, lethargy, poor temperature control, and respiratory distress.
- Hormone replacement is necessary throughout life.
- Parental education stresses the need for replacement hormone and close follow-up.

Congenital Adrenal Hyperplasia

- Congenital adrenal hyperplasia is the inability to produce cortisol in the adrenal glands that is caused by a defect in the enzyme 21-hydroxylase.
- It is autosomal recessive and affects 1 in 15,000 newborns in the general population, but 1 in 680 Eskimos (Bodamer, 2015).
- Hyperplasia of the adrenal gland develops.
- The result is excessive androgen production from the adrenal glands, leading to disorders of sexual identity in the child (Yang & White, 2017).

Galactosemia

- Galactosemia is a common enzyme deficiency that prevents the breakdown of galactose to glucose.
- Galactosemia can lead to mental retardation and failure to thrive.
- It is tested for in all 50 states and the District of Columbia.

Maple Syrup Disease

- Maple syrup disease is a rare autosomal recessive disorder common in those of Amish and Mennonite descent.
- Buildup of metabolic enzyme leads to severe ketoacidosis and encephalopathy.
- A protein-free diet must be implemented for the rest of the infant's life (Weiner, 2015).

Krabbe Disease

- Krabbe disease is an autosomal recessive genetic disorder that affects the brain and nervous system.
- It was first identified by Dr. Knud Krabbe in 1916 and affects 1 in 100,000 children (U.S. National Library of Medicine, 2016).
- Deletion of galactosylceramidase impairs the ability of the body to grow and repair the myelin sheath (protective lining of the nerve cell).
- Disease results in severe deterioration of mental and motor skills, resulting in muscle weakness, hypertonia, seizures,

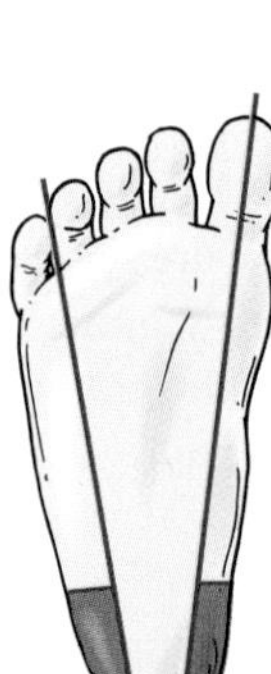

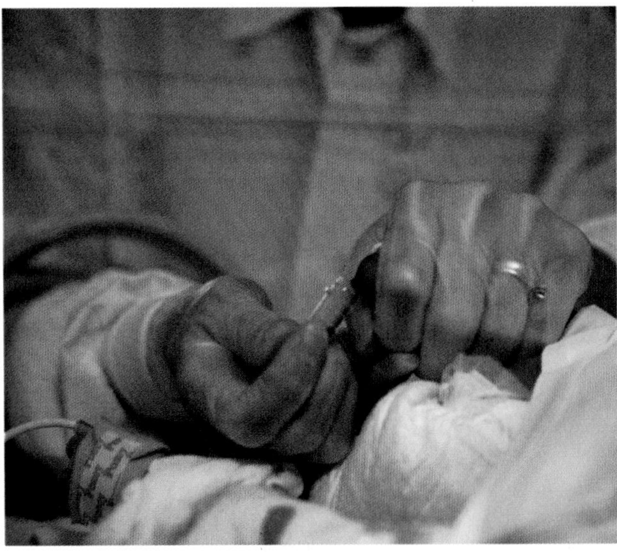

FIGURE 7–8 Heel stick of foot.

spasticity, fever, irritability, difficulty in swallowing, deafness, and vision loss (Langan, 2016).

- Due to the rareness of this disorder and the lack of treatment options, many states allow parents to opt out of testing (Rudd, 2017).

Sickle Cell Disease

Sickle cell disease is an inherited hematological disease in which red blood cells (RBCs) are sickled in shape, resembling the letter C rather than being round. RBCs carry oxygen and when they are misshapen, they become trapped in small areas such as joints, thus blocking blood flow. In the United States, sickle cell disease is more common in blacks and Hispanics, but throughout the world is common among people in Africa, the Caribbean, and Mediterranean areas.

This disease results in anemia, pain, infections, acute chest syndrome, vision issues, or stroke. There is no known cure for this disease, but stem cell treatments have been used with some success in limiting symptomology (March of Dimes, 2014).

Cystic Fibrosis

Cystic fibrosis is an exocrine gland disorder that results in problems with digestion and breathing. The disease produces thickened mucus that becomes trapped in the lungs and digestive system. Symptoms appear because of blockage in the respiratory system and often in the pancreas. These include coughing, mucus, lung infections, shortness of breath, salty skin, slow growth, and frequent loose, greasy stools.

Hepatic System Transition and Assessment

- The full-term neonatal liver is responsible for carbohydrate metabolism, iron storage, bilirubin conjugation, and blood coagulation. The stressed or immature infant is susceptible to alterations in these critical homeostasis maintenance mechanisms (Durham & Chapman, 2014).
- Iron stores in fetal liver are created in the last weeks of pregnancy. As RBCs are broken down, they are added to the liver stores until future RBCs are produced.
- Term infants who are breastfed do not need supplemental iron until 4 months of age.
- After 4 months of age in an exclusively breastfed infant, the baby should receive 1 mg/kg/day of a liquid iron supplement until iron-containing solids are introduced at 6 months of age (AAP, 2016a).
- Term infants who are bottle feeding require iron-fortified formula.
- After age 6 months, all infants require iron supplementation through supplements or iron-rich foods.

Coagulation

- Activation of clotting factors II, VII, IX, and X and prothrombin is influenced by vitamin K. At birth, maternal sources of vitamin K are removed. Intestinal flora needed to produce vitamin K are absent in the newborn until after the first feeding, which puts neonates at higher risk for coagulation issues.
- Infants receive a 1-mg intramuscular (IM) injection of vitamin K within 1 hour after birth to prevent vitamin K deficiency bleeding (Sankar et al., 2016).
- Infants who are breastfed, those deprived of oxygen at birth, or who have mothers who are treated with anticoagulants are at risk for decreased vitamin K levels (Durham & Chapman, 2014).
- Infants can be at risk for clotting delays and potential hemorrhage, called *hemorrhagic disease of the newborn.*
- Newborns have a higher hematocrit, slower bilirubin clearance, shorter RBC life span, and more immature liver conjugation processing. Conjugation is the process of converting lipid-soluble (nonexcreted or indirect) bilirubin into a water-soluble (excreted or direct) form (Ward & Hisley, 2015).

Hyperbilirubinemia

- Bilirubin pigment released from the breakdown of hemoglobin discolors the skin, sclera, and oral mucous membranes and is known as jaundice when it discolors these areas. Hyperbilirubinemia is an excessive amount of bilirubin in the blood, mainly due to the infant's immature liver.
- Unconjugated bilirubin (indirect bilirubin) is fat-soluble, nonexcretable, and binds to albumin. The liver must conjugate, or change, this form of bilirubin via liver enzymes into conjugated (direct) bilirubin so that it can be eliminated in the urine and stool (Figure 7–9).
- Increased levels of unconjugated bilirubin (indirect bilirubin) that saturate the albumin-binding sites cross the blood–brain barrier and can result in kernicterus, a life-threatening buildup of bilirubin in the brain and spinal cord. The total serum bilirubin (TSB) is the combination of direct bilirubin and indirect bilirubin.

Risk factors for hyperbilirubinemia include:

- Mother with diabetes
- ABO incompatibility: When mother and baby have different blood types—specifically, the mother has type O and the baby has type A or B—an immune system reaction occurs that results in excessive breakdown of RBCs and the release of bilirubin.
- Rh incompatibility: When the mother is Rh negative and the baby is Rh positive, the mother will produce antibodies against the baby's blood, and hemolysis of the neonate's blood will occur. Bilirubin levels rise dramatically, placing the infant at risk for kernicterus and erythroblastosis fetalis, as well as severe hemolytic anemia and jaundice. This condition is preventable with the administration of RhoGAM.
- Prematurity
- Delayed feeding, which delays the passage of bilirubin-rich meconium
- Birth trauma caused by accelerated breakdown of RBCs in bruising (e.g., cephalhematoma, asphyxia)
- Liver immaturity
- Stress in the neonate (cold stress, asphyxia, hypoglycemia)
- Use of Pitocin in labor

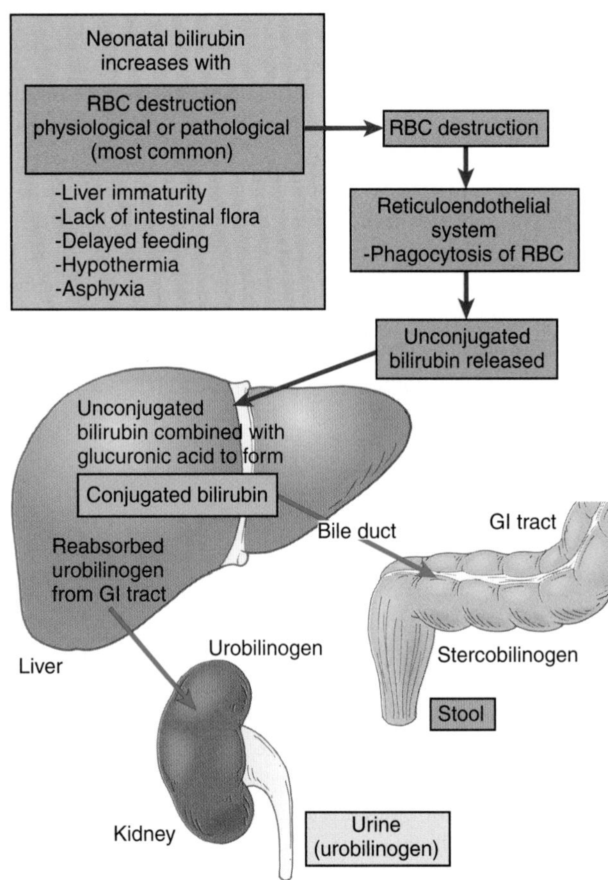

FIGURE 7–9 Physiological pathway for excretion of bilirubin. GI, gastrointestinal; RBC, red blood cell.

- East Asian, American Indian, or Mediterranean descent
- Sibling history of jaundice
- Breastfeeding

Nursing Interventions

Monitoring for hyperbilirubinemia includes the following measures:

- Observe the skin of the neonate; jaundice begins on the face and nose, then progresses down the trunk to the extremities (Han, Lui, & Zhang, 2017). However, this is not an accurate method of assessment, especially in darker-skinned infants.
- All neonates should be screened before discharge with a measurement of bilirubin levels and the assessment of clinical risk factors. Bilirubin levels are then plotted on the Bhutani nomogram, an hour-specific tool used for prediction in at-risk neonates who are more than 36 weeks' gestation, more than 2,000 g, and otherwise well with no ABO incompatibilities (Bhutani et al., 2013; Wong & Bhutani, 2016).
- Infants are rated as low, intermediate, or high risk for development of clinically significant hyperbilirubinemia.
- Severely at-risk infants are those with TSB levels greater than 95th percentile for age in hours (Bhutani et al., 2013).
- The Coombs' test is also used for monitoring.
  - A heel stick is performed with a sharp lancet to remove small drops of capillary blood to test for total, direct, and indirect serum bilirubin levels.
- Transcutaneous bilirubin (TcB) measurement: Noninvasive multiwavelength spectral skin monitoring of bilirubin levels in term or near-term infants via the upper part of the sternum. Up to 15 mg/dL, the TcB correlates with serum blood levels (Wong & Bhutani, 2016).

SAFE AND EFFECTIVE NURSING CARE: Clinical Pearl

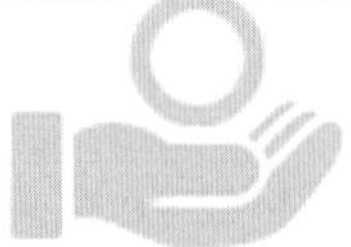

Coombs' Test

The Coombs' test is a measurement of antibodies attached to the newborn's RBCs that occur with Rh-negative mothers. Rh-negative mothers produce antibodies against the Rh-positive baby or in ABO incompatibilities. If there is an abnormal coating of the neonate's RBCs with an antibody globulin from the mother, it is considered a positive Coombs' test, and the neonate is at a higher risk for hemolytic disease of the newborn (Durham & Chapman, 2014; Wong & Bhutani, 2016).

Physiological Jaundice

- Transient rise in serum bilirubin levels within the first 24 to 48 hours of life
- Affects 60% of term newborns and 80% of preterm infants (Christensen & Yaish, 2015)
- Peak TSB levels in full-term infants result in phototherapy if the bilirubin level is at or above 15 mg/dL within the first 24 to 48 hours (Han et al., 2017)
- Peaks at 3 to 7 days of life
- Bilirubin levels are benign and usually do not exceed 15 mg/dL; levels from 17 to 18 mg/dL may be accepted as normal in term infants if they are older than 72 hours (Christensen & Yaish, 2015)

Evidence-Based Practice: Delayed Clamping of the Cord

American College of Obstetrician and Gynecologists. (2017). Delayed cord clamping after birth [Committee Opinion No. 684]. pp. 1–6. Retrieved from http://www.acog.org/-/media/Committee-Opinions/Committee-on-Obstetric-Practice/co684.pdf?dmc=1&ts=20170406T1645598732

McDonald, S. J., Middleton, P., Dowswell, T., & Morris, P.S. (2013). Effect of timing of umbilical cord clamping of term infants on maternal and neonatal outcomes. *Cochrane Database of Systematic Reviews, 7*, CD004074. doi: 10.1002/14651858.CD004074.pub3.

The American College of Obstetricians and Gynecologists (2017) has recommended the delayed clamping of the umbilical cord in vigorous term and preterm infants for 30 to 60 seconds after birth or until the cessation of cord pulsation (usually around 3 minutes). The optimum delay time is usually around 90 seconds. Delayed cutting of the cord results in increased levels of iron hemoglobin, decreased risk for anemia, decreased risk for intraventricular hemorrhage, and increased transfer of stem cells, and has no effect on bilirubin levels (McDonald, Middleton, Dowswell, & Morris, 2013).

Pathological Jaundice

- Pathological jaundice occurs within the first 24 hours of life.
- It results from excessive destruction of RBCs, infection, incompatibilities, or metabolic disorders.
- Consider if bilirubin levels are levels more than 15 mg/dL in term infant within the first 48 hours of life (Muchowski, 2014).
- Consider with bilirubin levels that increase by more than 5 mg/dL/day (Muchowski, 2014).
- There is no consensus on preterm infants and depends on clinical judgment, but phototherapy is usually begun when less than 1,000 g with levels of 5 to 7 mg/dL (Muchowski, 2014).
- Pathological jaundice is diagnosed with jaundice lasting longer than 1 week in a term newborn or more than 2 weeks in a premature infant (Bhutani et al., 2013).

Breast Milk Jaundice

- Affects 1% to 2% of breastfed babies (Centers for Disease Control and Prevention [CDC], 2016a)
- Early onset: poor feeding patterns; bilirubin levels may spike to 19 mg/dL (Bhutani et al., 2013)
- Late onset: peaks 2 to 3 weeks after birth, increased absorption of bilirubin resulting from a factor in breast milk that increases absorption of bilirubin from the intestines (Table 7–3; Bhutani et al., 2013; Ward & Hisley, 2015)

Nursing Interventions

- Identify infants at risk.
- Monitor bilirubin levels through close skin monitoring; digitally compress the skin.
- Monitor point-of-care heel sticks, TcB levels, and serum bilirubin levels.
- Support early and frequent feedings.
- Support and work with lactating mothers.
- Consult with lactation consultants.
- Monitor stooling and voiding patterns.
- Monitor and screen for lethargic or sleepy infants.
- Monitor for high-pitched cry and arching of the body.
- Maintain phototherapy.

CRITICAL COMPONENT

In phototherapy, the blue-green fluorescent light is absorbed into the skin, where it converts unconjugated bilirubin into bilirubin by producing lumirubin, which is water-soluble and thereby allows the infant to excrete bilirubin in the stool and urine (Muchowski, 2014). When conducting phototherapy, fluorescent lights should be calibrated periodically per the manufacturer's guidelines. The infant's eyes need to be covered to prevent cataracts because retinal damage can occur. Infants should be fully exposed, except for the diaper. Keep male scrotum covered and place the infant in a low-heat-setting isolette. Place the phototherapy lamp 45 to 50 cm away from infant, or 2 inches from the top of the isolette (Muchowski, 2014). The infant should be held only during feedings and then eye patches can be removed. The nurse needs to closely monitor temperature during phototherapy (Woodgate & Jardine, 2015). Never use lotions or ointments on the skin while the infant is under phototherapy.

Single phototherapy is the use of one light, double phototherapy the use of two, and triple phototherapy the use of three. The choice of methods depends on bilirubin levels and the rate of the rise of these levels (Figure 7–10). Dual therapy is often used with overhead bilirubin lights and a bilirubin blanket. The bilirubin blanket allows the infant to be removed from the lights and held for feedings. A fiberoptic blanket or band can be used at home and provides light similar to sunlight. Fluid requirements may increase during therapy because of insensible water loss; however, fluid supplementation is not supported in the literature if temperature homeostasis and fluid output are maintained (Hansen, 2016). Rebound bilirubin levels rise 1 to 2 mg/dL once phototherapy is discontinued. Partial-, single-, or double-volume-exchange blood transfusion may be necessary in a neonatal intensive care unit.

TABLE 7–3 Hyperbilirubinemia in Breastfeeding Jaundice Versus Breast Milk Jaundice

BREASTFEEDING JAUNDICE	BREAST MILK JAUNDICE
Early onset of jaundice (within the first few days of life)	Late onset (after 3–5 days)
Associated with ineffective breastfeeding	Gradual increase in bilirubin that peaks at 2 weeks of age
Dehydration can occur	Associated with breast milk composition in some women that increases the enterohepatic circulation of bilirubin
Delayed passage of meconium stool promotes reabsorption of bilirubin in the gut	**Treatment:** Continued breastfeeding in most infants. In some cases where bilirubin levels are excessively high, breastfeeding may be interrupted and formula feedings can be given for several days. This typically results in a decline of the bilirubin level. Breastfeeding is resumed when bilirubin levels decline.
Treatment: Encourage early, effective breastfeeding without supplementation of glucose water or other fluids.	

Source: Durham, R., & Chapman, L. (2014). Maternal-newborn nursing: Critical components of nursing care *(2nd ed.). Philadelphia: F.A. Davis.*

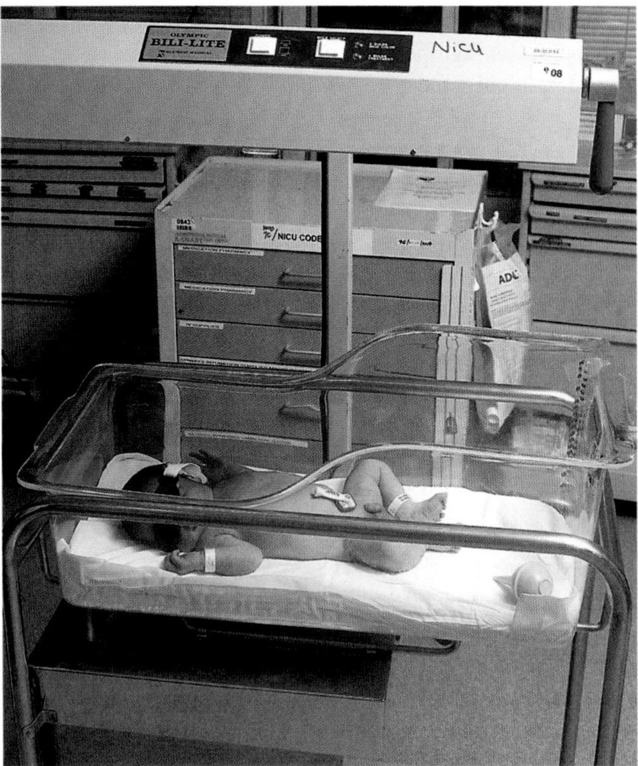

FIGURE 7–10 Phototherapy.

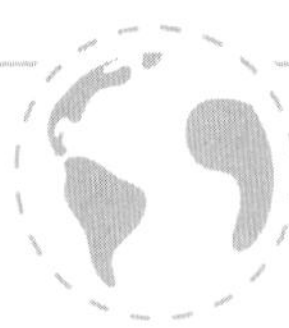

SAFE AND EFFECTIVE NURSING CARE: Cultural Competence

Communication and Client Teaching

Routine discharge teaching must be completed in the language spoken in the home. Teaching needs to be in both written and oral formats with patient-friendly information, including signs and symptoms of an infant's deteriorating status, follow-up monitoring instructions, and office contacts for questions (Nesrin et al., 2016).

Gastrointestinal System Transition and Assessment

The nurse should be aware of the following when performing gastrointestinal system assessment on a transitioning newborn (see Chapter 15 for further details):

- The abdomen should be cylindrical; a sunken abdomen should be reported.
- The stomach is immature but rapidly adjusts.
- Stomach capacity is 30 to 60 mL at birth and then rapidly increases.
- The infant may be in a quiet sleep state and uninterested in feeding.
- Both the desire for feeding and stomach size increase rapidly during infancy.
- Enzymes are present at birth to digest proteins, moderate fats, and simple sugars.
- Decreased esophageal sphincter pressure is present at birth but increases with age.
- The first stool is black and tarry, and is known as meconium. Meconium is formed starting around 16 weeks of gestation and usually is passed within 24 to 48 hours of age.
- Stool then becomes transitional around day 3 of life, with color and consistency dependent on feeding.
  - Breastfeeding stool beyond transitional is golden and semiformed.
  - Bottle-fed stool beyond transitional is drier and pale yellow or greenish black to brownish.
- A loose or green stool is considered diarrhea (Durham & Chapman, 2014). Most hospitalizations and deaths from diarrhea occur during the first year of life (National Institute of Diabetes and Digestive and Kidney Diseases, 2017).
- Breastfed babies eat more frequently because of the increased digestibility of breast milk. Breast milk is composed of 60% whey and 40% casein, whereas cow's milk has 20% whey and 80% casein. Casein forms a hard curd that is difficult to digest.
- Constipation does not occur in breastfed newborns.
- Breastfed babies often produce stool with every feeding, and by 1 month of age may progress to one stool every day or every other day.
- Bottle-fed babies may become constipated from improper formula mixing. Normal elimination patterns for bottle-fed infants are one or two stools a day.
- The AAP (2016a) recommends that newborns receive 400 IU of vitamin D per day after birth until the infant is taking 1 quart of whole milk at 1 year of age.
- After 4 months of age in an exclusively breastfed infant, the baby should receive 1 mg/kg/day of a liquid iron supplement until iron-containing solids are introduced at 6 months of age (AAP, 2016a).
- Mothers who are on strict vegetarian diets need to take an extra B-complex supplement when exclusively breastfeeding (AAP, 2014a).
- After the second month of life, stool increases in volume and decreases in frequency.
- Feedings for infants should be at least every 4 hours but may need to be more frequent in early infancy because of stomach emptying time. Breastfed newborns often want to go to the breast every 45 to 90 minutes, because their stomach capacity is only 20 to 30 mL.
- Infants progress from being able to suck, drink liquids, and be fed by a caregiver to become children who can feed themselves and digest solids.
- As the infant is weaned from the breast or bottle to solid foods, the consistency of the stool will change. It is not uncommon to see pieces of food in the stool.

Genitourinary System Transition and Assessment

See Chapter 16 for further details.

- Nephrons are fully functional at 34 to 36 weeks' gestation.
- The fetus produces urine within the first 3 months of gestation.

- The first urine output should occur within 24 hours after birth.
- In the first 1 or 2 days, urine may be stained orange or pink because of urate crystals.
- Newborns cannot concentrate or dilute urine in response to changes in intravascular fluid status, and therefore are at risk for dehydration or fluid overload.
- Infants are more prone to extracellular fluid loss than intracellular fluid loss.
- The term neonate is composed of 75% water (40% extracellular fluid, 35% intracellular fluid). Term neonates usually lose 5% to 10% of their weight in the first week of life, almost all of which is water loss.
- Fluid requirements during the first 2 days of life are 80 to 100 mL/kg/day, then increase to 100 to 150 mL/kg/day.
- The glomerular filtration rate decreases at birth.
- Specific gravity averages 1.001 to 1.010 during infancy.
- Infants cannot correct acid–base balance through bicarbonate and hydrogen ion concentration.
- Urine output should be 1 to 3 mL/kg/hr if monitored in the hospital to maintain adequate fluid maintenance.
- Strict input and output is essential in the nursing care of any infant in the hospital.
- By 3 months of age, infants can concentrate urine.
- Normal urine output is calculated based on weight.
- Six to 10 wet diapers per day is considered normal urine output (Table 7–4).

Genitalia

See Chapter 18 for further details.

- The normal male has descended testes and the urethral opening in the center of the penis.
- The scrotum at first appears edematous and disproportionately large.
- Hypospadias is when the urethral opening is on the underside (ventrum) of the penis. Epispadias is when the urethral opening is on the upper portion (dorsum) of the penis. In both conditions, circumcision is delayed so the prepuce can be used for surgical correction.

TABLE 7–4 Table of Fluid Intake

GENERAL GUIDELINES FOR A 24-HOUR PERIOD	FLUID INTAKE	BASED ON INCREMENTS OF 10 KG PER BODY WEIGHT
<10 kg	100 mL/kg	
>10 and <20 kg	1,000 mL for first 10 kg	+50 mL/kg for each kg >10 and <20
>20 kg	1,500 mL for first 20 kg	+20 mL/kg for each kg >20

Source: Durham, R., & Chapman, L. (2014). Maternal-newborn nursing: Critical components of nursing care *(2nd ed.). Philadelphia: F.A. Davis.*

- Circumcision is the surgical removal of the foreskin of the penis.
- In the normal female, the labia majora are larger than the labia minora.
- Observe for vaginal tags.
- Observe for ambiguous genitalia, a genetic defect in which the outward appearance of the genitalia does not resemble either a boy or a girl. The penis may be very small, the clitoris may be very large, or the labia may be fused, resembling a scrotum.
- Pseudomenstruation is a thin white or blood-tinged mucus that may be present because of withdrawal of maternal hormones.
- The breasts may be enlarged in both male and female infants at term birth. Breast tissue may be decreased in premature or postmature neonates.

Skin System Transition and Assessment

When assessing the newborn's skin, be aware of the following:

- Provide adequate lighting for assessment.
- Skin should be pink. Pale or dusky skin may indicate congenital heart disease (see Chapter 12). Color is influenced by ethnicity.
- Observe for jaundice; apply pressure and remove with your fingertip over bony prominences such as the nose, sternum, or sacrum.
- Observe for the presence of body hair, fine downy lanugo.
- Observe for acrocyanosis (normal and disappears with crying).
- Observe for petechiae, skin tags, breaks in the skin, forceps marks on the face or scalp, and electronic fetal monitoring marks on the scalp.
- Observe for milia (small white sebaceous cysts), usually present on the face.
- Vernix caseosa is a cheesy substance found mainly in the creases of the armpits and groin, but which may cover the entire body. This protective covering should not be removed because it provides an emollient effect to the skin.
- Erythema toxicum (newborn rash) are tiny pimples that disappear within the first few weeks.
- Baby acne consists of small red pimples on the face or body that appear at about 1 month of age.
- Grayish, dark blue, or black areas located over sacral region are called Mongolian spots (also referred to as congenital dermal melanocytosis); these are prominent in certain ethnic cultures from Asia, Africa, and Mediterranean areas (Figure 7–11).
- Observe for birthmarks, nevi, or stork bites (Figure 7–12).
- Cord begins to dry following the cutting of the cord. The cord clamp should be removed 24 to 48 hours after birth. Cord care includes keeping it dry. Some institutions leave the cord open to air, apply methylene blue to the cord as a drying agent, or apply alcohol to the cord. Keep the diaper below the cord. As it dries, the cord becomes black and hard, and it falls off within 2 weeks. Be aware that some cultures save the cord detachment (see Chapter 4). There should be no submersion in a tub of water until the cord has dried and come off; perform sponge baths only.
- Diapering can be with disposable or cloth diapers. Most parents choose disposable. The newborn infant should have between 6 and 10 wet diapers per day. Water should be used to clean

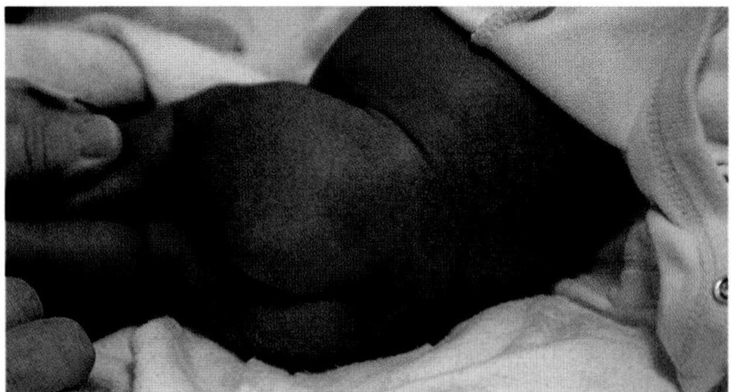

FIGURE 7–11 Mongolian spots.

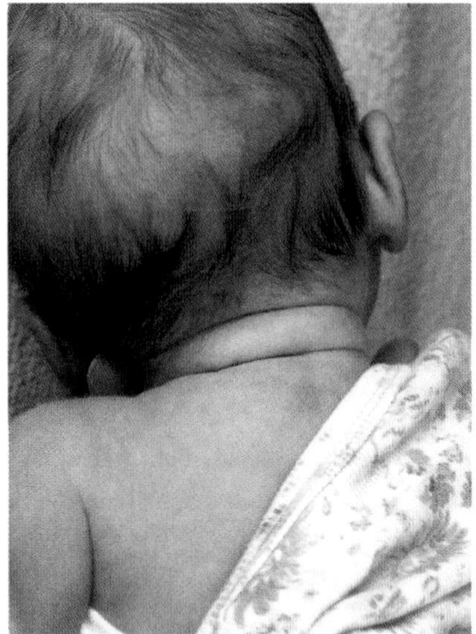

FIGURE 7–12 Stork bite.

the genital and rectal area, wiping in girls from front to back. Nurses need to instruct caregivers to wash their hands following every diaper change.

- Diaper rash consists of red and sore areas in the diaper region from urine and stool, often a result of candidiasis. Exposure to air helps.
- Heat rash or prickly heat is due to overdressing in warm weather.
- Cradle cap is scaly or crusty skin on the scalp due to a buildup of oils, scales, and dead skin. The head should be washed and dried every day.

See Table 7–5 for common newborn characteristics.

Evidence-Based Practice: Care of Neonatal Skin

Association of Women's Health, Obstetric, and Neonatal Nurses. (2016). Immediate and sustained skin-to-skin contact for the healthy term newborn after birth: AWHONN Practice Brief Number 5. *Journal of Obstetric, Gynecologic & Neonatal Nursing, 45*(6), 842–844. Retrieved from http://www.jognn.org/article/S0884-2175(16)30352-5/pdf

The AWHONN developed the "Immediate and Sustained Skin-to-Skin Contact for the Healthy Term Newborn After Birth: AWHONN Brief Number 5," an evidence-based practice guideline for the care of neonatal skin related to bathing, cord care, disinfectants, wound care, and the relationship between term infant and preterm infant skin care in the first 28 days of life.

This practice statement suggests that all stable 37-week 0-day infants born either by cesarean section or vaginal birth should be placed in skin-to-skin contact for at least the first hour of life or until breastfeeding has begun. It also indicates that infants of this same gestation age have skin-to-skin during all pain procedures such as vaccinations or blood sampling, and that during hospitalization the parents should have uninterrupted skin-to-skin contact as often as possible.

TABLE 7–5 Common Newborn Characteristics

CHARACTERISTICS	APPEARANCE	SIGNIFICANCE
Acrocyanosis	Hands and/or feet are blue	Response to cold environment Immature peripheral circulation
Circumoral cyanosis	A localized transient cyanosis around the mouth	Observed during the transitional period; if it persists it may be related to a cardiac anomaly
Mottling	A transient pattern of pink and white blotches on the skin	Response to cold environment
Harlequin sign	One side of the body is pink and the other side is white	Related to vasomotor instability

TABLE 7–5 Common Newborn Characteristics—cont'd

CHARACTERISTICS	APPEARANCE	SIGNIFICANCE
Mongolian spots	Flat bluish discolored area on the lower back and/or buttocks Seen more often in African American, Asian, Latin, and Native American infants	Might be mistaken for bruising Need to document size and location Resolves on own by school age
Erythema toxicum	A rash with red macules and papules (white to yellowish-white papule in center surrounded by reddened skin) that appears on different areas of the body, usually the trunk area Can appear within 24 hours of birth and up to 2 weeks after birth	Benign Disappears without treatment
Milia 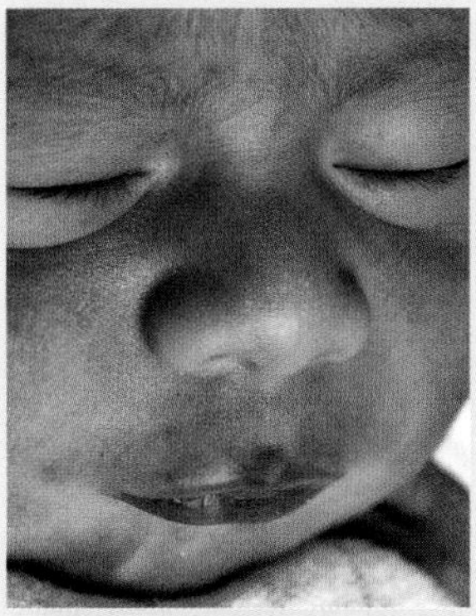	White papules on the face; more frequently seen on the bridge of the nose and chin	Exposed sebaceous glands that resolve without treatment Parents might mistake these for "whiteheads" Inform parents to leave them alone and let them resolve on their own
Lanugo 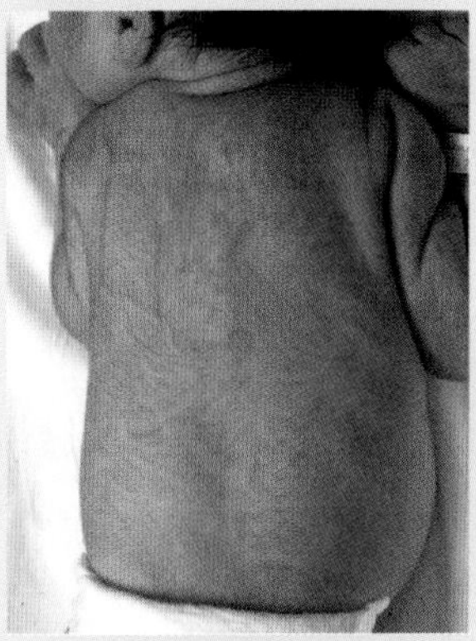	Fine, downy hair that develops after 16 weeks' gestation The amount of lanugo decreases as the fetus ages Often seen on the neonate's back, shoulders, and forehead	Gradually falls out The presence and amount of lanugo assist in estimating gestational age Abundant lanugo may be a sign of prematurity or a genetic disorder
Vernix caseosa 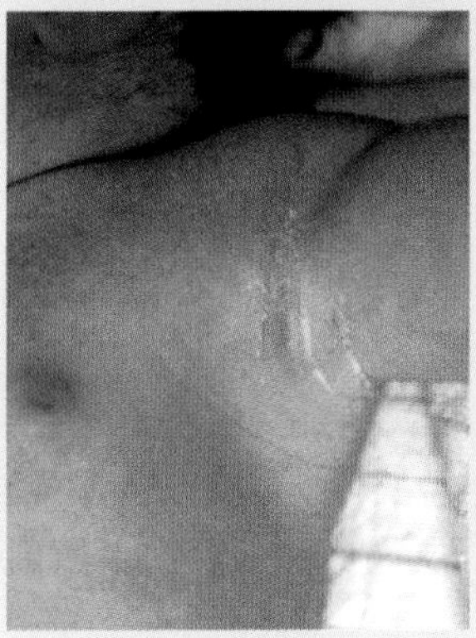	A protective substance secreted from sebaceous glands that covered the fetus during pregnancy It looks like a whitish, cheesy substance May be noted in the axillary and genital areas of full-term neonates	The presence and amount of vernix assist in estimating gestational age Full-term neonates usually have no vernix or only small amounts

Continued

TABLE 7–5 Common Newborn Characteristics—cont'd

CHARACTERISTICS	APPEARANCE	SIGNIFICANCE
Jaundice	Yellow coloring of the skin First appears on the face and extends to the trunk and eventually the entire body Best assessed in natural lighting When jaundice is suspected, the nurse can apply gentle pressure to the skin over a firm surface such as the nose, forehead, or sternum; the skin blanches to a yellowish hue	Jaundice within the first 24 hours is pathological; it is usually related to an immature liver (see Chapter 17) Jaundice occurring after 24 hours is referred to as physiological jaundice and is related to an increased amount of unconjugated bilirubin in the system (see Chapter 17)
Epstein's pearls	White, pearl-like epithelial cysts on gum margins and palate	Benign and usually disappear within a few weeks
Natal teeth	Immature caps of enamel and dentin with poorly developed roots Usually only one or two teeth are present	They are usually benign, but can be associated with congenital defects Natal teeth are often loose and need to be removed to decrease the risk for aspiration
Infant acne	Small red bumps or pimples on the infant's face or body that usually appear at 1 month of age	Usually benign but concerning to parents; parents should be taught to keep the infant's face or skin clean and not to apply creams or ointments to the skin, unless prescribed by the pediatrician

Source: Modified from Dillion, P. (2007) Nursing assessment: A critical thinking, case studies approach *(2nd ed, pp. 855–867) Philadelphia: F.A. Davis.*

Immune System Transition and Assessment

Nurses caring for transitioning neonates should be aware of the following aspects of immunity.

- The infant in utero is in a sterile environment.
- The infant is provided with maternal immunity through antibodies that bind to bacteria, viruses, and fungi that enter the body.
- Following birth, active humoral immunity is provided through acquired immunity from vaccination, or natural immunity from one's own production of antibodies in response to exposure to antigens.
- Temporary passive immunity is provided by those maternal antibodies that cross the placenta; the lymphocytes are T and B cells. Passive immunity is also provided by breast milk,

which contains all five immunoglobulins: IgG, IgA, IgD, IgM, and IgE.

- Immunoglobulins are maternal antibodies that cross the placenta and provide passive immunity—IgG, IgA, IgD, IgM, and IgE (Table 7–6).
- IgG is the only immunoglobulin that crosses the placenta during pregnancy and makes up 75% to 85% of all antibodies in the infant.
- IgA is primarily found in breast milk.
- IgM is primarily found in the lymph and bloodstream.
- IgD is primarily found in the abdomen and chest areas of the body.
- IgE is found in the lungs, skin, and mucous membranes.

- The infant's immune system is not fully developed until 6 months of age, and it begins to produce antibodies at about 2 to 3 months of age.
- There is no evidence that delaying the introduction of specific foods beyond 6 months of age prevents allergies (Chin, Chan, & Goldman, 2014). Recent research has indicated that early introduction of potentially allergic foods (at 4 to 6 months of age) might provide a form of protection and prevent allergy (Lerodiakonou et al., 2016).
- Infants are at risk for infection because of immature immune responses, lack of maternal antibodies, stress that depletes the immune system, and breaks in the skin due to invasive procedures that introduce bacteria or viruses.

Head and Neck Assessment

Aspects of head and neck assessment for this population include:

- The anterior and posterior fontanels (soft spots) should be assessed with the infant in an upright position.
  - The anterior fontanel is diamond shaped, averages 2 to 3 cm wide by 3 to 4 cm long, and closes at 12 to 18 months. You should be able to feel slight pulsations in this area. Abnormal findings are full or bulging fontanels, sunken fontanels, or closed suture lines. Assessment should be done when the baby is quiet.

CRITICAL COMPONENT

Microbiome Seeding

Infants born by cesarean section are not exposed to maternal vaginal microbiota but are exposed to *Staphylococcus* and *Streptococcus*. These bacteria predispose the cesarean-delivered infant to risks for immune and metabolic disorders (Dominguez-Bello et al., 2016). Infants who are born vaginally have gut, stomach, and skin bacteria that are enriched with vaginal bacteria for up to 30 hours after birth (Dominguez-Bello et al., 2016). The vaginal bacteria are "good" bacteria that are similar to what is carried on the skin throughout one's lifetime. Microbiome seeding of the baby occurs with bacteria from the mother's birth canal (through vaginal birth or in the future, wiping C-section babies with vaginal swabs taken from the mother), immediate skin-to-skin contact with mother or father, and breastfeeding (Dominguez-Bello et al., 2016). Some research also indicates that infant microbiota undergoes substantial reorganization based on body site, not necessarily the mode of delivery (Chu, Ma, Prince, & Antony, 2017).

  - The posterior fontanel is triangular, averages 1 to 2 cm wide, and closes in the second month of life.
- Bulging fontanels may occur with crying or increased intracranial pressure.
- Sunken fontanels indicate dehydration.
- Average head circumference is 35 cm but can range from 33 to 37 cm.
- Molding of the head occurs with normal vaginal deliveries, causing misshapen or elongated scalp.
- Bruising or swelling of the scalp may occur as the result of a difficult delivery or use of vacuum or forceps.
- Bleeding of the skull and its outer covering may cause a small bump, which will reabsorb in a few weeks.
- Caput succedaneum is the cone shape to the back of the head that crosses suture lines (Figure 7–13A). This shape occurs when blood and tissue become edematous from pushing against the mother's cervix.

TABLE 7–6 Classes of Immunoglobulins

NAME	LOCATION	FUNCTION
IgG	Blood Extracellular fluid	Crosses the placenta to provide passive immunity for newborns Provides long-term immunity after recovery or a vaccine
IgA	External secretions (tears, salvia, etc.)	Present in breast milk to provide passive immunity for breastfed infants Found in secretions of all mucous membranes
IgM	Blood	Produced first by the maturing immune system of infants Produced first during an infection (IgG production follows) Part of the ABO blood group
IgD	B lymphocytes	Receptors on B lymphocytes
IgE	Mast cells or basophils	Important in allergic reaction (mast cells release histamine)

Source: Scanlon, V., & Sanders, T. (2015). Essentials of anatomy and physiology *(7th ed., p. 370). Philadelphia: F.A. Davis.*

- Cephalhematoma is a swelling on one or both sides of the scalp that does not cross suture lines (Figure 7–13B). It is a result of bleeding over the skull bone or within the periosteum due to pressure against the pelvic bone. It can be life-threatening because of blood loss. It can increase jaundice as the blood is broken down.
- Craniosynostosis is the premature closure of one or more of the cranial sutures.
- Abnormalities in the head such as microcephaly (small head), intracranial calcifications, or other brain or eye abnormalities (glaucoma) may be present in the infant whose mother is Zika virus positive. Infants who present with these symptoms should have their urine and serum tested for the Zika virus RNA NAT (nucleic acid test) IgM antibodies. Ideally, these identified infants should be tested within 2 days after birth but can be tested weeks to months after birth with some success (CDC, 2017d).

Eyes

- The eyelids may be edematous from the birthing process; this resolves spontaneously.
- The iris should be grayish blue or gray-brown. The sclera should be blue or white. Jaundiced sclera is an abnormal finding.
- Pupils should be equal, round, and reactive to light activity. The cornea should be clear, and the red reflex should be present.
- Glaucoma can occur up to 3 months after birth in Zika-exposed infants (Ventura et al., 2016). Glaucoma in these infants is characterized with increased tearing, swelling, pain, and dullness of the iris (Ventura et al., 2016). Glaucoma can also occur in neonates not exposed to the Zika virus.

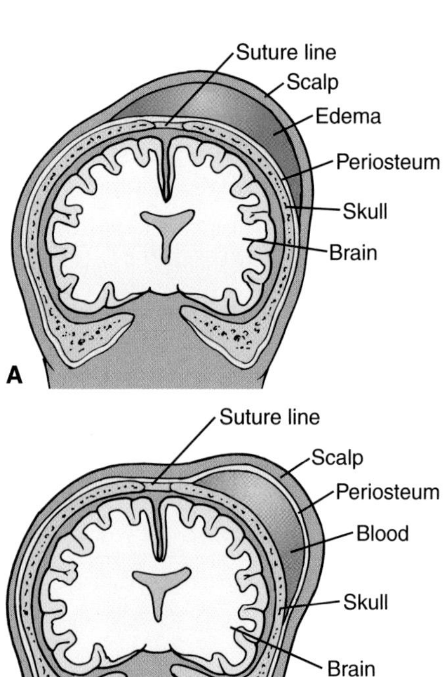

FIGURE 7–13 A, Caput succedaneum; **B,** cephalhematoma.

- Congenital cataracts can occur in the neonate causing clouding of the lens.
- The line from the inner epicanthal fold to the outer canthus to the top notch of the ear where it connects with the scalp should be symmetrical.
- Tears are not produced until the second month of life.
- Strabismus is an imbalance in ocular motor capacity.
- The visual acuity of a newborn is 20/400, improving in the first 2 years of life to 20/30.

Evidence-Based Practice: Red Reflex

American Academy of Pediatrics. (2016). Visual system assessment in infants, children, and young adults by pediatricians. Policy Statement. *Pediatrics, 137*(1), 28–30.

The red reflex is an important test in determining life-altering abnormalities such as cataracts, glaucoma, retinoblastoma, retinal abnormalities, and systemic abnormalities that may show signs or symptoms in the eye. A light is used to reflect off the ocular fundus of the eye and should result in a reddish-orange color. Obstructions can occur with mucus or abnormalities, and there are differences in the red reflex depending on race, ethnicity, and pigmentation of the fundus. A position statement by the AAP (2016e) indicates the need for a red reflex examination to be completed by a pediatrician or other trained primary care provider before discharge from the newborn nursery.

Ears

- Examine for position, structure, and function.
- Note absence of clefts, malformations, and cartilage or other abnormalities.
- The infant should startle to noise and move eyes to sound. The eyes seek the sound but cannot locate it directly.
- The infant should respond to soothing sounds.
- Unresponsiveness to noises should be investigated.

Nose

- Check the patency of the nares.
- Infants are obligatory nose-breathers.
- Monitor for nasal flaring.

Mouth

- The mouth should be symmetrical; the tongue should not protrude between the lips.
- The hard and soft palates should be intact and high arched.
- Epstein pearls are yellow or white fluid-filled papules on the palate of the mouth that spontaneously resolve.

Dental Development and Assessment

- Tooth buds are present during the third month of pregnancy.
- Natal teeth can be present at birth (usually lower central incisors without a root) and can interfere with breastfeeding.
- Teething is the eruption of the teeth through the gums. Teeth erupt at 4 to 10 months of age (usually around 6 months), starting with the two lower center teeth; the upper center teeth come in at about 8 to 12 months old. At the end of the first year, the child will have six to eight teeth.

- Signs and symptoms of teething including drooling, restlessness or difficulty falling asleep, sucking on the hands, and mild rash around the mouth because of drooling.
- Teething is not associated with generalized rash, fever, diarrhea, or prolonged fussiness. Numbing over-the-counter medications are brief in action and may also numb the throat and have a taste that is not pleasant for infants. Infants should never be given any medication with alcohol in the ingredients.
- The primary teeth are calcifying.
- The American Dental Association (ADA, 2017) recommends that the first dental visit occur at the time of the eruption of the first tooth, usually at age 6 months.
- A soft clean cloth should be used to clean the teeth as they erupt or to bite down on to decrease the pain of teething.

SAFE AND EFFECTIVE NURSING CARE: Clinical Pearl

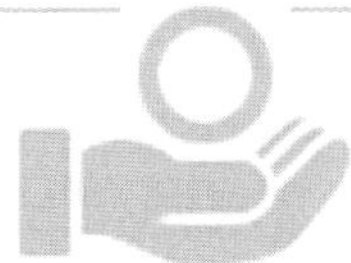

Dental Care for the Infant

- Feed only formula, breast milk, or water in a bottle.
- Juice should be delayed until the child is a toddler. If juice is introduced it should be delayed until 6 to 9 months of age, limited to 4 to 6 ounces, and given in a cup.
- Do not put infants to bed at night or for a nap with a bottle.
- Brush teeth with a soft cloth once they erupt.
- Do not use cold juice to soothe an infant's gums.
- Begin regular dental appointments by the first birthday (AAP, 2017d).

Cleft Lip and Palate

Cleft lip and palate are craniofacial deformities that occur early in pregnancy that can involve the soft and hard palate, the nose, the nasal septum, and the nasal and maxillary processes.

- The lip and palate develop separately in utero.
- Infants can have a cleft lip on only one side of the lip, usually the left side, or on both sides.
- The infant can also have a cleft palate that may be the only deformity, or it may be coupled with one-sided or bilateral cleft lip.
- Bilateral clefts are often associated with cleft palate.
- Cleft lip is more common than palate and occurs during the fourth to seventh week of gestation.
- A cleft lip is an opening in the formation of the lip and can vary from a slit to a large opening that can extend into the nose.
- It can occur on one side, both sides, or in the middle of the lip.
- Cleft palate results during the improper fusion of the roof or palate of the mouth during the 7th to 12th week of pregnancy.
- Incidence is higher in Asians, Latinos, and Native Americans.
- Boys have a higher incidence of cleft lip, whereas girls have a higher incidence of cleft palate (U.S. National Library of Medicine, 2017a).
- The deformity can occur in the hard palate, which is the roof of the front part of the mouth, or in the soft palate, which is at the back of the roof of the mouth, or both.

CRITICAL COMPONENT

Incidence

CDC statistics indicate that approximately 2,650 infants were born in the United States with cleft palate, and 4,440 infants were born with a cleft lip with or without a cleft palate (U.S. National Library of Medicine, 2017a). The causes of cleft lip and palate are unknown, but genetics and environment are thought to play a role. Deficiencies in folic acid intake during pregnancy, as well as alcohol consumption and smoking, have resulted in an increased incidence of cleft lip and palate. The use of certain medications during pregnancy, such as acne medications isotretinoin (Accutane) and antiseizure drugs phenytoin (Dilantin), have been shown to increase the incidence. Currently, the CDC is conducting a nationwide study on the causes and risks for genetic defects, known as the National Birth Defects Prevention Study.

Physical Assessment

- Cleft lip is visually apparent (Figure 7–14).
- Close inspection of the palate is necessary after birth for patency of the palate.

Nursing Interventions

- Feeding problems occur because of the opening in the palate of the infant.
- Saliva, formula, or breast milk can flow into the nasopharynx with resulting aspiration.
- Infants can have problems creating a seal around a nipple.
- An intact lip creates a negative pressure necessary to suck; however, an infant with a cleft lip and an intact palate will be able to breastfeed. Lactation consultants can help with obtaining a seal (Gallagher, McKinney, & Glass, 2017). "Cleft palates prevent the infant from isolating the oral palate from the nasal sinuses, which does not allow for a negative pressure vacuum needed to successfully draw milk from the breast" (Gallagher et al., 2017, p. 79).

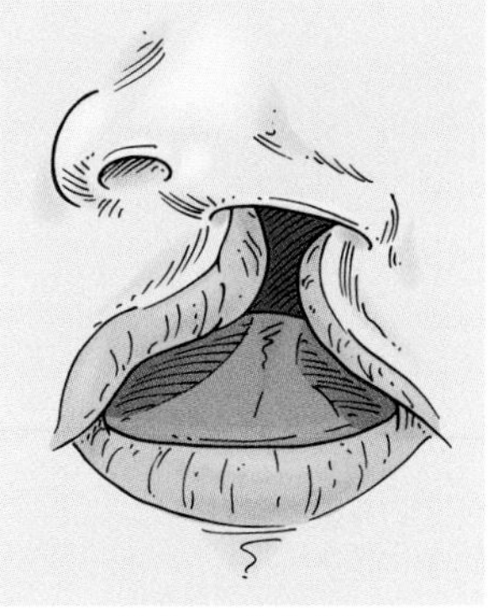

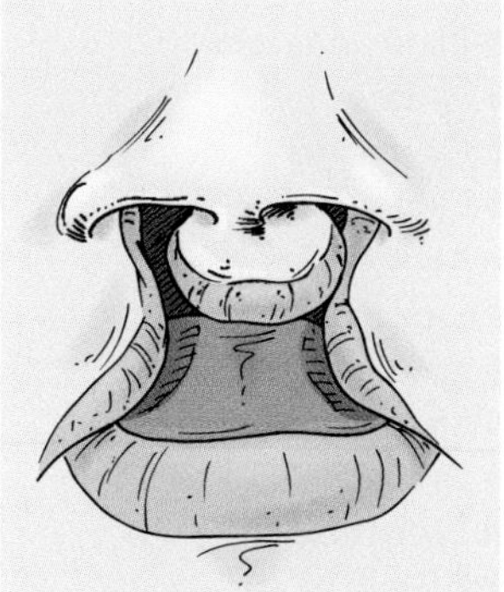

FIGURE 7–14 Cleft lip and palate.

- Most infants will require adaptive feeding methods (Gallagher et al., 2017), such as special nipples that are either longer to reach past the palate defect or are attached to an artificial palate that is placed into the infant's mouth, closing the defect. Specialized bottles are also used.
- Fluid intake and nutritional balance need to be maintained to support weight gain while nursing.
- Ear infections are common in children who have cleft palate due to the flow of saliva, milk, or breast milk into the middle ear.
- Repeated ear infections may increase the incidence of hearing loss because of scarring or damage to the Eustachian tubes.
- Speech issues in later life are also common.
- Dental issues in children with this defect include problems with dental malocclusions.
- There is a higher incidence of dental caries.
- Additional or missing development of dental eruptions may occur.

SAFE AND EFFECTIVE NURSING CARE: Clinical Pearl

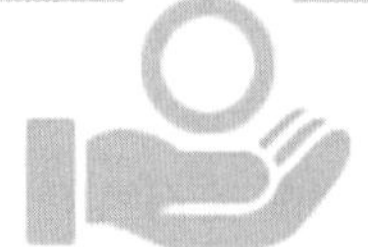

Psychosocial Problems With Cleft Lip and Palate

Children with cleft lip and/or cleft palate may experience psychosocial problems. They may have difficulty with speech or facial appearance issues. Parents may have bonding issues with the loss of the perfect baby, and mothers can have displaced guilt and feel that they have caused this defect. Other individuals can be cruel and stare or make fun of the child. Nurses may assist the parents and child with acceptance of the condition, encouraging bonding early and introducing the child to others with the condition, so they do not feel so different.

The nurse should discuss with the parents that this disorder is not anyone's fault and can happen to anyone. There is no one single cause of the disorder. The best support for families is to connect with a support group for parents with cleft lip and palate. Avoid internet sources because they often provide misinformation.

Treatment

A multidisciplinary treatment approach includes:

- Plastic surgeons
- Nurses
- Geneticists
- Oral surgeons
- Audiologists
- Otolaryngologists
- Speech therapists
- Social workers
- Psychologists
- Pediatricians
- Clergy

The repair is performed within 2 to 3 months of age up to 18 months with the goal of preventing speech and dental problems. Research indicates that correcting before 12 months results in better outcomes in terms of speech and the need for future corrections (Adu & Donkor, 2017; Patel, 2016). The infant must be gaining weight and be free of respiratory infections. Surgical repair involves a Z-plasty, which closes the palate in one procedure with a staggered suture line (Adu & Donkor, 2017). Multiple surgeries may be required depending on the extent of the defect.

Postoperative Nursing Care

- NPO immediately after surgery.
- Position infant on back or side.
- Assess respiratory status. Edema may cause an airway problem.
- Logan bow (a thin metal bar) or steristrips are taped to the face to maintain and keep the suture line intact, especially when the child is crying.
- The infant may be restrained for approximately 2 to 3 weeks with soft elbow restraints (splints), which are devices to keep his or her hands from disrupting the suture line.

SAFE AND EFFECTIVE NURSING CARE: Promoting Safety

Use of Restraints

Restraints on the child's arms should be removed every 2 hours, one arm at a time, to make sure the skin underneath and circulation are not compromised and to allow the infant to move his or her arm freely while the caregiver closely monitors the suture line.

- An infant with a cleft palate repair should not be suctioned orally. Infants are provided liquids with a cup and should avoid straws, pacifiers, and eating utensils to protect the suture line.
- A soft, rubber-tipped feeder or nipple is preferred and should be introduced in the side of the mouth to avoid the suture line.
- Breastfeeding during this time generally is avoided.

SAFE AND EFFECTIVE NURSING CARE: Clinical Pearl

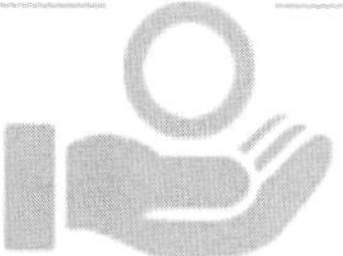

Feeding Devices

A variety of feeding devices are available to assist in feeding infants with cleft palate. A Ross Cleft Palate Nurser manufactured by Ross Laboratories and a Haberman feeder manufactured by Medula are two commercially available feeders (Wiet, 2015). In addition, a Breck feeder is a 10-mL syringe attached to a long, red rubber or soft rubber extended tube that is approximately 2 to 3 inches long. The purpose of the Breck feeder is to permit the elongated soft rubber end to extend beyond the defect. A soft, crosscut nipple and/or a Breck feeder is used to allow a faster flow of formula or expressed breast milk to be taken into the mouth. Care must be taken that the infant does not choke if the crosscut is large. Cup feeding is a safe alternative method of feeding that is recommended by the World Health Organization (WHO) in developing countries (Gallagher et al., 2017).

- Direct the flow of milk away from the defect and to the side.
- Feed the infant in an upright position and burp frequently.
- Clean the suture line after feeding; carefully observe for aspiration.
- Raise the head of the bed or place in a seat following feedings.
- Rinse the mouth with water after feedings.
- Clean the suture line often with half-strength hydrogen peroxide and water or normal saline per physician protocol.
- Some surgeons will order a topical antibiotic cream.
- Cleft palate repair is similar in postoperative care, although the infant may be placed on the abdomen to facilitate drainage if there is no cleft lip repair involved.

CRITICAL COMPONENT

Nursing Goals

1. Maintain the integrity of the suture line.
2. Assess respiratory status.
3. Promote bonding with the infant.
4. Promote optimal nutritional intake of the infant.
5. Manage pain.

Emergency Care

- Explain procedures to caregivers.
- Answer caregiver questions as needed.

Acute Care

- Instruct caregivers that children may require multiple surgeries, repairs, or gum grafts.
- Instruct caregivers to keep toys with protruding ends away from the infants, who may put them into their mouths and disrupt their suture lines.
- Teach caregivers to promote sucking between meals to help the children develop muscles that are not being fully used during feeding.

Chronic Care

- Instruct caregivers that psychological assistance may be required for children with facial abnormalities or for parent–infant bonding issues because of the lack of the perfect baby at birth.
- Instruct caregivers that children will need to see their dentists early, and that they often will require braces or dental prostheses.

SAFE AND EFFECTIVE NURSING CARE: Cultural Competence

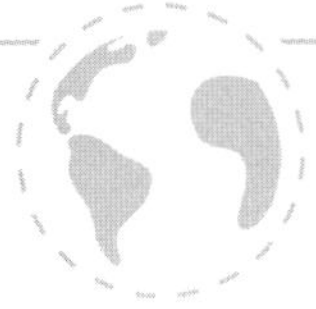

Pregnancy Superstitions

Many cultures have superstitions or beliefs about pregnant women and the effects of what they eat, see, or smell will have on the developing baby. Some cultures believe that if a pregnant woman encounters a rabbit during her pregnancy, then the baby will develop a harelip or cleft lip, whereas others believe that a cleft is caused by sins from a past life. These superstitions and beliefs may result in isolation and shame (Antiui-Kusi et al., 2015).

Neck

- The head should move freely from side to side.
- The infant should not move the head past the shoulder.
- The neck is short and thick; skin folds are present.
- No masses should be felt or observed.

Neurological Transition, Assessment, and Development

See Chapter 13 for further information on neurological development.

- The brain reaches 90% of its total size during infancy.
- All neurons are present by the end of the first year of life.
- Maturation follows cephalocaudal (head-to-toe), proximodistal (center-to-extremity) progression and mass to specific.
- Positional plagiocephaly (positional skull flattening) is treated by changes in position or physical therapy. Custom-fitted helmets are restricted to severe cases (Flannery et al., 2016).

Nurses who are conducting this assessment should be alert for:

- Uncoordinated movements
- Tremors in the extremities
- Poor muscle control or tone

Abnormalities are determined by testing the baby's reflexes; they need to be symmetrical on each side of the body. Asymmetry suggests abnormality or weakness. Reflexes present in the neonate include:

- Moro reflex or startle reflex: Occurs when the infant is startled with noise or rapid change in position; the infant throws the arms and legs out, cries, and then recoils the arms and legs. The neonate makes a C with the thumb and forefinger. This reflex disappears around 6 months of age.
- Rooting reflex: When the side of mouth is touched or stroked, the infant will turn its head and seek to suck. Disappears between 3 and 6 months of age.
- Sucking reflex: Reflex is present at birth but disappears at 10 to 12 months of age.
- Palmar grasp reflex: Grasping of a person's finger in the infant's hand; disappears at about 3 to 4 months of age and is replaced by the voluntary grasp.
- Plantar reflex: The infant's toes flex in a grasping motion in response to a thumb pressed against the ball of the foot; disappears at about 3 to 4 months of age.
- Tonic neck or fencing position reflex: The arm and leg are extended while the opposite side of the body is flexed; disappears around 4 to 6 months of age.
- Babinski reflex: The infant's toes flare when the foot is stroked in an upward motion; normal in children and disappears at 12 months of age.
- Stepping or dancing reflex: The neonate steps up and down in place when held upright; disappears at 3 to 4 weeks of age. See Table 7–7.

TABLE 7-7 Newborn Reflexes

REFLEX	AGE	HOW ELICITED	EXPECTED RESPONSE	ABNORMAL RESPONSE
Moro	Present at birth; disappears by 6 months	Jar the crib or hold the baby in a semi sitting position and let the head slightly drop back	Symmetrical abduction and extension of arms and legs, and legs flex up against trunk The neonate makes a C shape with the thumb and index finger	A slow response might occur with preterm infants or sleepy neonates An asymmetrical response may be related to temporary or permanent birth injury to clavicle, humerus, or brachial plexus
Startle	Present at birth; disappears by 4 months	Make a loud sound near the neonate	Same as Moro response	Slow response when sleeping Possible deafness Possible neurological deficit
Tonic neck	Present between birth and 6 weeks; disappears by 4–6 months	With the neonate in a supine position, turn the head to the side so that the chin is over the shoulder	The neonate assumes a "fencing" position with arms and legs extended in the direction in which the head was turned	Response after 6 months may indicate cerebral palsy
Rooting	Present at birth; disappears between 3 and 6 months	Brush the side of a cheek near the corner of the mouth	The neonate turns his or her head toward the direction of the stimulus and opens the mouth Instruct mothers who are lactating to touch the corner of the neonate's mouth with a nipple and the infant will turn toward the nipple for feeding	May not respond if recently fed Prematurity or neurological defects may cause weak or absent response
Sucking	Present at birth; disappears at 10–12 months	Place a gloved finger or nipple of a bottle in the neonate's mouth	Sucking motion occurs	May not respond if recently fed Prematurity or neurological defects may cause weak or absent response
Palmar grasp	Present at birth; disappears at 3–4 months	The examiner places a finger in the palm of the neonate's hand	The neonate grasps the finger tightly; if the neonate grasps the examiner's finger with both hands, the neonate can be pulled to a sitting position	Absent or weak response indicates a possible central nervous system defect or nerve or muscle injury
Plantar grasp	Present at birth; disappears at 3–4 months	Place a thumb firmly against the ball of the infant's foot	Toes flex tightly down in a grasping motion	Weak or absent response may indicate possible spinal cord injury
Babinski	Present at birth; disappears at 1 year	Stroke the lateral surface of the sole in an upward motion	Hyperextension and fanning of toes	Absent or weak response may indicate a possible neurological defect
Stepping or dancing	Present at birth; disappears at 3–4 weeks	Hold the neonate upright with feet touching a flat surface	The neonate steps up and down in place	Diminished response may indicate hypotonia

Source: adapted from Dillon, P. (2007). Nursing Health assessment: A Critical Thinking, Case Studies Approach (2nd ed.) *Philadelphia: F.A. Davis.*

PHYSICAL DEVELOPMENT

Physical development of the newborn is assessed to determine the gestational age of the newborn. Gestational age is calculated from the first start day of the mother's menstrual cycle to the current date or date of delivery. This age is based on the mother's history, prenatal ultrasounds, or neonatal maturation examination. It can be calculated using the Ballard scoring method.

Ballard Maturational Scoring consists of six areas of neuromuscular maturity and six areas of observed physical maturity, and is used to assess gestational age (Table 7–8). A score is assigned to each area. The physical maturity scoring should be completed within the first 2 hours of birth, and the neuromuscular scoring should be completed within the first 24 hours. Areas measured in Ballard Maturational Scoring include the following:

- Neuromuscular activity:
  - Posture: the position of the infant at rest, flaccid, or flexed
  - Square window: how far the infant's hand can be flexed toward the wrist
  - Arm recoil: how well the arms recoil back when flexed
  - Popliteal angle: how far the infant's knees can be flexed
  - Scarf sign: how far the infant's arm can be moved across the chest
  - Heel to ear: with the hips on the bed, how far the baby's feet can be moved toward the ear
- Physical maturity:
  - Skin: dryness, peeling, moisture
  - Lanugo: presence or absence
  - Plantar surfaces: presence or absence of creases and their depth
  - Breasts: normal 3 to 10 mm, nipples prominent
  - Ear/eyes: open or fused, amount of cartilage in the pinna; eyes need to be equal and symmetrical, and external canthus of the eyes need to line up with the top of the pinna
  - Genitalia: size of clitoris, labia minor, and labia majora; the urethral opening needs to be in the middle of the head of the penis with both testes palpable in the scrotum

The scores for these are plotted on a graph to provide a gestational age based on weight, length, and head circumference to determine whether the infant is appropriate for gestational age (AGA), SGA, or LGA. Term infants have higher scores than premature infants.

Weight

Infants who are AGA average between 2,500 g (5.5 lb) and 4,000 g (8.75 lb). The average birth weight is 7.5 lb. Categorizations include:

- AGA: between the 10th and 90th percentiles
- SGA: below the 10th percentile

TABLE 7–8 Ballard Maturational Assessment Tool

NEUROMUSCULAR MATURITY	PHYSICAL MATURITY
POSTURE Assess the position the neonate assumes while lying quietly on his or her back The more mature, the greater degree of flexion in the legs and arms	SKIN The examiner inspects the neonate's chest and abdominal skin areas for texture, transparency, thickness, and peeling and/or cracking A preterm neonate's skin is smooth, thin, and translucent (numerous veins visible) A full-term neonate's skin is thicker and more opaque, with some degree of peeling
SQUARE WINDOW Assess the degree of the angle created when the examiner flexes the neonate's hand toward the forearm The more mature, the greater the flexion	LANUGO The examiner assesses the amount of lanugo on the neonate's back Lanugo begins to form around the 24th week of gestation; it is abundant in preterm neonates and decreases in amount as the neonate matures
ARM RECOIL With the neonate in a supine position, the examiner fully flexes the forearm against the neonate's chest for 5 seconds The examiner extends the arms and releases them The more mature, the faster the arms return to the flexed position (recoil)	PLANTAR CREASES The examiner inspects the bottom of the feet for location of creases The more mature, the more creases over the greater proportion of the foot

Continued

TABLE 7–8 Ballard Maturational Assessment Tool—cont'd

NEUROMUSCULAR MATURITY	PHYSICAL MATURITY
POPLITEAL ANGLE With the neonate in a supine position and the pelvis flat, the examiner flexes the neonate's thigh to the abdomen; the leg is extended; the angle at the knee is estimated The more mature, the lesser the angle	BREAST TISSUE The examiner assesses the degree of nipple formation The size of the breast bud is measured by gently grasping the tissue with the thumb and forefinger and measuring the distance between the thumb and forefinger The more mature, the greater the degree of nipple formation and the size of the breast bud
SCARF SIGN With the neonate in a supine position, the examiner takes the neonate's hand and moves the arm across the chest toward the opposite shoulder The examiner notes where the elbow is in relationship to the midline of the chest The more preterm, the more the elbow crosses the midline	EAR FORMATION The examiner assesses the ear for form and firmness The more mature, the more defined and firmer the ear is
HEEL TO EAR With the neonate in a supine position, the examiner takes the neonate's foot and moves it toward the ear The more mature, the lesser the flexion (the further the heel is from the ear)	GENITALIA **Male:** The examiner palpates the scrotum for the presence of testis and inspects the scrotum for appearance The more mature, the greater the descent of the testis and the greater the degree of rugae (creases) **Female:** The examiner moves the neonate's hip one-half abduction and visually inspects the genitalia The more mature, the more the labia majora cover the labia minora and clitoris

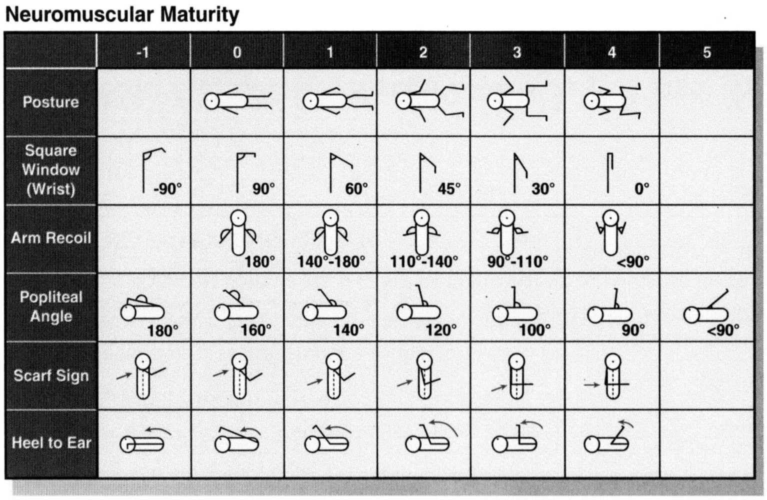

Neuromuscular Maturity

	-1	0	1	2	3	4	5
Posture							
Square Window (Wrist)	-90°	90°	60°	45°	30°	0°	
Arm Recoil		180°	140°-180°	110°-140°	90°-110°	<90°	
Popliteal Angle	180°	160°	140°	120°	100°	90°	<90°
Scarf Sign							
Heel to Ear							

TABLE 7–8 Ballard Maturational Assessment Tool—cont'd

Physical Maturity

Skin	sticky friable transparent	gelatinous red translucent	smooth pink visible veins	superficial peeling or rash, few veins	cracking pale areas rare veins	parchment deep cracking no vessels	leathery cracked wrinkled
Lanugo	none	sparse	abundant	thinning	bald areas	mostly bald	
Plantar Surface	heel-toe 40–50 mm:-1 <40 mm:-2	>50 mm no crease	faint red marks	anterior transverse crease only	creases ant. 2/3	creases over entire sole	
Breast	imperceptible	barely perceptible	flat areola no bud	stippled areola 1–2 mm bud	raised areola 3–4 mm bud	full areola 5–10 mm bud	
Eye/ear	lids fused loosely:-1 tightly:-2	lids open pinna flat stays folded	sl. curved pinna; soft; slow recoil	well-curved pinna; soft but ready recoil	formed and firm instant recoil	thick cartilage ear stiff	
Genitals (Male)	scrotum flat, smooth	scrotum empty faint rugae	testes in upper canal rare rugae	testes descending few rugae	testes down good rugae	testes pendulous deep rugae	
Genitals (Female)	clitoris prominent labia flat	prominent clitoris small labia minora	prominent clitoris enlarging minora	majora and minora equally prominent	majora large minora small	majora cover clitoris and minora	

Maturity Rating

Score	Weeks
−10	20
−5	22
0	24
5	26
10	28
15	30
20	32
25	34
30	36
35	38
40	40
45	42
50	44

Source: Reprinted from Journal of Pediatrics, *119:418, Ballard J, et al. Copyright 1991, with permission from Elsevier.*

- LGA: above the 90th percentile
- Low birth weight: 2,500 g or less (5.5 lb)
- Very low birth weight: 1,500 g or less (3.5 lb)
- Intrauterine growth restriction—growth of the fetus does not meet expected norms for gestational age
- Infants have a larger body surface area in comparison with their total weight

Height

The National Center for Health Statistics has developed growth charts used to compare a child's measurements with those of other children the same age, as well as specific growth charts for infants of Asian descent and those with Down syndrome. The average length at birth is 20 inches, and the best predictor of adult height is family history.

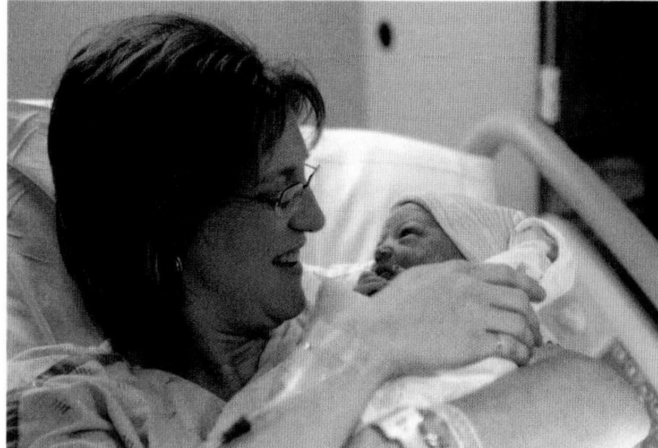

FIGURE 7–15 The mother and her newborn become acquainted during the first period of reactivity.

Head Circumference

Head and chest circumference are usually equal, with chest slightly smaller, usually 1 to 2 cm less than head. If the head is smaller than the chest, consider microcephaly, or small head. If the head is more than 1 inch larger than the chest, it can mean increased intracranial pressure or other issues.

Periods of Reactivity

- Initial period of reactivity (Figure 7–15)
  - Initial 30 minutes after birth
  - Active and very interested in environment
  - Bursts of eye movements
  - Responds to external stimuli
  - Excellent bonding time for family and infant
  - Eyedrops and ointment should be delayed (30 minutes) until family has made eye contact
  - Excellent time for breastfeeding
  - Heart rate, respiratory rate, and mucous production increase
  - Brief periods of tachypnea, tachycardia, apnea, cyanosis
- Period of relative inactivity
  - Begins 30 minutes to 2 hours after birth
  - Infant very sleepy and unresponsive to stimuli in the environment
  - Difficult period for feeding
  - Heart rate, respiratory rate, and mucous production decrease
- Second period of reactivity
  - Begins 2 to 8 hours after birth
  - Alert and responsive
  - Heart rate and respiratory rate increase

- Increased stooling
- Increased muscle tone

DEVELOPMENTAL MILESTONES

Infants achieve skills such as taking their first steps, rolling over, playing, speaking, and moving as they age. These skills are known as developmental milestones, and the timing of the appearance of these skills indicates whether the infant is developing at the normal rate consistent with his or her chronological age.

Birth to 3 Months

- Weight: gains 5 to 7 oz weekly during the first month and then 1 to 2 lb per month
- Feeding: Breastfed every 2 to 3 hours, formula-fed every 3 to 4 hours
- Height: grows 1 inch per month for first 6 months of life
- Head circumference: grows a half inch per month for first 6 months of life
- Motor skills:
  - Wobbly at first, but soon can lift head when on abdomen
  - Grasps an object, kicks vigorously, and turns head from side to side
  - Needs to have the head and neck supported
  - Can get their hands and thumbs to their mouths
  - Musculoskeletal and orthopedic disorders occur during fetal development; the most common of these disorders are talipes equinovarus (club foot) and developmental hip dysplasia (see Chapter 20 for details)
- Reflexes: primitive reflexes remain
- Hearing: should respond to parent's voice and respond to loud noises by blinking, startling, frowning, or waking from light sleep
- Vision: most newborns focus best on objects about 8 to 10 inches away, or the distance to your face during a feeding. Acuity is 20/100; they begin to recognize mother visually. Can track objects visually with more accuracy.
- Communication: sensitive to the way they are held, rocked, and fed. By age 2 months, the infant should smile on purpose (social smile), blow bubbles, and coo when spoken to. At 3 months the infant may laugh out loud and express moods.

Three to Six Months

- Birth weight doubles by 6 months of age
- Height increases 1 inch per month for first 6 months
- Can raise head (Figure 7–16) and support it by 4 months
- Reaches and grasps objects, plays with hands, moves objects to mouth, plays with toes
- Rolls from abdomen to back
- More stabilized sleeping patterns at 3 months
- Opens mouth for spoon
- Binocular vision: ability to see with both eyes coordinated
- Primitive reflexes begin to disappear
- Begins to drool, chew on toys as teething begins (6 months)
- Can sit when propped at 6 months (Figure 7–17)

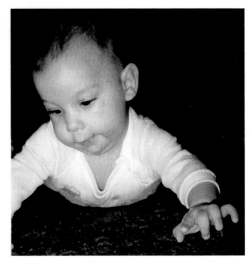

FIGURE 7–16 Infant lifting head up.

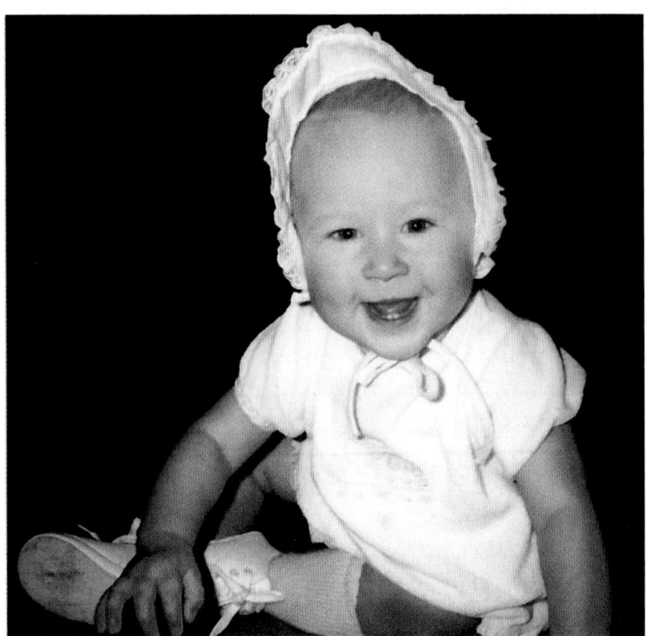

FIGURE 7–17 Infant sitting up.

- Can support some weight when held in a standing position
- Recognizes familiar objects and people, expresses displeasure when those objects or people are removed, babbles to self

Six to Nine Months

- All infants should be screened for developmental delays and disabilities at 9 months at the well-child visit (CDC, 2017b)
- Rolls from back to stomach and stomach to back
- Sits unsupported by 8 months
- Transfers objects from hand to hand, points at objects, and picks them up at 9 months
- Fine motor skills continue to develop

- Puts feet in mouth, plays pat-a-cake, loves to see own image in a mirror
- Develops and expresses taste preferences
- Begins to understand differences between inanimate and animate objects
- Displays stranger anxiety
- Develops object permanence
- Vocalizes with many-syllable vowel sounds and "m-m" with crying
- Around 9 months, says "Dada" and "Mama" and understands bye-bye and no
- Around 8 to 9 months begins to pull to stand, develops pincer grasp, crawls backward and then forward, and responds to own name (Figure 7–18)
- Understands where to look for an object that has been dropped; practices grasp-release movements
- Begins to test parent's responses, such as watching the parent while dropping food on the floor
- Distinguishes colors
- Distance vision
- Expresses emotions, including frustration and anger

Nine to Twelve Months

- Birth weight triples
- Birth length increases by 50%
- Head and chest circumference are equal
- Total of six to eight teeth
- Knows name
- Creeps along furniture
- Drinks from a cup; should be weaned from a bottle
- Stands alone for brief periods of time; raises arms when wants to be picked up

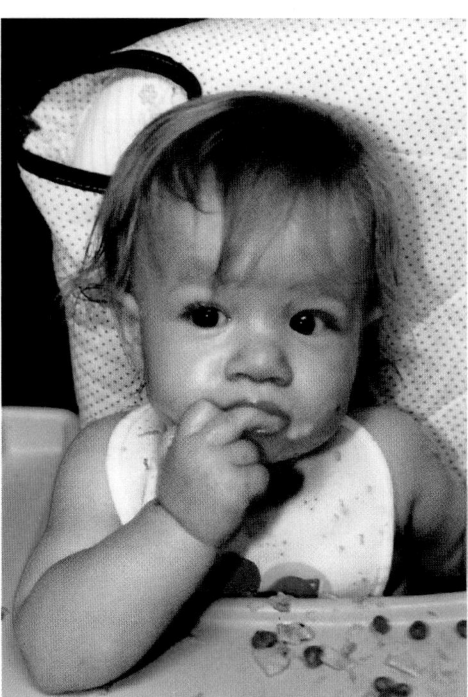

FIGURE 7–18 Infant with pincer grasp.

- May take first steps or walk alone
- Eats with spoon and cup but prefers fingers
- Enjoys familiar surroundings and people, expresses dissatisfaction with strangers or strange surroundings (stranger anxiety)
- May develop security objects such as favorite toys or blankets
- Enjoys books, especially board books
- Can understand simple communication or direction; says two or three words beyond Dada and Mama
- One or both feet may slightly turn in; the infant's lower legs are normally bowed
- At around 12 months of age can transition to whole cow's milk; do not use 1% or 2% because the infant needs the fat content for continuing brain development

COGNITIVE DEVELOPMENT

Cognitive development involves the infant's processing of information, conceptual processes, intelligence, language development, memory, and perceptual skills. Intellectual growth begins at birth and focuses on memory, problem solving, exploration of the environment, and understanding concepts. Primitive reflexes, which disappear within months after birth, are controlled by lower brain functions.

In this age group, cognitive development occurs quickly and may substantially vary from month to month. Infants develop on all levels and are influenced by cultural context, neurological development, and experience with others. Assessment models for infant cognitive development include the following:

- Brazelton Neonatal Behavioral Assessment Scale: Tests an infant's neurological development, behavior, and responsiveness. It is used only in the neonatal period.
- Gesell Developmental Schedules: Test for fine and gross motor skills, language, eye-hand coordination, imitation, object recovery, personal-social behavior, and play response.
- Denver Developmental Screening Test: Used to identify problems or delays. It measures personal/social, fine and gross motor, language, and social skills.
- Bayley Scales of Infant Development: Test the cognitive, behavioral, and motor domains of the infant. The assessment is used to identify infants with developmental disabilities. It is a highly reliable tool that uses mental, motor, and behavioral scales to rate an infant's functioning. The mental test screens for such items as whether the infant turns to a sound or looks for a fallen object. The motor test screens for gross and fine motor skill development.

Developmental Theorists

- Piaget (theory of cognitive development): In sensorimotor stage, infants use five senses to explore their world; the theory includes six substages that describe the infant's mental representation (see Chapter 6). Infants learn about their environments through their senses and begin to engage in goal-directed behaviors (Ward & Hisley, 2015).
- Vygotsky (social context of cognitive development): Describes how complex mental functioning originates in infants through

social interactions. Cultural factors influence attainment. There is a close correlation between language acquisition and the development of thinking (see Chapter 6).

- Erikson (psychosocial development): Highlights trust versus mistrust as the first psychosocial stage during the first year of life. This theory explains how the infant's personality develops.
  - Trust requires a feeling of physical comfort and a minimal amount of fear and apprehension about the future. It is a time where the infant has certain expectations about the predictability of the environment. If this stage is not attained, the infant feels insecure and learns mistrust (see Chapter 6).
  - Trust in infancy provides lifelong expectation that the world will be a good and pleasant place to live.
- Mahler (social development): Describes how an infant develops a sense of self through symbiosis and separation, or individualism (see Chapter 6).
- Kohlberg (moral development): Describes how moral reasoning aids in the development of ethical behavior and proceeds through six stages (see Chapter 6).

Sensory Development

- Vision: least-developed sense; infants are attracted to bright colors and black and white because of limited vision; objects appear two-dimensional with poor peripheral vision until 2 to 3 months of age
- Smell: well-developed sense; especially recognizes smell of own mother (Crenshaw, 2014)

Evidence-Based Practice: Soothing Odors

Hennet, T., & Borsign, L. (2016). Breastfed at Tiffany's. *Trends in Biochemical Sciences, 41*(6), 508–518.

Research has indicated that mothers pass on to their newborns chemosensory information that reveals her identity, the location of her breasts, and the composition of her milk. These pheromones help guide the newborn to finding the source of milk necessary for nutrition, fluids, and energy, and identify her to her newborn. Studies have shown that biologically meaningful odors such as amniotic fluid, colostrum, and breast milk are soothing to infants, particularly when obtained from the infant's own mother. These odors support successful mother–infant bonding and increase breastfeeding success.

- Taste: well-developed sense; sweet tastes are preferred
- Hearing: can hear beginning in the womb and can identify mother's voice; differentiates between male and female voices; hearing is critical for language development
  - Hearing test is administered before discharge, either through otoacoustic emissions or auditory brainstem response.
  - All 50 states, as well as Puerto Rico, Guam, and the District of Columbia, require hearing screening for newborns.
  - Tests are noninvasive, conducted before discharge by a trained professional, and performed in a quiet environment. Vernix, other fluids, and a withdrawing infant may affect the test.
  - Auditory brainstem response is a physiological measurement of the brainstem's response to sound. A clicking sound is produced, and the electrical activity response from the nerve is recorded as waveforms on a computer. This noninvasive test requires electrodes to be placed on the infant's scalp with adhesive and is conducted while the infant is sleeping (Chapman & Durham, 2014).
  - The otoacoustic emissions method uses an earplug that measures the responses of the cochlea to clicking sounds produced by a microphone. The infant is sleeping during the test. It is a noninvasive procedure (Figure 7–19).
  - Examination of the ears of an infant: Pull the pinnae straight back and down.
  - Communications with infants are similar in different cultures, with a higher-pitched voice used when attempting to get the infant's attention; deaf mothers use a slower pattern and sign more often.

SAFE AND EFFECTIVE NURSING CARE: Clinical Pearl

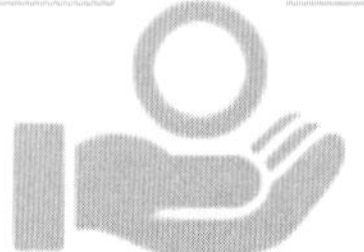

Hearing Screening at Birth

The U.S. Preventative Task Force, the CDC, and the AAP recommend that all newborn infants undergo screening at birth (AAP, 2017c). Some degree of hearing loss occurs in 3 out of 1,000 infants (AAP, 2017c). Any infant who does not pass the newborn hearing screening has the potential for a developmental emergency (AAP, 2016c). Initial newborn hearing screening occurs in the hospital setting by specially trained nursing staff with any necessary follow-up testing recommended in the pediatric medical home (AAP, 2017c). The State Early Hearing Detection and Intervention (EHDI) Laws and Regulations list the screening mandated by all 50 states and the District of Columbia (AAP, 2016d).

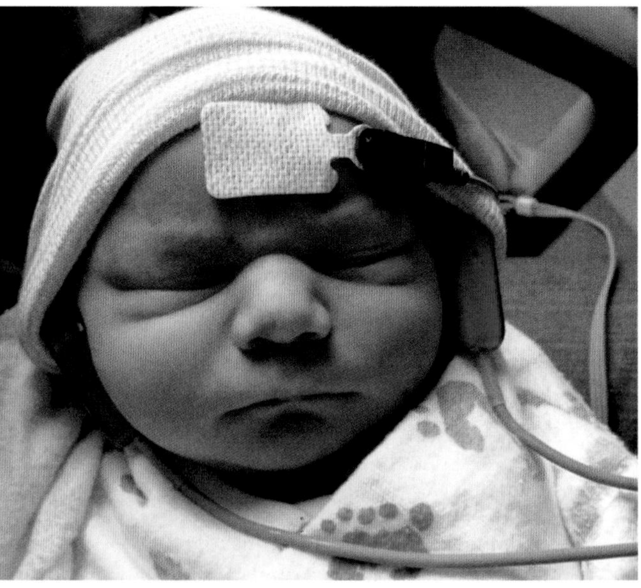

FIGURE 7–19 Neonatal hearing screening.

- Touch: Touch is extremely important for the newborn; gentle touch or massage is calming and pleasurable. Pain is a protective device; the infant responds by extending and retracting the extremities and crying.

Language Acquisition

Language acquisition is a partly innate and partly learned process. Linguist Noam Chomsky (nativist theory) describes the infant's acquisition of language as complex and not well understood; he coined the term *language acquisition device*. Vygotsky proposed the interactionist theory of language acquisition, which states that language is learned through socialization within the family context.

Early speech is evidenced by crying, babbling, and mimicking of repetitive vowel sounds such as *ma-ma-ma* and *da-da-da*. Single words are then used and accumulate into the infant's vocabulary. Children interact with other people and the environment, so favorable responses to speech encourage the infant to communicate.

Discipline

Although it is impossible to spoil an infant, discipline at this age should focus on setting limits for the child's safety and well-being.

- At 6 months of age, when the child is more mobile, use distraction to keep the child away from dangerous areas.
- Temper tantrums are the infant's way of expressing frustration, hunger, anger, illness, or fatigue.
- Reward good behavior.
- Remain calm, firm, and consistent.
- Maintain a set routine.

SAFE AND EFFECTIVE NURSING CARE: Promoting Safety

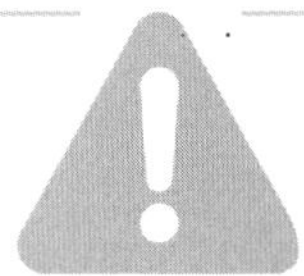

Corporal Punishment

Corporal punishment of children, such as spanking or hitting, has been found to have negative consequences and is less effective than other forms of discipline, such as the withdrawal of positive reinforcement (loss of privileges, time-outs). Spanking has been associated with a higher incidence of aggressive behavior in children, increased substance abuse, and higher rates of crime and violence in older children (Kilgore, 2015).

Colic

Some infants experience a great deal of intestinal gas, resulting in frequent crying known as colic. Colic usually happens at the end of the day. Usually no medical problem is present, but the infant should be assessed by a pediatrician if it continues. Parents of an infant with colic should be educated about the following:

- Make sure the infant is burped frequently.
- Parents should not change formula, unless directed by the pediatrician.
- If the infant is breastfed, the mother should decrease the intake of spicy or gaseous food; dairy and corn can also cause gastrointestinal disturbances.
- Infants tend to be sensitive to stimulation. Try a car ride, movement, infant massage, carrying the infant in a carrier, or creating a white noise environment.
- If a pacifier is used, it can help calm the infant; pacifiers have also been shown to decrease the incidence of sudden infant death syndrome (SIDS).
- Colic usually disappears by about 12 to 16 weeks of age.

CRITICAL COMPONENT

Diagnostic Criteria for Infant Colic

Colic is diagnosed under the following circumstances:

- Paroxysms of irritability, fussing, or crying that start or stop without obvious cause
- Crying is turbulent and dysphonic, with a higher pitch
- Episodes last 3 hours or longer and occur 3 days a week for at least 2 weeks, peaking at 6 weeks of age
- Infant thriving
- Diagnosis of exclusion (Desphande, 2015)

SAFE AND EFFECTIVE NURSING CARE: Clinical Pearl

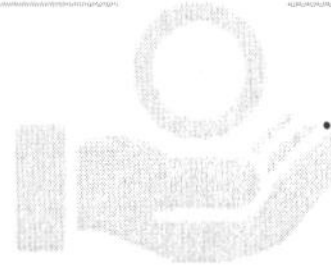

Care of the Infant With Colic

- Swaddle infant.
- Place in a safe area.
- Remove yourself from the infant for a 10-minute break once the child is secured in a safe place.
- Educate caregivers that colic is not a reflection of their caregiving skills.
- Realize that it is a heightened time of stress for caregivers.
- Simethicone drops have been prescribed to ease intestinal gas, but never give an infant an over-the-counter medication without consulting the child's pediatrician.

Play

Play is how infants learn about the world and themselves. Infants are primarily sensorimotor focused, so play should involve sensory stimulation. Infants explore the world with their mouths and imitate those around them. When choosing toys, safety is the number one consideration; avoid detachable or removable pieces or parts. Simple toys should be used because attention span is short. Opt for unbreakable mirrors, rattles, soft (nonremovable pieces) stuffed animals, large snap toys, and musical pull toys. Other tips for caregivers include:

- Place infants on their stomachs for supervised tummy time.
- Engage the infant with soothing tones and use of facial expressions.

- Use soothing music.
- If other siblings' toys are lying around, safety for the infant requires the caregiver to be aware of small pieces.
- Toys should help the infant in physical and fine motor development.
- Infants enjoy looking at themselves in mirrors.
- Play is essential in a hospitalized environment. The theorist Watson described the importance of positive play in fostering attachment between the infant and the caregiver. See Chapter 6 for further details.

NUTRITION

Parents of infants younger than 6 months can choose to either breastfeed or bottle-feed a commercially prepared formula. Because of the infant's developmental stage, he or she will push solids forward and out of the mouth. An objective of *Healthy People 2020* is to increase the proportion of breastfed infants from 74% to 81.99% (U.S. Breastfeeding Committee, 2017). The WHO recommends exclusive breastfeeding until the age of 6 months and to continue until the age of 2 years, with no supplementation of water, formula, or solids prior to this point (WHO, 2017). The decision to breastfeed versus bottle-feed is dependent on maternal knowledge, past exposure to breastfeeding, education level, perceptions of the benefits of breastfeeding, cultural factors, family and friend support, career barriers, husband or partner support, and support from health-care providers.

CRITICAL COMPONENT

Breastfeeding and Zika

No cases of Zika virus transmission have been associated with breastfeeding. The CDC and WHO recommend that the benefits of breastfeeding outweigh the risks of Zika virus transmission through breast milk (CDC, 2017).

For infants between 6 months and 1 year of age:

- Sufficient protein is needed to support growth and development.
- Fats are needed to provide calories and support brain development.
- Carbohydrates are needed to provide energy.
- Infants need 100 to 116 kcal/kg/day for basic growth and development.
- Adequate fluid and electrolyte intake is necessary.
- Fluids, mainly water, should total 120 to 150 mL/kg/day for infants.
- Supplemental iron is not necessary for breastfed infants before 6 months of age.
- All infants 6 months or older require iron supplementation. Iron can be supplied through lean red meats, fortified infant cereals, spinach, broccoli, green peas, or beans.
- Do not feed cow's milk until after 1 year of age.
- Soy formula is used for galactosemia, lactose intolerance, and allergies to cow's milk.

SAFE AND EFFECTIVE NURSING CARE: Clinical Pearl

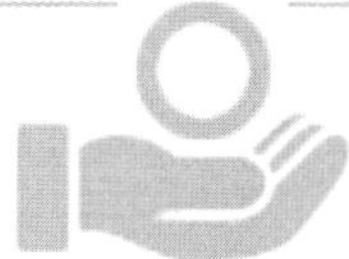

Soy Protein–Based Formula

Isolated soy protein–based formulas are safe and effective for normal growth and development of infants but are not to be used for preterm infants. Soy protein–based formulas have no advantage in the prevention of colic or as a supplement for breastfed infants (Bellaiche, Levy, & Camille, 2013).

Nonnutritive Sucking

- Nonnutritive sucking is a self-soothing or comforting measure used by infants.
- The infant's sucking ability is necessary for neurological development and survival.
- Pacifiers, fingers, or fists are used in self-sucking.
- Suckling, which the infant does at the breast, requires a different set of mouth movements than does bottle feeding or the use of fingers, fists, or a pacifier.
- Avoid using pacifiers in the early days of breastfeeding.
- Educate caregivers on the use of a pacifier, such as not using it as a substitute for feeding or holding.
- Never tie or clip the pacifier to the child's clothing because this can be a source of strangulation, even in older infants.
- Limit the use of the pacifier as the infant gets older to prevent creating a habit that will be difficult to break; distract the infant with an alternative.

Breastfeeding

Breastfeeding is the optimal method of feeding because it provides all necessary nutrients, minerals, and vitamins (Table 7–9).

- Should begin within the first hour after birth during the initial period of reactivity
- Infant should be fed on demand throughout the day and night
- Reduces costs and preparation time
- Promotes positive bonding between infant and mother
- Decreases risk for obesity

Composition of Breast Milk

Breast milk development begins early in pregnancy through the hormones of estrogen, progesterone, and prolactin. It is high in IgA and IgG, and contains higher levels of a protein with a laxative effect that aids in the passage of meconium. No immunoglobulins are found in formulas. Concentration of nutrients differs among women. Infant allergic responses to breast milk are rare. Components of breast milk include:

- Large water content; fat content accounts for 52% (Durham & Chapman, 2014)
- Carbohydrates (lactose, 42% of calories in breast milk)

TABLE 7–9 Selected Benefits of Breastfeeding

FOR MOTHERS	FOR INFANTS
• Decreased risk for breast cancer • Lactational amenorrhea (although breastfeeding is not considered an effective form of contraception) • Enhanced involution (due to uterine contractions triggered by the release of oxytocin) and decreased risk for postpartum hemorrhage • Enhanced postpartum weight loss • Increased bone density • Enhanced bonding with infant	• Enhanced immunity through the transfer of maternal antibodies; decreased incidence of infections, including otitis media, pneumonia, urinary tract infections, bacteremia, and bacterial meningitis • Enhanced maturation of the gastrointestinal tract • Decreased likelihood of development of insulin-dependent (type 1) diabetes • Decreased risk for childhood obesity • Enhanced jaw development • Protective effects against certain childhood cancers such as lymphoblastic leukemia, Hodgkin's disease (Karimi et al., 2016)

Source: Adapted from Ward, S. L., & Hisley, S. M. (2015). Maternal-child nursing care: Optimizing outcomes for mothers, children, & families *(2nd ed., p. 489). Philadelphia: F.A. Davis.*

- Protein, specifically whey (60% to 80%) and casein (20% to 40%), makes up approximately 6% of calories in breast milk (Durham & Chapman, 2014)
- Antibodies, bifidus factor (which stimulates the growth of lactobacillus)
- Lipase, amylase, and other enzymes
- Epidermal growth factor, nerve growth factor, other growth factors, and interleukins (Munblit et al., 2016)

Stages of Breast Milk

- Stage one: Colostrum, a yellowish fluid, is present in the first 2 to 3 days after birth and can also be secreted in the last trimester of pregnancy. Colostrum has higher concentrations of protein and lower levels of fat, carbohydrates, and calories than mature milk. It contains large amounts of IgA and IgG, and assists in the passage of the infant's first stool, known as meconium (WHO, 2016).
- Stage two: The milk transitions from colostrum to more mature milk at about 3 to 10 days after birth. It consists of increasing fat, carbohydrates, and calories (WHO, 2016).
- Stage three: Mature milk begins 10 days after birth. This mature milk has approximately 23 calories per ounce and is composed of foremilk and hind milk.
  - Foremilk is produced and released at the beginning of the feeding; it has a higher water and lactose content and a lower fat content.
  - The hind milk is released at the end of the feeding and has a higher fat content.

Production of Breast Milk

Lactation is the process of milk production (Figure 7–20). Once the baby is born, the levels of estrogen and progesterone are eliminated and prolactin becomes the predominant hormone. Infant stimulation influences supply and demand—as the infant demands, the woman's body supplies. Oxytocin is released from the posterior pituitary, which affects the breasts and the uterus. Oxytocin produces the letdown reflex, which forces milk into the lactiferous ducts of the breast. The letdown reflex is responsible for milk ejection. This reflex can occur during sexual stimulation, when hearing a baby cry, or when thinking of the infant. It can be inhibited by anxiety, stress, fatigue, and pain (Durham & Chapman, 2014). Infant cues and readiness to breastfeed are important adaptations that mother and infant need to make to facilitate the supply and demand.

Early Cues

- Rooting
- Head bobbing up and down
- Stirring and increased arm and leg movement
- Burying head in mattress or mother's chest

Late Cues

- Crying—extended crying can inhibit latching on to the breast
- Agitation

Latching On

Figure 7–21 illustrates breastfeeding positions. If placed on the mother's abdomen after birth, the infant will make crawling movements to reach the breast. The process of attaching the infant to the breast for feeding is as follows:

- Hold the breast like a sandwich with the thumb on the top and the other fingers underneath. The baby should be held close; as the baby's mouth is opened wide, place the breast fully (including the nipple and areola) into the baby's mouth (Figure 7–22).
- Encourage the infant's mouth to open by stimulating the rooting reflex.
- A successful latch is when the infant's mouth is around the areola with the nipple at the back of the mouth.

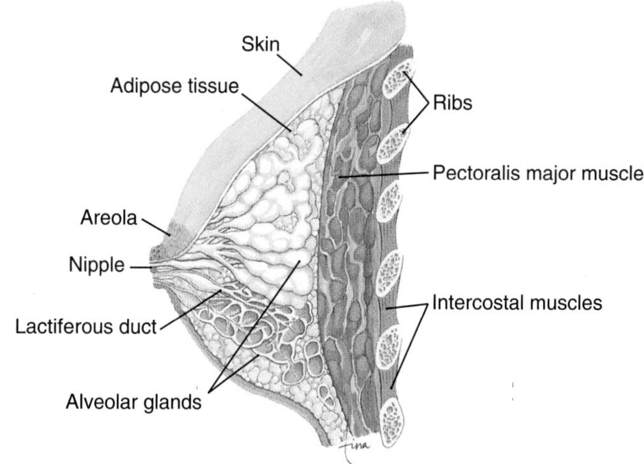

FIGURE 7–20 Mammary gland shown in midsagittal section.

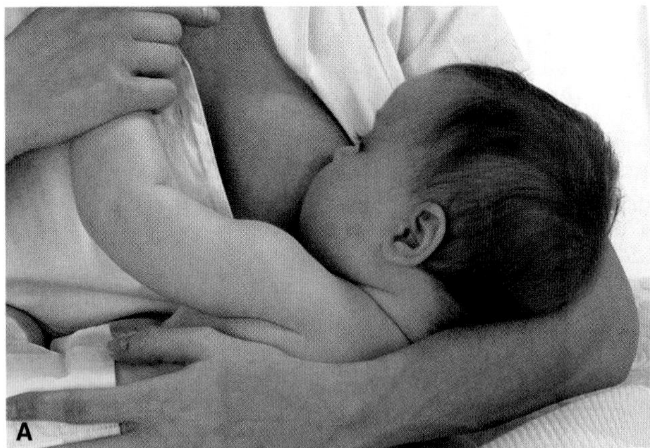

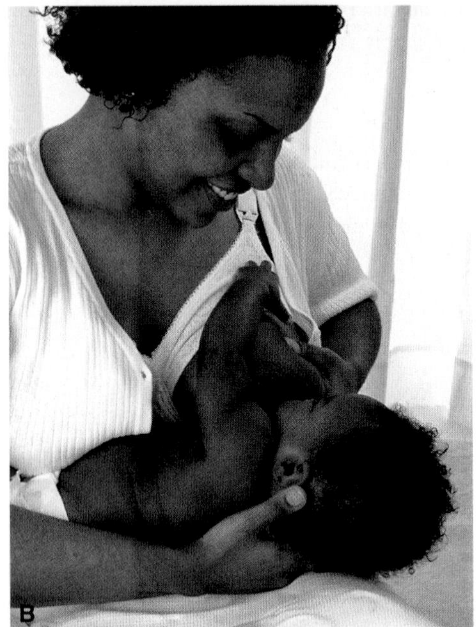

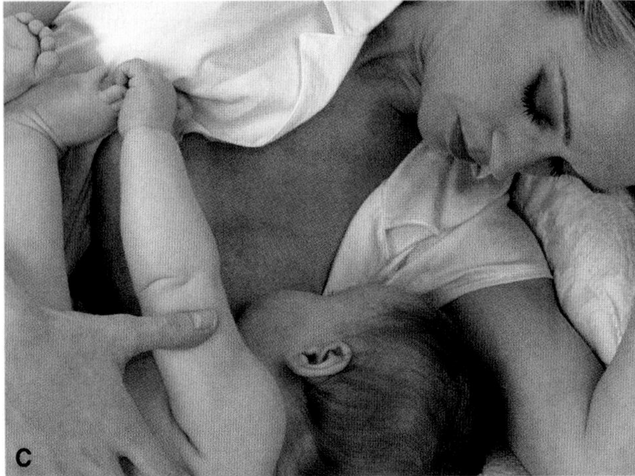

FIGURE 7–21 Common positions for breastfeeding. **A,** Cradle hold; **B,** football hold; **C,** side-lying position.

- The infant draws the milk forward in the breast.
- The tip of the nose, cheeks, and chin should be touching the breast. Align the breast with the infant's nose.
- Suck and swallow should follow.
- Often infants will feed from only one breast at a time for each feeding.
- Latch Scoring System can help determine a successful latch (Table 7–10)

Breastfeeding Success

- Feedings should last between 10 and 30 minutes—shorter times may indicate poor positioning or a sleepy infant; longer times can indicate nonnutritive sucking.
- Removing an infant from the breast is accomplished by inserting a clean finger into the corner of the infant's mouth to break the suction.
- Successful breastfeeding results in the infant gaining 1/2 to 1 oz per day (International Lactation Consultants Association, 2017).
- Expressed breast milk may be kept for 4 hours at room temperature, for 5 to 7 days in the refrigerator, and for 6 to 12 months in a deep freezer.
- Never reheat breast milk in a microwave or leave it on the counter to thaw or warm up.
- Thaw in the refrigerator.
- The AAP recommends breastfeeding for a full year.

CRITICAL COMPONENT

Lactation Consultant

A lactation consultant is a trained provider who is an expert in the field of lactation and breastfeeding. The AAP recognizes that assistance of lactation consultants helps to maintain a higher percentage of breastfeeding in the short and long term if their guidance is followed for 12 months. An International Board Certified Lactation Consultant (IBCLC) is a health-care professional who specializes in the clinical management of breastfeeding. IBCLCs are certified by the International Board of Lactation Consultant Examiners under the direction of the U.S. National Commission for Certifying Agencies (International Lactation Consultants Association, 2017).

Weaning an Infant

- Eliminate one feeding at a time.
- Observe for signs that the infant is having emotional or physical issues.
- Usually the last feeding to be eliminated is the nighttime feeding.

Bottle Feeding

Breast milk is the recommended method for infant feeding; however, if a mother chooses to bottle-feed her infant, never make her feel guilty for this choice. Often mothers may choose to bottle-feed and breastfeed, while waiting until they develop a milk supply. Commercially prepared formulas are nutritional appropriate if this is the parent's choice.

When feeding a newborn formula, carefully dilute with water based on the manufacturer's mixing instructions. Some preparations are ready to feed. Bottles and nipples must be washed thoroughly; use a dishwasher or boil all bottles, rings, and nipples. If formula needs to be heated, put it in a pan of hot water (not boiling) or use an electric warmer. Never microwave, because this can cause uneven heat distribution. Facilitate parent bonding by holding the infant close. Never prop a bottle because this can cause choking. Burp the infant frequently to prevent emesis.

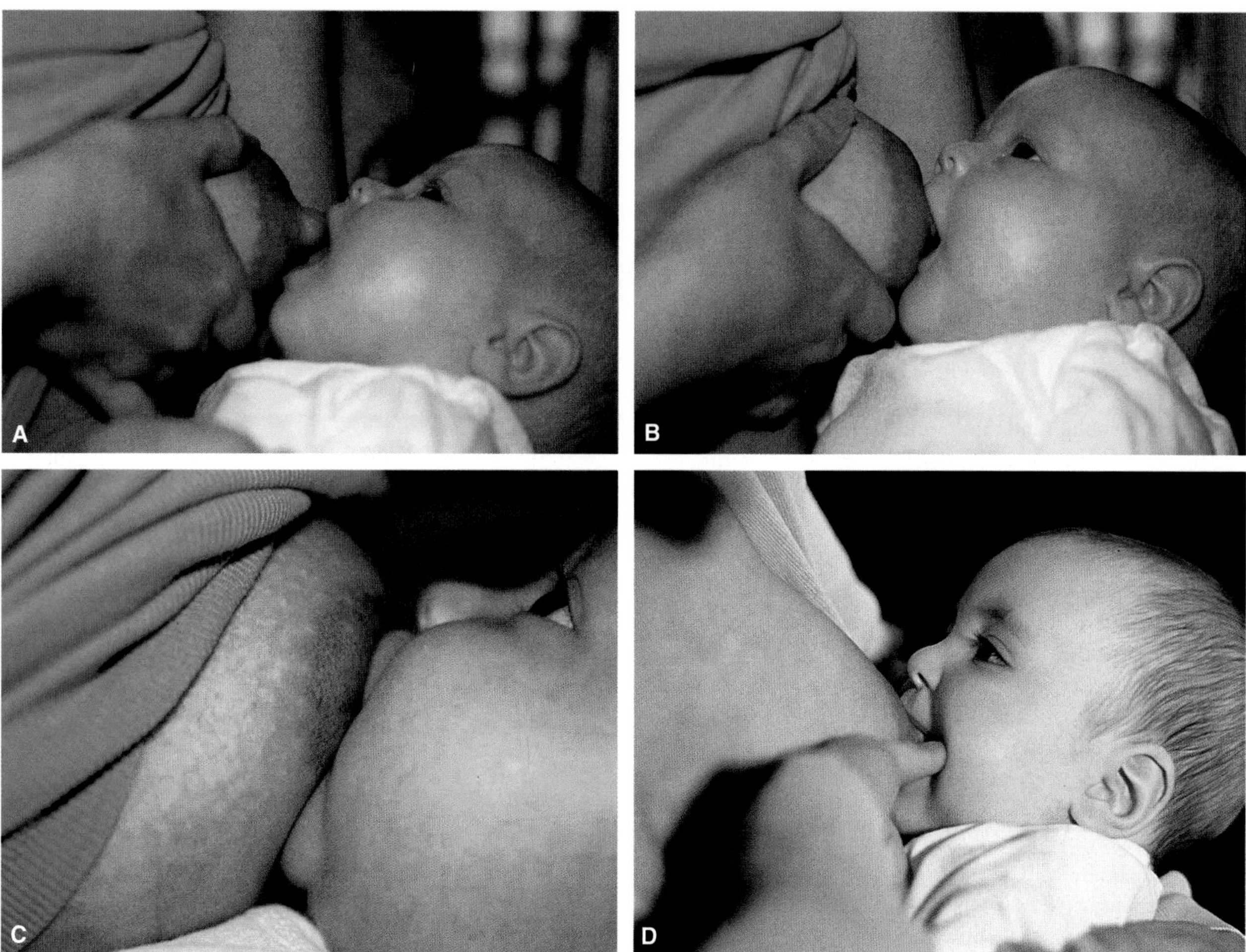

FIGURE 7–22 Infant latching on.

TABLE 7–10 Latch Scoring System

	0	1	2
L—Latch	Too sleepy or reluctant No latch achieved	Repeated attempts Hold nipple in mouth Stimulate to suck	Grasps breast Tongue down Lips flanged Rhythmic sucking
A—Audible swallowing	None	A few with stimulation	Spontaneous and intermittent <24 hours old Spontaneous and frequent >24 hours old
T—Type of nipple	Inverted	Flat	Everted (after stimulation)
C—Comfort (breast/nipple)	Engorged Cracked, bleeding, large blisters, or bruises Severe discomfort	Filling Reddened/small blisters or bruises Mild/moderate pain	Soft Tender
H—Hold (positioning)	Full assist (staff holds infant at breast)	Minimal assist (i.e., elevate head of bed; place pillow for support) Teach one side; mother does the other side Staff holds and then mother takes over	No assist from staff Mother able to position/hold infant

Source: Adapted from Jensen, D., Wallace, S., & Kelsay, P. (1994, January). LATCH: A breastfeeding charting system and documentation tool. Journal of Obstetric, Gynecologic, and Neonatal Nursing, *23(1), 27–32.*

Liquid formulas are sterile due to the manufacturing process. Powdered formulas are not sterile, and thereby increase the incidence of infections. Parents should be provided detailed instructions on hand hygiene, preparation, and equipment sterilization to prevent disease.

Advancing Feeding in Infants

An infant's requirement for calories is determined by size, rate of growth, activity, and energy needed for metabolic activities. Calorie needs per pound of body weight are higher during the first year of life than at any other time (Durham & Chapman, 2014). An infant is ready for solid foods at around 6 months of age. At this time, babies are able to move food around in their mouths. Breastfeeding should be on demand and average four to seven feedings per day; bottle feeding should average 24 to 32 oz of formula. No fruit juices should be given.

All foods should be placed on a spoon, not put in a bottle. Baby rice cereal is usually indicated for the first solid food (2 to 3 teaspoons) because it is iron fortified and associated with a decreased incidence of allergic reactions. At around 8 months, strained fruit, vegetables, and strained meats can be introduced. The caregiver should be taught to introduce a single type of food for 2 to 3 days to observe for reactions such as rashes, diarrhea, abdominal cramping, or vomiting. Use single-ingredient foods and do not add sugar, sweeteners, or corn syrup. The infant should receive only home-cooked food.

Self-feeding should begin when infants can sit up alone, hold their necks steady, draw in their lips when food is introduced into the mouth, and keep the food in their mouths and not push it back out. The extrusion reflex should be gone. Offer soft, mashed table food. Always cut up the infant's food into small pieces to prevent choking. The first teeth are biting teeth, not grinding teeth.

SAFE AND EFFECTIVE NURSING CARE: Promoting Safety

Choking Prevention

Foods that result in a decreased risk for choking in the infant include:

- Cooked macaroni
- Small pieces of cheese
- Soft cooked vegetables such as potatoes
- Small pieces of fruit such as bananas, peaches, or pears
- Small pieces of toast
- Grapes cut into fourths

Best practices to prevent choking include:

- Thoroughly cook and cut all foods into small pieces.
- Remove pits or seeds from fruit.
- Grind, mash, and add liquid to foods for younger infants.

When weaning the infant from a bottle at around 1 year of age, advance to a double-handled cup with a snap-on lid. The nighttime feeding is the last feeding to be removed because it is a source of comfort for the infant. Between 10 and 12 months, the infant will mimic the feeding habits of other family members. Do not feed an infant cow's milk until after 12 months of age. Cow's milk is deficient in iron, and the infant will experience development of anemia.

SAFE AND EFFECTIVE NURSING CARE: Promoting Safety

Avoiding *Clostridium botulinum* Contamination

Infants younger than 1 year should never be given honey or corn syrup because this may result in the ingestion of *Clostridium botulinum* bacteria, which is a spore-producing organism. The spores are found in improperly stored foods, home-canned foods, processed foods such as potato salad, restaurant-prepared foods, and bottled garlic (U.S. National Library of Medicine, 2017a).

SLEEP

Newborns sleep on average 8 to 9 hours per day and 8 hours at night. Infants normally do not sleep through the night until age 3 months, when their stomach size has increased so that they can take in more breast milk or formula. Infants, like adults, go through sleep periods of active and quiet sleep patterns (AAP, 2014). Newborn infants spend substantial time in rapid eye movement (REM) sleep indicative of rapid brain growth. At 3 months of age, REM sleep decreases and non-REM sleep occurs (AAP, 2014). Non-REM sleep has four stages:

- Stage 1: drowsiness
- Stage 2: light sleep
- Stage 3: deep sleep
- Stage 4: very deep sleep

Around 6 months of age, the infant may begin to sleep 8 to 12 hours at night. Sleep patterns for infants, as in adults varies, from infant to infant (AAP, 2014a).

Sudden Infant Death Syndrome

Sudden infant death syndrome (SIDS) and sudden unexplained infant death (SUID) are the leading cause of death from 1 month to 1 year of age, peaking between 2 and 4 months (CDC, 2017a). These are infant fatalities from an unknown cause and are not associated with infection, choking, vomiting, or abuse. SIDS/SUID occurs more often in male infants, in winter months, and in African American and American Indian infants. It is also more common among infants of mothers who did not have prenatal care and those who smoke. The "Safe to Sleep" program aims to prevent SIDS through caregiver education.

Evidence-Based Practice: Healthy Child Care America "Safe to Sleep" Campaign

Eunice Kennedy Shriver National Institute of Child Health and Human Development. (2015). Safe to sleep. Retrieved from https://www.nichd.nih.gov/news/releases/Pages/072015-podcast-safe-to-sleep.aspx

The "Safe to Sleep" campaign originally began in 1994 as the "Back to Sleep" program. This program highlighted how research had indicated that putting infants on their backs as the only sleeping position decreased the incidence of sudden infant death. This campaign evolved into a campaign highlighting safe sleeping practices in which the Academy of Pediatrics highlighted not only the position of the sleeping infant but the environment. The "Safe to Sleep" campaign highlights the following points:

- Always place babies to sleep on their backs during naps and at nighttime. Babies sleeping on their sides are more likely to accidentally roll onto their stomachs; the side position is not safe and is not recommended. Avoid products that prop the infant on their side such as wedges.
- Do not cover the heads of babies with a blanket or overbundle them in clothing and blankets.
- Avoid letting the baby get too hot, indicated by sweating, damp hair, flushed cheeks, heat rash, and rapid breathing. Dress the baby lightly for sleep. Infants placed in sleep sacks should not wear a hat; sleep sacks are sleeveless to prevent overheating, a risk factor for SIDS (AAP, 2016c).
- Place your baby in a safety-approved crib with a firm mattress and a well-fitting sheet. (Cradles and bassinets may be used, but choose those that are certified for safety by the Juvenile Products Manufacturers Association [JPMA].)
- Place the crib in an area that is always smoke free.
- Do not allow babies to sleep on adult beds, chairs, sofas, waterbeds, or cushions.
- Toys and other soft bedding, including fluffy blankets, comforters, pillows, stuffed animals, bumpers and wedges, should not be placed in the crib with the baby. These items can impair the infant's ability to breathe if they cover the infant's face.
- Breastfeed your baby. Experts recommend that mothers feed their children human milk at least through the first year of life.

SAFE AND EFFECTIVE NURSING CARE: Promoting Safety

Baby Boxes

In many U.S. states, new parents receive free "baby boxes." These boxes are portable, sturdy cardboard boxes that have firm foam mattresses with tight-fitting sheets, designed to encourage parents to place their infants on their backs to sleep. Most infants can sleep in the baby box until they outgrow it, usually at around 6 months of age. The highest incidence of sudden infant death is between 2 and 4 months of age. The AAP cautions that these boxes are not bassinets with firm frames and supports. Additional research on the impact on SIDS needs to be performed.

SAFE AND EFFECTIVE NURSING CARE: Promoting Safety

Bumper Pads

In 2016, the AAP reaffirmed that bumper pads never be used in the cribs of infants. This organization states that there is no clinical evidence that bumper pads prevent injuries, but they do pose a significant risk for suffocation or entrapment because infants do not have the motor skills to turn their heads.

- Newborns sleep from feeding to feeding; with age, the amount and length of wakeful periods increase. Newborns can sleep up to 17 hours a day in 3- to 4-hour intervals. Sleep deprivation is a factor for caregivers of newborns.
- By 3 months of age, the infant begins to sleep 6 to 8 hours a night.
- At 6 months, an infant takes two naps a day.
- At 1 year of age, the infant sleeps 15 hours a day—3 hours during the day and 11 hours at night.
- Infants' increase in sleep patterns is tied to growth spurts (Samson & Yetish, 2017).
- Infants, like adults, progress through REM and non-REM sleep cycles.
- The AAP and the U.S. Product Safety Commission recommend against co-bedding, or allowing the infant to sleep with parents/caregivers or siblings. No benefits were demonstrated through research on weight gain or vital signs.

SAFE AND EFFECTIVE NURSING CARE: Cultural Competence

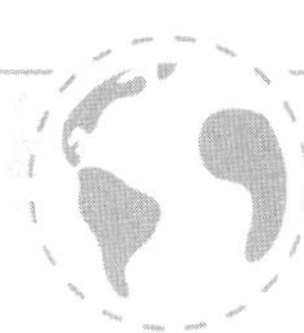

Co-bedding

Sleep patterns and behaviors are governed by cultural and societal norms (Williams et al., 2015). Co-bedding is practiced in many cultures (Lai, Foong, Foong, & Tan, 2016). The nurse can provide anticipatory guidance to safe sleep practices by encouraging room sharing of sleeping as a safe alternative to co-bedding. The risks of co-bedding should be discussed with the family.

CRITICAL COMPONENT

Infant Sleep and Parental Behavior

Infant sleep patterns undergo dramatic evolution during the first year of life. This process is driven by underlying biological forces but is highly dependent on environmental cues, including parental influences. There are links between infant sleep and parental behaviors, cognitions, emotions, and relationships, as well as psychopathology. Parental behaviors are closely related to infant sleeping patterns (Batra et al., 2016).

Evidence-Based Practice: Bedtime Routines

American Academy of Sleep Medicine. (2016). *Recharge with sleep: Pediatric sleep recommendations promoting optimal health.* Retrieved from http://www.aasmnet.org/articles.aspx?id=6326

Recommendations by the American Academy of Sleep Medicine (2016) have been made following "a 10-month project conducted by a Pediatric Consensus Panel of 13 of the nation's foremost sleep experts, and are endorsed by the AAP, the Sleep Research Society and the American Association of Sleep Technologists. The expert panel reviewed 864 published scientific articles addressing the relationship between sleep duration and health in children" (paras. 2–3).

"The Pediatric Consensus Panel found that sleeping the number of recommended hours on a regular basis is associated with overall better health outcomes including: improved attention, behavior, learning, memory, emotional regulation, quality of life, and mental and physical health" (para. 3). The recommendations in the consensus statement are as follows:

"Infants four to 12 months should sleep 12 to 16 hours per 24 hours (including naps) on a regular basis to promote optimal health" (para. 1).

NURSING PROCEDURES SPECIFIC TO NEWBORNS AND INFANTS

Nurses who care for neonates and infants perform specific functions such as assisting with circumcisions and administering medications.

Assisting With Circumcisions

Circumcision is the removal of the prepuce of the penis performed for religious, cultural, hygienic, or social reasons (Figure 7–23). There is no identified medical reason for circumcision. There are two main types of circumcision procedures: Gomco and plastibell (Figure 7–24). Infants with congenital hypospadias (the urethral opening is on the underneath portion of the shaft of the penis) or congenital epispadias (the urethral opening is on the top portion of the shaft of the penis) are not circumcised until after correction of the condition. Otherwise, circumcision is performed before the neonate is discharged from the hospital. Nursing functions when assisting with circumcisions include the following:

- Administer acetaminophen 1 hour before the procedure.
- Provide pain relief with a topical prilocaine-lidocaine (EMLA) cream applied to the distal half of the penis 60 to 90 minutes before the procedure. EMLA can be used for all painful procedures in children with a gestational age of 37 weeks or older.
- The infant is positioned on a circumcision board, which positions the arms and legs in a straddled position. The upper body should be covered to minimize heat loss.
- Suction should be available in case of emesis.
- Dorsal penile blocks are used.
- Small needles are used.
- Swaddling aids in increasing comfort.
- Sucrose (24% sugar water) solution can help to relieve pain.
- Nonnutritive sucking can also help to relieve pain.
- Decrease environmental stimuli (AAP, 2016b).
- Infant must be hospitalized for procedure if older than 1 month.

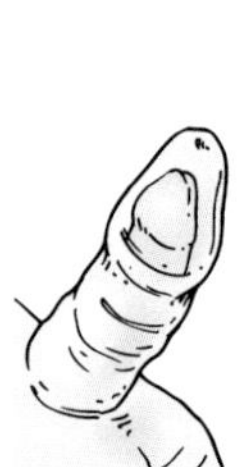
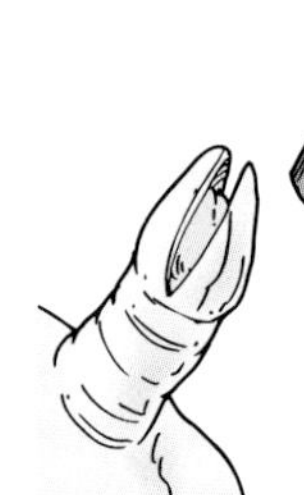
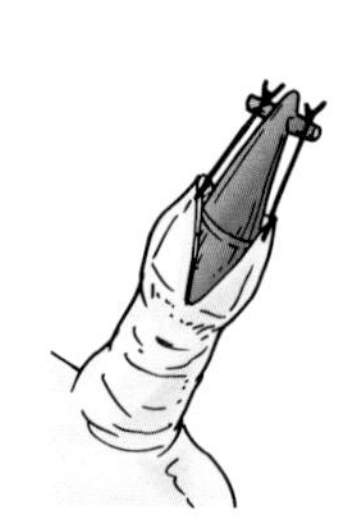

FIGURE 7–23 Removal of the prepuce during circumcision.

SAFE AND EFFECTIVE NURSING CARE: Understanding Medication

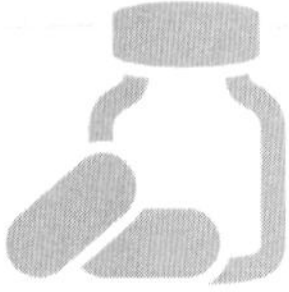

Sucrose Solution

Sucrose solution, which is 24% sucrose and water, provides analgesia for minor procedures.

- A pacifier, or a gloved finger if breastfeeding, used in conjunction with sucrose water enhances the analgesic effect.
- Do not use more than three doses during a single procedure.
- Do not use for infants who require ongoing pain relief; these infants will require acetaminophen or an opioid such as fentanyl or morphine.
- Although an infant may cry and show signs of pain when 24% sucrose water is used, studies have consistently shown that the sensation of pain and its negative effects will be diminished (Stevens, Yamada, Ohlsson, Haliburton, & Shorkey, 2016).
- The analgesic effect of 24% sucrose water appears to be reduced after 46 weeks' postconceptual age.
- Sucrose water needs to be ordered by a practitioner and documented as an administered medication.
- The administration of sucrose and the application of nonnutritive sucking are theorized to activate endogenous opioid pathways (natural pain relievers produced in the brain), with resulting calming and pain-relieving effects. The analgesic effects of nonnutritive sucking are thought to be activated through nonopioid pathways by stimulation of orotactile and mechanoreceptor mechanisms (Stevens et al., 2016).

- After the procedure, a petroleum gauze should be applied to the head of the penis to prevent irritation from the diaper.
- The penis is assessed every 15 minutes for the first hour and then every 2 to 3 hours depending on institution policy.

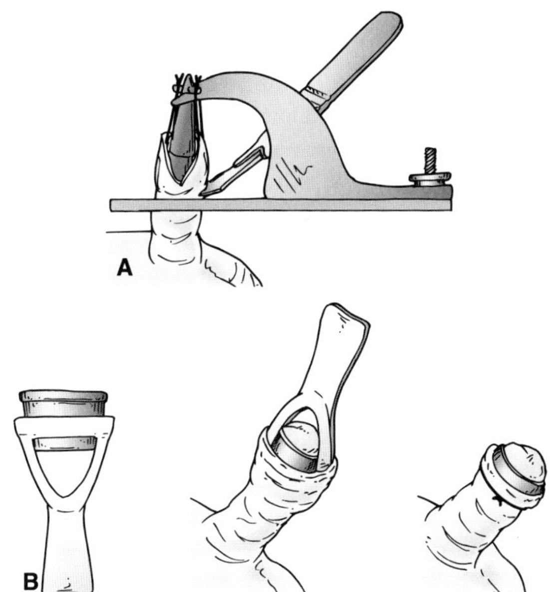

FIGURE 7–24 **A,** Gomco clamp; **B,** plastibell.

- The neonate should void within 24 hours of the procedure or before discharge.
- Instruct parents not to remove the gauze but to allow it to fall off, fasten diapers loosely, observe for bleeding every 4 hours during the first day, and observe for signs and symptoms of infection.
- Acetaminophen orally may be ordered every 4 to 6 hours for 24 hours after the procedure for pain (Figure 7–25).
- Educate caregivers that the healing penis develops a yellowish eschar, which should not be wiped off or removed because doing so will start the healing process over again.

SAFE AND EFFECTIVE NURSING CARE: Cultural Competence

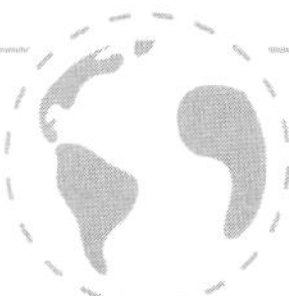

Circumcision and Culture

Circumcision has religious foundations dating to the Egyptians, who instituted the practice to ensure fertility, as a rite of passage, or for hygiene purposes. Jewish culture adopted circumcision as a religious ritual from prehistoric times into the modern world. In 2009, 55% to 65% of newborn infants in the United States and Canada were circumcised within 48 hours to 10 days following birth. Circumcision is more common in the United States, Canada, and the Middle East and is rare in Asia, South America, Central America, and Europe. Worldwide, one third of males are circumcised before adulthood (CircInfo, 2016). Prior to World War II, the male population in the United States was very infrequently circumcised. In recent years, the trend not to circumcise has witnessed a resurgence (Freedman, 2016). In 1997, the AAP and the American College of Obstetricians and Gynecologists reclassified circumcision from routine to elective (CIRP, 2011).

Discharge Care for the Circumcised Infant

Notify the physician in the case of:

- Persistent bleeding or blood on diaper (more than quarter-sized)
- Increasing redness
- Fever
- Other signs of infection, such as increased swelling or discharge, or the presence of pus-filled blisters
- Not urinating normally within 12 hours after the circumcision

Care of the Uncircumcised Male

- Do not force the foreskin over the penis.
- Make sure that the penis is cleaned meticulously to prevent infection.
- Do not insert any objects under the foreskin to clean it, such as cotton-tip applicators.

Medication Administration

Children are not little adults. Pediatric dosing must be precise to ensure adequate therapeutic levels; dosing is based on weight. When possible, caregivers should use syringes to measure and administer liquid medications. Caretakers should be discouraged from using household spoons because they may vary in size, which can lead to inaccurate dosing.

ANTICIPATORY GUIDANCE FOR THE FAMILY OF A NEWBORN

Psychological preparation of a caregiver is necessary to alleviate fears and anxiety in the care of the infant. Nurse education for caregivers must include information about the following:

- Developmental milestones
- Healthy and safe habits related to injury and illness prevention, such as childproofing the home
- Nutrition
- Oral health
- Family relationships and how they will change

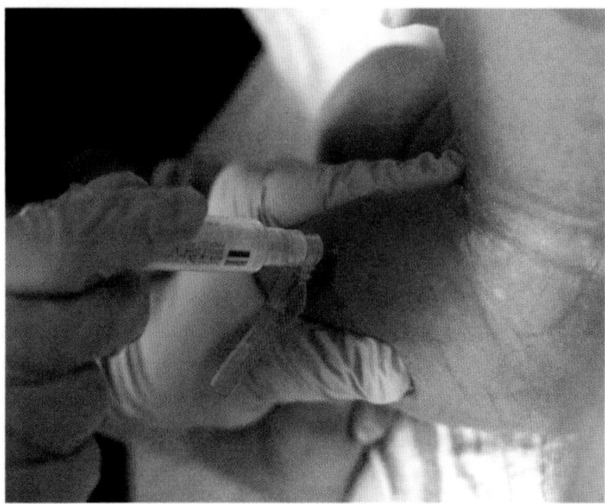

FIGURE 7–25 Medication administration.

SAFE AND EFFECTIVE NURSING CARE: Understanding Medication

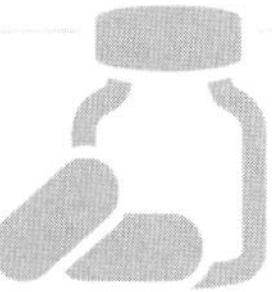

Neonates and Medication Administration

In neonates, there is an absence of hydrochloric acid, which may interfere with absorption of some medications.

- Variable weight and differences in body surface area affect medication administration.
- Infants are at greater risk for toxic levels that produce untoward effects.
- Infants have smaller amounts of pancreatic enzymes.
- Kidney function is immature in infants.

When administering medication to infants:

- Approach infant slowly, at eye level.
- Handle infant gently, keep infant on caregiver's lap, and use distraction.
- Do not put medications in a bottle of formula or breast milk because the infant must drink the entire amount to receive the appropriate dosage.
- Hold the infant in the nursing position, allowing him or her to swallow in between squirts of the medication in the buccal area of the mouth; do not lay the infant down until he or she swallows.
- Never give an infant over-the-counter medication. Instruct caregivers to call their practitioner with concerns.
- For rectal medications, lubricate the blunted end with water-soluble gel, insert approximately 1/2 inch, and hold the buttocks closed for approximately 10 minutes to allow for dissolution and absorption of the medication.
- For injections: In small infants, the nurse should use a 5/8-inch needle with up to 0.5 mL of fluid; with infants, a 1-inch needle with a maximum of 1 mL of fluid should be administered in the vastus lateralis. For adolescents, the nurse should use a 1- to 1.5-inch needle (22- to 27-gauge) up to 3 mL of fluid maximum.

- Sibling transition, including regressive behavior such as thumb sucking or bedwetting and aggressive behavior toward the infant (both normal responses); parents can address this transition by showing the child pictures of his or her new sibling, having someone other than the parents bring the new baby into the home, providing a gift from the infant to the sibling, and including the child in small tasks such as bringing the parent diapers
- Infant care
- Home infection-control measures, such as encouraging hand washing, limiting sick visitors, and keeping their infant in a car seat to limit handling by visitors; encourage all members of the household to get immunized for influenza and pertussis
- Parent–infant interactions, including playing, cuddling, the importance of talking to the child, and separation anxiety
- The importance of learning infant/child CPR

Pediatric Medical Home

The AAP developed the pediatric medical home model to deliver primary care to the child and family in a coordinated and comprehensive approach. This model delivers "primary care that is accessible, continuous, comprehensive, family-centered, coordinated, compassionate, and cultural effective for every child" (AAP, 2017a, para. 1). Medical homes coordinate care across the health-care spectrum and maximize continuous, uninterrupted, comprehensive care that addresses acute, chronic, and preventative care for the child from birth until adulthood (AAP, 2017a). A medical home integrates and coordinates care through interdisciplinary coordination with the child, family, primary physicians, specialists, hospitals, health-care systems, public health, and the community (AAP, 2017a).

Umbilical Cord Blood Banking

Umbilical cord blood banking is a fee-for-service option that stores cord blood obtained at the time of delivery to provide possible future reimplantation through the cryostorage of stem cells from the cord blood. Stem cells can produce cells that can be used in the future to replace bone marrow destroyed by disease, radiation, or chemotherapy. A strict protocol must be followed in stem cell recovery. Cord blood banking is not compatible with a delay in cord clamping; harvesting of the stem cells prevents them from returning to the infant.

Need for Immunizations

The benefits and risks associated with using immunobiologics should be discussed. Adult immunization behavior influences how these caregivers immunize their children. From a public health standpoint, encouraging immunization is good for society (Robinson & Osborn, 2017).

Evidence-Based Practice: Immunization Update

Frellick, M., & Barclay, L. (2017). ACIP releases pediatric vaccine schedule. *Medscape*. Retrieved from http://www.medscape.org/viewarticle/877092?nlid=113897_2709&src=wnl_cmemp_170410_mscpedu_peds&impID=1326206&faf=1

The 2017 immunization schedule has been updated to recommend that the hepatitis B vaccine now be given within 24 hours after birth, rather than in the first 2 weeks of life (Frellick & Barclay, 2017). Evidence has indicated that up to 90% of infants of chronically infected mothers could be infected. In addition, DTaP (diphtheria, tetanus, acellular pertussis) cannot be administered before the infant is 2 months of age.

Taking Temperature

- Instruct caregivers to take the infant's temperature if they suspect a fever.
- Digital, tympanic, or temporal thermometers are preferred over mercury-filled thermometers.

- Rectal temperatures are taken for children younger than 3 years only in the emergency department, newborn nursery, and pediatric units for accuracy. For rectal temperatures, lubricate the end with a water-soluble solution and insert the rectal thermometer no farther than 1/2 inch (2 to 2.5 cm) into the rectum. Hold buttocks and thermometer for safety. Parents are instructed not to take temperatures in this manner.
- For axillary temperatures, place the nonlubricated end in the armpit and hold the infant's arm at his or her side for approximately 1 minute; use with infants 3 months or older. This method can be 2 degrees lower than a rectal temperature.

Signs of Illness in the Newborn and Infant

Psychosocial and behavior assessments should be managed with a family-centered approach to include an evaluation of caregivers and social determinants of health (Swift & Barclay, 2017).

Parents should be instructed to notify the health-care practitioner with any of these concerns:

- Axillary temperature greater than 99.3°F or rectal temperature greater than 100.3°F
- Vomiting
- Decrease in the number of wet diapers
- Sunken or bulging fontanels
- Loss of appetite
- Foul odor or bleeding from the cord or circumcision
- Decreased level of consciousness; lethargy
- Increased irritability
- Blue or cool hands and feet
- Skin rash
- Drooling not associated with teething
- Refusal to lie down if 8 months of age or older

Sibling Rivalry

Sibling rivalry may occur because of changes in family structure and routine; it is not indicative of maladjustment or lack of preparation. However, preparation for these changes based on developmental age of the siblings can ease sibling rivalry. This can include the following measures:

- Encourage older children to attend sibling classes.
- Instruct caregivers to include siblings in the supervised care of the infant as appropriate.
- Do not leave the young infant alone with unsupervised young siblings.
- Foster opportunities for siblings to bond with the infant.
- Educate the caregiver on the need to spend alone/quality time with each of the siblings.

Milestone Concerns or Red Flags

Developmental concerns for this age group that require intervention by a health-care provider include the following:

- No attempts by the infant to lift head when lying facedown
- No improvement in head control
- Does not respond to loud noises
- Extreme floppiness
- Lack of response to sounds or visual cues, such as loud noises or bright lights
- Inability to focus on a caregiver's eyes
- Poor weight gain
- Does not crawl by 12 months

Fostering Positive Parenting Skills

Encourage parents of neonates to:

- Talk to the infant.
- Respond to infant's sounds by repeating and adding words.
- Read to the infant; this helps to develop and foster understanding of language and sounds.
- Sing to or play music for the infant.
- Praise the infant and give the infant attention.
- Spend time cuddling and holding the infant so that the infant feels cared for and secure.
- Play with the infant when he or she is alert and relaxed. Watch for signs of being tired or fussy so that the infant can take a break (CDC, 2012).

EMERGENCY CARE FOR THE INFANT AND NEWBORN

Nurses should provide parent education about the following emergency care measures:

- Stay calm—most serious illnesses provide warnings.
- Begin rescue breathing if infant is not breathing.
- Call 911.
- Apply pressure with a clean cloth to an area that is bleeding.
- If the infant is having a seizure, lower the infant to the floor, turn his or her head to the side, and do not put anything in the infant's mouth.
- Do not move a seriously injured infant unless he or she is in an unsafe situation, such as in a burning house, in a car, or underwater.
- Stay with the infant until help arrives.
- Bring all medication and/or poisons to the emergency department.
- Provide an accurate history of the preceding events, including the last time that the child ate and what was eaten.

HOSPITALIZED INFANT AND NEWBORN

Infancy is a period of rapid growth and development. When infants or newborns require hospitalization, the pediatric nurse must be able to care and develop nursing interventions that meet the unique needs of the infant and newborn in a hospital setting. By the age of 6 months, the infant becomes aware of the absence of their parent and can often sense anxiety in their parents as a result of the hospitalization. The pediatric nurse is in a unique position to attend not only to the needs of the infant or newborn, but to the family unit.

Nursing Care

When caring for a hospitalized infant, the nurse should:

- Encourage caregivers to room-in.
- Educate caregivers on the normal developmental milestones and stages, noting that a hospitalized infant may regress in behavior. Child life specialists are essential in describing developmental aspects related to play.
- Encourage caregivers to provide security items such as a favorite toy or blanket.
- Educate caregivers on safety risks in the hospital, such as lowered crib rails, the infant's crawling on the floor, or the presence of items that may not be in the infant's home.
- Reinforce the importance of therapeutic play.
- Perform the least invasive and least painful procedures first.
- Invasive procedures should be performed in the treatment room, not at the crib site.
- At 6 months of age, infants suffer separation anxiety and can be sensitive to caregiver cues.

CRITICAL COMPONENT

The Child Life Specialist

A child life specialist is a trained individual who works in a hospital or outpatient facility and is responsible for assisting in the stabilization of the psychological aspects of the child, the child's parents/caregivers, and the child's siblings in the health-care environment. The goal of the child life specialist is to reduce stress by explaining procedures, preparing the child for procedures, and comforting the child throughout procedures or hospitalizations. With infant patients, the specialist may focus on the family unit or the siblings. See Chapter 2 for further details.

Child Life Council, Inc., Rockville, MD (http://www.childlife.org).

Pain Management

Infants are exposed to a variety of painful stimuli, from blood draws to circumcision. Ongoing assessment is essential for type of pain, origin of pain, and behavioral responses to pain.

- Anything that would be painful to an adult will also be painful to an infant. Assessment of pain in the infant should be based on behavioral and physiological responses. Repeated exposure to painful stimuli can increase the response to noxious stimuli.
- Pain is assessed in newborns and infants by observing facial expressions such as bulged brow, eyes squeezed shut, open mouth, and quivering chin.
- Physiological responses are increased heart rate, respiratory rate, elevated systolic blood pressure, and decreased oxygen saturation.
- Pain causes increased fluid and electrolyte losses.
- Pain causes depression of the immune system through the depletion of mature white blood cells because of heightened stress responses.
- Gastric acid production increases.
- Dilated pupils and sweating may be observed.
- Newborns and infants are susceptible to the detrimental effects of pain because of their inability to communicate (Freedman, 2016).
- Pain relief for infants should be intravenous or oral; if administering opioids, closely monitor respiratory rate and pulse oximetry (Freedman, 2016).
- Use EMLA cream or similar topical anesthetics when starting IVs. EMLA requires a physician order and should be administered 60 minutes (90 minutes for darker skin) before the procedure.

Pain Scales

Several reliable infant pain scales may be used, including:

- Children's Hospital of Eastern Ontario Pain Scale (CHEOPS) (Table 7–11)
- Neonatal Infant Pain Scale (NIPS): measures five behavioral items and one physiological indicator
- FLACC: faces, legs, activity, crying, and consolability (Table 7–12)
- Riley Infant Pain Scale: based on similar criteria as FLACC; used on infants younger than 36 months and those with cerebral palsy
- Premature infant pain profile (PIPP): one of the most reliable and validated tools to assess pain in premature infants (Verklan & Walden, 2015)
- CRIES (Crying Requires Oxygen Increased Vital Signs Expression Sleep): a tool for measuring postoperative neonatal pain

Nonpharmacological Pain-Prevention Methods

- Breastfeeding
- Nonnutritive sucking
- Kangaroo care
- Swaddling
- Limiting environmental stimuli
- Attention to behavioral cues

ALTERNATIVE AND COMPLEMENTARY THERAPIES FOR THE INFANT AND NEWBORN

Alternative and complementary therapies are any healing therapies that are not part of mainstream medicine. Alternative therapies are used in place of conventional medicine, and complementary therapies are used in addition to conventional medicine therapies not as a replacement.

Infant Massage

A position statement by the American Massage Therapy Association in 2008 recognizes that newborns benefit from massage therapy, especially premature infants (Cooke, 2015). Infant massage:

- Stimulates organized sleep patterns
- Enhances growth
- May assist with colic in infants
- Promotes bonding with caregiver

TABLE 7–11 Children's Hospital of Eastern Ontario Pain Scale in Young Children

Overview

The Children's Hospital of Eastern Ontario Pain Scale (CHEOPS) is a behavioral scale for evaluating postoperative pain in young children. It can be used to monitor the effectiveness of interventions for reducing the pain and discomfort.

Patients

- The initial study was done on children 1–5 years of age.
- It has been used in studies with adolescents, but this may not be an appropriate instrument for that age group.
- According to Mitchell (1999), it is intended for ages 0–4.

Parameter	Finding	Points
Cry	No cry	1
	Moaning	2
	Crying	2
	Screaming	3
Facial	Smiling	0
	Composed	1
	Grimace	2
Child verbal	Positive	0
	None	1
	Complaints other than pain	1
	Pain complaints	2
	Both pain and nonpain complaints	2
Torso	Neutral	1
	Shifting	1
	Tense	2
	Shivering	2
	Upright	2
	Restrained	2
Touch	Not touching	1
	Reach	2
	Touch	2
	Grab	2
	Restrained	2
Legs	Neutral	1
	Squirming, kicking	2
	Drawn up, tensed	2
	Standing	2
	Restrained	2

Definitions

- No cry: child is not crying
- Moaning: child is moaning or quietly vocalizing silent cry

Continued

TABLE 7–11 Children's Hospital of Eastern Ontario Pain Scale in Young Children—cont'd

- Crying: child is crying, but the cry is gentle or whimpering
- Screaming: child is in a full-lunged cry; sobbing may be scored with complaint or without complaint
- Smiling: score only if definite positive facial expression
- Composed: neutral facial expression
- Grimace: score only if definite negative facial expression
- Positive (verbal): child makes any positive statement or talks about other things without complaint
- None (verbal): child not talking
- Complaints other than pain: child complains, but not about pain (e.g., "I want to see Mommy" or "I'm thirsty")
- Pain complaints: child complains about pain
- Both pain and nonpain complaints: child complains about pain and about other things (e.g., "It hurts"; "I want Mommy")
- Neutral (torso): body (not limbs) is at rest; torso is inactive
- Shifting: body is in motion in a shifting or serpentine fashion
- Tense: body is arched or rigid
- Shivering: body is shuddering or shaking involuntarily
- Upright: child is in a vertical or upright position
- Restrained: body is restrained
- Not touching: child is not touching or grabbing at wound
- Reach: child is reaching for but not touching wound
- Touch: child is gently touching wound or wound area
- Grab: child is grabbing vigorously at wound
- Restrained: child's arms are restrained
- Neutral (legs): legs may be in any position but are relaxed; includes gently swimming
- Squirming or kicking: definitive uneasy or restless movements in the legs and/or striking out with foot or feet
- Drawn up and tensed: legs tensed and/or pulled up tightly to body and kept there
- Standing: standing, crouching, or kneeling
- Restrained: child's legs are being held down

CHEOPS pain score = SUM (points for all six parameters)

Interpretation:
- Minimum score: 4
- Maximum score: 13

Sources: Adapted from McGrath, P. J., Johnson, G., Goodman, J.T., Schillinger, J., Dunn, J., Chapman, J. A., … Johnston, G. A. (1985). CHEOPS: A behavioral scale for rating postoperative pain in children. Advanced Pain Research Therapy, *9, 395–402; http://www.modernmedicine.com/sites/default/files/legacy/mm/Resource-Centers/Children%27s%20Hospital%20of%20Eastern%20Ontario%20Pain%20Scale%20%28CHEOPS%29.pdf.*

TABLE 7–12 FLACC Pain Scale

	SCORING		
Categories	**0**	**1**	**2**
Face	No particular expression or smile; disinterested	Occasional grimace or frown; withdrawn	Frequent to constant frown, clenched jaw, quivering chin
Legs	Normal position or relaxed	Uneasy, restless, tense	Kicking, or legs drawn up
Activity	Lying quietly, normal position, moves easily	Squirming, shifting back and forth, tense	Arched, rigid, or jerking
Cry	No cry (awake or asleep)	Moans or whimpers, occasional complaint	Crying steadily, screams or sobs, frequently complains
Consolability	Content, relaxed	Reassured by occasional touching, hugging, or talking to; distractible	Difficult to console or comfort

Each of the five categories—(F) face; (L) legs; (A) activity; (C) cry; (C) consolability—is scored from 0 to 2, which results in a total score between 0 and 10.

Source: Merkel, S. I., Voepel-Lewis, T., Shayevitz, J. R., & Malviya, S. (1997). The FLACC: A behavioral scale for scoring postoperative pain in young children. Pediatric Nursing, *23, 293–297. Adapted with permission from Sandra I. Merkel, MS, RN, Clinical Nurse Specialist. © 2002, The Regents of the University of Michigan.*

Music Therapy

Research supports the use of music to improve sucking, weight gain, sleep, and recovery from painful procedures, especially in premature infants (Loewy, Stewart, Dossler, Telsey, & Homel, 2013). Bonding and attachment develop through physical contact between infant and caregivers including touch, soothing measures, and vocal familiarity (Loewy et al., 2013). Music therapy promotes sleep patterns and circadian rhythms, and slows heart rate. Singing by a caregiver has positive emotional and physiological benefits that aid in communication and language acquisition, and assist in concentration.

Evidence-Based Practice: Music Therapy and Infants

Pool, J., & Macgee, W. L. (2016). Music in the treatment of children and youth with prolonged disorders of consciousness. *Frontiers in Psychology, 7*(202), PMC4756118.

Researchers and studies have shown that music therapy has the potential to improve cognitive development. Singing of lullabies by caregivers has a calming effect on infants, even if caregivers do not know the words to the songs. Playing soft and soothing music improves psychological well-being. Music has been shown to stimulate neurological growth and development, to calm, and to improve sleeping patterns in infants.

CHRONIC CARE FOR THE INFANT AND NEWBORN

Although most infants grow and thrive, some children die in infancy. For every 1,000 infants born, 6 will die before the age of 1 year (CDC, 2016b). The five leading causes of infant deaths or chronic care needs are complications of prematurity, birth defects, maternal complications during pregnancy, SIDS, and accidents or unintentional injuries (CDC, 2016b).

Premature Infants

Prematurity is the primary reason for low birth weight and carries a high risk for developmental and motor delay. Ballard scoring is 37 weeks or less. The multidisciplinary team focuses on maximizing the infant's long-term outcomes. Neonatologists, pediatricians, cardiologists, pulmonologists, social service workers, physical therapists, and pediatric neurologists are some of the specialists who may be involved. Developmental and neurological examinations are performed at routine and serial visits. Mortality and morbidity are influenced by numerous factors such as prenatal, intrapartum, and fetal issues. The lower the gestational age, the more complications that can occur.

Respiratory syncytial virus (RSV) is an acute infection limited to the lower respiratory tract and sometimes accompanied by fever in most healthy full-term infants. In 25% to 40% of RSV infections, the lower respiratory tract becomes infected, and bronchiolitis or pneumonia may develop. Very young infants, preterm infants, or high-risk infants with chronic conditions such as congenital heart disease or chronic lung changes are at increased risk for hospitalization (AAP, 2014b). The prevention for RSV is palivizumab (Synagis) prophylaxis immunization. There are significant benefits to premature infants and infants who are less than 35 weeks and 6 out of 7 days gestation with chronic diseases (AAP, 2014b). Palivizumab is given in no more than five monthly doses during RSV season (late October to late January) (AAP, 2014b).

Congenital and Acquired Conditions

A team of physicians, nurses, respiratory therapists, social workers, and other health professionals work together to meet the infant's needs and provide family-centered care.

See Chapters 17 and 18 for information on the endocrine system and genetics.

SAFETY MEASURES FOR INFANTS AND NEWBORNS

Accidents and injuries are the leading cause of death in children younger than 19 years (CDC, 2017c). Parents and caregivers are responsible for providing a safe environment for infants to decrease the incidence of these events. Injuries and accidents can include:

- Falls
- Car accidents
- Drownings
- Electrocution
- Suffocation
- Choking
- Burns

Anticipatory Guidance for Injury Prevention

- Make and keep infant appointments for medical checkups and vaccinations (2 months, 4 months, 6 months, 9 months, and 1 year).
- Immunizations are important because children are susceptible to many potentially serious diseases. Consult a local healthcare provider to ensure that childhood immunizations are up to date. Visit the CDC immunization Web site to obtain a copy of the recommended immunization schedule for U.S. children.
- Use "Safe to Sleep" positioning.
- Infants spend most of their time in cribs, which must be safe—no bumper pads, slats no more than 2-3/8 inches apart (JPMA approved).
- Prevent diaper rash with frequent diaper changes, and wipe front to back in girls.
- Childproof the home.

- Have doctor, police, fire, and poison control numbers at caregiver's fingertips.
- Use childproof locks, safety gates, and window guards to prevent accidents and falls. Encourage good hand washing for anyone in contact with the newborn or infant. This includes siblings.
- Keep anyone with a cough, cold, or infectious disease away from the infant.
- Call a physician if the infant appears to be sick.
- Call a physician if the infant has a fever, refuses to eat, or has vomiting and/or diarrhea.
- Call a physician if the infant is more fussy or quieter than usual, or looks jaundiced.
- Call the infant's physician or health-care provider if worried or have questions about the infant's growth or development.
- Keep the infant in a smoke-free area.
- Keep firearms in a locked cabinet.
- Never leave the child home alone or in an enclosed, nonrunning car. The temperature inside the car can change dramatically.
- Pay attention to product recalls of both infant equipment and toys.
- Install fire/smoke and carbon monoxide detectors on every level of the home.

Pets

Acclimate any pets to the new room setup before the baby is coming home. Make sure that the pet does not attempt to bite or unintentionally suffocate the infant, and never leave the infant alone with a pet.

Drowning

- Never leave the infant alone in water or near standing water.
- Do not leave the infant to answer the phone or doorbell.
- Keep toilet lids closed.
- Empty buckets immediately.

SAFE AND EFFECTIVE NURSING CARE: Clinical Pearl

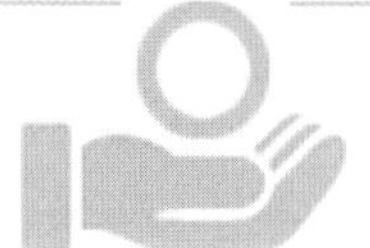

Safety Precautions Near Water

Parents and caregivers need to be advised that they should never—even for a moment—leave children alone or in the care of another young child while in bathtubs, pools, spas, or wading pools, or near irrigation ditches or other open standing water. Infant bath seats or supporting rings are not a substitute for adult supervision (WHO, 2016). Remove all water from containers, such as pails and 5-gallon buckets, immediately after use. To prevent drowning in toilets, young children should not be left alone in the bathroom, and unsupervised access to the bathroom should be prevented (WHO, 2016).

SAFE AND EFFECTIVE NURSING CARE: Promoting Safety

Limiting Submersion Time

Prolonged submersion in water, such as through infant swimming classes, increases the risk for water intoxication, as well as exposure to *Escherichia coli* contamination, both of which can be fatal. Many learn-to-swim programs limit an infant's pool time to 30 minutes. In addition, contamination of the pool from diapers may result in higher incidence of diarrhea (CDC, 2016c).

Burns

- Do not hold infant when smoking, drinking hot liquids, or cooking.
- Do not heat formula or breast milk in the microwave because it causes uneven heating and may also inactivate nutrients in breast milk.
- An infant's skin is very sensitive to the sun.
  - Keep infants out of direct sunlight to prevent sunburn.
  - Use sunscreen for infants older than 6 months.
  - Infants should wear hats when out in the sun.
- Turn pot handles away from the outside of the stove, where they can be pulled on by infants beginning to pull themselves to a standing position.
- Check the water temperature before putting a child in the tub.
- Reduce the water heater setting to less than 120°F to lessen the chance of an accidental burning.
- Keep electrical cords out of infant reach; cap electrical outlets.
- Use flame-retardant sleepwear for the infant.

Choking

- Do not attach pacifiers or other objects to the crib or body with a string or cord.
- Keep small objects away from infants, including toys or stuffed animals with small breakaway parts.
- Never leave plastic bags or wrappings where the infant can reach them.
- Keep objects that are choking hazards away from the infant, such as batteries (especially watch batteries), magnets, and balloons.
- Cut or remove pull cords on blinds and drapes.
- Anything smaller than an adult pinky finger can cause a choking situation. This includes foods such as hot dogs, whole grapes, raw carrots, raw celery, peanuts, popcorn, chips, candy, marshmallows, pretzels, and peanut butter.
- Cut all foods into small-sized bites.

Poisoning

- Keep the poison control number at every phone.
- Keep all medicines, cleaning products, nail polish remover, alcohol, and other household chemicals locked in their original containers and out of reach.
- Take all suspected poisons to the phone when poison control is called to be able to read the ingredients to the center.

- Remove lead paint from older cribs, infant furniture, walls, and window sills.
- Never leave an infant alone in a yard.
- Do not apply sunscreen or perfumed creams or lotions, because they will be absorbed in an infant younger than 6 months of age.
- Keep indoor plants out of the infant's reach.

Falls

- Never leave the infant alone on a changing table, couch, chair, or bed.
- Always keep a hand on the baby.
- Use gates at the top of stairwells.
- Do not use walkers; they have resulted in serious injuries and even death if they cause the infant to fall down stairs.
- Make sure that heavy furniture is secure and cannot be toppled over on top of an infant.
- Educate caregivers on how young children should hold an infant and protect their head and necks.

Car Seat Safety

- Each state has its own specific laws related to car seats.
- Always use a car seat when traveling in a car or airplane.
- Use approved car seats correctly.
- Check the age and weight limits for the seat.
- Put the car seat in the backseat of the car and secure it facing backward. Check state laws.
- Never put the infant in a front seat with a safety airbag.
- Rear-facing infant seats are used from birth up to 2 years of age, per 2017 AAP guidelines (AAP, 2017b).
- Parents can contact a certified child passenger safety technician (CPST) to correctly install infant car seats.
- Caregivers should never leave an infant in the car unattended.

Evidence-Based Practice: Car Seat Challenge Test

Davis, N. L. (2015). Screening for cardiopulmonary events in neonates: A review of the infants car seat challenge. *Journal of Perinatology, 35*(4), 235–240.

Physiological monitoring studies indicate that some preterm infants experience episodes of oxygen desaturation, apnea, or bradycardia when seated in standard car safety seats. The AAP recommends that all preterm infants younger than 37 weeks or less than 5 lb 8 oz should be assessed for cardiorespiratory stability in their car seat before discharge or the "car seat challenge." This article discusses how the emphasis should be on minimizing the amount of time that an infant spends in a car seat because of the risks for apnea, bradycardia, and desaturations.

Electrocution

- Keep cords unplugged when not needed.
- Watch for chewing marks on electrical cords.

Suffocation

- Remove excess bedding from crib.
- Remove stuffed toys from crib.
- Keep all plastic garbage bags, shopping bags, and dry cleaning bags out of reach of the infant.
- Monitor for issues in sling carriers; make sure that infant does not get wrapped up in clothing and that the head does not fall forward, cutting off the airway.

CHILD ABUSE CONSIDERATIONS

Abuse consists of intentional, improper actions that result in harm or injury and can be physical, sexual, or mental. Neglect is failure to provide the infant with his or her basic needs. The nurse's job in cases of suspected abuse is to advocate, protect, and care for the pediatric patient, not to investigate.

Shaken Baby Syndrome (Abusive Head Trauma)

With shaken baby syndrome, head trauma results from injuries caused by vigorously shaking a child. The anatomy of infants puts them at risk for injury from this kind of action.

- Most victims are infants younger than 1 year; the average age is between 3 and 8 months.
- Pay special attention when choosing a babysitter.
- Research suggests that teenage fathers are more likely to cause shaken baby syndrome.
- Contrecoup, injuries to the opposite side of the head, are common.
- Detached retinas may result.
- Permanent brain damage may result.
- Death may result.

SAFE AND EFFECTIVE NURSING CARE: Clinical Pearl

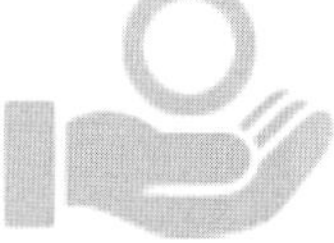

Daddy Boot Camp

These programs, taught by men for men, aim to support dads and foster improved relationships that translate into improved caregiving behaviors. Programs stress that babies cry and educate fathers about proper responses. For example, if frustrated, the father should place the infant in a safe place and remove himself from the room. Educators also:

- Instruct fathers-to-be and new fathers on the care and handling of the new infant.
- Explain importance of providing neck support, holding an infant correctly, and monitoring of soft spots.
- Discuss shaken baby syndrome and methods to deal with frustrations of new parenthood.
- Discuss postpartum depression.

Abduction Prevention

Educate the caregiver as follows:

- In the hospital, infants will be banded with electronic tags to prevent abduction.
- Hospital staff should be properly identified with hospital badges to identify that they have access to the postpartum and newborn areas.
- Be suspicious of casual acquaintances or strangers who attempt to befriend the parent.
- Learn hospital procedures for care after discharge if a visiting nurse is to come to your home.
- Demand positive identification before allowing anyone into your home.
- Do not post information about the infant on social media.
- Under no circumstances should the caregiver give the baby to a stranger.
- Do not allow casual acquaintances or strangers to babysit the infant.
- Never leave the infant alone at home.
- Do not place birth announcements in the newspaper.
- In shopping areas, do not turn your back on the infant. Make sure the infant is secured in a car seat that is buckled into a shopping cart.
- Place the infant in the car seat in the car, lock the doors, and then load your groceries or items from the store.
- Educate family members and friends who babysit the infant about infant security.
- Call police anytime you are suspicious or concerned about the infant's safety.

Sexual Abuse

Warning signs of sexual abuse in infants include:

- Stained or bloody diapers
- Genital or rectal pain, swelling, redness, or discharge
- Bruises or other injuries in the genital or rectal area
- Difficulty eating or sleeping
- Excessive crying
- Withdrawing from others
- Failure to thrive

Physical Abuse

Warning signs of physical abuse in infants include:

- Unexplained or repeated injuries such as welts, bruises, burns, fractured skull, and broken bones, especially spiral fractures
- Injuries in the shape of an object (e.g., belt buckle, electrical cord, cigarette)
- Injuries that are unlikely given the age or ability of the child, such as broken bones in a child too young to walk or climb
- Disagreement or inconsistency in parent/caregiver explanation of the injury
- Unreasonable explanation of the injury
- Fearful or detached behavior by the infant

Emotional Abuse

An infant may be subject to emotional abuse in the presence of these warning signs:

- Aggressive or withdrawn behavior
- Shying away from physical contact with parents or adults
- Basic needs of food, warmth, and cuddling not met

Neglect

Infant neglect may be indicated by:

- Consistent failure to respond to the child's need for stimulation, nurturing, encouragement, and protection, or failure to acknowledge the child's presence
- Actively refusing to respond to the child's needs, such as refusing to show affection
- Parents/caregivers expressing the fact that they are not going to spoil the baby or referring to the baby as evil
- Infant with malnourished appearance
- Obvious neglect of the child (e.g., dirty, undernourished, inappropriate clothes for the weather, lack of medical or dental care)
- Failure to provide necessary medications for chronic conditions, such as inhalers for children with asthma
- Delays in calling for help or taking infant to the doctor

Case Study

Anticipatory Guidance Regarding Breastfeeding

The Jones family had a baby girl 3 months ago. Mrs. Jones has been breastfeeding her little girl exclusively since birth, and both are satisfied with the breastfeeding process. Mrs. Jones, however, feels trapped in her home, and her little girl cries and will not eat for anyone else in the family. Mr. and Mrs. Jones want to be able to go out together for dinner and a movie, and the baby's grandma is a willing babysitter, but Mrs. Jones is feeling guilty because her baby will not eat for anyone else.

1. What anticipatory guidance can the nurse provide to the Jones family regarding the developmental stage of their baby daughter?
2. What information can the nurse provide to the Jones family in regard to making the transition to being able to go out for dinner and a movie?
3. What anticipatory guidance can the nurse provide to Mrs. Jones about her relationship with her daughter and her husband?
4. How can the nurse assist the Jones family to realize that the infant will be in capable hands during the dinner and movie?

REFERENCES

Adamkin, D. H., & Polin, R. (2016). Neonatal hypoglycemia: Is 60 the new 40? The questions remain the same. *Journal of Perinatology, 36*, 10–12.

Adu, E. K., & Donkor, P. (2017). Management of cleft lip and palate: A five year review. *Archives of Otolaryngology Rhinology, 3*(1), 023–026.

American Academy of Pediatrics (AAP). (2014a). *American Academy of Pediatrics recommendations for infant sleep patterns.* Retrieved from http://www.letmommysleep.com/blog/2014/09/04/aap-recommendations-infant-sleep-patterns

American Academy of Pediatrics (AAP). (2014b). Updated guidance for palivizumab prophylaxis among infants and young children at increased risk of hospitalization for respiratory syncytial virus infection. Committee on Infectious Diseases and Bronchiolitis Guidelines Committee. *Pediatrics, 134*(2), 415–420.

American Academy of Pediatrics (AAP). (2016a). Iron supplements for babies: AAP recommendations. Retrieved from https://www.healthychildren.org/English/ages-stages/baby/feeding-nutrition/Pages/Vitamin-Iron-Supplements.aspx

American Academy of Pediatrics (AAP). (2016b). Prevention and management of procedural pain in the neonate: An update. *Pediatrics, 137*(2), e20154271.

American Academy of Pediatrics (AAP). (2016c). SIDS and other sleep related infant deaths: Updated 2016 recommendations for a safe sleep environment. *Pediatrics, 138*(5), e20162938.

American Academy of Pediatrics (AAP). (2016d). State Early Hearing Detection and Intervention (EHDI) laws and regulations. Retrieved from https://www.aap.org/en-us/advocacy-and-policy/state-advocacy/Documents/EHDI%20State%20Requirements%20(2016).pdf

American Academy of Pediatrics (AAP). (2016e). Visual system assessment in infants, children, and young adults by pediatricians. Policy Statement. *Pediatrics, 137*(1), 28–30.

American Academy of Pediatrics (AAP). (2017a). *AAP agenda for children: Medical home.* Retrieved from https://www.aap.org/en-us/about-the-aap/aap-facts/AAP-Agenda-for-Children-Strategic-Plan/pages/AAP-Agenda-for-Children-Strategic-Plan-Medical-Home.aspx

American Academy of Pediatrics (AAP). (2017b). Car safety seats: 2017 guide for families, 1-48. Retrieved from https://drive.google.com/file/d/0B-H10w3hWogiV1JMNkU5eTRFYk0/view

American Academy of Pediatrics (AAP). (2017c). *Early Hearing Detection and Interventions (EHDI).* Retrieved from https://www.aap.org/en-us/advocacy-and-policy/aap-health-initiatives/PEHDIC/Pages/Early-Hearing-Detection-and-Intervention.aspx

American Academy of Pediatrics (AAP). (2017d). *Infant food and feeding.* Retrieved from https://www.aap.org/en-us/advocacy-and-policy/aap-health-initiatives/HALF-Implementation-Guide/Age-Specific-Content/pages/infant-food-and-feeding.aspx

American Academy of Pediatrics (AAP). (2017e). *Newborn screening.* Retrieved from https://www.aap.org/en-us/advocacy-and-policy/aap-health-initiatives/PEHDIC/pages/Newborn-Screening.aspx

American Academy of Sleep Medicine. (2016). *Recharge with sleep: Pediatric sleep recommendations promoting optimal health.* Retrieved from http://www.aasmnet.org/articles.aspx?id=6326

American College of Obstetrician and Gynecologists. (2017). Delayed cord clamping after birth [Committee Opinion No. 684]. pp. 1–6. Retrieved from http://www.acog.org/-/media/Committee-Opinions/Committee-on-Obstetric-Practice/co684.pdf?dmc=1&ts=20170406T1645598732

American Dental Association (ADA). (2017). Position statement on dental caries. Retrieved from http://www.mouthhealthy.org/en/babies-and-kids/healthy-habits

Antiui-Kusi, A., Addisson, W., Oti, A. A., Amuasi, A. A., Sabbah, D. K., ... Abu-Sakyi, J. (2015). Mothers of children with cleft lip and/or palate, perception about aetiology, social reaction and treatment of cleft. *Journal of Biosciences and Medicines, 3*, 98–101.

Association of Women's Health, Obstetric, and Neonatal Nurses (AWHONN). (2016). Immediate and sustained skin-to-skin contact for the healthy term newborn after birth: AWHONN Practice Brief Number 5. *Journal of Obstetric, Gynecologic & Neonatal Nursing, 45*(6), 842–844. Retrieved from http://www.jognn.org/article/S0884-2175(16)30352-5/pdf

Batra, E. K., Teti, D. M., Schaefer, E. W., Neumann, B. A., Meek, E. A., & Paul, I. M. (2016). Nocturnal video assessment of infant sleep environments. *Pediatrics, 138*(3), 1–9.

Bellaiche, M., Levy, M., & Camille, J. (2013). Treatment for colic. *Journal of Pediatric Gastroenterology and Nutrition, 57*, S27–S30.

Beyer, J. E., McGrath, P. J., & Berde, C. B. (1990). Discordance between self-report and behavioral pain measures in children aged 3–7 years after surgery. *Journal of Pain Symptom Management, 5*, 350–356.

Bhutani, V. K., Stark, A. R., Lazzeroni, L. C., Poland, R., Gourley, G. R., Kazmierczak, S., & Stevenson, D. K. (2013). Initial clinical testing evaluation and risk assessment for universal screening for hyperbilirubinemia screening group. Predischarge screening for severe neonatal hyperbilirubinemia identifies infants who need phototherapy. *Journal of Pediatrics,* 162(3), 477–482.

Bodamer, O. A. (2015). Approach to inborn errors of metabolism. In: Goldman, L., & Schafer, A. L. (Eds.), *Goldman's cecil medicine* (25th ed.). Philadelphia, PA: Elsevier Saunders.

Boucher, A. (2017). Nonopioid management of neonatal abstinence syndrome. *Advances in Neonatal Care, 17*(2), 84–90.

Centers for Disease Control and Prevention (CDC). (2012). *Child development.* Retrieved from http://www.cdc.gov/ncbddd/childdevelopment/positiveparenting/infants.html

Centers for Disease Control and Prevention (CDC). (2016a). *Advisory committee on immunization practices (ACIP).* Retrieved from https://www.cdc.gov/vaccines/hcp/acip-recs/vacc-specific/hib.html

Centers for Disease Control and Prevention (CDC). (2016b). *Jaundice and kernicterus.* Retrieved from https://www.cdc.gov/ncbddd/jaundice/index.html

Centers for Disease Control and Prevention (CDC). (2016c). *Protecting our next generation at a glance 2016.* Retrieved from https://www.cdc.gov/chronicdisease/resources/publications/aag/infant-health.htm

Centers for Disease Control and Prevention (CDC). (2017a). *About SUID & SIDS.* Retrieved from https://www.cdc.gov/sids/aboutsuidandsids.htm

Centers for Disease Control and Prevention (CDC). (2017b). *Developmental monitoring and screening.* Retrieved from https://www.cdc.gov/ncbddd/childdevelopment/screening.html

Centers for Disease Control and Prevention (CDC). (2017c). *Protect the ones you love: Child injuries are preventable.* Retrieved from https://www.cdc.gov/safechild/

Centers for Disease Control and Prevention (CDC). (2017d). Zika virus: Clinical guideline for healthcare providers caring for infants & children. Retrieved from https://www.cdc.gov/zika/hc-providers/infants-children.html

Centers for Disease Control and Prevention, National Center for Injury Prevention and Control, Division of Unintentional Injury Prevention (2016). *Unintentional drowning: Get the facts.* Retrieved from http://www.cdc.gov/HomeandRecreationalSafety/Water-Safety/waterinjuries-factsheet.html

Chandran, S., Rajadurai, V., Alim, A., & Hussain, K. (2015). Current perspectives on neonatal hypoglycemia, its management, and cerebral injury risk. *Research and Reports in Neonatology, 5*, 17–30.

Chin, B., Chan, E. S., & Goldman, R. D. (2014). Early exposure to food and food allergy in children. *Canadian Family Physician, 60*(4), 338–339.

Christensen, R. D., & Yaish, H. M. (2015). Hemolytic disorders causing severe neonatal hyperbilirubinemia. *Clinical Perinatology, 42*(3), 515–527.

Chu, D. M., Ma., J., Prince, A. L., & Antony, K. M. (2017). Mutation of the infant microbiome community structure and function across multiple body sites and in relation to mode of delivery. *Nature Medicine, 23*(3), 314–328.

CircInfo. (2016). *Rate of circumcision in adults and newborns.* Retrieved from http://www.circinfo.net/rates_of_circumcision.html

CIRP. (2011). *History of circumcision.* Retrieved from http://www.cirp.org/library/history/

Cooke, A. (2015). Infant massage: The practice and evidence-based to support it. *British Journal of Midwifery, 23*(3), 166–170.

Crenshaw, J. T. (2014). Healthy birth practice #6: Keep mother and baby together—it's best for mother, baby, and breastfeeding. *Journal of Perinatal Education, 23*(4), 211–217.

Davis, N. L. (2015). Screening for cardiopulmonary events in neonates: A review of the infants car seat challenge. *Journal of Perinatology, 35*(4), 235–240.

Desphande, P. G. (2015). Colic. *Medscape.* Retrieved from http://emedicine.medscape.com/article/927760-overview

Dillon, P. (2007). *Nursing assessment.* Philadelphia: F.A. Davis.

Dominguez-Bello, M. G., DeJesus-Laboy, K.M., Shen, N., Cox, L. M., Amir, A., Gonzelez, A., & Clemente, J. C. (2016). Partial restoration of the microbiota of cesarean-born infants via vaginal microbial transfer. *Nature Medicine, 22*(3), 250–253.

Durham, R., & Chapman, L. (2014). *Maternal-newborn nursing: Critical components of nursing care* (2nd ed.). Philadelphia: F.A. Davis.

Ehrenkranz, R. A., & Mercurio, M. R. (2017). Previable birth (limit of viability). *UpToDate.* Retrieved from https://www.uptodate.com/contents/periviable-birth-limit-of-viability

Eunice Kennedy Shriver National Institute of Child Health and Human Development. (2015). Safe to sleep. Retrieved from https://www.nichd.nih.gov/news/releases/Pages/072015-podcast-safe-to-sleep.aspx

Flannery, A., Tamber, M. S., Mazzola, C., Klimo, P., Baird, L. C., Tyagi, R., ... Nikas, D. (2016). Summary: Evidence-based guidelines for the treatment of pediatric positional plageocephaly. *Congress of Neurological Surgeons.* Retrieved from https://www.cns.org/guidelines/guidelines-management-patients-positional-plagiocephaly

Freedman, A. L. (2016). The circumcision debate: Beyond benefits and risks. *Pediatrics, 137*(5), e20160594.

Frellick, M., & Barclay, L. (2017). ACIP releases pediatric vaccine schedule. *Medscape.* Retrieved from http://www.medscape.org/viewarticle/877092?nlid=113897_2709&src=wnl_cmemp_170410_mscpedu_peds&impID=1326206&faf=1

Gallagher, E., McKinney, C., & Glass, R. (2017). Promoting breastmilk nutrition in infants with cleft lip and/or palate. *Advances in Neonatal Care, 17*(2), 79–80.

Han, J., Lui, X., & Zhang, F. (2017). Effect of the early intervention on neonate with hyperbilirubinemia and perinatal factors. *Biomedical Research, 28*(1), 58–60.

Hansen, W. R. (2016). Neonatal jaundice treatment and management. *Medscape.* Retrieved from http://emedicine.medscape.com/article/974786-treatment

Hennet, T., & Borsig, L. (2016). Breastfed at Tiffany's. *Trends in Biochemical Sciences, 41*(6), 508–518.

Institute for Patient- and Family-Centered Care. (2017). Advancing the practice of patient-and family-centered care in hospitals. How to get started. Retrieved from http://www.ipfcc.org/resources/getting_started.pdf

International Lactation Consultants Association. (2017). *Human lactation.* Retrieved from http://www.ilca.org/home

Jacobson, S. J., Kopecky, E. A., Joshi, P., & Babul, N. (1997). Randomised trial of oral morphine for painful episodes of sickle-cell disease in children. *Lancet, 350*, 1358–1361.

Jensen, D., Wallace, S., & Kelsay, P. (1994, January). LATCH: A breastfeeding charting system and documentation tool. *Journal of Obstetric, Gynecologic, and Neonatal Nursing, 23*(1), 27–32.

Jones, H. E., & Fielder, A. (2015). Neonatal abstinence syndrome: Historical perspective, current focus, future directions. *Preventative Medicine, 80*, 12–17.

Karimi, M., Haghighat, M., Dialamah, Z., Tahmasbi, L., Parand, S., & Bardestani, M. (2016). Breastfeeding as a protective effect against childhood leukemia and lymphoma. Iran Red Crescent Medicine Journal, 18(9), e2971. doi: 10.5812/ircmj.29771

Kilgore, C. (2015). AAP: Treat corporal punishment as a risk factor. *Family Practice News.* Retrieved from http://www.mdedge.com/familypracticenews/article/104080/pediatrics/aap-treat-corporal-punishment-risk-factor

Lai, N. M., Foong, S. C., Foong, W. C., & Tan, K. (2016). Co-bedding in neonatal nursery for promoting growth and development in stable preterm twins. *Cochrane Database of Systematic Reviews, 4*, CD008313. doi: 10.1002/14651858.CD008313.pub3

Langan, T. J. (2016). Krabbe disease. *UpToDate.* Retrieved from http://www.uptodate.com/contents/krabbe-disease

Lerodiakonou, D. Garcia-Larson, V., Logan, A., Groome, A., Cunha, S., Chivinge, J., ... Boyle, R. J. (2016). Timing of allergenic food introduction to the infant diet and risk of allergic or autoimmune disease: A systematic review & meta-analysis. *Journal of the Medical Association, 316*(11), 1181–1192.

Loewy, J., Stewart, K., Dossler, A., Telsey, A., & Homel, P. (2013). The effects of music therapy on vital signs, feeding, and sleep in premature infants. *Pediatrics, 131*(5), 902–918.

Ludington-Hoe, S. M. (2013). Kangaroo care as a neonatal therapy. *Newborn and Infant Nursing Reviews, 13*(2), 73–75.

March of Dimes. (2014). Sickle cell disease and your baby. Retrieved from http://www.marchofdimes.org/complications/sickle-cell-disease-and-your-baby.aspx

McDonald, S. J., Middleton, P., Dowswell, T., & Morris, P. S. (2013). Effect of timing of umbilical cord clamping of term infants on maternal and neonatal outcomes. *Cochrane Database of Systematic Reviews, 7*, CD004074. doi: 10.1002/14651858.CD004074.pub3

McGrath, P. J., Johnson, G., Goodman, J.T., Schillinger, J., Dunn, J., Chapman, J. A., ... Johnston, G. A. (1985). CHEOPS: A behavioral scale for rating postoperative pain in children. *Advanced Pain Research Therapy, 9*, 395–402.

McGrath, P. J., & McAlpine, L. (1993). Physiologic perspectives on pediatric pain. *Journal of Pediatrics, 122*, S2–S8.

McKee-Garrett, T. M., Weisman, L. E., & Duryea, T. K. (2017). Assessment of the newborn infant. *UpToDate.* Retrieved from http://www.uptodate.com/contents/assessment-of-the-newborn-infant

McQueen, K., & Murphy-Oikonen, J. (2016). Neonatal abstinence syndrome. *New England Journal of Medicine, 375*, 2468–2479.

Merkel, S. I., Voepel-Lewis, T., Shayevitz, J. R., & Malviya, S. (1997). The FLACC: A behavioral scale for scoring postoperative pain in young children. *Pediatric Nursing, 23*, 293–297.

Mitchell P. (1999). Understanding a young child's pain. *Lancet, 354*, 1708.

Muchowski, K. E. (2014). Evaluation and treatment of neonatal hyperbilirubinemia. *American Family Physician, 89*(11), 873–878.

Munblit, D., Treneva, M., Peroni, D. G., Colicino, S., Chow, L., Dissanayeke, S., ... Warner, J. O. (2016). Colostrum and mature human milk of women from London, Moscow, and Verona: Determinants of immune composition. *Nutrients, 8*(11), E695.

National Institute of Diabetes and Digestive and Kidney Disease. (2017). *Diarrhea.* Retrieved from https://www.niddk.nih.gov/health-information/digestive-diseases/diarrhea

Nesrin, A., Kavita, M., Sudersanadas, M., Senthilvel, V., Ghada, B. S., Malak, A., ... Lenna, W. H. (2016). Efficacy of patient discharge instructions: A pointer toward caregiver friendly communication methods from pediatric emergency personnel. *Journal of Family Community Medicine, 23*(3), 155–160. doi: 10.4103/2230-8229.189128

Patel, P. K. (2016). Cleft palate repair. *Medscape.* Retrieved from http://emedicine.medscape.com/article/1279283-overview

Patrick, S. W., Burke, J. F., Biel, T. J., Auger, K. A., Goyal, N. K., & Cooper, W. O. (2015). Risk of hospital readmission among infants with neonatal abstinence syndrome. *Hospital Pediatrics, 5*(10), 513–519.

Pool, J., & Macgee, W. L. (2016). Music in the treatment of children and youth with prolonged disorders of consciousness. *Frontiers in Psychology, 7*(202), PMC4756118.

Robinson, S. G., & Osborn, A. W. (2017). The concordance of parent and child immunization. *Pediatrics, 139*(5), 1–9.

Rozance, P. J., & Hay, W. W. (2016). New approaches to management of neonatal hypoglycemia. *Maternal Health, Neonatology and Perinatology, 2*, 3. doi: 10.1186/s40748-016-0031-z

Rudd, K. (2017). What is Krabbe? *Academy of Neonatal Nursing, 36*(2), 112–113.

Samson, D. R., & Yetish, G. M. (2017). Global and evolutionary perspectives on sleep: Sleep health request for papers. *Sleep Health, 3*(2), 73–74.

Sankar, M. J., Chandrasekaran, A., Kumar, P., Thurkal, A., Agarwal, R., & Paul, V. K. (2016). Vitamin K prophylaxis for prevention of vitamin K deficiency bleeding: A systematic review. *Journal of Perinatology, 36*, S29–S35.

Scanlon, V., & Sanders, T. (2011). *Essentials of anatomy and physiology* (6th ed.). Philadelphia: F.A. Davis.

Stevens, B., Yamada, J., Ohlsson, A., Haliburton, S., & Shorkey, A. (2016). Sucrose for analgesia in newborn infants undergoing painful procedures. *Cochrane Database of Systematic Reviews, 7,* CD001069. doi: 10.1002/14651858.CD001069.pub5

Swift, D., & Barclay, L. (2017). AAP releases recommended for preventative health care. *Medscape.* Retrieved from http://www.medscape.org/viewarticle/877090?nlid=114270_2713&src=wnl_cmemp_170424_mscpedu_nurs&uac=72056PG&impID=1334798&faf=1

Thornton, P. S., Stanley, C. A., DeLeon, D. D., Harris, D., Haymond, M. W., Hussain, K., & Wolfsdorf, J. I. (2015). *The Journal of Pediatrics, 167*(2), 238–245.

U.S. Breastfeeding Committee (USBC). (2017). *Health People 2020: Breastfeeding objectives.* Retrieved from http://www.usbreastfeeding.org/p/cm/ld/fid=221

U.S. National Library of Medicine. (2016). Krabbe disease. *NIH U.S. National Library of Medicine.* Retrieved from https:/ghr.nlm.nih.gov/condition/krabbe-disease

U.S. National Library of Medicine. (2017a). Cleft lip and palate. *NIH U.S. National Library of Medicine.* Retrieved from https://medlineplus.gov/cleftlipandpalate.html

U.S. National Library of Medicine. (2017b). Infant botulism. *NIH U.S. National Library of Medicine.* Retrieved from https://medlineplus.gov/ency/article/001384.htm

Vallerand, A. H., Sanoski, C. A., & Deglin, J. H. (2017). *Davis's drug guide for nurses* (15th ed.). Philadelphia: F.A. Davis.

Ventura, C. V., Maia, M., Bravo-Filho, V., Gois, A., & Belfort, R. (2016). Zika virus in Brazil and macular atrophy in a child with microcephaly. *Lancet, 387*(10015), 228.

Verklan, M. T., & Walden, M. (2015). *Core curriculum for neonatal intensive care nursing* (5th ed.). St. Louis, MO: Elsevier Saunders.

Ward, S. L., & Hisley, S. M. (2015). *Maternal-child nursing care: Optimizing outcomes for mothers, children, & families* (2nd ed.). Philadelphia: F.A. Davis.

Wassner, A. J., & Brown, R. S. (2013). Hypothyroidism in the newborn period. *Current Opinion in Endocrinology, Diabetes, and Obesity, 20*(5), 449–454.

Weiner, D. L. (2015). Inborn errors of metabolism. *Medscape.* Retrieved from http://emedicine.medscape.com/article/804757-overview

Wiet, G. J. (2015). Reconstructive surgery for cleft palate treatment and management. *Medscape.* Retrieved from http://emedicine.medscape.com/article/878062-treatment

Williams, N. J., Grandne, M. A., Snipes, A., Rogers, A., Williams, O., Airhihenbuwa, C., ... Jean-Louis, G. (2015). Racial/ethnic disparities in sleep health and health care: Importance of the sociocultural context. *Sleep Health, 1*(1), 28–35.

Wong, R. J., & Bhutani, V. R. (2016). Evaluation of unconjugated hyperbilirubinemia in term and late preterm infants. *UpToDate.* Retrieved from https://www.uptodate.com/contents/evaluation-of-unconjugated-hyperbilirubinemia-in-term-and-late-preterm-infants

Woodgate, P., Jardine, L. A. (2015). Neonatal jaundice: Phototherapy. *British Medical Journal Clinical Evidence, 2015,* 0319. Retrieved from http://reference.medscape.com/medline/abstract/25998618

World Health Organization (WHO). (2016). *Drowning.* Retrieved from http://www.who.int/mediacentre/factsheets/fs347/en/

World Health Organization Position Statement. (2017). *Exclusive breastfeeding for optimal growth, development and health of infants.* Retrieved from http://www.who.int/elena/titles/exclusive_breastfeeding/en/

Yang, M., & White, P. C. (2017). Risk factors for hospitalization of children with congenital adrenal hyperplasia. *Clinical Endocrinology, 86*(5), 669–673.

Zemel, B. S., Pipan, M., Stallings, V. A., Hall, W., Schgadt, K., Freedman, D. S., & Thorpe, P. (2015). Growth charts for children with Down syndrome in the U.S. *Pediatrics.* Retrieved from https://www.cdc.gov/ncbddd/birthdefects/downsyndrome/growth-charts.html

8

Toddlers and Preschoolers

Ludy Caballero, MSN, APRN, FNP-C, EMT-P
Diane M. Kocisko, MSN, RN, CPN

LEARNING OUTCOMES

Upon completion of this chapter, the student will be able to:

1. Identify normal growth and development for toddlers and preschoolers.
2. Discuss the nursing assessment of toddlers and preschoolers.
3. Identify safety risks for toddlers and preschoolers.
4. Discuss safety interventions to minimize risks.
5. Identify and discuss pain scales used with toddlers and preschoolers.
6. Identify appropriate nursing interventions and education regarding pain and safety for toddlers and preschoolers and their caregivers.
7. Identify and discuss different challenges faced by toddlers and preschoolers.

TODDLER GROWTH AND DEVELOPMENT (AGE 1 TO 3 YEARS)

According to the key theorists, stages related to toddler growth and development include:

- Erikson—autonomy versus shame and doubt. In Erikson's theory of psychosocial development, toddlers in this stage seek to attain autonomy by gaining more self-control in areas such as toileting and food and toy preferences. Success leads to self-confidence and self-control, whereas feelings of shame and doubt in these areas may lead to a sense of inadequacy.
- Piaget—preoperational. In Piaget's cognitive developmental theory, 2- to 7-year-olds are in the preoperational stage, which is characterized by magical thinking, the belief that their personal thoughts have a direct impact on the real world, and egocentrism, the inability to see things from another's perspective.
- Freud—anal stage (age 1 to 3 years). In Freud's psychosexual theory, toddlers are in the anal stage, which focuses on pleasure derived from the toddler's enjoyment of holding and releasing bowel movements.
- Kohlberg—preconventional. In Kohlberg's theory of moral development, 2- to 7-year-olds are in the stage of preconventional moral reasoning, and tend to follow set rules for fear of punishment.

Motor Development of a Toddler

Most children in this age group will be able to:

- Walk alone by 15 months
- Begin to run
- Stand on tiptoes
- Climb stairs while holding on to support by 21 months
- Build towers of four or more blocks by age 2 years
- Build towers of more than six blocks by age 3 years
- Kick a ball
- Climb on furniture by age 2 years

- Pull or carry toys while walking
- Run and jump by age 2 years
- Play on a riding toy (i.e., tricycle) by age 3 years (3 years to three wheels)
- Can turn a door knob

Language Skills of a Toddler

Developing language skills for this age group include:

- Pointing to objects when named by others
- Recognizing the names of well-known people and things
- Learning own name
- Understanding more than they can speak
- Repeating words that are overheard
- Saying five words by 12 months
- Saying 50 words by 18 months
- Speaking in two- to three-word sentences by age 2 years
- Converses using two to three sentences by age 3 years
- Uses words "I," "me," and "you" by age 3 years

Cognitive Skills of a Toddler

Key cognitive developments for this age group include:

- Finding objects that are hidden
- Beginning to identify and sort colors and shapes
- Beginning to play make-believe
- Beginning to scribble and show preference for one hand versus the other

CRITICAL COMPONENT

Promoting Self-Care

By 2 years of age, a child can follow simple instructions. A child can and should be encouraged to participate in self-care and the education process to some extent. Providing limited, appropriate choices for the child will allow for a sense of control. Routines and rituals are important.

Social and Emotional Milestones of a Toddler

Most children of this age:

- Imitate others
- Have awareness of self as separate from others
- Begin to enjoy spending time with other children
- Engage in parallel play, playing near other toddlers but not consistently interacting or playing together
- Show affection openly
- Begin to display defiance
- Display separation anxiety until approximately the end of the second year
- Express jealousy at the arrival of a new sibling

PRESCHOOLER GROWTH AND DEVELOPMENT (AGE 3 TO 5 YEARS)

Stages related to preschool growth and development include:

- Erikson—initiative versus guilt. Success in this stage involves initiative, wherein preschoolers begin to assert power and control over their environments; the opposite result is feelings of guilt and dependence on others.
- Piaget—preoperational. As described for toddlers, this stage of cognitive development (age 2 to 7 years) is characterized by magical thinking and egocentrism.
- Freud—phallic stage (age 3 to 6 years). The focus of this stage is pleasure derived from the genitals; childhood masturbation is common, and preschoolers may view the opposite-sex parent as a sexual object.
- Kohlberg—preconventional. As described for toddlers, this level of moral reasoning (age 2 to 7) involves an obedience/punishment mentality.

SAFE AND EFFECTIVE NURSING CARE: Clinical Pearl

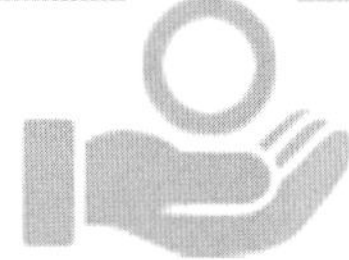

Providing Feedback

A child should be given feedback in relationship to his or her behavior. The child should be told "good job" instead of "good boy/good girl." Preschoolers cannot understand the process of disease transmission. The child may feel that an illness is a punishment for "being bad" (magical thinking).

Motor Development of a Preschooler

Most preschoolers are able to:

- Dress and undress self with assistance at age 3 years (later without assistance)
- Go up and down the stairs without assistance at age 3 years
- Draw squares, circles, and later triangles at age 3 years
- Begin learning to use utensils and drinking from a cup at age 3 years
- Hop and stand on one foot for 5 to 10 seconds at age 4 years
- Throw objects overhand at age 4 years
- Catch a bounced ball at age 4 years
- Draw stick figures with more than two body parts at age 4 years (later draws people with bodies)
- Use scissors at age 4 years

- Brush own teeth and go to the toilet without assistance at age 5
- Learn to skip, ride a bicycle, and swim at age 5

Language Skills of a Preschooler

Preschoolers typically:

- Speak clearly enough for strangers to understand (by age 5 years)
- Speak in three- to four-word sentences at age 3 years
- Speak in four- to five-word sentences at age 4 years
- Speak in sentences of five or more words at age 5 years
- Tell stories
- Use future tense
- Comprehend rhyming
- State full name and address (later in stage)
- Have concrete or literal interpretation of language

Cognitive Skills of a Preschooler

Children in this age group typically have the cognitive ability to:

- Recall parts of a story
- Count to 10, but no concept of numbers
- Correctly identify at least four colors
- Begin to understand the concept of time
- Know the meaning of *same* and *different*
- Begin to use imagination and creativity
- Ask "why" questions

Social and Emotional Milestones of a Preschooler

Preschoolers tend to:

- Be more independent
- Be proud of their abilities
- Show interest in new things
- Want to do things by themselves
- Obey rules
- Engage in role-play
- Play well with others; this is known as associative play
- Want to please and be like friends
- Try to negotiate problem solving
- Have trouble in differentiating between reality and fantasy (later preschoolers can tell the difference)
- Believe in monsters or be afraid of the dark
- Begin to understand gender and racial differences
- Begin to explore their genitalia through masturbation
- Can be demanding or eager to help
- Can be jealous over the arrival of a new sibling
- Place importance on body integrity

SAFE AND EFFECTIVE NURSING CARE: Clinical Pearl

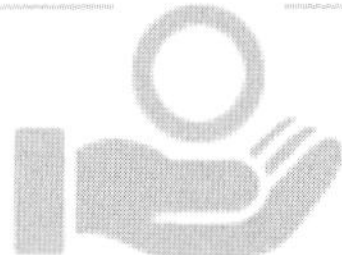

Fear of the Dark

Many preschoolers are afraid of the dark and may be afraid to sleep in a dark room. It is helpful to have a night-light that sheds minimal light to reduce fear. Providing a bedtime routine will decrease anxiety and provide a relaxing environment.

NURSING ASSESSMENT

Nursing assessments for children in this age group should include the elements discussed in the following subsections.

Health History

- Chief complaint: current signs/symptoms or events leading to visit
- Family medical history: genetic disorders, chronic diseases, childhood cancers
- Medical history: childhood illnesses, hospitalizations, surgeries, immunizations, and results of vision/hearing/developmental screens
- Medications: daily prescription, over the counter, and natural therapies
- Allergies: medications, foods, and environmental
- Review of systems: Are they eating, sleeping, and eliminating well?
- Social history: living arrangements, day care/preschool, and behavior

SAFE AND EFFECTIVE NURSING CARE: Clinical Pearl

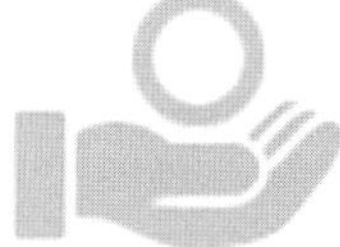

Head-to-Toe Assessment

Conduct head-to-toe assessment from least to most invasive/intrusive, leaving painful areas for last. The child will be more cooperative with the examination when performed in this order.

Physical Assessment

- Height: standing when able to stand. Recumbent for young toddler, because lordosis is common in this age group.
- Weight: minimal clothing, diaper, or underwear only preferred for accuracy. Include body mass index for children older than 2 years.

- Head circumference: measured for all children younger than 2 years. May be assessed after 2 years of age if difficulty with bone growth or issues identified that impact the growth of the head.
- Vital signs: heart rate, respiratory rate, temperature, pulse oximetry, and blood pressure (BP) within normal range (Table 8–1). Use an appropriate-size cuff to measure the BP (Fig. 8–1).

CRITICAL COMPONENT

Formula for calculating a child's BP: 70 + 2 × age in years = lower end of systolic BP; 90 + 2 × age in years = upper end of systolic BP (U.S. Department of Health and Human Services, National Institutes of Health, & National Heart, Lung, and Blood Institute, 2005).

General Assessment

- Appearance: appropriate cleanliness, dress, and behavior
- General: hearing, vision, and speech for difficulty or delay; appropriate interaction with caregiver
- Nutrition status: hair is evenly dispersed, child is visually not overweight or underweight, and skin is not overly dry
- Head: ears, eyes, nose, mouth, teeth, throat, and neck for symmetry, drainage, enlarged lymph nodes, and pain and/or abnormalities
- Torso: chest, back, and abdomen for variations of the skin, enlarged lymph nodes, masses, nodules, rashes, and pain and/or abnormalities
- Extremities: range of motion, strength, symmetry of length, variations of the skin, pain, and/or abnormalities of the hands, feet, or joints

CRITICAL COMPONENT

Physical Differences Between Children and Adults

Children are anatomically and physiologically different from adults:

- Proportionately larger heads as compared with bodies
- Greater ratio of body surface area to total weight
- Larger tongues and greater proportion of soft tissue in and around the airway
- Shorter, more narrow airway that is more elastic and collapsible
- More pliable chest
- Weaker abdominal muscles, creating the look of distention
- Belly breathers
- Higher metabolic rates
- Higher fluid requirements
- Higher total blood volumes

SAFE AND EFFECTIVE NURSING CARE: Clinical Pearl

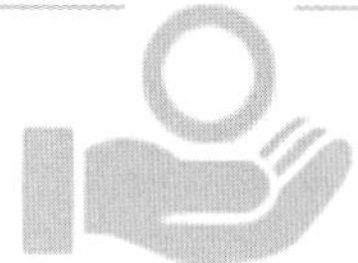

Child Participation and Comfort During Assessment

Use these best practices when assessing a toddler or preschool-age child.

- Allow the child to select which digit to put the pulse oximeter on.
- May demonstrate use on the caregiver's finger to show that it is a painless procedure.
- Allow child to select which arm to use for BP check when appropriate.
- Talk to the child and tell of the tight "hug" feeling to expect on the arm with BP check.
- Allow child to stay with caregiver so that respiratory rate and BP will not be falsely increased because of anxiety.
- Assess toddlers in their comfort zone, usually in a parent's lap.
- Remember to protect a preschooler's modesty.
- Approach children and get down to their eye level.
- Give praise whenever it is appropriate.

Visual Assessment

- Note the child's overall appearance.
- Look at the chest for labored respirations, accessory muscle use, and irregularity of breathing.
- Note the position of comfort the child places themselves when having difficulty breathing.
- Check skin for abnormal bruising, rash, or lesions.

Auscultation

- Lung sounds for clarity, wheezing, rhonchi, or crackles
- Neck sounds for stridor or snoring
- Heart sounds for regularity and murmur (listen apically for a full minute to assess thoroughly)
- Bowel sounds for abnormalities (absent, hypoactive, or hyperactive)

Palpation

- Abdomen for masses, organomegaly, and tenderness
- Pulses for quality; should be equal bilaterally and equal in upper and lower extremities
- Scalp for fontanels, which typically close by age 2 years

TABLE 8–1 Average Range for Toddler and Preschool Vital Signs

AGE GROUP	PULSE/HEART RATE (bpm)	RESPIRATION RATE (BREATHS/MIN)	SYSTOLIC BLOOD PRESSURE (mm Hg)	DIASTOLIC BLOOD PRESSURE (mm Hg)
Toddlers	70–110	20–30	90–105	55–70
Preschoolers	65–110	20–25	95–110	60–75

Source: Ward, S. L., & Hisley, S. M. (2010). Maternal-child nursing care. *Philadelphia: F.A. Davis.*

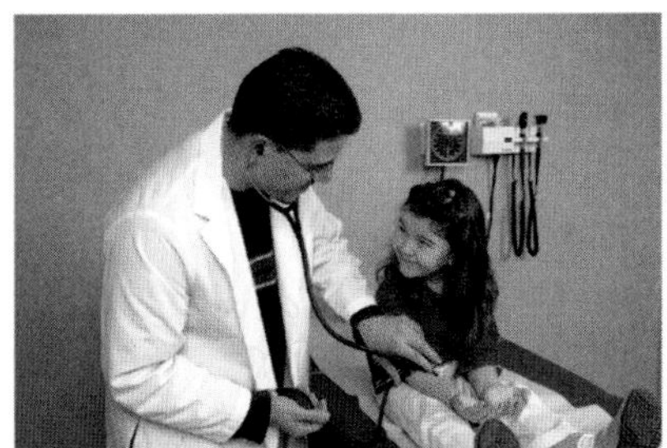

FIGURE 8–1 Taking vital signs: blood pressure.

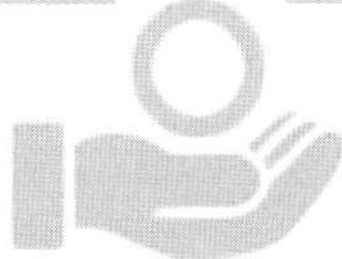

SAFE AND EFFECTIVE NURSING CARE: Clinical Pearl

Breath Assessment

The nurse may hold up an index finger and tell the child to pretend it is a candle. The child is then prompted to blow out the candle. After the child exhales and "blows," the nurse will lower the finger and tell the child that the candle was blown out. This brings fun and a gamelike atmosphere to the assessment. The child is then taking in deep breaths to adequately assess breath sounds.

Growth and Development Assessment Charts

See the Centers for Disease Control and Prevention (CDC, 2009) growth charts for typical heights and weights. At birth to 36 months, assess:

- Length for age and weight for age
- Head circumference for age and weight for length (done with preschoolers, 2 to 5 years)
- Weight for stature

The American Academy of Pediatrics (2017) recommends developmental screening at 9, 18, and 30 months for early detection of developmental problems. Screening tools include:

- Ages and Stages Questionnaire (ASQ), 4 to 60 months
- Denver Developmental Screening Test II (DDST-II), 1 month to 6 years
- Early Screening Inventory-Revised (ESI-R), 3 to 6 years
- Survey of Well-Being of Young Children (SWYC), 2 to 60 months

Many others can be found at the U.S Health and Human Services Web page titled Early Childhood Developmental Screening: A Compendium of Measures for Children Ages Birth to Five.

SAFETY

According to the CDC (2015), unintentional injury is the number one cause of death for all children in the United States.

- The top five leading causes of injury deaths in children aged 1 to 4 years are drowning, motor vehicle accidents, homicide, suffocation, and fires and/or burns (CDC, 2014).
- The leading causes of nonfatal injuries in children aged 1 to 4 years are falls, struck by/against an object, and bites/stings (CDC, 2015).
- Injury death rates were highest among American Indians and Alaska Natives, whereas rates for Caucasians and African Americans were approximately the same (CDC, 2015).
- Drowning was the leading cause of injury death for those 1 to 4 years of age (CDC, 2015).
- Falls and poisonings remain highest amongst children between 1 and 4 years of age (CDC, 2015).

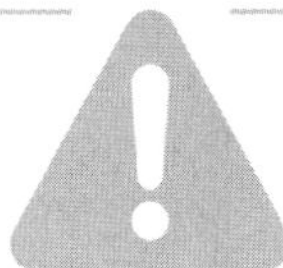

SAFE AND EFFECTIVE NURSING CARE: Promoting Safety

Drop-Side Cribs

In 2011, drop-side cribs were banned for sale and distribution in the United States because of multiple injuries. This style of crib may be passed down through friends and family, and thus still be used in homes. Discourage the use of this style of crib to promote injury prevention (Healthy Child Care America, 2011).

Nursing Interventions

When caring for children in this age group:

- Minimize falls risk by keeping the side rails on beds/cribs up.
- Remind caregivers to never leave the crib side if the rail is in the down position.
- Check equipment regularly—wire and cord placement to minimize entanglement, suction availability at crib side, and minimal equipment and crib attachments to decrease choking and suffocation hazards.
- Check temperature of water, food, and drinks to prevent burns.
- Explore any signs or symptoms that potentially may require a referral to child protective services. This is a legal requirement in most states that provides assistance for children and families of abuse. A child may experience abuse at any age.
- Educate caregiver on basic home, outdoor play, and car safety measures to ensure environmental safety for children.
- Install smoke and carbon monoxide detectors, and ensure they are operational by changing the batteries every 6 months.

SAFE AND EFFECTIVE NURSING CARE: Promoting Safety

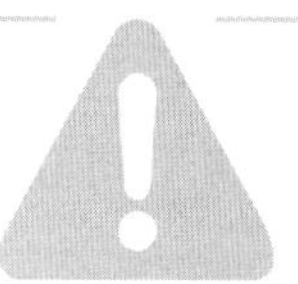

Evacuation Plans

A child may become scared and hide in fear during an emergency. Urge families to have an evacuation plan in case of fire or other emergency; the plan should include alternative exits and a meeting place outside of the home.

Safety Education for Caregivers

Educate parents and caregivers of children in this age group of the following:

- Do not carry hot liquids around children or while holding a child.
- Do not allow young children around stoves and fireplaces.
- Use the back burners on the stove and turn pot handles in toward back.
- Do not allow children around smaller hot appliances, such as irons, curling irons, and toasters.
- Set the temperature of hot water tanks to 120°F or lower to prevent scalds (CDC, 2016).
- Always check the temperature of water, food, and formula before use.
- Use safety gates to block stairs. If placed at top of staircase, secure to wall.
- Secure heavy furniture such as televisions and bookcases to walls to prevent tipping injuries.
- Keep windows closed. Screens will not hold children in and prevent falls.
- Do not leave young children alone on porches or balconies.
- Use night-lights.
- Keep all medications and poisonous products (e.g., hand sanitizer, laundry packets, household cleaners, and chemicals) in high places out of reach or in a locked cabinet.
- Have the number of local poison control center available or call the American Association of Poison Control Centers (AAPCC, 2017) at 1-800-222-1222. Keep poisonous materials in original containers so that the information on the labels can be accessed.
- Buy products with childproof tops.
- Clean up old, chipping paint around the house.
- Look for and take away small toys that could present a choking hazard.
- Buy age-appropriate toys.
- Throw away anything that is broken.
- Secure any loose cords from blinds, curtains, and clothing out of reach to minimize strangulation hazard.
- Keep up-to-date on recalled toys and furniture.
- Do not allow children to eat and play at the same time.
- Cut food into bite-size pieces and avoid foods such as nuts, hot dogs, hard candy, popcorn, and grapes that could cause choking.
- Do not allow children to play with coin money or latex balloons.
- Lock rooms that are not childproofed.
- Supervise children closely around all animals, including family pets.
- Do not leave water in the bathtub or cleaning buckets.
- Close bathroom doors.
- Never leave children alone near any basin of water.

SAFE AND EFFECTIVE NURSING CARE: Promoting Safety

Hand Sanitizer Danger

"While a child who licks a tiny amount of hand sanitizer off of his or her hands is unlikely to become sick, a child ingesting any more than a taste of hand sanitizer could be at risk for alcohol poisoning" (AAPCC, 2017).

SAFE AND EFFECTIVE NURSING CARE: Promoting Safety

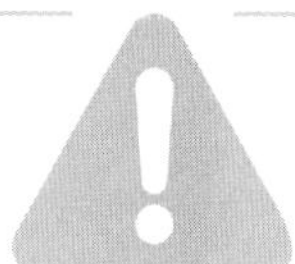

Medication Is Not Candy

Never tell a child medication is candy. Medication should be administered by an adult and kept in a place that is out of a child's reach. Child safety caps are not meant to be the primary prevention for accidental ingestion. Child safety caps are the last means of defense between the child and the medication. Caregivers should know how to measure the dosage accurately.

Outdoor Safety

- Childproof swimming areas, including access to pools, ponds, and lakes.
  - Never leave children unattended near swimming areas, even if they can swim.
  - Use flotation devices (Fig. 8–2).
  - Never leave toys in a pool because children may be tempted to retrieve them.
- Playgrounds and unfamiliar play areas post an increased risk for danger because of the unfamiliarity of the environment.
  - Teach playground and play area safety rules, such as no running near roped areas, no putting head through bars, and no trampoline use. Trampolines are a safety risk for children of all ages.
- Teach crosswalk safety, such as how to cross correctly; running into the street for toys is not allowed; playing in the street is not allowed.
- Children should always wear a bicycle helmet and never ride bicycles in the street.
- Always use child safety/booster seats and place children in the backseat.
  - Required U.S. child restraint laws by state are available from the Insurance Institute for Highway Safety and Highway Loss Data Institute (2017).

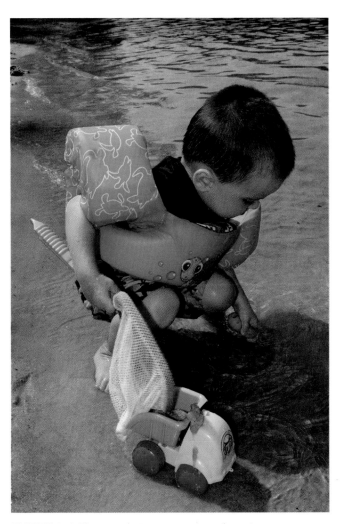

FIGURE 8–2 Flotation devices can prevent drowning.

PAIN

Pain assessment can be difficult in this age group because of age, developmental delay, and chronic illness. The nurse should ask for caregiver opinion without them influencing the child's response, ask preschool-age children questions about the quality of their pain, and avoid making assumptions on the level of pain the child "should" be experiencing (Nash, 2012). Young toddlers do not have the cognitive ability to convey the pain they are feeling, but this capability begins at about age 2 years. Assess for causes of pain such as infection, injury, surgical/procedural, or disease, as well as for elevated heart rate, BP, and respiratory rate. (Reminder: These alone are considered poor indicators of pain.) Observe specific behaviors children display in reaction to pain, such as facial expression, movement, and vocalization (Fig. 8–3), including:

- Furrowed brow and open-mouth-type grimace, or lack of expression
- Restlessness or sleeping and withdrawal (ways to cope with pain)
- Wariness/fear of movement
- Irritability/agitation
- No vocalization to harsh/high-pitched cry

Choose the appropriate pain scale. There are 16 published postoperative pain scales for use with infants, toddlers, and preschool-age children (Table 8–2). When in doubt, assume pain is present and treat accordingly. Evaluate and document for efficacy of all pain-control interventions, including medication, repositioning, and/or consolation measures.

SAFE AND EFFECTIVE NURSING CARE: Clinical Pearl

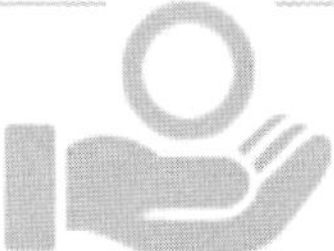

Medical Play

Use medical play to explain and prepare for medical procedures. A child life specialist may assist with this preparation with the nurse. Medical play allows the child to use concrete thinking to understand upcoming events. The medical play items prepare the child for how equipment may feel and sound. The preparation will help to eliminate some fear of the unknown. Whenever possible, allow children to keep comfort items (e.g., stuffed animals and blankets) with them during procedures (Fig. 8–4).

CRITICAL COMPONENT

Provide Appropriate Choices When Giving Medications

Never give children the choice of taking a medication or not. Instead, give them a choice in medication form, such as liquid or chewable, or a choice in what to take the medication with, such as water, juice, or applesauce.

FLACC Pain Scale

Scoring			
Categories	0	1	2
Face	No particular expression or smile; disinterested	Occasional grimace or frown; withdrawn	Frequent to constant frown, clenched jaw, quivering chin
Legs	Normal position or relaxed	Uneasy, restless, tense	Kicking, or legs drawn up
Activity	Lying quietly, normal position, moves easily	Squirming, shifting back and forth, tense	Arched, rigid, or jerking
Cry	No cry (awake or asleep)	Moans or whimpers, occasional complaint	Crying steadily, screams or sobs, frequent complaints
Consolability	Content, relaxed	Reassured by occasional touching, hugging, or talking to; distractible	Difficult to console or comfort

A

Each of the 5 categories—(F) Face; (L) Legs; (A) Activity; (C) Cry; (C) Consolability—is scored from 0 to 2, which results in a total score between 0 and 10.

From: FLACC Pain Scale, from The FLACC: A behavioral scale for scoring postoperative pain in young children, by S. Merkel et al, 1997, Pediatr Nurse 23(3), pp. 293–297. Copyright 1997 by Jannetti Co., University of Michigan Medical Center. Reprinted with permission.

Wong-Baker FACES™ Pain Rating Scale

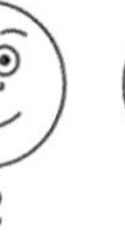

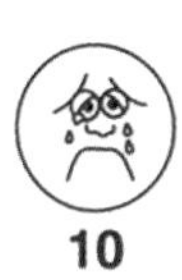
0
No Hurt
2
Hurts Little Bit
4
Hurts Little More
6
Hurts Even More
8
Hurts Whole Lot
10
Hurts Worst
B

FIGURE 8–3 Pediatric pain scales. **A,** FLACC Pain Scale. **B,** Wong-Baker FACES Pain Scale. *(**A**, FLACC Pain Scale, from Merkel, S., et al. [1997]. The FLACC: A behavioral scale for scoring postoperative pain in young children.* Pediatric Nurse, *23[3], 293–297. Copyright 1997 by Jannetti Co., University of Michigan Medical Center. Reprinted with permission; **B**, Wong-Baker FACES™ Pain Scale, © 1983, Wong-Baker FACES™ Foundation, http://www.WongBakerFACES.org. Used with permission.)*

TABLE 8–2 Pain Scales Tested in Toddlers and Preschoolers

ABBREVIATED NAME OF PAIN SCALE	NAME OF SCALE	APPROPRIATE AGE USE	DESCRIPTION
CHEOPS	Children's Hospital of Eastern Ontario Pain Scale	Study done on children aged 1–5 years; intended for age 0–4 years; can be used on children up to 7 years of age	A behavioral scale that gives a number value for cry intensity, facial expression, child verbalization of pain, torso position, touch, and leg movement
CHIPPS	Children and Infants Postoperative Pain Scale	Studied in infants and children aged 0–5 years; recommended for children aged 0–3 years	A behavioral scale that assigns a number value for cry intensity, facial expression, trunk position, leg movement, and restlessness
FACES	Wong-Baker FACES Pain Rating Scale	Recommended for children aged 3–7 years; several studies are unable to support reliability for children younger than 5 years	A self-reporting rating scale that assigns a number value to a facial expression to be chosen by a child

TABLE 8–2 Pain Scales Tested in Toddlers and Preschoolers—cont'd

ABBREVIATED NAME OF PAIN SCALE	NAME OF SCALE	APPROPRIATE AGE USE	DESCRIPTION
FLACC	Faces, Legs, Activity, Cry, Consolability Observational Tool	Studied in children aged 2 months to 7 years; recommended for age 1–5 years or any preverbal child	A behavioral scale that assigns a number value for facial expression, leg movement, activity/restlessness, cry intensity/continuity, and consolability
DEGR	Douleur Enfant Gustave Roussy	Studied on children with cancer aged 2 to 6 years	A behavioral scale in which an observer assigns a score of 0 for none to 4 for extreme on 16 different scale items
TPPPS	Toddler-Preschooler Postoperative Pain Scale	Recommended for children aged 1 to 5 years	A behavioral scale that assigns a number value for verbal response, facial expression, and body language

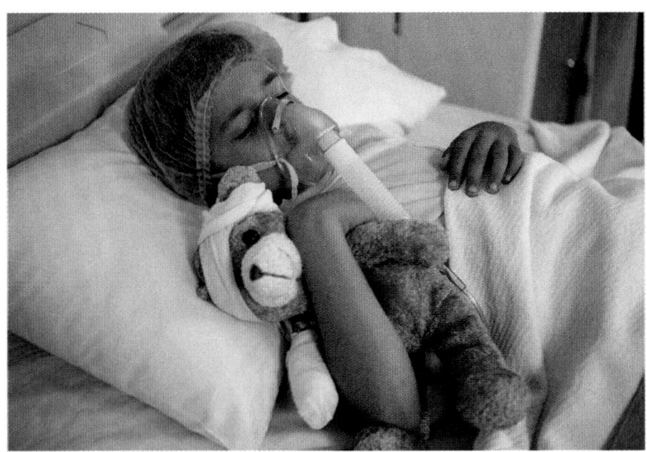

FIGURE 8–4 Kindergartner before surgery.

SAFE AND EFFECTIVE NURSING CARE: Cultural Competence

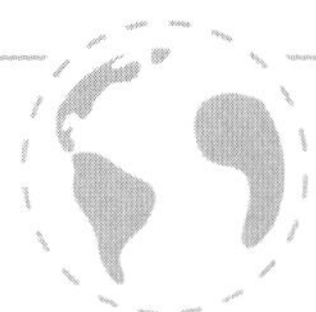

Pain Scales Are Not Reliable for All Cultures

Some pain scales may not be reliable for children of different cultures because of cultural influence on pain response. Nash (2012) discusses the Oucher scale, which provides seven versions for five different ethnicities and both sexes.

Evidence-Based Practice: Pediatric Pain Scales

Cohen, L. L., Lemanek, K., Blount, R. L., Dahlquist, L. M., Lim, C. S., Palermo, T. M., ... Weiss, K. E. (2008). Evidence-based assessment of pediatric pain. *Journal of Pediatric Psychology, 33*, 939–955.

Cohen et al. (2008) reviewed the evidence-based practice of the use of pediatric pain scales. Many scales have been validated and are considered strong measures for assessing pain in children, which gives medical professionals options to meet the needs of the patient. However, it is more important to identify why the particular scale is being used. Some scales have been used in specific environments and for different types of pain. The nurse must choose a pain scale that is most appropriate for each individual child. Cohen et al. (2008) maintain that "future directions in pain assessment have been identified, such as highlighting culture and the impact of pain on functioning...This review examines the research and characteristics of some of the commonly used pain tools in hopes that the reader will be able to use this evidence-based approach and the information in future selection of assessment devices for pediatric pain."

AGE GROUP CHALLENGES

Common challenges for children in this age group include those discussed in the following subsections.

Potty Training

Toilet training usually begins between the ages of 2 and 3 years. Signs of readiness include:

- Ability to have dry diaper for a few hours at a time or during a nap

- Regularly timed bowel movements
- Interest in the potty or going to the potty with others
- Physical ability to get to potty and pull up/down pants
- Ability to follow simple directions
- Unhappiness with the feeling of a wet or dirty diaper
- Ability to vocalize when they went and/or if they have to go

When the child begins to display readiness, caregivers should:

- Have the child practice sitting on the potty for a few minutes at a time.
- Practice hand washing; encourage the child to sing a song to wash for the appropriate amount of time.
- Teach proper use of hand sanitizer: must cover hands and dry completely; do not place hands in mouth (can be toxic to children).
- Teach girls to wipe front to back to minimize risk for urinary tract infections.
- Teach boys to urinate in the sitting position first. Once mastered, then move on to standing. May use flushable toilet targets for teaching purposes (do not put toys in the toilet for this purpose).
- Provide encouragement in the form of praise and celebration, along with rewards and incentives such as treats, stickers, and new underwear.
- Do not be severe or punitive when accidents happen.

A child who shows resistance to toilet-training attempts is likely not ready. Rushing a child into potty training will only make the process more lengthy and frustrating. Parents should avoid potty training during stressful times, such as a move or new baby arrival.

Separation Anxiety

Distress caused by a fear of abandonment, separation anxiety is a normal stage of development that can begin as early as 8 months of age and end as late as 3 years of age, but peaks between 10 and 18 months (HealthyChildren.org, 2015). Over time, this fear lessens as the child learns that parents will come back. To reduce separation anxiety, parents/caregivers should:

- Distract the child, say goodbye, and leave quickly. The quicker you leave, the quicker the episode will end.
- Practice leaving at home by going to another room and saying you will be back soon.
- Stay calm, be consistent, and give reassurance that you will be back.

Tantrums and Discipline

Most common in children aged 1 to 4 years, tantrums are a way for children to express anger and frustration. Episodes are characterized by:

- Whining and crying to screaming
- Hitting and kicking to scratching and biting
- Breath holding

Tantrums are often triggered by:

- Hunger
- Tiredness
- Being uncomfortable/sick
- Being overstressed
- Attention seeking
- Other problems (mental, physical, or emotional)

When faced with a tantrum, caregivers need to stay calm and collected; venting frustration verbally or physically can worsen the situation. Consequences should follow poor behavior and can include a time-out in a quiet place until the child is calm. Parents should establish and maintain routines to prevent acting out. Tantrums usually decrease in number with increase in language skills.

Sibling Rivalry

Sibling rivalry includes jealousy, competition, and fighting among siblings, often to gain attention from parents or to show dominance over one's brother or sister. Some level of quarreling is normal, including fighting over toys (especially for toddler), name calling, and telling on each other. Parents should encourage them to resolve the problem themselves but intervene if the situation is unsafe. When intervention is necessary, parents should:

- Separate the children to their own spaces.
- Set rules, such as no name calling, no pushing, and no slamming things.
- Avoid choosing sides.
- Assist with proper expression of feelings of anger and frustration.
- Teach them to be kind to each other by encouraging apologizing, sharing, and comforting each other when hurt.

Nutrition

Toddlers eat approximately seven times a day, consuming more meals than snacks. Preschoolers only eat approximately three meals a day with quite a few snacks throughout the day. Serving larger portions than recommended and/or pressuring a child to eat or clean his or her plate can lead to overeating and increased risk for childhood obesity. Allow children to self-regulate intake while providing healthy, nutrient-filled choices. Children should also be allowed to graze throughout the day, as toddlers may not sit for three meals. Toddlers are also known to have "food jags," preferring to eat only one food over and over.

At age 1 year, toddlers transition to whole milk. Children 1 to 2 years of age need two to three servings of whole milk or milk products (i.e., yogurt, cheese) per day (KidsHealth, 2014). Children older than 2 years should drink two servings of skim or low-fat milk or other milk product (KidsHealth, 2014). Some toddlers may still be breastfeeding. Support the breastfeeding mother by allowing privacy and bonding during feedings.

Although protein is important for children in this age group (the recommended daily allowance is 13 g/day for age 1 to 3 years and 19 g/day for age 4 to 8 years), many sources of protein are also common allergens:

- Dairy products
- Seafood
- Nuts
- Soy products

Snacks should be healthy enough to provide part of a child's total nutrient intake for the day. Good choices include:

- Fruits and vegetables
- Milk, yogurt, and cheese
- Whole-grain crackers and cereal
- Nuts and peanut butter

CRITICAL COMPONENT

Serving Sizes

According to the Academy of Nutrition and Dietetics (Hayes, 2017), an appropriate serving size for a child who is 2 to 3 years of age is half of an adult serving or 1,000 to 1,200 calories per day.

Caregivers should encourage self-feeding both to reinforce self-regulation of intake and to improve motor function. Because appetite fluctuates in toddlers and preschoolers, the amount of intake can vary with each meal. Children should be transitioned to cups and utensils by age 2 years. Although preschoolers may have difficulty sitting at the table because of short attention spans, they should be encouraged to do so at mealtimes even when not eating to promote routine and good eating habits.

Nutrition challenges for this age group include the following:

- Difficulty consuming enough iron and zinc. The recommended daily allowance (RDA) for iron is 7 mg for age 1 to 3 years and 10 mg for age 4 to 8 years. The RDA for zinc is 3 mg for age 1 to 3 years and 5 mg for age 4 to 8 years. Providing a list of iron- and zinc-rich foods to choose from may help remedy this problem.
- Difficulty fostering healthy eating habits
  - Finicky eaters
  - Normal to play with food
  - Learning about different textures and tastes
  - May prefer to eat only from a few selected foods
- Difficulty decreasing amount of intake of juice and sweet drinks
  - Juice and sweetened drinks should be limited to 4 to 6 oz/day.
  - The ideal drink choice is plain water.

CRITICAL COMPONENT

Avoiding Dental Caries

Drinking from a bottle throughout the day or at night increases the risk for dental caries (Fig. 8–5). It may also decrease appetite for solid food, and thus increase risk for malnutrition. The American Dental Association (2017) recommends that a child see the dentist from first tooth to age 1, then every 6 months throughout life.

Dental Caries

Dental caries in children are a serious public health problem that rapidly progresses, can have lifelong implications, has significant impact on families and communities, and often goes untreated (Colak, Dulgergil, Dalli, & Hamidi, 2013).

- Dental caries cause pain and infection, which can affect children's eating, sleeping, learning, and growth. These effects can continue into adolescence and adulthood, affecting behavior, mood, and social skills.
- The increased cost associated with multiple dental care visits, emergency department visits, and restorations can affect families and communities.
- There is also a relationship between dental caries and child mistreatment and/or neglect at the family level (Colak et al., 2013).

Parents can prevent dental caries with appropriate hygiene practices:

- For children 1 to 3 years old, use a smear of toothpaste the size of a grain of rice, and for 3 to 6 years old, use a pea-size amount of fluoride toothpaste in the morning and at night.
- Start flossing once a day when child has two teeth that touch together.

GROWING INDEPENDENCE

Caregivers should foster the growing independence of toddlers and preschoolers while taking measures to keep them safe. This includes:

- Teaching toddlers:
  - Rules and responsibilities
  - How to be safe

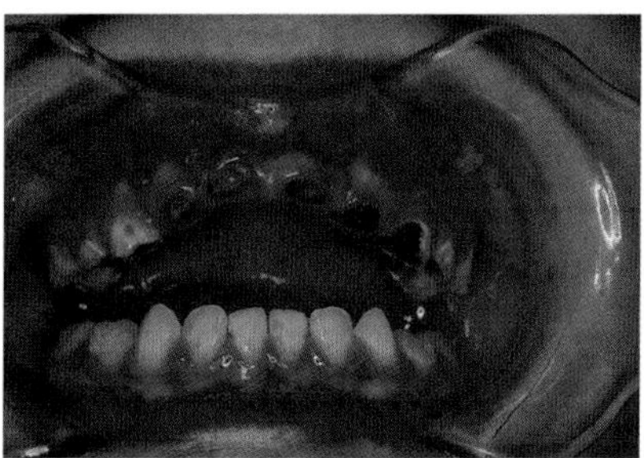

FIGURE 8–5 Baby-bottle caries.

- How to be a good friend by sharing, being kind, and not hitting others
- How to establish and keep routines so they can begin to do these routine things on their own
- Giving toddlers age-appropriate chores: allowing them to help teaches responsibility.
- Taking time to listen
  - Ask them open-ended questions.
  - Provide eye contact to show that attention is being given.
- Encouraging children to bathe and dress themselves or assist in these tasks

CAREGIVER SUPPORT

Nurses can provide valuable support for parents and caregivers of children in this age group.

In Hospital (Acute and Chronic Care)

When caring for a child in a hospital setting:

- Orient caregivers to unit.
- Explain all procedures in a step-by-step manner.
- Review the plan of care with caregivers daily or as it changes.
- Encourage families to stay informed by asking for test results, updates on patient care, and changes in patient status.
- Encourage caregivers to ask questions and express concerns.
- Instruct caregivers to ask for further explanation when needed.
- Urge caregivers to learn about the child's medications.
- Encourage involvement in decision making.
- Reassure caregivers that it is normal to feel scared, helpless, overwhelmed, guilty, sad, worried, confused, frustrated, angry, alone, and tired.
- Remind caregivers to care for themselves. Reassure them that it is fine to go home for a while, whether to relieve stress, take a shower, go to sleep, and/or take care of other responsibilities.

In Home

Caregivers should have emergency phone numbers readily available:

- Nurse advice line
- Number for health-care provider on call
- Poison control line
- 911 availability

Educate about signs and symptoms of common childhood infections:

- Fever accompanied by
  - Moist, productive cough
  - Green or blood-tinged nasal discharge
  - Pulling at ears

Teach caregivers how to care for children at home when they have a fever:

- Have a thermometer at home.
- Give medication with dosage appropriate to the weight of the child
- Use patient cooling techniques
- Promote dehydration prevention
  - Small, frequent sips of fluids
  - Electrolyte-replacement beverages
  - Broths
  - Popsicles
- Diet advancement (as tolerated)
  - Clear liquids
  - May begin with a BRAT diet (bananas, rice, applesauce, and toast) and quickly advance to soft foods; the BRAT diet by itself does not provide the proper nutrition intake.
  - Soft/bland foods
  - Solids: when able, it is best for the child to resume a well-balanced diet to ensure proper nutrition intake

> **CRITICAL COMPONENT**
>
> **Assessing for Child Abuse**
>
> Nurses are required to report suspected abuse by law. The nurse cannot keep a "secret" shared by a child when abuse is suspected. Be aware of:
>
> - Bruises in areas that are not typically bruised during play
> - Symmetry of bruises
> - Bruising that looks like an object
> - Bruises in different stages of healing
> - History of multiple broken bones
> - Caregiver speaks up when nurse asks how a bruise occurred
> - Caregiver's story does not fit the identified injury or developmental ability of the child
> - Multiple hospitalizations and child does not have a chronic health problem

Simple First Aid

- Wound cleansing
- Use of Band-Aids
- Topical antibiotics

Signs and Symptoms of Respiratory Distress

- Tachypnea
  - Breathing rapidly
  - Unable to complete sentences
- Retractions
  - Ability to see ribs during inhalation
- Nasal flaring
  - Nares flare out in an effort to take in air
- Accessory muscle use
  - Use of shoulders and abdomen to breathe
- Tripod positioning
  - Sitting with head up and out to stent the airway open
- Stridor, wheezing, and sonorous respirations
  - Cool mist humidifier
  - Warm steam bath

See Chapter 11 for additional respiratory information.

When to Call the Primary Care Provider

- Follow instructions as provided.
- Call if there has been a negative change from what the primary care provider (PCP) has first assessed.
- It is best to call the PCP whenever there is immediate information that the provider needs to know.
- Bring to the PCP if the child is no longer able to perform a skill that he or she was once able to perform.
- Bring to PCP whenever the caregiver believes the child is ill or his or her behavior has changed and there is suspicion that something is wrong.

When to Call 911

- Call 911 for all emergencies.
- Child is not breathing properly or adequately.
- Child's face is blue or extremities are blue.
- Child has decreased responsiveness
- Child becomes injured and has excessive bleeding
- Call for all perceived emergencies.

PEDIATRIC DISASTER PLANNING

More attention has been brought to disaster planning since the New York terrorist attacks on September 11, 2001. All hospitals are not equipped to provide extensive critical care to pediatric patients. Equipment standards may vary among first responders (U.S. Department of Health and Human Services, 2010). Weight-based single-dose medications are more difficult to stockpile than adult standard-dose medications. Children need to be transported to facilities that can care for their immediate needs. Hospitals that care for children are required to have appropriate-size equipment with health-care providers who can address the child's immediate needs. Child safety is the responsibility of all adults; however, it is a nurse's duty to advocate for the best care and safety of all pediatric patients.

Caregivers should have a disaster plan that includes the children. For example, children should have a place to meet and phone numbers of significant family members to contact in an emergency.

CASE STUDY

Mary is divorced and cares for her 2-year-old and 18-year-old sons. She tells you that she is not sure if her child is eating enough each day. The 18-year-old regularly brings home fast food and shares with the 2-year-old sibling. Both children can regularly be found drinking pop. The younger child enjoys drinking out of a cup with a straw and is frequently crying for French fries and doughnuts. The mother knows that this food is not good for either child, but appreciates the convenience of not having to cook. She is concerned that the younger child will not grow properly and become overweight. The mother further explains that she is a single parent and must work to support her family. It is challenging to pay the monthly bills and have food left over for groceries. She admits to buying items that are on sale and that are inexpensive to be able to feed her family for the week. She feels guilty not giving her kids what they want when she spends less time with them during the day. When she comes home from work, she doesn't feel much like cooking, let alone preparing a highly nutritious meal.

1. What information can assist the nurse to determine whether the child is eating a well-balanced diet?
2. What physical assessment data will assist the nurse to determine whether the child is eating too much?

REFERENCES

American Academy of Pediatrics. (2017). *Children with disabilities: Description and policy.* Retrieved from https://www.aap.org/en-us/about-the-aap/Committees-Councils-Sections/Council-on-Children-with-Disabilities/Pages/Description-and-Policy.aspx

American Dental Association. (2017). *Baby teeth.* Retrieved from http://www.mouthhealthy.org/en/az-topics/b/baby-teeth

American Association of Poison Control Centers (AAPCC). (2017). *Hand sanitizer.* Retrieved from http://www.aapcc.org/alerts/hand-sanitizer/

Centers for Disease Control and Prevention (CDC). (2009). *Clinical growth charts.* Retrieved from http://www.cdc.gov/growthcharts/clinical_charts.htm

Centers for Disease Control and Prevention (CDC). (2014). 10 Leading causes of injury deaths by age group highlighting unintentional injury deaths, United States—2014 Rank. Retrieved from https://www.cdc.gov/injury/wisqars/pdf/leading_causes_of_injury_deaths_highlighting_unintentional_injury_2014-a.pdf

Centers for Disease Control and Prevention (CDC). (2015). *Protect the ones you love: Child injuries are preventable.* Retrieved from http://www.cdc.gov/safechild/Child_Injury_Data.html

Centers for Disease Control and Prevention (CDC). (2016). *Protect the ones you love: Child injuries are preventable: Burn prevention.* Retrieved from https://www.cdc.gov/safechild/burns/

Cohen, L. L., Lemanek, K., Blount, R. L., Dahlquist, L. M., Lim, C. S., Palermo, T. M., ... Weiss, K. E. (2008). Evidence-based assessment of pediatric pain. *Journal of Pediatric Psychology, 33*, 939–955.

Colak, H., Dulgergil, C. T., Dalli, M., & Hamidi, M. M. (2013). Early childhood caries update: A review of causes, diagnosis, and treatments. *Journal of Natural Science, Biology and Medicine, 4*(1), 29–38.

Hayes, D. (2017). What and how much should my preschooler be eating? *Academy of Nutrition and Dietetics.* Retrieved from http://www.eatright.org/resource/food/nutrition/dietary-guidelines-and-myplate/size-wise-nutrition-for-preschool-age-children

Healthy Child Care America. (2011). *Crib regulations.* Retrieved from http://www.healthychildcare.org/CribRegulations.html

Healthy Children.org. (2015). *How to ease your child's separation anxiety.* Retrieved from https://www.healthychildren.org/English/ages-stages/toddler/Pages/Soothing-Your-Childs-Separation-Anxiety.aspx

Insurance Institute for Highway Safety and Highway Loss Data Institute. (2017). *Safety belts.* Retrieved from http://www.iihs.org/iihs/topics/laws/safetybeltuse

KidsHealth. (2014). *Nutrition guide for toddlers.* Retrieved from https://kidshealth.org/en/parents/toddler-food.html?WT.ac=p-ra#

Nash, L. (2012). How to assess pain in children and young people. *Emergency Nurse, 20*(2), 19–22.

U.S. Department of Health and Human Services. (2010). *Emergency medical services and pediatric transport*. Retrieved from http://archive.ahrq.gov/prep/nccdreport/nccdrpt4.htm

U.S. Department of Health and Human Services, National Institutes of Health, & National Heart, Lung, and Blood Institute. (2005). The fourth report on the diagnosis, evaluation, and treatment of high blood pressure in children and adolescents (NIH Publication No. 05-5268). Retrieved from https://www.nhlbi.nih.gov/files/docs/resources/heart/hbp-ped.pdf

Ward, S. L., & Hisley, S. M. (2010). *Maternal-child nursing care*. Philadelphia: F.A. Davis.

9

School-Age Children

Daniel C. Rausch, BSN, RN

LEARNING OUTCOMES

Upon completion of this chapter, the student will be able to:

1. Describe growth and development during the school-age years.
2. Identify age-specific physical assessment approaches for school-age patients.
3. Explain medication approaches for school-age patients.
4. Explain variations in nursing procedures for school-age patients.
5. Describe strategies for assessing health promotion practices among school-age patients.
6. Describe emergency care considerations for school-age patients.
7. Identify strategies to support school-aged adolescents.
8. Integrate chronic care concepts and considerations specific to the school-age population.
9. Integrate home-care concepts and considerations specific to the school-age population.
10. Recognize complementary and alternative therapies used by school-age patients.
11. Recognize child abuse considerations relevant to school-age patients.

INTRODUCTION

Children 6 to 12 years old are considered "school age" (Fig. 9–1). During these years, children are growing at a slower rate than before but still accomplishing important developmental milestones. A wide variety of both physical and behavioral changes can be observed among children in this age group. The younger school-age child will be similar to the late-stage preschooler, whereas the older school-age child will be more similar to an adolescent. Each child will move through this stage at a different pace. Careful assessment and adaptability on the part of the nurse are required in caring for patients of this age group.

GROWTH AND DEVELOPMENT

Physical assessment of this age group should include the following components:

- Vital signs (Table 9–1): Attainment of vital signs should not be difficult with this population. Explain the procedures to the child and allow him or her to choose, as appropriate, which side blood pressure will be taken, oral versus axillary temperature, and which finger to use for pulse oximetry.
  - Pulse oximetry values should be the same as adult values (93% to 100%).

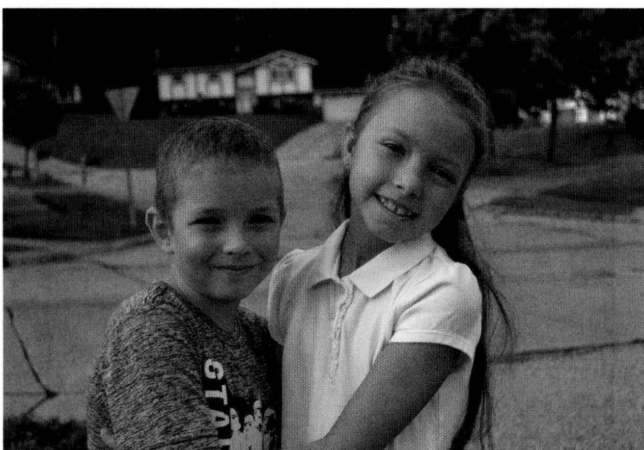

FIGURE 9–1 School-age children.

- Pulse oximetry values may be different if there is an underlying cardiac or pulmonary diagnosis.
- A fever is generally considered to be a temperature greater than 101.4°F or 38.5°C. Fevers do not cause seizures, although a sudden increase in body temperature may result in a febrile seizure. High fevers greater than 104°F or 40°C in children do not indicate that the infection is more serious, as they may in adults, because less-refined pediatric immune systems may produce higher fevers than needed (Children's Health Team, 2015).

- Height/weight: The Centers for Disease Control and Prevention (CDC) provides sex- and age-specific grids on which height and weight can be plotted (CDC, 2016). Weight and height should be taken standing unless the child has a condition that does not allow him or her to stand. Children in this age group should:
  - Gain 3 kg/year in weight
  - Gain 5 cm/year in height
  - Experience a growth spurt at age 10 to 12 years for girls and around age 12 years for boys
- Daily fluid requirements: Daily intake requirements are based on weight (Box 9–1), whereas normal urine output is based on patient age and calculated by weight (Box 9–2).
- Pain assessment: The nurse can choose between a few different pain scales depending on age and developmental level. Each pain assessment begins by explaining how the pain scales work and assessing the child's ability to properly use the scale. Make sure to specifically ask the child about pain level, not how he or she feels; being sick and in the hospital may cause the child to give a higher rating than is accurate.
  - The FACES scale may be used for younger school-age children. (See Chapter 8 for information on the FACES scale.)
  - This age group can also point to where it hurts and describe the pain with words like *stabbing* or *burning*.
  - The FACES scale has been proved over time to correlate highly with the visual analog scale (Thrane, Wanless, Cohen, & Danford, 2016).
  - One downside noted with the FACES scale is that some children will choose the smile face because that is the most desirable. In addition, if a child is feeling pain, he or she may automatically be drawn to the crying face, number 10. Educate the child to point to the face that reflects the level of pain he or she is experiencing.
  - Older school-age children may be able to use a visual analog scale or numeric of 1 to 10. As children grow older, increased vocabulary increases their ability to describe pain.
  - Parents or the child's primary caregiver will be able to assist in the assessment of pain. They will notice minute differences in their children that the nurse may not immediately notice.
  - Facial expression as a sole means of determining pain is not recommended.

SAFE AND EFFECTIVE NURSING CARE: Cultural Competence

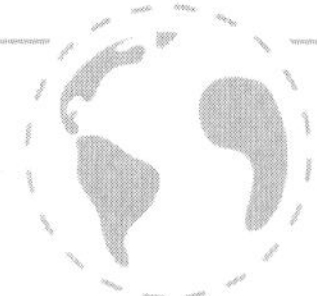

Language Differences in Pediatric Pain

There are many Spanish-speaking individuals in the United States, including among the pediatric population. However, Spanish-language tools for pediatric pain reporting have not received much research attention. There are many different dialects of the Spanish language. Individuals who identify themselves as Hispanic may be of many different countries, including Mexico, Puerto Rico, Cuba, and nations of South or Central America. Pain may be defined or explained differently among individuals for these countries. Besides Spanish, Arabic and Urdu are the fastest-growing languages used in the United States. About 21% of U.S. residents speak a language other than English in the home (Camarota & Zeigler, 2015).

TABLE 9–1 Vital Signs Typical for Age

AGE	TEMPERATURE	PULSE	RESPIRATIONS	SYSTOLIC BP	DIASTOLIC BP
6 years	98.6°F	95	20–25	95	55–70
9 years	98.1°F	95	17–22	105–110	60–75
12 years	97.8°F	85	17–22	118–120	62–76

BP, blood pressure.

Adapted from National Institutes of Health. (2008). Pediatric blood pressure charts. *Retrieved from https://www.nhlbi.nih.gov/files/docs/guidelines/child_tbl.pdf.*

BOX 9–1 | Fluid Requirements by Weight

WEIGHT	FLUID REQUIREMENT (mL/kg/day)
11–20 kg	1,000 mL + 50 mL for each kg above 10 kg
>20 kg	1,500 mL + 20 mL for each kg above 20 kg

Source: Adapted from Guid (n.d.).

BOX 9–2 | Expected Urine Output

AGE	EXPECTED URINE OUTPUT
6–7 years	1–2 mL/kg/hr
8–12 years	0.5–1 mL/kg/hr

Source: Patient.co.uk (2010).

General Survey

In the general survey for the pediatric patient, determine developmental history, family composition, and school performance. Somatic complaints without verified diagnostic clinical data—such as chronic pain, dizziness, sweating, headaches, chest pain, shortness of breath, gastrointestinal issues, nausea, vomiting, diarrhea, or back or joint pain—may be an indication of school or home avoidance/problems, anxiety and stress, or depression (Kaneshiro, Zeive, & Ogilvie, 2014) (see Chapter 14). Yearly health maintenance visits with a primary care provider are recommended for school-age children (American Academy of Pediatrics [AAP], n.d.).

- Annual assessments check height, weight, body mass index (BMI), blood pressure, hearing, vision, and anemia. Immunizations should also be given as recommended by the schedule updated each year in January at the CDC Web site (see Chapter 22). The nurse should also assess the following areas:
- Skin
  - Assess for signs of child abuse, such as bruises in various stages of healing, bruises on unusual parts of the body, and cigarette burns.
  - Assess for dryness, rashes, eczema, abrasions, and contusions or scratches.
  - Abused children in this age group may fear that they have done something wrong or that they somehow deserve what is happening to them. Primary caregivers should make sure that children understand good touch/bad touch and the danger of engaging with strangers. Caregivers should listen to children's concerns, ask questions about the adults/peers at school/activities, and monitor for changes in mood or behavior, which may indicate that abuse has taken place. After-school time should be supervised and structured.
- Head
  - Assess for lice (Fig. 9–2).
  - Assess hair for dryness and brittleness that can indicate nutrition status.

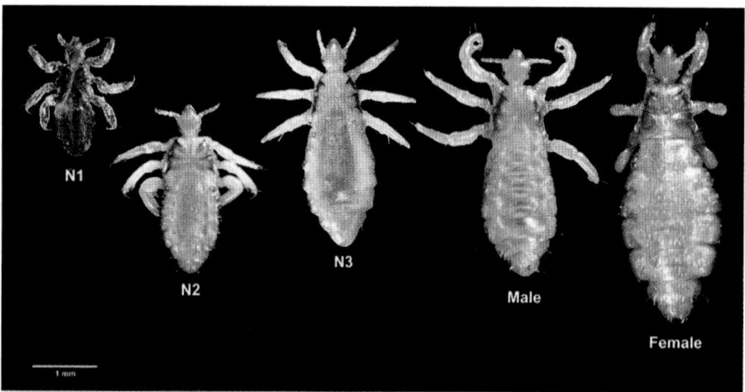

FIGURE 9–2 Pediculosis (head lice).

  - Assess for open lesions/signs of trauma.
  - Assess for symptoms or recent history of head trauma, including headaches, difficulty concentrating, or loss of consciousness.
- Eyes
  - Assess for use of glasses/contacts.
  - Assess visual acuity.
  - Assess for broken blood vessels, jaundice, and dryness.
- Ears
  - Assess for hearing aid use and hearing acuity.
  - Assess for buildup of earwax, which can impair hearing.
  - Assess for an excess buildup of fluid in the canal.
- Mouth/Teeth
  - Loss of primary (baby) teeth and eruption of new adult teeth starting with 6-year molars
  - Orthodontic treatment
  - Promotion of good dental hygiene, especially as children of this age begin independent self-care
  - Dental checkups every 6 months, with fluoride treatments if fluoride in the water supply is low (AAP, n.d.), or more often for children with increased risk for tooth decay, improper hygiene, or unusual growth patterns
  - Loose teeth or removable orthodontic appliances that may need to be removed or observed during an emergency

SAFE AND EFFECTIVE NURSING CARE: Cultural Competence

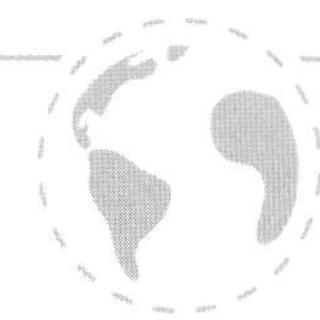

Belief in the Tooth Fairy

The tooth fairy is a modern U.S. construct with origins in Norse mythology and Northern European traditions (Saunders, 2016). Do not assume that the "tooth fairy" visits every home because this is influenced by culture.

- Throat
  - Ensure the trachea is midline.
  - Inspect and palpate for an enlarged thyroid (goiter).
  - Assess for difficulty swallowing.

- Nose
  - Assess for a blue or "boggy" appearance of the nasal mucosa, which indicates allergies.
  - Assess for allergic rhinitis and treatments, including oral or nasal medications, over-the-counter treatments, and saline nasal irrigation. The latter has been found to have a positive impact on allergic rhinitis, although adoption is slow (Ryan, 2016). Educate parents about use of saline, distilled, or other approved water over the use of tap water because of risk for infection.
  - Assess for frequent nosebleeds and mucosal dryness.
  - Assess for airflow, which may be restricted because of acute or chronic sinusitis.
- Cardiovascular
  - Assess for any congenital cardiac anomalies by history and auscultation.
  - With corrected cardiac defects, the patient may have scars on the chest such as a midline incision or chest tubes.
  - Innocent heart murmurs are very common in school-age children. Some cardiologists estimate that up to 90% of children aged 4 to 7 years have heart murmurs, often a result of turbulent blood flow at the aorta or pulmonary artery (Cincinnati Children's Hospital, 2014).
  - Heart sounds should have normal S1 and S2.
- Respiratory
  - Assess for a history of asthma, the most prevalent chronic illness in children.
  - Lungs should sound clear.
  - Check for signs/symptoms of chronic respiratory issues such as barrel chest and clubbed fingers.
  - Abnormalities may include crackles, rhonchi, wheezing, retractions, grunting, and nasal flaring (see Chapter 11).
  - Assess skin color to note any oxygenation issues, such as pallor or cyanosis that can be related to respiratory or cardiac issues.
- Gastrointestinal/Genitourinary
  - Assess for enuresis, or urine incontinence (see Chapter 3).
  - Assess for encopresis, the deliberate withholding of stool (see Chapter 15). Evacuation of a small amount of stool may indicate encopresis.
  - Assess for constipation/diarrhea, acute or chronic, and any treatments the patient may be receiving.
- Reproductive
  - Girls may experience menarche, the start of menses, near the end of this stage. (For information on puberty, see Chapter 10.) Primary caregivers should be prepared to support the child during this emotional and potentially scary time. Early discussions with the child will help her prepare.
  - Refer to the Tanner stages to identify the child's current stage of puberty (see Chapter 10).
  - Some children may experience precocious puberty (defined as experiencing puberty before age 7 years for girls and before age 9 years for boys) (Kaneshiro et al., 2014). Make sure that appropriate support is available because this can be very difficult for children who are affected. Although a child's primary caregiver may intend to discuss menarche with his or her daughter, precocious puberty may come before this discussion takes place.
  - The onset of puberty in boys will be accompanied by increased upper body mass, increased amount and thickness of hair on the body and genitalia, and nocturnal emissions, or the release of semen during sleep. This is a normal part of puberty and may be seen in the late stage of school age, but is more likely in adolescence.
- Neurovascular/Musculoskeletal
  - Increased coordination
  - Increased fine motor skills
  - Increased balance
  - The ability to do complex tasks, such as riding a bike
  - Scoliosis checks beginning at age 12 years (see Chapter 10)
- Cognitive
  - Piaget's cognitive developmental theory (see Chapter 6)
  - Mastery of mathematics and reading skills
  - Classification and serialization of numbers
  - Understanding cause and effect
  - The ability to decenter (see the perspectives of others)
- Psychological
  - Freud's psychosexual development theory—age 6–12 years: latency stage (see Chapter 6)
  - Erikson and psychosocial development—age 6 to 12 years: industry versus inferiority (see Chapter 6)
- Social
  - Kohlberg's theory of moral development: preconventional level (see also Chapter 6)
  - Likes to forms clubs with rules and requirements
  - Likes to do favorite activities with a best friend
  - Usually socializes primarily with children of the same gender
  - Follows rules and understands consequences
  - Enjoys playing games
  - Enjoys having a collection of items, such as video games

PHYSICAL ASSESSMENT APPROACHES

School-age children should be cooperative with the physical assessment. Ask the child whether he or she would like the parent or primary caregiver present during the assessment. Typically, younger school-age children will like to have the primary caregiver present and older school-age children may or may not want the primary caregiver present during the entire assessment. Speak and ask questions directly to the child. Give the child rationales for all actions you perform (Kaneshiro et al., 2014).

SAFE AND EFFECTIVE NURSING CARE: Clinical Pearl

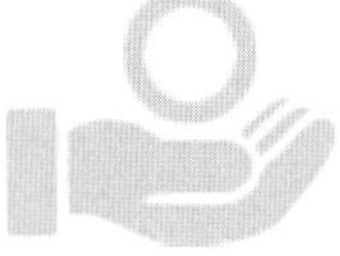

Good Touch/Bad Touch

Use inspection of the genital area during the physical assessment as a springboard for discussing good/bad touches. Indicate which areas the child should report to a trusted adult if anyone touches them, including the breasts, buttocks, and genitals.

Approaches to Medication Administration

School-age children should be able to assist in the medication administration process.

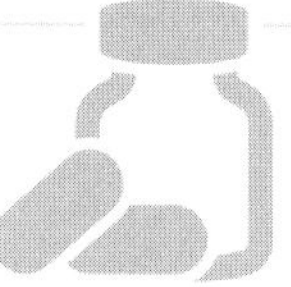

SAFE AND EFFECTIVE NURSING CARE: Understanding Medication

Medication Dosing

Medications should have weight-based dosing to provide an appropriate dose for pediatric patients. A child has a faster metabolic rate than an adult. Weight-based dosing ensures that the child will receive adequate medication to produce therapeutic results. Typically, children older than 14 years and more than 50 kg should receive a standard adult dose. This is a just a guide to ensure that the obese child does not receive a medication dose greater than the recommended adult dose.

- Basing medication dosage on weight gives an accurate and safe dose for each patient.
- Medication dosing should not be based on age because patient size may vary.

Oral Medications

Younger school-age children may choose to take oral liquids from an oral syringe or a medicine cup. If appropriate, the nurse may choose food or drink as a reward. If the medication tastes bad, you can offer a "chaser," numb the child's tongue beforehand with a popsicle, or have the child pinch his or her nose while ingesting the medication. The child's caregiver may administer medications, under nursing supervision, when appropriate. Be sure to monitor all administration of medication to the child.

Oral medications can often be prepared in a flavored liquid provided by the pharmacy. Use caution with flavorings that taste like candy, and educate parents to store medications in a safe area so younger children cannot access them.

CRITICAL COMPONENT

How Children Take Oral Medications

A small number of children in this age group may start swallowing pills. Be sure to assess how the child prefers to take oral medications, and give a choice when possible.

Subcutaneous Medications

When administering subcutaneous medications, use eutectic mixture of local anesthetics (EMLA) medicated cream when appropriate. This is used to prevent pain associated with needle insertion, IV cannulation, and superficial surgery on the skin and genital mucous membranes. Assess the depth of adipose tissue and muscle mass to ensure use of an appropriate needle size and depth to place the medication subcutaneously, not intramuscularly.

If the patient has a history of diabetes, his or her caregiver may be experienced at administering subcutaneous injections. Older school-age children with diabetes may be starting to administer their own injections. This must occur under parental/caregiver supervision.

IV Medications

With this age group, medical play can be helpful when IV medications are required. A child life specialist can help explain procedures in an age-appropriate manner. Older children may be more compliant if they can make appropriate decisions, such as on which side to insert the IV. Remember that the patient will still need to perform age-appropriate activities such as coloring for younger children and writing, homework, or crafts for older children; if possible, place the IV in the non-dominant hand. Distractions, such as discussions about something other than the current procedure, can be helpful if they are perceived by the child as authentically calm and positive, with signifiers such as a rising tone and happy expressions (Thrane et al., 2016).

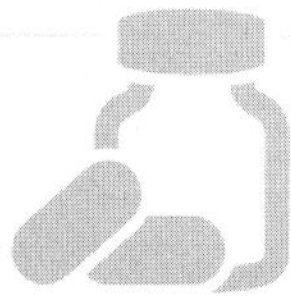

SAFE AND EFFECTIVE NURSING CARE: Understanding Medication

Eutectic Mixture of Lidocaine and Prilocaine (EMLA) Cream

EMLA is a medicated cream applied to the skin before painful procedures. The mixture contains 2.5% lidocaine and 2.5% prilocaine. It should be in place at least 45 minutes. The longer it is in place, the deeper it will penetrate; 2 hours is best for intramuscular injection. After 4 hours, it begins to lose its effectiveness and should be removed. Another product, called ELA-Max, absorbs into the skin more quickly than EMLA. When using these medications:

- Assess for allergic reaction to the medication.
- Apply a large "glob" of the medication to the skin.
- Do not rub it in.
- Apply an occlusive dressing over the medication.
- Do not rub, massage, or disturb the area until ready to perform the procedure.
- Advise the patient's primary caregiver to watch the medicated area so the child does not disturb the cream, pull off the dressing, or consume the cream.
- When dressing is removed, wipe remainder of medication from the skin before cleaning for the procedure (Hazard Vallerand, Sanoski, & Hopfer Deglin, 2017).

Variations on Nursing Procedures

When caring for this age group, it is important to gain the trust of the child before beginning assessment or procedures. Explain procedures in an age-appropriate way. Do not lie if a procedure will be uncomfortable or painful; this will cause you to lose the child's trust.

Tell the child and the parents/caregivers what you will be doing before doing it. Try the following approach:

- Look: Assess the child's appearance, muscle tone, and skin.
- Talk: Discuss with the child and the parents/caregivers any recent history or problems. Listen to what the child tells you.
- Touch: Be nonthreatening by avoiding sudden movements and staying at the level of the child whenever possible.
- Allow for privacy.
- Appropriate rewards such as stickers or small toys may be given after the examination.
- If a procedure must be performed, have the instruments ready and inform the child immediately before the procedure. The longer a child is aware that a painful or uncomfortable procedure is coming, the greater the stress that can occur.
- Do the least invasive parts of an examination first. If part of the examination is invasive or painful, this will make the child fearful of further, even noninvasive, painless parts of the examination.

HEALTH PROMOTION

Health promotion for this age group includes the topics discussed in the following subsections.

Safety

School-age children are very physically active in biking, sports, and other activities. Unintentional injury, including head injury, is the leading cause of death in this age group.

- Head injury prevention
  - Studies show that parents' knowledge of head injuries is limited (LaBond, Barber, & Golden, 2014).
  - The school nurse can be very helpful in giving information to parents on treatment and symptoms to watch for (LaBond et al., 2014).
  - Because there are currently no tests to determine the extent of brain injury, parents may not realize that symptoms such as headache and problem with concentration are caused by a "mild" traumatic brain injury (LaBond et al., 2014).
- Bike/scooter/skateboard/sports safety: Assess for and educate on use of helmets and pads (Fig. 9–3). The child should be taught to put these on correctly and do so independently.
- Pedestrian safety (Fig. 9–4): This includes walking on sidewalks, looking both ways when crossing streets, and walking against traffic for safety.
- Need for adult supervision
  - Children are starting to have independence at this age and may be able to do many activities with less direct supervision.
  - Children are able to play alone with adults nearby but should not be left unsupervised for any extended period.

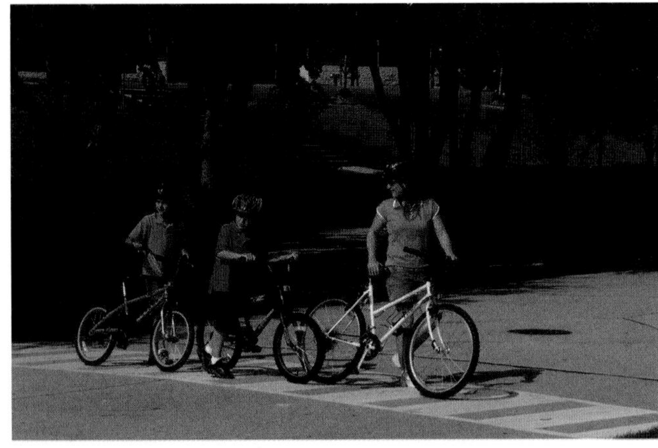

FIGURE 9–3 Children wearing bike helmets and walking bikes across the street in a cross walk.

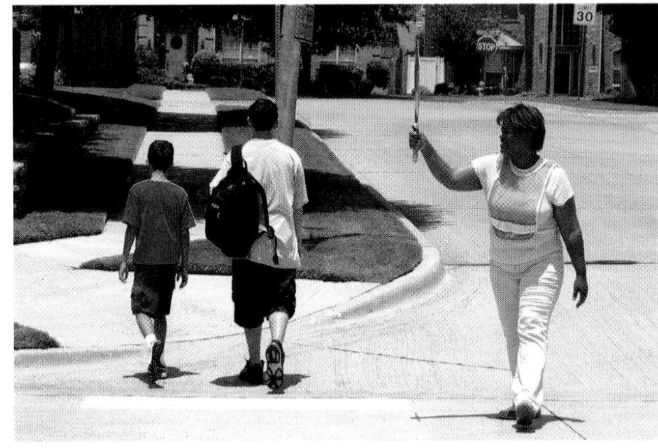

FIGURE 9–4 Children walking across the street with a crossing guard.

  - By the end of this phase, children will engage in unsupervised activities, such as staying home while their parents/primary caregivers run errands. Readiness to be left unsupervised will vary by developmental level.
  - In addition, older school-age children may start babysitting.
  - Children will try to be more independent and try more "exciting" and dangerous activities.
  - School-age children will be more involved in team activities, such as football, baseball, swimming, and cheerleading.

SAFE AND EFFECTIVE NURSING CARE: Promoting Safety

As children begin to babysit, they should learn about and be comfortable with creating and maintaining a safe environment for the children they supervise and themselves. This includes:

- Knowledge of fire safety
- Care for and observation of children in various stages of growth and development
- Basic first aid and possibly CPR
- Many of these skills are taught in babysitting classes offered by hospitals and other organizations, such as the YMCA

Nutrition

School-age children have a decreased caloric requirement compared with previous stages of development. This is an important time to teach children and primary caregivers about proper nutrition. During the next stage, adolescence, the child's nutrition requirements will increase again.

Approximately 17.4% of school children are obese, BMI is defined as greater than the 95th percentile by the CDC, and another 18% are overweight (CDC, 2014). A high BMI in children is linked with increased lipid levels, insulin levels, and blood pressure; these can lead to higher risks for atherosclerosis and obesity in adulthood. In addition, overweight children have a greater chance of being overweight as adults. The health consequences of obesity in children will have a negative effect on their morbidity and mortality as adults. Modeling and directed communication about the importance of a healthy diet should carry over into adulthood (Scheinfeld & Shim, 2017).

Exercise

Children should have at least 1 hour of physical activity a day (Kaneshiro et al., 2014). Nurses and caregivers should support this by:

- Encouraging normal school-age activities, such as ball, jumping rope, bike riding, skating, and using playground equipment
- Encouraging participation in school exercise programs and available sports

As with nutrition, early education and experience with exercise can help to form good habits that can last a lifetime.

School

The nurse should assess for school avoidance/refusal/phobia. Signs among this age group include the following:

- Child displays somatic symptoms such as a "stomachache" without any clinical basis, but only on school days.
- Child refuses to attend school.

In the case of school avoidance, an interdisciplinary approach should involve teachers, school counselors, parents or primary caregivers, and health-care professionals. Homeschooling may be an option until the issue is resolved.

Bullying

Bullying is an aggressive interaction between individuals or between an individual and a group. The interaction is unsolicited and unwanted by the individual being harassed. The interaction brings about psychosocial distress and is meant to bring ill feelings and fear to an individual. The person being bullied may feel that he or she is being targeted for having different beliefs and attitudes, for dressing in a certain style of clothing, or for absolutely no reason at all. The aggressive behavior may occur once or repeated multiple times. The aggressors aim to implant fear and power over an individual. Bullying, which occurs in most cultures and countries to some degree, is significantly more prevalent in the school-age group than in the adolescent group. Various factors are associated with being a bully, a victim, or both, including:

- Age
- Lower socioeconomic status
- Parents and caregivers with a high school or lower educational level
- Poor health status, increased health needs, and mental health issues
- Physical appearance
- Poor academic achievement or social adjustment
- Sexual orientation

Many schools now have programs to deal with bullying and a zero-tolerance anti-bullying policy. The nurse caring for a school-age child should:

- Assess for both physical and psychological signs of bullying.
- Help caregivers find resources to assist with bullying.
- For children with special needs, assess the resources available at the school.

Substance Use and Sexual Activity

Health-care providers should assess for and discourage the use of alcohol, tobacco, and drugs. Many schools have substance abuse prevention programs, such as DARE. Parents have the strongest influence on teaching children to avoid drugs.

The health-care provider should also assess children in this age group for understanding and knowledge of sex. Children may be more willing to discuss this topic privately, without their parents present. Sex education in schools often starts during this age range. The nurse should:

- Assess whether the caregivers have started to discuss sex with older school-age children.
- Be aware that discussing this subject can be difficult for caregivers.
- Help caregivers find resources to teach their children and creative ways to open the discussion.

Sexting

The practice of sending nude or explicit photos, videos, or messages through a smartphone or other device, sometimes called *sexting*, is increasingly prevalent and may begin in this age group. Sexting has been linked with an increased likelihood of risky sexual behaviors in middle school students (Rosenberg, 2014). Children can suffer emotional and legal consequences for sharing this type of photo with peers. Caregivers should ask their children about sexting and be aware of their child's online activity.

EMERGENCY CARE

Unintentional injuries and cancer are the two leading causes of death for children 5 to 14 years old (CDC, 2016). When a child has been injured, the family often sees the physician as the point person, but he or she is often unavailable to talk with the family during the crisis while providing and directing care. For this reason, child life specialists, social workers, and chaplains should be available to the child and family during this time. Family-centered care remains a priority (Fig. 9–5).

ACUTE-CARE HOSPITALIZATION

When a child requires acute care, the environment of care depends on the facility. In any situation, it is beneficial to allow the child and family an area for their own items. The room should be a safe area for the child, with all invasive and painful procedures performed in a treatment room. This helps prevent child and caregiver fear when clinicians enter the room. Educate parents/caregivers as to the reason for the use of the treatment room. When possible, older school-age children can decide whether they want to go to the treatment room or have the procedure at the bedside. When caring for a pediatric patient in acute care, the nurse should:

- Encourage caregivers to have an active role in caring for the child.
- Encourage caregivers to bring items from home that help the child feel more comfortable and reduce stress. Depending on facility policy, children may feel more comfortable wearing their own clothes or pajamas in the hospital.
- Allow walks with caregivers when possible based on the child's diagnosis and facility policy.
- Encourage visitation of siblings to promote a normal environment, provided siblings are free of illness. Siblings can participate in activities with the sick child whenever possible.
- Ensure that siblings admitted together get a double room or are placed in rooms next to each other to facilitate care for the primary caregivers and help the children cope with hospitalization.

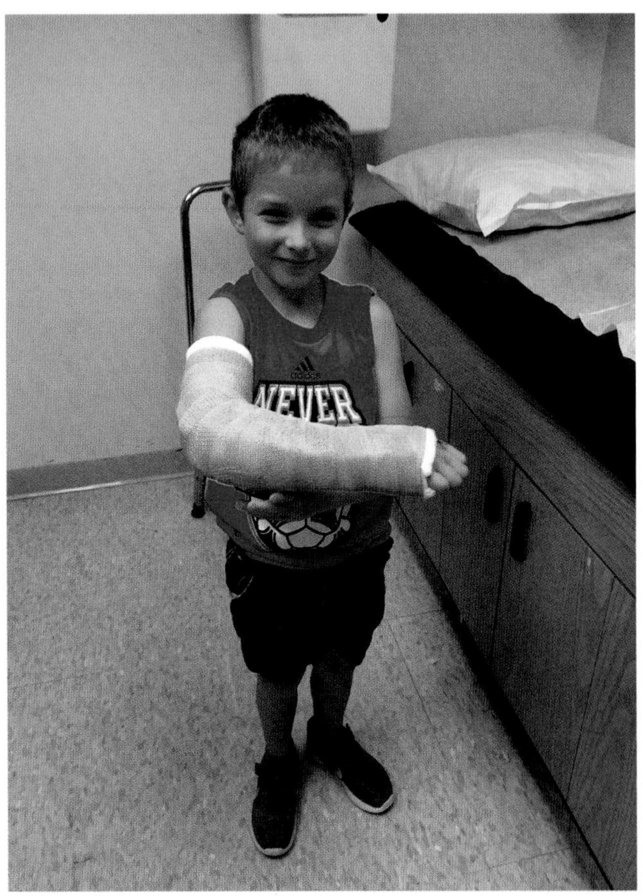

FIGURE 9–5 Child with cast after emergency department visit.

Evidence-Based Practice: Early Warning Systems

Glasper, A. (2016). Keeping sick children in the hospital safe from harm. *British Journal of Nursing, 25*(20), 1144–1145.

During routine assessment in the hospital, it is important to evaluate whether a patient is becoming more acutely ill. For pediatric patients, the use of the Pediatric Early Warning System (PEWS) is a good tool to improve earlier identification of a deteriorating condition (Table 9–2). This system evaluates the heart rate, respiratory rate, and behaviors of the patient and scores them from 0 (normal for age) to higher numbers with increasing severity from baseline. Not only is this evaluation needed, but communication to the interdisciplinary team is critical for early intervention (Glasper, 2016). Communication with a multidisciplinary team early on can identify issues earlier. The use of a rapid response team is recommended.

Role of the Child Life Specialist

Child life specialists offer a variety of services for children who are hospitalized and their families. These include:

- Preparation for medical procedures, including medical play: For example, using a doll to help a child act out a planned procedure can significantly decrease his or her anxiety; this is known as therapeutic play.
- Accompanying a school-age child to a procedure or test to provide distraction and coaching
- Planning celebrations for children who are in the hospital for a major milestone, such as a birthday or holiday
- Offering music or art therapy to provide distraction and a creative outlet for stress
- Offering therapeutic puppetry featuring characters to whom children can relate: For example, Rainbow Babies and Children's Hospital in Cleveland, Ohio, has a puppet mascot named Buddy who can visit children and host shows on the hospital's closed circuit television channel.
- Coordinating an activity room where children can play with toys and games or participate in organized activities: Children who are in isolation may have toys brought to their rooms. All toys should be able to be cleaned with water and disinfectant.

TABLE 9–2 Pediatric Early Warning System (PEWS) Scale

COMPONENTS	0	1	2	3	SCORE
Behavior	Playing/ Appropriate	Sleeping	Irritable	Lethargic/Confused OR Reduced response to pain	
Cardiovascular	Pink or capillary refill 1–2 seconds	Pale or capillary refill 3 seconds	Gray or capillary refill 4 seconds OR Tachycardia of 20 above normal rate	Gray and mottled or capillary refill 5 seconds or above OR Tachycardia of 30 above normal rate or bradycardia	
Respiratory	Within normal parameters, no retractions	>10 above normal parameters, using accessory muscles OR 30+% FiO_2 or 3+ L/min	• >20 above normal parameters • Retractions OR • 40+% FiO_2 or 6+ L/min	• 5 below normal parameters with retractions • Grunting OR • 50% FiO_2 or 8+ L/min	

Score 2 extra for quarter hourly nebulizers or persistent vomiting after surgery.

Adapted with the author's permission from Tucker, K. M., Brewer, T. L., Baker, R. B., Demeritt, B., & Vossmeyer, M. T. (2009). Prospective evaluation of a pediatric inpatient early warning scoring system. Journal for Specialists in Pediatric Nursing, 14, 79–85.

Pediatric Care Preferences

School-age children express individual preferences and personalities. Nurses can help patients in this age group make appropriate choices; offering a choice the child does not have, such as whether to take medication, can result in a loss of trust. Older school-age children seek more autonomy and may want to assist with their own care. All children in this age range will be curious about their care. Nurses should answer questions honestly at an age-appropriate level. Keep in mind that the younger children in this age group are concrete thinkers, so avoid using inaccurate terms like "a little stick" for a needle.

CARE WHEN CHRONICALLY ILL

Nursing care for the chronically ill pediatric patient should consider normalization of lifestyle, limitations, and reaching milestones. Children with chronic illnesses should be praised for attaining milestones and may do so later than peers. Resources such as physical and occupational therapy can assist in these accomplishments.

Role of the Primary Caregiver

Most caregivers will have a very active role in the care of their chronically ill child and possess extensive knowledge of his or her conditions, treatments, and medications. As in other areas of nursing, family-centered care is paramount. Children with chronic conditions may be unable to communicate in the same manner or to the same extent as other children. Caregivers will notice changes in their child that nurses may not.

Caregiver fatigue is common among families with a child who has a chronic illness. These parents must devote significantly more time to caring for their child than those who care for healthy children, often at great time, effort, and expense. These factors can have a significant negative effect on the family and be very stressful for the caregiver. Marital stress and divorce may be more common with a family who has a child with special needs (Stannard, 2016). To combat the effects of caregiver fatigue, caregivers must have a good support network and ability to participate in activities that promote stress relief.

Home-Care Considerations

Chronically ill school-age children who are receiving care at home still need to have some control over their time and activities. School work should be kept up to date, and time for interaction with peers, either in person or over the phone or internet, should be allotted daily.

- Examples of home care needs include:
  - Tracheostomy
  - Vent-dependent child that requires continuous care
  - Immunosuppressed children without the immunity to be around other children
  - Nasogastric/Gastric tube feedings
  - Ostomy care
  - Oxygen
  - IV antibiotic administration
  - Total parenteral nutrition
  - Urinary catheterization
  - Dressing changes
  - Diabetic care
    - Blood sugar testing
    - Insulin administration
    - Care when sick
- School considerations include:
  - Most children can be cared for at school with the school nurses. Medications for asthma and diabetes are commonly administered by the school nurse.
  - Many children have a personal caregiver who cares for them in school.
  - School nurses provide straight catheterizations and tube feedings.
  - Individualized care plans are developed to address the child's individual needs at school.
  - Homeschooling can be considered for children who cannot attend a school outside the home.
  - Many states have online public education available that can be used for children who cannot leave the home for school.

CRITICAL COMPONENT

School for Hospitalized Children

Children in acute care who are well enough to study should do so to avoid falling behind. Some facilities have a dedicated teacher who works with the child's school to receive his or her current assignments.

CASE STUDY

Assessing Child Abuse

Patrick, a 9-year-old patient with cerebral palsy, is admitted to your unit. His parents state that he has been vomiting with feeds and having increased periods of inconsolability. Both parents work and they have three other children aged 15, 12, and 1 years. The parents state that life is very busy around the house and they do not have a lot of time to provide the extra attention that Patrick requires. The parents have been paying an unemployed friend of the family to watch Patrick during the day while they are at work and help with the other children. While performing your admission head-to-toe assessment, you note the patient is mentally delayed and is around a toddler level of development. The patient is nonverbal. Patrick has contractions in all four extremities and a gastric tube in place that is patent. He appears unkempt and dirty. While performing your skin assessment, you note that there are bruises in various states of healing on his forearms and legs. You also notice a few healing burns about 1 cm in diameter on his arms and torso.

1. What concerns do you have?
2. What actions should you perform?
3. What resources should you enlist to assist with this patient?
4. As a nurse, what is your responsibility in reporting any concerns you may have from this assessment?

REFERENCES

American Academy of Pediatrics (AAP). (n.d.). Bright future guidelines for middle childhood 5 to 10 years. Retrieved from http://brightfutures.aap.org/pdfs/Guidelines_PDF/17-Middle_Childhood.pdf

Camarota, S., & Zeigler, K. (2015). One in five U.S. residents speaks foreign language at home. Center for Immigration Studies, October, 2015. Retrieved from https://cis.org/sites/default/files/camarota-language-15.pdf

Centers for Disease Control and Prevention (CDC). (2016). *Child health.* Retrieved from https://www.cdc.gov/injury/images/lc-charts/leading_causes_of_death_age_group_2016_1056w814h.gif

Centers for Disease Control and Prevention (CDC). (2016). *Clinical growth charts.* Retrieved from https://www.cdc.gov/growthcharts/cdc_charts.htm

Children's Health Team. (2015). *When a child's fever becomes a serious problem.* Retrieved from https://health.clevelandclinic.org/2014/01/when-a-childs-fever-becomes-a-serious-problem-infographic/

Cincinnati Children's Hospital. (2014). *Pediatric heart murmur.* Retrieved from https://www.cincinnatichildrens.org/health/h/murmurs

Glasper, A. (2016). Keeping sick children in the hospital safe from harm. *British Journal of Nursing, 25*(20), 1144–1145.

Guid, F. D. (n.d.). *Pediatric fluid and electrolyte requirements.* Retrieved from https://www.pediatriccareonline.org/

Hazard Vallerand, A, Sanoski, C. A., & Hopfer Deglin, J. (2017). *Davis's drug guide for nurses* (15th ed.). Philadelphia: F.A. Davis.

Kaneshiro, N. K., Zieve, D., & Ogilvie, I. (2014). *School age children development.* Retrieved from https://medlineplus.gov/ency/article/002017.htm

LaBond, V., Barber, K., & Golden, I. (2014). Sports-related head injuries in students: Parents' knowledge, attitudes, and perceptions. *NASN School Nurse, 29*(4), 194–199.

Monaghan, A. (2005). Detecting and managing deterioration in children. *Paediatric Nursing, 17*, 32–35.

National Institutes of Health. (2008). *Pediatric blood pressure charts.* Retrieved from https://www.nhlbi.nih.gov/files/docs/guidelines/child_tbl.pdf

Patient.co.uk. (2010). *Dehydration in children.* Retrieved from http://www.patient.co.uk/doctor/Managing-Dehydration-in-Children-Paediatric-Fluid-Regimes.htm

Rosenberg, J. (2014). Sexting is positively linked to sexual experience among middle school students. *Perspectives on Sexual and Reproductive Health, 46*(4), 242.

Ryan, D. (2016). How to identify and manage seasonal allergic rhinitis. *Journal of Community Nursing, 30*(2), 54–60.

Saunders, M. J. (2016). A small trip through tooth lore, or where did the tooth fairy come from? *Generations, 40*(3), 16–18.

Scheinfeld, E., & Shim, M. (2017). Understanding eating behaviors through parental communication and the integrative model of behavioral prediction. *American Journal of Health Behavior, 41*(3), 228–239.

Stannard, M. (2016, December). 5 Ways to advocate for a child with special needs during a divorce. *EP Magazine.* Retrieved from https://www.eparent.com/money-uncategorized/5-ways-advocate-child-special-needs-divorce/

Thrane, S., Wanless, S., Cohen, S., & Danford, C. (2016). The assessment and non-pharmacologic treatment of procedural pain from infancy to school age through a developmental lens: A synthesis of evidence with recommendations. *Journal of Pediatric Nursing, 31*, K23–K32.

Tucker, K. M., Brewer, T. L., Baker, R. B., Demeritt, B., & Vossmeyer, M. T. (2009). Prospective evaluation of a pediatric inpatient early warning scoring system. *Journal for Specialists in Pediatric Nursing, 14,* 79–85.

10

Adolescents

Courtney Kwapinski, MSN, RN
Ludy Cabellero, MSN, APRN, FNP-C, EMT-P

LEARNING OUTCOMES

Upon completion of this chapter, the student will be able to:

1. Describe the growth and development that occur during adolescence.
2. Identify age-specific physical assessment approaches for adolescents.
3. Explain medication approaches for adolescent patients.
4. Explain variations in nursing procedures for adolescent patients.
5. Describe strategies for assessing health promotion practices among adolescents.
6. Describe emergency care considerations for adolescent patients.
7. Identify strategies to support hospitalized adolescents.
8. Integrate chronic-care concepts and adolescent-specific considerations.
9. Integrate home-care concepts and adolescent-specific considerations.
10. Recognize complementary and alternative therapies used by adolescents.
11. Recognize child abuse considerations relevant to adolescents.

GROWTH AND DEVELOPMENT

Adolescence is the transition period between childhood and adulthood (Fig. 10–1). It is considered to have three stages:

- Early adolescence (age 11 to 14 years)
- Middle adolescence (age 15 to 17 years)
- Late adolescence (age 18 to 21 years)

Although adolescence is often regarded as a period of extreme personal turmoil, most adolescents experience only mild difficulties during this time of life. Developmental warning signs during adolescence include school failure and/or absenteeism and aggressive behavior. The outcomes of this stage of maturity include the development of:

- Advanced cognitive abilities
- Autonomy
- Self-identity

Cognitive

According to Piaget's cognitive developmental theory (see also Chapter 6), adolescents are in the following stages of cognitive development:

- Age 10–11 years: concrete operations
- Age 12 years and older: formal operations

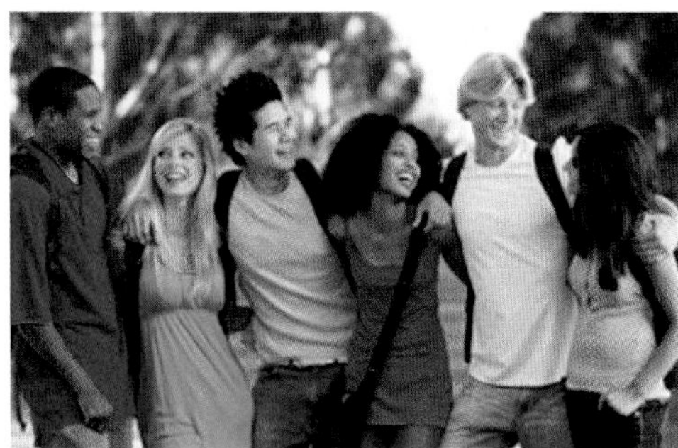

FIGURE 10–1 Adolescents.

The prefrontal cortex of the adolescent brain, the area associated with critical thinking and decision making, is still developing. During this stage, the adolescent:

- Develops analytic thinking
- Develops abstract thinking
- Shows concern for politics and social issues
- Becomes able to think long term and set goals
- Compares self with peers
- Begins to have some awareness of personal limitations
- Becomes able to predict outcomes and consequences

Psychological

Adolescents are engaged in the following stages based on Freud's theory of psychosexual development (see also Chapter 6):

- Age 10–12 years: latency stage
- Age 12–18 years: genital stage

Erikson's theory of psychosocial development (see also Chapter 6) indicates that adolescents embark on stages of identity uncertainty and identity crisis (Becht et al., 2016) with the goal of forming a stable identity and sense of self (Knight, 2017). These stages include:

- Age 10–12 years: industry versus inferiority
- Age 12–18 years: identity versus role confusion
- Age 19 years: intimacy versus isolation

Characteristics of adolescent psychology include the following:

- Self-conscious
- Compares own body with others
- Interested in sexuality and gender roles
  - Emergence of sexual feelings and experimentation
  - Has a need for privacy
  - "Tries on" different styles of dress, communication, and personae
- Develops personal values
- Wants to be an adult but still needs the support of the family/caregiver
- Self-image is dependent on what others think
- Has mood swings
- Feels as if "onstage" with others around and paying special attention
- Believes that he or she is special and unique
- Has a sense of invincibility
- Is impulsive
- Assumes that others have the same perspective
- Has unrealistic career goals
- Tests limits and rules
- Develops a sense of conscience
- Knows right from wrong
- Can compromise with others when desired

BIOPSYCHOSOCIAL ASSESSMENT

Adolescence is a period of rapid physical, cognitive, psychological, and social growth. It is the process of becoming an adult. The experience of adolescence is unique for each person. Therefore, growth and development should be assessed individually. Adolescents of the same chronological age may be at different developmental stages. Stressors, such as trauma, loss, illness, and environmental factors, can slow or reverse growth and development processes.

General Survey

Nurses assessing the adolescent patient should be aware of the following:

- Sense of physical awkwardness is normal.
- Determine developmental history, family composition, and school situation.
- Yearly health maintenance visits with a primary care provider are recommended for adolescents between ages 11 and 21 years (American Academy of Pediatrics [AAP], 2017).
- Annual assessments include:
  - Height
  - Weight
  - Body mass index
  - Blood pressure
  - Hearing
  - Vision
- Cholesterol screening should take place once during late adolescence (normal range for age 11 to 20 years is less than 170 mg/dL) (Van Leeuwen & Bladh, 2015).
- Tuberculosis screening is recommended for at-risk adolescents, including those who are from countries outside of the United States, who are HIV positive, and who are incarcerated or homeless (AAP, 2017).
- Immunizations should be based on the schedule from the Centers for Disease Control and Prevention (CDC) website. (See also Chapter 22.)

Physical

- Vital sign parameters reach adult values during adolescence.
  - Heart rate of 55 to 100 bpm
  - Respiratory rate of 15 to 20 breaths/minute
  - Systolic blood pressure less than 120 mm Hg (Dillon, 2016)

- Height/weight can be plotted on sex- and age-specific grids available at the CDC Web site.
  - Adolescents, particularly girls, may be sensitive to height/weight measurements.
- Daily fluid requirement is 1,500 mL plus 20 mL for every kilogram above 20 kg.
- Normal urine output is 0.5 to 1 mL/kg/hour.
- Use a numeric or visual analog scale for pain assessment (Fig. 10–2).
- General somatic complaints without verified diagnostic clinical data—such as chronic pain, dizziness, sweating, headaches, chest pain, shortness of breath, gastrointestinal issues/pain such as nausea/vomiting/diarrhea, and back/joint pain—may be an indication of school or home avoidance/problems, anxiety and stress, or depression (see Chapter 14).

When performing a physical assessment for this population, the nurse must:

- Respect privacy.
- Inform the adolescent of your actions and explain the rationales.
- Focus on the positive aspects of the individual.
- Address the adolescent's concerns directly.
- Be cautious about pointing out physical abnormalities.
- Examine the genitals last.
- Use the correct words for anatomy.

SAFE AND EFFECTIVE NURSING CARE: Clinical Pearl

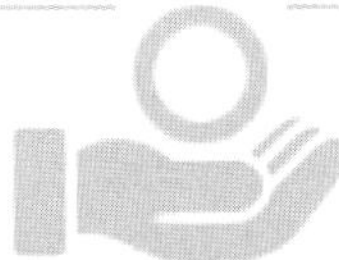

Privacy and Confidentiality

Assess the adolescent without the caregiver being present to ensure maximum privacy and confidentiality.

Skin

- The adolescent skin becomes thicker and tougher.
- Hormone changes during puberty cause an increase in sweat secretion and oily skin, especially on the face, back, axillae, breasts, and anus.
- Acne may develop (see Chapter 21).
- Daily washing is important.
- Assess sunscreen use.
- Document birthmarks.
- Check for bruises and burns that could indicate child abuse.
- Check for scratches and eraser burns that could indicate self-harm.

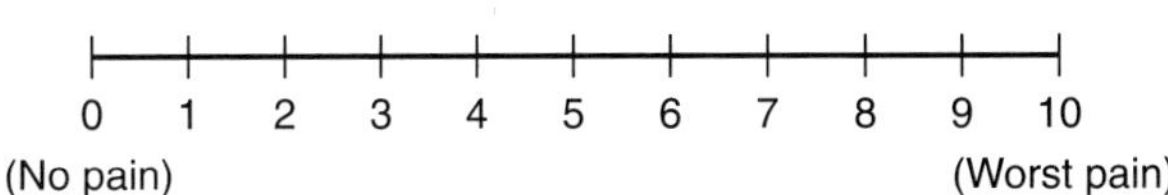

FIGURE 10–2 Numeric scale.

- Document tattoos and piercings.
- Assess and document birthmarks, moles, needle marks, or other skin aberrations.

SAFE AND EFFECTIVE NURSING CARE: Promoting Safety

Body Piercings

Around 25% to 35% of adolescents have a body piercing other than the ear lobes (Desai, 2016). Research shows as association with body piercings and participation in other high-risk behaviors, such as tobacco and drug use or sexual activity (Desai, 2016). Nurses need to educate adolescents and caregivers on the risks associated with body piercing, such as infection, allergic reaction to metal piercings, excessive bleeding, nerve damage, keloids, and dental complications (oral piercing).

Head

- Head reaches adult size during adolescence.
- Assess for migraines/stress headaches.
- Hair might be brittle and dry if subjected to frequent dyeing or heat styling.

Eyes

- Visual acuity testing should be done at ages 12 and 15 years (AAP, 2017).
- Assess for glasses and contact lens use, including the use of colored contact lenses for cosmetic purposes.
- Look for signs and symptoms of infection from excessive use of eye makeup.

Ears

- Assess for external ear trauma, piercings/gauges, and signs of infection.
- Assess for evidence of hearing loss, such as not responding to questions or tilting the head to a certain side.
- Assess for use of hearing aids.
- Hearing testing should be done once between ages 11 and 14, 15 and 17, and 18 and 21 years (AAP, 2017).

Mouth, Throat, and Teeth

- Inspect mouth for ulcers that might indicate inhalant or smokeless tobacco use.
- Assess for tongue/lip piercing.
- Dental checkup and tooth cleaning is recommended every 6 months (American Academy of Pediatric Dentistry, 2013).
  - Red gums may be an indication of periodontal disease.
  - Check for dental erosion, tooth loss, and cavities.
- Tooth erosion could indicate that patient has been inducing vomiting.

- The third molars (wisdom teeth) erupt between ages 17 and 21 years.
- Bruxism, which is teeth grinding, may be present because of stress.
- Malocclusion, which is crowded or misaligned teeth, is common between age 8 and 16 years and may require orthodontic correction.
- Check the cervical lymph nodes for enlargement and fixation.
- Palpate the thyroid to check for enlargement.

Nose

- Check for nose piercing.
- The nose may appear too large for the face during early adolescence.

Cardiovascular

- The heart grows in strength and size during adolescence.
- Assess for innocent murmurs (see Chapter 9).
- Screen for iron-deficiency anemia only if risk assessment is positive (AAP, 2017).

Respiratory

- The length and diameter of the lungs increase during adolescence.
- Assess for a history of asthma, which is the number one chronic illness in children.
- Lungs should sound clear.
- Check for signs/symptoms of chronic respiratory issues. Chronic cough that affects sleeping and shortness of breath are the most common. Signs such as barrel chest and clubbed fingers are rarely seen in children.

For more information on respiratory disorders, see Chapter 11.

Gastrointestinal

- Assess nutritional status.
- Assess constipation/diarrhea/vomiting.
- Assess for chronic abdominal pain, which could be an indication of stress/anxiety.

Renal

- Assess hydration status.
- Assess for enuresis.
- Assess signs/symptoms of urinary tract infection, particularly among sexually active adolescents.

Reproductive

Standard assessments include the following:

- Breast self-examination monthly
- Clinical breast examination yearly
- First gynecological examination should occur between ages 13 and 15 years for external examination only, pelvic examinations are only completed when problems arise such as pain or abnormal bleeding, and Pap tests are no longer conducted until the age of 21 years (American Congress of Obstetricians and Gynecologists, 2015)
- Testicular self-examination monthly
- Hernia checks for boys, especially for athletes
- Assess for signs and symptoms of sexually transmitted infections (STIs), such as genital discharge or rash (see Chapter 18)
- Assess for signs and symptoms of abuse, such as bruises and skin tears in the genital and anal areas (see Chapter 14)

Puberty is the process of becoming reproductively mature. The onset and timing of puberty are highly individual, with many factors contributing to these variations. The most influential of these factors is genetics. Although onset varies, the stages of puberty are predictable.

- Girls: Puberty begins between ages 8 and 13 years and is completed in about 4 years (Fig. 10–3).
- Boys: Puberty begins between ages 9 and 14 years and is completed in about 3.5 years.
- During puberty, the secretion of sex hormones increases.
  - Estrogen
  - Progesterone
  - Androgens
- Boys and girls will experience a growth spurt that lasts 24 to 36 months.
  - Girls will have a growth spurt at age 10 to 12 years.
  - Boys will have a growth spurt at age 12 to 14 years.
- Lean body mass will decrease in girls and increase in boys.
- Adipose body mass will increase in girls and decrease in boys.
- Both sexes will develop coarse hair in the pubic area and under the arms.
- Female breast development begins at age 8 to 10 years.
  - One breast may develop faster than the other.
  - Breast tenderness is common.

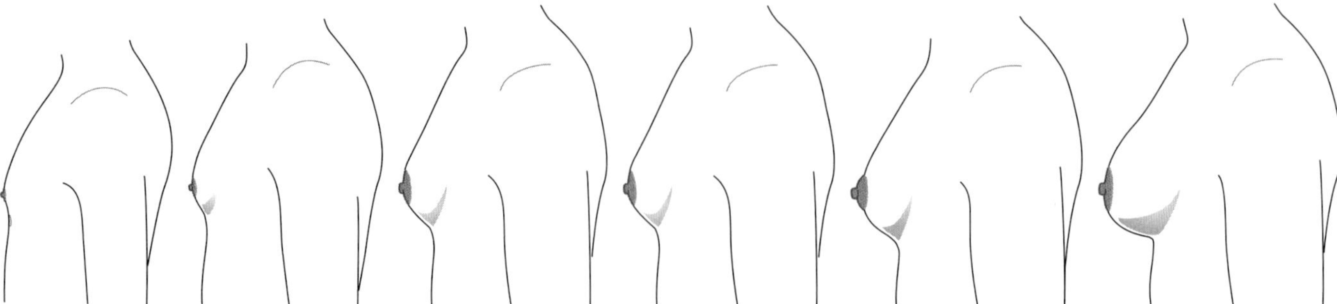

FIGURE 10–3 Breast development.

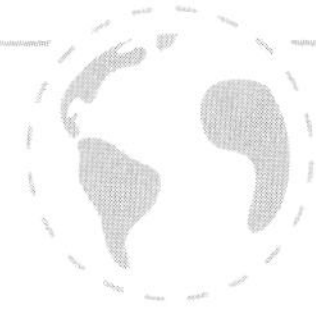

SAFE AND EFFECTIVE NURSING CARE: Cultural Competence

Breast Development

Breast development can start earlier in African American girls than in girls of other ethnicities (Weir, 2016), typically around age 7 or 8 years. Unfortunately, there is not any scientific research or reason to explain this trend.

- Gynecomastia refers to abnormal breast development in boys.
  - This is a self-limiting condition.
  - It may be related to the increase in sex hormones.
  - It is more common in overweight boys.
- Girls begin menstruation, the shedding of the uterine lining, approximately 2 years after the onset of breast development.
  - Leukorrhea, a thick white discharge from the vagina, is seen 3 to 6 months before menarche.
  - Periods may be irregular for up to 1 to 2 years after a girl first begins menstruating.
  - Periods will become more regular over time.
  - Girls can become pregnant after the first menstruation.
  - Assess for symptoms of premenstrual syndrome, such as irritability, anxiety, depression, crying, mood swings, feeling bloated, breast tenderness, and fatigue.
- Assess for precocious puberty (onset before age 8 years) or late-onset puberty (after age 14 years).
- Assess for the cessation of menstrual periods after an established pattern of regularity, which could indicate a drop in body fat because of excessive exercising, deliberate food restriction/eating disorder, or illness.
- Secondary sex characteristics develop (Tables 10–1 and 10–2).
- Male and female voices deepen.
  - Boys develop a more pronounced Adam's apple.
  - Pubic hair increases and becomes dark and coarse.
  - Hair also grows under arms and on legs.
  - The scrotum and the penis enlarge in boys.

See Chapter 18 for additional reproductive information.

Neurovascular

- The brain is in a period of rapid development. Judgment is sometimes impaired as the frontal lobe remains underdeveloped until the mid-20s.
- Check for equal strength left to right via hand grasps.
- Check deep tendon reflexes (Fig. 10–4).

Musculoskeletal

- Muscles grow during puberty.
- Feet, hands, arms, and legs grow before the torso, causing adolescents to become prone to clumsiness.
- The shoulders and chest increase in breadth.
- The female pelvis widens during puberty.
- Growth plates at the end of long bones (epiphyses) close by age 20 years.

TABLE 10–1 Tanner Staging (Male Secondary Sex Characteristics)

STAGE	PUBIC HAIR	PENIS	TESTES AND SCROTUM
1. Preadolescent	No pubic hair except for fine body hair similar to that on abdomen	Same size and proportions as in childhood	Same size and proportions as in childhood
2.	Sparse growth of long, slightly pigmented, downy hair, straight or only slightly curled, chiefly at the base of penis	Slight or no enlargement	Testes larger; scrotum larger, somewhat reddened and altered in texture

Continued

TABLE 10-1 Tanner Staging (Male Secondary Sex Characteristics)—cont'd

STAGE	PUBIC HAIR	PENIS	TESTES AND SCROTUM
3.	Darker, coarser, curlier hair spreading sparsely over pubic symphysis	Larger, especially in length	Further enlarged
4.	Coarse and curly hair, as in adult; area covered greater than in stage 3 but not as great as in adult	Further enlarged in length and breadth, with development of glands	Further enlarged; scrotal skin darkened
5.	Hair same as adult in quantity and quality, spreading to medial surfaces of thighs but not up over abdomen	Adult in size and shape	Adult in size and shape

Source: Dillon, P.M. (2016) Nursing Health Assessment: A Critical Thinking, Case Studies Approach (3rd ed., p. 296) Philadelphia, PA: F.A. Davis

- Fractures in the epiphyses before closure jeopardize the long-term growth of long bones.
- Check knuckles for Russell's sign: abrasions or cuts from sticking fingers down throat to induce vomiting.
- Begin scoliosis checks at age 10 to 12 years (Fig. 10–5).

Social

Adolescents are in the conventional level of Kohlberg's theory of moral development (see also Chapter 6). Based on this theory, the adolescent:

- Challenges the values, traditions, and beliefs of the family
- Develops own value system
- Wants independence from caregivers
- Conflicts with caregivers
- Resists adult supervision
- Depends on family in times of crisis
- Has best friend
- Idealizes friendships
- Socializes in cliques of the same sex
- Compares self with others
- Strives for peer acceptance
- Conforms to the norms of the peer group
- Is influenced by peer pressure
- Is prone to gang membership because of the desire for peer acceptance
- May be employed
- Is focused on activities outside of the home
- Explores gender roles
- Seeks out information about sex
- Experiences emergence of sexual feelings
- Explores sexual orientation
- Starts to develop intimate relationships
- Romances are usually brief but can be very intense

TABLE 10–2 Maturation States in Females (Secondary Sex Characteristics)

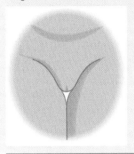

Stage 1 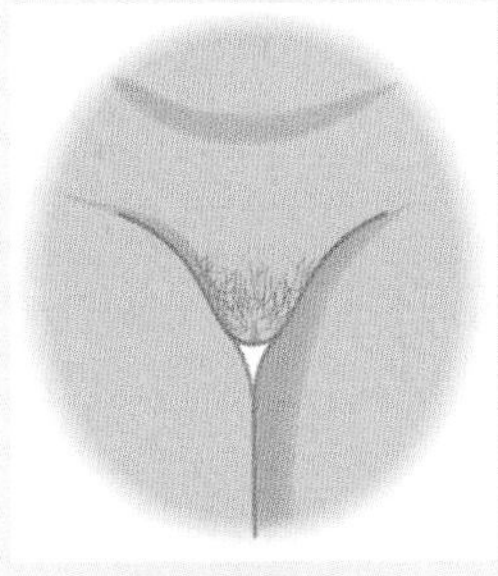	Preadolescent: no pubic hair except for fine body hair similar to hair on abdomen
Stage 2 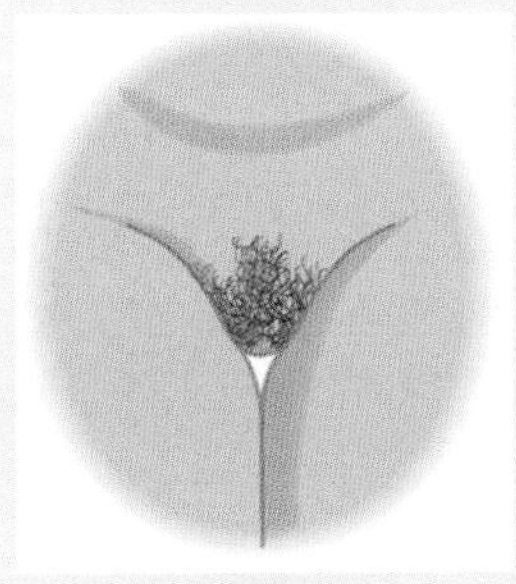	Sparse growth of long, slightly pigmented, downy hair, straight or only slight curled, mostly along labia
Stage 3 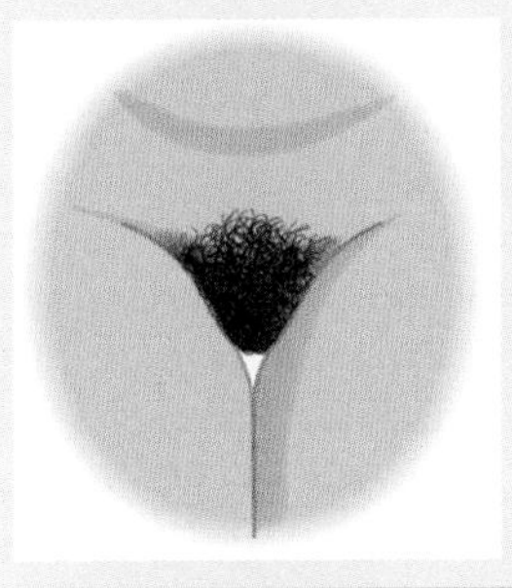	Hair becomes darker, coarser, and curlier and spreads sparsely over pubic symphysis
Stage 4	Pubic hair is coarse and curly as in adults; covers more area than in stage 3 but not as much as in adults
Stage 5 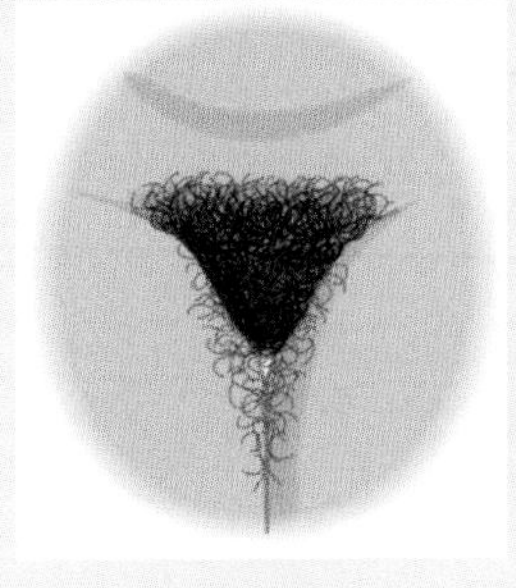	Quality and quantity are consistent with adult pubic hair distribution and spread over medial surfaces of thighs but not over abdomen

Source: Dillon, P.M. (2016) Nursing Health Assessment: A Critical Thinking, Case Studies Approach (3rd ed., p. 276) Philadelphia, PA: F.A. Davis

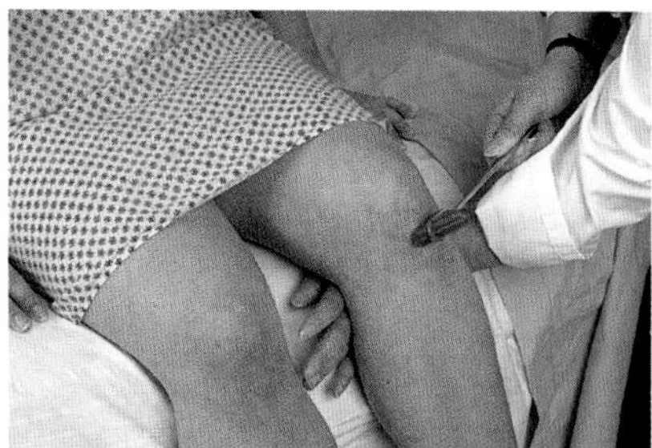

FIGURE 10–4 Deep tendon reflexes.

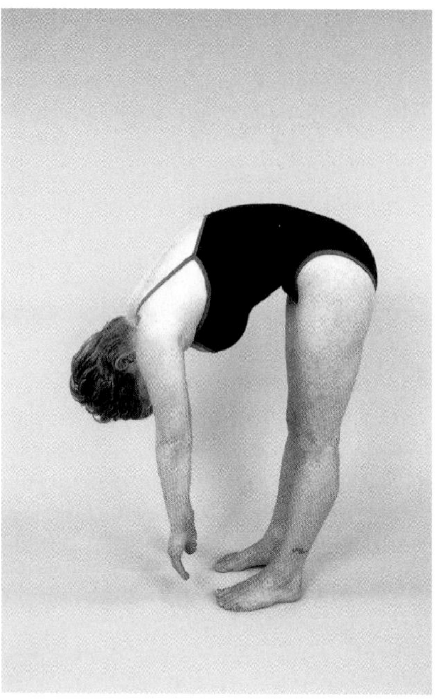

FIGURE 10–5 How to perform a scoliosis check.

- May have feelings of being in love
- Has romantic fantasies
- Lesbian, gay, bisexual, transgender, and questioning (LGBTQ) youth are more likely to engage in risky behaviors and to have psychiatric problems than heterosexual youth (Levine, 2013).

SAFE AND EFFECTIVE NURSING CARE: Promoting Safety

Internet Safety

Internet safety is important for adolescents. Social networking Web sites have increased adolescents' potential exposure to unsafe persons. Signs that an adolescent is engaging in risky online behavior include spending a large amount of time online, initiating or receiving calls from individuals unknown to the caregiver, receiving mail/gifts from an unknown person, and quickly changing the monitor screen when the caregiver approaches the computer. More information about internet safety for adolescents and caregivers is available at the Federal Bureau of Investigation Web site.

CRITICAL COMPONENT

Sexual Identity

Some adolescents identify themselves as gay, lesbian, or bisexual. When communicating with adolescents, do not assume heterosexuality. The nurse should not focus on the adolescent's orientation because some adolescents may have had a same-sex experience and not be gay, and teens who identify as gay may have never had a same-sex experience (Tulloch & Kaufman, 2013). Instead, the goal is to create an environment that makes the adolescent feel comfortable to discuss their concerns with you.

Spiritual

- Adolescents may start to question or disagree with the religious beliefs of the family.
- Adolescents understand the permanence of death and may ask questions about an afterlife (see Chapter 5).

SAFE AND EFFECTIVE NURSING CARE: Cultural Competence

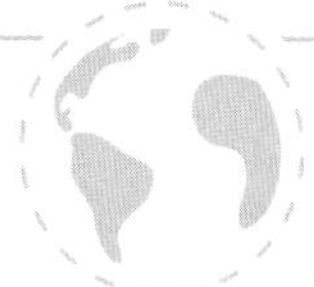

Religious Ceremonies

For some, adolescence is a time of religious ceremonies that require significant preparation time/activities on the part of the individual, such as the bar or bat mitzvah among Jewish youth and confirmation for Catholics or Lutherans.

APPROACHES TO MEDICATION ADMINISTRATION

More than 80% of medications are not approved for use in pediatric patients. Due to recent pediatric drug studies, more than 80 new drugs are now labeled for pediatric use (U.S. Food and Drug Administration [FDA], 2016). However, the legalities of testing medications in children through large randomized clinical drug trials mean that most medications are used off label in pediatrics.

- Medications obtain a pediatric label through surveying of prescribers.
- Some medications are labeled for use in adolescents older than 12, 13, or 17 years.

Eyedrops, Nasal Sprays, and Ear Drops

- Encourage self-administration.
- Pull the pinna back and up for otic medications.

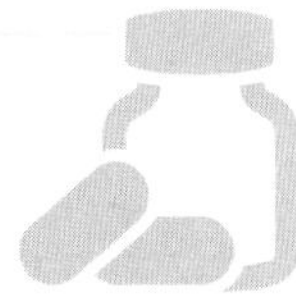

SAFE AND EFFECTIVE NURSING CARE: Understanding Medication

Changing Drug Labels

Several recent changes to medications that affect adolescents include:

- Loratadine (Claritin) syrup: 10 mg dose recommended for adolescents to treat allergies and hives.
- Fentanyl (Duragesic) transdermal patch: Used for pediatric patients who have been chronically taking opioids to manage chronic pain.
- Fluvoxamine maleate (Luvox) tablets: Suggest giving adult dose for adolescents to treat obsessive-compulsive disorder. Girls aged 8 to 11 years may require a lower-than-recommended dose.
- Midazolam hydrochloride syrup and injection: Has high risk for serious adverse events with patients who have congenital heart disease and pulmonary hypertension. Recommended to use as a sedative and begin dosing at a lower-than-recommended dose to prevent life-threatening respiratory problems.
- Gabapentin (Neurontin) capsules and oral solution: Recommended for pediatric patients aged 3 to 12 years to help treat partial seizures. Neuropsychiatric adverse events have been reported in this age range.
- Famotidine (Pepcid) tablets, injection, and oral suspension: Used for gastroesophageal reflux disease. No concern for pediatric patients older than 3 months.
- Sevoflurane (Ultane) volatile liquid for inhalation: Used for pediatric patients for general anesthesia. Reported rare side effect includes seizures.

(FDA, 2016)

Oral Medications

- Tablets and capsules may need to be crushed because some adolescents are not able to swallow these types of pills.
- An alternative preparation of the medication may be available.
  - Suspension
  - Oral disintegrating tablets
- Most adolescents master pill swallowing through repeated attempts.
- Learning to swallow pills can lead to a sense of control and ownership over one's own health care.

Medications via Gastrostomy or Nasogastric Tube

Encourage self-administration of medications via gastrostomy or nasogastric tube.

Rectal Medications

Encourage self-administration of rectal medications.

Subcutaneous Medications

Use eutectic mixture of lidocaine and prilocaine (EMLA) cream when available.

IV Medications

Use EMLA cream when available.

Pharmaceutical Warnings

Developmental changes affect medication absorption, metabolism, and elimination.

- Specifically, the metabolism of medications is affected by puberty.
- Most medications are metabolized faster by a patient in puberty.
- After puberty, medication metabolism decreases to adult levels.
- Nurses cannot rely on symbols or phrases to warn adolescents of medicine-related risks.
- Adolescents have the best understanding of medication warnings when directly informed verbally by health-care personnel.

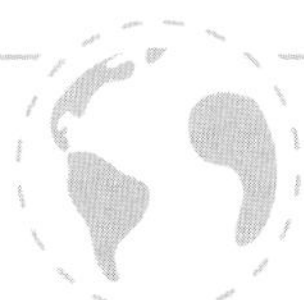

SAFE AND EFFECTIVE NURSING CARE: Cultural Competence

Biocultural Implications of Medication Metabolization

Different ethnic groups may have a significant pharmacogenetic variant; this field distinguishes people of Asian descent as metabolizing some medications slower than average and may need lower and less frequent doses of medication to achieve optimum therapeutic effect (Lee, Kwok, Wong, & Lui, 2017).

VARIATIONS IN NURSING PROCEDURES

When caring for an adolescent patient, the nurse must:

- Obtain guardian consent.
- Obtain assent from patient (see Chapter 2).
- Explain rationales to family and patient.
- Show equipment ahead of time.
- Be honest about the potential for discomfort/pain.
- Maintain patient confidentiality.
- If performing procedures in a setting where multiple adolescents are "lined up" to receive care, such as scoliosis/eye/hearing/

lice checks at a school, ensure privacy for each individual and do not announce results in front of others.

HEALTH PROMOTION AND EDUCATION

Health-care encounters provide an opportunity for the nurse to assess and educate adolescents about health promotion.

CRITICAL COMPONENT

HEADSS

Areas of health promotion for which adolescents should be assessed and educated can be summarized with the acronym HEADSS (Goldering & Cohen, 2004):

H—Home

E—Education

A—Activities

D—Drugs/Diet

S—Sexuality

S—Suicide/Safety

Home Assessment

- Assess the caregiver–adolescent relationship.
- Assess relationships with siblings.
- Assess support of the extended family.
- Assess where the adolescent lives.
- Ask about substance use in the home.
- Ask about violence in the home.
- Ask about the safety of the neighborhood.
- Ask about community supports and resources.

Education Assessment

- Assess school performance, a strong indicator of the adolescent's overall well-being.
- Ask about school absenteeism.
- Assess feelings regarding teachers and classmates.
- Assess for bullying.
  - Behaviors that are aggressive, repeated, and involve a power imbalance (Gower & Borowsky, 2013)
  - Acts of perpetration and victimization (Gower & Borowsky, 2013)
  - Physical actions and verbal threats (Wang & Iannotti, 2012)
  - Cyberbullying through electronic media (Carter & Wilson, 2015)
  - Results in academic, psychosocial, and health-related problems (Gower & Borowsky, 2013)
- Refer to a mental health professional if the adolescent admits to negative thoughts or feelings surrounding school.
- Assess vocational/career aspirations.

Activities Assessment

- Assess knowledge of injury prevention.
  - Leading causes of death in adolescence are motor vehicle accidents, homicide, and suicide.
  - Type and severity of injuries are closely related to developmental stage, psychological needs, and cognitive skills.
  - Practice safe driving, including wearing seat belt, minimizing the number of passengers, not driving when under the influence of alcohol or drugs, and not driving while using a cell phone for texting or talking.
  - Practice gun safety.
  - Practice water safety.
  - Sports injuries: Wear protective gear such as helmet and pads.
- Assess for the presence of violence.
  - Assess for emotional, physical, and sexual abuse.
  - Assess for intimate partner violence.
  - Assess for neighborhood safety.

Drugs/Diet Assessment

- Screen for tobacco use.
  - Tobacco use includes cigarettes and smokeless "chew."
  - The NAPNAP position paper discusses the prevention of tobacco use in the pediatric population. Specifically, it examines the serious health hazards associated with smoking, smokeless (electronic) cigarettes, and secondhand smoke. The paper encourages smoking cessation in all youth and explores NAPNAP endeavors to prevent tobacco use.

SAFE AND EFFECTIVE NURSING CARE: Clinical Pearl

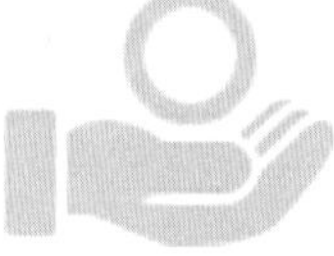

Substance Use

If an adolescent admits to cigarette smoking, ask about the use of other substances. Nicotine is usually the first drug used by an adolescent and is believed to be a gateway to stronger substances such as alcohol and marijuana (Nkansah-Amankra & Minelli, 2016). Cigarette smoking predicts more than a 30% chance of the willingness to try a flavored electronic cigarette (Clarke & Lusher, 2017). The use of electronic cigarettes is more appealing to adolescents because of the variety of flavors, such as fruits and chocolate (Clarke & Lusher, 2017). This causes equivalent danger as cigarettes because of the addictive properties of the nicotine and tobacco.

- Assess alcohol/substance use.
  - Illegal substances
  - Prescription drugs
  - Over-the-counter medications
  - Herbal/dietary supplements
  - Propellants/inhalants

Evidence-Based Practice: Prescription Drug Abuse Research

Partnership for Drug-Free Kids. (2017). Heroin, fentanyl & other opioids: From understanding to action. Retrieved from http://drugfree.org/article/heroin-other-opioids-from-understanding-to-action/

The increased trend in abusing prescription painkillers is causing an epidemic that is leading to heroin and fentanyl abuse. Between 2010 and 2015, there was a 328% increase in deaths from heroin (http://www.drugfree.org/wp-content/uploads/2011/04/PATS-Teens-Full-Report-FINAL.pdf)

Nearly 90% of addictions start in the adolescent years (Partnership for Drug-Free Kids, 2017b). In a 2012 report from the Partnership Attitude Tracking Study, 45% of adolescents agreed with the statement that "movies and TV shows make drugs seem like an okay thing to do."

Therefore, it is very important that we teach this age group the harmful effects of these drugs, assess for and address any risk factors, and encourage strong family relationships that include parenting skills with appropriate and consistent discipline (National Institute on Drug Abuse, 2014).

SAFE AND EFFECTIVE NURSING CARE: Clinical Pearl

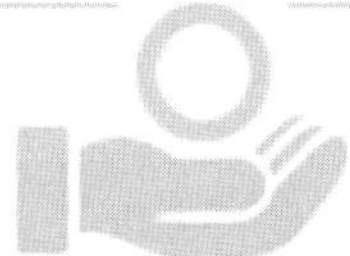

Screening for Substance Use

In a comparison of three alcohol/substance use screening tools, CRAFFT was found to be the most reliable and valid for use with adolescents (Center for Adolescent Substance Abuse Research, 2016):

1. Have you ridden in a **C**ar driven by someone (including yourself) who had been drinking or using drugs?
2. Do you use alcohol or drugs to **R**elax, feel better about yourself, or fit in?
3. Do you use alcohol or drugs when you're by yourself, **A**lone?
4. Do you **F**orget things you did while using alcohol or drugs?
5. Do your family or **F**riends tell you that you should cut down on your drinking or drug use?
6. Have you gotten into **T**rouble while using alcohol or drugs?

Nutrition Assessment

- Adolescents have an increased caloric need because of rapid growth.
  - For most adolescent boys, 2,800 calories per day is recommended (AAP, 2016).
  - For most adolescent girls, 2,200 calories per day is recommended (AAP, 2016).
- It is recommended that vitamins and minerals be obtained by eating a well-rounded diet rather than from dietary supplements (AAP, 2016).
- Encourage healthy dietary habits.
- Assess for vegan/vegetarian diets and provide education or refer to dietician.
- Eighty percent of obese adolescents will be obese as adults (American Academy of Child and Adolescent Psychiatry, 2016).
- Obese adolescents are prone to development of hypertension, type II diabetes, dyslipidemia, ankle sprains/fractures, gastroesophageal reflux, sleep apnea, and fatty liver disease.
- Encourage safe weight management.
  - Watch for signs of eating disorders such as vomiting, fasting, fad diets, and use/abuse of diet pills and laxatives (see Chapter 14).
  - Assess type and frequency of fast-food consumption.
  - Encourage a low-fat diet, reduced-calorie substitutions, keeping a food log, eating at the table instead of in front of the television, and focusing on the development of a positive self-image.
  - Of 12- to 21-year-olds, 50% get no regular physical activity (President's Council on Fitness, Sports & Nutrition, n.d.). It is recommended that adolescents participate in 60 minutes or more of physical activity every day (U.S. Department of Agriculture, 2016).
  - Encourage stretching before vigorous exercise to prevent muscle injury.

Sexuality Assessment

- Assess safe sex practices:
  - Abstinence
  - Birth-control options
  - Number of partners
  - STIs
  - Assess condom use
  - Assess engagement in oral/anal sex and educate about risks such as acquiring STIs via oral and anal routes; oral/anal sex is often considered "safe" by adolescents
  - STI testing as appropriate
  - HIV testing as appropriate
- For pregnant adolescents:
  - Assess pregnancy history.
  - Assess feelings about the pregnancy.
  - Encourage patient to tell caregiver about pregnancy.
  - Educate patient about options, such as adoption and terminating the pregnancy.
  - Provide agency information if considering adoption.
  - Educate patient about finding a skilled provider if adolescent is considering abortion.
  - Assist the adolescent in finding an appropriate health-care provider or agency.
  - Encourage early prenatal care.
  - Encourage the attendance of a parenting class if adolescent is planning to assume parenting role.
  - Seek out support resources for pregnant adolescents such as the Women, Infants, and Children program, Medicaid, teenage pregnancy classes, groups, and Web sites.

Suicide/Safety Assessment

- Screen for depression/suicidal ideation/self-harming behavior.
- Assess for stressors such as transitioning from high school to college.
- Teach stress management/relaxation techniques (see Chapter 14).

EMERGENCY CARE

Common adolescent emergency injuries/issues include:

- Traumatic injury due to risk-taking behaviors, a sense of immortality, and a lack of connection between cause and effect
- Injuries related to accidental or intentional alcohol/substance overdose
- Motor vehicle accidents (passenger or driver)
- Sports injuries
- Sexual assault
- Mental health emergencies

Primary Assessment

- Ability to recite ABCs
- Pain
- Skin for evidence of drug use
- Do not resuscitate (DNR) status (see Chapter 2)
- Identification of the patient's guardian
- Identification of the patient's legal status, such as mature/emancipated minor (see Chapter 2)
  - Under the Emergency Medical Treatment and Active Labor Act of 1986, adolescents who require emergency care may be treated regardless of whether caregiver consent has been obtained.
- Contextual information related to the injury/condition
- Family/social history
- Immunization status
- Transportation availability if being discharged from the emergency department

Additional Considerations

- Availability of age- and size-appropriate medical equipment, such as blood pressure cuffs and precalculated emergency drug cards
- Education of nurse in advanced cardiac life support (ACLS) and pediatric advanced life support (PALS) protocols
- Speak with the adolescent privately and ensure confidentiality of the conversation, unless doing so directly threatens the well-being of the adolescent or another person
- Allow adolescents and caregivers to decide together whether to have family members present during procedures such as diagnostic tests or resuscitation
- Some adolescents have the capability and desire to make some medical decisions, which should be encouraged and supported
- Be a patient advocate
- Provide education of the patient/family
- Sensitively convey "bad news" to caregivers, who may or may not be present (see Chapter 5)
- Facilitate conversations between the adolescent and caregiver(s) regarding sensitive subjects
- Consider the assistance of a chaplain and/or ethics committee if the adolescent and the caregiver(s) disagree about treatment
- Child protective services will need to be called if the caregiver refuses lifesaving treatment
- Prepare for the possibility of transferring the patient to a more appropriate facility
- Ask the adolescent for a secure e-mail address or phone number if providing sensitive follow-up information

ACUTE-CARE HOSPITALIZATION

When caring for an adolescent who has been hospitalized for an acute condition:

- Establish nurse–patient relationship (see Chapter 3).
- Define roles and establish boundaries.
  - The nurse is not the adolescent's friend, but a professional helper.
  - Be consistent and set expectations and consequences for language and behavior.
  - Be respectful.
  - Be nonjudgmental.
  - Develop trust.
  - Understand the unique concerns of adolescents.
  - Use humor appropriately.

Environment of Care

- The care environment should provide a sense of control and reduce feelings of anxiety. Orientation materials and visitation hours should be different for adolescents than for younger patients.
- Posters of rock stars, popular actors, and famous athletes are preferred over cartoon characters.
- Adolescents prefer a more homelike setting rather than a hospital-like setting.
- Physical space should promote privacy, socialization, and education.
- Comfortable furniture should be provided, with extra chairs for when family and peers visit.
- Visible medical equipment in patient rooms is disturbing to adolescents and can increase anxiety; leave only necessary equipment in the patient room or put away in a dresser or closet when not using.
- Allow for privacy by implementing curtains between bed spaces and locks on the bathroom door.
- Offer a variety of age-appropriate leisure (nonmedical) reading material for distraction, such as teen-oriented magazines.
- Offer age-appropriate video or computer games and television shows.
- Offer access to games that release physical energy, such as pool tables, air hockey tables, and table tennis.
- Provide a separate area for adolescent patients if possible. For example, perhaps the patient lounge could become teens only for an hour every evening.
- A separate teen activity area allows adolescents to feel a sense of control over a space within the hospital unit and decreases the risk for regression to more childlike activities and behaviors.
- Allow adolescents to leave the unit for brief periods if feasible based on condition.

- Offer private telephone access.
- If not on a diet or activity restriction, offer kitchen access so that the adolescent can obtain beverages and snacks independently.
- Adolescents prefer other adolescents as roommates. Avoid wide variation in ages during roommate selection.

Nursing Interventions

- Provide treatments in private.
- Cluster activities to leave periods of free time for relaxation, homework, or visiting with family and friends.
- Encourage the adolescent's active participation in meeting health-care needs.
- Provide appropriate patient education.
- Show the patient equipment ahead of time.
- Be honest about pain and side effects.
- Use pediatric assessment tools when needed.
- Use size-appropriate blood pressure cuffs.
- Use age-appropriate pain assessment tools, such as a numeric scale.
- Use an age-appropriate falls risk tool, such as the Humpty Dumpty Falls Risk Scale.

CARE WHEN CHRONICALLY ILL

Nurses caring for chronically ill adolescent patients should keep the following best practices in mind.

Physical Care

- Ensure that family and adolescent understand condition/treatments.
- Educate families and adolescents on how to minimize exacerbations of the condition.
- Assure medical control and involvement.
- Assess caregiver burden.
- Promote self-care and functional independence.
- Promote appropriate use of health-care services.
- Coordinate services between health-care providers, school, and home.
- Follow up with families and adolescents after transitioning to adult-focused care.
- Refer families and adolescents to appropriate internet resources.
- Advocate for chronically ill adolescents.

> **CRITICAL COMPONENT**
>
> **Sexual Activity Among Chronically Ill Adolescents**
>
> Do not assume that chronically ill adolescents are asexual. Assess for sexual activity and safe sex practices.

Psychosocial/Spiritual Care

- Use developmental rather than chronological age when caring for chronically ill adolescents, because there may be some developmental delays.
- Allow for adolescent completion of tasks as able.
- Promote self-esteem and confidence.
- Foster realistic expectations in parents regarding the adolescent's future personal, academic, and career potential.
- Ensure continued academic success with tutors or other resources.
- Support an adolescent's desire for a vocation/career.
- Assess for grief of losing friends with the same disease (see Chapter 5).
- Assess for fear of facing own premature death.
- Involve in individual and group therapy as appropriate.
- Refer caregivers and adolescents to support groups.
- Refer to chaplain as desired.

HOME-CARE CONSIDERATIONS

There is a growing shift to home care from medical inpatient facilities for adolescents with complex medical conditions. Advances in therapies have decreased the need for hospitalization. In addition, home care decreases financial costs, travel costs, and caregiver burden. Nurses should facilitate the transition from hospital to home. The National Association of Children's Hospitals and Related Institutions offers a tool for families to use when selecting a home-care agency. Note the following home-care considerations:

- Home care allows collaboration with the adolescent's medical team and increases family satisfaction.
- Adolescents may have increased opportunities for socializing with peers and participating in school/extracurricular activities because of having health-care needs met in the home.
- Caregivers may feel anxious about administering treatments/medications and responsibility for scheduling health-care appointments.

ADOLESCENTS AND INFORMATION HEALTH TECHNOLOGY

Many believe that encouraging adolescents to get involved in their own health and wellness can be challenging. According to a survey conducted by Northwestern University (2015), 84% of teens have obtained health information online. However, the internet is the fourth leading source of health information behind parents, school health class/teachers, and medical providers (Northwestern University, 2015).

Due to the growing number of adolescents using health information technology, research of the benefits of the use of electronic health record (EHR) among teens is also growing. The use of EHR among adolescents has shown to improve care for attention deficit-hyperactivity disorder and depression, increase vaccination rates, and reduce antibiotic misuse (Gray et al., 2014).

Capturing the attention of this age group by providing them with the means of communicating directly with their provider via a patient portal or other means of communication technology while maintaining adolescent confidentiality (meaning without inadvertently disclosing information protected by law to parents), may improve outcomes, decrease health disparities, and increase accessibility (Gray et al., 2014).

CRITICAL COMPONENT

Telemedicine

Telemedicine provides an opportunity to deliver home care and health advice via telephone/videoconferencing technologies (Blake, Roberts, & Stanulewicz, 2015).

COMPLEMENTARY AND ALTERNATIVE THERAPIES

Nearly 16% of adolescents use complementary and alternative medicine (CAM) therapies (National Center for Complementary and Integrative Health, 2016). Herbal and dietary supplements are not regulated by the FDA and have wide variation in content and dose across manufacturers. Although many of these substances are beneficial, interactions with prescription and over-the-counter medications can lead to toxic or subtherapeutic effects. Family and peer use of CAM influence adolescent use.

SAFE AND EFFECTIVE NURSING CARE: Clinical Pearl

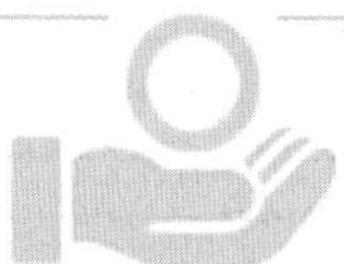

Use of Complementary and Alternative Medicine

Adolescents are often reluctant to discuss their use of CAM. Start out by asking the adolescent about family and peer use of CAM. If the adolescent reports use by a close family member or peer, then he or she is most likely also using CAM.

- Commonly used herbs/dietary supplements among adolescents:
  - Fish oil supplements, glucosamine, chondroitin, melatonin, creatine, probiotics, vitamins (Clarke, Black, Stussman, Barnes, & Nahin, 2015)
- Commonly used home remedies among adolescents:
  - Honey, lemon, green tea, chamomile tea
- Commonly used alternative therapies among adolescents:
  - Faith healing/prayer, massage therapy, deep-breathing exercises, acupuncture, yoga, tai chi, essential oils/aromatherapy (Clarke et al., 2015)

Evidence-Based Practice: Complementary and Alternative Medicine

Oren-Amit, A., Berkovitch, M., Bahat, H., Goldman, M., Kozer, E., Ziv-Baran, T., & Bbu-Kishk, I. (2017). Complementary and alternative medicine among hospitalized pediatric patients. *Complementary Therapies in Medicine,* 31, 49–52. doi:10.1016/j.ctim.2017.02.002

Oren-Amit et al. (2017) conducted a study on children at the Assaf Harofeh Medical Center in Israel. The study included children aged 18 years and younger and was performed between January and July of 2015. The objective was to identify whether the medical staff were aware of children's use of CAM. Children and parents were asked to participate in this study, and there was a 96% response rate.

This study found that more than half of the children used CAM and did not report the use to the provider caring for the child. This study reported that only 3% to 4% of patients were even asked about CAM.

According to Bailey, Gahche, Thomas, and Dwyer (2013), 31% of children use dietary supplements, with 41% reporting use for overall health improvement, whereas those 16 to 19 years of age reporting they use these supplements to gain more energy. Less than 1% reported supplement use for specific health conditions such as weight loss, sleep aid, or allergies (Bailey et al., 2013).

Nurses must ask what medications the patient is currently taking and ask whether CAM is being used. Both studies show that CAM is being used in the pediatric population. Many nurses and patients are not familiar with the potential drug interactions or adverse effects with the use of CAM. Questions about CAM use should be included with each contact with the provider.

CHILD ABUSE CONSIDERATIONS

Adolescents may be the victims of physical, emotional, or sexual abuse.

- Adolescents and young adults have higher rates of sexual assault than any other age group (Park, Scott, Adams, Brindis, & Irwin Jr., 2014).
- Adolescents are less likely to report abuse than adults because of worry that parents will not let them attend social events anymore, guilt, or lack of memory about the event because of substance use.
- Boys are less likely to report sexual abuse than girls.
- Adolescents with developmental disabilities are more likely to become victims of sexual abuse.
- Alcohol and substance use place an adolescent at greater risk for becoming a victim of sexual assault.

- There is an increasing ability to obtain date-rape drugs, such as flunitrazepam (Rohypnol), hydroxybutyrate (GHB), and ketamine. As a result, the use of these substances in adolescent acquaintance-rape assaults is on the rise (Office of Women's Health, U.S. Department of Health and Human Services, 2012).
- Adolescents are less likely to be physically injured in the attack than adults.
- Nonspecific physical complaints could be an indication of sexual abuse (see Chapter 14).
- Adolescents with a history of sexual abuse are more likely to engage in risky behaviors such as sexual promiscuity and alcohol/substance use.
- Sexually abused adolescents have increased rates of mental health problems, such as depression, anxiety, and post-traumatic stress disorder (see Chapter 14).
- See Chapter 14 for care of the sexual assault victim.

SAFE AND EFFECTIVE NURSING CARE: Promoting Safety

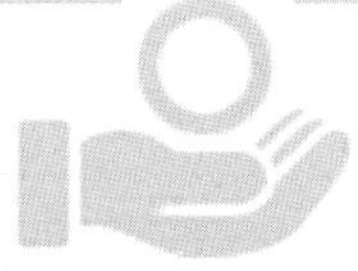

Sexual Assault Prevention

Nurses should reinforce safety strategies for avoiding sexual assault, such as going out with a group of friends, staying in public places, and avoiding alcohol/substance use.

Human Trafficking

Human trafficking is the act of recruiting, transporting, or harboring individuals through the use of force, coercion, abduction, or deception for the purpose of prostitution, forced labor, or slavery (Chaffee & English, 2015; Chung & English, 2015). Victims can include children, women, and men. Human trafficking can occur in any location, within country borders as well as across borders. According to the National Human Trafficking Resource Center (2015), California, Texas, Florida, Ohio, and New York were the top five states in the United States reporting human trafficking. Perpetrators often commit this crime in Ohio because of access to five major highways that transport to other states and Canada (Ohio Human Trafficking Task Force, 2012).

- About 33% of human trafficking victims are minors (Chaffee & English, 2015).
- Average age is 12 to 15 years (Chaffee & English, 2015).
- Poor health conditions among this population include STIs; urinary tract infections; multiple pregnancies, abortions, and/or miscarriages; and mental health issues with depression, anxiety, and suicide attempts (Chung & English, 2015).
- Health-care providers play an important role in identifying victims and assessing their needs (Chaffee & English, 2015).

CASE STUDY

Shannon is a 16-year-old girl who had her wisdom teeth removed by a local dentist 3 weeks ago. Today, she is at her primary care provider's office. Shannon was prescribed opioids to help manage the pain after surgery and is being seen today because she is still reporting pain. The assessment completed by the physician showed no evidence of infection in her mouth. The nurse tries to engage Shannon in conversation about school, peers, and hobbies, but she changes the subject and complains about stress and anxiety with working a summer job. Shannon says she needs something to calm her down and "take the edge off."

Shannon had recently had an abrupt change in friends. Her mother has voiced concern to Shannon and the provider. Shannon's responses are short, and she consistently tells her mother that she doesn't ever like any of her friends. The mother shares that she does not trust them and that Shannon is a completely different person when she is around them

1. Referring to the physical, social, and emotional domains of Shannon, describe any evident concerns.
2. Identify the signs of substance abuse in the case study.
3. What information obtained from the above questions should be shared with the primary care provider?

ADDITIONAL RESOURCES

Internet resources for CAM and adolescents include the National Institutes of Health National Center for CAM Web site (http://www.nccam.nih.gov) and the National Institutes of Health Office of Dietary Supplements Web site (http://ods.od.nih.gov).

REFERENCES

American Academy of Child and Adolescent Psychiatry. (2016). *Obesity in children and teens.* Retrieved from https://www.aacap.org/AACAP/Families_and_Youth/Facts_for_Families/FFF-Guide/Obesity-In-Children-And-Teens-079.aspx

American Academy of Pediatric Dentistry. (2013). Guideline on periodicity of examination, preventive dental services, anticipatory guidance/counseling, and oral treatment for infants, children, and adolescents. *Clinical Practice Guidelines.* Retrieved from http://www.aapd.org/media/policies_guidelines/g_periodicity.pdf

American Academy of Pediatrics (AAP). (2017). *Recommendations for preventive pediatric health care.* Retrieved from https://www.aap.org/en-us/Documents/periodicity_schedule.pdf

American Academy of Pediatrics (Committee on Nutrition). (2016). *Healthy children: A teenager's nutritional needs.* Retrieved from http://www.healthychildren.org/English/ages-stages/teen/nutrition/pages/A-Teenagers-Nutritional-Needs.aspx

American Congress of Obstetricians and Gynecologists. (2015). *Your first gynecological visit (especially for teens).* Retrieved from https://www.acog.org/Patients/FAQs/Your-First-Gynecologic-Visit-Especially-for-Teens

Bailey, R. L., Gahche, J. J., Thomas, P.R., & Dwyer, J. T. (2013). Why U.S. children use dietary supplements. *Pediatric Research, 74*(6), 737–741.

Becht, A. I., Nelemans, S. A., Branje, S. J., Vollebergh, W.A., Koot, H.M., Denissen, J.J., & Meeus, W. H. (2016). The quest for identity in adolescence: Heterogeneity in daily identity formation and psychosocial adjustment across 5 years. *Developmental Psychology, 52*(12), 2010–2021.

Blake, H., Roberts, A., & Stanulewicz, N. (2015). Telemedicine and mHealth interventions for children and young people with type one Diabetes (T1DM).

Journal of Endocrinology and Diabetes Research, 1(1), 1–18. Retrieved from https://www.researchgate.net/publication/299845523_Telemedicine_and_mHealth_Interventions_for_Children_and_Young_People_with_Type_One_Diabetes_T1DM

Carter, J. M., & Wilson, F. L. (2015). Cyberbullying: A 21st century health care phenomenon. *Pediatric Nursing, 41*(3), 115–125.

Center for Adolescent Substance Abuse Research. (2016). *The CRAFFT screening tool.* Retrieved from http://www.ceasar-boston.org/CRAFFT/

Chaffee, T., & English, A. (2015). Sex trafficking of adolescents and young adults in the United States: Healthcare provider's role. *Current Opinion in Obstetrics and Gynecology, 27*(5), 339–344.

Chung, R., & English, A. (2015). Commercial sexual exploitation and sex trafficking of adolescents. *Current Opinion in Pediatrics, 27*(4), 427–433.

Clarke, T. C., Black, L. I., Stussman, B. J., Barnes, P. M., & Nahin, R. L. (2015). Trends in the use of complementary health approaches among adults: United States, 2002-2012. *National Health Statistics Reports, 79,* 1–16.

Clarke, T. N., & Lusher, J. M. (2017). Willingness to try electronic cigarettes among UK adolescents. *Journal of Child & Adolescent Substance Abuse, 26*(3), 175–182.

Desai, N. (2016). Body piercing in adolescents and young adults. *UpToDate.* Retrieved from http://www.uptodate.com/contents/body-piercing-in-adolescents-and-young-adults

Dillon, P. M. (2007). *Nursing health assessment: A critical thinking, case studies approach* (2nd ed.). Philadelphia: F.A. Davis.

Dillon, P. M. (2016). *Nursing health assessment* (3rd ed.). Philadelphia: F.A. Davis.

Goldering, J. M., & Cohen, E. (2004). Getting into adolescent heads: An essential update. *Contemporary Pediatrics, 5,* 75–90. Retrieved from http://contemporarypediatrics.modernmedicine.com/contemporary-pediatrics/news/clinical/pediatrics/getting-adolescent-heads-essential-update

Gower, A. L., & Borowsky, I. W. (2013). Associations between frequency of bullying involvement and adjustment in adolescence. *Academic Pediatrics, 13*(3), 214–221.

Gray, S. H., Pasternak, R. H., Gooding, H. C., Woodward, K., Hawkins, K., Sawyer, S., & Anoshiravani, A. (2014). Recommendations for electronic health record use for delivery of adolescent health care. *Journal of Adolescent Health, 54*(4), 487–490.

Knight, Z. G. (2017). A proposed model of psychodynamic psychotherapy linked to Erik Erikson's eight stages of psychosocial development. *Clinical Psychology & Psychotherapy, 24*(5), 1047–1058.

Lee, Y. F., Kwok, R. C. C., Wong, I. C. K., & Lui, V. W. Y. (2017) The pharmacogenomic era in Asia: Potential roles and challenges for Asian pharmacists. *Journal of Pharmacogenomics and Pharmacoproteomics, 8,* 164. doi: 10.4172/2153-0645.1000164

Levine, D. A. (2013). Office-based care for lesbian, gay, bisexual, transgender, and questioning youth. *Pediatrics 132,* e297–e313. doi: 10.1542/peds.2013-1283

National Center for Complementary and Integrative Health. (2016). *The use of complementary and alternative medicine in the United States.* Retrieved from https://nccih.nih.gov/research/statistics/2007/camsurvey_fs1.htm

National Human Trafficking Resource Center. (2015). National Human Trafficking Resource Center (NHTRC) data breakdown: United States report. Retrieved from https://humantraffickinghotline.org/sites/default/files/NHTRC%202015%20United%20States%20Report%20-%20USA%20-%2001.01.15%20-%2012.31.15_OTIP_Edited_06-09-16.pdf

National Institute on Drug Abuse. (2014). *Advancing addiction science and practical solutions.* Retrieved from https://www.drugabuse.gov/publications/drugs-brains-behavior-science-addiction/advancing-addiction-science-practical-solutions

Nkansah-Amankra, S. & Minelli, M. (2016). "Gateway hypothesis" and early drug use: Additional findings from tracking a population-based sample of adolescents to adulthood. *Preventative Medicine Reports, 4,* 134-141. doi: 10.1016/j.pmedr.2016.05.003

Northwestern University. (2015). *Teens, health, and technology: A national survey.* Chicago: Center on Media and Human Development School of Communication Northwestern University. Retrieved from http://cmhd.northwestern.edu/wp-content/uploads/2015/05/1886_1_SOC_ConfReport_TeensHealthTech_051115.pdf

Office of Women's Health, U.S. Department of Health and Human Services. (2012). *Date rape drugs fact sheet.* Retrieved from https://www.womenshealth.gov/publications/our-publications/fact-sheet/date-rape-drugs.html

Ohio Human Trafficking Task Force. (2012). *Recommendations to Governor John R. Kasich.* Retrieved from http://slpaud.ohio.gov/pdfs/Task%20Force%20Report%20on%20Human%20Trafficking.pdf

Oren-Amit, A., Berkovitch, M., Bahat, H., Goldman, M., Kozer, E., Ziv-Baran, T., & Bbu-Kishk, I. (2017). Complementary and alternative medicine among hospitalized pediatric patients. *Complementary Therapies in Medicine, 31,* 49–52.

Park, M. J., Scott, J. T., Adams, S. H., Brindis, C. D., & Irwin Jr., C. E. (2014). Adolescent and young adult health in the United States in the past decade: Little improvement and young adults remain worse off than adolescents. *Journal of Adolescent Health, 55*(1), 3–16.

Partnership for Drug-Free Kids. (2017a). *Heroin, fentanyl & other opioids: From understanding to action.* Retrieved from http://drugfree.org/article/heroin-other-opioids-from-understanding-to-action/

Partnership for Drug-Free Kids. (2017b). *Risk factors and why teens use.* Retrieved from https://drugfree.org/article/risk-factors-why-teens-use/

President's Council on Fitness, Sports & Nutrition. (n.d.). *Facts and statistics.* Retrieved from https://www.fitness.gov/resource-center/facts-and-statistics/

Tulloch, T., & Kaufman, M. (2013). Adolescent sexuality. *Pediatrics in Review, 34*(1). Retrieved from http://pedsinreview.aappublications.org/content/34/1/29

U.S. Department of Agriculture. (2016). *How much physical activity is needed?* Retrieved from https://www.choosemyplate.gov/physical-activity-amount

U.S. Food and Drug Administration (FDA). (2016). *Drug research and children.* Retrieved from https://www.fda.gov/drugs/resourcesforyou/consumers/ucm143565.htm

Van Leeuwen, A. M., & Bladh, M. L. (2015). *Davis's Comprehensive handbook of laboratory & diagnostic tests with nursing implications* (6th ed.). Philadelphia: F.A. Davis Company.

Wang, J., & Iannotti, R. J. (2012). Bullying among U.S. adolescents. *The Prevention Researcher, 19*(3), 3–6.

Weir, K. (2016). The risks of earlier puberty. *Monitor on Psychology, 47*(3), 40. Retrieved from http://www.apa.org/monitor/2016/03/puberty.aspx

UNIT 4

Common Illnesses or Disorders in Childhood and Home Care

11

Respiratory Disorders

Jill Morinec, RN, BSN, CCRN

LEARNING OUTCOMES

Upon completion of this chapter, the student will be able to:

1. Identify normal assessment of anatomy and physiology of the pediatric respiratory system.
2. Identify differences in the anatomy and physiology of the pediatric and adult patient.
3. Identify the clinical presentation and nursing care of the pediatric patient with respiratory disorders.
4. Describe common tests used in diagnosing and treating pediatric respiratory disorders.
5. Identify areas of education for caregiver of a child with a respiratory disorder.

ANATOMY AND PHYSIOLOGY

The upper airway is a passageway that includes the nasopharynx and oropharynx (Fig. 11–1), and is connected to the ears by the eustachian tubes. The nose, pharynx, and larynx are separated from the lower airway by the trachea. The larynx is covered by the epiglottis. Cilia and mucus in the nostrils warm, clean, and humidify the air. The lower airway includes the trachea, bronchi, bronchioles, and alveoli.

The left lung has two lobes and the right has three lobes. From the top, the two bronchi split into branches called *bronchioles*. The lobular bronchiole splits into terminal bronchioles. The terminal bronchioles end in sacs called *alveoli*, surrounded by capillaries where oxygen and carbon dioxide diffuse. Surfactant is a phospholipid in the alveoli that keep alveoli pliable, preventing them from collapsing completely at the end of each expiration.

The lungs are protected by the ribcage, which is surrounded by muscles in the thoracic cavity and separated by the diaphragm muscle from the abdominal cavity. The diaphragm contracts, creating a negative pressure that pulls air into the lungs. The lungs and chest wall actively expand on inspiration but passively return to resting state with expiration. There are two pleural membranes, normally separated by only enough fluid to lubricate for painless movement:

- Parietal pleura lines thoracic cavity, and adheres to ribs and superior aspect of diaphragm.
- Visceral pleura surrounds each lung; when lungs are inflated, it lies directly against parietal pleura.
- Normal breathing is involuntary; the central nervous system controls rate and volume of respiration.
- Signals sent by receptors in the lungs and chemoreceptors (pH, $Paco_2$, Pao_2) in the arterial blood alert the brain.
- Adjustments are made in respirations and heart rate and output to maintain adequate gas exchange.
- Adequate gas exchange requires equal ventilation and blood distribution.
- Oxygen diffuses across the alveolocapillary membrane and dissolves in plasma (pressure measured as Pao_2).
- Oxygen is then bound and transported by hemoglobin to the cells for metabolism.
- Conversely, carbon dioxide produced by cellular metabolism dissolves in the plasma ($Paco_2$) or as bicarbonate.
- Carbon dioxide travels back to the lungs and across the alveolocapillary membrane.

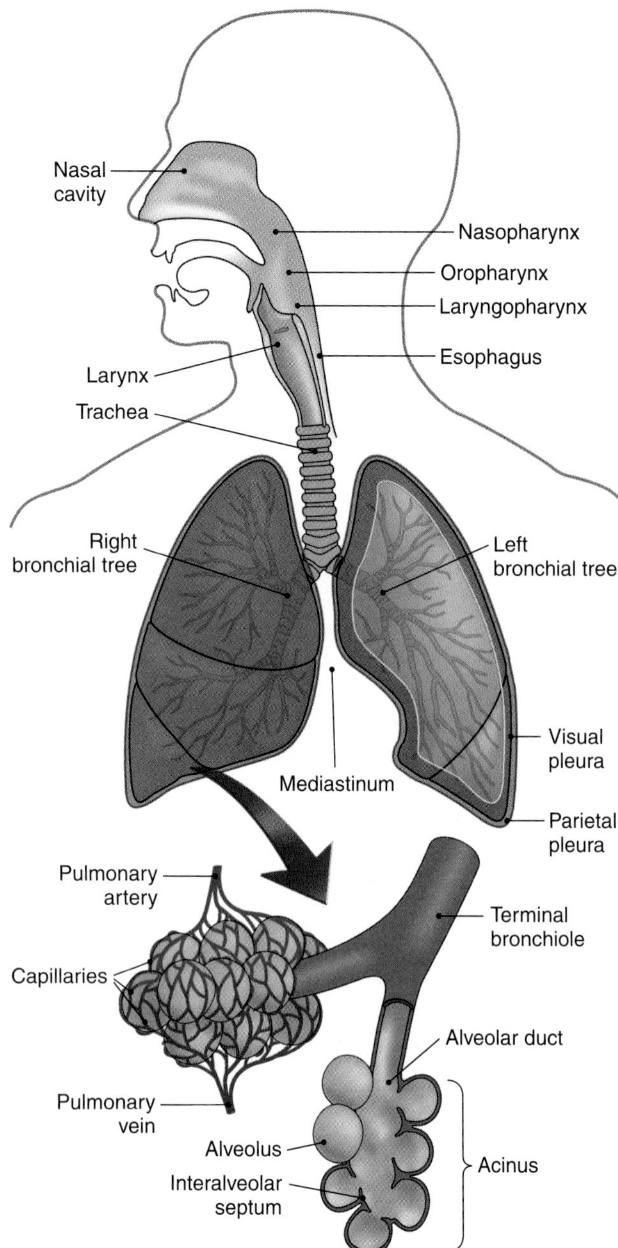

FIGURE 11–1 Structures of the respiratory tract.

DEVELOPMENTAL DIFFERENCES IN THE RESPIRATORY SYSTEM

The nurse caring for a pediatric patient with respiratory issues should be aware of the following key differences between child and adult respiratory systems:

- A child's upper airway is shorter and narrower than an adult's.
  - Newborn airways are approximately 4 mm in diameter compared with 20 mm for the average adult's airway.
  - Inflammation 1 mm in circumference would decrease a child's airway diameter 50%, but only 20% for an adult.
- Newborns are obligatory nose breathers until 4 weeks of age.
- Only ethmoid and maxillary sinuses are present at birth, not aerated until 4 months; sphenoid and frontal sinuses develop later in childhood and continue to mature to adolescence.
- The child's larynx is more flexible than an adult's and easily stimulated to spasm.
- The child's intercostal muscles are not fully developed; pronounced abdominal wall movement with respiration is normal until 6 years old.
- Periods of apnea (the absence of respiration) that last up to 15 seconds are normal in the newborn period.
- A child's metabolic rate is higher than that of an adult's, creating a higher oxygen demand. Newborns use 4 to 8 L of oxygen a minute, and adults use 3 to 4 L per minute. A child's respiratory rate is thus faster, with an irregular pattern.
- Newborns do not have the defense of bronchospasms or constriction to trap foreign irritants because smooth muscles are not fully developed until about 5 months of age.
- At birth, an infant has about 25 million alveoli; by age 3 years, this increases to 200 million. As the lungs become more complex, alveoli reach 300 million by adulthood.
- In children, the bifurcation of the right and left bronchi occurs higher in the airway and the right bronchus enters the lung at a steeper angle than an adult's bronchi.
- A child's cartilage surrounding the trachea is more flexible and can compress the airway if the head is not positioned properly.
- Eustachian tubes are shorter and more horizontal in children than in adults.
- A child's lung volume is proportional to chest size; lung growth continues through adolescence.
- A child's tonsils and lymphoid tissues are larger than an adult's.
- Anterior-to-posterior diameter of chest is equal at birth but decreases with age.

RESPIRATORY DISORDERS

Respiratory disorders can be classified as upper airway, lower airway, or other. When assessing a pediatric patient with a respiratory disorder, consider the factors discussed in the following subsections.

General History

- Gestational age
- Medical history including onset of current symptoms, pattern of recurrent sore throats, eczema, respiratory problems at birth
- Detailed family history, including chronic respiratory conditions such as asthma
- Exposure to environmental irritants, pets, and smokers in household
- Feeding and sleeping patterns
- Growth and reaching milestones
- International travel or adoption

Physical Assessment

- Chest diameter, anterior-to-posterior diameter
- Work of breathing, respiratory effort
- Flaring, tachypnea, retractions, paradoxical breathing (Fig. 11–2)

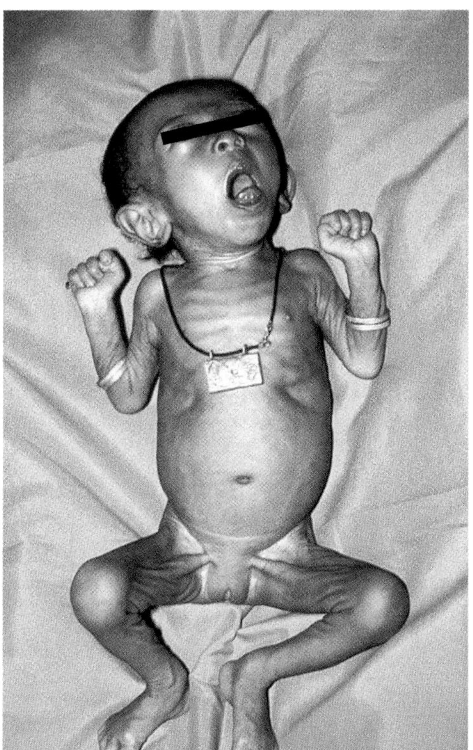

FIGURE 11-2 Flaring of nostrils during respiratory effort of breathing.

- Optimal chest expansion when positioned supine with head of bed elevated at a 45-degree angle
- Position of comfort
  - Tripod, jaw thrust, or insistence on sitting upright are signs of air deficiency
- Symmetrical chest rise
  - Asymmetrical may indicate tension pneumothorax
- Color of skin, mucous membranes, nail beds, lips, tip of nose
  - Acrocyanosis normal up to 48 hours after birth
- Simultaneous abdomen and chest rise
- Cough quality, productivity
- Nasal flaring—widening of nares with inspiration
  - Sign of air hunger
- Clubbing of fingertips: loss of 160-degree angle of nail bed
  - May be a sign of chronic hypoxia such as seen in cystic fibrosis (CF) and similar chronic respiratory disorders
- Hydration status
  - Mouth breathing, tachypnea, fever, and anorexia all contribute to dehydration

SAFE AND EFFECTIVE NURSING CARE: Clinical Pearl

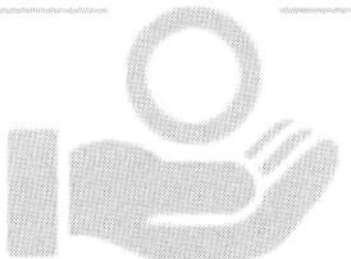

Barrel Chest

A child's anterior-to-posterior diameter is equal until about the age of 2 years. In older children, this characteristic may signify a chronic obstructive lung condition known as "barrel chest," typically observed in CF or asthma.

SAFE AND EFFECTIVE NURSING CARE: Cultural Competence

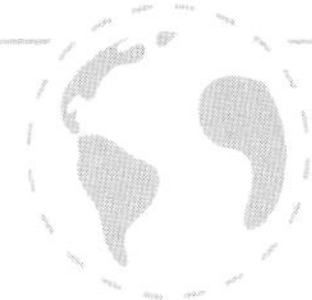

Assessing Differences in Skin Color

In dark-skinned infants and children, determine the normal skin color and assess for differences. Erythema will appear violet or dusky red, cyanosis will appear black, and jaundice will appear darker than normal skin. In Asian and dark-skinned infants, jaundice is best assessed as a yellow imprint when pressure is applied to infant's forehead or tip of nose and then removed. The infant is jaundiced if skin appears yellow before blood returns to area.

Auscultation

- Anterior and posterior chest, and bilateral mid-axillary for aeration
- Respiratory rate varies based on child's age
- Heart rate depends on age; increases with fever, dehydration
- Adventitious breath sounds
- Crackles (rales): fine cracking noises heard on inspiration
  - Air moves through fluid-filled alveoli as in pneumonia
  - May not change after coughing
  - Simulate sound by rolling hair between your fingers
- Snoring (rhonchi): low-pitched sounds heard throughout respiration
  - Air passes through thick secretions
  - May clear after coughing
- Stridor: high-pitched sound heard on inspiration in the upper airway in conditions such as croup
- Wheezes: high-pitched musical sounds heard throughout respiration
  - Air passing through constricted bronchioles or narrowed smaller airways as in asthma

SAFE AND EFFECTIVE NURSING CARE: Clinical Pearl

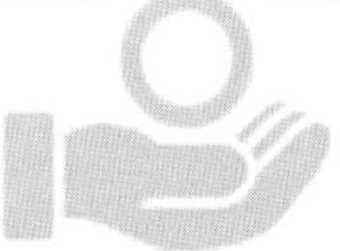

The Skill of Suctioning

Suctioning is essential to maintain the airway patency of infants and children.

Nurses must know how and when to suction a child or infant. Most pediatric respiratory conditions produce secretions that the child may be too young or ill to cough up or remove by nose-blowing. The suctioning procedure may frighten both parents and child because you must secure the child tightly and it temporarily takes his or her breath away, startling them and often causing tears. Providing emotional support and verbal explanation of the procedure to both child and parent is crucial for establishing a good rapport.

Percussion

- Lung should resonate when percussed
  - Flat or dull sounds in consolidated area
  - Tympany with pneumothorax
  - Hyperresonance may be heard with the presence of asthma.

Palpation

- Lymph nodes in head and neck may be enlarged because of infection.
- Assess sinuses in older children for tenderness.
- Tactile fremitus, the vibrations made during speech or making sounds, will increase with pleural effusion and pneumonia.
  - Absent in atelectasis or pneumothorax or barrel chest
- Pulses should be equal when comparing peripheral pulses with central pulses.
  - Severe respiratory distress and decreased perfusion result in weaker peripheral pulses.
- Respiratory distress can progress to respiratory failure; symptoms of each are listed in Box 11–1.
- Signs of respiratory failure: Muscles of ventilation are fatigued, and greater metabolic and oxygen requirements.
  - Body can no longer compensate and maintain adequate oxygen and carbon dioxide exchange
  - Can occur if respiratory center is depressed, such as during an overdose of narcotics
  - Emergent interventions imminent

Diagnostic Tests

The following subsections describe diagnostic tests are used when a respiratory issue is suspected.

Arterial Blood Gas

- Evaluates ventilation by measuring pH and partial pressure of oxygen (PaO_2) and carbon dioxide ($PaCO_2$).
- PaO_2 is the amount of oxygen in lungs available to diffuse into blood.
  - Decreased because of hypoventilation, ventilation-perfusion mismatch, or shunting
- $PaCO_2$ is the amount of carbon dioxide in blood that can diffuse out of the blood.
  - Increased because of hypoventilation, marked ventilation-perfusion mismatch
  - Decreased because of increased alveolar ventilation
- pH reveals acid–base balance, normally about 7.4 on a 1 to 14 scale.
  - Acidotic below 7.4, alkalotic above 7.4
  - Changes because of respiratory or metabolic dysfunction
  - Identify respiratory or metabolic compensation mechanisms
- Obtaining an arterial blood gas (ABG) is invasive and anxiety provoking for child and parents. This procedure is avoided if possible unless the child is critically ill or injured.

Venous/Capillary Blood Gas

- Less invasive and less painful than arterial sample
- Good correlation with pH and PCO_2 in arterial blood

Chest X-Ray

- Judicious use, radiation exposure
- Identify thoracic structures
- Take different views: anteroposterior (AP), lateral, or oblique
- Lead protection over gonads

BOX 11–1 | Signs of Respiratory Distress

SIGNS OF RESPIRATORY DISTRESS

- Tachypnea
- Dyspnea
- Hypernea
- Nasal flaring
- Use of accessory muscles
- Retractions: intercostal—mild distress, suprasternal, subcostal, and supraclavicular seen in moderate distress
- Sitting with head of bed elevated
- Coughing: intermittent
- Adventitious breath sounds
- Tachycardia
- Dusky nail beds
- Hypercapnia
- Hypoxia: ability to speak full sentences
- Crying: strong

SIGNS OF RESPIRATORY FAILURE

- Mental status change, extreme irritability
- Circumoral cyanosis or mottled skin color
- Lethargy, change in mental status
- Grunting
- Head bobbing
- Coughing continuously
- Retractions: moderate along with the use of accessory muscles
- "Quiet" breathing
- Sitting forward with arms, knees for support, tripod
- Normal or shallow respirations
- Seesaw respirations
- Hypopnea
- Hypoxemia, lower than normal oxygen in the blood, that is persistent with supplemental oxygen administered
- Weak or absent cry
- Tachycardia: further elevated

Computed Tomography

- More sensitive, more radiation exposure than chest x-ray (CXR)
- Three-dimensional picture
- Contrast medium may be used
  - NPO for 4 to 6 hours
  - Child may need sedation

Ultrasound

- Uses sound waves, no radiation exposure
- Identifies structures, organs, and spaces in between
- Portable, done at bedside

Magnetic Resonance Imaging

- Identifies structures and any obstruction of blood flow in blood vessels and tissue
- A powerful magnet is used; ensure that there is no metal in or on the body before obtaining magnetic resonance imaging (MRI)
- Child may need sedation to stay still during the imaging

Bronchoscopy

- Allows direct visualization of trachea, upper parts of bronchi.
- Collect secretion samples, brush or lesion biopsy, or remove foreign objects.
- Child should have an empty stomach before bronchoscopy.
- The child should have nothing by mouth at least 4 to 6 hours before this test to prevent aspiration.

Pulmonary Function Test

- Measures lung volumes, flow rates, and compliance by measuring expirations
- Children 5 years old or older
- Pulmonary function test uses expiratory flow rates calculated
- Assesses respiratory impairment, effectiveness of therapy

Sweat Test

- Pilocarpine is used to stimulate sweat glands to measure the amount of sodium and chloride produced to identify CF.

Nasal/Throat Swab

- Identifies pathogens
- Invasive, uncomfortable

Sputum Culture

- Identifies pathogens
- Collect in early morning
- Nasal or gastric washings for children too young to produce sputum

Pulse Oximetry

- Measures amount of oxygen in blood; supplemental oxygen may be needed (Table 11–1).
- Finger clip or tape with infrared light

TABLE 11–1 Oxygen Flow Rates

OXYGEN DELIVERY SYSTEM	O_2 CONCENTRATION DELIVERED (%)	FLOW RATE (L/MIN)
Nasal cannula	22–40	0.25–4
Simple mask	35–50	6–10
Partial rebreather	60–95	>6
Nonrebreather	Approaches 100	10–15
Venturi mask	24–50	Variable
Oxygen hoods	Approaches 100	>10
Oxygen tents	Up to 50	>10

Oxygen flow rate (L/min) of supplemental oxygen does not *equal the concentration of oxygen delivered to the child. Oxygen concentration delivered is dependent on the system that is used.*

UPPER AIRWAY INFECTIOUS DISORDERS

The infectious disorders discussed in this section are confined to the upper portion of the respiratory system, consisting of the sinuses, structures of the ears, and throat.

Otitis Media

- Often caused by bacteria
  - *Streptococcus pneumoniae*, *Haemophilus influenza*, and *Moraxella catarrhalis*
  - Most common reason children receive antibiotics, accounts for 15 million prescriptions per year (Boatright, Holcomb, & Replogle, 2015)
- Can be caused by viruses
  - Most commonly, respiratory syncytial virus (RSV), rhinoviruses, influenza viruses, and adenoviruses
  - One of most common childhood illnesses
- Short, immature upper respiratory tract eustachian tubes connected to nasopharynx (Fig. 11–3)
  - Bottle feeding infant supine can cause reflux of formula from nasopharynx into eustachian tube

Assessment

- Earache, pulling at the ears
- Bulging, red, or opaque eardrum
- Yellow or green or purulent foul-smelling drainage
- May be accompanied by other nonspecific signs of infection
- Fever
- Anorexia
- Crying
- Sleep disturbances
- Vomiting

- Diarrhea
- Lymph glands enlarged

Otitis Media With Effusion

Otitis media with effusion (OME) is a common clinical condition diagnosed at least once in approximately 80% of preschool children, 30% to 40% of whom have recurrent episodes (Principi, Machisio, & Esposito, 2016).

- Collection of fluid in middle ear with or without symptoms of acute infection
- Decreased mobility of eardrum
- Eardrum appears retracted, either yellow or gray
- Tinnitus
- Feeling of fullness
- Hearing loss
- Mild inability to maintain balance

Otitis Externa

Often called swimmer's ear, otitis externa (OE) is an inflammation of the external ear canal that may involve the pinna or tympanic membrane with pruritus and/or erythema (Fig. 11–4).

- Tenderness is the hallmark sign, tragus and/or pinna
- Purulent drainage
- Almost exclusively bacterial infection
- Rapid onset of symptoms

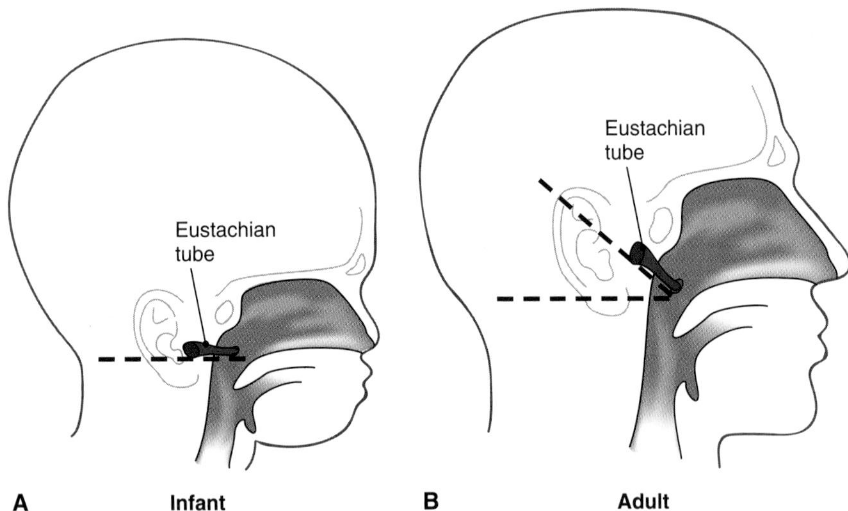

FIGURE 11–3 Differences in (**A**) infant and (**B**) adult ear canal angle.

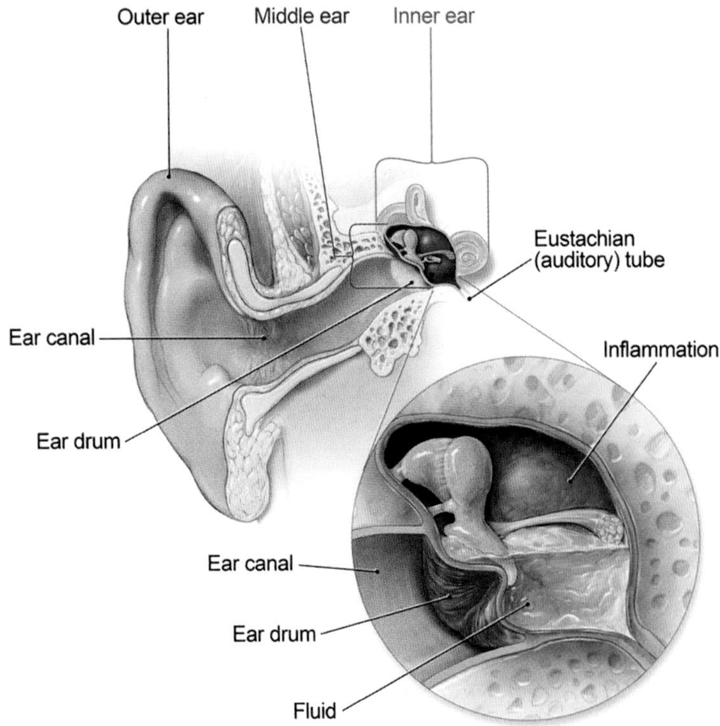

FIGURE 11–4 Ear infections.

Diagnosis of Otitis Media, Otitis Media With Effusion, and Otitis Externa

- Based on history, signs and symptoms
- Otoscopy (visualization) or pneumatic otoscopy
- Tympanometry (measured movement of eardrum)

Nursing Interventions

- Management based on discernment of otitis media (OM) versus OME
- Antibiotics as prescribed conservatively
- Topical antibiotics, an acidifying agent and steroid preparation for OE
- Supportive care such as analgesics, antipyretics, and adequate hydration
  - According to Casey and Pichichero (2015), the updated American Academy of Pediatrics guidelines on OM and OME recommend that if a child older than 23 months is not in severe discomfort and fever is lower than 102.2°F, observation for 48 to 72 hours is an important option (Casey & Pichichero, 2015). This option is cost-effective and decreases over use of antibiotics that leads to resistant strains of pathogens (Sun, McCarthy, & Liberman, 2017).

Caregiver Education

- Feed infant in upright position.
- Avoid exposure to tobacco smoke.
- Avoid propping the bottle in infant's mouth.
- Discontinue use of pacifier after 6 months.
- Stress importance of immunizations, pneumococcal and influenza vaccines.
- Only bacterial infections require antibiotics.
  - Stress importance of completing antibiotics as prescribed.
- Improvement should begin within 48 hours.
  - Myringotomy: incision in eardrum to relieve pressure, drain fluid
  - Tympanostomy: a tube placed through eardrum to relieve pressure
    - Usually falls out spontaneously within a year

Sinusitis

Sinusitis is an inflammation of the sinuses due to virus, bacteria, or allergens. The inflammation creates mucus that is subsequently blocked from draining into the nose and acts as a pool for pathogens (Fig. 11–5).

Assessment

- Facial pain
- Headache in older children
- Low-grade fever
- Coldlike symptoms lasting up to 14 days
- Postnasal drip, bad breath, nausea, vomiting
- Thick yellow-green nasal discharge
- Swelling around eyes
- Fatigue, irritability

Evidence-Based Practice: Flu Vaccine Safety for Children With Egg Allergy

Turner, P. J., Southern, J., Andrews, N.J. Miller, E., & Erlewyn-Lajeunesse, M. (2015). Safety of live attenuated influenza vaccine in young people with egg allergy: Multicentre prospective cohort study. *BMJ, 351*, h6291. doi:10.1136/bmj.h6291

Influenza is the major cause of morbidity and mortality in children worldwide. Many people cite an egg allergy as the reason for not getting annual influenza vaccines. Turner, Southern, Andrews, Miller, and Erlewyn-Lajeunesse (2015) conducted an open-label IV intervention study during the flu season 2014–2015 in children 2 to 18 years of age with an egg allergy. A total of 779 children were enrolled in the study, 34.7 % of whom had previous anaphylaxis to egg. None of the participants had egg in their diets. The live attenuated influenza vaccine (LAIV) product information list cites egg allergy as a contraindication to receiving the vaccine. Vaccination was deferred for acute febrile illness, wheezing in the past 72 hours, acute asthma symptoms, or use of antihistamines in previous 4 days. Baseline vital signs were done including pulse oximetry; then LAIV was administered. The children were observed for 30 minutes after the vaccination for signs of local or systemic allergic reactions. A phone call was made 72 hours after vaccination to inquire about each child having any delayed allergic reaction. Seventeen adverse events were reported within 2 hours of vaccination. No participants experienced a systemic reaction to the LAIV. It is unlikely that LAIV is a trigger for systemic allergic reactions in children with egg allergy. A more expensive, recombinant trivalent influenza vaccine that has no egg protein may be given instead of LAIV. Parents and children should not defer influenza vaccine for fear of an allergic reaction (Turner et al., 2015).

Diagnosis

- Clinical presentation

Nursing Interventions

- Supportive care
- Internasal steroid
- Antihistamine and/or leukotriene receptor antagonist
- Antibiotics as prescribed
- Saline nasal drops or decongestants

Caregiver Education

- Teach sinusitis prevention during a cold or allergy attack.
- Use oral decongestants or nasal sprays.
- Have child blow nose, one side at a time, blocking the other.
  - Can attempt this method when the child is developmentally around 2 years of age
- Warm compresses to facial sinus areas
- Cool mist humidifier

Pharyngitis

- Inflammation of throat mucosa and underlying structures
- Triad of sore throat, fever, and pharyngeal inflammation
- Multitude of causes: viruses, bacteria, fungi, noninfectious agents

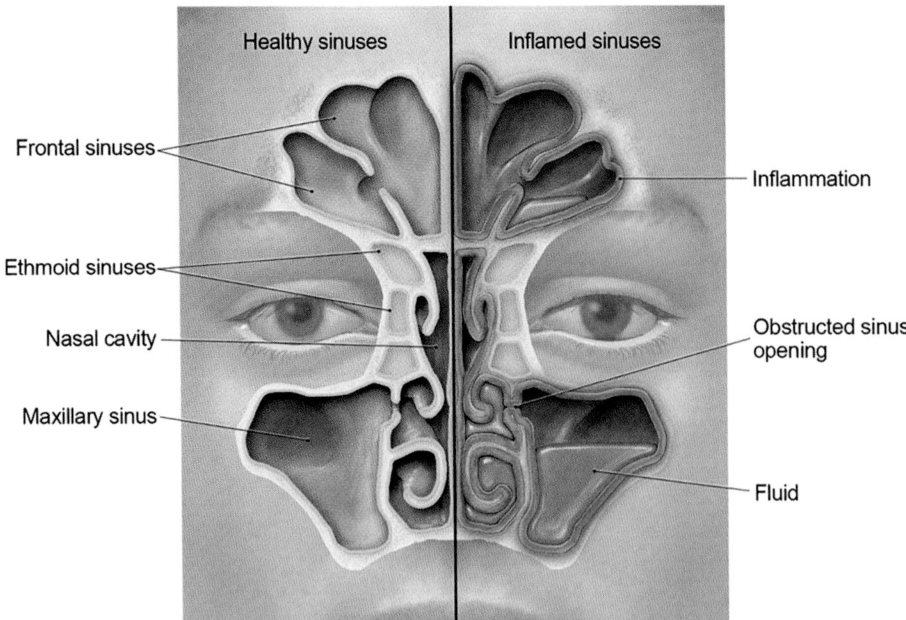

FIGURE 11–5 Sinusitis.

- Viral causative factors; may present with conjunctivitis, coryza, oral ulcers, cough, and diarrhea
- Adenovirus: most common cause when pharyngitis occurs in the late fall or winter

Nasopharyngitis

- Inflammation of the nasal and throat mucosa caused by bacteria or virus
- Rhinovirus, enterovirus, adenovirus, metapneumovirus
- Occurs in the cold months and lasts 4 to 10 days
- Nasal congestion present
- Bacterial infection often with sore throat

Diagnosis of Pharyngitis or Nasopharyngitis

- Clinical presentation
- Nasal or throat swab to identify the organism causing the illness

Nursing Interventions

- Monitor respiratory status
- Supportive care
- Antibiotics as ordered

Influenza

- Viral infection spread through contact or inhalation of droplets
- Contagious 1 to 2 days before onset of symptoms and usually affects the upper respiratory tract
- Multiple strains of influenza
- December to February is peak season in the United States
- Vaccination significantly decreases infections
  - *Haemophilus influenza*—childhood schedule for type B
  - Annual flu shot vaccine for estimated dominant influenza
  - First seasonal vaccine for children 6 months to 8 years of age given by two injections at two separate times, at least 28 days apart
  - Not protected until 2 weeks after second vaccine
- Secondary bacterial infections are common with influenza

Assessment

- Abrupt onset
- Fever
- Chills
- Headache
- Flushed cheeks
- Cough

SAFE AND EFFECTIVE NURSING CARE: Understanding Medication

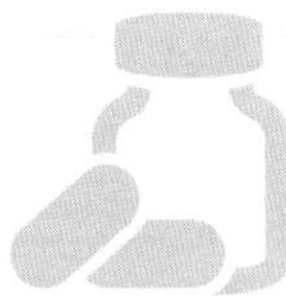

Parent Education: Over-the-Counter Medications

Over-the-counter medications treat only symptoms. Parents need to know that medication labeled "pediatric" has been exclusively studied for effectiveness and side effects in children. Parents should read the label to identify active ingredients and use only as directed. Children are more sensitive than adults to medication and may have an increase in paradoxical effects. Some drugs, such as aspirin, can cause serious illness or death if given to a child with chicken pox or flu-like symptoms. Cold medicine should not be used in children younger than 4 years. Although acetaminophen can be used for infants for fever, ibuprofen should not be used until after 6 months of age.

- Malaise
- Cold symptoms
- Possible dry or sore throat, erythematous rash, and diarrhea
- Wheezing may occur if bronchitis is present

Diagnosis for Influenza Types A or B

- Viral culture of nasopharyngeal or throat samples
- Rapid influenza diagnostic tests
- Immunofluorescence or enzyme-linked assays

Diagnosis for Avian Influenza

- Blood culture
- Complete blood cell count with differential
- Electrolyte panel
- Liver enzyme assay
- Blood urea nitrogen/creatinine
- Rapid influenza diagnostic tests

Nursing Interventions

- Supportive care of symptoms
- Antipyretics
- Cough suppressants
- Oral or IV hydration
- Antiviral medication such as oseltamivir may reduce symptoms if started within 48 hours of onset of symptoms
  - If suspected or confirmed avian influenza, start oseltamivir as soon as possible.
- Annual vaccinations recommended for age 6 months and older

Caregiver Education

- Supportive care
- Prevention is best; decrease respiratory symptoms and decrease contact to prevent the spread of the virus.
- Frequent hand washing at home, cover your cough, and limit visitors.
- Encourage fluids to liquefy secretions and prevent dehydration.
- Antiviral medications may cause nausea and exacerbate asthma.
- Provide rest and quiet, diversional activities.

Tonsillitis

- Inflammation of palatine tonsils, a major component of lymphoid tissue in oropharynx
- Adenoiditis is inflammation of the pharyngeal tonsils on posterior wall of nasopharynx
  - Either bacterial or viral
- Incidence of pharyngitis and tonsillitis is highest in children 4 to 7 years of age
- Palatine tonsil size is graded in relation to how much airway obstruction protruding from either side of the oropharynx (Fig. 11–6)
  - A grade of +1 or +2 is normal tonsil size

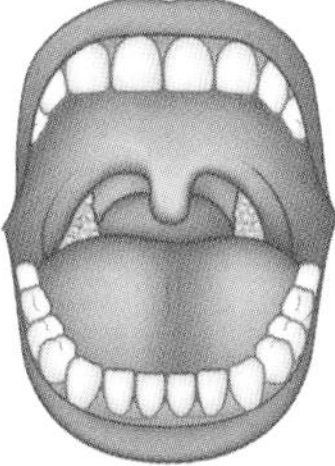

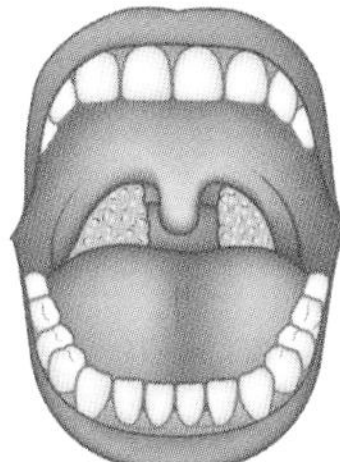

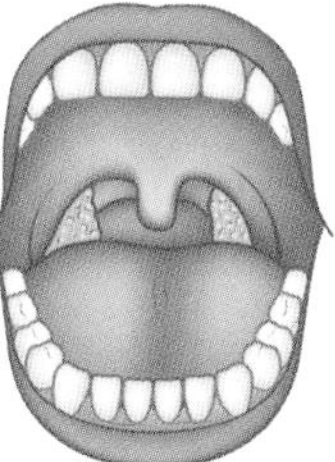

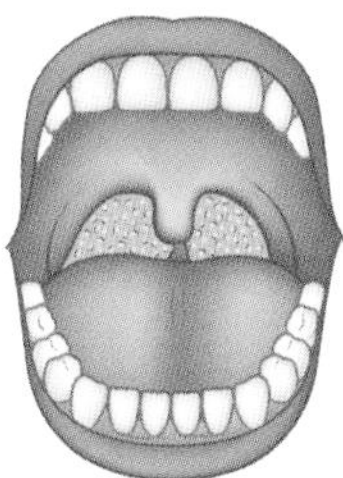

FIGURE 11–6 Tonsil grading scale.

  - A grade of +3 is enlarged tonsils seen with infection
  - A grade of +4 is seen with significant, almost touching or "kissing"

Assessment

- Sore throat
- Enlarged tonsils, may be red or covered with exudate
- Difficulty swallowing
- Mouth breathing with halitosis
- Enlarged adenoids may affect speech and cause child to mouth breath, snore, or have obstructive sleep apnea

Diagnosis

- History of present illness and physical assessment of pharynx
- Serum analysis reveals leukocytosis
- Throat culture may identify bacterial cause

Nursing Interventions

- Supportive care
- Antibiotics as ordered
- Tonsillectomy and possible adenoidectomy for chronic inflammation
  - After tonsillectomy, place in side-lying or prone position to drain secretion until child awakens.
- Gentle oral assessments, avoiding disruption of surgical site
  - Assess for hemorrhage, restlessness, tachycardia, thread pulse, pallor, or frequent swallowing.
- Avoid coughing, using a straw, or blowing nose to prevent the risk for bleeding
- Encourage popsicles and ice chips while avoiding acidic foods
- Dark brown (old) blood-tinged secretions are normal, bright red blood is not
- Child may be nauseated from drainage

- Avoid vomiting, minimize crying
- Adequate pain relief is essential to optimize oral intake
  - Encourage child to take pain medicine or obtain an order to change oral medications to IV pain medications.

CRITICAL COMPONENT

Bleeding Post-tonsillectomy

A child who is post-tonsillectomy and is continually swallowing is most likely bleeding. Assess for restlessness, frank red blood in the mouth and nose, and increased pulse rate.

Family Education

- Instruct parent to report any bleeding immediately. Postoperative hemorrhage could occur anytime from immediately after the procedure up to 10 days later.
- Instruct caregivers and child that child should avoid acidic, highly seasoned, hard, or sharp foods like tortilla chips for 2 weeks.
- Instruct caregivers and child that child should avoid coughing, clearing throat, gargling, or disturbing tonsils with toothbrush.
- Reinforce the importance of taking pain medicine before ingesting fluids or food.

Tracheitis

- Rare but life-threatening bacterial inflammation of trachea
- Most frequently caused by *Staphylococcus aureus*, but also *Streptococcus pneumoniae*, group A *Streptococcus*, and *Moraxella catarrhalis*
- Occurs in natural or artificial airways, such as endotracheal intubation after an infection
- Preceded by upper airway infection, trauma, or intubation
- Symptoms mimic croup and epiglottitis
- Does not improve with corticosteroids and nebulized epinephrine

Assessment

- Thorough history, onset of stridor, precipitating factors
- Stridor at rest
  - Inspiratory stridor, blockage above vocal chords
  - Expiratory stridor, blockage below vocal chords
    - This could be a sign of a foreign body aspiration.
  - Biphasic stridor, blockage at or below vocal chords
- Hypoxia, increased work of breathing
- Substernal and intercostal retractions

Diagnosis

- History of trauma, prodromal upper airway infection, trauma, intubation
- No improvement with corticosteroids and nebulized epinephrine
- Direct visualization, bronchoscopy, or intubation
- Edema, erythema of subglottis, mucopurulent secretions, pseudomembrane formation, and sloughing may obstruct airway
- Rapid clinical deterioration in 2 to 10 hours to complete airway obstruction

Nursing Interventions

- Monitor for acute respiratory distress utilizing continuous pulse oximetry and frequent respiratory reassessments.
- Provide supplemental oxygen as ordered if hypoxic.
- Keep child calm; allow child to sit in caregiver's lap and/or assume position of comfort.
- Delay painful or anxiety-producing procedures such as an IV start or throat examination.
- Prepare for intubation with respiratory failure.
- Prepare for endoscopic removal of membranes obstructing airway.
- Administer antibiotics as ordered.

Caregiver Education

- Provide emotional support.

UPPER AIRWAY NONINFECTIOUS DISORDERS

The disorders included in this section are noninfectious and confined to the sinuses, throat, or structures of the ears. Some are congenital abnormalities in the structures that form part of the upper airway.

Esophageal Atresia and Tracheoesophageal Fistula

- Spectrum of malformations of esophagus predominantly associated with communication with trachea
- Usually seen together, rare to have tracheoesophageal fistula alone

Assessment

- Respiratory distress within minutes, days, or weeks of birth
- Excessive oral secretions
- Cyanosis
- Coughing spells
- Abdominal distention
- Upper airway instability

Diagnosis

- Prenatal ultrasonography
- Polyhydramnios in utero
- X-rays, tracheoscopy, echocardiography, and ultrasound

Nursing Interventions

- Prepare for surgical repair hours to days after birth
- Administer surfactant to assist in lung maturity
- Assist with extracorporeal membrane oxygenation (ECMO)

- Presurgical/Postsurgical care
  - Prevent aspiration, constant oral suction, nasogastric (NG) tube for feeds
  - NPO before surgery
  - Elevate head of bed 30 degrees
  - Oxygen, mechanical ventilation
  - Monitor for respiratory distress, ABGs

Caregiver Education

- Prevent aspiration, feeding, positioning
- Importance of adherence to frequent follow-up appointments

Laryngomalacia

With this congenital laryngeal cartilage abnormality, tissue is soft and floppy. It collapses in on itself, obstructing the upper airway.

Assessment

- Inspiratory stridor within first 2 weeks of life
- Crowing noise with respirations
- Normal vital signs and oxygen saturation
- Mild tachypnea
- Suprasternal retractions may be present
- Stridor increases when child is supine, crying, feeding, experiencing emotional stress

Diagnosis

- History and clinical symptoms that increase with feeding
- Flexible laryngoscopy

Nursing Interventions

- Symptoms usually resolve by age 2 years without intervention
- Monitor height and weight, assess development for age
- Rare intubation or tracheostomy
- Monitor for acute respiratory distress, stridor, retractions or dyspnea, feeding difficulty
- Position the neck with slight hyperextension to optimize airflow in flexible airway
- Postsurgical care of child
- Only 20% of cases are severe enough to require surgical intervention (Van der Heijden, Frederik, & Halmos, 2016).

Caregiver Education

- Teach signs and symptoms of baseline versus worsening sounds.
- Monitor feeding for difficulty sucking or choking.
- Smaller, frequent feeds may ensure adequate intake.
- Reassure parents that most children outgrow this disorder by age 2 years.

Subglottic Stenosis

Subglottic stenosis is the narrowing of the airway within the rigid cricoid cartilage. It can be congenital or result from prolonged intubation.

Assessment

- Stridor: inspiratory, expiratory, or both
- Adventitious breath sounds and decreased air movement post-extubation
- Increased work of breathing
- History of recurrent or croup to identify any additional edema
- Presence of gastroesophageal reflux that may contribute to airway irritation and inflammation

Nursing Interventions

- Close monitoring of respiratory status
- Supplemental oxygen
- Monitor intermittent obstructive episodes
- Medications
  - Oral, IV, or inhaled steroids
  - Inhaled epinephrine
- Prepare for possible surgical intervention, tracheostomy, laryngotracheal reconstruction

Caregiver Education

- Tracheostomy care
- Monitor breathing
- Suctioning to prevent or clear mucous plug

Croup Syndromes

Croup is a general term referring to the inflammatory process. See Table 11–2 for a summary of viral croup disorders.

Acute Laryngitis

- Viral or bacterial inflammation of the larynx
- Can present as sole disorder or be one of multiple respiratory symptoms
- Viral laryngitis alone resolves without treatment
- Loss of voice, hoarseness, pain with speaking, pain/difficulty swallowing
- Rest voice for 24 hours, encourage oral fluids
- Self-limiting

Acute Spasmodic Laryngitis (Spasmodic Croup)

- Viral laryngitis affects children 3 months to 3 years of age
- Pattern of seal-like cough worse at night, may be absent by day

Assessment

- History of previous attacks lasting 2 to 5 days followed by uneventful recovery
- Nighttime barky, seal-like cough
- Afebrile
- Mild respiratory distress
- Stridor scoring to assess difficulty of breathing

Diagnosis

- Clinical signs
- Direct examination, edema, erythema, and vascular engorgement of vocal chords

TABLE 11–2 Summary of Viral Croup Syndrome

	ACUTE SPASMODIC LARYNGITIS	LARYNGOTRACHEOBRONCHITIS	LARYNGOTRACHEITIS	EPIGLOTTITIS
Risk	Least serious	Most common	Serious	Most serious
Age of occurrence	3 months to 3 years	3 months to 8 years	3 months to 8 years	2–8 years
Onset	Abrupt, peaks and recurs at night	Gradual onset, progressive	Gradual onset, progresses to marked respiratory distress	Abrupt, progresses rapidly to complete occlusion
Symptoms	Barky, seal-like cough, afebrile, mild respiratory distress	Early, low-grade fever, hoarseness, characteristic croupy cough, upper respiratory infection symptoms, moderate distress	Early, low-grade fever, hoarseness, harsh barking cough, stridor, retractions, cyanosis	Sudden high fever, drooling, dysphonia, dysphagia, stridor

Nursing Interventions

- Close monitoring of respiratory status, can progress rapidly
- Keep child calm, promote a calm environment, and allow the child to maintain a position of comfort with parent
- Cool mist or going out into cold night air may relieve spasms
- Supplemental, highly humidified oxygen if saturation less than 94%
- Hydration, NG, or IV fluids
- Beta-adrenergics (racemic epinephrine)
  - Aerosolized, rapid acting, decrease inflammation and mucus, temporary
  - Onset 30 minutes, lasting 2 hours
  - Can lead to tachycardia, hypertension, headache, and anxiety
- Corticosteroids (dexamethasone): longer acting, 36- to 54-hour half-life
  - May lead to hypertension and elevated glucose levels

Caregiver Education

- Encourage resting voice
- Importance of hydration

Laryngotracheitis

Laryngotracheitis is viral inflammation of the glottis and subglottic region, and is the most common form of croup.

Laryngotracheobronchitis

- Viral inflammation of larynx, trachea, and bronchioles
- Usually symptoms peak 3 to 5 days, resolve in 4 to 7 days
- Most common in children 3 to 36 months of age, incidence dramatically decreases by 6 years of age
- RSV and parainfluenza virus are most common and can occur in all seasons
- Influenza A and B infections occur in winter and early spring
- Rhinovirus, human metapneumovirus, coronavirus, and adenovirus

Assessment

- Inspiratory stridor
- Fever
- Restlessness
- Hoarseness and air hunger
- History of prodromal upper respiratory infection (URI), coryza, nasal congestion, cough for 2 to 3 days, then harsh, "barklike" cough
- Stridor usually at night, often awakens child
- Variable degrees of respiratory distress
- Mild expiratory wheezing on auscultation to inspiratory stridor at rest with nasal flaring and suprasternal and intercostal retractions
- Hypoxemia: lethargy or agitation
- Tachypnea, tachycardia

Diagnosis

- Clinical presentation
- AP CXR displays a funnel-shaped narrowing of glottis and subglottic area

Nursing Interventions

- Close monitoring of respiratory status, can progress rapidly
- Keep child calm, promote a calm environment, and allow the child to maintain a position of comfort with parent
- Cool mist or going out into cold night air may relieve spasms
- Supplemental, highly humidified oxygen if saturation less than 94%
- Hydration, NG, or IV fluids
- Beta-adrenergics (racemic epinephrine)
  - Aerosolized, rapid acting, decrease inflammation and mucus, temporary
  - Help to control symptoms within 30 minutes and may last up to 2 hours
  - Can lead to tachycardia, hypertension, headache, and anxiety
- Corticosteroids (dexamethasone): longer acting, 36- to 54-hour half-life
  - May lead to hypertension and elevated glucose levels

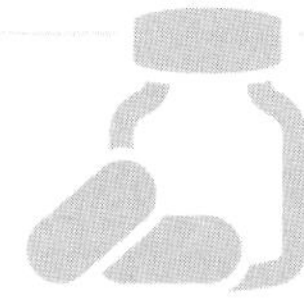

SAFE AND EFFECTIVE NURSING CARE: Understanding Medication

Oral Steroids

Oral corticosteroids are the treatment of choice for mild-to-moderate croup, whereas inhaled corticosteroids and inhaled epinephrine are used for severe respiratory distress.

Epiglottitis

This acute, rapidly progressing inflammation of the larynx and epiglottis can be life-threatening.

- Affects 2- to 8-year-olds
- Usually caused by bacteria
- Most often due to *Haemophilus influenza* type B

CRITICAL COMPONENT

Inspection for Epiglottitis

If you suspect a child has epiglottitis, don't inspect the mouth or throat without emergency personnel and intubation supplies on hand. Inspection of oropharynx could stimulate bronchospasm and lead to complete airway occlusion and death.

Assessment

- Previously healthy child quickly becomes very ill
- Sudden high fever
- Severe sore throat
- Symptoms characterized by the four Ds and an S: drooling, dysphagia, dysphonia, distressed inspiratory air movement, stridor
- Restlessness, anxiety
- Tachycardia, tachypnea with high fever
- Child may be sitting up and forward with lower jaw thrust forward, tripod position, head held in sniffing position

Diagnosis

- Clinical symptoms
- Lateral neck x-ray-narrowed airway, thickening of epiglottis at base of tongue, appears as inverted thumb
- Suspected epiglottitis is contraindication for visual inspection of mouth and throat
- If airway secured, throat culture, treat for gram-positive results until cultures return

Nursing Interventions

- Monitor respiratory status closely, prepare for intubation
- Encourage child not to cry, avoid laryngospasms
- Medications as prescribed
- Hydration, IV fluids
- Emotional support for frightened family
- Supportive treatment

Family Education

- Proper administration of antibiotics
- Encourage oral hydration
- With the *Haemophilus influenzae* type B vaccine, epiglottitis is a rare condition in the United States (Udeani, 2016)

LOWER AIRWAY INFECTIOUS DISORDERS

The infections included for discussion in this section begin with the trachea and end with the alveoli, including the lungs, bronchi, and bronchioles.

Bronchitis

- Acute inflammation of bronchi (Fig. 11–7)
- Causes wheezing in children 12 to 36 months of age
- Most frequently caused by rhinovirus but can be caused by other viruses

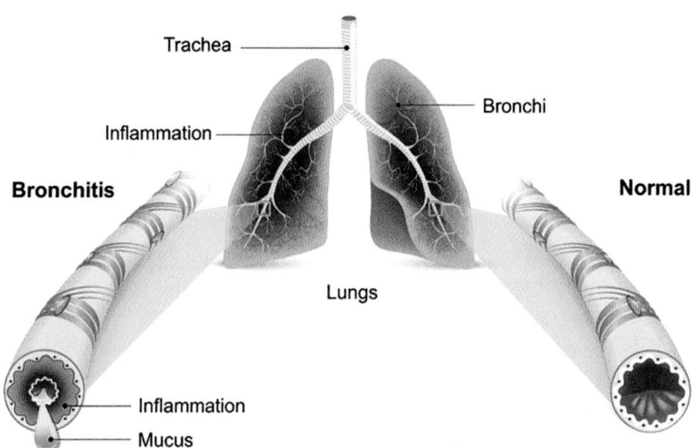

FIGURE 11–7 Bronchitis.

Bronchiolitis

- Acute inflammation of bronchioles
- Term used in the United States for children younger than 24 months with wheezing
- In Europe, refers to children younger than 12 months with first episode of wheezing
- Most often caused by either a virus or bacteria: RSV, rhinovirus, parainfluenza, human metapneumovirus, adenovirus, human bocavirus, and influenza viruses
- About 3% of infants diagnosed with bronchiolitis will require hospitalization for supportive care such as suctioning (Meissner, 2016)
- Viruses enter mucosal cells and rupture these cells, creating debris and increased mucous production and causing bronchospasms and obstruction
- Air trapped in alveoli is absorbed by blood, causing atelectasis
    - Reduced lung compliance
    - Ventilation: perfusion mismatch is increased, which causes hypoxemia and hypercapnia
    - Risk for pneumonia increases because of tissue damage in alveoli

Assessment

- Mucus may produce wheezing and crackle sounds
- Apnea, especially in premature infants
- Nasal congestion
- Low-grade fever
- Dry, nonproductive cough
- Wheeze and/or crackles or reduced air sounds because of air trapping and hyperinflation
- Tachypnea often greater than rate of 60 breaths per minute
- Can progress to severe respiratory distress, exhaustion, and failure

Diagnosis

- History and clinical signs
- CXR: pattern of hyperinflation
- Polymerase chain reaction (PCR) assay, PCR

Nursing Interventions

- Cardiorespiratory monitoring
- Supportive therapy via supplemental oxygen
- NG or IV fluids
- High flow or positive pressure humidified oxygen if saturation less than 90%
- Good hand hygiene is essential
- Surfactant administration
- Contact and airborne precautions, prevent spread of organisms
- Nebulized hypertonic saline
- Pulmonary hygiene: chest physiotherapy, postural drainage, suctioning
- Palivizumab: prophylactic RSV vaccine for premature or high-risk infants

SAFE AND EFFECTIVE NURSING CARE: Understanding Medication

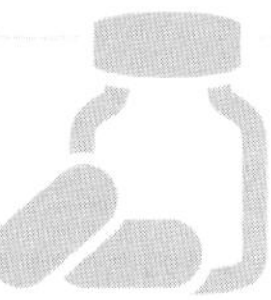

Palivizumab

Bronchiolitis is the most common cause of hospitalizations of children with high direct and indirect costs for the health-care system and families. RSV is the most common cause of bronchiolitis (National Institute for Health and Care Excellence, 2015). Treatment is largely supportive with hydration and supplemental oxygen. Palivizumab is a humanized monoclonal antibody vaccine used as prophylaxis for RSV. A study done by Farber et al. (2016) supported the practice guidelines for use of palivizumab in preterm infants less than 36 weeks' gestation, providing decreased RSV hospitalizations, decreased severity of symptoms, and shorter length of time requiring oxygen support. It is given as an IM injection before the start of RSV season (usually October to May depending on geographical area) and every month for a total of five injections during RSV season at the cost of about $1,000 for the smallest single dose.

Before administering, determine normal partial thromboplastin time, prothrombin time, and international normalized ratio and platelet levels. High-risk groups recommended to receive the RSV vaccine include infants 29 to 35 weeks' gestation who are 3 months or younger at the start of RSV season, infants and children younger than 2 years with congenital heart defects, and infants 35 weeks' gestation with chronic lung disease or neuromuscular disorders (Ralston et al., 2014).

Caregiver Education

- Use of bulb syringe
- Avoid spread of RSV with hand washing, alcohol hand rubs
- Hydration, oral, and nasal saline drops to liquefy secretions
- Monitor temperature, antipyretics
- Maintenance of RSV vaccine schedule
- Avoid exposure to tobacco smoke and air pollution
- Assess for respiratory distress, changes in symptoms
- Symptoms may linger for 2 to 3 weeks
- Cluster care to allow for rest period
- Teach when they should notify physician
    - Worsening respiratory distress in a high-risk infant younger than 1 year old, indicated by increased retractions, increased respiratory rate, or adventitious respiratory sounds
    - Child appearing more ill; not eating, drinking, or sleeping

Pneumonia

- Inflammation of lung parenchyma leading to consolidation
    - Caused by viruses, bacteria, mycoplasma, fungus, or aspiration
- Invading organism travels to lungs via upper respiratory tract or systemically

SAFE AND EFFECTIVE NURSING CARE: Clinical Pearl

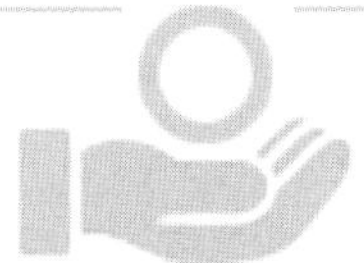

Importance of Hand Hygiene

Hands contaminated with respiratory secretions are the major mode of spread of respiratory infections. Bacteria and viruses can live for 20 minutes to months on surfaces. Most people wash their hands inadequately. Antibacterial soap and warm water are needed. First, wet your hands; then work up a generous lather for about 30 seconds or the time it takes to sing "Happy Birthday" twice. Be sure to wash in between fingers and fingernails. Rinse thoroughly with ends of fingers pointing downward as not to splash or contaminate anything. Dry hands with paper towels and turn faucet off with paper towel. Avoid cross contamination of patients separated in different rooms. Strict attention to maintaining physician-ordered respiratory or contact precautions is vital to prevent cross contamination.

- Virus causes cellular destruction and accumulation of debris in bronchioles and alveoli, leading to patchy infiltrates
    - Bacteria cause fluid accumulation and cellular debris in bronchioles and alveoli, causing consolidation
    - Impaired gas exchange due to atelectasis and inflammatory response with both viruses or bacteria

Assessment

Viral

- Often influenza viruses and RSV: 80% to 85% of all pneumonias
- Retractions
- Tachypnea with a respiratory rate greater than 50 breaths per minute
- Variant fever, low to high
- Cough crackles
- Wheezing, more common with RSV
- General malaise, fatigue
- Headaches and stomachaches
- CXR: hyperinflation or consolidation
- Duration: 5 to 7 days

Bacterial

- Recent history of URI
- High fever, chills
- Cough
- Abnormal or decreased breath sounds
- Retractions
- Older children may have chest pain, gastrointestinal symptoms
- Tachypnea with a respiratory rate of greater than 50 breaths per minute
- Respiratory distress and restlessness
- CXR: consolidation

Diagnosis

- Pulse oximetry normal or decreased
- CXR consolidation
- Chest ultrasound
- White blood cell count slightly elevated in viral (less than 20,000/ mm^3) but much higher in bacterial, erythrocyte sedimentation rate, C-reactive protein
- Sputum culture: children who are able to follow directions can cough up secretions and spit them into a specimen container
- Nasal washing: most children younger than 3 years

Nursing Interventions

- Supportive care for viral pneumonia
- Supplemental oxygenation and hydration
- Monitor respiratory status, pulse oximetry
- Antibiotics as prescribed for bacterial

Caregiver Education

- Avoidance of aspiration
    - Elevate head of bed 30 degrees.
    - Avoid overfeeding.
    - Burp frequently during a bottle feed.
- Teach administration of antibiotics as ordered
- Inform caregiver that fatigue and cough may linger for a few weeks
- Pneumococcal vaccine

Pertussis (Whooping Cough)

- Highly contagious, bacterial infection by *Bordetella pertussis*
- Occurs mainly in children younger than 10 years
- Global burden with 16 million cases and 195,000 childhood deaths annually (CDC, 2017b)
- Peak occurrence in spring and summer months
- Decreased incidence with pertussis vaccine
    - DTaP (diphtheria, tetanus, [acellular] pertussis) in infants and children up to age 6 years
    - Tdap (tetanus, diphtheria, [acellular] pertussis) in children aged 7 years and older and adults
    - Vaccines are highly effective for 3 years, protection wanes after 4 years (Schwartz et al., 2016).
- Paroxysmal coughing attacks occur most frequently at night; intense effort to expel thick mucus, post-tussive emesis, and exhaustion is common
- May not appear ill in between coughing episodes

Assessment

- In the United States, epidemics are seen in unvaccinated babies and vaccine-lapsed teenagers
- Characteristic whooping sound after a cough episode, gasping for air

- Three stages:
  - First stage presents as URI: nasal congestion coughing, rhinorrhea, watery eyes, sneezing, lasts 1 to 2 weeks.
  - The second stage is marked by intense coughing fits, lasts about a week. Young infants may not exhibit classic whoop sound but become apneic from partial airway closure; lasts 1 to 6 weeks.
  - The third stage is chronic cough lasting up to 10 weeks or longer.
- Known as 100-day cough

Diagnosis

- Clinical presentation
- History of incomplete or absent pertussis vaccine
- Nasopharynx or throat culture is gold standard
- PCR from nasopharyngeal swab 0 to 3 weeks after onset of cough
- Nasopharyngeal culture

Nursing Interventions

- Drug therapy as prescribed
- Monitor respiratory status and give supplemental, humidified oxygen
- Droplet precautions
- Maintain hydration
- Supportive care

Caregiver Education

- Importance of DTaP vaccination
- Prevent spread of infection
- Inform caregiver that child may have persistent cough up to 10 weeks after the infection

Tuberculosis

According to the World Health Organization's (WHO's) Global Tuberculosis Report of 2016, one million children developed tuberculosis (TB) and 170,000 children died of TB. This excludes children with HIV (WHO, 2017).

- Inhaled droplets of *Mycobacterium tuberculosis*, an acid-fast bacillus, cause immune response in alveoli
- Droplets transmitted through speaking, coughing, or sneezing
- Once in alveoli, bacillus triggers immune response
- Macrophages form hard tubercles around bacilli
- Tubercles can remain dormant or progress to active TB; not as prevalent in children as in adults
- Bacilli may spread via the lymphatic or circulatory systems to other sites
- Difficult to diagnose because sputum specimens are nonconclusive and symptoms are vague compared with adults
- Latent TB infection: no symptoms and not contagious, but can be activated to develop into disease.

SAFE AND EFFECTIVE NURSING CARE: Cultural Competence

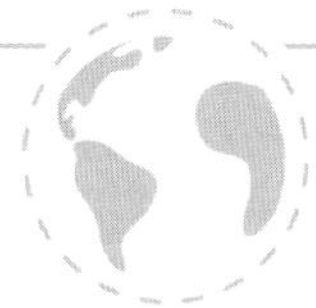

Prevalence of Tuberculosis in Developing Nations

TB is most prevalent in developing countries, a result of challenges such as HIV epidemics, population growth and migrations, poverty, and sociopolitical instabilities. The diagnosis and treatment is long, intensive, and costly, with many potential side effects. The WHO Global Tuberculosis Report of 2016 reported 49 million deaths between 2000 and 2015; TB is one of the top 10 leading causes of death worldwide. In 2015, 10.4 million people fell ill with TB and 1.8 million died; more than 95% of these deaths occurred in low- and middle-income countries. Children were reported to be 15% to 20% of the TB cases worldwide. In the United States, there were only 495 cases of TB, and children accounted for only 5% of those cases (WHO, 2016). In 2017, the highest incidence of TB has been in the African and Asian regions (WHO, 2017).

Assessment

- Latent TB: no symptoms, positive skin test, not contagious, can be activated
- Active TB, persistent cough more than 3 weeks
- Weight loss or inability to gain weight
- Fatigue
- Fever higher than 38°C/100.4°F for more than 2 weeks
- Anorexia
- Night sweats
- Wheezing or decreased breath sounds may be heard in infants
- Lymphadenopathy can be massive, compressing airways

Diagnosis

- Clinical examination usually nonspecific for lower respiratory tract infection in combination with history
- Clinical symptoms of TB
- Positive tuberculin skin test or blood interferon gamma release assay test
- CXR with TB pattern
- History of contact with person infected with TB
- Challenging, symptoms nonspecific, vary and dependent on age of child
  - Children 5 to 10 years of age may not have clinical symptoms but x-ray is TB pattern positive
  - Laboratory tests less likely to be positive in children, diagnosis often without laboratory confirmation
  - Screening questions for identifying at-risk children:
    - Close contact with person infected with TB?
    - Immigrant or adopted from endemic area?
    - Low income or homeless?

    - Immunocompromised?
    - Younger than age 5 years?
- Tuberculin skin test
- Interferon gamma release assay
- Sputum culture
    - Serial specimens collected early in a.m.
    - Takes 4 weeks to confirm
    - Used in children 10 years and older who can produce sputum
    - Expectorated or nasopharyngeal aspiration in younger children
- Gastric lavage: early-morning collection after fasting overnight
- CXR-AP and lateral: TB pattern
    - Upper and posterior lobes of lungs, nodules, cavities, atelectasis
    - Presence of tubercles seen in older children
- Computed tomography (CT) scan: tree in bud pattern

Nursing Interventions

- Drug therapy and supportive care
- Encourage nutrition and rest
- Monitor respiratory status
- Droplet precautions
- Hydration
- For active TB, give anti-TB chemotherapy
    - Given in combination for 6 months
    - Isoniazid, rifampicin, ethambutol, streptomycin
- Bacillus Calmette–Guérin (BCG) vaccine—not generally used in the United States

Caregiver Education

- Promote nutrition and overall health to avoid infections
- Prevent exposure and spread of TB
    - Take TB medication for at least 2 weeks before exposing noninfected people
    - Family and close contacts should take preventive medication
    - If traveling abroad, the individual should get BCG vaccine
    - Wash hands or use sanitizer after exposure to respiratory secretions
    - Infected person should cover mouth and nose with coughs or sneezes
- Direct observation therapy: routine person directly observes and ensures the child is taking medications
- BCG vaccine: live attenuated strain of *Mycobacterium bovis*
    - Not widely used in the United States: less risk for infection
    - Provides incomplete protection
    - Better protection for children than adults

LOWER AIRWAY NONINFECTIOUS DISORDERS

Noninfectious disorders of the lower airway involve the trachea, lungs, bronchi, bronchioles, or alveoli. They are noninfectious but include major lung diseases frequently requiring hospitalizations and/or daily medications.

Respiratory Distress Syndrome

Respiratory distress syndrome is an inflammatory process of the alveolar-capillary membrane that is related to underdeveloped lungs and surfactant deficiency, primarily occurring in preterm infants earlier than 34 weeks. Nearly all infants born at 28 weeks or earlier have respiratory distress syndrome.

- Dysfunctional, decreased surfactant production
- Alveolar edema and accumulation of cellular debris
- Increased airway resistance
- Alveoli collapse at end expiration and cannot remain open
- Pulmonary blood is shunted to systemic circulation
- Altered surface tension causes fluid and protein leak from capillaries
    - Producing hyaline membrane
    - Atelectasis
    - Hypoperfusion to the lung
    - Results in hypoventilation, increased $Paco_2$, and decreased Pao_2 and pH
    - Hypercapnia and hypoxia cause arterial vasoconstriction, resulting in further hypoperfusion
- Infants with diabetic mothers, second-born twins, those delivered by cesarean section, and those with pneumonia or perinatal asphyxia are at higher risk
- Incidence decreases significantly with increased gestational age
- If infants still require oxygen at gestational due date, this condition is diagnosed as bronchopulmonary dysplasia (BPD)

Assessment

- Signs of respiratory distress present within minutes to several hours after birth
- Tachypnea
- Intercostal and subcostal retractions
- Nasal flaring
- Cyanosis
- Grunting
- Fine rales and diminished breath sounds
- CXR looks like ground glass, bronchial tree visible, dark

Diagnosis

- Respiratory distress starting a few minutes to hours after birth
- CXR: ground-glass appearance
- ABG: hypoxemia variable, metabolic acidosis

Nursing Interventions

- Vigorous respiratory monitoring, support, and pulmonary hygiene
- Early administration of positive airway pressure, nasal continuous positive airway pressure, or mechanical ventilation
- Support and maintain mechanical ventilation
    - Nitric oxide, selective pulmonary vasodilator
    - High-frequency jet ventilation
    - ECMO: artificial heart and lung machine
- Administration of surfactant and antenatal steroids

- Maintain normothermia
- Supportive care, nutrition, fluid electrolyte balance, prevention of infection

Caregiver Education

- Signs and symptoms of respiratory distress
- Oxygen use and safety measures
- Home oxygen use usually weaned off by end of first year

Congenital Diaphragmatic Hernia

- Syndrome consisting of incomplete diaphragm formation
- Associated with pulmonary hypoplasia in utero and pulmonary hypertension
- Most often affects the left side; affected lobes may not be fully developed
- Respiratory distress occurs immediately after birth or within first days of life
- Can be life-threatening

Assessment

- Tachypnea, nasal flaring, and retractions
- Circumoral and nail-bed cyanosis
- Tachycardia, heart sounds may be heard on right side of chest
- Irregular chest wall movements
- Decreased breath sounds on affected side
- Bowel sounds heard in the chest
- Visibly sunken abdomen or decreased fullness perceived when palpating abdomen

Diagnosis

- Ultrasound in utero
- MRI in utero
- Scaphoid abdomen
- CXR
- MRI helpful in determining position of organs

Nursing Interventions

- Immediate respiratory support
- Place child in semi-Fowler's position on affected side, head of bed elevated
- Place and maintain patency of NG tube
- Monitor IV fluids
- Monitor and maintain mechanical ventilation, ECMO
- Preoperative/postoperative care
- Monitor for signs of infection and respiratory distress
- Provide for increased calorie needs and monitor for feeding intolerance
- Provide support for parents who may be mourning loss of perfect child

Caregiver Education

- Positioning head and thorax higher than abdomen
- Prescribed feeding techniques
- Encourage breastfeeding moms to pump and freeze milk
- Wound care
- Prevention of infection
- Importance of nutrition
- Refer family to community support groups

Cystic Fibrosis

- Autosomal recessive disorder of exocrine glands marked by increased mucous production and decreased pancreatic enzyme production
- Deletion in chromosome 7 at the cystic fibrosis transmembrane regulator (CFTR)
  - Absence of gene decreases chloride-ion and water transport at cellular level
- Affects multiple organ systems
- One of the most common causes of childhood death
- Cystic Fibrosis Foundation (CFF) cites occurrence of 1 in 1,600 Caucasian births, 1 in 13,000 African American births, and 1 in 50,000 Asian American births
- 30,000 children and adults in the United States have CF, and another 12 million carry the trait (Katkin, 2017)
- Excess mucous production in lungs often leads to secondary bacterial infections; chronic infection leads to tissue damage and, over time, respiratory failure
- Digestive system effects include:
  - Thick mucus in pancreatic ducts block enzymes responsible for the digestion of nutrients, resulting in loss of ability to absorb fat, proteins, and carbohydrates
  - Decreased or no release of amylase, trypsin, and lipase
  - Hepatic bile ducts, gallbladder, submaxillary, and intestinal glands are obstructed by thick mucus and eosinophilic debris
- Metabolic system is affected by excess sodium chloride production by sweat glands, causing hyponatremia
- Ovarian ducts and vas deferens are blocked with mucus, causing sterility in the majority of children

Assessment

- History of episodes of recurrent respiratory infections, pneumonia, bronchitis
- Eating behaviors, pulmonary screening, and current therapies
- Parents report salty taste on child's skin
- Crackles, wheezes or diminished breath sounds, or prolonged expiration
- Digital clubbing indicates hypoxia; increased rounding and loss of angle at base of nail bed is a late sign
- Barrel chest
- Voracious appetite from lost nutrients in undigested food
- Protruding abdomen with thin extremities
- Stool history of malabsorption, bulky stools, or steatorrhea, as well as pain with bowel movement, presence of blood in stool, constipation, or foul odor
- Girls may have vaginal itching, discharge
- Edema: cardiac or liver failure
- Distended neck veins or heave: cor pulmonale

- Older children may report chronic pain in later stages of the disorder
  - Headaches from hypoxia and hypercarbia, sinusitis
  - Musculoskeletal pain from accessory muscle use

Diagnosis

- Prenatal: DNA testing of amniotic fluid for deletion of delta F508 chromosome, evaluate if decreased
- Newborn screening routinely in all 50 U.S. states
  - Serum immunoreactive trypsinogen
  - DNA assay: test for CFTR mutation
- Clinical symptoms consistent with CF in at least one organ system *and* evidence of CFTR dysfunction
  - Evidence of CFTR dysfunction
  - Elevated sweat chloride results dependent on age (on two occasions)
  - Presence of two disease-causing mutations in CFTR, one from each parental allele
  - Abnormal nasal potential difference
- Sweat chloride test: two to five times normal level of sodium and chloride, must be repeated to confirm
  - Sweat chloride concentration of greater than 50 mEq/L is suspicious
  - Positive if increased sodium and chloride greater than 60 mEq/L on two occasions
- CXR: hyperinflation, atelectasis, infiltrates, bronchial wall thickening
- Detailed pulmonary evaluation, including pulmonary function test, respiratory culture, bronchioalveolar lavage, and exclusionary testing
  - Decreased forced vital capacity (FVC)
  - Decreased forced expiratory volume (FEV)
  - Increased residual volume
- Laboratory tests
  - Fecal elastase suggests pancreatic insufficiency
  - Fecal fat: 72-hour collection, increased fat and decreased albumin
  - Serum albumin to assess nutritional status

SAFE AND EFFECTIVE NURSING CARE: Clinical Pearl

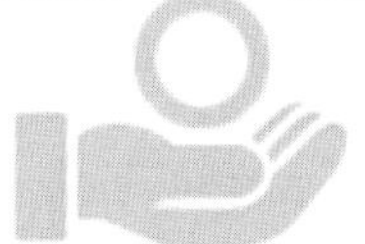

Patient-Centered Care for Cystic Fibrosis

Cystic fibrosis (CF) is a chronic and life-shortening disease. Adolescents and children with CF often have a sense of vulnerability, loss of independence, isolation, and disempowerment. It is important that a multidisciplinary patient-centered care is implemented. This promotes shared decision making, control, and self-efficacy in treatment management and physical and social functioning, which can lead to optimal treatment, health, and quality of life. Encourage children to be involved and active in decisions about their health care. Remind children that they are more than the disease.

Nursing Interventions

- Maintain airway, pulmonary hygiene
- Chest physiotherapy (CPT) includes postural drainage, chest percussion, vibration, and coughing with deep breathing exercises to mobilize/eliminate secretions, re-expand lung tissue, and promote efficient respiratory muscle use. CPT is contraindicated with chest wall trauma, lung contusion or abscess, pneumothorax, and hemoptysis.
  - Postural drainage: sequential positioning of patient to allow gravity to work and encourage secretions in the alveolar periphery to move toward the bronchioles and bronchi to be coughed or suctioned out
  - Percussion: using cupped hands to clap on the chest or motorized device; may be done with vibration
  - Vibration: done manually using hands or a motorized handheld massager; used with percussion or as an alternative to percussion in patients with chest trauma or severe pain, or who are too frail to tolerate percussion
  - Teach breathing and coughing techniques: autogenic drainage, active cycle breathing, and incentive spirometry
    - Can be performed by older children without the aid of another person
  - Vest: oscillating wrap that encircles the chest and can go over the shoulders (Fig. 11–8)
    - Uses air pressure to inflate and deflate
    - Often used in patients with asthma and CF

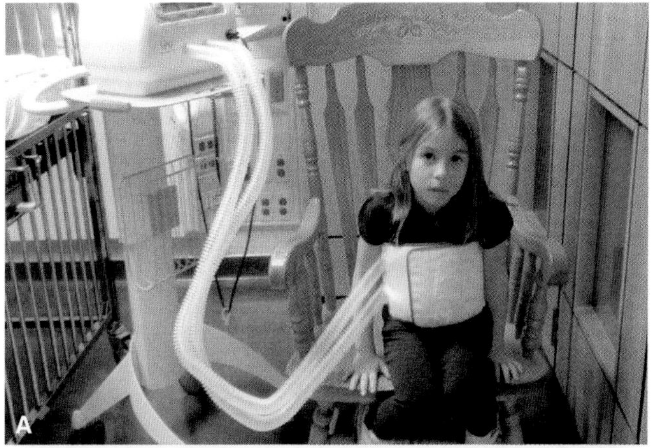

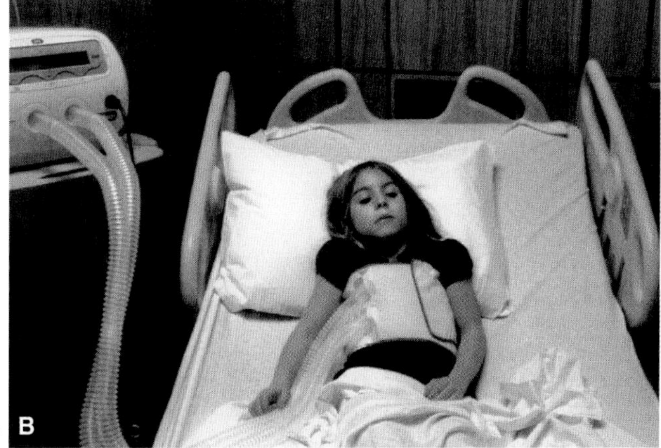

FIGURE 11–8 **A** and **B,** Vest for chest physiotherapy.

- Alternative use, similar action on lungs as percussion and vibration
- Forced exhalation and incentive spirometry
  - Used in combination to mechanically mobilize/eliminate secretions, re-expand lung tissue, and promote efficient respiratory muscle use
  - Prevents or manages atelectasis and pneumonia
- Aerosolized agent to promote airway clearance, hypertonic saline, mucolytic agents, and bronchodilators
  - Dornase alfa, genetically engineered pulmonary enzyme
  - Administered via nebulizer, thins mucus, improves lung function, and decreases risk for infection
- Low-flow, humidified supplemental oxygen: if too high can depress respirations in child with chronic hypoxia
- Monitor respiratory status, and assess for signs and symptoms of infection
- Antibiotics for acute and chronic infections
  - Require higher doses because children with CF have higher drug clearance
  - *Staphylococcus aureus* is the most prevalent chronic bacteria, then *Haemophilus influenza* and *Pseudomonas aeruginosa*
- Short-term use of anti-inflammatory agents: ibuprofen, glucocorticoids, cromolyn
- Individualized dietary modifications and pancreatic enzyme, multivitamin, and caloric supplements
  - Prevent gastrointestinal blockages with adequate fluid, fiber, and stool softeners
  - Fat-soluble A, D, E, and K supplements
  - High-protein diet
- Routine monitoring and nutrition care
  - Administer pancreatic enzymes.
  - Measure height and weight.
- Ivacaftor: use with certain mutations for children older than 6 years; decreases mucous production
- Promote a normal lifestyle for family
- Postoperative care with single or double lung transplant

SAFE AND EFFECTIVE NURSING CARE: Understanding Medication

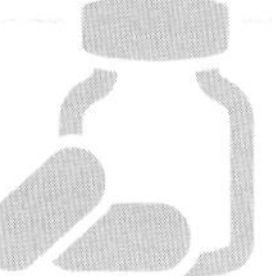

Antihistamine Use for Patients With Cystic Fibrosis

Use of antihistamines is contraindicated for patients with CF because these drugs have a drying effect, making expectoration of mucus more difficult.

Caregiver Education

- CPT technique is critical.
  - Performed three to four times daily.
  - May induce bronchospasm; precede with intermittent positive pressure breathing, aerosol, or nebulizer.
  - Avoid percussing over the spine or internal organs.
  - Cover chest with lightweight shirt or infant blanket.
  - Place child in different positions and perform cupped-hand percussion on areas of chest for at least 2 minutes. It should sound like popping when performed correctly.
  - Finish therapy by using base of hand and straightened arm to vibrate the lower lobe segment as the child exhales at least five times.
  - Avoid chest physiotherapy immediately after eating.
- Avoid hospitalization.
- Teach vest therapy, correct positioning, and use.
- Teach postural drainage and sequential repositioning, which use gravity to help peripheral pulmonary secretions move to bronchi and trachea for expectoration.
- Avoid exposure to infections; immediately report increase in cough, change in sputum, or fever.
- Genetic counseling: Screening confirms diagnosis and identifies carriers.
- Stress importance of daily physical activity to loosen secretions and promote optimal lung expansion.
- Demonstrate correct performance of nebulizer treatments and inhalers.
- Review high-calorie foods and high-protein foods.
- Encourage adequate hydration, addressing activity and seasonal changes.
- Encourage daily fat-soluble vitamin supplements.
- Review administration of supplemental pancreatic enzymes before all meals, snacks, and daily vitamins.
- Teach parents and child not to restrict salt in the diet; in hot weather a supplement may be needed.
- Provide emotional and mental health support resources such as a family's religious leader or a psychologist trained in chronic illness.
- Provide information on community resources, Cystic Fibrosis Foundation, American Lung Association, and a list of home health-care referrals with visiting nurses and respiratory therapists.
- Annual influenza vaccines are recommended for children with CF and family.

SAFE AND EFFECTIVE NURSING CARE: Understanding Medication

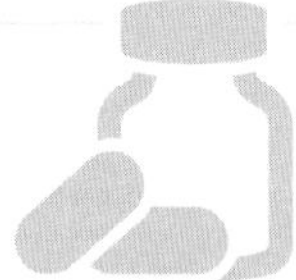

Pancreatic Enzymes

Pancreatic enzymes are effective for only 45 to 60 minutes after administration. This medication must be given at the start of a meal or snack to promote digestion and absorption of vitamins.

Asthma

Asthma is a chronic, obstructive inflammatory disorder caused by hyper-responsiveness of airways, airway edema, narrowing, and mucous production.

- Genetic, environmental, intrinsic, and extrinsic factors affect asthma.

- Approximately 5 million U.S. children had asthma in 2015: 6.4% of children aged 0 to 4 years and 9% to 10% of children aged 5 to 17 years. Statistically, 14% of African American children, 13.2% of multiracial children, and 7.4% of Caucasian children have asthma (Clinical Key, 2015).
- Care aims to reduce impairment by symptoms and reduce risk for adverse outcomes with exacerbation and ongoing treatment.
- Asthma triggers are irritants that stimulate inflammation of the airways. Some of these triggers are regularly found in the home.
  - Cold air
  - Smoke
  - Viral infections
  - Stress
  - Pet dander
  - Exercise
- Bronchospasm may occur from constriction of smooth muscle.
- Inflamed and edematous mucous membranes may cause an accumulation of secretions.
- Immediate or delayed response:
  - Immediate: Sensitized airway mast cells activate immunoglobulin E, causing release of mediators. Histamine, leukotriene, and prostaglandin mediators cause bronchoconstriction shortly after exposure that resolves within 1 to 2 hours.
  - Delayed response: Chemical mediators attract immune system cells (eosinophils, basophils, and neutrophils), infiltrate these cells, and release additional inflammatory materials. This damages smooth muscles cells, causing further edema and mucous obstruction of small airways.
  - Bronchoconstriction can recur and last for several hours.
  - Airway hyper-responsiveness can last for weeks or months.
- Blood flows equally to the obstructed alveoli, as well as open alveoli, creating a ventilation–perfusion mismatch, decreased Po_2, and hypoxia.
- Airway obstruction: Contraction of smooth muscles of airway, swelling, and mucus can cause obstruction.
  - Circumferential narrowing significantly obstructs airflow.

Assessment

- Cough, nonproductive, progressing to frothy, worse at night
  - May present with sole symptom of cough.
  - Night cough may signify need for advancing therapy.
- Shortness of breath
- Chest pain, tightness
- Wheezing
- Prolonged expiration
- Careful history of exposure to possible food allergies and triggers
  - High prevalence of asthma in food-allergic children
  - Egg and tree nut allergies are most prevalent
- History of allergic rhinitis, atopic dermatitis
- Mild retractions, accessory muscle use, infants may head bob
- Coarseness or absence of breath sounds ominous
- Percussion reveals hyper-resonance
- Barrel chest if chronic asthma
- Exposed to cigarette smoke
  - Cigarette smoke exacerbates and compounds treatment
  - Increases symptoms, severity, lowers lung function

Diagnosis

- Detailed history and physical examination on at least two occasions, with focus on excluding other causes of symptoms
- Considerable breathlessness and either coughing, wheezing, or both
- Detailed focused questions on presenting symptoms and precipitation of symptoms
- Family history: parental smoking, asthma, eczema, eosinophilia, any evidence of genetic predisposition to hypersensitivity reactions
- Dermatological signs: atopic dermatitis
  - Allergic shiners
  - Nasal creases
  - Pebbled conjunctiva
- Tachypnea with prolonged expiratory phase
- Pulse oximeter may be low even with mild symptoms
- CXR reveals hyperinflation
- ABGs reveal hypoxemia and hypercapnia
- Pulmonary function tests, spirometry can confirm diagnosis or eliminate others
  - Used in children at least 5 years old
  - Measure FVC, complete exhalation, and FEV over 1 second (FEV1) before and after inhalation of short-acting beta-adrenergic agonist (SABA)
  - The two numbers are used as a ratio FEV1/FVC to determine severity
    - Risk for exacerbation identified
- Peak flow meter: portable, handheld device measures ability to push air out of the lungs
  - Not diagnostic
  - Used to monitoring therapy
  - Below personal best: best level measured when in optimal health
  - Action plan, interventions based on color zones
- Allergy testing to identify triggers
- The National Heart, Lung, and Blood Institute (NHLBI) and WHO established a Global Initiative for Asthma in 1993, with the last revision in 2016 (Table 11–3).
  - Practical approach for asthma management, prevention, and education
  - Asthma management adjusted based on clinical presentation
    - Mild, well controlled with steps 1 to 2 (as needed SABA or low-dose inhaled corticosteroids [ICSs])
    - Moderate, well controlled with step 3 (low-dose ICSs/long-acting beta-adrenergic agonist [LABA])
    - Severe, requires step 4/5 (moderate- or high-dose ICSs/LABA +add on treatments)

TABLE 11–3 Determining Asthma Therapy: Global Initiative for Asthma

	STEP 1	STEP 2	STEP 3	STEP 4	STEP 5
Preferred control medication		Low-dose ICS with as needed SABA	≥12 years old: low-dose ICS/LABA ***or*** ICS/formoterol 6–11 years old: medium-dose ICS	≥12 years old: combination low-dose ICS/formoterol as maintenance with reliever ***or*** Combination medium-dose ICS/LABA 6–11 years old: refer to expert	Referral to specialist and add on tiotropium with exacerbations, omalizumab for patient with allergic asthma, or mepolizumab for eosinophilic asthma
Other control medication	Consider low-dose ICS	LTRAs ***or*** Combination low-dose ICS/LABA ***or*** Episodic ICS for purely seasonal allergic asthma (stop 4 weeks after end of pollen season)	≥12 years old: increase ICS dose or add LTRAs or theophylline 6–11 years old: add LABA	≥12 years old: tiotropium by mist inhaler for exacerbations, trial high-dose combination ICS/LABA, increase dosing frequency (budesonide agents), add on LTRA or low-dose theophylline	Add low-dose oral corticosteroids
Reliever medication	As needed inhaled SABA	As needed SABA	As needed SABA or low-dose ICS/formoterol	Maintenance with reliever beclomethasone/formoterol or budesonide/formoterol As needed SABA	As needed SABA or low-dose ICS/formoterol
	Classify by symptoms less than twice a month, and no risk for exacerbations, short duration	Before stepping up, check inhaler technique, adherence, confirm diagnosis	Before stepping up, check inhaler technique, adherence, confirm diagnosis		Phenotype-guided treatment Sputum-guided treatment in specialized center Aspirin may exacerbate respiratory disease

ICS, inhaled corticosteroids; LABA, long-acting beta$_2$-agonist; LTRA, leukotriene receptor antagonist; SABA, short-acting beta$_2$-agonist.

Adapted from National Heart, Lung, and Blood Institute & World Health Organization. (2016). Global initiative for asthma (GINA). *Retrieved from https://www.chicagoasthma.org/wp-content/uploads/2016/07/Whats-new-in-GINA.*

- Step down when symptoms are well controlled longer than 3 months
- Prepare to step down with continued symptom diary and asthma action plan

Nursing Interventions

- Detailed respiratory assessment
  - Location of wheeze during a breath
  - Ratio of inspiration to expiration
- Assess severity and control of symptoms
- Teach/reinforce inhaler skills and adherence
- Health-care team approach to care of the child
- Elimination or management of triggers
- Assist in balance between good control with medications (Table 11–4)
  - Rescue medication use should be rare and daily medications used with minimal side effects
  - Stepwise escalation of care as necessary
  - Use a calm approach for child and family, who may be frightened
  - Spacers/aerochambers offer faster delivery time and deposit 50% more medication in airway than mouth inhaler (Fig. 11–9).
- Assist the parents in educating school teachers, administrators, and sport coaches (Fig. 11–10)
- Obesity should be managed concomitantly with asthma

Evidence-Based Practice

Centers for Disease Control and Prevention. (2015). *Prevalence of obesity among adults and youth: United States.* Retrieved from https://www.cdc.gov/nchs/data/databriefs/db219.htm

Vijayakanthi, N., Greally, J. M., & Rastogi, D. (2016). Pediatric obesity-related asthma: The role of metabolic dysregulation. *Pediatrics, 137*(5), e20150812. doi:10.1542/peds.2015-0812

Den Dekker, H. T., Ros, K. P., Jongste, J. C., Reiss, I. K., Jaddoe, V. W., & Duijts, L. (2017). Body fat distribution and interrupter resistance, fractional exhaled nitric oxide and asthma at school age. *Journal of Allergy and Clinical Immunology, 139*(3), 810–818. doi:10.1016/j.jaci.2016.06.022

Body mass index has long been the measure of obesity. Childhood asthma and obesity have reached epidemic proportions worldwide. The National Health and Nutrition Examination Survey (NHANES) conducted by the CDC (2015) reported that 17.2% of U.S. children are obese and 16.2% are overweight. Obesity has been studied as the precursor to asthma and diabetes, particularly the mechanical effect of fat deposits on respiratory compliance and the role of nutrients, antioxidants, insulin resistance, and saturated fats. Studies have shown that obesity asthma is different from normal-weight asthma in children.

Although obesity is an independent risk factor for asthma, not all obese children experience development of asthma. A meta-analysis by Vijayakanthi, Greally, and Rastogi (2016) focused on the mechanisms underlying obesity-related asthma including role of diet, sedentary lifestyle, mechanical fat load, and adiposity-mediated inflammation. The immunomodulatory effects of obesity, mediated proinflammatory markers, adipocytokines, including interleukin-6 and leptin, are causing hyper-responsiveness and bronchial constriction. This in turn decreases lung volume, which has been identified in asthma and are associated with insulin resistance, dyslipidemia, and metabolic syndrome. Obese asthma has shown to be resistant to standard care regimens. But because not all obese children have asthma, these factors only play a role in developing asthma. Body mass index has long been the measure of obesity.

Vijayakanthi et al.'s (2016) study was supported by another study done by Den Dekker et al. (2017). This study revealed a correlation of truncal or peritoneal fat to eosinophil-driven airway inflammation causing wheezing, airway restriction, and increased exhaled nitic oxide in obese children, not seen in android/gynoid (waist and hip) fat/mass ratio or subcutaneous (generalized) fat distributions. Truncal adiposity poses a mechanical disadvantage to the diaphragm and is associated with decreased functional residual capacity of the lungs and reduced residual volume and expiratory reserve volume. Obese children have increased forced expiratory capacity and volume compared with normal-weight counterparts. The mechanical restriction of the diaphragm with fat deposits and low lung volumes predispose obese children to lower FEV1/FVC ratio.

Hispanics and African Americans bear a higher burden of obesity-related asthma and have greater truncal adiposity for same body weight Caucasians. Studies have shown that weight loss in obese-related asthma has improved clinical and quality-of-life parameters. Increased intake of processed food has been associated with asthma and is linked to systemic inflammation. Conversely, the Mediterranean diet, high in fruits, vegetables, and omega-3 fatty acids, has been protective. Vitamins A, C, E, and D are being studied as to their role in childhood obese asthma. Obese children tend to have a sedentary lifestyle; an increase in television and video games has been directly correlated to asthma. Obese children are influenced by parental routines surrounding food. The review of all of the studies confirms the complex nature of obese asthma in children related to inflammation, metabolic dysregulation, and pulmonary function. Obese asthma should be managed differently than asthma in nonobese children.

TABLE 11–4 Asthma Medications

LONG-TERM CONTROL	QUICK RELIEF
ICS: anti-inflammatory, decrease hyper-responsiveness, inhibit inflammatory cell migration and activation, block late reactions to allergen, decrease exacerbations Examples: beclomethasone, budesonide	SABA: relaxes smooth muscles in the airway, increases water into mucus, promoting clearance, effects seen in 5–10 minutes. Drug of choice acute therapy, nebulizer, or metered dose inhaler Examples: albuterol, terbutaline, levalbuterol
LABA: relaxes smooth muscles in airway, duration of action at least 12 hours, used in combination with ICS Examples: salmeterol, famoterol	Corticosteroids: decrease airway inflammation, enhance bronchodilation effects of SABA, use in moderate-to-severe persistent asthma with SABA Examples: methylprednisone, IV or PO
Leukotriene modifiers: decrease inflammation cascade, alternate choice for mild persistent asthma, used with ICS for moderate-to-severe asthma Examples: Montelukast, Zafirlukast	Anticholinergics: inhibit bronchoconstriction, decrease mucous production, used with SABA in acute exacerbation
Mast cell inhibitors: interfere with chloride channels, stabilize mast cells, alternative for mild persistent Examples: cromolyn sodium, nedocromil	
Anti-immunoglobulin E antibody: children ≥12 years old with sensitivity to dust mites, cockroaches, dogs, and cats; used in moderate-to-severe persistent asthma; anaphylaxis may occur	
Methylxanthines: relax smooth muscles in airway, continuous airway dilation Examples: PO theophylline, IV aminophylline, monitor serum levels	

ICS, inhaled corticosteroids; LABA, long-acting beta$_2$ agonist; SABA, short-acting beta$_2$-agonist.

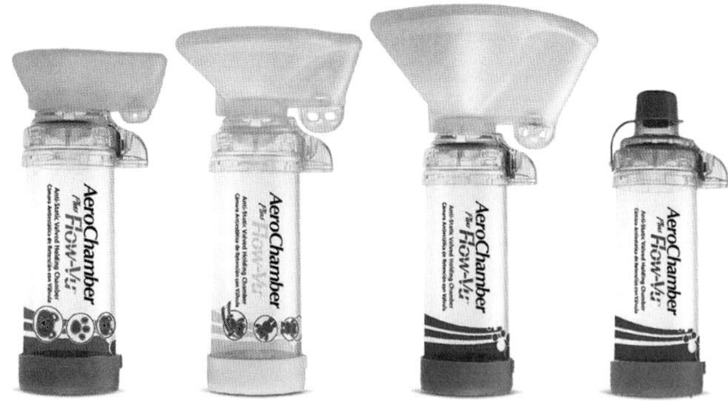

FIGURE 11–9 Aerochamber and mask.

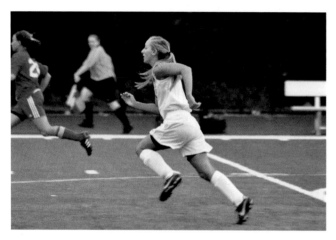

FIGURE 11–10 Playing soccer, and other vigorous physical activity, is a potential trigger for asthma.

Caregiver Education

- Basic facts about asthma, the role of medications, and patient skills
- Adherence to follow-up health-care visit
- Guided self-management: written action plan, self-monitoring, and regular medical review
  - Development of a personal, age-appropriate, written plan based on peak flow meter readings and symptoms, instructing child specifically what medications to take and whom to call if asthma symptoms get worse
- Correct use of inhalers and aerochambers
  - Metered dose inhaler (MDI) with age-appropriate spacer device to ensure proper dosing
  - Breath actuated pressurized MDI and dry powder inhalers
- Importance of reducing obesity, age-appropriate nutrition
- Consider stepping down after 3 months of good symptom control
- Importance of using medication as prescribed
  - Take regular prevention medication, even when symptom-free.
  - Avoid overuse of short-acting beta-adrenergic blockers.

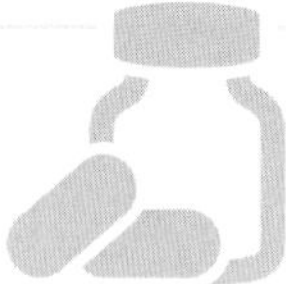

SAFE AND EFFECTIVE NURSING CARE: Understanding Medication

Inhaled Asthma Medications

Short-acting $beta_2$ agonist inhalers should be used no more than twice a week, because overuse can exacerbate symptoms. ICSs are most beneficial in low doses; escalation is arbitrary. High-dose ICSs can lead to osteoporosis.

OTHER NONINFECTIOUS DISORDERS

The disorders included in this discussion vary in their causes and treatment but represent a dysfunction in the respiratory system frequently requiring prompt medical attention.

Foreign Body Aspiration

Solid or liquid inhalation into the respiratory tract is most frequently seen in infants 6 months old to 5 years of age. It commonly occurs:

- At 8 to 10 months of age when infants are curious, developing pincher grasp
- At 1 to 2 years of age when toddlers start walking and climbing and have increased mobility

Assessment

- Coughing
- Wheezing
- Stridor
- Gagging
- Possible cyanosis
- May be asymptomatic for hours or weeks; eventually irritation, edema, and obstruction will develop, producing symptoms
- Usually small toy, tree nuts, peanuts, coin, or latex balloon

Diagnosis

- History and clinical signs
  - May have unwitnessed or unrecognized coughing or choking spell
- CXR, CT or MRI, bronchoscopy

Nursing Interventions

- Assess respiratory status and work of breathing
- Dependent on degree of respiratory impairment
- Allow child to assume position of comfort
- Prepare for removal of object at the bedside or in surgery
- After object removal, observe for laryngeal edema, respiratory distress

- Antibiotics only if there is a bacterial infection
- Cool mist and bronchodilators or corticosteroids for 24 to 48 hours

Caregiver Education

- Age-appropriate toys and foods
- Cut table food into small pieces
- Choking interventions
  - Back blows, abdominal thrusts with head lower than chest for infants
  - Heimlich maneuver is used for older children

Bronchopulmonary Dysplasia

Bronchopulmonary dysplasia (BPD) is a chronic respiratory disorder in premature infants that is treated with a high concentration of oxygen and possible mechanical ventilation.

- Most common chronic lung disease of infancy; 5,000 to 10,000 cases each year according to NHLBI (2015)
- Usually requires hospitalization for several weeks and home oxygen for months to years
- Short-term and long-term consequences
  - Assisted ventilation can injure lungs: a child has less functional surface area with reduced capillary in growth to alveoli, ventilation–perfusion mismatch
  - Pulmonary hypertension, increased lung fluid, interstitial fibrosis, and smooth muscle hypertrophy
- Forty-five percent of preterm infants less than 29 weeks' gestation have BPD (Stoll et al., 2015)
- Immature lungs have fewer alveoli because the alveolar sacs develop between 26 and 28 weeks' gestation
- Hyperinflation of immature lungs produces inflammation and scarring in lungs
- Milder forms of BPD can heal, remodel lungs close to normal
- Contributing factors: infection, patent ductus arteriosus, malnutrition

Assessment

- Increased work of breathing, accessory muscle use
- Tachypnea, respiratory rate increased by 20 to 40 breaths per minute
- Circumoral cyanosis and nail beds
- Retractions, beginning as subcostal and substernal with mild distress and continuing with intercostal and suprasternal as distress worsens
- Atelectasis
- Prolonged exhalation and use of accessory muscles
- Weight loss or poor weight gain, poor feeding
- Wheezing, coughing
- Hyperextending the neck
- Nasal flaring
- Right-sided heart failure

> **CRITICAL COMPONENT**
>
> **Feeding and Activity Intolerance**
>
> Feeding and activity intolerance among infants with BPD makes them prone to malnutrition, resulting in arrested growth and development. Nursing care should cluster necessary tasks and take a hands-off approach.

Diagnosis

- Clinical presentation, if infant requires oxygen for more than 28 days after birth
- CXR: bronchiolar metaplasia, interstitial fibrosis

Nursing Interventions

- Promoting and monitoring respiratory function
- INSURE strategy: **in**tubation, **sur**factant, **e**xtubation; this should be followed by continuous, nasal positive pressure oxygen to decrease the risk for prolonged oxygen requirement and lung damage
- Supplemental oxygen initially, prepare for intubation
- Assist parental coping with intubated child who may remain intubated for weeks
- Mechanical ventilation pressures at lowest effective settings
  - Positive end expiratory pressure 6 to 7 cm H_2O
  - Slightly longer inspiratory time
- Drug therapy as prescribed
  - Surfactant
  - Vitamin A: associated low levels, affects growth and bone development
  - Fluid restriction, diuretics, decrease interstitial edema
  - Bronchodilators
  - Caffeine to stimulate the respiratory center and central nervous system (Abdel-Hady, Nasef, Shabaan, & Nour, 2015)
  - Palivizumab injections to prevent RSV
  - Optimizing nutritional intake, calories, and vitamins
- Monitor intake and output and electrolyte balance
- Cluster nursing care
- Encourage parental interaction with infant, provide support, and increase confidence

Caregiver Education

- Oxygen administration
- Signs and symptoms of respiratory distress
- Stringent hand washing
- Ventilator management
- Medication administration
- High-calorie feedings
- Monitor intake and output

Apnea

Apnea is the cessation of breathing for longer than 20 seconds, or any cessation accompanied by cyanosis, bradycardia, pallor, and hypotonia.

- Inverse relationship found with apnea of prematurity for both birth weight and gestational age
  - As ultra-premature birth has expanded in the United States, so has the incidence of apnea
- Apnea of prematurity occurs in most infants less than 28 weeks' gestation
  - Occurs in 50% of infants 30 to 31 weeks' gestation; if born at 32 to 33 weeks, the risk is 14%; if born 34 to 35 weeks, risk is 7 % (Rocker, 2015)
  - Usually resolves by 36 weeks' post-conceptual age
- Affected by maternal drug use, thermal instability, infection, conditions of insufficient oxygen delivery, metabolic and central nervous system disorders
- Treatment of choice is noninvasive positive airway oxygenation
- Can be early sign of sepsis, respiratory illness, or patent ductus arteriosus
- Obstructive sleep apnea: partial or complete airway obstruction while asleep
  - Treatment of choice is continuous positive airway pressure
  - May be caused by tonsil enlargement
  - Leads to hypoventilation, hypoxia, hypercapnia, hypertension
  - Increasing incidence parallels increasing childhood obesity
  - Craniofacial abnormalities may be a factor
- Central apnea: condition affecting the brain's respiratory center, medulla oblongata
  - May occur if the child has had intraventricular hemorrhage, meningitis, seizures, congenital myopathies
  - Different from normal periodic breathing of newborns

Assessment

- Observed cessation of breathing
- Observe infant startle awake from sleep
- Snoring
- Mouth breathing
- Daytime sleepiness
- Hypoventilation, nail-bed cyanosis
- Nasal or oral obstruction: enlarged tonsils or tongue
- Obesity

Diagnosis

- Sleep history
- Evaluate upper airway and respiratory status
- Apnea monitor
- Polysomnogram
- Sleep apnea significant if child has more than 10 episodes a night, or 1 or more episodes an hour while asleep

Nursing Interventions

- Cardiorespiratory monitoring with continuous pulse oximetry
- Position head and neck to keep airway patent
- Supportive care for medical management
  - Prematurity: administer caffeine, methylxanthines, and doxapram
  - Continuous positive airway pressure ventilation
  - Tonsillectomy
  - Weight reduction
  - Tracheostomy

Caregiver Education

- Safe sleep practices
- Correct application/use of apnea monitor
- Record episodes in diary or calendar
- Optimal head and neck positions for airway patency

SAFE AND EFFECTIVE NURSING CARE: Promoting Safety

Safe Sleep

The infant should sleep in the same room as but not in bed with the parents. The infant should sleep in a crib or bassinette with fitted sheet and dressed in a sleep sack for warmth. No toys or puffy, soft bedding should be in the crib. The infant should sleep on his or her back. The infant may have a pacifier, but it should not be tethered to clothing. Parents should remember the ABCs: "Alone, on my Back, in a Crib."

Apparent Life-Threatening Event, Also Known as Brief Resolved Unexplained Event

An apparent life-threatening event (ALTE) or brief resolved unexplained event (BRUE) is a frightening episode of apnea that affects infants younger than 4 months with gestational age of 37 weeks or older.

- Apnea is accompanied by color change, hypotonia, and choking.
- Fifty percent of ALTE cases occur during wake times (Choi & Kim, 2016).
- Potential causes include gastroesophageal reflux, acute respiratory infection, seizures, feeding aspiration, heart defects, and child abuse.

Assessment

- Careful history and history of events just before event

Diagnosis

- Process of elimination of all other differential diagnoses

Nursing Interventions

- Cardiopulmonary monitoring with continuous pulse oximetry
- Emotional support for family

Caregiver Education

- Use of apnea monitor
- Optimal feeding position
- Safe sleep practices

Pneumothorax

- Extravasation of air from parenchyma into the pleural space because of trauma to chest wall or respiratory tract
- Positive pressure in the chest cavity can cause alveoli to rupture
- Blood in pleural space is hemothorax
- Tension pneumothorax: life-threatening emergency
  - Air enters chest with inspiration but cannot exit on expiration
  - Accumulation of air compresses the lung
  - Mediastinal structures displaced to contralateral side and impair venous return to heart, decreasing cardiac output

Assessment

- Decreased or absent breath sounds on affected side
- Decreased chest wall movement and paradoxical breathing
- Sudden or gradual onset of tachypnea
- Retractions, nasal flaring, or grunting depending on amount of air trapped in the pleura
- Decreased oxygen saturation
- Pallor or cyanosis
- Auscultate for tachycardia and breath sounds, absent or diminished on affected side
- Hemothorax: symptoms can be less conspicuous depending on blood loss from cardiac and vascular injuries

Diagnosis

- CXR
- Clinical presentation

Nursing Interventions

- Oxygen administration
- Cardiopulmonary monitoring with continuous pulse oximetry
- Assist with needle aspiration and/or chest tube placement

Caregiver Education

- Condition is temporary
- Managed in hospital setting

Sudden Infant Death Syndrome or Sudden Unexplained Death of an Infant

Sudden infant death syndrome (SIDS) is the sudden, unexpected death during sleep of an infant younger than 1 year, in which the cause is undetermined even after thorough investigation.

- The number of SIDS cases has declined from 1990 to 2015 (CDC, 2017a).
- Peak incidence of SIDS is 2 to 4 months of age.
- The caregiver finds the infant after a nap or nighttime sleep not breathing and with no pulse. Autopsy reveals pulmonary edema, but no other cause of death is identifiable.
- Studies show 13% of SIDS cases include history of apnea,
- More than 80% of cases occur between midnight and 6 a.m.

Nursing Interventions

- Resuscitation as ordered
- Guide to counseling and community resources, empathy, support
- Prevention of SIDS through safe sleep practices
  - ABCs: "Alone, on my Back, in a Crib"
  - Discuss before going home from hospital and every visit
  - Firm mattress, fitted sheet, avoid loose bedding or toys in crib

Caregiver Education

- Risk factors
  - Mother younger than 20 years
  - Low-birth-weight neonate
  - Premature birth
  - Multiple pregnancy
  - Use of a pacifier with clip
  - Lack of breastfeeding
  - Family history of SIDS
  - Maternal smoking
  - Infant co-sleeping with mother and/or another child

Case Study

You enter the room, where Amy, an 11-year-old girl, neatly dressed with very tight-fitting clothes, is sitting with her mother. The odor of cigarette smoke fills the room. You notice that her abdomen is protruding beneath her shirt and sticking out above her pants. She tells you that she is at the pediatrician's office for a follow-up asthma visit. You greet her and she is smiling while you take her temperature. You ask her to take her shoes off and step on the scale to measure her weight. Suddenly Amy is visibly upset; she starts crying and says "I have been riding my bike and trying to take walks, but nobody ever wants to go with me because I am fat!"

1. How would a nurse set aside any personal feelings concerning smoking and obesity and respond appropriately to Amy?
2. How might this insight help to best support Amy and guide interventions?
3. What are some questions to consider asking Amy?
4. What are some age appropriate activities that you can suggest for Amy?

REFERENCES

Abdel-Hady, H., Nasef, N., Shabaan, A. E., & Nour, I. (2015). Caffeine therapy in preterm infants. *World Journal of Clinical Pediatrics, 4*(4), 81–93. doi: 10.5409/wjcp.v4.i4.81

Boatright, C., Holcomb, L., & Replogle, W. (2015). Treatment patterns for pediatric acute otitis media: A gap in evidence based theory and clinical practice. *Pediatric Nursing, 41*(6), 217–276.

Casey, J. R., & Pichichero, M. E. (2015). Acute otitis media: Update 2015. *Contemporary Pediatrics, 32*(3), 15–18.

Centers for Disease Control and Prevention. (2015). *Prevalence of obesity among adults and youth: United States.* Retrieved from https://www.cdc.gov/nchs/data/databriefs/db219.htm

Centers for Disease Control and Prevention. (2017a). Sudden unexpected infant death and sudden infant death syndrome. Retrieved from https://www.cdc.gov/sids/data.htm

Centers for Disease Control and Prevention. (2017b). *Tuberculosis.* Retrieved from http://www.cdc.gov/tb/topic/populations/tbinchildren/default.htm

Choi, H. J., & Kim, Y. H. (2016). Apparent life-threatening event in infancy. *Korean Journal of Pediatrics, 59*(9), 347–354. doi:10.3345/kjp.2016.59.9.347

Clinical Key. (2015.) Asthma in children. *First Consult.* Retrieved from https://www.clinicalkey.com/asthma-in-children

Den Dekker, H. T., Ros, K. P., Jongste, J. C., Reiss, I. K., Jaddoe, V. W., & Duijts, L. (2017). Body fat distribution and interrupter resistance, fractional exhaled nitric oxide and asthma at school age. *Journal of Allergy and Clinical Immunology, 139*(3), 810–818. doi:10.1016/j.jaci.2016.06.022

Faber, H. J., Buckwold, F. J., Lachman, B., Simpson, J. S., Buck, E., Arun, M., Valadez, A. M., & Glomb, W. B. (2016). Observed effectiveness of palivizumab for 29-36 week gestation infants. *Pediatrics, 138*(2), 1–8. doi:10.1542/peds.2016-0627

Katkin, J. P. (2017). Cystic fibrosis: Clinical manifestations and diagnosis. *Up To Date.* Retrieved from https://webmail.metrohealth.org/gw/webacc?User.context=83cfb91b355a3713df4b06cd115

Meissner, C. H. (2016). Viral bronchiolitis in children. *New England Journal of Medicine, 374,* 62–72. doi:10.1056/NEJMral1413456

National Heart, Lung, and Blood Institute (NHLBI). (2015). *Cystic fibrosis.* Retrieved from https://www.cdc.gov/excite/ScienceAmbassador/ambassador_pgm/lessonplans/CysticFibrosis-Fact-Sheet

National Heart, Lung, and Blood Institute & World Health Organization. (2016). *Global initiative for asthma (GINA).* Retrieved from https://www.chicagoasthma.org/wp-content/uploads/2016/07/Whats-new-in-GINA

National Institute for Health and Care Excellence. (2015). *Bronchiolitis: diagnosis and management of bronchiolitis in children.* Retrieved from https://www.nice.org.uk/guidance/ng9/chapter/1-Recommendations#management-of-bronchiolitis

Principi, N., Marchisio, P., & Esposito, S. (2016). Otitis media with effusion: Benefits and harms of strategies in use for treatment and prevention. *Expert Review of Antiinfective Therapy, 14*(4), 415–423. doi: 10.1586/14787210.2016.1150781

Ralston, S. L., Lieberthal, A. S., Meissner, H. C., Alverson, B. K., Baley, J. E., Gadomski, A. M., ... Hernandez-Cancio, S. (2014). Clinical practice guideline: The diagnosis, management and prevention of bronchiolitis. *Pediatrics, 134*(5), e1474–e1502.

Rocker, J. A. & Isreal J. (2018). Pediatric apnea. *Medscape.* Retrieved from http://emedicine.medscape.com.article/800032-overview

Schwartz, K. L., Kwong, J. C., Deeks, S. L., Campitelli, M. A., Jamieson, F. B., Marchand-Austin, A., & Crowcroft, N. S. (2016). Effectiveness of pertussis vaccination and duration of immunity. *Canadian Medical Association Journal, 188*(16), E399–E406. doi:10.1503/cmaj.160193

Stoll, B. J., Hansen, N. I., Bell, E. F., Walsh, M. C., Carlo, W. A., Shankaran, S., ... Higgins, R. D. (2015). Trends in care practices, morbidity, and mortality of extremely preterm neonates, 1993-2012. *JAMA, 314*(10), 1039–1051. doi:10.1001/jama.2015.10244

Sun, D., McCarthy, T. J., & Liberman, D. B. (2017). Cost-effectiveness of watchful waiting in acute otitis media. *Pediatrics, 139*(4), e20163086. doi:10.1542/peds.2016-3086

Turner, P. J., Southern, J., Andrews, N.J. Miller, E., & Erlewyn-Lajeunesse, M. (2015). Safety of live attenuated influenza vaccine in young people with egg allergy: Multicentre prospective cohort study. *BMJ, 351,* h6291. doi:10.1136/bmj.h6291

Udeani, J. (2016). Pediatric epiglottits. *Medscape.* Retrieved from http://emedicine.medscape.com/article/963773

Van der Heijden, M., Dikkers, F. G., & Halmos, G. B. (2016). Treatment of supraglottoplasty vs. wait and see policy in patients with laryngomalacia. *European Archives of Otolaryngology, 273,* 1507–1513. doi:10.1007/s00405-016-3943-3

Vijayakanthi, N., Greally, J. M., & Rastogi, D. (2016). Pediatric obesity-related asthma: The role of metabolic dysregulation. *Pediatrics, 137*(5), e20150812. doi:10.1542/peds.2015-0812

World Health Organization. (2016). *Global tuberculosis report 2016.* Retrieved from http://apps.who.int/iris/bitstream/handle/10665/250441/97?sequence=1

World Health Organization. (2017). *Tuberculosis.* Retrieved from http://www.who.int/mediacentre/factsheets/fs104/en/

12 Cardiovascular Disorders

Kathryn Rudd, DNP, MSN, BSN RN, C-NIC, C-NPT

LEARNING OUTCOMES

Upon completion of this chapter, the student will be able to:

1. Identify the normal assessment of the anatomy and physiology of the pediatric cardiovascular system.
2. Identify the physical assessment components of pediatric clients with cardiovascular disease.
3. Identify the anatomic features, clinical presentation, stabilization, emergent, and long-term care of the pediatric client with cardiovascular disease.
4. Identify the nursing interventions necessary to educate the caregiver to care for a child with cardiovascular disease.
5. Describe the common diagnostic tests used in diagnosing and treating cardiovascular diseases in the pediatric population.
6. Develop a nursing care plan for a child with a cardiac condition.

HEART ANATOMY AND PHYSIOLOGY

The heart is located in the center of the chest and is about the size of a child's fist. Heart rate varies with the age of the child from 60 to 160 beats/min (bpm); the child's heart pumps as hard as an adult's heart. The heart is composed of four chambers: right and left atria, and right and left ventricles (Fig. 12–1).

- The right atrium collects deoxygenated blood from the entire body, except for the lungs.
- The right ventricle pumps deoxygenated blood to the lungs via the pulmonary artery.
- The left atrium collects oxygenated blood from the capillary beds of the lungs through the pulmonary veins.
- The left ventricle pumps oxygenated blood through the aorta to the systemic circulation.

Heart Valves

Four valves prevent blood from regurgitating. The atrioventricular (AV) valves connect the atria and ventricles (Fig. 12–2). These include the tricuspid (three-leafed) valve that connects the right atria and right ventricle, and the bicuspid (two-leafed) valve that connects the left atria and left ventricle. The aortic and pulmonic valves (semilunar or half-moon shaped—three leaves each) include the pulmonic valve that connects the right ventricle and pulmonary artery, and the aortic valve that connects the left ventricle and ascending aorta.

Heart Vessels

- The vena cavae carries blood to the right atrium (Fig. 12–3).
  - The superior vena cava lies above the heart and carries blood from the head, arms, and upper body.
  - The inferior vena cava carries blood from the legs, abdominal cavity, and lower part of the body to the right atrium. It lies below the heart.
- The pulmonary artery carries deoxygenated blood from the right ventricle to the lungs to be oxygenated.
- The pulmonary vein carries oxygenated blood from capillary beds of the lungs to the left atrium and left ventricle.
- The aorta is a large vessel that carries oxygenated blood from the left ventricle to the rest of the body.

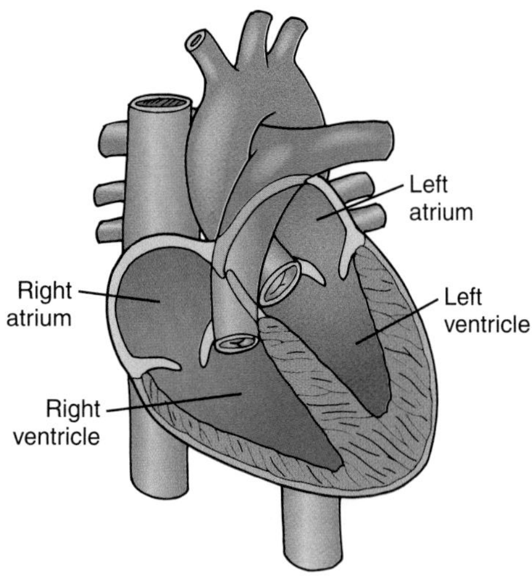

FIGURE 12–1 Chambers of the heart.

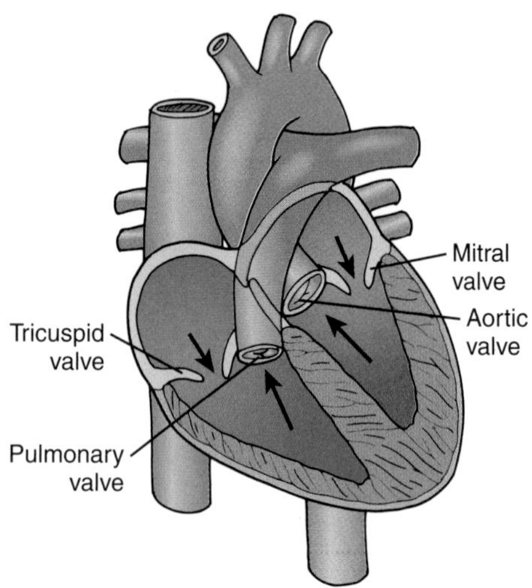

FIGURE 12–2 Valves of the heart.

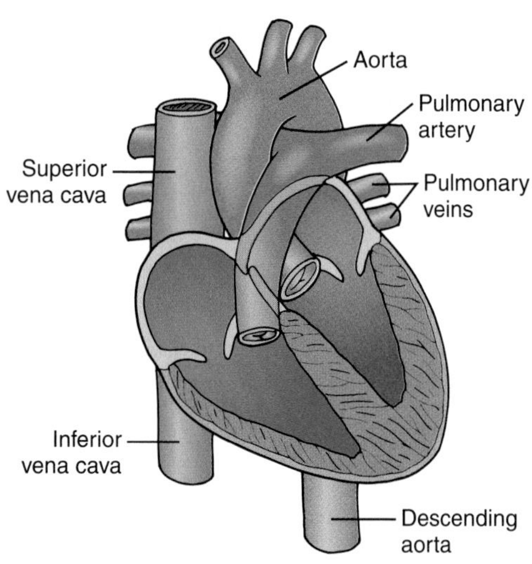

FIGURE 12–3 Vessels of the heart.

Normal Blood Flow

Unoxygenated blood enters the heart through the right atrium and passes through the tricuspid valve into the right ventricle. This unoxygenated blood is pumped through the pulmonary artery, carrying unoxygenated blood to the lungs. Carbon dioxide is exchanged in the lungs and replaced with oxygen. Oxygen-enriched blood is returned to the heart via the pulmonary veins to the left atrium. It passes out of the left atrium through the mitral valve into the left ventricle. Oxygenated blood is then pumped out of the heart through the aortic valve into the aorta and delivered to all of the body's tissues. This oxygenated blood carries the oxygen via hemoglobin to the tissues, which is necessary for cell function (Fig. 12–4).

Cardiac Output

Tissue perfusion is achieved with sufficient cardiac output, the amount of blood ejected from the right or left ventricle per minute. Cardiac output is calculated by multiplying stroke volume × heart rate (measured in L/min).

Stroke Volume

Stroke volume is the amount of blood pumped out of the left ventricle per minute, which is altered by the size of the heart and the heart rate. The Fick calculation is an accurate method to measure stroke volume (Fig. 12–5).

Pressure Gradients

Pressure gradients are necessary for adequate circulation to lungs and body. They are disrupted if the cardiac structures fail to develop or close, are transposed, or become narrowed.

Electrical Conduction

The conduction of the electrical impulses through the heart results in an electrical discharge across the myocardium and is

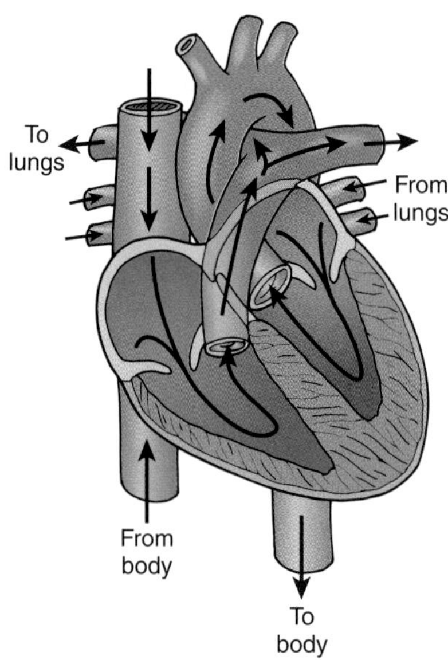

FIGURE 12–4 Normal blood flow.

$$\text{Pulmonary flow } (Q_p) = \frac{Vo_2}{C_{PV} - C_{PA}}$$

$$\text{Systemic flow } (Q_s) = \frac{Vo_2}{C_{AO} - C_{MV}}$$

FIGURE 12–5 Fick calculation.

measured by an electrocardiogram (EKG). The sinoatrial (SA) node in the right atrium, known as the pacemaker of the heart, fires at end of diastole to cause depolarization and contraction of the atria (Fig. 12–6). This results in blood being pumped into the ventricles. It is measured as the P wave on the EKG. The electrical signal moves down to the AV node located between the atria and ventricles.

- The P-Q interval on the EKG reflects slowed conduction to allow the right and left ventricles to fill with blood.
- Electrical impulses move across the fibers called the bundle of His located in the walls of the ventricles.
- Fibers then divide into the right and left bundle branches, Purkinje fibers, in the cell walls of the right and left ventricles. Contraction begins in the walls of the ventricles and is shown in the Q wave of the EKG.
- The left ventricle contracts just before the right ventricle, with the R wave indicating left ventricular contraction and the S wave indicating right ventricular contraction.
- The ventricles then relax and wait for the next signal, which is seen as the T wave on the EKG.

Fetal Circulation

- Before birth, 90% of blood bypasses the lungs; the placenta is the organ of respiration (Fig. 12–7).
- Oxygenated blood is returned via the umbilical vein to the inferior vena cava and to the right atrium.
- Oxygenated blood crosses from the right atrium to the left atrium via the patent foramen ovale (PFO) and is pumped by the left ventricle.
- Deoxygenated blood flows from the superior vena cava to the right atrium and then to the right ventricle, the pulmonary artery, the patent ductus arteriosus (PDA), and the aorta.
- Upon birth and first breath, the foramen ovale and ductus arteriosus close.

CONGENITAL OR ACQUIRED HEART DEFECTS

Heart defects are classified as congenital heart defects or acquired heart defects. Congenital heart defects are genetic, meaning the child is born with the disorder. These defects affect 6 to 8 in 1,000 live births, or 40,000 live births per year (Tsuda, 2016; U.S. Library of Medicine, 2017). Defects can either be a single lesion or multiple abnormalities.

Cyanosis occurs when blood flow to the lungs is insufficient or there is a lack of oxygen in the blood. A large portion of deoxygenated blood is pumped into the systemic circulation when hemoglobin is less than 5 mg/dL (Tsuda, 2016). A decrease in oxygen saturation to 85% with normal hemoglobin levels will result in cyanosis (Ward & Hisley, 2015) (Tables 12–1 and 12–2).

Classifications of Congenital Heart Defects

- Increased pulmonary blood flow—abnormal connection through the septa or the great vessels; increased blood volume on right side of heart with increased pulmonary blood flow and decreased systemic blood flow
  - PDA
  - Atrial septal defects (ASDs)
  - Ventricular septal defects (VSDs)
- Decreased pulmonary blood flow—pulmonary blood flow is obstructed within the right ventricular outflow; desaturated blood shunts from right to left across an ASD or VSD into systemic circulation, and the neonate is likely desaturated and cyanotic
  - Tetralogy of Fallot (TOF)
  - Tricuspid atresia
  - Eisenmenger syndrome
- Obstructive disorders
  - Coarctation of the aorta (COA)
  - Aortic stenosis (AS)
  - Pulmonary stenosis (PS)
  - Pulmonary atresia (PA)
  - TOF with PA
- Mixed disorders—blood from systemic and pulmonary circulations is mixed in the heart chambers, desaturation of blood occurs, and cardiac output decreases because of increased volume load on ventricles
  - Transposition of the great vessels
  - Truncus arteriosus
  - Total anomalous pulmonary venous return (TAPVR)
  - Hypoplastic left heart
  - Ebstein's anomaly

CRITICAL COMPONENT

Genetic Factors in Congenital Cardiac Malformations

Genetic factors are the most common causes of congenital cardiac malformations and account for approximately one-fourth of all congenital malformations (Haroun, 2017). The remainder of congenital malformations have no known cause. The most common type of congenital defects is septal defects such as VSDs or ASDs, followed by valve stenosis, atresia, or regurgitation.

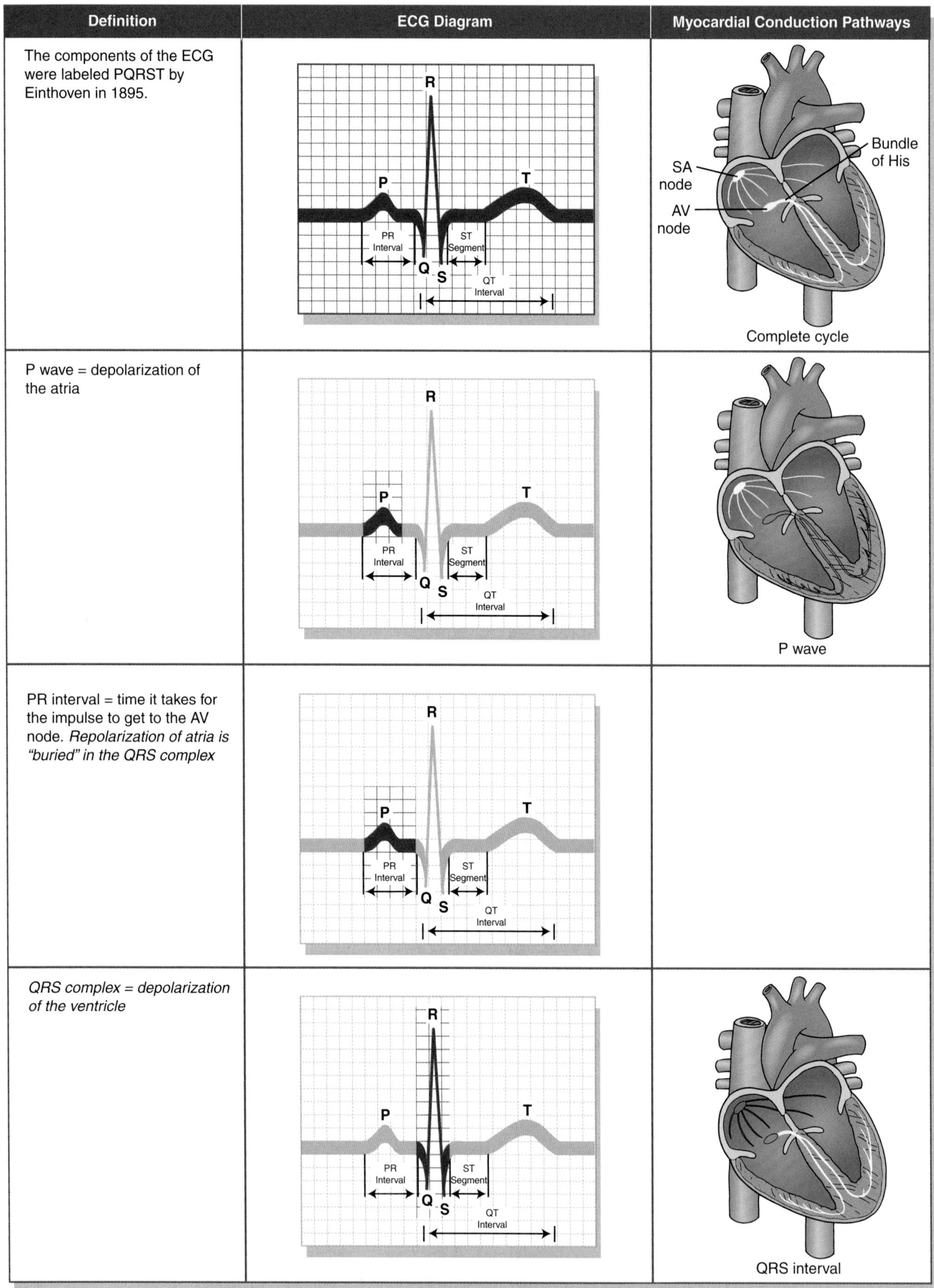

Definition	ECG Diagram	Myocardial Conduction Pathways
The components of the ECG were labeled PQRST by Einthoven in 1895.	R P T PR Interval ST Segment Q S QT Interval	SA node AV node Bundle of His Complete cycle
P wave = depolarization of the atria	R P T PR Interval ST Segment Q S QT Interval	P wave
PR interval = time it takes for the impulse to get to the AV node. *Repolarization of atria is "buried" in the QRS complex*	R P T PR Interval ST Segment Q S QT Interval	
QRS complex = depolarization of the ventricle	R P T PR Interval ST Segment Q S QT Interval	QRS interval

FIGURE 12–6 Conduction of the heart.

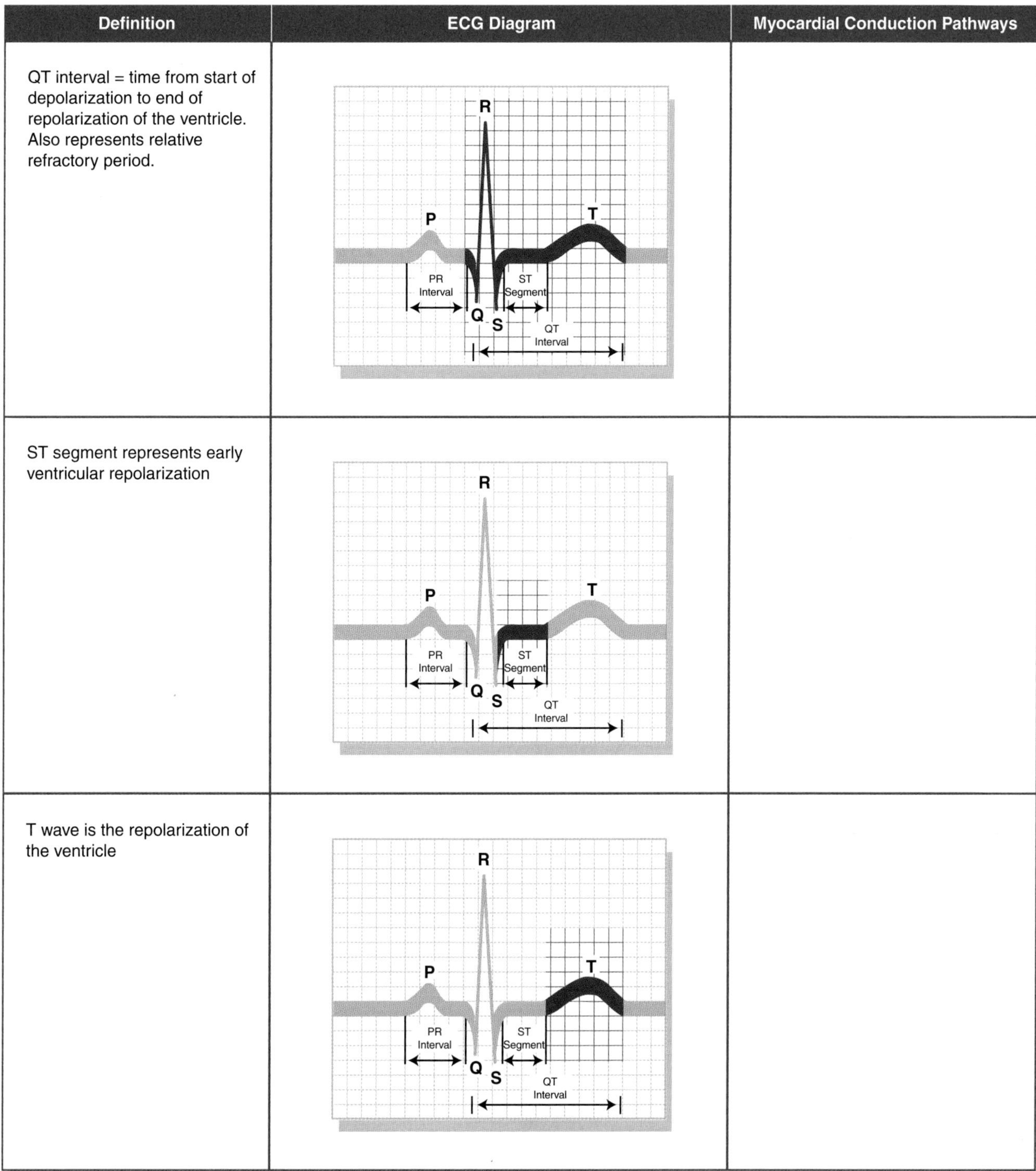

FIGURE 12-6—cont'd

Acquired Heart Disease

- Acquired heart disease can occur in the normal heart or in the heart with a congenital defect. Acquired heart disease is most often due to:
  - Infections
  - Autoimmune factors
  - Genetic factors
  - Teratogens: any inhaled, ingested, or absorbed agent that has the possibility of altering genetic structure or function; these agents are classified as physical, chemical, infectious agents, or maternal conditions
  - Chemical agents: alcohol, angiotensin-converting enzyme (ACE) inhibitors, chemotherapeutic agents, smoking,

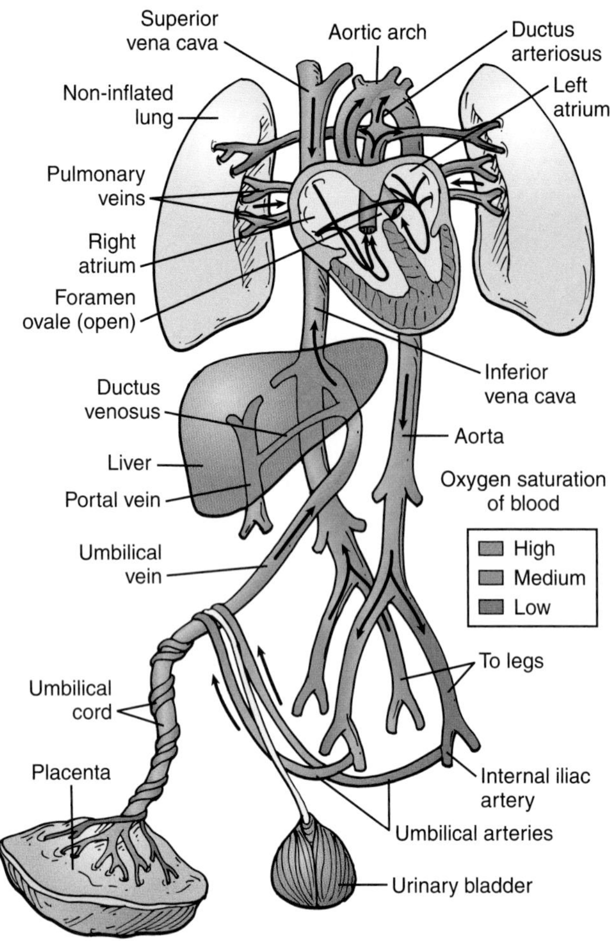

FIGURE 12-7 Fetal circulation.

isotretinoin (Accutane), lithium, cocaine, thalidomide, warfarin (Coumadin), phenytoin (Dilantin), vitamin A, and others

- Infectious agents: cytomegalovirus, rubella, varicella, HIV, toxoplasmosis, herpes, varicella (Hill, 2017)
- Maternal factors: such as infant of a diabetic mother, which can increase risk for neural tube defects, malnutrition, and thyroid disorders (Hill, 2017)
- Physical agents that cause hyperthermia are teratogens: these include exposure of the pregnant women to saunas, hot tubs, or infections in which her body temperature increases to 102°F or higher; this can result in central nervous system disorders or abdominal wall defects (Hill, 2017)

ASSESSMENT

Congenital heart defects often present with vague or no symptoms and may be detected during a general physical assessment.

General History

History for a pediatric client with a cardiovascular disorder should include:

- Comprehensive history and physical examination
- Detailed family history, including history of congenital heart disease or genetic disorders
- Prenatal history, including rapid or slow heart rate in utero, diabetes, or lupus

TABLE 12-1 Classification of Cardiac Defects

CLASS	NAME	PREVALENCE RATE (% OF ALL DEFECTS)	TYPES OR FORMS	ASSOCIATED DEFECTS
L–R shunt	Atrial–septal defect	5–10 (50–100)	Secundum or primum or sinus venosus	PAPVR or MVP
	VSD	20–25 (200–250)	Perimembranous, muscular, multiple	PDA, CoA, AV prolapse
	PDA	5–10 (50–100)	Large shunt or small	
	AV canal	0.02 (0.20)	Complete or partial; balanced or unbalanced	AV regurgitation; 30% of cases occur with Down syndrome
	Partial anomalous pulmonary venous return	<1 (10)	TAPVR	ASD
Obstructive lesions	PS	5–8 (50–80)	Valvular, subvalvular, supravalvular (PA)	VSD, Noonan syndrome
	AS	0.05 (0.50)	Valvular, subvalvular, supravalvular	Bicuspid aortic valve, Williams syndrome, IHSS

TABLE 12-1 Classification of Cardiac Defects—cont'd

CLASS	NAME	PREVALENCE RATE (% OF ALL DEFECTS)	TYPES OR FORMS	ASSOCIATED DEFECTS
	CoA	5–10 (50–100)	Preductal, postductal, ascending aorta, descending aorta	Bicuspid AV, aortic hypoplasia, VSD, PDA, abnormal MV
	Interrupted aortic arch	0.01 (0.10)	Type of coarctation: types A, B, C	PDA, VSD, bicuspid AV, MV deformity, truncus arteriosus, subaortic stenosis
Cyanotic defects	TGA	0.05 (0.50)	D-type, L-type	ASD, VSD, PDA, PS
	Tetralogy of Fallot	0.10 (1.00)	PS or PA or absent PV with PS	May be cyanotic or acyanotic if PS is mild
	TAPVR	0.01 (0.10)	Supracardiac, cardiac draining into right atrium, cardiac draining into the coronary sinus, infracardiac, obstructive	ASD or PFO
	Tricuspid atresia	1–2 (10–20)		ASD, VSD, PDA, CoA, TGA
	PA	<1 (10)	Variable RV sizes	ASD, PFO, or PDA
	Ebstein's anomaly	<1 (10)	Variable degrees of displacement	Wolff-Parkinson-White syndrome, RA hypertrophy, ASD
	Truncus arteriosus	<1 (10)	Types I–IV showing various placements of PA arising from the aorta	Large VSD, right aortic arch, DiGeorge syndrome
	Single ventricle	<1 (10)	DILV or RV	ASD, PS, PA, CoA, VSD, asplenia, polysplenia, TGA
	Double-outlet RV	<1 (10)	Types are by the position of the VSD: subaortic VSD, subpulmonary VSD, remote VSD, subaortic VSD with PS, doubly committed VSD	VSD, PS
	Splenic syndromes	<1 (10)	Asplenia and polysplenia	Various redundant cardiac structures or absence of structures

The numbers in parentheses indicate the number of infants born with defects out of 100,000 live births.

AS, aortic stenosis; ASD, atrial septal defect; AV, atrioventricular; CoA, coarctation of the aorta; DILV, double inlet left ventricle; IHSS, idiopathic hypertrophic subaortic stenosis; MV, mitral valve; MVP, mitral valve prolapse; PA, pulmonary atresia; PAPVR, partial pulmonary venous return; PDA, patent ductus arteriosus; PFO, patent foramen ovale; PS, pulmonary stenosis; PV, pulmonary value; RA, right atrium; RV, right ventricle; TAPVR, total anomalous pulmonary venous return; TGA, transposition of the great arteries; VSD, ventricular septal defect.

Source: Adapted from Judith M. Marshall, 2006.

- Detailed history of exposure to infections, exposure to environmental teratogens such as alcohol, cocaine, phenytoin, or lithium
- Gestational age at birth
- Feeding history, weight gain
- Diaphoresis
- Attainment of developmental milestones
- Respiratory status
- Pain
  - Chest pain is a rare symptom in the pediatric cardiac client.
  - Myocardial infarction (MI) can occur in disease processes such as Kawasaki disease.
  - Chest pain is often due to other conditions, such as costochondritis, musculoskeletal discomforts, skin conditions, or pleural pain.

TABLE 12–2 Syndromes Associated With Cardiac Disease

SYNDROME/DISEASE/ CHROMOSOMAL ABERRATIONS	CARDIAC DEFECT/ CONDITION	OTHER PHYSICAL FINDINGS
Down syndrome	AV canal, VSD	Down's facies, developmental delay
Noonan syndrome	Pulmonic valve stenosis, LVH	Elfin facies, pectus deformity, joint laxity, undescended testes, spine abnormalities, hypotonia, seizures
Williams syndrome	Supravalvular AS, PA stenosis	Williams facies: small, upturned nose, long philtrum (upper lip length), wide mouth, full lips, small chin, and puffiness around the eyes Hypercalcemia, dental abnormalities, renal problems, sensitive hearing, hypotonia, joint laxity, overly friendly personality
DiGeorge or velocardiofacial chromosome	Interrupted aortic arch, truncus arteriosus, VSD, PDA, TOF	Decreased immune response, low-set ears, palate problems, hypoparathyroidism, hypocalcemia
Duchenne's muscular dystrophy	Cardiomyopathy	Generalized weakness and muscle wasting first affecting the muscles of the hips, pelvic area, thighs, and shoulders; calves are often enlarged
Marfan syndrome	Aortic aneurism, aortic and/or mitral regurgitation	Arms disproportionately long, tall, and thin with laxity of joints, dislocation of lenses, spinal problems, stretch marks, hernia, pectus abnormalities, restrictive lung disease
Trisomy 18	VSD, PDA, PS	Multiple joint contractures, spina bifida, hearing loss, radial aplasia (underdevelopment or missing radial bone of forearm), cleft lip, birth defects of the eye
Trisomy 13	VSD, PDA, dextrocardia	Omphalocele, holoprosencephaly (an anatomic defect of the brain involving failure of the forebrain to divide properly), kidney defects, skin defects of the scalp
CHARGE	TOF, truncus arteriosus, vascular ring, interrupted aortic arch	*C*oloboma of the eye, *h*eart defects, *a*tresia of the choanae, *r*etardation of *g*rowth and development, and *e*ar abnormalities and deafness
Fetal alcohol syndrome	VSD, PDA, ASD, TOF	Growth deficiencies, skeletal deformities, facial abnormalities, kidney and urinary defects, central nervous system handicaps, organ deformities: genital malformations
VATER (VACTERLS)	VSD and others	*V*ertebral anomalies, vascular anomalies, *a*nal atresia, *c*ardiac anomalies, *t*racheo–esophageal (T–E) fistula, *e*sophageal atresia, *r*enal anomalies, radial dysplasia, *l*imb anomalies, *s*ingle umbilical artery
Turner syndrome	CoA, ASD, AS	Kidney problems, high blood pressure, overweight, hearing difficulties, diabetes, cataracts, thyroid problems, lack of sexual development, "webbed" neck, low hairline at the back of the neck, drooping of the eyelids, dysmorphic, low-set ears, abnormal bone development, multiple moles

AS, aortic stenosis; ASD, atrial septal defect; AV, atrioventricular; CoA, coarctation of the aorta; LVH, left ventricular hypertrophy; PA, pulmonary atresia; PDA, patent ductus arteriosus; PS, pulmonary stenosis; TOF, tetralogy of Fallot; VSD, ventricular septal defect.

CRITICAL COMPONENT

Family History and Congenital Heart Defects

A family history, especially of siblings, with heart defects indicates a greater risk for congenital heart defects (American Heart Association [AHA], 2015a). Up to a fourth of congenital heart defects are attributed to genetic syndromes and teratogens.

Physical Examination

When caring for pediatric clients with cardiovascular disease, nurses should be aware of the factors discussed in the following subsections.

Possible Indicators of Heart Disease in Children

- Failure to thrive (FTT)
- Small for gestational age
- Poor weight gain
- Dysmorphic features
- Infants who have congenital defects are more likely to have developmental disabilities (Diane & Mvongo, 2017).
- Chest wall deformities, which are a feature of congenital heart disease due to increase in cardiac size, activity, and left-to-right shunting
- Scoliosis is common in adolescents with congenital heart disease
- Clubbing and erythema in fingers and toes (Fig. 12–8)
  - May result from longstanding cyanosis due to increased formation and enlargement of the capillaries in the periphery to improve circulation
  - Excessive growth of soft tissue in fingers and toes
  - Result of chronic hypoxia
  - Polycythemia is an increase in red blood cell mass that increases blood viscosity and limits the body's ability to perfuse the tissues

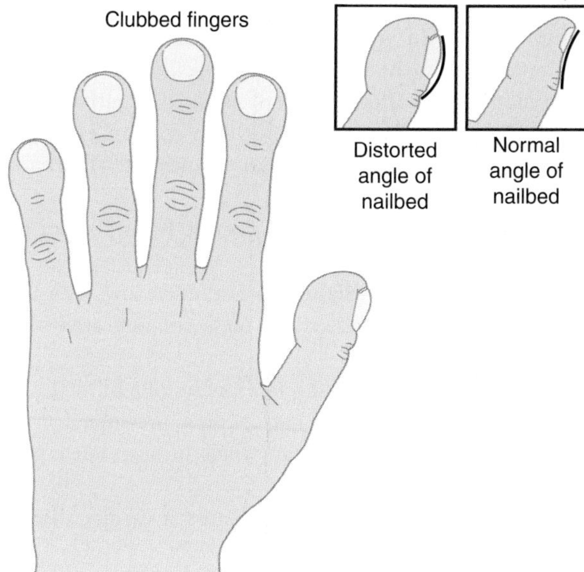

FIGURE 12–8 Clubbing of the fingers.

  - Polycythemia predisposes the child to stroke and clot formation (Nagalla, 2016)

Respiratory System

- Close evaluation of the respiratory rate and evidence of retractions is important in assessing whether the child has a primary respiratory disorder or cardiac disease.
- Shallow, rapid respirations with a rate more than 60 breaths per minute in a content infant are abnormal and need to be investigated because this may indicate a left-to-right shifting of blood in the heart (Slodki, Respondek-Liberska, Pruetz, & Donofrio, 2016).
- Children with congenital heart disease often have respiratory tract infections, resulting in dyspnea with activity and fatigue (Tsuda, 2016).
- Observe closely the infant who develops respiratory distress and cyanosis during feedings or crying because this indicates that the body is not able to deliver the oxygen needed to the tissues during these times of increased demand.
- Respiratory symptoms that may indicate pulmonary edema include increased work of breathing, grunting, nasal flaring, and retractions (Tsuda, 2016).

SAFE AND EFFECTIVE NURSING CARE: Clinical Pearl

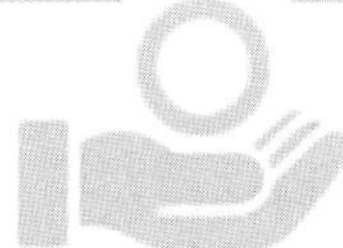

Hyperoxia Test

The hyperoxia test, also known as an oxygen challenge test, is used to determine whether the cyanosis experienced by the neonate is cardiac or respiratory in nature. An arterial blood gas is obtained from the right radial artery when the infant is breathing room air, then obtained again following the placement of an infant in 100% oxygen for 10 minutes. The infant with cardiac disease will have a 25 to 40 mm Hg Pao_2 in room air that will not significantly rise in 100% oxygen, because of continued mixing of oxygenated and nonoxygenated blood. In an infant with pulmonary disease, the PaO_2 will generally rise to more than 80 mm Hg unless there is significant pulmonary hypertension present. This is a screening test only, with exceptions that may occur (Acute Care of At-Risk Newborns Neonatal Society, 2009).

Cardiovascular System

See Table 12–3 for cardiac assessment techniques. The nurse should assess for:

- Level of alertness, activity, and tone
- Chest symmetry and pulsations
- Capillary refill
  - Pressing a central location (sternum or forehead)
  - Normal is less than or equal to 3 seconds
  - Prolonged capillary refill indicates poor cardiac output and perfusion (Oster et al., 2016)

TABLE 12–3 Cardiac Assessment Techniques

ASSESSMENT TECHNIQUE	WHAT TO LOOK FOR	NORMAL FINDINGS	ABNORMAL FINDINGS	RATIONALE
Inspection	Skin color, shape, and symmetry of chest, clubbing	Pink, symmetrical chest	Pallor, cyanosis, asymmetry of chest shape and movement, hyperdynamic precordium	Poor cardiac output; deoxygenated circulating blood, ventricular failure or hypertrophy, tachycardia
Palpation	Skin and body temperature, moisture, chest movement, point of maximal impulse (PMI)	Warm, dry, symmetrical movement, PMI at 4th or 5th intercostal space (ICS) at midclavicular line	Cold extremities, dry flaky skin, diaphoresis, thrills or heaves	Poor circulation, heart failure, ventricular hypertrophy
Percussion	Heart shape and size	Normal size and shape for age and weight	Enlarged heart, axis deviation	Heart failure and hypertrophy
Auscultation	Murmurs, other sounds	No murmurs, innocent murmurs; quiet precordium	Murmurs, clicks, rubs, snaps	Structural defects, increased workload of heart, and volume overload

Source: Judith M. Marshall, 2006.

Pulses

- Pulse volume is rate from 0 to 4: 0 = absent, 1+ = weak, 2+ = average, 3+ = strong, 4+ = bounding.
- When normal, usually easy to feel in a child.
- Heart for infants is 160 beats/min, preschool children 120 beats/min, and adolescents 100 beats/min.
- Include radial, carotid, brachial, and femoral pulses.
- Should be equal in strength between right and left arms and upper and lower extremities.
- Pulses that are bounding in upper extremities and decreased in lower extremities may indicate COA.
- Pulses that are bounding may suggest systemic hypertension or PDA.
- Cardiac pulsations are seen in subaortic stenosis.
- Peripheral pulses are indicators of cardiac output, systolic pressure, and diastolic pressure.
- Pulses that are difficult to palpate may indicate poor cardiac output, shock, or obstructive outflow lesions (Slodki et al., 2016).
- Bounding pulses indicate excessive fluid volume.
- Pedal pulses are found on the top of the foot (dorsalis pedis) and the medial malleolus (posterior tibial).
- Peripheral edema is the measurement of edema in the extremities. Edema is rated from +1, slight edema less than one-quarter inch and disappears immediately; +2 edema, which is less than one-half inch and disappears in 10 to 15 seconds; +3 edema, which is less than 1 inch and disappears in 1 to 2 minutes; and +4 edema, which is more than 1 inch and disappears after 2 to 5 minutes (Kumarasinghe & Carroll, 2015).
- Thrills—palpation of vibrating sensations due to rapid flow blood from an area of higher pressure to an area of lower pressure; always an abnormal finding (Oster et al., 2016).
- Temperature of the extremities—cold feet or hands in comparison with torso suggests poor perfusion beyond 8 hours after birth (Tsuda, 2016).

Blood Pressure

- Blood pressure (BP) should be assessed by Doppler with the proper size of cuff.
- Use a nonthreatening approach; the child may sit on parent's lap depending on age.
- BP varies with gestational age, weight, or postnatal age.
- In newborns, the mean arterial pressure is measured in millimeters of mercury (mm Hg) and is usually the newborn's completed age in weeks. BP is not a routine part of the neonatal assessment in the normal newborn (Durham & Chapman, 2014). If taken, the BP is taken on either the arm or leg. Normal BPs range from 50 to 75 mm Hg systolic and 30 to 45 mm Hg diastolic in the neonate (Durham & Chapman, 2014).
- In older children, the minimum systolic BP is 70 mm Hg + (2 × age in years).
- Wide pulse pressures—diastolic pressures are low, with a wide gap between diastolic and systolic pressures; indicative of such processes as PDA.
- Poor cardiac output will result in a low systolic BP with a high diastolic pressure, creating a narrow pulse pressure.
- Noninvasive BPs are less accurate when the heart rate is greater than 200 bpm.
- Four limb extremity BPs are indicated if cardiac disease is suspected or murmur is present.
- Distended or pulsating neck veins require investigation (American Academy of Pediatrics [AAP], 2017).

- Hepatomegaly, where the liver is felt more than 3 cm below the right costal margin, indicates increased right arterial pressure and is highly suggestive of congestive heart failure (CHF) (Postma, Bezzina, & Christoffels, 2016).

SAFE AND EFFECTIVE NURSING CARE: Clinical Pearl

Critical Congenital Heart Defects

In 2011, newborn critical congenital heart defects screening was added to the U.S. Recommended Screening Panel and is performed in all states and the District of Columbia (Oster et al., 2016). This test is used to screen for seven major congenital heart defects: hypoplastic left heart syndrome, PA, TOF, TAPVR, transposition of the great vessels, tricuspid atresia, and truncus arteriosus. This test is performed on all newborns to detect hypoxemia using pulse oximetry with the newborn being older than 24 hours. One pulse oximeter probe is placed on the right hand (preductal) and one on either foot (postductal). If either reading is less than 90% it is considered a failure (Oster et al., 2016). If either reading is greater than or equal to 95% and the difference between the two readings is less than or equal to 3%, the result is considered a pass (Oster et al., 2016). Results outside of these ranges require a repeat within 1 hour up to two additional times (Oster et al., 2016). Pulse oximetry is not a replacement for a complete history and physical examination (AHA, 2015b).

SAFE AND EFFECTIVE NURSING CARE: Clinical Pearl

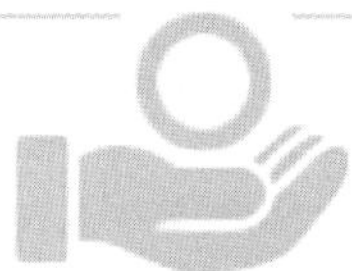

Blood Pressure Cuffs

BP cuffs should measure 25% greater than the width of the extremity. Undersized BP cuffs will give the nurse a falsely high BP reading, whereas an oversized cuff will give the nurse a falsely low BP reading (Jahangir, 2015). BPs should be compared between the upper and lower extremities because a BP 20 mm Hg greater than that of the lower extremity is indicative of aortic arch abnormalities (Jahangir, 2015).

Color

- Cyanosis is the bluish discoloration of the skin, nail beds, tongue, or mucosa.
- Cyanosis is always an abnormal finding. Cyanosis is also influenced by anemia (low hematocrit) or polycythemia (high hematocrit).
- Central cyanosis seen by bluish discoloration of mucous membranes, tongue, circumoral, or core body is due to problems with the heart or lungs.
- Elevated levels of deoxygenated hemoglobin, which is blue, are present.
- Peripheral cyanosis (acrocyanosis) is often due to interruption in blood flow to the extremity. Acrocyanosis is normal during the transition of the newborn.
- Shock can be seen with a prolonged capillary refill time, and pallor is associated with poor perfusion (AAP, 2017).
- Pulse oximeter readings of 78% or lower with normal hemoglobin levels will result in outward signs of cyanosis (AAP, 2017).
- Anemia may not show cyanosis because of decreased levels of hemoglobin; polycythemia may show cyanosis with a smaller amount of deoxygenated hemoglobin.
- Quiet pericardium combined with cyanosis is often an indicator of congenital heart disease (Altman, 2017).
- Skin that is pale, mottled, or gray in appearance indicates poor perfusion.
- Urine output is indicative of perfusion to the kidneys.

SAFE AND EFFECTIVE NURSING CARE: Clinical Pearl

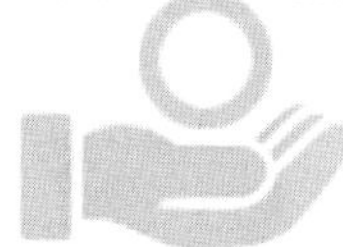

Acrocyanosis

Acrocyanosis can occur when blood flow is interrupted because of constriction (BP cuff or tourniquet) or vasoconstriction caused by temperature changes. Acrocyanosis is very common at birth during the period of transition of the newborn and is seen as bluish discoloration of the hands and feet (Dani, Drovandi, Bertini, Poggi, & Pratesi, 2017).

Auscultation

- Heart sounds heard with diaphragm and bell of the stethoscope (Fig. 12–9)
  - S_1 (lub sound) is heard at the 4th or 5th intercostal space at the midclavicular line—the closure of the mitral (heard at apex of heart) and tricuspid valve (heard at left sternal border) (Ward & Hisley, 2015).

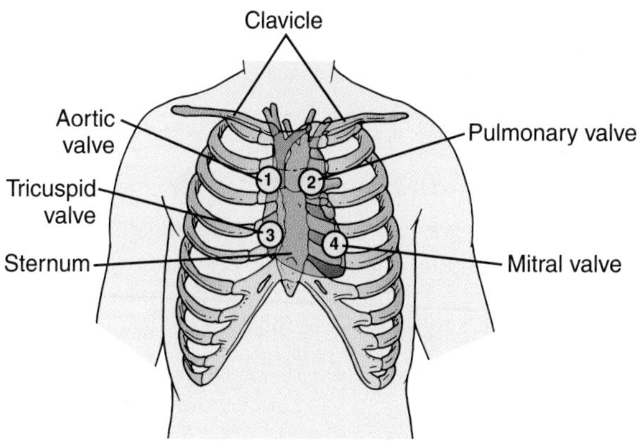

FIGURE 12–9 Cardiac auscultation landmarks.

- S_2 (dub sound) is heard at the closure of the pulmonic and aortic valves. May be split. Single S_2 is due to absent flow or obstruction in flow to aortic or pulmonic valves (Ward & Hisley, 2015).
- S_3, S_4 gallop—considered normal before the age of 20 years (Altman, 2017).
- Point of maximum impulse—area of most intense pulsation heard by a stethoscope
  - In children younger than 7 years, located at left midclavicular line and 4th intercostal space
  - In children older than 7 years, located along the left sternal border in the 5th intercostal space
- Hyperactive precordium (during auscultation the heart sounds are magnified) or shift in the point of maximum impulse indicates consideration of dextrocardia or pneumothorax (Tsuda, 2016)
- Precordial activity
- Tachycardias—fast heart rates
- Bradycardias—slow heart rates
- Distant or muffled heart sounds
- Murmurs are heart sounds that are due to turbulent blood flow; assess for intensity, location, duration, and quality
- Diastolic and continuous murmurs are usually pathological (Shea, 2016)
- Innocent murmurs (e.g., systolic, vibratory, musical) are present in many children (Table 12–4) due to thin chest walls in the child and hyperactive heart sounds (Shea, 2016)

TABLE 12–4 Murmurs

Murmurs grade 1–6 (1 being softest, 6 being loudest). Not every murmur is a sign of valve disease (AHA, 2016b).

Holosystolic	Shunting of blood from an area of higher pressure to an area of lower pressure such as in a ventricular septal defect, which are harsh murmurs, and atrioventricular regurgitation, which are soft murmurs
Ejection systolic	As blood flow increases in systole there is turbulence through restricted flow patterns, such as in pulmonary stenosis or aortic stenosis
Diastolic	Regurgitation of blood flow from the aorta or pulmonary artery into the ventricles because of pulmonary or aortic insufficiency; always abnormal
Systolic and diastolic	Result of pressure differences between two structures, such as in patent ductus arteriosus
Pansystolic	Heard with congestive heart disease or severe regurgitation of mitral or tricuspid valves
Continuous	Heard with patent ductus arteriosus or atrioventricular malformations

Adapted from American Heart Association. (2016). Heart murmurs and valve disease. *Retrieved from http://www.heart.org/HEARTORG/Conditions/More/HeartValveProblemsandDisease/Heart-Murmurs-and-Valve-Disease_UCM_450616_Article.jsp#.WQ9T4vkrKiQ*

Diagnostic Tests

- Diagnostic tests for pediatric clients with cardiovascular issues may include chest x-ray, blood gases, EKG, echocardiogram, angiography, cardiac catheterization, biopsy of the myocardium, and pulmonary artery banding.

Chest X-ray

Chest x-rays, including anteroposterior and lateral views indicate:

- Pulmonary vascularity
- Cardiac size and shape
- Lung vascular markings
- Position of the stomach

Blood Gases

- Metabolic acidosis shows as a decrease in pH and an increase in base excess.
- Base excess is the accumulation of metabolic acids in the blood.
- It is monitored by arterial, venous, or capillary blood.
- In cardiac disease, the partial pressure of carbon dioxide is generally within normal ranges.

Electrocardiogram

- Useful to determine conduction issues
- Needs to be evaluated by a cardiologist

Echocardiogram

- Ultrasound of the heart
- Noninvasive test that indicates structure, size, flow patterns, function, and the blood vessels attached to the heart

Angiography

- Visualizes the structure and function of the ventricles
- Dye injected via a catheter

Cardiac Catheterization

Nurses must provide caregiver education about the procedure, in which small catheters or small, flexible tubes are inserted through small incisions in the neck or groin and threaded to the heart. These small tubes allow for blood samples to be taken, x-rays (fluoroscopy) to be done, and small instruments to be carried to the heart if repairs are needed (Ward & Hisley, 2015).

- Invasive diagnostic procedure that takes place in a cardiac catheterization laboratory
- Cannulization of a vein, usually in the groin or neck area, to pass a catheter into the heart or major vessels of the heart after the child is anesthetized
- Advanced with the use of x-ray fluoroscopy
- Interventional catheters used to open valves or septum in the heart
- Diagnostic catheters used to measure internal pressures or to visualize circulation
- Electrophysiological catheters used to evaluate conduction pathways or alter accessory pathways to avoid surgical intervention; can be used to measure pressures within the ventricles and vessels

- Cardiac catheterization can be used to perform myocardial biopsies
- Temporary measures to delay reparative surgeries

Biopsy of the Myocardium

- Frequent in heart transplants
- Monitors for rejection

Pulmonary Artery Banding

- Palliative measure to decrease pulmonary blood flow
- Prevents pulmonary hypertrophy and pulmonary hypertension
- Precursor to cardiac surgery, such as in large VSDs

SAFE AND EFFECTIVE NURSING CARE: Promoting Safety

Nursing Care During Cardiac Catheterization

Cardiac catheterization is used to obtain pressures in the child's heart and vessels, to take x-rays of the heart, to obtain myocardial biopsies, or to perform corrective procedures.

- Nursing care is aimed at alleviating preprocedure and post-procedure anxiety and complications.
- Preparation and postoperative care depends on developmental age and parent involvement.
- A sedative will be administered before the procedure to make the child sleepy, and a local anesthetic will be injected in the femoral vein or artery site before cannulization of the catheter.
- In catheterization with contrast dye, nursing care should emphasize intake and output.
- Keep extremities straight for 4 to 6 hours with no movement; child should be positioned flat on the back; a sandbag may be used on the extremity.
- A Foley catheter may be used.
- Check pulses above and below catheter site.
- Monitor for bleeding with a pressure dressing for 24 hours, then dry occlusive dressing.
- Auscultate for abnormal heart rate or rhythm and compare with preoperative assessment.
- Monitor for temperature changes or color changes in the arm or leg that is used for the catheterization.
- No tub baths for several days; showers are fine.
- Observe for signs and symptoms of infections such as redness, fever, pain, thrombus formation, dysrhythmias, bleeding, and perfusion. Fever is common following catheterization but should not last longer than 24 hours or go above 100°F.
- Avoid strenuous activity such as lifting, sports, or physical education, although school is appropriate.
- Notify the physician if there is any yellow or green drainage or chest pain.
- Regular diet can be consumed.
- Return to school within 3 days.
- Follow-up appointments are essential.

(AHA, 2017)

Caregiver Education

The nurse should discuss limitations in physical activity for the pediatric cardiology client with the physician, child, and caregiver. Emotional support may be required because the child may feel different from peers because of frequent hospitalizations; this may result in feelings of isolation, sadness, or abnormality. Behavioral issues may occur because of extreme illness or jealous sibling interactions.

The nurse should provide education to the child and caregiver about the need for follow-up by a cardiologist for the rest of the child's life. The need to transition to an adult cardiologist should be discussed with teens. Endocarditis prevention is necessary for some children prior to many dental or medical procedures. Teen girls should be counseled by nurses and physicians related to birth control, because certain congenital heart defects can predispose a teen to higher risks from birth control pills and intrauterine devices. People with certain congenital heart defects may be at a higher risk of having children with congenital heart defects.

SAFE AND EFFECTIVE NURSING CARE: Promoting Safety

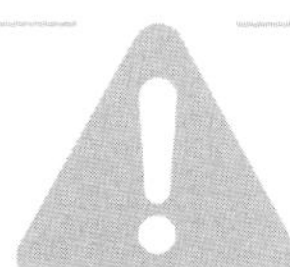

To prevent bacterial endocarditis, antibiotics need to be prescribed for all dental and surgical procedures with high-risk valvular clients, including prosthetic valvular repairs. The child and caregivers must notify their health-care providers of their valvular history (Nishimura et al., 2017; Sexton, 2017).

CONGENITAL HEART DISEASE WITH INCREASED PULMONARY BLOOD FLOW

Congenital heart defects that increase blood flow to the lungs, often resulting in pulmonary edema, include patent ductus arteriosus, atrial septal defect, and ventricular septal defect.

Patent Ductus Arteriosus

The ductus arteriosus connects the aorta to the pulmonary artery outside of the heart. Left-to-right shunting occurs through the duct that will then connect the pulmonary artery (nonoxygenated) with the aorta (oxygenated) (Fig. 12–10; for blood flow, see fetal circulation in Fig. 12–7). The pulmonary artery and the cardiac ducts are lined with smooth muscle tissues that normally close within a few hours to days after birth. Most ducts close nearly 100% within 72 hours with full-term infants, and the incidence of them staying open or opening increases as the gestational age of the infant decreases (Prescott & Keim-Malpass, 2017). In preterm infants, 10% of infants

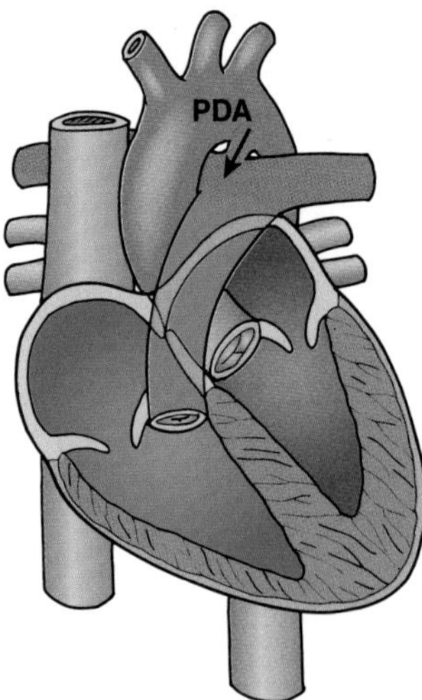

FIGURE 12–10 Patent ductus arteriosus (PDA).

born between 30 and 37 weeks' gestation and 80% of preterm infants between 25 and 28 weeks remain open after 4 days of life (Benitz, 2016).

In fetal life, pulmonary vascular resistance is high due to fluid in the lungs rather than air because the placenta is the organ of respiration in the fetus. Prostaglandins produced by the placenta and decreased partial pressure of oxygen in fetal circulation maintain open ducts in utero (Prescott & Keim-Malpass, 2017).

Following birth, peripheral vascular resistance decreases and the ducts close because of the production of bradykinin in the lungs and an increase in neonatal blood oxygen levels (Prescott & Keim-Malpass, 2017). Increase in oxygen levels causes muscular constriction around the ducts (Prescott & Keim-Malpass, 2017). The severity of the disease depends on the gestational age of the neonate, the size of the ductal opening, and the degree of pulmonary vascular resistance.

SAFE AND EFFECTIVE NURSING CARE: Promoting Safety

Preventing Bacterial Endocarditis

PDA predisposes the child to the development of bacterial endocarditis caused by irritation of the smooth muscle tissue of the pulmonary artery resulting in a more favorable medium for bacterial growth (Nishimura et al., 2017). Preventive antibiotics are used to prevent the development of bacterial endocarditis before procedures. These procedures may be dental, oral, or respiratory.

Assessment

PDA may be indicated by:

- Heart murmur—systolic murmur, mid- to lower-left sternal border, washing machine sound
- Some infants will have no murmur
- "Wet"-sounding breath sounds known as crackles
- Tachypnea
- Increased work of breathing, or apnea
- Poor feeding
- Poor weight gain and growth pattern
- Fatigue
- Sweating with feeding
- Excessive fluid weight gain

Diagnostic Tests

- Wide pulse pressures—low diastolic pressures
- Increased vascular markings on the chest x-ray are a late sign due to enlarged heart
- Poor oxygen saturation
- Bounding pulses
- Enlarged heart
- Prolonged capillary filling time
- Hyperactive precordium
- An echocardiogram will show increased enlargement of left heart chambers (Ward & Hisley, 2015)

Nursing Interventions

- Provide postoperative care after coil embolization or ligation.
- Decrease work of breathing by providing frequent rest periods that maximize oxygen delivery to the tissues
- Provide frequent rest periods.
- Do not cluster care because clustering care can result in an increased oxygen demand during the clustering.
- Provide strict intake and output fluid restrictions and diuretics as ordered.
- Dopamine may be required.
- Administer digoxin (Lanoxin) as ordered.
- Maintain indomethacin and ibuprofen administration, which is dependent on weight, renal function, and gestational age.
- Monitor urine output.
- Monitor laboratory tests for thrombocytopenia.
- Monitor daily weights.
- Monitor tolerance of feedings.
- Provide preparation of child for surgical closure.
- Monitor closely following postsurgical closure.
- Monitor wound care.

Evidence-Based Practice: Clustering Care

Valizadeh, L., Avazeh, M., Hosseini, M. B., & Jafarabad, M. A. (2014). Comparison of clustered care with three and four procedures on physiological responses of preterm infants: Randomized crossover clinical trial. *Journal of Caring Science, 3*(1), 1–10. doi:10.5681/jcs.2014.001

Clustering care is effective in promoting the circadian and homeostatic equilibriums of sleep during acute critical care. Recent studies indicate that clustering care over the long term may actually reduce the neonate's and infant's periods of growth and adaptability to pain. The decision to cluster care is dependent on the diagnosis of the heart defect and may or may not be beneficial.

Medical Management

Medical management includes using NSAIDS that inhibit cyclooxygenase-1 (COX-1) or COX-2.

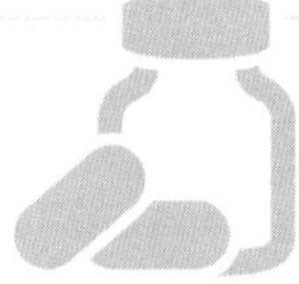

SAFE AND EFFECTIVE NURSING CARE: Understanding Medication

Ibuprofen, Indomethacin, and Paracetamol

Ibuprofen results in complete cessation of ductal flow by facilitating necrosis of the intima of the ductus arteriosus. Side effects of ibuprofen include pulmonary hypertension, kidney damage, or retinopathy of prematurity (Prescott & Keim-Malpass, 2017). Indomethacin has been the conventional drug of choice, but some clients have more adverse side effects than with ibuprofen (Prescott & Keim-Malpass, 2017). Side effects of indomethacin include renal insufficiency, necrotizing enterocolitis, gastrointestinal bleeding, gastrointestinal perforation, or bleeding disorders (Prescott & Keim-Malpass, 2017; Vallerand, Sanoski, & Deglin, 2017).

Acetaminophen (Paracetamol) is an alternative to ibuprofen and has been shown in studies to have similar closure of the PDA rates as ibuprofen with a decreased need for extra oxygen, a decreased risk for hyperbilirubinemia, and possibly fewer side effects (Ohlsson & Shah, 2015).

Surgical Management

- Ligation of the duct through a posterior-lateral thoracotomy for infants requiring increasing respiratory or cardiovascular support
- A stainless-steel coil occlusion of the PDA is also used through cardiac catheterization

Child and Caregiver Education

- Closely monitor oral intake.
- Closely monitor diapers for urine output.
- Monitor for signs and symptoms of irritability and/or lethargy.
- Keep cardiology appointments.
- Continue diuretics.

Atrial Septal Defect

ASDs occur between the right and left atrium when the two septal walls fail to form (Fig. 12–11). The septal walls normally close between weeks 4 and 8 of fetal development but may remain open up to 1 year (Ward & Hisley, 2015). This defect allows more blood to flow into the right side of the heart from the left atrium, increasing pulmonary blood flow to the lungs through a hole in the atria. This defect may result in pulmonary hypertension with right atrial enlargement that can lead to right ventricular hypertrophy. A left-to-right mixing or shunting of blood may occur at the PFO (a necessary fetal structure) or through the septal defect. This may increase the incidence of stroke in unrepaired ASDs and

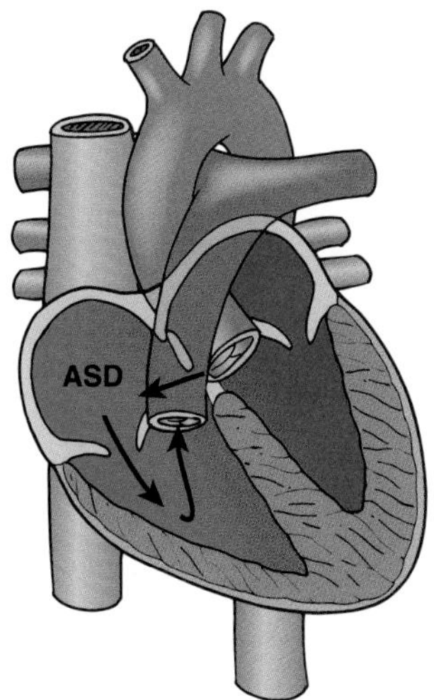

FIGURE 12–11 Atrial septal defect.

produces a fixed split-second heart sound caused by right ventricular overload.

Assessment

- Heart murmur known as ejection systolic murmur because of blood being forced through pulmonary valve
- Atrial dysrhythmias
- Higher incidence of emboli
- Recurrent respiratory infections
- Few symptoms in children
- Shortness of breath
- Tires easily with playing
- Poor feeding
- Poor growth if CHF develops due to left-to-right shunting
- Liver enlargement or congestion

Diagnostic Tests

- Echocardiogram shows enlargement of right atrium and right ventricle.
- EKG shows thickening of the heart muscle.
- Chest x-ray shows enlargement of the heart and an increase in blood flow to the lungs.
- Transesophageal ultrasound takes a picture of the heart to visualize blood vessels or heart disease or conditions.

Medical Management

- Administer medications, such as digoxin and diuretics, to decrease the load on the right side of the heart.
- Surgical closure may increase the incidence of pulmonary hypertension, resulting in dysrhythmias, and surgical clients may experience a greater mortality risk.
- Provide pain medications as ordered to decrease oxygen consumption.

Surgical Repair

- Closure with cardiac catheterization—trans-septal closure across the defect with transthoracic echocardiography

- Surgical repair can also be performed by patching with the child's own tissue, bovine tissue, or artificial structures

Nursing Interventions

- Monitor feeding tolerance; offer small, frequent feedings with infants and small children.
- Monitor for signs and symptoms of CHF.
- Monitor for increased work of breathing, grunting, retractions, and flaring.
- Monitor growth patterns.

Caregiver Education

- Educate on care of the child after cardiac catheterization, which includes monitoring for bleeding at the catheter insertion site.
- Surgical closures with a patch may result in arrhythmias.
- Monitor for increase in temperature and changes in color or temperature of the catheterized extremity.
- The child may need to be prescribed blood thinners for several months after the procedure.
- Educate on risk for embolization because of dislodgement of the patch.
- The child may need to take antibiotics for dental work after treatment (Nishimura et al., 2017).
- Monitor for cyanosis, poor weight gain, respiratory distress, lethargy, and bleeding at insertion site after the procedure.
- Provide caregiver information related to the schedule of yearly close follow-up appointments with cardiologist.

Ventricular Septal Defect

VSD is the most common overall congenital heart disease (Fig. 12–12). This defect forms at weeks 4 to 8 of fetal development (Ward & Hisley, 2015). The degree of clinical presentation is dependent on the size of the defect, with up to 75% of small defects closing spontaneously (AHA, 2016f). VSD results in right ventricular hypertrophy with left-to-right shunting that produces an increase in pulmonary blood flow that decreases pulmonary compliance. This results in stiffening of the lungs with ineffective ventilation. This defect can occur anywhere on the ventricular septum either in one defect or several (also known as Swiss cheese VSD) (Ward & Hisley, 2015).

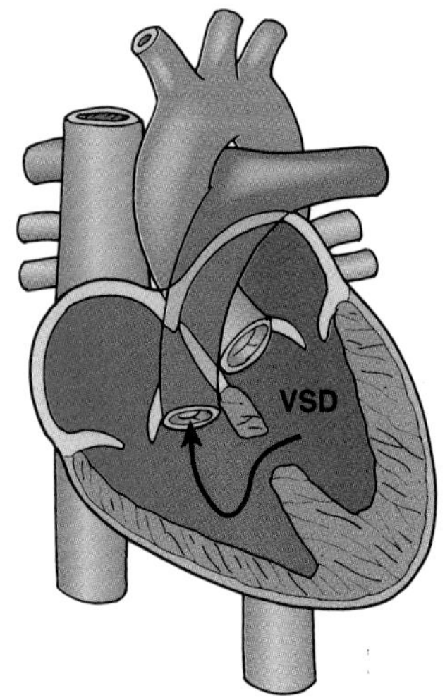

FIGURE 12–12 Ventricular septal defect (VSD).

Assessment

- Often asymptomatic or with a heart murmur
- Shortness of breath
- Feeding difficulties
- Murmur
- Systolic thrill in lower left sternal border
- FTT
- Recurrent respiratory infections (Ward & Hisley, 2015)

Diagnostic Testing

- Echocardiogram—large left atrium
- Chest x-ray—cardiomegaly of left heart and increased pulmonary vascularity
- Cardiac catheterization

Surgical Repair

Occurs through suturing if the defect is small or patching through a surgical sternotomy. The defect is repaired within the first 6 to 12 months of life and when the infant weighs more than 2,000 g. Complications from the surgery can include dysrhythmias.

Nursing Interventions

- Same as for ASD

Caregiver Education

- Similar to that for ASD
- Manage postoperative care

SAFE AND EFFECTIVE NURSING CARE: Clinical Pearl

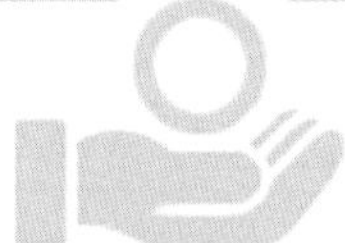

Ventricular Septal Defects

In VSDs, chest x-rays show the shunting of blood from the left ventricle into the right ventricle. Increased pulmonary blood flow is indicated by an increase in pulmonary vascular markings. The right ventricle of the heart will indicate hypertrophy and cardiomegaly, which is an abnormal enlargement of the heart.

CONGENITAL HEART DISEASE WITH DECREASED PULMONARY BLOOD FLOW

Congenital heart defects that decrease or interrupt the amount of blood flow to the lungs include tetralogy of Fallot, tricuspid atresia, and Eisenmenger syndrome.

Tetralogy of Fallot

TOF is the third most common lesion and is classified as a non-ductal cyanotic heart defect (Fig. 12–13) (Centers for Disease Control and Prevention [CDC], 2016c). This defect is associated with 22 deletion chromosome disorders such as DiGeorge and Down syndromes. TOF occurs more frequently in males than females (CDC, 2016c). This cardiac defect results in right-to-left shunting of blood in the heart, which recirculates venous blood to the body without it being oxygenated in the lungs. Tetralogy (or "tetra") means "four"; this type of cyanotic heart disease comprises four separate defects:

- VSD between right and left ventricles
- Obstructive right ventricular outflow—PS or obstruction
- Overriding aorta lies directly over VSD and takes blood from both the right and left ventricles; permits oxygenated blood to rest of body
- Secondary thickening of right ventricle (right ventricular hypertrophy) due to restrictive outflow

Assessment

- Right-to-left shunting
- "Tet" spells—sudden, marked increase in cyanosis; syncope; can lead to hypoxic brain injury and death
- Pink tet spells are due to left-to-right shunting
- Increased cyanosis with irritability and crying
- Increased irritability because of lack of oxygen
- Clubbing of fingers
- Poor growth in response to chronic lack of oxygen

SAFE AND EFFECTIVE NURSING CARE: Clinical Pearl

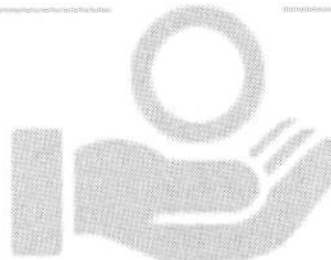

"Tet" Spells

Children may squat during a tet spell to improve blood flow from legs back to brain and vital organs, increasing systemic vascular resistance (Bhimji, 2016).

Clinical Indicators

The following clinical indicators may be present at birth or within first year of life:

- PDA causes increased blood flow to lungs
- Profound cyanosis is rare
- Heart murmur may be soft to loud
- Failure to gain weight
- Fainting
- Dyspnea on exertion
- Polycythemia
- Boot-shaped heart, right ventricular hypertrophy, and small pulmonary artery
- As PDA closes, cyanosis increases

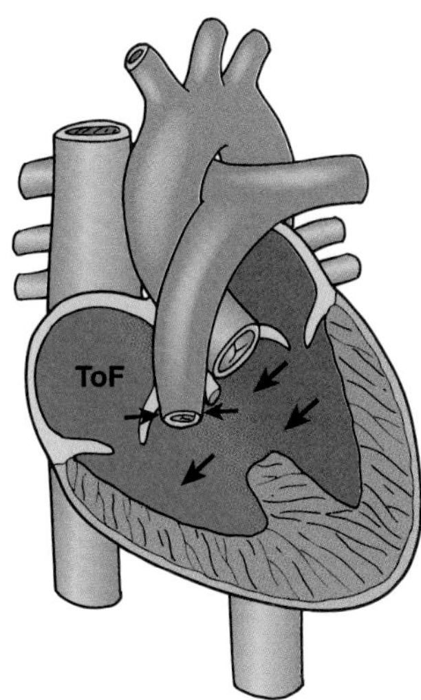

FIGURE 12–13 Tetralogy of Fallot (TOF).

- Degree of cyanosis is dependent on restriction of blood flow to lungs
- Child remains pink with a low degree of mixing; known as "pink tet" (Bhimji, 2016)

Nursing Interventions

- Improve oxygenation through clustering care to allow for adequate rest periods. The nurse should continue sedative or morphine sulfate to decrease agitation and prevent inconsolable crying, which will decrease pulmonary blood flow and increase the incidence of tet spells. The nurse should maintain fluid balance to prevent fluid overload, which increases the workload on the heart.
- Provide oxygen to reduce pulmonary vasoconstriction, but note that this will not improve oxygen saturation or alleviate the cyanosis.
- The nurse should maintain vasopressors to increase systemic vascular resistance and prostaglandin E1 drip as ordered to keep PDA open (Table 12–5).
- The nurse should prepare the family for possibility of multiple surgeries, beginning with a VSD patch and resection to alleviate the PS, and the possibility of additional procedures such as a modified Blalock–Taussig procedure if the infant has severe PS or PA.

Caregiver Education

- Teach the family to calm the infant by holding the infant over the caregiver's shoulders with the child's knees drawn up toward the chest. This will increase the blood flow to the lungs.
- Support the family in asking questions related to physical activity restrictions and pharmacological regimen.
- Support the caregiver's access to a pediatric cardiologist for the child's lifelong care.

Tricuspid Atresia

Tricuspid atresia is a heart condition in which the tricuspid valve is either defective or missing (Fig. 12–14). This defect blocks the

SAFE AND EFFECTIVE NURSING CARE: Understanding Medication

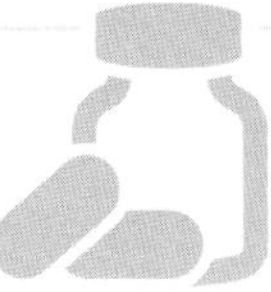

Prostaglandin E1

Prostaglandin E1 is a potent vasodilator on smooth muscle tissue that keeps the foramen ovale and the ductus arteriosus open. Action is within a few minutes and results in improved pulmonary and systemic blood flow. Nursing interventions include watching for respiratory depression or apnea, flushing, bradycardia, irritability, and diarrhea, and monitoring for bleeding. Dilation is not specific to the smooth muscle tissue in the heart and occurs systemically. This drug needs to be administered by continuous infusion and requires a separate IV site. The dosage is usually 0.05 to 0.1 mcg/kg/min IV infusion (Vallerand et al., 2017).

blood flow from the right atrium to right ventricle, diminishing the blood flow to the lungs. If there is no VSD, then systemic blood flow is shunted across the right atrium through an ASD or the PFO.

Assessment

- Cyanosis
- Shortness of breath

TABLE 12–5 Prostaglandin E1 Medication

Drug	Prostaglandin (Alprostadil)
Dosage	Neonatal initial dose: 0.05–0.1 mcg/kg/min IV Maintenance dosage: 0.01–0.4 mcg/kg/min IV Infuse IV into large vein or umbilical cord
Actions	Relaxes smooth muscle of the ductus arteriosus, leading to increased pulmonary blood flow with increased blood oxygenation and lower body perfusion; increases Spo_2 and Pao_2
Contraindications	Respiratory distress syndrome
Precautions	Apnea, seizures, fever, hypotension, leukocytosis, fever, and pulmonary overcirculation Infants are usually intubated Prolonged use in hypoplastic left-heart syndrome, third spacing: monitor blood oxygenation, arterial pressure

From Vallerand, A. H., Sanoski, C. A., (2017). Davis's drug guide for nurses *(16th ed.). Philadelphia, PA: F.A. Davis*

Tricuspid Atresia

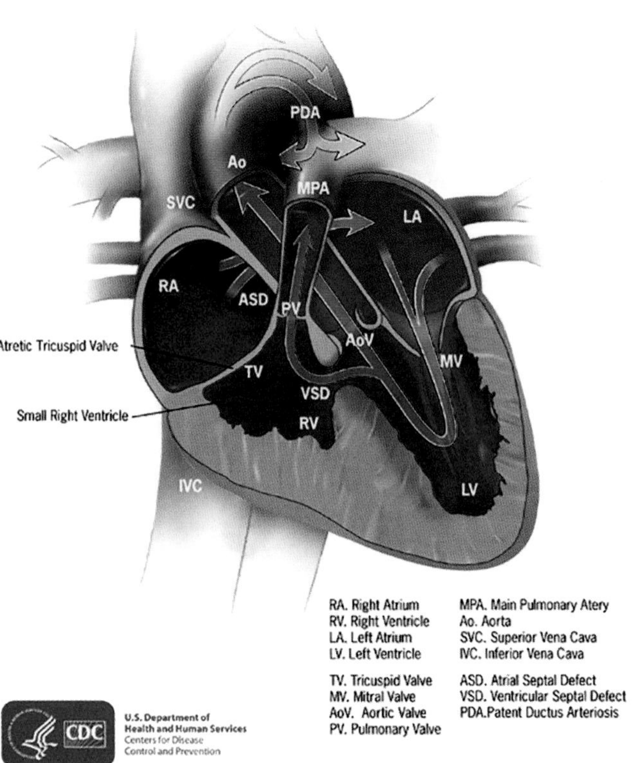

FIGURE 12–14 Tricuspid atresia.

- Delayed growth and poor weight gain
- Murmur due to ASD that is usually present
- Often associated with PS
- Clubbing of fingertips in older children

Diagnostic Tests

- Echocardiogram
- EKG
- Chest x-ray
- Cardiac catheterization

Nursing Interventions

- Prepare child for surgery.
- Prepare family for a series of corrective surgeries. Tricuspid atresia requires emergency interventions for survival of the infant. The nurse needs to sustain prostaglandin E1 administration to maintain blood flow to the lungs and then a balloon septostomy is performed. Eventually, stage II surgery is the Glenn stage, with stage III surgery known as the Fontan procedure (Ward & Hisley, 2015).
- Prepare family for possibility of heart transplant procedure if needed.

Caregiver Education

- Counsel family that child will need lifelong cardiology care.
- Inform caregivers that further surgeries may be required.

- The child will need to transition to an adult cardiologist.
- Monitor for signs and symptoms of fluid retention, fast heart rate, and chronic diarrhea.
- Monitor for signs of shortness of breath, bluish skin color, or slow growth (Ward & Hisley, 2015).

Eisenmenger Syndrome

Eisenmenger syndrome occurs with a PDA, VSD, or ASD (Fig. 12–15) as a result of a hole in the atria (ASD), where high pressures push nonoxygenated blood from the right atrium into the left atrium due to right ventricular hypertrophy, or as a result of a hole in the ventricles (VSD), which pushes nonoxygenated blood into the left ventricle, bypassing the lungs. This congenital defect increases pulmonary vascular resistance that exceeds left ventricular pressure, resulting in pulmonary hypertension with right-to-left shunting.

Assessment

- Shortness of breath
- Fatigue
- Chest pain
- Cyanosis
- Increased red blood cell production

Diagnostic Tests

- Echocardiogram
- Chest x-ray

Nursing Interventions

- Monitor the child's BP and administer hypertensive medications, anticoagulants, and antidysrhythmics.
- Maintain pulmonary vascular dilation.
- Prepare child and family for bypass (extracorporeal membrane oxygenation [ECMO]).

Caregiver Education

- Provide teaching related to treatment issues, such as bypass information.
- Prepare child/caregiver for possible transfer to another facility for bypass treatment.
- The child can have sponge baths but should not take long showers or be submerged in a tub or pool for several weeks after surgery. Children can resume normal activities except for rough or vigorous play. The family should be counseled to notify the surgeon if their child develops a fever, has chest pain, difficulty breathing, or redness, swelling, or excessive drainage of any color from the incision site. The family must be counseled that they will need follow-up visits with their surgeon and cardiologist.

CONGENITAL HEART DISEASE WITH OBSTRUCTIVE DISORDERS

Congenital heart defects that obstruct the flow of blood within or outside of the heart include COA, AS, PS, PA, and TOF with PA.

Coarctation of the Aorta

COA is a critical congenital heart defect that results in a narrowing of the aorta between the upper body and the lower extremities, usually distal to left subclavian artery (Fig. 12–16). COA is usually distal to the carotid arteries with VSDs common, and is classified as preductal, ductal, and postductal (Ward & Hisley, 2015). COA results in increased BP in the upper extremities and head, and reduction of BP in the lower extremities. Abnormalities in renin-angiotensin-aldosterone mechanisms and aortic valve abnormalities often accompany this disorder. This disorder is often associated with Turner's syndrome.

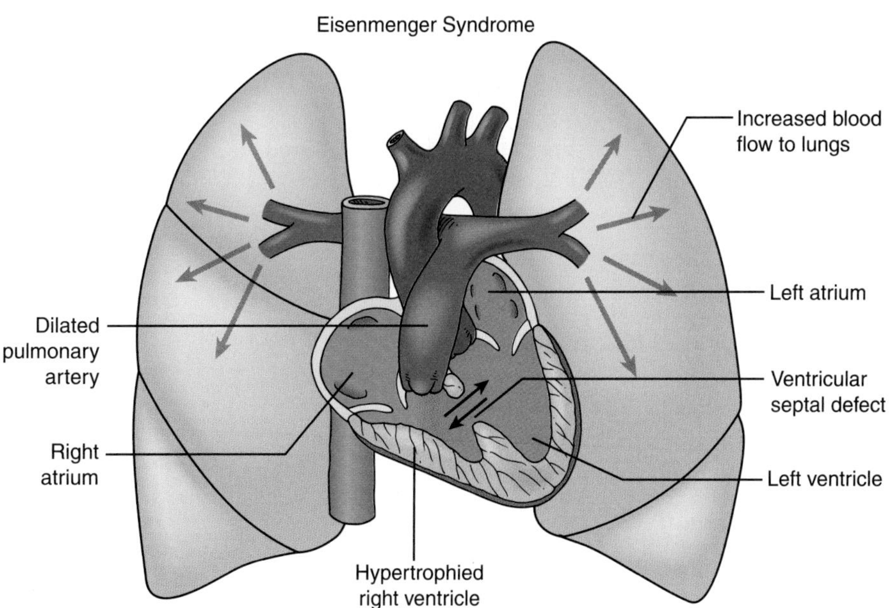

FIGURE 12–15 Eisenmenger syndrome.

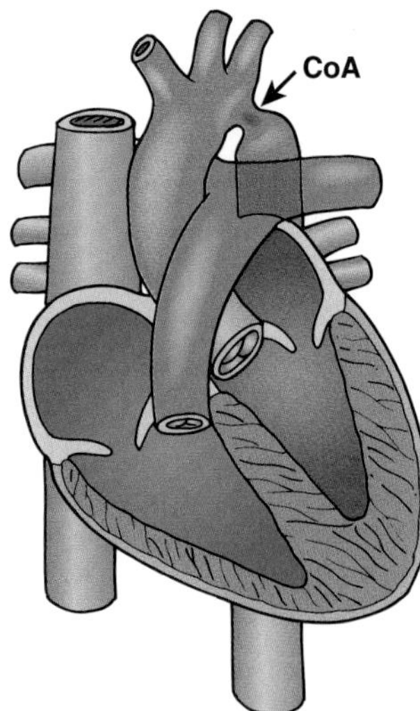

FIGURE 12–16 Coarctation of the aorta (CoA).

Assessment

- Few symptoms
- Systolic ejection murmur
- Decreased femoral pulses
- Cardiomegaly and right-sided heart failure secondary to aortic constriction
- In adolescents, may present as hypertension
- Headache
- BPs are higher in the upper extremities than in the lower—BP in lower extremities is more than 20 mm Hg less than in the upper extremities (Jahangir, 2015)
- If necessary to check only one extremity, use the right arm with the lower extremity, which is preductal (Ward & Hisley, 2015)
- Hypertension
- Shortness of breath
- Poor feeding, growth, and development
- Signs and symptoms of CHF (Ward & Hisley, 2015)

Diagnostic Tests

- Chest x-ray or esophagram will show "3 sign" or reverse 3 ("E sign") is due to poststenotic dilation of the aorta arch and the left subclavian artery (Gaillard, 2017)
- Cardiac catheterization
- Rib notching may be present because of collateral vessels eroding the adjacent bones (Ward & Hisley, 2015)
- Balloon dilation
- Stint placement

Nursing Interventions

- Monitor medications for CHF—Digoxin, Lasix.
- Monitor perfusion.
- Obtain four extremity BPs.
- Provide postsurgical care following cardiac catheterization or surgery with graft from a cadaver or resection.

Caregiver Education

- Continue to monitor BP as ordered by the cardiologist, usually monthly.
- May need to restrict strenuous activity.
- Educate on bacterial endocarditis prevention.

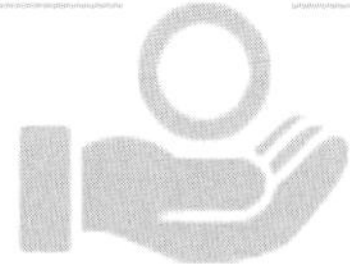

SAFE AND EFFECTIVE NURSING CARE: Clinical Pearl

Assessment of Pulses

Evaluation of pulses for COA would demonstrate normal or elevated pulses in the upper extremities and decreased pulses in the lower extremities. It is important in this assessment that the right brachial artery be palpated, because the subclavian artery may be involved in giving a false reading on the left brachial artery (Patnana, 2015).

Aortic Stenosis

AS is the obstruction of blood flow from the left ventricle to the aorta (Fig. 12–17). Causes include valve stenosis or a narrowing of the aorta above the valve from age or congenital disease. Stenosis or narrowing increases the workload of the myocardium of the left ventricle, leading to hypertrophy. Scarring of the aortic valve occurs from rheumatic fever caused by group A *Streptococcus.*

Assessment

- Chest pain
- Fatigue
- Syncope
- Murmur—systolic ejection
- Shortness of breath
- Narrow pulse pressure with decrease in systolic pressures (Ward & Hisley, 2015)
- Exercise intolerance, which may result in sudden death
- Increased pressure load on left ventricle

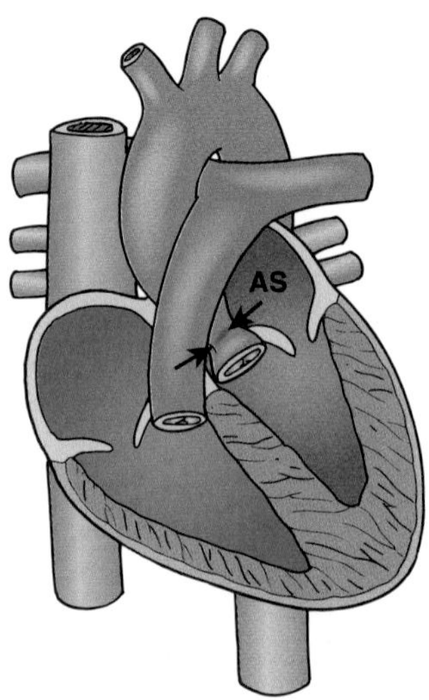

FIGURE 12–17 Aortic stenosis (AS).

Diagnostic Tests

- EKG—thickening of the septum and mitral valve abnormalities
- EKG—inverted T waves
- Chest x-ray—cardiomegaly, dilated ascending aorta
- Cardiac catheterization
- Balloon valvuloplasty

Nursing Interventions

- Monitor for signs and symptoms of CHF.
- Prepare for emergency measures for atrial fibrillation.
- Provide caregiver teaching on procedures.
- Provide caregiver home-care teaching.
- Maintain pain management for chest discomfort and prostaglandin E1 drip to maintain a PDA until surgery.

Caregiver Education

- Provide bacterial endocarditis information.

Pulmonary Stenosis

PS results in narrowing of the opening in the pulmonary artery or pulmonary valve (Fig. 12–18).

Assessment

- Increased workload of right ventricle
- CHF
- Hepatomegaly
- Often associated with other disorders, such as Noonan syndrome or TOF
- Murmur
- Shortness of breath
- Cyanosis

SAFE AND EFFECTIVE NURSING CARE: Clinical Pearl

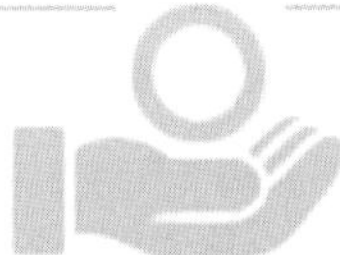

Noonan Syndrome

Noonan syndrome is an autosomal dominant (chance is 1 out of 2) chromosomal defect that mimics Turner syndrome in the webbing of the neck and barrel-shaped chest wall (McGovern, 2017).

Diagnostic Tests

- Echocardiogram
- Cardiac catheterization

Nursing Interventions

- Continue nursing care after catheterization or surgical repair, providing a calm environment to decrease oxygen requirements.
- Closely monitor BP.

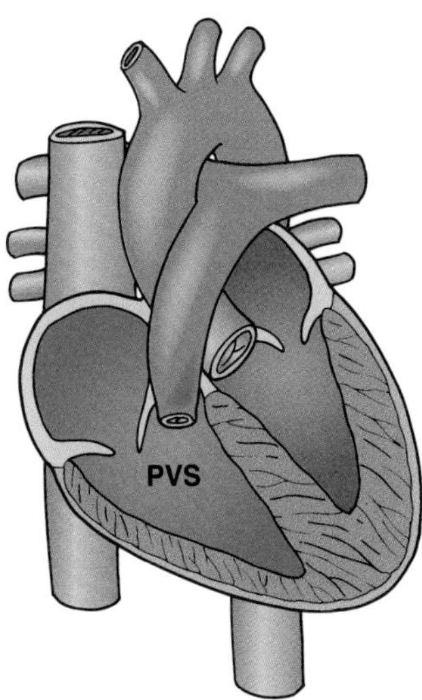

FIGURE 12–18 Pulmonary vein stenosis.

Caregiver Education

- The child will be hospitalized, and balloon angioplasty or valvuloplasty may be needed.
- The child must return to cardiologist frequently for follow-up, and caregivers should be provided information on the recurrence of symptoms that may occur because of restenosis.

Pulmonary Atresia

PA is a congenital defect in which the pulmonary valve or pulmonary artery does not form properly (Fig. 12–19) (CDC, 2016b). PA has no known causes and may also occur with VSDs. It is often associated with PDA (CDC, 2016b). To survive, the child must have a PDA or PFO.

Assessment

- Shortness of breath
- Severe cyanosis at birth
- Fatigue

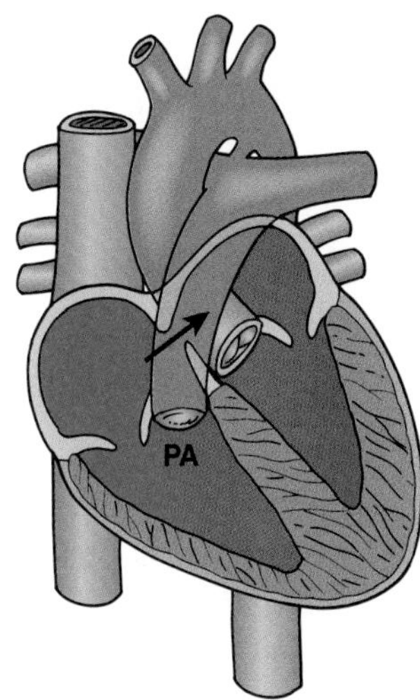

FIGURE 12–19 Pulmonary atresia (PA).

- Tachypnea
- Poor feeding and weight gain

Diagnostic Tests

- Murmur associated with the VSD or PDA
- EKG
- Echocardiogram
- Chest x-ray
- Pulse oximeter
- Cardiac catheterization used to determine the atresia (Lui, Li, Lui, Wu, & Xu, 2016)

Nursing Interventions

- Maintain prostaglandin E1 drip to keep the ducts open, and permit a mixing of the oxygenated and nonoxygenated blood.
- Provide postoperative stabilization if a balloon atrial septostomy is used to keep the foramen ovale open.
- Surgical care may be indicated after surgery (Fontan procedure) to repair or replace the valve, or a heart transplant may be necessary (Lui et al., 2016).

Tetralogy of Fallot With Pulmonary Atresia

- Occurs with chromosome arm 22q11 deletion (Pettersen, 2015)
- Associated with VATER syndrome
  - V—vertebral anomalies
  - A—anal anomalies
  - T–E—tracheo-esophageal anomalies
  - R—renal anomalies (Pettersen, 2015)
- May result from maternal diabetes, maternal phenylketonuria, maternal ingestion of retinoic acid
- Symptomatic within a few hours of birth
- Severe cyanosis after PDA closes
- In the arteriopulmonary collateral circulation, cyanosis is not as severe (Pettersen, 2015)

Assessment

- Profound cyanosis
- Peripheral pulses and BP stable until pulmonary blood flow results in bounding pulses
- Normal first heart sound, single second heart sound (Pettersen, 2015)
- PDA murmur may be heard
- Delayed growth and development

Diagnostic Tests

- Complete blood count, arterial blood gases
- Echocardiogram, EKG
- Cardiac catheterization with angiography
- Surgical repair with modified Blalock–Taussig procedure and balloon dilation of the stenotic pulmonary valve (Pettersen, 2015)

Nursing Interventions

- Monitor for pain, hemorrhage, and thrombospasms.
- Maintain oxygenation through monitoring of pulse oximetry and hydration through strict intake and output recordings (Pettersen, 2015).

Caregiver Education

- Explain importance of follow-up with pediatric cardiologist and the need for future procedures and catheterizations.
- Exercise capacity is limited.
- Maintain caloric intake.
- Monitor for signs and symptoms of heart failure.
- Educate on bacterial endocarditis prophylaxis.

SAFE AND EFFECTIVE NURSING CARE: Clinical Pearl

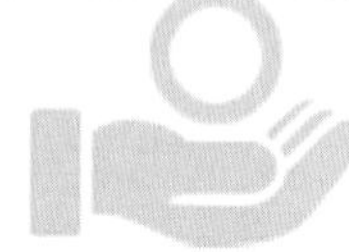

Nutrition Supplementation

Children who are in cardiac failure because of pulmonary overcirculation require specific nutritional supplementation to maintain sufficient weight gain. Caloric intake may require up to 150 kcal/kg/day (Mozaffarian, 2016).

CONGENITAL HEART DISEASE WITH MIXED DISORDERS

Mixed disorders occur when blood from systemic and pulmonary circulation is mixed in the heart chambers. Desaturation of blood occurs and cardiac output decreases because of increased volume load on ventricles.

Transposition of the Great Vessels

Transposition of the great vessels occurs when the two great vessels of the aorta and pulmonary artery are reversed; nonoxygenated blood thus flows to the brain, resulting in damage (Fig. 12–20). This defect creates two separate circulatory systems—systemic and pulmonary—that do not mix. The aorta receives nonoxygenated blood from the right ventricle that then goes out to the systemic circulation without going to the lungs to become oxygenated. The pulmonary artery receives oxygenated blood from the left ventricle that then goes back to the lungs. The survival of the infant requires a mixing of oxygenated and unoxygenated blood at the ductus arteriosus or through an arterial septal defect or VSD.

Assessment

Transposition of the great vessels usually presents within the first 24 hours after birth and is a cardiac emergency. The upper

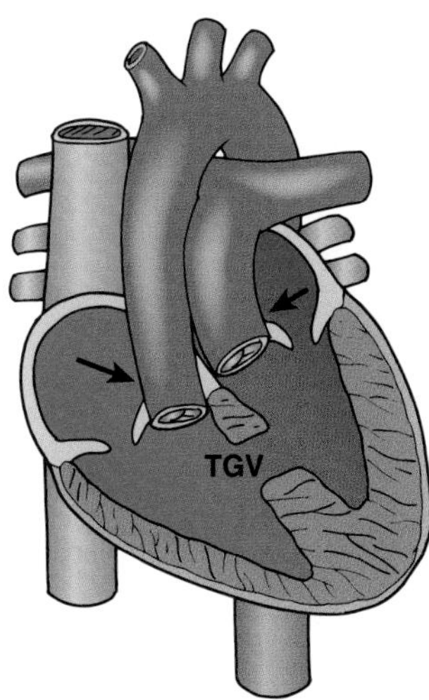

FIGURE 12–20 Transposition of the great vessels (TGV).

extremities have decreased oxygen saturation versus the lower extremities, especially in the right arm. The infant presents with profound cyanosis, especially with crying. The infant will have tachypnea or quiet tachypnea, heart murmur, and signs and symptoms of CHF (Charpie, 2017).

Diagnostic Tests

- Negative hyperoxygenation test (Charpie, 2017)
- Chest x-ray—"egg on a string" visualization, which may be absent in neonates (Ward & Hisley, 2015)
- Cardiac catheterization
- Echocardiogram

Nursing Interventions

- Oxygen saturations in right arm greater than 75% need to be sustained to decrease pulmonary vascular resistance (Charpie, 2017).
- The nurse must safely administer medications that are ordered to treat CHF or prostaglandin E1 drip to maintain fetal circulation.
- Monitor children prescribed captopril/enalapril to relax the coronary arteries.
- Provide postoperative care after corrective Jatene arterial switch procedure.
- Provide postoperative care after Rashkind balloon atrial septostomy (Charpie, 2017).

Caregiver Education

- The child will be hospitalized and atrial septostomy surgery performed to maintain mixing.
- The child will need to return to cardiologist frequently for follow-up. Parents will also be encouraged to follow their child's neurological development because risks for neurological and developmental complications are high after the arterial switch procedure.

Truncus Arteriosus

Truncus arteriosus occurs when a single great artery from both ventricles has an overriding VSD. The truncal valve is stenotic or incomplete. The incidence increases in children of women who are exposed to German measles or viral infections, and it is associated with DiGeorge syndrome, 22q11 deletion disorder, infants with Down syndrome, infants of diabetic mothers, and infants of mothers with excessive alcohol consumption during pregnancy (CDC, 2016d) (Fig. 12–21).

Assessment

- Mixing of oxygenated and nonoxygenated blood—cyanosis
- Tachypnea
- Diaphoresis
- Increased blood flow leads to increased pulmonary congestion and CHF (Ward & Hisley, 2015)
- Wheezing, grunting, and retractions
- Wide pulse pressures
- Difficulty in feeding
- Loud pansystolic murmur (regurgitating murmur heard throughout systole) and single S_2 (CDC, 2016d; McElhinney, 2015)

SAFE AND EFFECTIVE NURSING CARE: Clinical Pearl

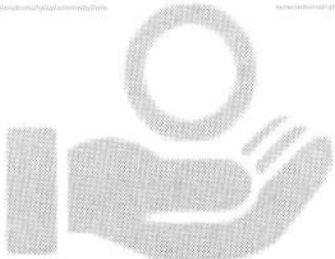

Pansystolic Murmur

A pansystolic murmur is turbulence that is heard throughout systole, from the first heart sound to the second heart sound. Blood can be heard flowing between the right and left sides of the heart because of the differences in systolic pressures.

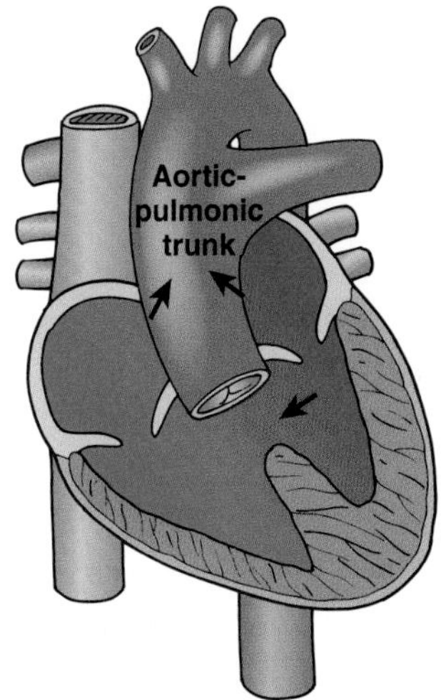

FIGURE 12–21 Truncus arteriosus.

Diagnostic Tests

- Chest x-ray indicates enlarged heart with hazy lung fields
- Echocardiogram shows a single vessel from the right and left ventricles
- Cardiac catheterization

Nursing Interventions

- Avoid supplemental oxygen, which decreases pulmonary vascular resistance and leads to excessive pulmonary blood flow (CDC, 2016d).
- Monitor child closely with mechanical ventilation.
- Monitor invasive lines; provide inotropes to maximize cardiac function (Ward & Hisley, 2015).
- Maintain nutritional intake.
- Complex surgical repair involves separation of aorta and pulmonary artery with a possible VSD repair.
- Monitor for stabilization of vital signs and the weaning of oxygen.

Caregiver Education

- Teach signs and symptoms of CHF.
- Educate on importance of follow-up appointments with cardiologist.
- Surgery with the Rastelli operation dramatically improves outcomes.
- Monitor for signs and symptoms of tissue changes.

Total Anomalous Pulmonary Venous Return

In TAPVR, pulmonary veins with oxygen-rich blood follow an abnormal route back to the right atrium instead of the left atrium, making it difficult to distinguish between TAPVR and ASDs (Fig. 12–22) (Viola, 2015). This condition can be obstructive or nonobstructive, and often occurs with DiGeorge syndrome (Viola, 2015). It includes three separate types:

- Interruption occurs beyond the left subclavian artery.
- Interruption occurs between left carotid artery and left subclavian artery.
- Interruption occurs between innominate artery and left carotid artery (Viola, 2015).

Assessment

- While PDA is open, the child has few symptoms.
- When PDA closes, profound cyanosis, severe shock, and CHF result (Ward & Hisley, 2015).

Diagnostic Tests

- "Snowman sign" or figure-of-eight will appear on chest x-ray (Viola, 2015)
- Normal or small heart
- Pulmonary edema on x-ray
- Oxygen saturation levels
- Echocardiogram

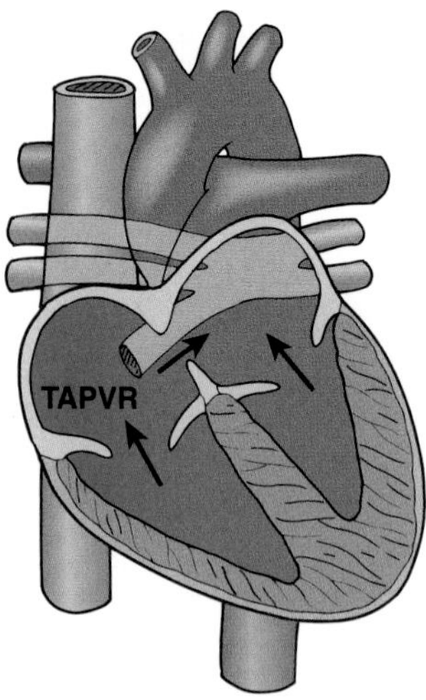

FIGURE 12–22 Total anomalous pulmonary venous return (TAPVR).

Nursing Interventions

- Maintain a patent airway.
- Monitor strict intake and output through diuretics for CHF.
- Monitor arterial blood gases.
- Provide postsurgical care related to valvular repair.

Caregiver Education

- Educate caregiver on signs and symptoms of restricted blood flow caused by continued stenosis (Ward & Hisley, 2015).
- Educate on importance of long-term follow-up with pediatric cardiologist.

Hypoplastic Left Heart

Hypoplastic left heart is the second most common congenital heart defect, caused by underdevelopment of the left side of the heart, aorta, aortic valve, left ventricle, and mitral valve. This leads to pulmonary venous congestion and edema (Fig. 12–23; Ohye, 2016). As the PDA is open, blood reaches the aorta through this duct; symptoms then appear when the PDA closes. This defect is associated with the absence of corpus callosum (Ohye, 2016).

Assessment

- Asymptomatic until ducts close
- Skin ashen in color
- Rapid and difficult breathing
- Difficulty feeding (Ohye, 2016)
- Usually fatal within the first days or months of life unless treated

Diagnostic Tests

- As PDA closes, baby will become very dusky and ashen
- Single S_2, gallop (Ohye, 2016)
- Echocardiogram
- Chest x-ray

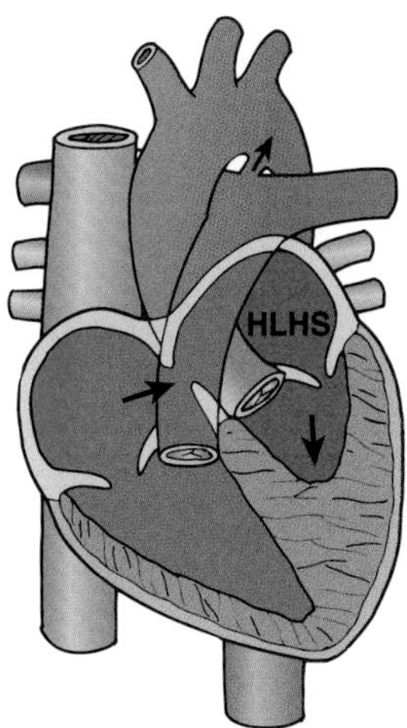

FIGURE 12–23 Hypoplastic left-heart syndrome (HLHS).

Nursing Interventions

- Maintain prostaglandin E1 infusion to keep PDA open.
- Provide nursing preparation for surgery—Norwood three-stage procedure to increase ventricular function (Ohye, 2016).
- Provide caregiver preparation for severity of condition.
- Anticipate possible transport out of the facility for heart transplant.

Caregiver Education

- Surgical correction or transplantation
- Lifelong follow-up with pediatric cardiologist
- Long-term heart medications
- Bacterial endocarditis protocols (Nishimura et al., 2017)

Ebstein's Anomaly

Ebstein's anomaly is a rare defect that has an increased incidence with maternal lithium use (Fig. 12–24). This disorder results in displacement of the tricuspid valve into right ventricle with an enlarged right atrium and cardiomegaly, and is associated with other congenital heart defects and dysrhythmias, such as ASD and Wolff-Parkinson-White syndrome (WPW; cardiac dysrhythmia) (Postma et al., 2016). This anomaly is present at birth, but if minor, symptoms may not appear until the child is a teenager or an adult.

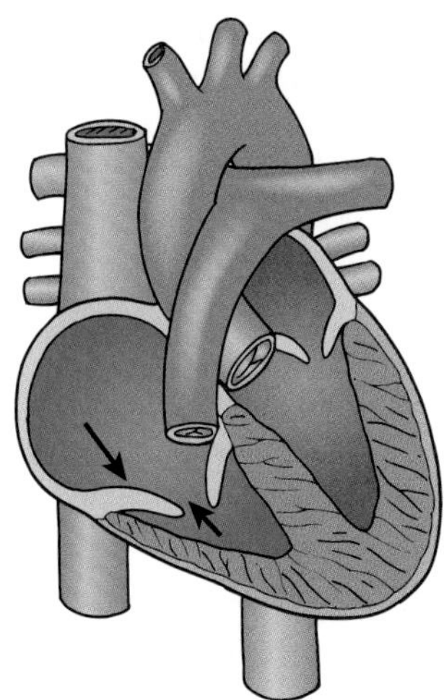

FIGURE 12–24 Ebstein's anomaly.

Assessment

- Mild-to-severe cyanosis related to incompetence of tricuspid valve and the blood flow to the lungs
- Often no murmur
- Hepatomegaly
- Splenomegaly
- Feeding problems
- The child may need immediate surgery
- A gallop heart murmur may be heard

Diagnostic Tests

- Chest x-ray will show enlarged, balloon-shaped heart
- Decreased pulmonary vascular markings
- May predispose child to electrical conduction issues from right atrium to the right ventricle through the bundle of Kent
- Results in increased incidence of WPW syndrome and supraventricular tachycardia dysrhythmias
- Cardiac catheterization for conclusive diagnosis (Postma et al., 2016)

Nursing Interventions

- Monitor for stabilization of the child's vital signs.
- Continue the administration of oxygen and the maintenance of prostaglandin E1 to improve oxygenation through the ducts.
- Continue ordered inotropes such as dopamine or dobutamine to increase BP.
- Prepare child/caregiver for surgery on an emergent basis—Fontan procedure or transplant.

Caregiver Education

- The earlier the symptoms present, the greater the long-term consequences for the child.
- Close monitoring by cardiologist is necessary.
- Depending on leaky valve, the child may be restricted during sports.

ACQUIRED CONGENITAL HEART DISEASE

Acquired congenital heart defects can occur during childhood. Although acquired heart disease is more common in adults, heart disease can develop in children as a complication of conditions such as rheumatic fever and Kawasaki disease.

Cardiomyopathy

Cardiomyopathy is a chronic progressive disease that occurs within the heart muscle itself (primary or a genetic defect) or as a result of another disease or toxin that affects all organs, including the heart, such as infections, low blood flow to the heart, decreased oxygen levels, or high BP (AHA, 2017).

- There are three types of cardiomyopathy: dilated, hypertrophic, and restrictive.
  - Dilated or congested—enlarged heart, weak and ineffective pump
    - Most common form
    - Carnitine deficiency
    - Develop heart failure
    - Blood clots due to slow blood flow
    - Dysrhythmias
  - Hypertrophic—most common inherited heart defect in the absence of other cardiac disease with left ventricle enlarged; found in infants of diabetic mothers, Noonan and Pompe syndromes (AHA, 2017)
    - Enlarged heart
    - Diastolic dysfunction
    - Exercise intolerance
    - Fainting
    - Leaking valves caused by increase septal and ventricle muscle
  - Restrictive—heart muscle becomes rigid and fails to relax; rarest type
    - Diastolic dysfunction
    - Fatigue
    - Shortness of breath
- Ventricles are primarily affected and become enlarged, thickened, and stiff.
- Child is born with normal heart anatomy.
- Heart muscle loses the ability to pump effectively; heart failure and cardiac dysrhythmias occur (AHA, 2017).
- Cardiomyopathy is not gender, race, or geographically dependent.
- This is the leading cause of heart transplants in children despite being relatively rare. Causes include:
  - Chemotherapy
  - Viral infections such as Coxsackie B
  - Genetic factors—fatty acid oxidation
  - Metabolic disorders (AHA, 2017)
  - Persistent rhythm abnormalities

Assessment

- CHF
- Sweating with feedings
- Dizziness
- Weight loss
- Murmur—gallop
- Hepatomegaly with venous congestion
- Fatigue
- Frequent colds, pneumonia
- Dysrhythmias

Diagnostic Tests

- Murmur
- Chest x-ray shows thickening of the cardiac musculature and enlargement
- EKG indicates the degree of enlargement
- Echocardiogram reveals right- or left-sided enlargement
- Cardiac catheterization
- Cardiac dysrhythmias

Nursing Interventions

During the acute phase, nursing interventions include:

- The nurse should continue IV fluids, endotracheal intubation, ventilator, ECMO/artificial heart-lung machine, diuretics, and anticoagulation therapy (AHA, 2017).
- ACE inhibitors have positive inotropic properties and are used because they inhibit the chemical angiotensin, which constricts arteries (AHA, 2017). These ACE inhibitors may have to be taken for the rest of the child's life.
- Beta blocker therapy, calcium channel blockers, and nutritional supplementation with carnitine may also be warranted (Ward & Hisley, 2015).
- Provide valve replacement therapy postoperatively.
- Provide heart transplant care if warranted.

During the chronic phase:

- Anticipate major complications that can include arrhythmias and CHF.
- Anticipate tachycardias (fast heart rates) or bradycardias (slow heart rates).
- Monitor for tachycardias, which can develop into fibrillation.
- Provide nutritional supplementation with carnitine.
- Monitor children prescribed ACE inhibitors. Captopril/enalapril relaxes the coronary arteries, which may cause diarrhea, muscle cramps, high potassium levels, and kidney and liver abnormalities (AHA, 2017).
- Maintain diuretics except for hypertrophic cardiomyopathy (Tayal, Prasad, & Cook, 2017).
- Monitor potassium levels with the use of diuretics.
- Monitor children receiving Lasix/Aldactone to reduce excess fluid in the lungs.
- Monitor children receiving digoxin (Lanoxin), which is used to improve cardiac function in those children with a dilated cardiomyopathy by enhancing the pumping effort of the heart (Tayal et al., 2017).
- Lanoxin (Digoxin) or verapamil should not be considered for treating sustained tachycardia until ventricular tachycardia has been ruled out (Houston & Stevens, 2015).
- Monitor for bradycardias when the conduction is interrupted or totally blocked and the child may need to have a pacemaker.
- Monitor for thromboembolus, which may occur because of interrupted blood flow (Houston & Stevens, 2015; Tayal et al., 2017).
- An internal cardioverter/defibrillator (ICD) is capable of shocking life-threatening dysrhythmias (Tayal et al., 2017).
- During the critical phase, those with irreversible heart damage and persistent poor function may require a heart transplant.

Caregiver Education

- Aimed at the intensive care necessary for a child with a life-threatening condition
- Possible terminal status of the child

- Frequent echocardiograms to monitor size and function of the heart
- Psychological as well as physical preparation
- Activity restrictions to prevent overstimulation of the heart
- Allow the child to discuss feelings, such as concerning the restriction of activity in the previously active child
- Encourage participation in cardiomyopathy programs (Ooi, 2016)
- Anticipatory grieving of the parents is expected in this life-threatening situation

CRITICAL COMPONENT

Implanting Internal Cardioverter/Defibrillator

The AHA (2016d) recommends that before a client is considered as a candidate for an ICD, the dysrhythmia in question must be life-threatening and doctors have ruled out correctable causes of the dysrhythmia. Clients with ICD should be aware of their surroundings with potential disruption of the device by strong magnetic fields that prevent the device from working (AHA, 2016). Since 2015, the U.S. Food and Drug Administration has approved a wearable life vest that detects abnormally fast heart rates (ventricular tachycardia) or irregular heartbeat (ventricular fibrillation) and delivers a shock when this is registered.

SAFE AND EFFECTIVE NURSING CARE: Understanding Medication

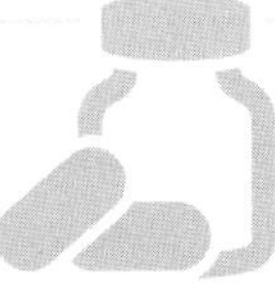

Medications for Attention Deficit-Hyperactivity Disorder

The Pediatric Drug Advisory in 2006 issued a Black Box warning to be applied to attention deficit-hyperactivity disorder (ADHD) medications. Children with structural defects, cardiomyopathy, or heart rhythm disorders who are administered these medications may be at risk for sudden death (Berger, 2016). Joint statements by the AAP and the AHA show that children with heart conditions have a higher incidence of ADHD, but that medications used to treat ADHD have not been shown in most cases to cause heart disease or result in sudden cardiac death (CDC, 2016; Magellan Health, 2016a).

Congestive Heart Failure

With CHF, the heart cannot supply enough oxygenated blood to meet the metabolic needs of the body tissues either at rest or work (Ward & Hisley, 2015). The heart may fail with high afterloads (COA, AS), valvular regurgitation, or impaired myocardial contractility, as in cardiomyopathy. CHF in pediatric clients with congenital heart disease will depend on whether the child has a ductal-dependent lesion, which will most likely present with cyanosis in the newborn period as the ducts begin to close. Left-to-right shunting such as in VSDs may not show CHF until

SAFE AND EFFECTIVE NURSING CARE: Understanding Medication

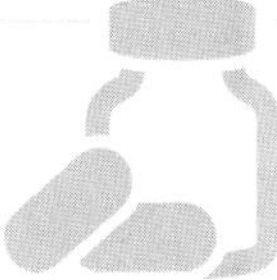

Digoxin (Lanoxin)

Daily dosing for children with normal renal function:

- Age 1 to 24 months: (IV/IM) digitalizing dose—30 to 50 mcg/kg given at 50% of the dose initially and one-fourth of the initial dose in each of two subsequent doses at 6-to 12-hour intervals
- Age 2 to 5 years: (IV/IM) Digitalizing dose—25 to 35 mcg/kg given as 50% of the dose initially and one-fourth of the initial dose in each of two subsequent doses at 6- to 12-hour intervals
- Age 5 to 10 years: (IV/IM) digitalizing dose—20 to 30 mcg/kg given at 50% of the dose initially and one-fourth of the initial dose in each of two subsequent doses at 6- to 12-hour intervals
- Older than 10 years: (IV/IM) digitalizing dose—8 to 12 mcg/kg given at 50% of the dose initially and one-fourth of the initial dose in each of two subsequent doses at 6- to 12-hour intervals.

The nurse should also note the following:

- Be aware of the child's baseline parameters, including peripheral pulse, BP, and heart rate.
- Administer 1 hour before or 2 hours after meals; if child vomits dose, do not repeat dose.
- Take apical pulse for a full minute. Instruct parents that changes in heart rate, especially bradycardia, are one of the first signs of digoxin toxicity in infants and children. Educate family on how to assess infant's apical pulse rate and to notify the health-care practitioner if the heart rate is out of the range set by the health-care provider.
- Note rate, rhythm, and quality. If changes occur, take an EKG and notify the physician.
- Monitor baseline and periodic ongoing potassium, magnesium, and calcium levels.
- Monitor for signs and symptoms of digoxin toxic effects, including anorexia, nausea, vomiting, diarrhea, and visual disturbances.
- Closely monitor for digoxin toxicity with antibiotic therapy caused by changes in intestinal flora.
- Digoxin (Lanoxin) has a narrow therapeutic range. Medication errors with digoxin include miscalculation of doses and insufficient monitoring of digoxin levels. A second nurse should check the original order and dose calculations (Vallerand et al., 2017).
- Monitor for intake and output in children with renal disorders (Vallerand et al., 2017).

Caregiver education for administration of Lanoxin includes:

- Administer medication at the same time every day and at the correct frequency. Do not double up for a missed dose.
- Notify your physician for advice before administering any over-the-counter medications.
- Do not breastfeed without contacting your physician if you are taking this medication (Vallerand et al., 2017).

several weeks after birth as a result of chronic pulmonary edema (AHA, 2015f).

- Right-sided heart failure—right ventricle cannot pump blood into the pulmonary artery, resulting in increased pressure in the right atrium and the systemic venous system.
- Left-sided heart failure—blood is backed into the left atrium and the pulmonary veins, resulting in increased lung congestion.

Assessment

- Edema of the face, hands, and feet, or weight gain
- Cardiac enlargement
- Gallop rhythm, changes in heart rate
- Tachycardia
- When completing four limb blood pressures, the blood pressure will be higher in the arms than the legs.
- Cyanosis
- Tachypnea
- Shortness of breath
- Crackles
- Fatigue
- Poor appetite
- Poor growth, FTT
- Sweating with minimal activity

Diagnostic Tests

- History and physical examination
- Chest x-ray indicates an enlarged heart, increase in pulmonary vascularity, and edema
- Echocardiogram defines anatomy and physiology
- EKG indicates an enlarged atrium
- Urine and blood tests evaluate blood gas, anemia, and electrolyte balance

Nursing Interventions

- Maintain oxygenation by elevating the head of the bed.
- Decrease oxygen consumption by minimizing stimulation and decrease work of breathing.
- Monitor intake and output daily weights at the same time, with the same scale, with the same clothes.
- Monitor breath sounds.
- Provide supplemental oxygen.
- Cluster care to decrease oxygen consumption.
- Use of high-caloric formula or the use of medium-chain triglycerides that enhances the calories without providing additional fluid volume.
- Administer pharmacological therapy—Lanoxin therapy, diuretic therapy, and inotropic agents—to maximize cardiac output and eliminate excess fluid.

Caregiver Education

- Surgery may need to be performed to correct congenital heart defects.
- Provide discharge instructions on observation for tachypnea and increased work of breathing.
- Maintain diuretics as ordered (Table 12–6).
- Avoid high-salt-content foods.
- Monitor weight: same scale, same time of day, same clothes.
- Elevate the head of the bed.
- Provide frequent rest periods by clustering care.

HYPERLIPIDEMIA

Hyperlipidemia, in which the blood has high concentrations of low-density lipoprotein (LDL) and low concentrations of high-density lipoprotein, is a high-risk factor for cardiovascular disease.

- May be present early in life.
- Comorbid with high BP, type I or II diabetes, smoking, overweight, and inactivity
- National Cholesterol Education Program (NCEP) guidelines indicate that if the pediatric client's LDLs are greater than or equal to 130 mg/dL, the client has an increased risk for complications resulting from hyperlipidemia (Rohrs, 2015b).
- Dietary and behavioral changes are necessary for long-term benefits in reduction of cholesterol and prevention of complications.
- Dietary recommendations will only decrease the cholesterol levels by a small percentage.
- Controllable factors need to be addressed throughout life: weight, smoking, hypertension, and inactivity.
- Noncontrollable factors are hereditary factors that significantly impact the incidence of hyperlipidemia.
- Treatment is aimed at controlling manageable factors and the use of statins and niacin for hereditary factors.

CRITICAL COMPONENT

Screening for Hyperlipidemia

The National Heart, Lung, and Blood Institute recommends screening children aged 9 to 11 and 17 to 21 years regardless of family history or risk factors for high cholesterol or premature cardiac disease (Rohrs, 2015b).

Evidence-Based Practice: Lipid Screening

U.S. Preventive Services Task Force; Bibbins-Doming, K., Grossman, D. C., Curry, S. J., Davidson, K. W., Epling, J. W., Jr., . . . Siu, A. L. (2016). Screening for lipid disorders in children and adolescents. US Preventative Services Task Force recommendation statement. *Journal of the American Medical Association, 316*(6), 625–633. doi: 10.1001/jama.2016.9852

Cholesterol levels vary by age and sex throughout childhood. Total cholesterol levels increase at birth, stabilize around age 2, peak before puberty, and slightly decrease in adolescence. Elevated cholesterol levels in childhood do not necessarily track into adulthood. Selective screening is based on family history of hyperlipidemia or premature cardiovascular disease. There are no universally accepted criteria for the diagnosis of familial hypercholesterolemia. Pharmacological treatment of hyperlipidemia is recommended for children older than 10 years whose LDL cholesterol is greater than 190 mg/dL (Rohrs, 2015a).

TABLE 12-6 Diuretics Used to Treat Congestive Heart Failure

ACTION ADMINISTER IN THE MORNING	NURSING INTERVENTIONS	FAMILY/CAREGIVER EDUCATION
SPIRONOLACTONE (ALDACTONE) Potassium-sparing diuretic antagonizes aldosterone receptors of distal convoluted tubule (DCT)	Monitor kidney function with strict intake and output (I&O); watch for alterations in potassium level	Notify physician if child develops diarrhea, vomiting, or signs of dehydration Give missed dose as soon as discovered Do not double up on the doses. Monitor for rash which may be Stevens-Johnson syndrome.
HYDROCHLOROTHIAZIDE (DIURIL) Inhibits carbonic anhydrase in the (DCT) Inhibits the cotransport of sodium (Na) and chloride (Cl), thus decreasing sodium chloride (NaCl) reabsorption from the kidneys	Give with meals to prevent gastric upset	Avoid exposure to sunlight Take with food Notify physician if child is dehydrated; vomiting and diarrhea Avoid NSAIDs, as they decrease the effectiveness of this drug Administer medication in the morning. Monitor for rash which may be Stevens-Johnson syndrome.
FUROSEMIDE (LASIX) Loop diuretic—acts mainly by inhibiting sodium and chloride reabsorption in the nephron at the thick ascending limb of Henle's loop. Increases excretion of water, sodium, chloride, magnesium, potassium, and calcium.	Monitor electrolyte levels, especially potassium; monitor for ototoxicity; may develop renal calculi with prolonged use.	May be instructed to feed foods that are high in potassium, such as bananas Give with food—if given once a day, give with breakfast; if twice a day, give at evening meal but not close to bedtime to prevent the need for repeated bathroom trips Report signs of dehydration, allergic responses, shortness of breath. Monitor for rash which may be Stevens-Johnson syndrome.
BUMETANIDE-BUMEX Loop diuretic—acts mainly by inhibiting Na reabsorption in the nephron at the thick ascending limb of Henle's loop	Monitor for electrolyte imbalances, especially potassium; may potentiate ototoxic drugs such as aminoglycosides	Report signs of dehydration, vomiting, and diarrhea Avoid exposure to sun May be instructed to feed foods high in potassium, such as bananas

From Vallerand, A. H., Sanoski, C. A., & Deglin, J. H. (2017). Davis's drug guide for nurses *(15th ed.). Philadelphia, PA: F.A. Davis*

CRITICAL COMPONENT

Dietary Recommendations

- Refer to a dietician for nutritional support.
- The AHA (2016a) recommends the following dietary recommendations for fat intake for healthy children as 30% to 35% for 2 to 3 years of age and 25% to 35% for 4 to 18 years of age in which the fats should be polyunsaturated and monounsaturated fats.
- 7% of calories from saturated fat
- 10% from monounsaturated fat
- Less than 200 mg of cholesterol per day
- Avoid trans fats

(Rohrs, 2015a)

HYPERTENSION

Pediatric hypertension is now a common occurrence and is a common cause of morbidity and mortality in the pediatric population. The Task Force on Blood Pressure Control in Children was commissioned by the National Heart, Lung, and Blood Institute (Rodriquez-Cruz, 2017). The AHA (2016a) recommends that children older than 3 years have yearly BP measurements. BP is dependent on the child's age, gender, and weight.

- Systolic BP in infants is between 70 and 90 mm Hg; adolescents reach adult levels.
- BP is the force of the blood hitting against the artery walls during contraction of the heart (systole) and during relaxation of the heart (diastole).

- Routine monitoring should begin around age 3 years.
- Diagnosis of hypertension is not made from one reading.
- Hypertension is diagnosed when BP is more than 95% for age, weight, height, and sex (Rodriquez-Cruz, 2017).
- Primary hypertension—child is usually less than 10 years of age. This is a disease of exclusion.
- Secondary hypertension—daytime diastolic BP elevations and nighttime BP elevations. May indicate renal or organ involvement.
- Risk factors include genetic causes, obesity, and secondary hypertension issues related to renal perfusion or structural anomalies.
- Syndrome X is the triad of insulin resistance, hypertension, and hyperlipidemia. In recent years, this has resulted in a dramatic increase in obesity in young children.
- Systolic and diastolic BPs are preferred measurements used to diagnose hypertension.
- True BP is measured over a period of time.
- Monitor for correct position for BP reading: seated, relaxed, uncrossed arms and legs (Rodriquez-Cruz, 2017).

CRITICAL COMPONENT

Blood Pressure Percentiles

- Normal BP: less than 90th percentile
- Prehypertension: 90th to 95th percentile with a BP of 120 mm Hg
- Stage I hypertension: 95th to 99th percentile +5 mm Hg
- Stage II hypertension: >99th percentile +5 mm Hg
- "White coat" hypertension is when BP is >95th percentile in the doctor's office but is normal outside the doctor's office (Rodriquez-Cruz, 2017)

SAFE AND EFFECTIVE NURSING CARE: Cultural Competence

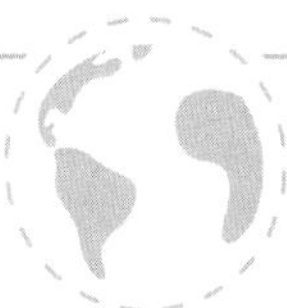

Hereditary Risk Factors for Hispanic Americans

Hereditary factors related to heart disease, hypertension, and stroke are the number one killers of Hispanic Americans (Ewald & Haldeman, 2016). Compared with non-white Hispanics, Hispanics have higher circulating triglycerides and lower high-density lipoproteins, as well as higher levels of inflammatory markers represented by C-reactive protein levels (Ewald, 2016). Recognizing these genetic and hereditary factors can allow the nurse to identify those children who may be at risk for heart disease, hypertension, and stroke.

Assessment

- The left side of the heart works harder and may thicken.
- Hypertension can result in stroke and often affects the child's vision because of increased pressure in the blood vessels of the eye.

SAFE AND EFFECTIVE NURSING CARE: Cultural Competence

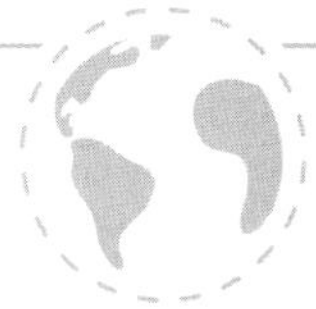

Metabolism of Antihypertensive Medications

Racial differences are associated with enzyme polymorphisms in the metabolism of antihypertensives. Nurses should consider the risks for impaired drug metabolism for hypertension based on ethnic or racial affiliation (Chen, Simonsen, & Liu, 2015).

Diagnostic Tests

- Monitored at well-child visits

Nursing Interventions

- Aim is for reduction of the BP to less than 95% and resolution of end-organ dysfunction.
- Encourage routine exercise.
- Encourage weight loss if indicated.
- Educate the child/caregiver on healthy meal choices with lower intake of salt, saturated fat, trans-fatty acids, cholesterol, and carbohydrates, and increased dietary fiber intake.
- Emergency treatment of acute hypertension is the administration of labetalol (0.1 mg/kg) (Vallerand et al., 2017).
- Chronic hypertension is usually treated with ACE inhibitors.

RHEUMATIC HEART DISEASE

Rheumatic heart disease is systemic inflammatory disease that occurs in response to a group A beta-hemolytic streptococcal infection, such as strep throat, rheumatic fever, or scarlet fever, that starts in the throat. Left untreated or only partially treated, the infection spreads into bloodstream, usually 20 days after the onset of the illness (Ward & Hisley, 2015; Chin, 2017). If the infection remains untreated, it can lead to bacterial or fungi clumps that can break off and travel to the lungs, brain, kidneys, or other organs (rheumatic fever). Damage to the heart valves ensues, which is rheumatic heart disease.

- Antibodies are produced in response to the organism, and lesions develop in the heart and joints.
- The disease is familial.

- It often occurs in children between 5 and 15 years of age who are in lower socioeconomic situations (Ward & Hisley, 2015).
- It is prevalent in the northeastern part of the United States in winter and early spring.

Assessment

- Abdominal pain
- Nosebleeds
- Chest pain and heart palpitations
- Waking from sleep with the need to sit or stand up (paroxysmal nocturnal dyspnea)

Diagnostic Tests

- Jones criteria—first established in 1944 and continually updated. States that there must be two of the major criteria or one of the major and two of the minor criteria present with a streptococcal infection (Gewitz et al., 2015; Special Writing Group of the Committee on Rheumatic Fever, Endocarditis, and Kawasaki Disease of the Council on Cardiovascular Disease in the Young of the American Heart Association, 1992). Revised Jones criteria are as follows:
    - Major criteria include symptoms such as polyarthritis, carditis, subcutaneous nodules, nonpruritic ring rash on the trunk or arms, and subcutaneous nodules (Gewitz et al., 2015; Special Writing Group of the Committee on Rheumatic Fever, Endocarditis, and Kawasaki Disease of the Council on Cardiovascular Disease in the Young of the American Heart Association, 1992).
    - Minor criteria include a history of rheumatic heart disease, increase in C-reactive protein, fever greater than or equal to 38.5°F, and evidence of heart block (Gewitz et al., 2015; Special Writing Group of the Committee on Rheumatic Fever, Endocarditis, and Kawasaki Disease of the Council on Cardiovascular Disease in the Young of the American Heart Association, 1992).
- Physical assessment
- Blood tests for the presence of exposure to strep infection
- EKG
- Echocardiogram
- Enlarged heart and CHF per chest x-ray

Nursing Interventions

- Maintain administration of inflammatory medications and antibiotics.
- Prepare child for admission to hospital and/or surgery.
- Provide detailed education to family regarding prevention, treatment, and reoccurrence of symptoms.

Caregiver Education

- Educate families on the screening of school-age children for sore throats.
- Educate families on the need for completion of antibiotic regimen or prophylaxis as ordered.
- Prepare caregiver for possible hospitalization or heart valve surgery.
- Encourage regular check-ups with cardiologist.
- Encourage immunizations and the annual flu shot.
- Provide education related to prophylaxis antibiotic therapy for dental work.

SUBACUTE BACTERIAL ENDOCARDITIS

Subacute bacterial endocarditis results from a bacterial infection or the introduction of an infective agent through any invasive procedure such as surgery or through a dental cleaning (Ward & Hisley, 2015). Rarely, it can occur through a noninfective source such as severe CHF, renal disease, or severe anemia. Entry of organisms can occur with simple cuts, dental work, teeth brushing, respiratory infections, or catheter placement. The endocardium of the heart becomes inflamed with *Viridans streptococcus*, *Streptococcus mutans*, *Streptococcus sanguis*, or *Staphylococcus*. Bacteria or fungi that have entered the body through the mouth, respiratory system, or bloodstream invade and attach themselves to damaged areas of the endocardium that allow the bacteria to easily attach and multiply. Healthy hearts do not develop endocarditis, but those children with damaged heart valves or heart disease are more susceptible (Friedewald, 2016). Endocarditis can be life-threatening.

Assessment

- Vague symptoms such as low-grade fever; a high fever indicates an acute illness
- Fatigue
- Cough
- Heart murmur
- Chills
- Shortness of breath
- Joint pain
- Loss of appetite and weight loss
- Flank pain
- Petechiae

Diagnostic Tests

- History and physical examination
- Can mimic other infections
- Blood cultures
- Roth spots—round or oval white spots sometimes seen in the retina in the early stages
- Janeway lesions—flat, painless, red to bluish red spots on palms and soles of feet (Friedewald, 2016)
- Osler nodes—painful, red, raised lesions on the palms and soles due to immune complex (Friedewald, 2016); Osler and Roth spots arise because of immune-mediated vasculitis (Brusch, 2016)
- Splinter hemorrhages—black or brown lines under the nails (Friedewald, 2016)
- Complete blood cell count

- Echocardiogram
- Transesophageal echocardiogram—to assess valvular function or vegetation growth

Nursing Interventions

- If untreated, can lead to bacterial or fungi clumps that can break off and travel to the lungs, brain, kidneys, or other organs.
- Monitor for stroke, poor pumping action.
- Maintain intensive antibiotic therapy.
- Monitor for fluid imbalances caused by nausea, vomiting, and diarrhea from antibiotics.
- Monitor for CHF symptoms such as shortness of breath, poor weight gain, and edema.
- Monitor for valve failures and cardiac failure.
- Monitor for septic emboli to the lungs.
- Prepare the child for transplanted valves.

Caregiver Education

- High-risk children with past valve damage, repairs, or defects are at an increased risk and may be treated with prophylactic antibiotics.
- Prepare caregiver for possibility of surgery for valvular replacement.
- Maintain dental health through regular checkups starting as soon as the child's teeth begin to erupt.

Evidence-Based Practice: Dental Procedures for Children With Heart Disease

American Heart Association. (2016). *Infective endocarditis.* Retrieved from http://www.heart.org/HEARTORG/Conditions/CongenitalHeartDefects/TheImpactofCongenitalHeartDefects/Infective-Endocarditis_UCM_307108_Article.jsp#.WQ5C1vkrKiQ

If a child requires dental work and has congenital heart disease, the AHA (2016c) recommends prophylactic antibiotics for dental procedures that involve manipulation of gingival tissue or perforation of the oral mucosa. Children with the highest risk for infective endocarditis include those with the following characteristics:

- A prosthetic heart valve
- A history of endocarditis
- A heart transplant
- Certain congenital heart defects including those birth defects with decreased oxygen levels or those not fully repaired including shunts and conduits
- A congenital heart defect that has been corrected for the first 6 months after the repair
- Repaired congenital heart disease that has residual defects, such as with persisting leaks or abnormal flow

KAWASAKI DISEASE

Kawasaki disease, also known as mucocutaneous lymph node syndrome, is the leading cause of acquired heart disease in children in the developed world. This is a multisystem disease that affects the cardiovascular system and can lead to coronary artery aneurysm (Ward & Hisley, 2015). This childhood polyarteritis nodosa results in acute febrile inflammation of the vasculature and primarily affects children younger than 5 years, with a peak incidence in children younger than 2 (Ward & Hisley, 2015). This disease is not contagious or congenital, and is thought to be caused by an infective organism seen seasonally in certain geographic locations, with a higher incidence in late winter and early spring. Mortality in children results from scarring, stenosis of the main coronary arteries, or MI due to coronary thrombosis. This disease often mirrors other infectious diseases such as measles and scarlet fever.

Assessment

- Kawasaki disease diagnosis is a diagnosis of exclusion.
- Signs and symptoms that last longer than 5 days include high fever greater than 101.3°F (38.5°C), plus a minimum of four of the clustered symptoms in Box 12–1.

Diagnostic Tests

- Diagnosis is through exclusion because it often mimics other diseases such as scarlet fever, toxic shock syndrome, infectious mononucleosis, and mycoplasma.
- Initial laboratory results will indicate an increased white blood cell count.
- Lymphocytosis and thrombocytosis occur.
- High fever that is not resolved with antibiotics or antipyretic therapy may develop.
- A life-threatening complication of Kawasaki disease is the development of coronary artery aneurysms. Baseline echocardiogram 6 to 8 weeks after the onset of symptoms is used to rule out this complication.

BOX 12–1 | Symptoms of Kawasaki Disease

Persistent fever (5 days or more spiking to 104°F (40°C) and the child has four of the following five signs:

- Bilateral conjunctivitis without exudate
- Painful joints
- Red lips, strawberry tongue, congested oral pharynx
- Enlarged lymph nodes—cervical lymphadenopathy (one lymph node larger than 1.5 cm) (Tang, Gao, Shen, Sun, & Yen, 2016)
- Nonspecific groin rash
- Edematous and red (erythema) of hands and feet
- Mimics scarlet fever rash—diffuse polymorphous rash
- Increased white blood cell count
- Extreme irritability
- Cardiac involvement—myocarditis, pericarditis, coronary artery aneurysm, valvular regurgitation, systemic artery aneurysms (Tang et al., 2016)

- Complications include myocarditis, pericarditis, leaking of the valves, pericardial effusion, and CHF.
- MI occurs in 73% of children within the first year of diagnosis (Scheinfeld, 2016).
- Neurological complications can occur, as well as gastrointestinal complications such as hydrops of the gallbladder (Scheinfeld, 2016).

Nursing Interventions

- Maintain anti-inflammatory medications such as high-dose salicylate therapy, which can also be continued for 6 to 8 weeks as an antiplatelet therapy.
- IV gamma globulin is given for the first 10 days after the onset of the symptoms to prevent coronary aneurysms.
- Monitor the child's cardiac status closely for signs and symptoms of CHF.
- Nursing care is aimed at symptom relief (Ward & Hisley, 2015).

Caregiver Education

- Encourage professional intervention in an infant or child with unresolved fever.
- Kawasaki disease is usually self-limiting.

SAFE AND EFFECTIVE NURSING CARE: Promoting Safety

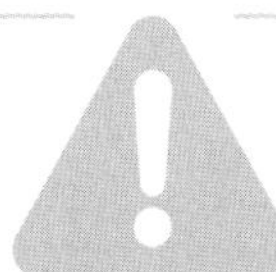

Safety education for caregivers of children with Kawasaki disease should include:

- Loose clothing
- Cool cloths
- Lip and mouth care
- Clear liquids that are tepid and soft foods to minimize irritation of the oral mucosa
- Parental support for inconsolable child
- Discharge teaching aimed at understanding the progression of the disease
- Prolonged irritability
- Peeling of hands and feet
- Arthritis of weight-bearing joints—stretching and passive range of motion
- Defer live immunizations such as measles, mumps, rubella, chickenpox
- Educate on lifelong possibility of development of cardiac disease.
- CPR training (Scheinfeld, 2016)

HEART TRANSPLANTATION

The replacement of diseased heart with a healthy one is indicated for children who have serious heart dysfunction, congenital heart disease, or cardiomyopathy. The United Network for Organ Sharing (UNOS) is responsible for transplant organ distribution in the United States. People in most urgent need of a transplant are placed highest on the list and are given priority when a donor heart becomes available; the list is assessed daily. Healthy hearts are given by organ donors or parents of critically ill children.

Diagnostic Tests

- Blood tests
- Echocardiogram
- EKG
- Cardiac catheterization

Nursing Interventions

- Provide preparation of children for surgery.
- Provide preparation of caregiver for surgery.
- Provide detailed education on medications, signs and symptoms of rejection, and follow-up care.

Caregiver Education

- When organ is available, child will be called to hospital.
- Final blood work will be done to ensure match to organ.
- Child will go to the operating room.
- Transplant will take several hours.
- Long-term medication will be necessary for cardiac management, to reduce risk for organ rejection, and to decrease the load on the heart.
- Educate caregiver on antirejection drugs.

SAFE AND EFFECTIVE NURSING CARE: Clinical Pearl

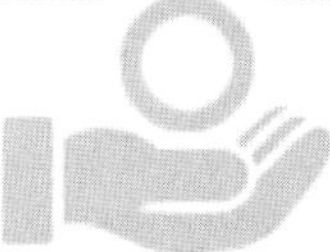

After an organ has been transplanted, the body's immune system may identify this organ as a foreign object and will develop antibodies to attack the donor heart.

Common Signs and Symptoms of Heart Transplant Rejection

- Fever
- Decreased urine output or fewer wet diapers than usual
- Elevated heart rate
- Fast breathing rate
- Weight gain
- Fatigue
- Irritability
- Poor appetite
- Random episodes
- Palpitations
- Anxiety
- Lightheadedness

CARDIAC DYSRHYTHMIAS

Cardiac dysrhythmias are problems with the rate or rhythm of the heartbeat; heart rates that are too fast or too slow affect cardiac output to the brain, heart, and other organs. This is a medical emergency.

Tachycardia

There are two primary types of tachycardia: supraventricular tachycardia and ventricular tachycardia.

Supraventricular Tachycardia

- Occurs in the atria of the heart
- Heart rate greater than 220 bpm
- Treatment
  - Stimulate vagal response through nasal suctioning.
  - Apply crushed ice to the forehead.
  - Adenosine (Adenocard)—rapid IV push in a proximal site, repeat within 2 minutes with no response (Valleran et al., 2017).
  - Older children may be asked to bear down as if having a bowel movement, which stimulates the vagus nerve to slow the heart rate.

Ventricular Tachycardia

- Occurs in the ventricles
- Loss of consciousness
- Sudden death

Torsades de Pointes

- Inherited or induced disorder of the electrical system with prolonged QT intervals
- The QT interval represents repolarization of a cardiac cell
- Affects approximately 1 in 5,000 people (Ward & Hisley, 2015)
- Sudden, unexpected, life-threatening type of ventricular tachycardia
- Causes include inherited factors, diarrhea, malnutrition, hypomagnesium, hypokalemia, and hypocalcemia, and it may be drug induced, such as from anti-arrhythmics or some forms of antibiotic use
- Rapid decline in BP, fainting, ventricular fibrillation, and death
- Treatment includes removing the causes, such as the drugs; treating the abnormalities, such as with administration of magnesium or potassium; and unsynchronized defibrillation for ventricular fibrillation because of the polymorphic nature
- Implantation of a defibrillator may be needed

Bradycardia

- Conduction moves to the SA node down a specific path to reach the ventricles
- Passes through specialized conducting tissue called the AV node
- Sinus bradycardia is when a QRS wave follows a P wave
- Doesn't transmit = heart block or AV block
- Blocks classified by level of impairment: first-degree heart block, second-degree heart block, or third-degree (complete or AV heart block)
- Congenital, injury, or postsurgical
- A pacemaker may be necessary

Wolff-Parkinson-White Syndrome

- Electrical stimulation reaches the ventricles too soon
- Pre-excitatory syndromes
- Tachycardia
- Syncope
- Chest palpitations
- Death
- Ablation with radiofrequency to treat

SHOCK

Shock is the inability of the body to maintain adequate blood flow and oxygen supply to the tissues needed for metabolism.

- Shock is the leading cause of childhood morbidity and mortality in the world (Pasman, 2015).
- The underlying cause is often difficult to diagnose.
- The three types of shock are hypovolemic, cardiogenic, and septic or distributive (Lee et al., 2017)
  - Hypovolemic—profound dehydration or loss of blood with decrease in hemoglobin; chest x-ray shows normal heart
  - Cardiogenic—damage to the heart muscle resulting in a failure of the pump (Lee et al., 2017)
  - Septic or distributive—shifting of fluids from the intravascular space to the extracellular space; caused by blood vessel dilation, often due to sepsis
- Shock can affect any end organs in the body.
- This is a medical emergency and is fatal if not treated right away.
- Treatment is dependent on identified cause, fluids, blood and blood products, antibiotics, and inotropes to increase BP and delivery of oxygen to the tissues (Colleti & Werther, 2017; Lee et al., 2017).

Assessment

- Confusion or lack of alertness
- Loss of consciousness
- A sudden, rapid heartbeat
- Sweating
- Pale skin
- A weak pulse
- Rapid breathing
- Decreased or no urine output
- Cool hands and feet

Diagnostic Tests

- Monitoring of BP
- Chest x-ray
- Echocardiogram
- Arterial blood gases

Nursing Interventions

- Provide emergency interventions.
- Maintain medications, IV access, and fluids to increase volume and BP.
- Maintain oxygen supplementation.

Caregiver Education

- Provide education to call 911 for signs and symptoms of shock.
- Provide education related to intake and output of the child.

Case Study

Obesity and Hypertension

Maria, age 8, is the fourth child of a single-mother household. Maria is in the third grade, is 50 inches, and weighs 75 pounds. Maria does well in school and has many friends her age. Her three older siblings are of average height and weight. Maria's body mass index (BMI) is 21.1, and she is in the 95th percentile for BMI. Maria is classified as obese. Maria's healthy weight should be between 51 and 66 pounds. Her BP this morning was 120/80 mm Hg.

Childhood obesity has been linked with adverse health outcomes including cardiovascular disease, diabetes, and some cancers (Simmonds, Llewellyn, Owen, & Woolacott, 2016). Cultural factors in the Hispanic community often view thinness in their children as a sign of poor parenting (Simmonds et al., 2016). Obesity is the number one risk factor in the development of hypertension.

1. What does it mean that Maria's BMI is in the 95th percentile?
2. What type of anticipatory guidance can the nurse provide to Maria's mother to address her weight issues?
3. What is the DASH eating plan?
4. What other risk factors can be modified in the hypertensive child?

REFERENCES

Acute Care of at-Risk Newborns Neonatal Society (ACoRN). (2009, September). 2010 Update. Vancouver, British Columbia: Author.

Altman, C. A. (2017). Identifying newborns with critical congenital heart disease. *UpToDate.* Retrieved from https://www.uptodate.com/contents/identifying-newborns-with-critical-congenital-heart-disease

American Academy of Pediatrics (AAP). (2017). *Congenital Heart Public Health Consortium: Fact sheets.* Retrieved from https://www.aap.org/en-us/advocacy-and-policy/aap-health-initiatives/chphc/Pages/Fact-Sheet.aspx

American Heart Association (AHA). (2015a). *CHD's impact on children.* Retrieved from http://www.heart.org/HEARTORG/Conditions/Congenital-HeartDefects/TheImpactofCongenitalHeartDefects/CHDs-Impact-on-Children_UCM_307115_Article.jsp#.WQiNkfnyuiQ

American Heart Association (AHA). (2015b). *Facts about critical congenital heart defects.* Retrieved from https://www.cdc.gov/ncbddd/heartdefects/cchd-facts.html

American Heart Association (AHA). (2015c). *The impact of congenital heart defects.* Retrieved from http://www.heart.org/HEARTORG/Conditions/CongenitalHeartDefects/TheImpactofCongenitalHeartDefects/The-Impact-of-Congenital-Heart-Defects_UCM_001218_Article.jsp#.WQiNGvnyuiQ

American Heart Association (AHA). (2016a). *Dietary recommendations for children.* Retrieved from http://www.heart.org/HEARTORG/HealthyLiving/HealthyKids/HowtoMakeaHealthyHome/Dietary-Recommendations-for-Healthy-Children_UCM_303886_Article.jsp#.WQ4La_krKiQ

American Heart Association (AHA). (2016b). *Heart murmurs and valve disease.* Retrieved from http://www.heart.org/HEARTORG/Conditions/More/HeartValveProblemsandDisease/Heart-Murmurs-and-Valve-Disease_UCM_450616_Article.jsp#.WQ9T4vkrKiQ

American Heart Association (AHA). (2016c). *Infective endocarditis.* Retrieved from http://www.heart.org/HEARTORG/Conditions/CongenitalHeartDefects/TheImpactofCongenitalHeartDefects/Infective-Endocarditis_UCM_307108_Article.jsp#.WQ5C1vkrKiQ

American Heart Association (AHA). (2016d). *Implantable cardioverter defibrillatory (ICD).* Retrieved from http://www.heart.org/HEARTORG/Conditions/Arrhythmia/PreventionTreatmentofArrhythmia/Implantable-Cardioverter-Defibrillator-ICD_UCM_448478_Article.jsp#.WQ3zN_krKiQ

American Heart Association (AHA). (2016e). *Pediatric cardiomyopathies.* Retrieved from http://www.heart.org/HEARTORG/Conditions/More/Cardiovascular-ConditionsofChildhood/Pediatric-Cardiomyopathies_UCM_312219_Article.jsp#.WQzeePnyuiQ

American Heart Association (AHA). (2016f). *Ventricular septal defect (VSD).* Retrieved from http://www.heart.org/HEARTORG/Conditions/Congenital-HeartDefects/AboutCongenitalHeartDefects/Ventricular-Septal-Defect-VSD_UCM_307041_Article.jsp#.WQudl_nyuiQ

American Heart Association (AHA). (2017). *Cardiac catheterization.* Retrieved from http://www.heart.org/HEARTORG/Conditions/HeartAttack/SymptomsDiagnosisofHeartAttack/Cardiac-Catheterization_UCM_451486_Article.jsp#.WQuBd_nyuiR

Berger, S. (2016). Cardiac evaluation of patients receiving pharmacotherapy for attention deficit hyperactivity disorder. *UpToDate.* Retrieved from http://www.uptodate.com/contents/cardiac-evaluation-of-patients-receiving-pharmacotherapy-for-attention-deficit-hyperactivity-disorder

Benitz, W. E. (2016). Patent ductus arteriosus in preterm infants. *Pediatrics, 137*(1), e20153730. doi: 10.1542/peds.2015-3730

Bhimji, S. (2016). Tetralogy of Fallot treatment and management. *Medscape.* Retrieved from http://emedicine.medscape.com/article/2035949-treatment#d14

Brusch, J. L. (2016). Infective endocarditis clinical presentation. *Medscape.* Retrieved from http://emedicine.medscape.com/article/216650-clinical

Centers for Disease Control and Prevention (CDC). (2016a). *Attention-deficit/hyperactivity disorder (ADHD).* Retrieved from https://www.cdc.gov/ncbddd/adhd/guidelines.html

Centers for Disease Control and Prevention (CDC). (2016b). *Facts about pulmonary atresia.* Retrieved from https://www.cdc.gov/ncbddd/heartdefects/pulmonaryatresia.html

Centers for Disease Control and Prevention (CDC). (2016c). *Facts about tetralogy of Fallot.* Retrieved from https://www.cdc.gov/ncbddd/heartdefects/tetralogyoffallot.html

Centers for Disease Control and Prevention (CDC). (2016d). *Facts about truncus arteriosus.* Retrieved from https://www.cdc.gov/ncbddd/heartdefects/truncusarteriosus.html

Charpie, J. R. (2017). Transposition of the great arteries. *Medscape.* Retrieved from http://emedicine.medscape.com/article/900574-overview

Chen, L., Simonsen, N., & Lui, L. (2015). Racial differences of pediatric hypertension in relation to birth weight and body size in the U.S. *PLoS ONE, 10*(7), e0132606. doi: 10.1371/journal.pone0132606

Chin, T. K. (2017). Rheumatic heart disease. *Medscape.* Retrieved from http://emedicine.medscape.com/article/891897-overview

Colleti, J., & Werther, B. (2017). Vasoactive drugs in pediatric shock: In search of a paradigm. *Pediatric Critical Care Medicine, 18*(2), 202–203. doi: 10.1097/PCC.0000000000001040

Dani, C., Drovandi, L., Bertini, G., Poggi, C., & Pratesi, S. (2017). Unexpected episodes of cyanosis in late preterm and term neonates prompted admission to a neonatal care unit. *Italian Journal of Pediatrics, 43*(35), 1–5. doi: 10.1186/s13052-017-0349-9

Diane, V., & Mvongo, N. (2017). Congenital heart disease and impact on child development. *Pediatric Cardiologists, 6*(Suppl. 2). doi: 10.4172/2329-6607-C1-003

Durham, R. & Chaptman, L. (2014). *Maternal Newborn Nursing: The Critical Components of Nursing Care* (3rd ed.). Philadelphia, Pa: FA Davis.

Ewald, D. R., & Haldeman, L. A. (2016). Risk factors in adolescent hypertension. *Global Pediatric Health, 3,* 2333794x15625159. doi: 10.1177/2333794x15625159

Friedewald, V. E. (2016). Infective endocarditis (subacute bacterial endocarditis/SBE). *Clinical Guide to Cardiovascular Disease,* 771–787. doi: 10.1007/978-1-4471-7293-2_55

Gaillard, F. (2017). Figure 3 sign. *Radiopoedia.* Retrieved from https://radiopaedia.org/articles/figure-3-sign

Gewitz, M. H., Baltimore, R. S., Tani, L. Y., Sable, C. A., Shulman, S. T., Carapetis, J., & Kaplan, E. L. (2015). Revision of the Jones criteria for the diagnosis of acute rheumatic fever in the era of Doppler echocardiography. *Circulation, 131,* 1806–1818. doi: 10.1161/CIR.0000000000000205

Haroun, H. (2017). Teratogenicity and teratogenic factors. *Anatomy & Physiology, 3*(1), 1–5. doi: 10.15406/mojap.2017.03.00082

Hill, M.A. (2017). Abnormal development—Teratogens. *Embrology.* Retrieved from https://embryology.med.unsw.edu.au/embryology/index.php/Abnormal_Development-Teratogens

Houston, B. A., & Stevens, G. R. (2015). Hypertrophic cardiomyopathy: a review. *Clinical Medicine Insights: Cardiology, 8*(Suppl. 1), 53–65. doi: 10.4137/CMC.S15717

Jahangir, E. (2015). Blood pressure assessment. *Medscape.* Retrieved from http://emedicine.medscape.com/article/1948157-overview

Kumarasinghe, G., & Carroll, G. (2015). A guide to peripheral oedema. *Medicine Today, 16*(6), 26–34.

Lee, E., Hsia, S., Lin, J., Chan, O., Lee, J., Lin, C., & Wu, H. (2017). Hemodynamic analysis of pediatric septic shock and cardiogenic shock using transpulmonary thermodilution. *BioMedical Research International, 2017,* 3613475. doi: 10.1155/2017/3613475

Lui, J., Li, H., Lui, Z., Wu, Q., & Xu, Y. (2016). Complete preoperative evaluation of pulmonary atresia with ventricular septal defect with multi-detector computed topography. *PLoS ONE, 11*(1), e0146380. doi: 10.1371/journal.pone.0146380

Magellan Health. (2017). Appropriate use of psychotropic drugs in children and adolescents: A clinical monograph. *Magellan Healthcare & Magellan Rx Management,* 1–62. https://www.magellanhealth.com/media/445492/magellan-psychotropicdrugs-0203141.pdf

McElhinney, D. B. (2015). Truncus arteriosus clinical presentation. *Medscape.* Retrieved from http://emedicine.medscape.com/article/892489-clinical

McGovern, M. M. (2017). Noonan syndrome. *Medscape.* Retrieved from http://emedicine.medscape.com/article/947504-overview

Mozaffarian, D. (2016). Dietary and policy priorities for cardiovascular disease, diabetes, and obesity. *Circulation, 133,* 187–225. doi: 10.1161/CIRCULATIONAHA.115.018585

Nagalla, S. (2016). Secondary polycythemia clinical presentation. *Medscape.* Retrieved from http://emedicine.medscape.com/article/205039-clinical

Nishimura, R. A., Otto, C. M., Bonow, R. O., Carabello, B. A., Erwin, J. P., Fleisher, L. A., ... Thompson, A. (2017). 2017 AHA/ACC focused update of the 2014 AHA/ACC guideline for the management of patients with valvular heart disease: A Report of the American College of Cardiology/American Heart Association Task Force on Clinical Practice Guidelines. *Circulation, 135*(25), e1159–e1195. doi: 10.1161/CIR.0000000000000503

Ohlsson, A., & Shah, P. S. (2015). Paracetamol (acetaminophen) for patent ductus arteriosus in preterm or low-birth-weight infants. *Cochrane Database of Systematic Reviews, 3,* CD010061. doi: 10.1002/14651858CD010061.pub2

Ohye, R. G. (2016). Current therapy for hypoplastic left heart syndrome and related single ventricle lesions. *Circulation, 134,* 1265–1279. doi: 10.1161/CIRCULATIONAHA.116.022816

Ooi, H. H. (2016). Heart failure guidelines. *Medscape.* Retrieved from http://emedicine.medscape.com/article/2500037-overview

Oster, M. E., Aucott, S. W., Glidewell, J., Hackell, J., Kochilas, L., Martine, G. R., ... Kemper, A. R. (2016). Lessons learned from newborn screening for critical congenital heart defects. *Pediatrics, 137*(5), e20154573. doi: 10.1542/peds.2015-4573

Pasman, E. A. (2015). Shock in pediatrics. *Medscape.* Retrieved from http://emedicine.medscape.com/article/1833578-overview

Patnana, S. R. (2015). Coartation of the aorta. *Medscape.* Retrieved from http://emedicine.medscape.com/article/895502-clinical

Pettersen, M. D. (2015). Tetralogy of Fallot with pulmonary atresia. *Medscape.* Retrieved from http://emedicine.medscape.com/article/899368-overview

Postma, A. V., Bezzina, C. R., & Christoffels, V. M. (2016). Genetics of congenital heart disease: The contribution of the noncoding regulatory genome. *Journal of Human Genetics, 61,* 13–19. doi: 10.1038/jhg.2015.98

Prescott, S., & Keim-Malpass, J. (2017). Patient ductus arteriosus in the preterm infant. *Advances in Neonatal Care, 17*(1), 10–18. doi: 10.1097/ANC.0000000000000375

Rodriquez-Cruz, E. (2017). Pediatric hypertension. *Medscape.* Retrieved from http://emedicine.medscape.com/article/889877-overview

Rohrs, H. J. (2015a). Pediatric lipid disorders in clinical practice workup. *Medscape.* Retrieved http://emedicine.medscape.com/article/1825087-workup

Rohrs, H. J. (2015b). Pediatric lipid disorders in clinical practice treatment and management. *Medscape.* Retrieved from http://emedicine.medscape.com/article/1825087-treatment

Scheinfeld, N. S. (2016). Kawasaki disease. *Medscape.* Retrieved from http://emedicine.medscape.com/article/965367-overview

Sexton, D. J. (2017). Patient education: Antibiotics before procedures (Beyond the basics). *UpToDate.* Retrieved from http://www.uptodate.com/contents/antibiotics-before-procedures-beyond-the-basics

Shea, M. J. (2016). Cardiac auscultation. *Merck Manual.* Retrieved from https://www.merckmanuals.com/professional/cardiovascular-disorders/approach-to-the-cardiac-patient/cardiac-auscultation

Simmonds, M., Llewellyn, A., Owen, C. G., & Woolacott, N. (2016). Predicting adult obesity from childhood obesity: A systematic review and meta-analysis. *Obesity Review, 17*(2), 95–107. doi: 10.1111/obr.12334

Slodki, M., Respondek-Liberska, M., Pruetz, J. D., & Donofrio, M. T. (2016). Changing the definition of critical heart disease in the newborn. *Journal of Perinatology, 36*(8), 575–580. doi: 10.1038/jp.2016.20

Special Writing Group of the Committee on Rheumatic Fever, Endocarditis, and Kawasaki Disease of the Council on Cardiovascular Disease in the Young of the American Heart Association. (1992). Guidelines for the diganosis of acute rheumatic fever: Jones Criteria, 1992 update. Journal of the American Medical Association, 268, 2069–2073.

Tang, Y., Gao, X., Shen, J., Sun, L., & Yen, W. (2016). Epidemiological and clinical characteristics of Kawasaki disease and factors associated with coronary artery abnormalities in east China: Nine years experience. *Journal of Tropical Pediatrics, 62*(2), 86–93. doi: 10.1093/tropej/fmv077

Tayal, U., Prasad, S., & Cook, S. A. (2017). Genetics and genomics of dilated cardiomyopathy and systolic heart failure. *Genome Medicine, 9*(1), 20. doi: 10.1186/s13073-017-0410-8

Tsuda, T. (2016). Lectures series of congenital heart disease. Cyanotic congenital heart disease. *Journal of Heart and Cardiology, 2*(1), 1–5. doi: 10.15436/2378-6914.16.014

U.S. Library of Medicine. (2017). *Congenital heart defects.* Retrieved from https://medlineplus.gov/congenitalheartdefects.html

U.S. Preventive Services Task Force; Bibbins-Doming, K., Grossman, D. C., Curry, S. J., Davidson, K. W., Epling, J. W., Jr., ... Siu, A. L. (2016). Screening for lipid disorders in children and adolescents. US Preventative Services Task Force recommendation statement. *Journal of the American Medical Association, 316*(6), 625–633. doi: 10.1001/jama.2016.9852

Valizadeh, L., Avazeh, M., Hosseini, M. B., & Jafarabad, M. A. (2014). Comparison of clustered care with three and four procedures on physiological responses of preterm infants: Randomized crossover clinical trial. *Journal of Caring Science, 3*(1), 1–10. doi: 10.5681/jcs.2014.001

Vallerand, A. H., Sanoski, C. A., & Deglin, J. H. (2017). *Davis's drug guide for nurses* (15th ed.). Philadelphia, PA: F.A. Davis & Co.

Viola, N. (2015). Surgical approach to partial and total anomalous pulmonary venous connection. *Medscape.* Retrieved from http://emedicine.medscape.com/article/902981-overview

Ward, S. L., & Hisley, S. M. (2015). *Maternal-child nurse care: Optimizing outcomes for mothers, children, & families* (2nd ed.) Philadelphia: F.A. Davis Co.

13

Neurological and Sensory Disorders

Tina Goodpasture, MSN, RN, FNP

LEARNING OUTCOMES

Upon completion of this chapter, the student will be able to:

1. Identify the normal assessment of the pediatric nervous system.
2. Describe normal growth and development of the brain and spinal cord.
3. Identify disorders that can result in intellectual and developmental delays in children.
4. Identify common neurological congenital abnormalities of the nervous system.
5. Recognize seizure disorders and treatment for seizure types.
6. Recognize disorders resulting in temporary loss of consciousness.
7. Identify headache disorders in children.
8. Identify neurocutaneous disorders in children.
9. Identify common movement disorders in children.
10. Identify common causes of pediatric stroke.
11. Identify neuromuscular disorders in children.
12. Identify types of neuropathy that occur in children.
13. Identify types of infections that affect the neurological system.
14. Identify common behavioral concerns in children.

ANATOMY AND PHYSIOLOGY

The nervous system has two parts: the peripheral nervous system and the central nervous system. The neuron is the central component of the nervous system. Myelin is a protective covering that provides insulation for electrical impulses from nerve cells.

Peripheral Nervous System

The peripheral nervous system has two parts: the somatic or voluntary nervous system and the autonomic or involuntary nervous system. The somatic system has two kinds of nerves: afferent and efferent nerves.

- Afferent nerve fibers carry information from receptors in the body to the brain.
- Efferent nerve fibers carry information from the brain to the body.

Autonomic Nervous System

The autonomic nervous system is responsible for involuntary nerve actions that control body functions, such as heart rate, breathing, digestion, perspiring, urination, salivation, and sexual arousal. The two divisions of the autonomic nervous system are the sympathetic and parasympathetic nervous systems.

- The sympathetic system is responsible for action, such as the fight-or-flight response.
- The parasympathetic system is responsible for rest and recuperation of the body systems.

Central Nervous System

The central nervous system is composed of the brain and the spinal cord. The brain is divided into three main sections: cerebrum, cerebellum, and brainstem.

Brain

- The cerebrum, the largest section of the brain, is responsible for complex functions such as actions and thoughts (Fig. 13–1).
  - The cerebrum is divided into two hemispheres and four lobes.
  - The hemispheres are separated by the longitudinal fissure and communicate with each other via the corpus callosum.
  - The four lobes are named for the bones that cover them.
- The surface of the brain is a layer of gray matter called the cerebral cortex.
  - There are three types of functional areas in the cerebral cortex: motor areas that control voluntary movement, sensory areas that control conscious awareness of sensation, and association areas that integrate information.
  - Conscious behavior involves the entire cortex. There is no functional area that acts independently.
  - Below the gray matter is a layer of white matter, which is composed of bundles of myelinated nerve cells that carry nerve impulses to neurons.
- Each brain hemisphere is divided into four lobes: the frontal lobe, the parietal lobe, the temporal lobe, and the occipital lobe.
  - The frontal lobe is responsible for managing emotions, judgment, impulse control, social behavior, and some motor functions.
  - The parietal lobe is responsible for perception and interpretation of touch, pressure, temperature, and pain, as well as some muscular movements.
  - The temporal lobe is responsible for perception and recognition of auditory information, memory, and speech.
  - The occipital lobe is responsible for processing visual information.
- Hemispheres act in a contralateral fashion, which means that they control the opposite side of the body.
- The cerebellum is a small structure that lies under the larger cerebrum and serves to coordinate motor activity and equilibrium.
- The brainstem is the lower portion of the brain.
  - The brainstem connects with the spinal cord and houses the connections between the motor and sensory portions of the brain and the rest of the body.
  - It houses 10 of the 12 pairs of cranial nerves.
  - It controls automatic behaviors necessary for the body to survive.
  - It contributes to the regulation of the heart rate and respirations, as well as the body's ability to manage consciousness and sleep patterns.

Cranial Nerves

There are 12 pairs of cranial nerves (Table 13–1). All but two pairs emerge from the brainstem. Some cranial nerves are involved in the function of special sensory functions (such as vision and hearing), whereas others control motor movements in the face and neck.

Ventricles and Meninges

- The ventricles are cavities in the brain that produce cerebrospinal fluid (CSF).
- CSF serves to provide nourishment and cushioning to the brain and the spinal cord.
- The meninges are the system of membranes that make up the covering of the central nervous system and are composed of three layers: dura mater, arachnoid, and pia mater.
  - The dura mater—means "tough mother"; a thick, strong membrane that surrounds the venous system that takes blood from the brain to the heart

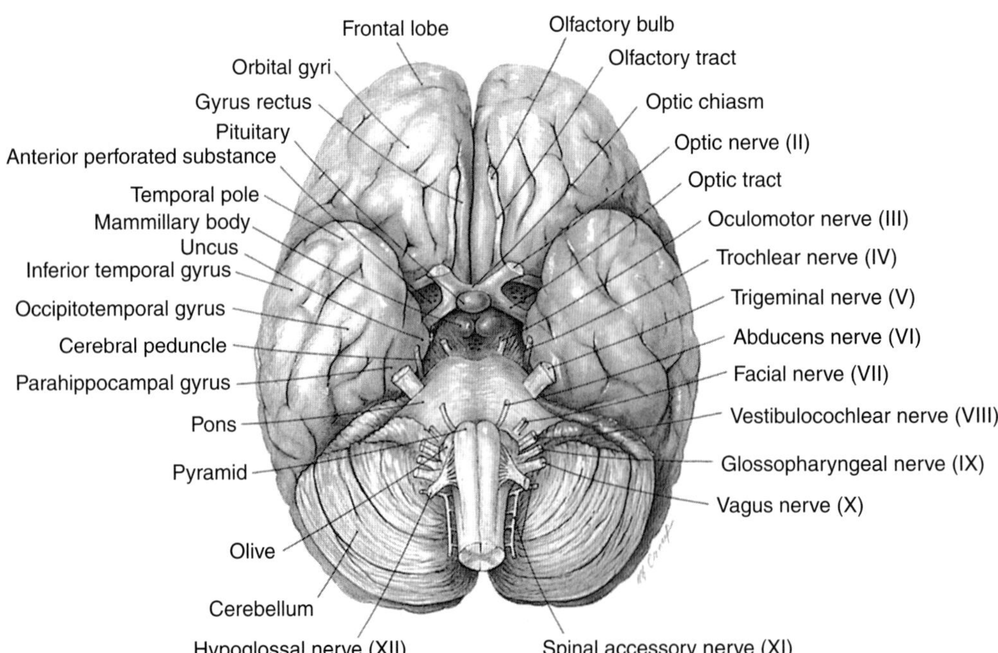

FIGURE 13–1 Ventral surface of the human brain.

TABLE 13–1 Cranial Nerves

CRANIAL NERVE	FUNCTION
Olfactory (I)	Sensory—smell
Optic (II)	Sensory—vision and visual reflexes
Oculomotor (III)	Motor—extraocular eye movement, eyelids, papillary constriction, accommodation of lens
Trochlear (IV)	Motor—extraocular eye movement
Trigeminal (V)	Sensory—facial sensation, corneal reflex, chewing Motor—biting and jaw movements
Abducens (VI)	Motor—extraocular eye movement
Facial (VII)	Sensory—facial sensation, taste Motor—facial expression, salivation, lacrimation
Vestibulocochlear (VIII)	Sensory—equilibrium and hearing
Glossopharyngeal (IX)	Sensory—sensation of middle ear; pharynx, palate, and posterior tongue; taste from posterior tongue Motor—swallowing, salivation
Vagus (X)	Sensory—pharynx, larynx, thorax, abdomen Motor—swallowing and speech, heart rate, gag reflex Autonomic—parasympathetic response to thorax and abdomen
Spinal accessory (XI)	Motor—head rotation, shoulder muscles
Hypoglossal (XII)	Motor—tongue

- The arachnoid—has a thin and spidery appearance; a loose-fitting sac that serves to help cushion and protect the central nervous system
- The pia mater—means "soft mother"; a thin membrane that completely covers all of the surfaces of the brain and spinal cord, holding blood vessels and capillaries

Spinal Cord

- The spinal cord is protected by the bones of the vertebrae and is divided into five sections: cervical, thoracic, lumbar, sacral, and coccygeal (Fig. 13–2).
  - Cervical—nerves in the neck that supply movement and feeling to top of the head, base of the skull, neck muscles, shoulders, elbows, arms, wrists, hands, fingers, esophagus, heart, coronary arteries, lungs, chest, breast, and diaphragm
  - Thoracic—nerves in the upper back that supply blood to the head, brain, eyes, ears, nose, sinuses, mouth, esophagus, heart, lungs, breast, gallbladder, liver, diaphragm, stomach, pancreas, spleen, kidneys, small intestines, uterus, appendix, buttocks, and colon
  - Lumbar—nerves in the lower back that control and provide regulation for the uterus, large intestines, buttocks, groin, reproductive organs, colon, upper legs, knees, and sciatic nerve
  - Sacral—nerves that control and regulate the buttocks, reproductive organs, bladder, prostate, sciatic nerve, lower legs, ankles, feet, and rectum
  - Coccygeal—nerves that control and regulate the rectum
- The spinal cord is covered by meninges and has five layers:
  - Dura mater
  - Subdural space
  - Arachnoid space
  - Subarachnoid space
  - Pia mater
- The spinal cord has gray matter in the center of the cord and white matter in the outer aspect.
  - The spinal cord gray matter functions to provide communication between the peripheral and central nervous systems.
  - Spinal cord gray matter is not covered by a myelin sheath.
  - The spinal cord white matter functions to hold columns or tracts that carry information to and from the brain.
    - The ascending tracts carry sensory information toward the brain.
    - The descending tracts carry motor information from the brain to the body.

Reflexes

Reflexes are involuntary movements that occur in response to a stimulus. They occur at the brainstem or spinal cord level.

- Deep tendon reflexes occur at the level of the spinal cord (Table 13–2).
  - Provide information about the communication between the central nervous system and the peripheral nervous system.

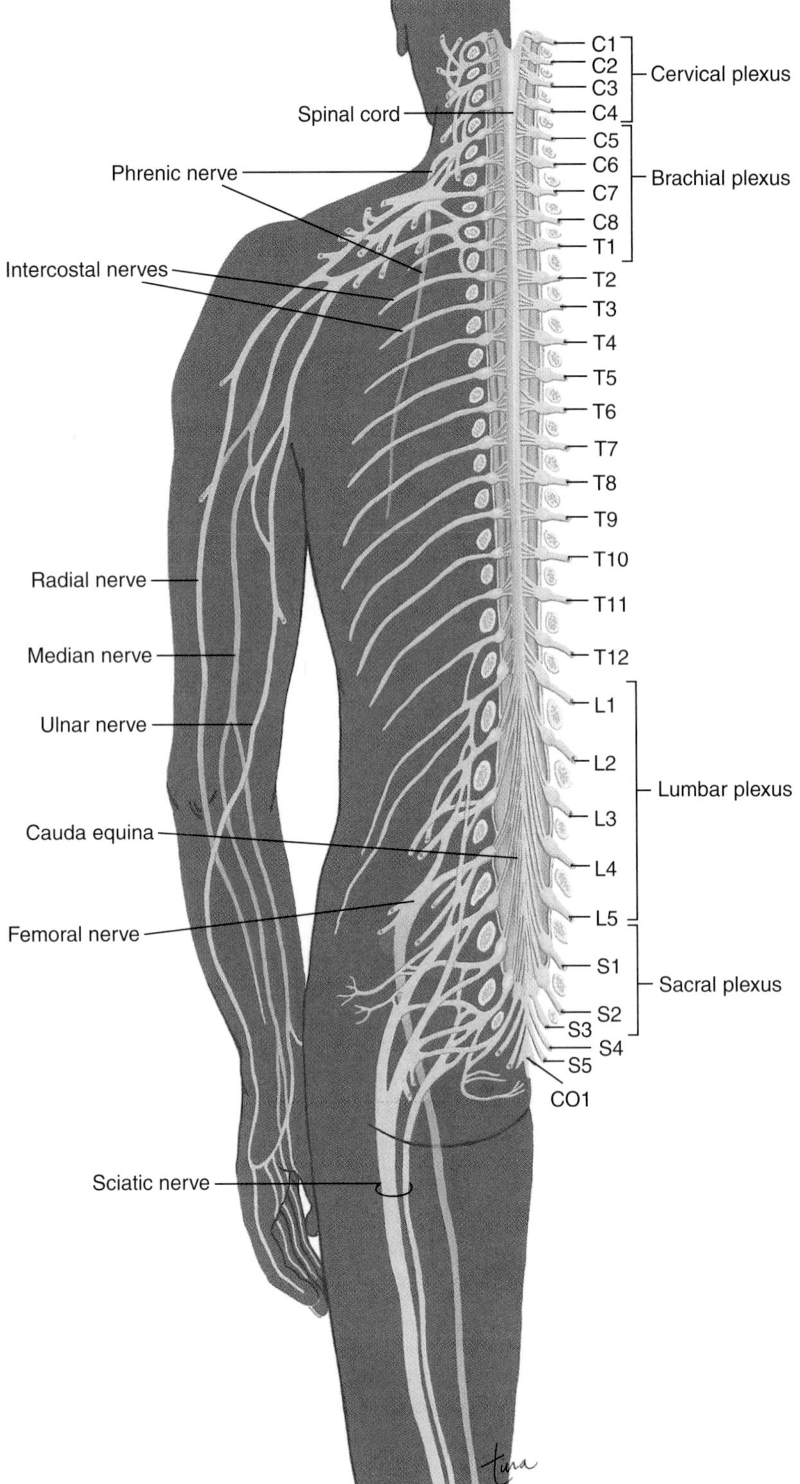

FIGURE 13–2 The spinal cord and vertebral bodies.

- A decreased reflex response usually indicates a problem with the peripheral nervous system.
- A brisk or exaggerated reflex response indicates a problem with the central nervous system.
- The deep tendon reflexes are sometimes called stretch reflexes.
- The deep tendon reflexes are controlled by the spinal nerves.

● Primitive reflexes are controlled by the brainstem (Table 13–3).
- Primitive reflexes are also called survival reflexes or newborn reflexes.
- They are automatic, stereotyped movements in infants.
- Primitive reflexes are present at birth in full-term newborns, and most disappear in the first months of life.
- In premature infants, some primitive reflexes are not present or are suppressed by treatment necessary for them to survive.
- Some primitive reflexes remain throughout life, such as blinking.
- Absent primitive reflexes indicate interruptions in sensory and motor processes in the brain and spinal cord.

TABLE 13-2 Deep Tendon Reflexes

REFLEX	SOURCE SPINAL NERVES
Biceps reflex	C5, C6
Brachioradialis reflex	C5, C6, C7
Extensor digitorum reflex	C6, C7
Triceps reflex	C6, C7, C8
Patellar reflex or knee-jerk reflex	L2, L3, L4
Achilles reflex or ankle-jerk reflex	S1, S2
Babinski reflex or plantar reflex	L5, S1, S2

- If primitive reflexes persist past the age at which they should disappear, it indicates that the child will have problems with normal development, because the frontal lobe of the brain has not inhibited these reflexes and the cerebral cortex has not assumed the role of directing more complex, voluntary functions.
- In patients with brain injury, the primitive reflexes may resurface if the frontal lobe is no longer suppressing them. This is called the frontal release sign.

NEUROLOGICAL DEVELOPMENT

Neurological development begins during the embryonic period and continues on a fairly predictable schedule through adolescence. This predictable pace of development is known as developmental

TABLE 13-3 Primitive Reflexes

REFLEX	ONSET	ACTION	EXPECTED AGE OF DISAPPEARANCE
Asymmetrical tonic neck reflex or "fencing" reflex 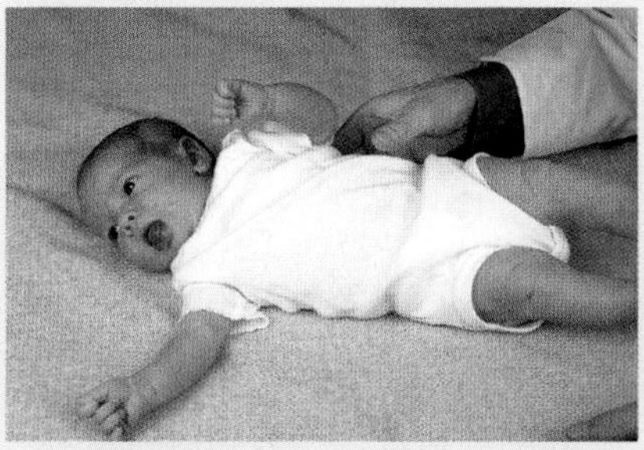	Birth	When the infant is lying in a supine position and the head is turned to the side, the infant responds by extending the arm and leg outward on the side to which the head is turned; the arm and leg on the opposite side remain flexed	At 6 months when the child is awake Abnormal if the infant holds the posture for more than a few seconds or if it is present after 6 months of age Indicates a lesion in the hemisphere of the brain opposite the direction to which the face is turned
Palmar grasp reflex 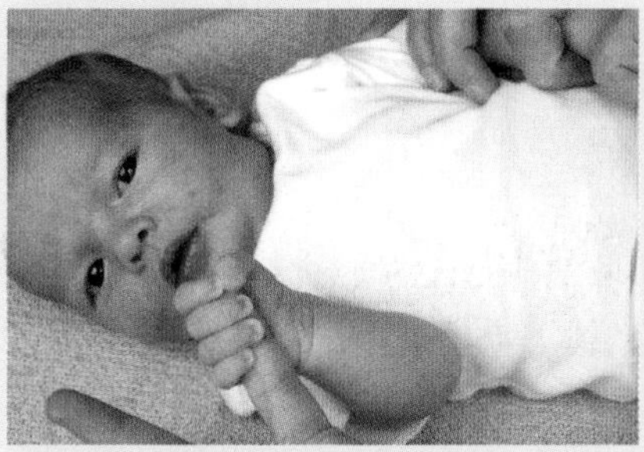	Birth	A finger or small object placed in the infant's hand elicits an involuntary flexion or grasp; the grasp tightens when the finger or object is moved away	Weakens by 3 months Should be completely absent by 6 months of age Abnormal if the grasp is asymmetric or if it persists past 6 months
Placing reflex	Birth	When the infant is held upright and the foot is allowed to touch a firm surface, the hip and foot will flex as the infant withdraws the foot	Disappears by 5 months of age Abnormal if asymmetric or persists past 5 months of age

Continued

TABLE 13-3 Primitive Reflexes—cont'd

REFLEX	ONSET	ACTION	EXPECTED AGE OF DISAPPEARANCE
Moro reflex or startle reflex 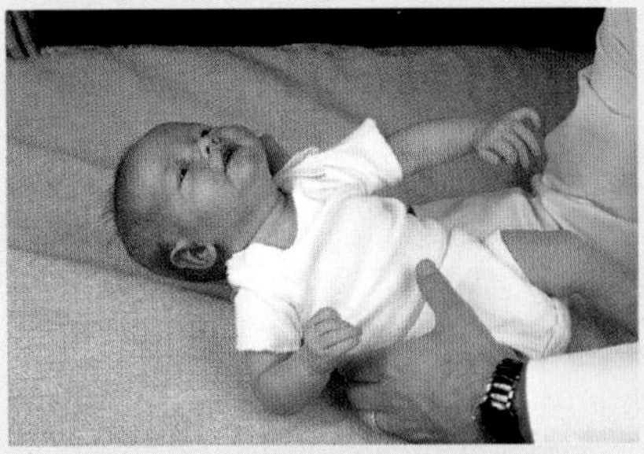	Birth	Occurs with sudden movement, noise, or change of light The back arches, the arms flex and move away from the body, and then return to the body; often accompanied by crying	Typically disappears by age 6 months Abnormal if absent Abnormal if asymmetric and may indicate birth trauma to the nerves of the arm
Blinking (glabellar) 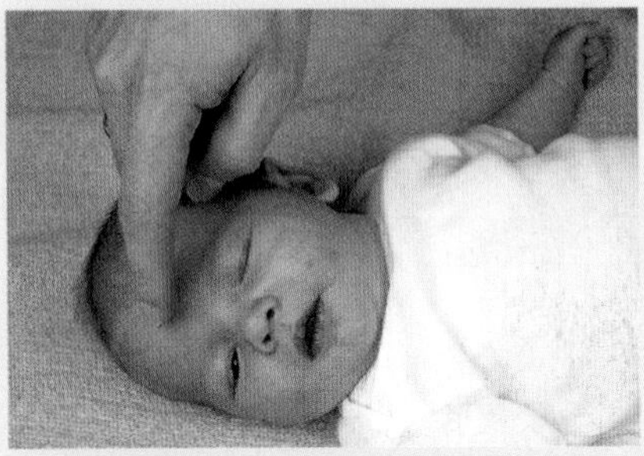	Birth	A light puff of air will result in the infant closing the eyes	Should be a permanent reflex
Babinski sign 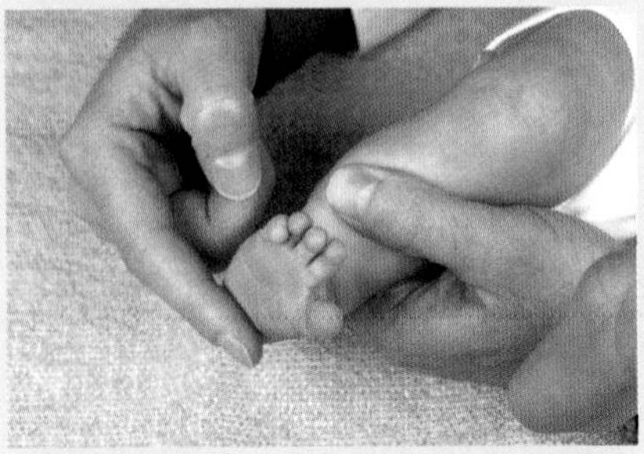	Birth	When the sole of the foot is stroked upward, the toes fan out	Should disappear between 9 and 12 months of age
Rooting reflex 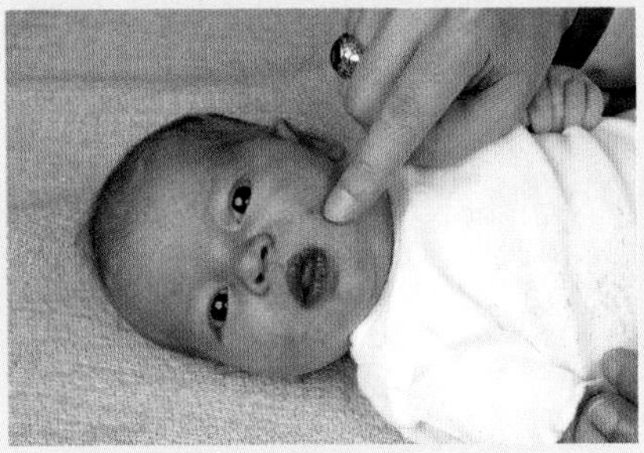	Birth	When the cheeks or side of the mouth is touched, the infant turns the head and begins sucking	Disappears by 3–4 months of age

TABLE 13–3 Primitive Reflexes—cont'd

REFLEX	ONSET	ACTION	EXPECTED AGE OF DISAPPEARANCE
Stepping 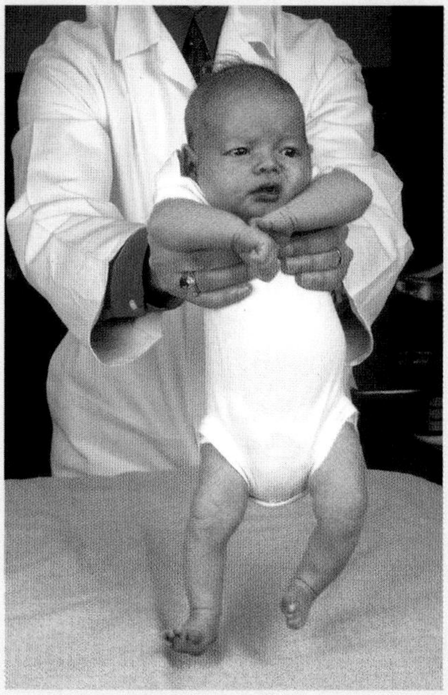	Birth	Infant held above surface and feet lowered to touch surface moves feet as if to walk	Disappears after 3–4 months
Swimming reflex	Birth	When placed facedown in water, makes coordinated swimming movements	Disappears by 6 months
Sucking reflex 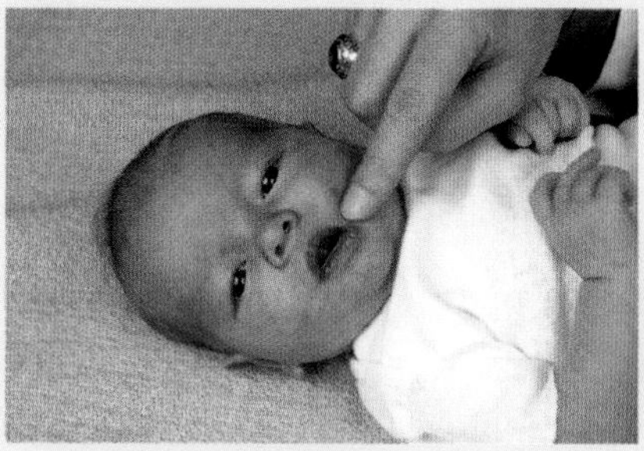	Birth	When an object touches the mouth, the infant should suck automatically	Disappears after 3–4 months
Parachute reflex	By 10 months of age	When the infant is held in the prone position and the body is moved abruptly, headfirst in a downward direction, the infant extends both arms and legs symmetrically	Should persist Abnormal if this fails to develop or if it is asymmetric
Traction (pull to sit) 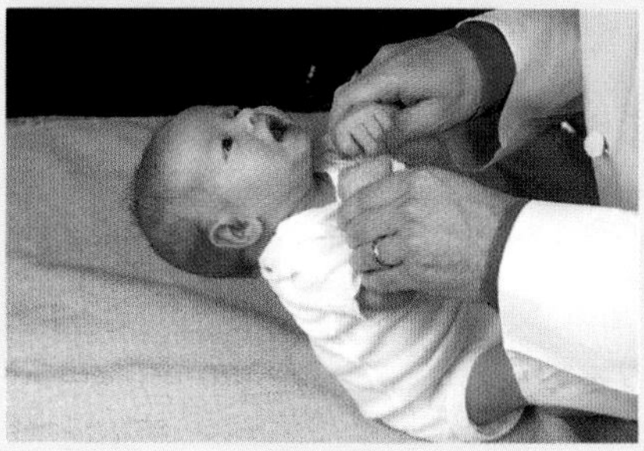	By 5 months of age	When the infant is pulled by the hands to a sitting position from a supine position, the infant should resist by pulling against the examiner and raise the head	Should persist Abnormal if there is head lag

Continued

TABLE 13–3 Primitive Reflexes—cont'd

REFLEX	ONSET	ACTION	EXPECTED AGE OF DISAPPEARANCE
Trunk righting	By 8 months of age	While sitting, the infant is gently but firmly pushed to one side, past midline; the infant should flex the trunk toward the force of the push and extend the arm and hand away from the force	Should persist Abnormal if this fails to develop or if it is asymmetric
Head righting	By 4 months of age	When the infant is gently swayed from side to side in a vertical position, the head should remain vertical despite the body's change in position	Should persist Abnormal if this fails to develop or if it is asymmetric

From Dillon, P. M. (2016). Nursing health assessment: the foundation of clinical practice *(3rd ed.). Philadelphia: F.A. Davis.*

milestones. Most changes occur in infancy and early childhood, until about 6 years of age. Development continues at a slower pace through adolescence.

Disruptions in Neurological Development

Disruptions in the neurological development of infants and children can have various causative factors:

- Genetic
- Metabolic
- Infectious
- Trauma
- Degenerative disorders
- Anatomic brain malformations

Associated conditions include:

- Seizures
- Sensory impairments
- Problems with physical growth
- Psychiatric and behavioral disorders

INTELLECTUAL AND DEVELOPMENTAL DELAY

Developmental delay is primarily a descriptive term, not a specific diagnosis, and is used for situations in which the child is not meeting age-appropriate milestones as expected in one or more areas of development:

- Fine motor skills, which are small muscle movements, usually movements of the fingers that require hand–eye coordination
- Gross motor skills, which are large muscle movements associated with movement of the entire body
- Language (both receptive and expressive language)
- Social skills, which are appropriate social interactions such as bonding and then separating from parents and age-appropriate play with others
- Adaptive skills, which are skills needed for independence such as feeding, dressing, bathing, and toileting

Types of developmental delays may include:

- An individual milestone
- Mixed milestones
- Global developmental delay in which all milestones are delayed

The presentation of developmental delay is age dependent. The most common parental concern is delayed development of expressive language.

ASSESSMENT

When evaluating a child with a suspected neurological disorder or delay in development, the nurse needs to have knowledge of typical child development and awareness of available child screening tools, as well as the ability to interview the parent or caregiver in a nonthreatening, supportive manner. The nurse must listen to parent concerns, assess for cultural differences and values, and personalize the assessment to the child and family. The following subsections describe data that should be gleaned from the parent/child interview and assessment.

General History

- Detailed medical and social history of the child
- History of the mother's pregnancy, labor, and delivery
  - Exposure to Zika or other viral infections
- Child's birth history
  - Gestational age
  - Birth weight
  - Apgar scores

- General health of the child
  - Accidents
  - Illnesses
  - Surgical history
  - Ages when milestones were achieved
  - History of regression of milestones
- Concerns regarding behavior
  - Interaction with others
  - Aggression
  - Repetitive behaviors
  - Attention
  - Activity level
- Social history
  - Parenting variations
    - Loss of parent through abandonment, incarceration, or death
    - Alterations in parenting through separations and divorce
    - Foster parenting
    - Professional parenting, such as group homes
    - Adoptive parents
    - Elderly parents (grandparents)
    - Adolescent parents
- Socioeconomic issues
  - Homelessness
  - Poverty
  - Availability of medical services (rural health)
  - Race and ethnicity
  - Cultural differences
  - Literacy of parents

Physical Examination

- Head circumference abnormalities
  - Microcephaly—the head circumference is more than two standard deviations below average for the child's age, sex, race, and period of gestation.
  - Macrocephaly—the head circumference is more than two standard deviations above average for the child's age, sex, race, and period of gestation.

SAFE AND EFFECTIVE NURSING CARE: Cultural Competence

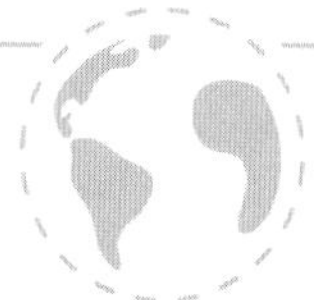

Differences in Head Circumference

Average head circumference may vary among different populations. For instance, infants from China, Vietnam, Thailand, and Southeast Asia tend to have a smaller head circumference and overall growth rate. The nurse must select the appropriate chart for the child he or she is screening, and observe for the presence or absence of growth in the percentile for the child's age and sex (Centers for Disease Control and Prevention [CDC], 2017b).

- Muscle tone abnormalities
  - Increased muscle tone: hypertonia
  - Decreased muscle tone: hypotonia
- Muscle atrophy or wasting
- Large or clustered skin lesions, called neurocutaneous lesions
- Dysmorphic features, such as low-lying ears, flattened nose, or abnormal eyelid creases
- Abnormalities in the cranial nerves, such as decreased vision or hearing, or inability to use the tongue
- Documentation of the presence of physical findings of known genetic disorders, such as facial or hand features of a child with Down syndrome

Achievement of developmental milestones in infants and children is best screened by using a standardized developmental screening tool (Table 13–4). This helps to improve early detection

TABLE 13–4 Developmental Screening Tools

NAME OF DEVELOPMENTAL SCREENING TOOL	AGES	DESCRIPTION
Ages and States Questionnaire (ASQ)	Infants to 5 years	A parent-completed questionnaire to assess developmental, social, and emotional milestones
Denver Developmental Screening Test–II (DDST-II)	1 month to 6 years	Used by professionals to screen children for possible developmental problems, to confirm suspected problems with an objective measure, and to monitor children at risk for developmental problems
Early Screening Inventory–Revised (ESI-R)	3 months to 6 years	A brief developmental screening tool used by educators to identify children who may need special education services in school
Bayley Infant Neurodevelopmental Screen (BINS)	3–24 months	Used by professionals to identify infants who are developmentally delayed or who have neurological impairments

Continued

TABLE 13–4 Developmental Screening Tools—cont'd

NAME OF DEVELOPMENTAL SCREENING TOOL	AGES	DESCRIPTION
Brigance Screens	21–90 months	Nine separate screens—one for each 12-month age range—to evaluate speech-language, motor, readiness, general knowledge, social-emotional skills; typically used by professionals and educators
Battelle Developmental Inventory	Birth to 8 years	Screens receptive and expressive language, fine and gross motor, adaptive, personal-social, and cognitive/academic to identify children at risk for delay
Child Development Inventories or Child Development Review	3–72 months	Screens child's development in major developmental areas by parent report of child's behavior
Child Development Review—Parent Questionnaire (CDR-PQ)	18 months to 5 years	Parent-completed questionnaire along with professional-completed child development chart that measures social, self-help, motor, and language skills
Infant Development Inventory (IDI)	0–18 months	Parent-completed questionnaire; measures social, self-help, motor, and language skills
Parent Evaluations of Developmental Status (PEDS)	Birth to 8 years	A screening and surveillance tool to assess developmental issues, behavioral, and mental health problems; used by professionals and educators
The Bzoch-League Receptive-Expressive Language Test (REEL-2)	Infants to 3 years	A screening tool used by professionals to measure and analyze emergent language

Adapted from First Signs. (2014). Recommended screening tools. *Retrieved from http://www.firstsigns.org/screening/tools/rec.htm.*

of children at risk for developmental delay and to determine the direct intervention required.

SAFE AND EFFECTIVE NURSING CARE: Clinical Pearl

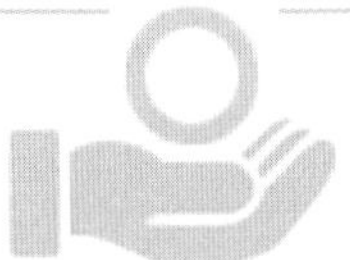

Assessment of Motor Skills

Watch children at play before attempting to examine or interact with them. Information about their fine motor, gross motor, and adaptive skills can be observed during play. Offer age-appropriate toys as part of the assessment to see whether the child manipulates the toy appropriately.

Diagnosis

- Chromosome testing
- Metabolic screening
- Thyroid function screening
- Magnetic resonance imaging (MRI) in the following situations:
  - Dysmorphic features
  - Sudden loss or regression of skills
  - Traumatic injury
  - Multiple developmental delays without obvious cause (Moeschler, Shevell, & Committee on Genetics, 2014)

Treatment

- Multidisciplinary approach
  - Physical therapy
  - Occupational therapy
  - Speech therapy
  - Educational services
  - Audiology
  - Psychology
  - Social work
  - Child life specialist
- Treatment of any associated condition, such as thyroid disorders and failure to thrive, will also be indicated.
- When a child with an intellectual disability requires treatment in any health-care setting, the nurse must individualize instructions and care that is sensitive to his or her level of understanding. The child should be approached with respect and included in the treatment plan. The nurse should not assume that the child will not understand or comply simply because he or she has intellectual delay.

SAFE AND EFFECTIVE NURSING CARE: Promoting Safety

Pediatric Magnetic Resonance Imaging Safety Measures

Nurses should consider the following when caring for a pediatric patient for whom an MRI has been ordered.

- The child will be given age-appropriate sedation for the MRI, because no movement is permitted to obtain clear images.
- Nursing care is aimed at alleviating anxiety and complications. Age-appropriate teaching about the procedure should be provided to the child before the administration of sedation.
- Any metallic piercings or jewelry must be removed from the child before the procedure.
- Vital signs must be monitored and compared with presedation values.
- Level of alertness and safety must be monitored as the child awakens from sedation.
- Intake and output must be monitored. The child should be able to drink adequate liquids and demonstrate sufficient urinary output before discharge.
- Parents must be taught what to expect after sedation. Often children cry and react paradoxically to sedatives.

- The family of a child with developmental delay requires additional support due to stressors:
  - Time
  - Emotion and grief
  - Finances

CRITICAL COMPONENT

Early Diagnosis of Developmental and Behavioral Disabilities

In the United States, 17% of children have a developmental or behavioral disability. Unfortunately, fewer than 50% of these children are identified before school age. By this time, considerable delays have already occurred, and thus treatment begins much later in life than is optimal for the best outcome (CDC, 2017b).

CONGENITAL ABNORMALITIES OF THE NERVOUS SYSTEM (NEURAL TUBE DEFECTS)

Congenital abnormalities of the nervous system are called neural tube defects (NTDs) (Fig. 13–3). They occur in the brain and spinal cord during the fetal period and are thought to be due to folic acid deficiency in pregnant women. It is recommended that all women of child-bearing age take folic acid supplements before and during pregnancy. Normally, the closure of the neural tube occurs around the 28th day after fertilization. The two most common defects are spina bifida, in which the spinal column does not close completely, and anencephaly, in which most of the brain does not develop (Ellenbrogen & Roberts, 2015).

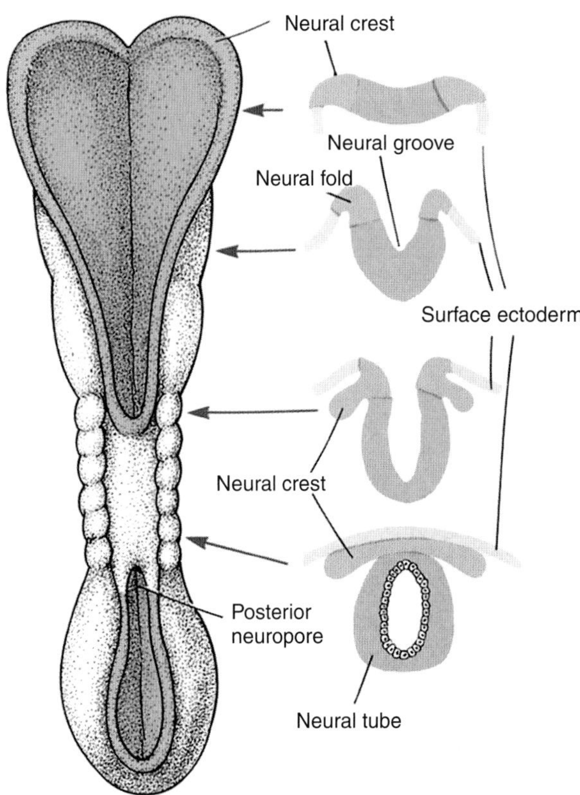

FIGURE 13–3 The neural tube.

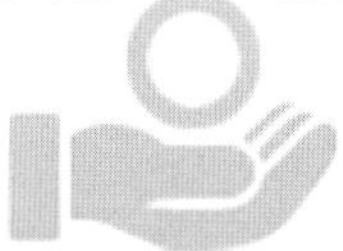

SAFE AND EFFECTIVE NURSING CARE: Clinical Pearl

Folic Acid Supplements

Because neural tube closure occurs before most women even know they are pregnant, it is important to teach adolescent girls to begin taking folic acid supplements of at least 0.4 mg/day before pregnancy occurs (Ellenbrogen & Roberts, 2015). This is especially important for girls who take potentially teratogenic medications, such as anticonvulsants.

Spina Bifida

- Children with spina bifida can have paralysis of the legs. This is dependent on the severity of the defect, but includes flaccid muscles with varying degrees of sensory loss.
- Problems with control of the bowel and bladder are also common.

- Types of spina bifida
  - Spina bifida cystica—a section of the spinal cord and the nerves that come from the cord is exposed and visible on the outside of the body.
    - Also called myelomeningocele
    - Causes partial or complete paralysis below the spinal opening (Ellenbrogen & Roberts, 2015)
    - Can be removed surgically but does not correct any deficit
  - Meningocele—the membrane that surrounds the spinal cord is enlarged, creating a cyst-like sac.
    - The sac that is present usually on the lower back contains meninges, which is the membrane covering the spinal cord
    - May not be visible on examination, but seen by ultrasound or MRI
    - Can be removed surgically but does not correct any deficit
    - Does not always cause disability (Jallo & Kao, 2015)
  - Spina bifida occulta—a section of the spinal vertebrae is malformed, but the spinal cord and nerves are normal.
    - The defect is not visible, although newborns may display dimpling, hair, or hemangioma in the lumbar sacral area.
    - It is usually found accidentally. This defect sometimes occurs in association with dimpling, hair tufts, or a hemangioma in the sacral area.
    - A version of spina bifida occulta is tethered cord syndrome, in which tissue attachments limit the movement of the spinal cord within the spinal column (National Institute of Neurological Disorders and Stroke [NINDS], 2017d).

CRITICAL COMPONENT

Protection of Open Spinal Cord Defects

When a child is born with an open spinal cord defect, the nurse must exercise caution to keep the defect covered and protected until surgical correction can occur (Verklan & Walden, 2015). Using aseptic technique, the nurse should cover the defect with a sterile dressing moistened with warm sterile normal saline. The child should be positioned prone and lying on an open diaper.

Treatment

- Treatment is based on the degree of the spinal cord defect that is present. Surgical correction closes the protrusion and prevents further harm to the delicate tissues, but does not repair damage to the nerves and spinal cord.
- A multidisciplinary approach to treatment will be necessary and must include services such as:
  - Neurosurgery
  - Neurology
  - Pediatrics
  - Physical therapy
  - Occupational therapy
  - Speech therapy
  - Social work
  - Education
  - Child life specialist

Other Types of Neural Tube Defects

In addition to defects in the neural tube that occur in the spine, some defects occur in the region of the brain. These defects can be incompatible with life, such as anencephaly, or have no symptoms, such as Chiari malformation type 1.

Anencephaly

Anencephaly is a neural cord defect in which most of the brain does not develop. The child can be missing both portions of the brain and skull. Anencephaly occurs in approximately 3 pregnancies out of 10,000 in the United Sates. Those affected are usually stillborn or die shortly after birth. The rate of anencephaly has declined by 28% since the United States began fortifying grains with folic acid. Women of child-bearing age should receive 400 mg of folic acid daily either by supplements or diet to help prevent NTDs such as anencephaly (CDC, 2017d).

Encephalocele

With encephalocele, a portion of the brain protrudes through an opening in the skull. The severity varies depending on the size and location. Common locations include:

- A groove in the middle of the skull
- Between the forehead and nose
- On the back side of the skull

Chiari Malformation

A Chiari malformation is a structural defect in the cerebellum, the part of the brain that controls balance (NINDS, 2017a). The bony space at the lower portion of the skull is smaller than normal. The cerebellum and brainstem are pushed downward. The pressure on the cerebellum can block the flow of spinal fluid. Symptoms may include:

- Dizziness
- Muscle weakness
- Numbness
- Vision problems
- Headaches
- Problems with balance and coordination

Types of Chiari Malformation

- Type 1
  - Usually no symptoms
  - Frequently diagnosed by accident during an evaluation for another condition
- Type 2
  - Also known as Arnold-Chiari malformation
  - Larger, downward herniation of the cerebellum and possibly the brainstem through the foramen magnum to the spinal column
  - May be accompanied by a myelomeningocele

- Type 3
  - Associated with occipital encephalocele, in which a portion of the brain protrudes through an opening on the back of the head (CDC, 2017d)
- Type 4
  - Associated with an incomplete or underdeveloped cerebellum, called cerebellar hypoplasia. This condition is now more commonly referred to as cerebellar hypoplasia and the name Chiari type 4 is considered obsolete.
  - The cerebellum is typically in the correct position, but parts of the cerebellum are missing and portions of the skull or spinal cord may be visible.
  - Children with Chiari type 4 do not survive infancy.

CRITICAL COMPONENT

Decompression for Chiari Malformation

When a Chiari malformation has been discovered on an imaging study of the brain, the child should be evaluated by neurosurgery to determine whether a decompression procedure is necessary. Surgical correction is indicated if the degree of protrusion of the cerebellum to the spinal cord results in compression of the cerebellar tonsils. The decompression procedure creates more space for the protrusion of the cerebellum, thereby minimizing the symptoms that the child experiences and protecting the delicate cerebellar tissues.

Diagnosis

- A Chiari malformation is diagnosed with an MRI of the brain, where the abnormal protrusion of the cerebellum to the spinal cord can be seen. This protrusion of the cerebellum is called cerebellar tonsils.
- The amount of protrusion is measured in millimeters; the greater the protrusion, the more severe the condition as the cerebellar tonsils become compressed in the small space.
- When Chiari malformation is present, potential exists for a cyst to form in the spinal column, called a syrinx or syringomyelia. When a syrinx is present, the child usually experiences numbness in the lower extremities. Surgical intervention is typically required if the child is symptomatic.

Treatment

- Treatment of a Chiari type 1 malformation is usually not required, unless there is progression of the tonsillar protrusion as the child grows.
- Chiari type 2 may or may not require treatment depending on the degree of protrusion. If the protrusion is greater than 5 mm, surgery may be necessary to make more space in the area where the cerebellar tonsils are compressed.
- Chiari types 3 and 4 may require surgical intervention depending on the degree of malformation. Children with Chiari types 3 and 4 generally have serious to profound neurological deficits.
- Nursing intervention is based on the type of Chiari malformation, the child's symptoms, and whether surgical decompression is required.

SAFE AND EFFECTIVE NURSING CARE: Promoting Safety

Activity Recommendations With Chiari Malformation

Children with Chiari malformation should be allowed to attend school, play, and participate in most sports with their peers. Contact sports are generally avoided because there can be differences in the amount of spinal fluid present to help protect the brain and spinal cord in a high-velocity impact. This is particularly true if a syrinx is present because there is less room in the spinal column.

CONGENITAL MALFORMATIONS

Congenital malformations usually occur during fetal development. They can be caused by:

- Genetic influences
- Exposure to medications known or suspected to cause birth defects, also known as teratogens
- Infections
- Radiation
- Maternal drug and alcohol use during pregnancy
- Unknown cause

Types of Congenital Malformations

Congenital malformations can occur in the brain or in the bony structures of the skull and face. Notable congenital malformations include the following:

- Agenesis of the corpus callosum—the structure or bridge that connects the two hemispheres of the brain is partially or completely missing (National Organization for Rare Diseases [NORD], 2017)
  - The most common brain malformation
  - Children with agenesis of the corpus callosum can have normal intelligence with only mild differences in learning or may display severe mental retardation, hydrocephalus, and seizures.
  - This defect can occur by itself or in conjunction with other defects of the brain. It can also occur with other defects, such as facial malformations.
- Dandy Walker malformation—malformation of the cerebellum and the fluid-filled spaces around it (National Institutes of Health [NIH], 2017a)
  - There is enlargement of the fourth ventricle and increased intracranial pressure.
  - Agenesis of the corpus callosum is frequently associated with Dandy Walker malformations.
  - There are often malformations of the heart, face, limbs, fingers, and toes as well.

- Lissencephaly, which means "smooth brain"
  - Absence of the folds, grooves, and fissures in the brain
  - Severe neurological impairment
- Microcephaly—the circumference of the head is more than two standard deviations below normal
  - The brain has not developed properly or has stopped growing.
  - May be present at birth or may develop when the child grows, but the head does not.
  - Associated with Down syndrome, chromosomal abnormalities, metabolic processes, maternal substance abuse, maternal cytomegalovirus, Zika virus infection, rubella, or chicken pox exposure.
  - Often causes cognitive, motor, and speech delays.
  - Can cause dysmorphic facial features, growth retardation or dwarfism, hyperactivity, and seizures.
- Schizencephaly—the presence of abnormal slits or clefts in the hemispheres of the brain (Close & Smirniotopoulos, 2015)
  - Clefts in both hemispheres will usually result in developmental delays and problems with purposeful movement, including paralysis.
  - Clefts in one hemisphere will usually result in paralysis on one side of the body, but the child may have normal intelligence.
  - May be associated with microcephaly, hydrocephalus, poor muscle tone, and seizures.
- Craniosynostosis—premature closure of sutures on infant's head that results in abnormal head shape (see Chapter 7 for further details).
  - Often associated with facial deformities.
  - Surgical correction is performed in infancy.

Assessment

- General physical examination
- Documentation of dysmorphic features or obvious malformations
- Assess presence or absence of developmental milestones

Diagnosis

- In addition to physical examination, an MRI of the brain is necessary for diagnosis.
- X-rays and computed tomography (CT) scan of the skull and facial bones are used in craniosynostosis to determine the location of premature closure of the sutures and to plan for surgical correction.

Treatment

- The treatment and prognosis of these disorders depend on the particular disorder.
- Some children may require surgery, such as shunts or surgeries to repair craniofacial problems.
- Others may require supportive care, such as medications to treat seizures or physical and speech therapy, to help them achieve developmental milestones.
- Parents may need support in the following areas, because parenting children with NTDs can cause stress.
  - Time
  - Emotions
  - Grief
  - Finances

HYDROCEPHALUS

Hydrocephalus occurs when CSF collects in an abnormal pattern in the brain (Fig. 13–4). This can cause an enlargement in the ventricles called ventriculomegaly, which in turn may cause harmful pressure on the other fragile tissues of the brain. Four ventricles in the brain are connected by narrow channels that allow the CSF to drain and be reabsorbed into the bloodstream. If there is an increase in the normal amount of CSF, the result is hydrocephalus.

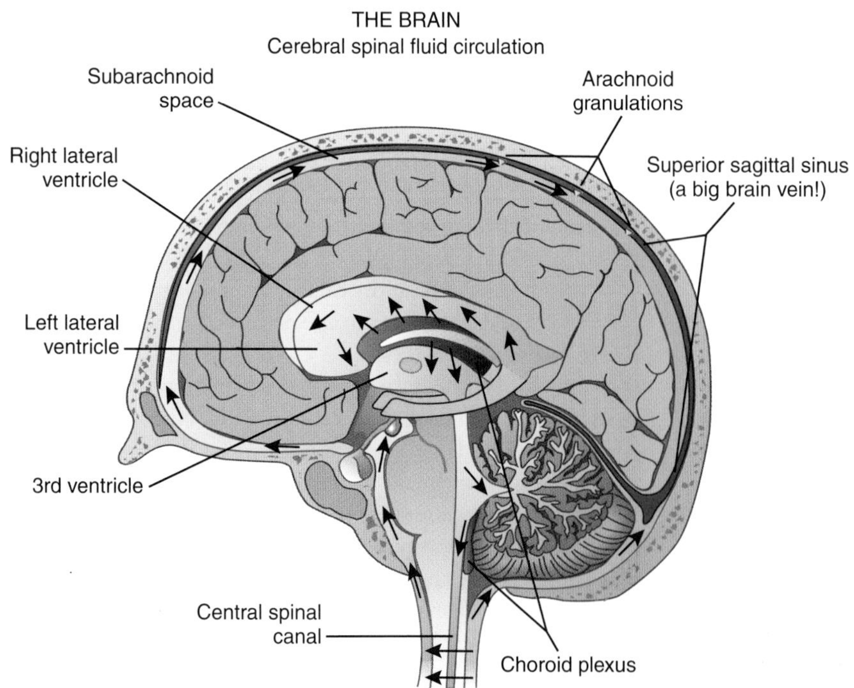

FIGURE 13–4 The circulation of spinal fluid.

Types of Hydrocephalus

There are two types of hydrocephalus, congenital and acquired.

- With congenital hydrocephalus, the blockage occurs before birth and is evident on prenatal ultrasound studies.
- Acquired hydrocephalus occurs at or after birth. Types of acquired hydrocephalus include:
  - Communicating hydrocephalus—the flow between the ventricles is not impaired and the cerebrospinal flow is blocked after it leaves the ventricles.
  - Noncommunicating hydrocephalus—the CSF flow is blocked at some point along the narrow channels that drain the ventricles. This can also be called obstructive hydrocephalus (Nelson, 2016).
  - Hydrocephalus ex vacuo—occurs after injury to brain tissue, for example, after problems such as cancer, brain infection, stroke, or trauma. It can cause the brain tissue to shrink.
  - Normal pressure hydrocephalus—most common in the elderly and causes significant problems with walking, memory, and bladder control.

Symptoms of Hydrocephalus

Symptoms of hydrocephalus vary according to the age of onset and based on how rapidly and severely CSF accumulation occurs. Infants can tolerate increased CSF and ventricular enlargement better than adults because the bones of the skull have not fully closed, thus allowing the body to better accommodate the building pressure. Symptoms in infants may include:

- Rapid increase in head circumference or an unusually large head size
- Depending on the age of the infant, a bulging fontanel may be present
- Vomiting
- Lethargy
- Irritability
- A high-pitched, shrill cry
- Seizures
- A downward deviation of the eyes called "sunsetting" (Fig. 13–5)
- Pupils can be sluggish in response to light; an unequal response is also possible
- Bradycardia may be present initially with tachycardia occurring as the intracranial pressure increases
- Hypertension
- Apnea can occur in infants as an early symptom; this worsens as the intracranial pressure increases
- If the hydrocephalus is not corrected and the intracranial pressure continues to worsen, opisthotonos can occur. This is an abnormal posture with rigidity and severe arching of the back, with the head thrown back.

Children and adolescents have different symptoms, which may include:

- Headache: an early-morning headache that is relieved by vomiting can occur, as well as a relentless headache that is not relieved by any usual measures

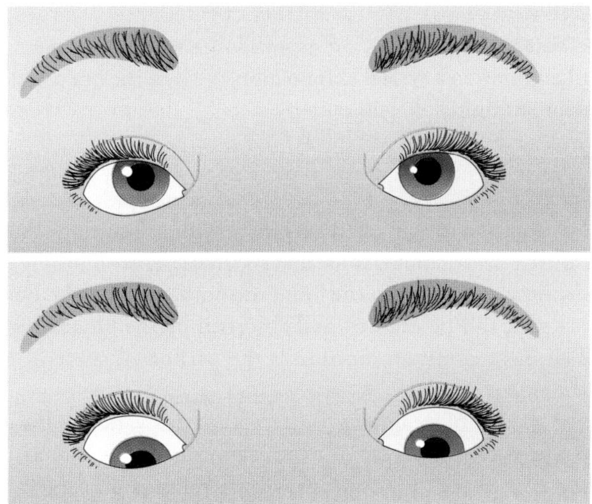

FIGURE 13–5 "Sunsetting" eyes in hydrocephalus.

- Vomiting: can increase to projectile as the intracranial pressure in the head increases
- Papilledema (swelling of the optic disc)
- Blurred or double vision
- Sunsetting eyes
- Lethargy
- Problems with balance
- Slowed developmental progress or changes in memory
- Irritability
- New onset of urinary incontinence
- Bradycardia can occur initially, with tachycardia occurring as the intracranial pressure increases
- Hypertension can occur
- If the hydrocephalus is not corrected and the intracranial pressure continues to worsen, opisthotonos can occur.

Assessment

- General physical examination
- Documentation of dysmorphic features
- Assess presence or absence of developmental milestones
- Serial head circumference measurements are required to monitor head growth; rapid or linear head growth is an indicator of developing hydrocephalus

SAFE AND EFFECTIVE NURSING CARE: Clinical Pearl

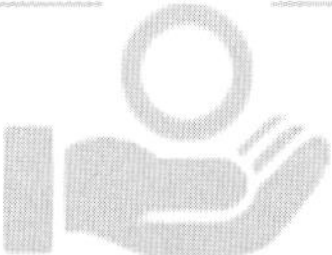

Measuring Head Circumference

Head circumference should always be measured at the fullest part of the head, above the eyebrows and ears, and around the back of the head (Dillon, 2016).

Diagnosis

- In addition to physical examination, MRI of the brain is necessary for initial diagnosis.

Treatment

- Hydrocephalus is treated surgically with a shunting system called a ventriculoperitoneal (VP) shunt. This shunt diverts the flow of CSF from the brain to another part of the body, where it can be drained and absorbed by the bloodstream. The most common location is the peritoneal space of the abdomen.
- The success of treatment for hydrocephalus varies and is dependent on the severity of the malformation as well as the cause. In some cases, such as when a shunt is implanted because of a brain tumor, the outcome is not favorable.
- Preoperative nursing care of an infant with hydrocephalus includes:
  - Teaching the parent about the condition and the proposed operative procedure
  - Frequent assessment of the head circumference, fontanelles, and cranial sutures
  - Assessment of vital signs
  - Assessment of level of consciousness and behavior
  - Encouraging parent/child bonding if the infant is a newborn
- Preoperative care of an older child includes:
  - Teaching the child and parent about the condition and the proposed operative procedure
  - Frequent assessment of vital signs
  - Assessment of level of consciousness and behavior
  - Emotional support
- Postoperative care of a child who has undergone a shunt implant procedure includes:
  - Assessment for signs of increased intracranial pressure as was performed preoperatively
  - Assessment of pain level and administering analgesics as indicated
  - Teaching the child and parents about home care with a VP shunt
- Postoperative nursing care for a VP shunt includes:
  - Monitor the child for signs of shunt failure or infection such as rapid onset of vomiting, severe headache, irritability, lethargy, and fever.
  - Monitor the wound site for redness or drainage. Depending on the surgical technique, there can be two or three incision sites on the scalp and trunk.
- The nurse will monitor for signs of increased pressure, as well as signs of the shunt draining the ventricles too aggressively. Symptoms of overdrainage include headache, nausea, and dizziness.
- Overdrainage of the ventricles can lead to slit ventricle syndrome.
  - The ventricles become accustomed to a very small or slitlike configuration.
  - This limits the ability of the ventricles to tolerate variations in increased intracranial pressure.

SAFE AND EFFECTIVE NURSING CARE: Clinical Pearl

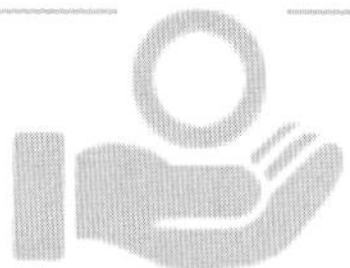

Shunt Catheters and Hydrocephalus

- If a child has an implanted VP shunt but develops symptoms of hydrocephalus, a CT scan of the brain with x-rays of the chest and abdomen must be performed to assess the patency and function of the shunt catheters.

CRITICAL COMPONENT

Symptoms of Shunt Infection or Malfunction

The nurse caring for a patient who has had a VP shunt implant should be alert to signs and symptoms of shunt infection or malfunction. These can include rapid onset of vomiting, severe headaches, irritability, lethargy, fever, redness at the surgical wound sites, or leaking CSF at the head along the shunt valve area (Wright, Larrew, & Eskandari, 2016). The nurse should also assess for a halo sign on the bed linens, which is a blood-tinged spot encircled by a lighter ring. This is indicative of CSF leakage at the incision site.

Home Care of a Ventriculoperitoneal Shunt

The nurse should provide the child and parents with the following information for care of a VP shunt at home:

- Sutures or staples are typically removed 7 to 14 days postoperatively.
- At first, the area on the scalp where the shunt was implanted may seem large or swollen. As the site heals and hair growth occurs, this is less noticeable. A small raised area behind the ear about the size of a quarter is typical. This area should not be pushed or pressed with the fingers.
- When shunt infections occur, they usually appear within the first 2 months after surgery. *Staphylococcus aureus* is the most common organism.
- Parents should be taught signs of shunt infection and malfunction, and provided with instructions on how to contact the surgeon after leaving the hospital. Typical signs of shunt infection or malfunction include:
  - Fever
  - Lethargy
  - Abdominal pain or bloating
  - Headache
  - Anorexia
  - Irritability
  - Redness, swelling, or discharge from an incision site
  - Vomiting
  - High-pitched cry in infants

- Bulging fontanels or cranial sutures in infants
- Seizures

- The child should not bathe, soak in water, or swim until the surgeon gives approval. A sponge bath is necessary until the skin at the incision sites has completely healed.
- The child can usually resume most activities (other than swimming and contact sports).
- An infant can be held and handled as usual.
- Some children have some incision-site pain for a few days after the surgery. Parents should be taught how to manage pain with appropriate dosages of acetaminophen or ibuprofen.
- As the child grows, shunt revisions are often needed until approximately 80% of adult height has been reached. If the shunt is functioning normally, most children have a revision due to growth once or twice every 10 years. A shunt revision due to growth is a planned, scheduled procedure, whereas shunt failure or infection requires urgent intervention.

SLEEP DISORDERS

Sleep disorders in children are common and affect not only the child's rest, but behavior and learning ability as well. Most children stop these behaviors as they mature, but while they occur, they are disruptive to both the child and the family, including parents and other siblings. Types of sleep disorders in children include:

- Problems with going to sleep (insomnia); can be transient or chronic
- Problems with staying asleep (sleep arousals during the night or awakening very early in the morning)
- Sleeping at inappropriate times
  - Hypersomnia—excessive sleepiness
  - Narcolepsy—excessive sleepiness along with daytime sleep attacks
- Obstructive sleep disorder: sleep apnea
  - Obstructive sleep apnea is the most common reason for tonsillectomy and adenoidectomy in children.
  - Because of childhood obesity rates, obstructive sleep apnea is occurring more commonly in obese children and adolescents than in previous years.
- Limb movements in sleep
  - Periodic limb movement disorder—unusual limb jerking that limits restfulness
  - Restless leg syndrome—leg discomfort such as pain or crawling sensations that limit sleep
- Parasomnias—abnormal behaviors associated with sleep arousals such as night terrors, sleepwalking, rapid eye movement (REM) sleep behavior disorder, and nightmares
  - Night terrors—awakening in the first one-third of the night, usually between midnight and 2 a.m., screaming in fear, disoriented upon awakening; parents unable to comfort the child (Spratt, 2016)
    - May be triggered by fever, emotional stress, or sleep deprivation.
    - The child does not recall the event the following day.
    - Most common in boys aged 5 to 7 years but can occur in all children aged 3 to 7 years.
    - Can also occur in older children and adolescents with emotional stress and with alcohol intake.
  - Sleepwalking
    - Can include other physical activity during sleep, even complex activity such as dressing or undressing
    - Occurs in non-REM, stage 3 or 4 sleep
    - Occurs early in the night
    - Tends to run in families
    - Most common at age 4 to 8 years
    - The child looks awake and eyes are open
    - May have nonsensical speech
    - Is usually brief, lasting just a few minutes, but can last up to 30 minutes
    - If awakened, the child will be confused and disoriented
    - May go back to sleep in an unusual place
  - REM sleep behavior disorder
    - Acting out dreams violently
    - Tends to occur near morning
  - Nightmares
    - They occur in the early morning.
    - The child remembers details of the dream.
    - The child is not confused upon awakening (Chiu, 2016).

Assessment

- A general physical assessment should be performed to evaluate for conditions that would cause disruptions in sleep, such as abrupt changes in blood sugar, gastroesophageal reflux disease (GERD), and seizures.
- A careful history of the child's habits should be obtained.
  - Prior sleep habits
  - Daytime napping
  - Stressors such as the death of a loved one, bullying at school, anxiety
  - Caffeine intake
  - Medications that cause sleep disturbance
  - Weight gain and obesity

CRITICAL COMPONENT

Screening for Sleep Disorders

All children should be screened for sleep disorders, and children who are obese should have specific screening for sleep apnea. Parents may report heavy snoring or choking sounds during sleep, as well as daytime fatigue, irritability, or learning problems in school.

Diagnosis

- A diagnosis can be made from a thorough history in most cases.
- A polysomnogram or sleep study may be necessary to evaluate the problem.

SAFE AND EFFECTIVE NURSING CARE: Clinical Pearl

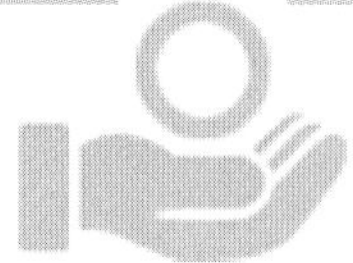

Ruling Out Other Causes of Sleep Disorders

A preverbal infant or nonverbal older child should be assessed to rule out discomfort causing sleep disturbance, such as GERD or ear infection.

Treatment

- Treatment is aimed at the cause of the problem.
- Sleep hygiene or habits to promote sleep should be instituted, including:
  - Going to bed at the same time each night and getting up at the same time each morning, even on weekends.
  - The child should only sleep in bed. Using electronic devices, playing video games, and watching TV while lying on the bed should be avoided so that the brain associates the bed only with sleep.
  - The bedroom should be dark, quiet, and cool. If a night light must be used, choose the lowest wattage possible.
  - If a child has an alarm clock, it should be turned to the wall so that the child cannot see the time.
  - Establish a bedtime routine such as brushing teeth, putting on pajamas, and reading a story. This routine helps to train the brain to know that time for sleep is coming.
  - Dim lights and turn off electronics such as TVs, stereos, video games, computers, and phones at least 30 minutes before bedtime. The child can engage in quiet, relaxing activities but not stimulating play before bedtime. Similarly, for older children and adolescents, exercise should not occur just before bedtime.
- Hypnotic sleep aids should not be used in children.
- Safety measures should be instituted for sleepwalking behaviors, such as blocking stairways and clearing walkways to prevent falls.
- There is no treatment for sleepwalking, but children can be injured during sleepwalking behaviors. For this reason, the earlier safety measures should be instituted.

SEIZURE DISORDERS

Seizures occur because of sudden abnormal electrical activity in the brain. A single seizure, or convulsion, is a symptom of abnormal electrical activity in the brain. Recurrent seizures, particularly when accompanied by electroencephalogram (EEG) findings of persistent abnormal brain activity, are diagnostic of epilepsy. The types of seizures are classified according to the origination of the seizure in the brain and the effect on the child. Some children and adults experience an aura warning that a seizure is going to occur. This could include a premonitory feeling, an odor only the person smells, a pain in their head or a limb, or other events lasting between a few seconds and a few minutes. Most people have no warning of a seizure. The most common seizure trigger in any age person is sleep deprivation, but other events that can trigger seizures are stress, use of alcohol or other substances, and for those with known seizure disorders, not taking their antiepileptic medication.

Table 13–5 describes the types of seizures.

Assessment

- General physical examination
- Note the presence of any dysmorphic features
- Document presence or absence of developmental milestones

Diagnosis

- The diagnosis of a seizure disorder is first made on the history of the event: what happened before, during, and after the seizure.
- An EEG should be performed with the child awake and asleep.
- An MRI of the brain should be performed if the EEG is abnormal, showing an irritable focus in the brain.

CRITICAL COMPONENT

Performing an Electroencephalogram

It is best to do an EEG on an infant or young child at naptime when possible. Children must be very quiet and cooperative during the EEG recording, and performing the study at naptime will help to ensure that the recording will not produce scalp muscle artifact. This is a situation in which normal movements of the scalp muscles, particularly if the child is struggling or resisting the procedure, are recorded and camouflage the brain waves that the examiner is attempting to find. The EEG will also indicate whether there is a relationship between sleep and the seizure activity, and whether further EEG studies such as a prolonged or overnight EEG need to be performed. The child's hair should be shampooed after the EEG has been performed to remove the electrode adhesive.

Treatment

- Treatment is aimed at the frequency and type of seizures.
- Antiepileptic medications may be used to reduce the seizure frequency and severity.
- For febrile seizures, it is important to identify the source of the infection causing the fever and adequately treat the fever at its inception in susceptible children.
- If a seizure lasts longer than 2 minutes and includes loss of awareness, parents can be taught to administer rectal diazepam gel (Diastat) or intranasal midazolam (Versed) at home to attempt to stop the seizure.
- If the seizure does not respond to the administration of rectal diazepam gel and continues longer than 5 minutes, the parents should call 911 to summon help.
- Lengthy seizures may require IV medications to stop the seizure.
- Lengthy seizures may also require respiratory support and administration of supplemental oxygen.

TABLE 13–5 Seizure Types

GENERALIZED SEIZURES	SYMPTOMS
Caused by Electrical Impulses Moving Through the Entire Brain	
Tonic-clonic, also known as grand mal	Rhythmic jerking of the extremities with muscle rigidity and loss of consciousness, incontinence
Absence	Brief loss of consciousness
Myoclonic	Brief, isolated jerking movements
Clonic	Repetitive, rhythmic jerking movements
Tonic	Muscle rigidity
Atonic	Loss of muscle tone
PARTIAL SEIZURES	**SYMPTOMS**
Caused by Abnormal Electrical Impulses Moving Through a Small Part of the Brain	
Focal	Motor symptoms—jerking, muscle rigidity, spasms, head turning Sensory symptoms—unusual sensations affecting vision, hearing, smell, taste, or touch Psychological—alterations in memory of the appropriate response for emotions All occur without loss of consciousness
Complex partial	Automatisms such as lip smacking, chewing, sucking, repetitive and involuntary movements, walking, restlessness Consciousness is altered but the person remains awake
Partial secondary generalization	Partial seizure symptoms that evolve into loss of consciousness and convulsive movements

Nursing Interventions

- The child should be turned to his or her side when experiencing a seizure to help the airway remain open and allow fluids or emesis to drain from the mouth. Turning the person to the left side is preferable if she is pregnant to avoid compression of the inferior vena cava by the gravid uterus.
- Nothing should be placed in the mouth of a person having a seizure.
- The child should not be restrained during the seizure.
- Clothing that is tight around the neck should be loosened when the child is experiencing a seizure.
- The child should be protected from injury caused by the movements of the seizure.
- The child should be comforted and allowed to rest after the seizure has ended.
- Children may be incontinent of urine or stool during the seizure.
- Some children may vomit during or after the seizure.
- Brief periods of confusion may occur after the seizure.
- Many children report headache after a seizure.
- Prolonged seizures that last longer than 5 minutes may require emergency care, such as respiratory support and IV medication to abort the seizure. It is important to time the seizure from the onset of jerking, loss of consciousness, or other involuntary behaviors to the end of the behaviors. The post-ictal period, in which the child may be in a deep sleep, is not part of the seizure behavior and does not need to be timed.
- If the child in the hospital is at risk for seizure, there should be oxygen and suction at the bedside and IV access should be established. Some institutions provide bumper pads around the inner aspect of the bed's side rails.
- If the child has epilepsy or recurrent seizures, antiepileptic medication may be administered. These medications are selected based on the seizure type and frequency (Table 13–6).

SAFE AND EFFECTIVE NURSING CARE: Promoting Safety

Nurses should help parents plan for safety in the event of seizures, such as ensuring children wear helmets and protective gear when playing sports.

- The nurse should promote water safety by instructing parents to allow children to bathe with supervision (with unlocked doors and within earshot of parents), and teens should not be allowed to shower or bathe unless another responsible person is in the home.
- Swimming should never occur without direct supervision.
- Instruct parents to provide a bed of lower height for the child with seizures if possible—sleeping on an upper-level bunk bed should be avoided.

(Text continued on page 274)

TABLE 13–6 Antiepileptic Medications

DRUG	INDICATION	BRAND NAME	DOSAGE	SIDE EFFECTS	MONITORING
Acetazolamide	Menstrual-related seizures	Diamox	5 mg/kg/day, titrating up to 20 mg/kg/day (tablets)	Anorexia, weight loss, sleepiness, tingling in the hands and feet, increased urination, headache	Blood urea nitrogen (BUN), creatinine, complete blood count (CBC) at baseline and at least every 6 months thereafter
ACTH, corticotropin	Infantile spasms	Acthar gel	5–40 U/day IM for 1–6 weeks, 40–160 U/day IM for 3–12 months if indicated (injectable)	Increased appetite, weight gain, irritability, edema, hypertension, risk for infections	Monitor food intake and weight Monitor glucose and electrolytes weekly during therapy
Carbamazepine	Partial and tonic-clonic seizures	Carbatrol, Epitol, Tegretol	10–20 mg/kg/day, titrating up to 35 mg/kg/day (tablets, chewable tablets, long-acting tablets, liquid suspension)	Sleepiness, rash, ataxia, headaches, nausea and vomiting, aplastic anemia, agranulocytosis, changes in liver function, hyponatremia, syndrome of inappropriate antidiuretic hormone (SIADH), water intoxication	Monitor CBC, liver enzymes, BUN, creatinine, urinalysis, and lipid panel Monitor for depression, suicidality, behavior changes May make absence and myoclonic seizures worse
Clobazam	Tonic-clonic, complex partial, myoclonic seizures, Lennox-Gastaut	Onfi	<30 kg: 5 mg/day, titrating up to no more than 20 mg/day (tablets, oral suspension) 30 kg or greater: 5 mg every 12 hours, titrating up to no more than 40 mg/day	Ataxia, sleepiness, diplopia, dysarthria, may affect liver function	Monitor liver enzymes before initiating therapy and periodically during therapy
Clonazepam	Tonic-clonic, partial, absence, and myoclonic seizures; Lennox-Gastaut syndrome; infantile spasms	Klonopin	25 mcg/kg, titrating up to 1–2 mcg/kg/day (tablets, oral dispersible tablets)	Sleepiness and sedation common Irritability, aggression, and restlessness can occur	Tolerance can develop—monitor administration carefully
Diazepam	Status epilepticus	Diastat	0.2 mg/kg (gel, rectal delivery system)	Sedation, ataxia, blurred vision	Used for emergency treatment of prolonged seizures
Divalproex (valproic acid, valproate)	Absence, tonic-clonic, partial, and myoclonic seizures	Depakote, Depacon Depakene Depakote ER	10–15 mg/kg/day, titrating up to 30–60 mg/kg/day (tablets, liquid suspension, capsules, injectable)	Weight gain, hair changes/loss, changes in liver function, rash, elevated ammonia level, tremor, anemia, low platelets	CBC and liver function tests at baseline and monthly thereafter Ammonia levels if lethargy occurs Monitor weight Birth defects if taken in pregnancy

TABLE 13-6 Antiepileptic Medications—cont'd

DRUG	INDICATION	BRAND NAME	DOSAGE	SIDE EFFECTS	MONITORING
Ethosuximide	Absence seizures	Zarontin	7.5 mg/kg, titrating up to 45 mg/kg/day; maximum of 1.5 g/day if necessary (capsules, liquid suspension)	Nausea, vomiting, headache, drowsiness, rash, anemia	CBC at baseline and at least every 6 months thereafter
Felbamate	Partial seizures and tonic-clonic seizures in Lennox-Gastaut syndrome	Felbatol	15 mg/kg/day, titrating up to 45 mg/kg/day; maximum 3,600 mg/day (tablets, liquid suspension)	Aplastic anemia, liver failure, anorexia, weight loss, nausea and vomiting, headache, dizziness, insomnia	CBC and liver enzymes at baseline and monthly thereafter
Fosphenytoin sodium	Status epilepticus seizures or IV substitution for oral phenytoin in some cases	Cerebyx	Load with 15–20 mg PE/kg, then administer 3 mg PE/kg/min up to 150 mg PE/min IV for status epilepticus Can be given 4–6 mg PE/kg/day IM or IV in divided doses for short-term therapy (injectable only, measured in PE)	Nystagmus, dizziness, headache, sleepiness, ataxia, itching, tingling sensations, cardiac arrest, hypotension, central nervous system depression	BP, EKG, respirations continuously during and every 20 minutes after loading CBC, liver enzymes, folate if prolonged treatment Also monitor for depression, suicidality, behavior changes
Gabapentin	Partial seizures	Neurontin	10–15 mg/kg/day, titrate to 50 mg/kg/day (tablets and capsules)	Sleepiness, dizziness, ataxia, fatigue, rash, behavior changes, peripheral edema	Creatinine at baseline Monitor for depression, suicidality, behavior changes
Lamotrigine	Partial seizures, tonic-clonic seizures in Lennox-Gastaut, primary generalized tonic-clonic seizures	Lamictal, Lamictal ODT, Lamictal XR	0.15 mg/kg/day, titrate up to 3 mg/kg/day in divided doses (tablets, chewable tablets, oral dispersible tablets)	Rash, dizziness, sleepiness, headache, diplopia, blurry vision, nausea, and vomiting May worsen myoclonus	Rash usually occurs within the first 6 weeks of treatment Need to titrate dose slowly More common if taken along with Depakote
Levetiracetam	Partial seizures, juvenile myoclonic epilepsy, primary generalized tonic-clonic seizures	Keppra, Keppra XR, Spritam	20 mg/kg/day, titrate up to 60 mg/kg/day (maximum 3,000 mg/day) (liquid suspension, tablets)	Dizziness, tiredness, weakness, increased infections, anger, irritability, anorexia, agitation, diplopia, ataxia, rash, depression, thoughts of suicide	Creatinine at baseline Monitor for depression, behavior changes, suicidality

Continued

TABLE 13–6 Antiepileptic Medications—cont'd

DRUG	INDICATION	BRAND NAME	DOSAGE	SIDE EFFECTS	MONITORING
Lorazepam	Status epilepticus	Ativan	0.05–0.1 mg/kg IV, may repeat 0.05 mg/kg ×1 after 10–15 minutes if seizures continue (injectable, tablets)	Sleepiness, irritability, hyperactivity, cognitive slowing, blurred vision, confusion, respiratory depression, blood dyscrasias	Respirations (when given IV for status epilepticus), CBC, liver enzymes for prolonged treatment
Oxcarbazepine	Partial seizures	Trileptal, Oxtellar, Oxtellar XR	16–20 mg/kg/day to start, titrate up to maximum of 60 mg/kg/day (tablets and liquid suspension)	Dizziness, sleepiness, fatigue, tremor, diplopia, headache, nausea, vomiting, abdominal pain, ataxia, visual changes, hyponatremia, rash, confusion, cognitive slowing	Creatinine at baseline, sodium levels periodically Monitor for depression, behavior changes, suicidality
Phenobarbital	Primary generalized tonic-clonic seizures, status epilepticus	Phenobarbital	3–5 mg/kg/day for infants 5–8 mg/kg/day for young children For status epilepticus, 10–20 mg/kg IV, then 5–10 mg/kg IV every 15–30 min Maximum 40 mg/kg IV (injectable)	Sleepiness, cognitive and behavior changes, rash, liver function changes, anemia	CBC and liver function at baseline and at least every 6 months thereafter
Phenytoin	Tonic-clonic seizures, complex partial seizures, status epilepticus	Dilantin, Phenytek	Dosage based on age, start with 5 mg/kg/day and titrate accordingly (capsules, chewable tablets, injectable)	Rash, ataxia, diplopia, slurred speech, confusion, gingival complications, coarsening of facial features, changes in liver function, anemia	CBC, liver enzymes, folate at baseline and at least every 6 months thereafter
Pregabalin	Partial seizures	Lyrica	Not applicable for children May use in older adolescents 50 mg to start, titrate up to 600 mg/day (capsules)	Dizziness, sleepiness, ataxia, peripheral edema, weight gain, blurred vision, diplopia, rash, confusion, dry mouth, tremor, thrombocytopenia, rhabdomyolysis, suicidality	Creatinine at baseline Monitor for depression, suicidality, behavior changes
Primidone	Seizure disorder	Mysoline	15–20 mg/kg/day, may increase up to 250 mg three times per day (tablets)	Ataxia, vertigo, nausea, vomiting, fatigue, irritability, emotional labiality, diplopia, rash, drowsiness, osteopenia, thrombocytopenia, megaloblastic	Creatinine at baseline, CBC, metabolic panel, drug levels, folate every 6 months Monitor for suicidality

TABLE 13–6 Antiepileptic Medications—cont'd

DRUG	INDICATION	BRAND NAME	DOSAGE	SIDE EFFECTS	MONITORING
				anemia, lupus erythematosus, suicidality	
Rufinamide	Lennox-Gastaut syndrome	Banzel	10 mg/kg/day, titrating up to 45 mg/kg/day (tablets)	Sleepiness, ataxia, tremor, diplopia, nystagmus, nausea, and vomiting	Suicidal thoughts, shortened QT interval—do EKG at baseline and with dose changes
Tiagabine	Partial seizures	Gabitril	Start at 4 mg/day titrating up to 2–56 mg/day For use in children >12 years old (tablets)	Dizziness, abdominal pain, nausea, vomiting, diarrhea, rash, irritability, tremor, depression, confusion, weight gain, cognitive slowing, status epilepticus, central nervous system depression, incapacitating weakness, suicidality	Monitor for depression, behavior changes, suicidality, weight gain
Topiramate	Partial seizures, primary generalized tonic-clonic and tonic-clonic seizures in Lennox-Gastaut syndrome	Topamax, Trokendi XR, Qudexy XR	1–3 mg/kg/day to start, titrating up to 5–9 mg/kg/day; maximum 400 mg/day (tablets)	Anorexia, weight loss, tingling in hands and feet, cognitive slowing, kidney stones, acute glaucoma, heat stroke	BUN, creatinine, sodium bicarbonate at baseline and every 6 months thereafter Monitor weight and adequate hydration Monitor for depression, behavior changes, suicidality
Lacosamide	Partial seizures	Vimpat	Not applicable for children May start with 50 mg twice a day, titrating up to 400 mg/day in older adolescents (tablets)	Dizziness, headache, diplopia, nausea, vomiting, fatigue, sleepiness, tremor, nystagmus, diarrhea, depression, cognitive slowing, itching, PR prolongation, atrial fibrillation, atrial flutter, syncope, suicidality	Creatinine and EKG at baseline, then periodically thereafter Monitor for depression, behavior changes, suicidality
Zonisamide	Partial seizures	Zonegran	Not applicable for children May use in adolescents >16 years old; start with 100 mg/day, titrating up to maximum of 600 mg/day (capsules)	Sleepiness, dizziness, fatigue, anorexia, nausea, headache, irritability, agitation, cognitive slowing, depression, diplopia, ataxia, tingling, rash, weight loss, dry mouth, kidney stones, pancreatitis, rash, constipation, depression, suicidality	Sodium bicarbonate, BUN, creatinine at baseline and every 6 months thereafter, CBC at least annually Monitor for depression, behavior changes, suicidality

ACTH, adrenocorticotropic hormone; BP, blood pressure; EKG, electrocardiogram; PE, phenytoin equivalents.

Adapted from Vallerand, A. H., Sanoski, C. A. & Deglin, J.H. (2017). Davis's drug guide for nurses *(15th ed.). Philadelphia: F.A. Davis.*

SAFE AND EFFECTIVE NURSING CARE: Clinical Pearl

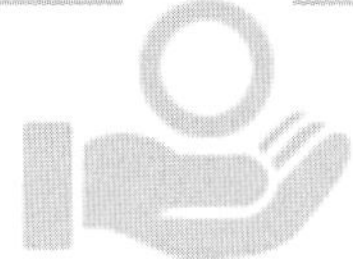

Seizure Action Plan

Nurses can help parents to feel more in control by helping them to develop a seizure action plan (Fig. 13–6). This is a medical plan of treatment and recovery that can be used by parents, caregivers, and teachers (Epilepsy Foundation, 2015b).

Types of Seizures

Some of the most prevalent types of seizure disorders that affect pediatric patients are focal seizures, temporal lobe epilepsy, juvenile myoclonic epilepsy, benign rolandic epilepsy, Dravet syndrome, Panayiotopoulos syndrome, Landau-Kleffner syndrome, electrical status epilepticus in sleep, generalized seizures, Lennox-Gastaut epilepsy, infantile spasms, and status epilepticus.

Focal Seizures

Focal seizures are also known as partial seizures. They begin in just one part of the brain and spread to other regions.

- The symptoms of focal seizures vary according to the location of origin of the seizure and the area to which the seizure spreads.
- Focal seizures are usually brief and confined to small movements with no or mild loss of awareness.
- Sometimes this seizure can spread widely throughout the brain and become secondarily generalized, meaning that tonic-clonic (alternating periods of rigidity and jerking) movements and loss of consciousness occur after the focal seizure behavior spreads.

Focal seizure types include:

- Simple focal seizures, also known as simple partial seizures
    - Mild twitching of one body part or clonic (jerking) movements of an extremity without loss of consciousness
    - Unusual smells, tastes, or tingling sensations
    - Feelings of emotional distress, such as feelings of fear
- Complex focal seizures—also known as complex partial seizures
    - The same symptoms as simple focal seizures with the addition of loss of awareness, confusion, and sometimes automatisms
        - Automatisms are small involuntary behaviors such as lip smacking, mumbling, repetitive tapping, fumbling with the fingers, or picking at something.

Temporal Lobe Epilepsy

Temporal lobe epilepsy is the most common partial seizure or localization-related epilepsy (Ko, 2014). Temporal lobe seizures are often resistant to treatment with medication, so this condition is sometimes called drug-resistant epilepsy. Temporal lobe epilepsy is associated with a specific lesion in the medial aspect of the temporal lobe called hippocampal sclerosis. This condition is characterized by neuronal cell loss and gliosis (formation of a lesion) in the hippocampus, which leads to scarring in the temporal lobe.

There are two types of temporal lobe sclerosis based on the location of the scarring: medial, the internal aspect of the temporal lobe, and neocortical, the outer portion of the temporal lobe. Approximately 80% of temporal lobe epilepsy occurs from medial temporal sclerosis. The abnormality in the temporal lobe can be a congenital brain malformation or a lesion that develops in the temporal lobe. Other causes of temporal lobe sclerosis are early childhood head trauma that resulted in loss of consciousness, history of complex or prolonged febrile seizures, and infections such as encephalitis or meningitis.

- Onset is usually age 10 to 20 years.
- Some children benefit from surgical intervention, if the lesion can be located and dissected without significant damage to adjacent areas.
- Children with temporal lobe epilepsy are at higher risk for memory and mood disorders.
- Diagnosis is made by history of the seizure events, MRI of the brain, and an EEG, which reveals anterior temporal spike and sharp waves, which can occur both awake and asleep.

Juvenile Myoclonic Epilepsy

Juvenile myoclonic epilepsy is an epilepsy syndrome in which myoclonic seizures or rapid brief jerks of the arms and legs occur, most frequently in the early morning soon after awakening (Selph, 2016). These seizures can be photosensitive, or triggered by flickering light, such as strobe lights, television, video games, sunlight shining through trees, or sunlight reflecting off snow or water. The EEG shows a specific pattern of spikes and waves. Flashing lights are often shown to children undergoing an EEG to test for this pattern.

- One of the most common epilepsy syndromes in children
- Some children have staring behavior or absence seizures with the myoclonic seizures
- Some go on to have a tonic-clonic seizure after the myoclonic seizures
- Surfaces between late childhood and early adulthood, usually around puberty
- More common in children who experience absence seizures
- More common in children with family members who have generalized seizures

Benign Rolandic Epilepsy

Benign rolandic epilepsy is an epilepsy syndrome in children between the ages of 3 and 13, most often occurring between 6 and 8 years.

- More common in boys than girls
- More common in children with close relatives with epilepsy
- The child exhibits twitching, numbness, or tingling in the face and tongue
    - The seizure interferes with speech.
    - Drooling may occur as well.
    - The seizure lasts less than 2 minutes.
    - The child remains fully conscious.

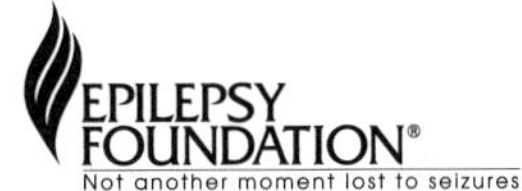

Seizure Action Plan

Effective Date

This student is being treated for a seizure disorder. The information below should assist you if a seizure occurs during school hours.

Student's Name | Date of Birth

Parent/Guardian | Phone | Cell

Other Emergency Contact | Phone | Cell

Treating Physician | Phone

Significant Medical History

Seizure Information

Seizure Type	Length	Frequency	Description

Seizure triggers or warning signs:

Student's response after a seizure:

Basic First Aid: Care & Comfort

Please describe basic first aid procedures:

Does student need to leave the classroom after a seizure? ❐ Yes ❐ No

If YES, describe process for returning student to classroom:

Basic Seizure First Aid

- Stay calm & track time
- Keep child safe
- Do not restrain
- Do not put anything in mouth
- Stay with child until fully conscious
- Record seizure in log

For tonic-clonic seizure:

- Protect head
- Keep airway open/watch breathing
- Turn child on side

Emergency Response

A "seizure emergency" for this student is defined as:

Seizure Emergency Protocol
(Check all that apply and clarify below)

❐ Contact school nurse at ______
❐ Call 911 for transport to ______
❐ Notify parent or emergency contact
❐ Administer emergency medications as indicated below
❐ Notify doctor
❐ Other ______

A seizure is generally considered an emergency when:

- Convulsive (tonic-clonic) seizure lasts longer than 5 minutes
- Student has repeated seizures without regaining consciousness
- Student is injured or has diabetes
- Student has a first-time seizure
- Student has breathing difficulties
- Student has a seizure in water

Treatment Protocol During School Hours (include daily and emergency medications)

Emerg. Med. ✓	Medication	Dosage & Time of Day Given	Common Side Effects & Special Instructions

Does student have a **Vagus Nerve Stimulator?** ❐ Yes ❐ No If YES, describe magnet use:

Special Considerations and Precautions (regarding school activities, sports, trips, etc.)

Describe any special considerations or precautions:

Physician Signature ______ **Date** ______

Parent/Guardian Signature ______ **Date** ______

DPC772

FIGURE 13–6 Seizure action plan.

- Tonic-clonic seizures may occur, usually during sleep.
- The EEG shows a pattern of spikes, called centrotemporal spikes; this epilepsy syndrome is also known as benign childhood epilepsy with centrotemporal spikes.

SAFE AND EFFECTIVE NURSING CARE: Clinical Pearl

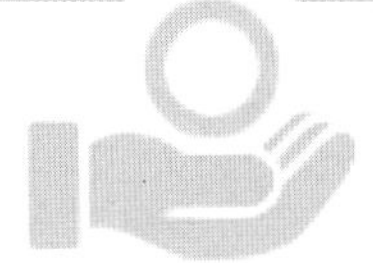

Post-Ictal Paralysis

A phenomenon known as Todd's paresis or post-ictal paralysis may occur after a seizure. This is a weakness on one side of the body that may last between 30 minutes and 36 hours. The paralysis can be partial, affecting only one limb, or it can be complete, affecting the entire side of the body. It is not known why this temporary paralysis occurs; it is more common after generalized seizures and febrile convulsions, but can also occur after focal motor seizures. It is important for the nurse to be alert to this phenomenon. The child's affected limbs should be protected from injury until the paralysis has resolved, and the parents will need to be reassured that the condition is temporary.

Dravet Syndrome

Dravet syndrome is a rare, genetic epileptic encephalopathy, formerly called severe myoclonic epilepsy in infancy, that begins in the first year of life in an otherwise healthy infant and continues throughout life. Development is fairly normal until age 2 years, when the child begins regressing in developmental milestones. About 80% of children with this syndrome have a genetic mutation in the way that ion channels in the brain function. Seizures can occur as generalized tonic-clonic, myoclonic, absence, atypical absence, atonic, partial, and nonconvulsive status epilepticus. Seizures are typically refractory to treatment (Epilepsy, 2014).

Treatment

Treatment for Dravet syndrome is aimed at finding some combination of medications that provide seizure control and prevent seizure emergencies such as status epilepticus. Sodium channel blockers should be avoided because they worsen seizure frequency and severity in Dravet syndrome.

- The ketogenic diet is helpful for some patients with Dravet syndrome.
- The vagal nerve stimulator may be helpful for some patients with Dravet syndrome.
- Medical cannabis is helpful for some patients with Dravet syndrome.

Panayiotopoulos Syndrome

Panayiotopoulos syndrome is early-onset occipital epilepsy that usually manifests between 3 and 10 years of age. Seizures begin as partial or focal seizures that may or may not spread to a generalized seizure. This condition is sometimes misdiagnosed as encephalitis, syncope, migraine, cyclic vomiting, motion sickness, sleep disorder, or gastroenteritis.

- The child may look pale, report nausea, and vomit. Eye deviation to one side and tonic-clonic movements may also occur.
- More than half of the seizures begin in sleep, especially within the first hour after falling asleep.
- Seizures can be prolonged, sometimes lasting 20 to 60 minutes.
- An EEG reveals abnormal spikes in one or both occipital lobes. Centrotemporal spikes may also be seen.
- A fixation sensitivity may be seen on the EEG. Epileptiform discharges are seen when the eyes are closed or not focused on an object. When the eyes are open or focused on an object, the discharges on the EEG disappear.
- Because seizures in Panayiotopoulos syndrome can be infrequent, sometimes treatment is not necessary. When seizures are frequent, anticonvulsant medications such as oxcarbazepine, carbamazepine, levetiracetam, gabapentin, zonisamide, and lacosamide are used to reduce the frequency of the seizure occurrences.
- Because the seizures in Panayiotopoulos syndrome can be prolonged, the child may need rescue medications such as diazepam or midazolam to break the seizure (Epilepsy, 2015a).

SAFE AND EFFECTIVE NURSING CARE: Understanding Medication

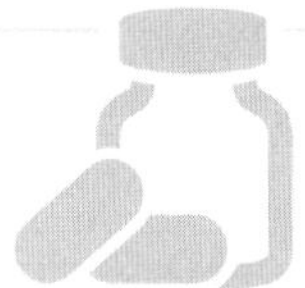

Rescue Medication for Seizures

When rescue medication is needed because of prolonged seizures, parents should be taught how to administer the medications, what to do if the seizure continues after administration, and how to monitor the child for potential side effects such as respiratory depression. Parents should have a plan of action when seizures occur so that they are prepared to administer the correct amount of medication for a seizure emergency.

Landau-Kleffner Syndrome

With Landau-Kleffner syndrome, seizures are infrequent and typically occur during sleep. Simple partial seizures are most common, but atypical absence and tonic-clonic seizures may also occur. The age of onset is 3 to 7 years. Language disorder is present, affecting either receptive or expressive speech. The hallmark is an acquired aphasia, in which there is loss of language that was formerly present. The clinical course of this disorder fluctuates and sometimes disappears on its own as the child gets older. Most children with Landau-Kleffner syndrome do not experience seizures after age 10 years. Some children continue to have permanent language difficulties despite treatment (Epilepsy Foundation, 2013).

Electrical Status Epilepticus in Sleep

Electrical status epilepticus in sleep, also called continuous spike wave of slow sleep, occurs in mid-childhood in children with known epilepsy. The first symptom most commonly reported is a significantly slowed rate of learning. Many children also exhibit receptive and/or expressive dysphasia. This means that they have difficulty understanding and using speech. Children with this syndrome can have many types of seizures, including absence, myoclonic, and focal seizures, particularly during sleep.

- An overnight EEG provides the definitive diagnosis by revealing continuous spike and wave discharges during sleep. An EEG while awake may be normal.
- Treatment is by administration of an anticonvulsant medication such as ethosuximide, valproate, and clobazam.
- Steroids, adrenocorticotropic hormone, or IV immunoglobulin (IVIG) may be prescribed for children who do not respond to anticonvulsant medications.
- Supportive treatments such as speech and occupational therapies should be provided.

Generalized Seizures

Generalized seizures are seizures in which both cerebral hemispheres are involved and the person suffers a loss of awareness or loss of consciousness. As with all seizures, the condition is diagnosed by obtaining the history of the event and performing an EEG study. There are four main types of generalized seizures: generalized tonic-clonic seizures, myoclonic seizures, atonic seizures, and absence seizures.

- Generalized tonic-clonic seizures used to be called grand mal seizures and are characterized by abnormal disorganized activity on both sides of the brain. The patient usually experiences tonic (rigid) as well as clonic (bilateral rhythmic jerking of the extremities) movements, with total loss of awareness.
  - Generalized tonic-clonic seizures may occur once in response to an event such as trauma, severe sleep deprivation, as an adverse effect of medication, illicit drug or alcohol abuse, or related to another condition such as a metabolic disorder.
  - When generalized tonic-clonic seizures occur more than once, that typically indicates the presence of an epilepsy syndrome.
  - Seizures that occur as a result of an epilepsy syndrome are usually treated with antiepileptic medications.
- Myoclonic seizures are sudden, brief jerks of muscle groups, experienced as rapid involuntary movements of the limbs (usually the arms). Loss of consciousness may be brief and go unnoticed by parents or caregivers. Myoclonic seizures may occur in clusters, either several in a row or several in a day.
  - Myoclonic seizures sometimes do not require treatment if the seizures are infrequent and brief.
  - Myoclonic seizures that occur frequently or in clusters are usually treated with antiepileptic medication.
- Atonic seizures produce a rapid loss of muscle tone. The child may simply drop his head, or may have sudden loss of posture and collapse. This seizure has been referred to as "drop attacks."
  - Because of the falls that occur with the sudden loss of muscle tone, many of these patients wear helmets to protect their head if they fall.
  - The seizure is usually brief, lasting seconds to minutes.
  - Atonic seizures are treated with antiepileptic medication.
- Absence seizures used to be called petit mal seizures and are characterized by loss of awareness but no tonic-clonic movements.
  - When absence seizures occur in childhood, it is called childhood absence epilepsy.
  - The child appears to be staring into space or daydreaming.
  - Sometimes small movements may be present with absence seizures such as:
    - Subtle lip movements or lip smacking
    - Small chewing motions
    - Fluttering eyelids
    - Small twitches or movements of the hands or fingers
  - Absence seizures usually last only a few seconds but may occur hundreds of times per day.
  - There is no known cause of absence seizures, but they can be provoked by hyperventilation.
  - Absence seizures are dangerous because the lapse in awareness can result in injury.
  - The child may have problems with learning because he or she misses information in school when seizures occur.
  - Absence seizures are frequently not recognized by teachers or parents, and the child may be punished for daydreaming.
  - Absence seizures can be controlled with antiepileptic medication.
  - Most children outgrow these seizures by their teen years, but about 50% of children with absence seizures will experience development of juvenile myoclonic epilepsy.
  - Complications of absence seizures include:
    - Progression of the seizure disorder to lifelong disorder
    - Absence status epilepticus, in which the child has a prolonged absence seizure that lasts minutes instead of a few seconds

Febrile Seizures

Febrile seizures are convulsions triggered by a rise in body temperature. These seizures are common in children 3 months to 5 years of age and are twice as common in boys as in girls. These seizures are infrequent, last less than five minutes, and typically do not cause brain injury or increase the risk for epilepsy. When febrile seizures are prolonged, this condition is called febrile status epilepticus. When a child has episodes of febrile status epilepticus, there is risk for development of hippocampal sclerosis and temporal lobe sclerosis. These conditions can lead to temporal lobe epilepsy. Parent/caregiver education should include treating a fever at its beginning.

Lennox-Gastaut Epilepsy

Lennox-Gastaut epilepsy is a type of epilepsy characterized by multiple types of seizures.

- Tonic seizures and atonic seizures are common.
- The seizures are often intractable, or difficult to control.
- The EEG shows a characteristic pattern of background slowing along with spike and wave bursts.
- Most children with Lennox-Gastaut epilepsy exhibit some degree of intellectual disability.
- The cause is not usually identified.
- The syndrome persists from childhood through adulthood, with some subtle changes in the types of seizure.

Infantile Spasms

Infantile spasms are a type of myoclonic epilepsy that occurs in infants from 3 to 12 months of age.

- Consists of sudden flexor or extensor movements of the neck, trunk, and extremities.
- The EEG shows a characteristic pattern called hypsarrhythmia.
- Usually occurs upon awakening or going to sleep.
- Seizures can occur 100 or more times per day.
- The cause is not always known.
- The standard of care is to start treatment within 4 weeks of onset of seizures.
- West syndrome is a syndrome that encompasses infantile spasms, the EEG pattern of hypsarrhythmia, and mental retardation.

Status Epilepticus

Status epilepticus is a condition in which the brain is in a state of constant seizure. Some evidence suggests that seizures that last 2 minutes or longer may be unable to stop on their own and progress to status epilepticus (Ochoa & Riche, 2016). Children who experience status epilepticus events in early life are at risk for hippocampal sclerosis and temporal lobe epilepsy.

- Generally described as a seizure that lasts 30 minutes or longer
- Can also be described as recurrent seizures without regaining consciousness between seizures for greater than 30 minutes (or less than 30 minutes if treatment has been given to stop the seizures)
- Always considered a medical emergency
- More common in very young children and in the elderly

SAFE AND EFFECTIVE NURSING CARE: Clinical Pearl

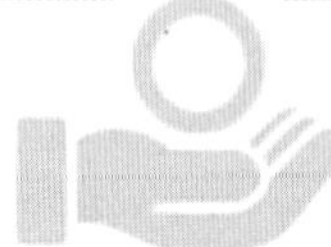

Assessing Movements

For young infants, to determine whether movements are normal-for-age tremulous movements or seizure activity, check for subtle signs of seizures such as lip smacking, tongue thrusting, or REMs. The nurse can also gently grasp the extremity; tremulous movements will stop, seizure activity will not.

SYNCOPE

Syncope, or fainting, is a common condition that affects children and adolescents in which a brief loss of consciousness and posture occurs, caused by a temporary decrease in blood flow to the brain.

- Fainting has many possible causes. If blood does not circulate properly or if the autonomic nervous system does not work properly, changes in blood pressure and heart rate can cause fainting.
- The child regains consciousness and becomes alert quickly, but may have a few moments of confusion after a syncopal event.
- Types of syncope:
  - Vasovagal syncope—the most common type of syncope; blood pressure drops quickly, reducing the blood flow to the brain. Standing results in a flow of blood in the lower extremities, and the autonomic nervous system needs to act in conjunction with the heart to normalize blood pressure. Also known as neurocardiogenic syncope.
  - Postural tachycardia syndrome (POTS)—characterized by a rapid heartbeat and then fainting when the person stands up from a seated position. Because of the complex nature of this condition, it is managed by both neurology and cardiology.
  - Orthostatic hypotension or orthostatic intolerance—occurs when the body has slowed responses to changes in position or in response to exercise, heat intolerance, or stress.
  - Cardiac syncope—loss of consciousness because of a heart condition that interferes with blood flow to the brain.
    - Abnormal heart rhythms
    - Obstructed blood flow in the heart or cardiac blood vessels
    - Heart valve disease
    - Aortic stenosis
    - Heart failure
  - Psychogenic syncope—a person faints in response to anxiety or panic.
  - Metabolic syncope—a person faints in response to metabolic conditions such as hypoglycemia or hyperventilation (EBMedicine, 2014).

Assessment

- General physical examination
- Detailed history of the event

Diagnosis

- Diagnosis can sometimes be made based on the history of the event.
- An EEG and electrocardiogram (EKG) should be performed to evaluate for other conditions.
- Blood tests to evaluate for metabolic problems such as diabetes should be performed.
- In about 30% of cases, the cause cannot be determined.

Treatment

- Treatment is aimed at supportive care.
- Prevention of future syncope events is also important.

HEADACHES AND MIGRAINES

Headaches are a common pediatric report. About 75% of children will experience a headache before age 15 years. About 10% occur before the age of 10 years (Migraine Research Foundation, 2017). Headaches in children are usually benign, but they can still frighten the child and parents. They account for missed participation in school, sports, and social activities, as well as parents missing days from work to care for the child.

Types of Headaches

- Primary headaches
  - The headaches occur spontaneously, and not because of any other health problem or trauma
  - Include migraine and tension headaches (Robertson, 2016)
- Secondary headaches occur because of another condition, such as:
  - Infection
  - Head injuries such as concussions
    - A concussion is a closed head injury in which there is a blow to the head that may or may not result in loss of consciousness.
    - Following the head injury, headache and changes in cognitive function are the most common symptoms.
    - Recovery from concussion may take days, weeks, or months. The child must refrain from activities, such as sports, that put him or her at risk for a second concussion until the first concussion has completely resolved.
    - There is risk for a lethal condition known as second impact syndrome, in which the brain swells rapidly and the person succumbs quickly, if a second concussion occurs before the first concussion has resolved.
  - Chronic sinus disease
  - Problems with blood vessels in the head (such as aneurysms)
  - Tumors
  - Other medical conditions, such as diabetes (Robertson, 2016)

SAFE AND EFFECTIVE NURSING CARE: Clinical Pearl

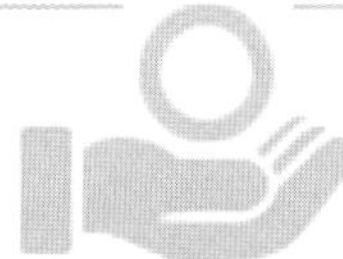

History of Headaches

It is important to gather a complete history of the headaches, because the headache presentation is often the best clue to their source. Information such as time when the headaches occur, whether headaches awaken the child from sleep, whether sudden vomiting without nausea occurs, whether the child has had a recent injury, and whether the headache is accompanied by a fever or stiff neck are all sources of vital information when assessing a child's history of headaches.

Tension Headaches

- Feelings of tightness or pressure around the head
- A steady pain as opposed to a pounding or throbbing pain
- Mild or moderate pain
- Do not usually prevent children from participating in their usual activities
- Are not usually associated with any other symptom, such as nausea or vomiting
- Some children report increased sensitivity to noise
- Typically last 30 minutes to a few hours, but can also be chronic and occur every day
- Usually lessen during school holidays

Migraine Headaches

- Migraine headaches are severe and have disabling symptoms of severe throbbing or pounding unilateral pain.
- They worsen with exertion.
- Sensitivity to light and sound is common.
- Nausea, vomiting, and stomach pain can occur.
- Some children have an aura or warning that the headache is going to occur.
  - Flashing lights
  - Colored spots in their vision
  - Blurry vision
  - Dizziness
  - Vague feeling of malaise
- Headaches may last from a few hours to several days.
- They may be an inherited family condition.
- Sleep may be needed for the headache to be fully relieved.
- Sometimes patterns can be noted, such as occurrence after prolonged exertion in athletes or with menstrual cycles (Robertson, 2016).
- Treatment is aimed at supportive care and identification of migraine triggers.

Abdominal migraines are migraine variants that occur in children.

- Unknown cause
- More common in girls
- Symptoms
  - Acute, severe midline abdominal pain
  - Nausea
  - Vomiting
  - Pallor
  - Anorexia
- Duration of 1 hour to 3 days

Cyclic vomiting is a migraine variant characterized by recurrent attacks of violent or prolonged vomiting.

- No headache is associated with cyclic vomiting.
- May last for hours.
- Amitriptyline, a tricyclic antidepressant, is helpful in preventing cyclic migraines in some children (Robertson, 2016).

Assessment

- A general physical assessment should be performed.
- A detailed history of the headache should be obtained.

Diagnosis

- Diagnosis is often made based on the history of the event.
- Headache diaries are helpful in assessing the frequency and severity of the headaches.
- Headache diaries may also help identify potential headache triggers.
- An MRI or CT scan of the brain is not indicated unless there is an abnormal finding on the examination of the child.
- A serum lactate level can exclude a mitochondrial disorder in children with cyclic vomiting, because the level is elevated in mitochondrial disorders and normal in cyclic vomiting.

Treatment

Treatment is aimed at supportive care and at prevention of the headaches. Patients should be counseled to avoid headache triggers when possible. Common headache triggers in children include:

- Skipping meals, most commonly breakfast
- Inadequate fluid intake
- Sleep deprivation
- Stress

Parents and children are encouraged to keep a diary of the headaches to better classify the headaches and identify potential triggers.

Some children have a significant headache disorder and need prescription medications aimed at prevention of migraines. These include:

- Beta blockers such as propranolol
- Seizure medications such as valproate (Depakote) or topiramate (Topamax)
- Antidepressants such as amitriptyline, nortriptyline (Pamelor), or venlafaxine (Effexor HCL)

Some children need prescriptions to treat severe migraines. These include:

- Triptan medications such as sumatriptan (Imitrex), zolmitriptan (Zomig), and rizatriptan (Maxalt)
- Anti-emetics such as promethazine (Phenergan) and ondansetron (Zofran)
- Analgesic medications such as acetaminophen and ibuprofen

Some children need to stop activities and go to sleep for the headache to completely resolve.

SAFE AND EFFECTIVE NURSING CARE: Clinical Pearl

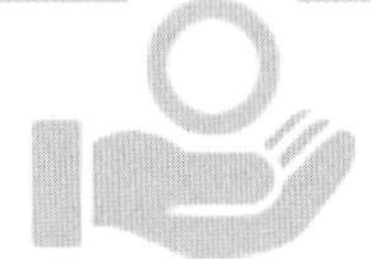

Headache Diary

A diary of the child's headaches is valuable for identifying triggers, determining the headache type, and helping the child to feel in control of the condition. The diary includes time and dates of the headaches, the severity of the headache, what treatment was done, and how long it took to resolve. Grading the severity of the headache on an approved age-appropriate pain scale is recommended.

NEUROCUTANEOUS DISORDERS

Neurocutaneous syndromes are disorders in nerve cells that lead to abnormal growth of tumors in various parts of the body. They are caused by the abnormal development of cells in the embryonic stage. Neurocutaneous syndromes are characterized by distinctive neurocutaneous lesions. Some of these conditions can be diagnosed at birth but may not cause problems until later in life. Neurocutaneous disorders in infants and during childhood include neurofibromatosis and ataxia telangiectasia, among others.

Neurofibromatosis

Neurofibromatosis is one of the most common neurocutaneous syndromes. With this condition, tumors called neurofibromas grow on nerve cells (NINDS, 2017c), causing skin changes, bone deformities, and eye problems. Seizures can also occur because of lesions that may occur in the brain.

- Neurofibromatosis is usually inherited, but up to half of cases occur because of spontaneous changes or mutations within a person's genes.
  - The child of a parent with neurofibromatosis has a 50% chance of inheriting the disorder.
- The two different forms of this disorder are neurofibromatosis type 1 (NF1) and type 2 (NF2).
  - NF1 accounts for approximately 90% of all cases and is also known as von Recklinghausen disease.
  - The classic sign of NF1 is skin pigment findings known as café-au-lait spots (Dillon, 2016).
    - These light brown or coffee-colored patches may be present at birth and can look like freckles at first.
    - Axillary freckling in a young child is high suspicious for NF1 (Hsieh, 2016)
    - The lesions increase in size and number during the first few years of life.
    - A child diagnosed with NF1 will usually have at least six café-au-lait spots that are larger than 1/2 inch in diameter.
    - The lesions are flat, do not cause pain, and do not progress to tumors.
  - Lisch nodules may also be found in patients with NF1 (Hsieh, 2016).
    - The nodules are tiny, benign tumors found on the iris of the eye.
    - In some cases, tumors can develop along the optic nerves and affect vision.

Assessment

- General physical examination
- Thorough skin examination
- Measurement and documentation of skin lesions

SAFE AND EFFECTIVE NURSING CARE: Clinical Pearl

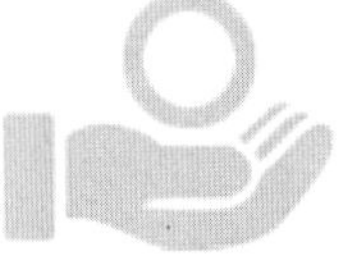

Measuring Lesions

A small clear ruler is helpful for measuring the size of lesions such as café-au-lait spots without obscuring the mark.

Diagnosis

- Diagnosis is based on clinical findings.
- A baseline MRI of the brain should be performed and then repeated as the child grows to monitor for tumors.
- An MRI of the brain and optic nerve should be performed in children with Lisch nodules.
- An EEG should be performed if seizures occur.
- A blood test can be performed to evaluate for a defect in the NF1 gene.

Treatment

- Treatment focuses on managing the symptoms.
- Sometimes the neurofibromas are surgically removed if they are causing pain or causing problems with a vital organ.
- Seizures usually can be controlled with medication.
- A child may need specialized educational plans if learning is a problem.
- Psychological therapy may be needed for children and adolescents with self-esteem problems because of the visible tumors (see Chapter 18 for further details).

Ataxia Telangiectasia

Ataxia telangiectasia is a progressive degenerative disease that ultimately involves most body systems (NORD, 2016). It is a recessive genetic disease, which means that both parents carry the gene, but they do not have the disorder. Ataxia telangiectasia is typically diagnosed when the child is approximately 2 years old. This condition progresses until the child is unable to sit or stand unsupported. Cerebellar degeneration occurs, causing ataxia and slurred speech.

Most children require a wheelchair for mobility.

- Telangiectasias are tiny red veins that appear in the corners of the eyes or on the exposed ears and cheeks when the child is in sunlight.
- The appearance of the veins is a significant symptom in the diagnosis of this disease.
- Disruptions in the immune system are extremely common in children with ataxia telangiectasia.
- Recurrent respiratory infections and pneumonia are common.
- Some cancers are more common in this population, particularly leukemia.

Assessment

- General physical examination
- Thorough skin examination
- Evaluation of presence or absence of developmental milestones

Diagnosis

- Diagnosis is based on clinical findings.
- A baseline MRI of the brain should be performed.
- A blood test can be performed to evaluate for a genetic marker.

Treatment

- The treatment focuses on managing the symptoms.
- Screening for other health problems should be performed.
- A multidisciplinary approach is needed because of the complex nature of this disorder.

Other Neurocutaneous Disorders

- Sturge-Weber syndrome—angiomas develop on the thin membrane that surrounds the brain and spinal cord and the skin of the face, usually in the ophthalmic and maxillary divisions of the trigeminal nerve (The Sturge-Weber Foundation, 2017).
- Tuberous sclerosis—tumors grow in the brain, kidneys, heart, lungs, eyes, and on the skin (NIH, 2017c).

MOVEMENT DISORDERS IN CHILDREN

The two main types of movement disorders in children are excessive or hyperkinetic movement and diminished or bradykinetic movement. Hyperkinetic movement is more common in the pediatric population, characterized by abnormal, repetitive, and involuntary movements that include:

- Tics—sudden, repetitive, involuntary movements
- Tremors—involuntary trembling movements
- Dystonia—muscle contractions cause twisting movements of the muscle groups, resulting in abnormal postures
- Chorea—muscle contractions result in quick, rhythmic movements that resemble dancing movements.

Tics

Movement disorders are thought to be caused by disorder in the communication from the brain to the muscles that results in unintentional movements. Children with tics, the most common pediatric movement disorder, do not intend to blink their eyes rapidly or clear their throats excessively, but communication occurs from the brain that causes them to do so. Motor tics are most frequently seen.

- These sudden, brief involuntary moments may include:
  - Eye blinking
  - Grimacing
  - Neck jerks
  - Movements of the shoulder
  - Nose twitches
  - Grinding of the teeth
  - Tensing of the muscles of the chest or abdomen
- A child may have complex motor tics with more than one body part involved.

Vocal tics may also occur.

- These may include sounds such as:
  - Sniffing
  - Clearing of the throat
  - Grunting
  - Squeaking

- Humming sounds
- Clicking the teeth together
- Sucking sounds
- Complex vocal tics may be repetition of words or syllables, spoken syllables or words, shouts, or obscenities.
- Complex motor and vocal tics are often mistakenly thought to be voluntary by the public and can be disturbing to the family of the child (Association for Children's Mental Health, 2017).
- Parents often assume that their child has Tourette's syndrome, a more complex tic disorder, when the child actually has a condition known as transient tic of childhood.
- The distinction between these two conditions is noted by the length of time the tic has been present and the type of tic seen.
  - Transient tic of childhood is typically a disorder of motor or vocal tics that may last for several months but not greater than 1 year.
  - Tourette's syndrome is a disorder of complex motor and vocal tics that have been present for more than 1 year and began before the child's 18th birthday (Hawley, 2015).
- It is possible for motor tics to become chronic in some children, whereas chronic vocal tics are rare.
- If the child has only one type of tic for more than 1 year, it is termed a chronic tic disorder, not Tourette's syndrome (which requires both motor and vocal tics to be present).
- Tics usually appear before the age of 10 years, with the most common age at diagnosis being 6 to 7 years.
- The most common motor tic is eye blinking.
- The most common vocal tic is sniffing or clearing of the throat, often misdiagnosed as an allergy manifestation.
- Tics may worsen at around age 12 years and usually disappear completely by age 18.
- Tics will worsen with anxiety in most children.
- Tics can sometimes occur as a secondary symptom as a result of:
  - Infections—particularly streptococcal infections
  - Medication effects—tics are common side effect to neurostimulants such as methylphenidate (Ritalin) or Adderall (amphetamine, dextroamphetamine mixed salts) for ADHD
  - Developmental—such as the transient tic of childhood; this is usually a simple tic that appears between the ages of 3 and 9 years, and lasts for less than 1 year
  - Genetic disorders—often Tourette syndrome is familial
  - Neurocutaneous disorders—such as tuberous sclerosis
  - Degenerative disorders—such as Rett syndrome
  - Stroke—thought to be caused by damage to the basal ganglia
  - Head trauma—thought to be caused by damage to the basal ganglia
- Most children learn to manage the tic on their own, with supportive parents and teachers who do not focus on the behavior.
- By their mid-teens, most have developed social relationships with people who show acceptance of the tic as part of the person.
- The behavior tends to diminish until it is absent by the time the child is 18 years old.

Bradykinetic movements are less common in children than in adults, such as the very slow and rigid movements of a person with Parkinson's disease. Ataxia and spasticity are classified as motor dysfunctions, not motion disorders.

Assessment

- General physical examination
- In evaluating a movement disorder, ask:
  - Whether the frequency of the movement in question is abnormal
  - If the character of the movement is abnormal
  - If anything in the environment is causing the disorder (such as a foreign body in the eyes of a child, thus causing the ticlike movement of the eyes)
  - Whether the movement can be voluntarily suppressed

Diagnosis

- Diagnosis is based on clinical findings and history of the tics.

Treatment

- Treatment focuses on supportive care.
- Most children learn to manage the tic on their own, with supportive parents and teachers who do not focus on the behavior.
- By their mid-teens, most have developed social relationships with people who show acceptance of the tic as part of the person.
- Medications to suppress the tic can be considered if the tic is emotionally distressing to the child or if the tic causes pain or discomfort.
- Screening for other health problems should be performed.

PEDIATRIC STROKE

Stroke or cerebrovascular accidents are more common in adults but can occur in children in utero, during or shortly after birth, or as a result of trauma or illness.

- Neonatal hemorrhages are unfortunately common in premature infants due to the fragile nature of their neurovascular networks (Fig. 13–7).
- Malformations of brain structures or blood vessels are often the cause of strokes in young children.
- Infections or illnesses, such as meningitis, encephalitis, and sickle cell disease states, may also cause strokes.
- The effects can be mild, with only some mild weakness in an extremity, or devastating, with profound and severe neurological impairment (American Stroke Association, 2017; National Stroke Association, 2017).

Assessment

- A thorough examination and vigilance on the part of the nurse are necessary to assess for subtle changes in motor or sensory function.

Diagnosis

- Diagnosis is made based on areas of bleeding in the brain verified by CT or MRI imaging.
- For premature infants and neonates, hemorrhages in the brain can be seen on cranial ultrasound.

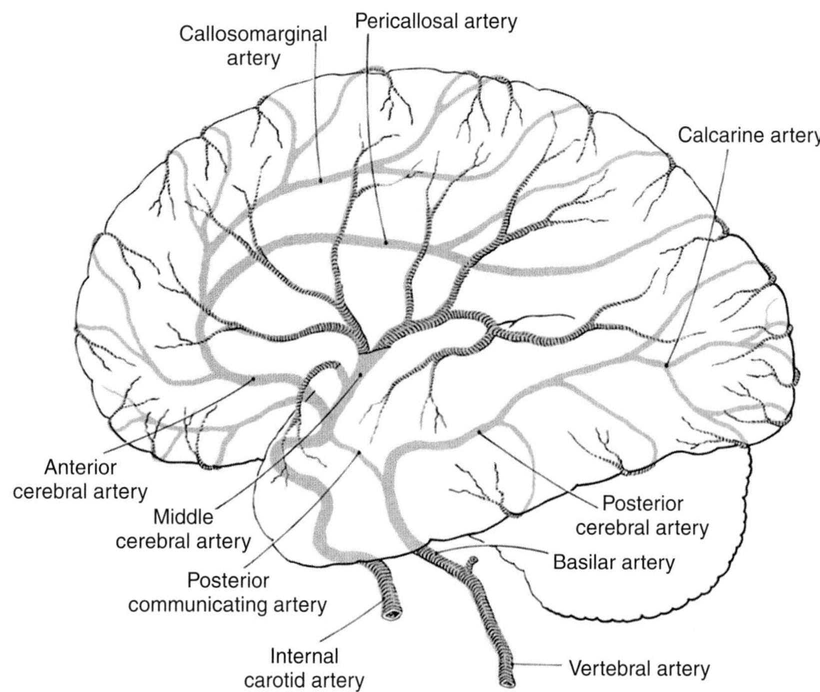

FIGURE 13–7 Arteries in the brain.

Treatment

- Treatment is aimed at the cause of the stroke, as well as its symptoms and residual effects.
- Intensive physical, occupational, and speech therapies are required.
- An individualized education plan should be initiated if a stroke occurs in a young child.
- The family needs support, because caring for children with these conditions is emotionally, physically, and financially exhausting. A social work referral should be included in the plan of care.
- Screening for the development of hydrocephalus in indicated, because this is a common complication of pediatric stroke.

INFECTIONS OF THE NERVOUS SYSTEM

Infections of the nervous system have four main causes: bacterial, viral (aseptic), fungal, or parasitic.

Meningitis

The most common infection is meningitis, which affects the coverings of the brain and spinal cord called the meninges (CDC, 2017e) (Fig. 13–8). Meningitis can be a life-threatening infection, and thus must be treated as a medical emergency.

- Can be a precursor to encephalitis, which is an acute inflammation of the brain.
- Brain abscess can occur.
- Symptoms include:
  - Severe headache
  - Stiff neck
  - Sudden high fever
  - Photosensitivity
  - Bulging fontanel in infants
  - Altered mental status
    - Infants and young children may exhibit more subtle symptoms such as irritability and sleepiness.
    - If a rash is present, it can indicate the existence of a specific bacterial infection such as *Neisseria meningitides*. This infection results in a purpuric rash, often combined with sepsis. Death can occur in hours after the rash appears.

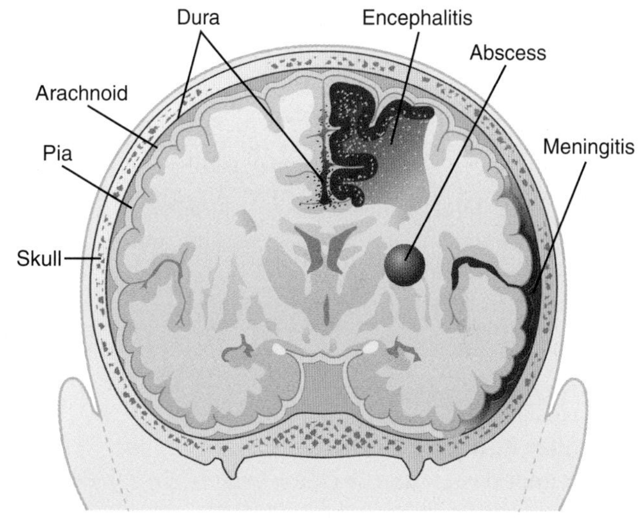

FIGURE 13–8 Major sites of infection in the brain.

Assessment

- Thorough physical examination
- Thorough history of the child's illness

- Physical signs of neck rigidity
  - Kernig's sign: With the child lying on his or her back, flex the hip and knee 90 degrees. If the Kernig's sign is positive, pain will prevent the child from extending the knee (Dillon, 2016).
  - Brudzinski's sign: Flexion of the neck causes involuntary flexion of the knee and hip (Dillon, 2016).

Diagnosis

- Diagnosis is made based on symptoms and laboratory data.
- Complete blood count shows elevation in white blood cell count.
- Lumbar puncture or spinal tap is performed to obtain spinal fluid for testing. This should always be done before the administration of an antibiotic.
- CSF is tested for the presence of protein and white blood cells, and cultured to identify a causative agent. This varies according to the child's age. In newborns, the typical causative agent is group B *Streptococcus* and *E. coli*. In older children and adolescents, *Streptococcus pneumonia*, *Neisseria meningitides*, and *Haemophilus influenzae* type b are the common causes of meningitis.
  - An elevated white blood count (>1,000/mm^3), elevated protein count (greater than 50 mg/dL), and low glucose level (<40% of serum glucose) in spinal fluid indicate bacterial meningitis (Caserta, 2015). The CSF will also be cloudy in appearance.
  - The white blood count is variable, is normal to elevated (>50 mg/dL), and the glucose count is low (<40% of serum glucose) in fungal meningitis.
  - The white blood count is low (<100/mm^3), the protein count is normal to elevated (>50 mg/dL), and the glucose level is normal to high (>60% of serum glucose) in viral meningitis (Ward, 2014). The CSF is clear.

CRITICAL COMPONENT

Lumbar Puncture

The nurse will need to help the child to be properly positioned for a lumbar puncture. Because of the degree of flexion needed for access to the lumbar spine, the nurse should be alert to respiratory compromise in the infant or child. Positions for infants and children include a lateral, side-lying position with the hips and neck flexed, as well as a sitting position with the hips and neck flexed. The position chosen for the procedure will be based on the child's condition and age at the time of the procedure. It is important for the nurse to prevent the child's movement during the procedure.

After the lumbar puncture has been completed, the nurse will apply a dry dressing to the puncture site. The child should remain flat in bed for 4 to 24 hours and should be well hydrated with amounts as indicated for the child's age and weight. The nurse should assess the puncture site for signs of CSF leakage or hematoma formation, should monitor the vital signs and neurological status of the child at least every 4 hours for 24 hours, or as indicated by the child's condition, and should assess the child for adequate urinary elimination within 8 hours of the procedure.

Treatment

- Treatment is aimed at rapid recognition of the cause of the infection.
- Broad-spectrum antibiotics may be administered.
- Supportive care of the child is important.
- Rapid deterioration is possible in patients with meningitis.
- The nurse must be vigilant to recognize even the subtlest symptoms.
- As the causative agent is identified, the treatment is revised to be more specific to that organism.
- Infection-control measures, such as airborne or droplet precautions, are indicated for 24 hours after the antibiotic treatment has been started.
- Meningitis of any type can leave children with deficits.
  - Hearing loss (sensorineural)
  - Learning problems
  - Seizures
  - Mental retardation (intellectual disability)
- Bacterial meningitis is fatal if untreated. About 5% to 20% of newborn infants die of bacterial meningitis, even with treatment (Caserta, 2015).
- Even when treated, bacterial meningitis may have grave effects, depending on the age of the child and the causative organism.
- Viral meningitis is rarely fatal and usually resolves without antiviral medications.
- Fungal meningitis can be fatal without treatment, and unfortunately the treatment is not without its own risk to the child.
- Protozoan or parasitic infections can be treated with some specific medications, such as antimalarial drugs, as well as some antibiotics.
- Prevention of nervous system infections is possible in some cases.
- A vaccine is available for some types of bacterial meningitis. At this time, *Haemophilus influenzae* type b, pneumococcal, and meningococcal vaccines are available.
- In the case of infants being born to mothers known to be infected with specific organisms, prophylactic antibiotics are considered the standard of care.
- Prevention of infection by protozoan organisms should be implemented when possible.
- For close contacts of patients with some types of bacterial meningitis, appropriate antibiotic therapy should be administered. The most commonly used antibiotics for prophylactic treatment for family members in the same household are rifampin, ciprofloxacin, and ceftriaxone. The dosage and length of therapy should be based on the age and condition of the family member, and should be monitored by an infectious disease provider.

CRITICAL COMPONENT

Fever and Lethargy as Symptoms of Meningitis

Meningitis should always be suspected in acutely ill infants and children with fever and lethargy until proven otherwise (Muller, 2016). Work-up in the emergency department should include lumbar puncture and blood cultures. Most children will be admitted to the hospital for further evaluation, treatment, and monitoring.

Acute Flaccid Myelitis

Acute flaccid myelitis is a neurological disorder characterized by sudden onset of limb weakness, loss of muscle tone, and loss of deep tendon reflexes (Patel, 2017).

- Associated symptoms include weakness in the face or eyelids, difficulty moving the eyes, slurred speech, and difficulty swallowing.
- In severe cases, respiratory failure can occur.
- Sometimes diagnosis is difficult, because symptoms are similar to other conditions such as acute flaccid paralysis, some genetic disorders, and Guillain–Barré syndrome.
- Acute flaccid myelitis has been a relatively rare occurrence, but pediatric cases have steadily risen in the last few years. In 2016, the CDC confirmed 144 cases in 37 states and the District of Columbia (American Academy of Pediatrics, 2017).
- It is thought to be related to a viral infection such as enterovirus, adenovirus, and West Nile virus.
- There is no specific treatment other than supportive care and therapies.

Encephalitis

Encephalitis is an acute infection of the brain related to viral infections such as the herpes simplex virus and West Nile virus.

- Symptoms of encephalitis in children and adults are similar to those of the flu and can last for a few days to a few weeks.
- Symptoms of encephalitis in infants are irritability, poor feeding, bulging fontanels, vomiting, and body stiffness. These symptoms are always considered a neurological emergency in infants.

Zika Virus

Zika virus exposure in pregnant women can be devastating to the developing infant.

- The Zika virus is transmitted through mosquito bites.
- Symptoms of the Zika virus in the mother can include fever, rash, joint pain, and red sclera, but some people have no symptoms.
- If a pregnant woman is infected with the Zika virus, she can pass the infection to the child during pregnancy or at the time of birth, potentially causing congenital Zika syndrome.
- Congenital Zika syndrome is characterized by five distinct features:
  - Severe microcephaly in which the skull has partially collapsed
  - Decreased brain tissue with a specific pattern of brain damage, including subcortical calcifications
  - Damage to the back of the eye, including macular scarring and focal pigmentary retinal mottling
  - Congenital contractures such as clubfoot or arthrogryposis, a condition in which the infant is born with multiple joint contractures throughout the body
  - Hypertonia restricting body movement soon after birth
- There is no treatment for congenital Zika syndrome other than supportive care.

SAFE AND EFFECTIVE NURSING CARE: Promoting Safety

Zika Virus Education

The primary way that the Zika virus is transmitted is through mosquito bites. The nurse should educate parents about measures to help prevent mosquito bites, such as using an appropriate insect repellent, to cover exposed skin, and to sleep in either an air-conditioned room or in a bed covered with insect-proof netting around it. Infants younger than 2 months should not have insect repellent applied to their skin, and some insect repellants are not appropriate for children younger than 3 years. Pregnant women should avoid travel to areas known to have outbreaks of the Zika virus.

NEUROMUSCULAR DISORDERS

Neuromuscular disorders are the cause of muscular weakness and abnormal tone in infancy and childhood. These disorders are diagnosed based on which area of the neuromuscular system is affected. The most common neuromuscular disorders are:

- Cerebral palsy
- Muscular dystrophy
- Myasthenia gravis
- Spinal muscle atrophy (SMA), a degenerative disorder of the anterior horn cell of the spinal cord

Cerebral Palsy

Cerebral palsy is the name given to a group of conditions that affect motor development in children. It can be quite mild, with abnormal tone and weakness in one extremity, or severe, affecting all extremities, growth and development, and the intellectual capabilities of the child.

Cerebral palsy is a result of damage to the brain before, during, or after the child is born. If the damage occurs before or during birth, it is called *congenital* cerebral palsy. If it occurs afterward, due to injury or illness, it is called *acquired* cerebral palsy.

Types of Cerebral Palsy

- Spastic—most common; about 70% of affected children have this type
  - Spastic diplegia/diparesis—stiffness in the legs with difficulty walking as stiffness in the hips causes a scissor-like gait
  - Spastic hemiplegia/hemiparesis—stiffness on one side of the body, usually in the arm more than the leg
  - Spastic quadriplegia/quadriparesis—stiffness in all of the limbs of the body, the trunk, and the face; often associated with difficulty with swallowing, intellect, sight, and hearing

- Athetoid/dyskinetic—difficulty controlling movements of the body and can have sudden, uncontrollable changes in muscle tone
  - Athetoid—involuntary movements that typically alternate between hypotonic and hypertonic movements; these movements can have a writhing quality at times
  - Choreoathetoid—sudden involuntary movements, particularly of the fingers and toes, combined with writhing movements
  - Dystonic—slow rotational movements, particularly of the torso, arms, and legs
- Ataxic—problems with balance and coordination, especially with purposeful movements like writing or reaching for objects
- Mixed—some people have more than one type. The most common combination is spastic/dystonic cerebral palsy, but any of the types can be combined in any child. Sometimes one limb is affected more than the others, and sometimes one limb is spared more than the other limbs. The nurse must approach each child with cerebral palsy as an individual and carefully assess the child's ability to independently move his body.

Screening for Cerebral Palsy

- Infants and young children not meeting developmental milestones should be screened.
- Infants and young children with hypertonia or hypotonia should be screened.
- Infants and young children who have had accidental or nonaccidental trauma or a central nervous system infection should be screened.

Treatment

There is no cure for cerebral palsy. Treatment is aimed at early intervention and aggressive institution of physical, occupational speech, and educational therapies. Treatment is lifelong to reduce disability and maximize the child's potential for independent functioning.

Muscular Dystrophy

Muscular dystrophy is a disorder that results in muscular weakness and a decrease in muscle tone over time through gradual progressive degeneration of symmetrical groups of skeletal muscles (Ward, 2014). The protein dystrophin is produced by the short arm of the X chromosome. In cases of muscular dystrophy, a gene mutation causes a reduction or absence of dystrophin production. Dystrophin is important to muscle membrane integrity and when inadequate, destruction of muscles occurs. Dystrophin is also present in cardiac and smooth muscles. This lack of dystrophin is most devastating in Duchenne muscular dystrophy.

There are several types of muscular dystrophy.

- Becker muscular dystrophy
  - Inherited disorder that causes progressive weakness in the pelvis and legs over time
  - Symptoms usually noted around age 12 years
  - Disability tends to occur at a fairly slow rate
  - Cardiomyopathy, or weakness in the heart muscles, can occur
- Duchenne muscular dystrophy
  - More rapidly progressing
  - Usually diagnosed before the age of 6 years
  - An X-linked recessive inheritance through the mother and expressed in male children
  - A leading cause of rapid disability in young children
  - Cardiomyopathy, or weakness in the heart muscles, can occur
  - Death usually occurs in the twenties and is usually caused by respiratory or cardiac failure
  - A classic finding is Gowers' sign, which is seen when children who are in a squatting position have to use their hands and arms to "walk up" their own bodies, pushing as they go, in order to stand; this is due to weakness in the proximal muscles (the hips and thighs) of the lower limbs (EpoMedicine, 2016)
- Facioscapulohumeral muscular dystrophy
  - This condition is less disabling than other neuromuscular disorders.
  - Diagnosis is based on weakness in the shoulder and facial muscles.
  - Weakness can occur in the limbs, but this is less common and tends to occur only later in life as the condition worsens.
  - It is also a genetic disorder.

Myasthenia Gravis

Myasthenia gravis is an autoimmune disorder in which antibodies block acetylcholine receptors at the neuromuscular junction or the site where the neuron causes muscles to react (Howard, 2015). It affects voluntary muscles in the eyes, mouth, throat, and extremities. There are three types of myasthenia gravis:

- Congenital
  - The rarest form is congenital; in this disorder, genes must be transmitted from each parent for the child to have the disorder (autosomal recessive). Symptoms begin in infancy and do not go into remission.
- Transient neonatal
  - This form occurs when a woman with myasthenia gravis gives birth.
  - The baby has symptoms of the disease as a result of myasthenia antibodies crossing the placenta to the fetus.
  - This occurs in about 10% to 15% of babies born to mothers with myasthenia gravis and disappears without recurrence in the first few weeks of life (Bodamer & Miller, 2016).
- Juvenile
  - Juvenile myasthenia gravis is most common in female adolescents, particularly Caucasians.
  - This lifelong condition is usually diagnosed in the midteens and continues as the adolescent goes into and out of remission.
  - About 10% of all cases of myasthenia gravis begin as juvenile myasthenia (Myasthenia Foundation, 2014).

Assessment

- The symptoms of myasthenia gravis are predominantly weakness and fatigue.
- Persons with this disorder are unable to keep their eyelids raised and develop a condition called ptosis, or drooping eyelids.
- Mouth and throat muscles are weakened, affecting the ability to smile responsively and to drink liquids through a straw.
- Swallowing becomes difficult in untreated cases.

SAFE AND EFFECTIVE NURSING CARE: Clinical Pearl

Symptoms of Myasthenia Gravis

Parents often report that the child looks tired or sad. These are cues to screen for myasthenia gravis, as the child may be developing ptosis of the eyelids or the inability to smile.

Diagnosis

- A blood test is performed to evaluate serum acetylcholine receptor antibodies.
- Electromyography (EMG) may be performed to confirm muscle activity.
- A Tensilon test may be performed, in which a medication called edrophonium chloride is injected IV to determine whether myasthenia gravis symptoms temporarily resolve (Ward, 2014).

SAFE AND EFFECTIVE NURSING CARE: Understanding Medication

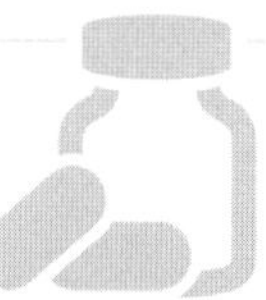

Medications and Myasthenia Gravis

Some medications can exacerbate weakness in a child with myasthenia gravis. These drugs include aminoglycosides, procainamide, quinidine, curare, succinylcholine, some channel blockers, and beta blockers. The nurse should have a thorough awareness of medications that are being administered to the child (Bird, 2016).

Treatment

- Treatment is aimed at supportive care.
- Cholinesterase inhibitors may be used, which act to prevent the acetylcholine receptor from being blocked or broken down, thus allowing it to act as a neurotransmitter.
- Immunosuppressants can also be used in some cases if the patient is unresponsive to or intolerant of cholinesterase inhibitors.
- Sometimes a surgical procedure is required to remove the thymus gland, which works to provide T cells that are necessary for autoimmunity. The thymus loses most of its function after adolescence, so this procedure is usually done in adulthood.

CRITICAL COMPONENT

Respiratory Function

Nurses must be alert to respiratory function changes in children with myasthenia gravis. Thorough assessment of breath sounds, respiratory rate, and oxygenation is critical (Bird, 2016). A primary feature of myasthenia gravis is muscle weakness, which can affect the ability of the child to keep the airway open. In addition, because of the weakness in the airway and throat muscles, aspiration occurs as a result of the resultant dysphagia.

Spinal Muscle Atrophy

SMA is a degenerative disorder of the anterior horn cells of the spinal cord (Muscular Dystrophy Association, 2017) that results in weakness and wasting of voluntary muscles. SMA is the most common recessive genetic disorder that is lethal in children (Muscular Dystrophy Association, 2017). In milder forms, it is the second most common neuromuscular disorder in childhood. A characteristic initial finding is often proximal lower extremity weakness. Recent research has indicated that there may be a genetic component because of an abnormality on chromosome 5. There are three types of SMA:

- SMA type 1 is also known as Werdnig-Hoffman disease.
  - This is the most severe form.
  - It begins in utero or early infancy.
  - Infants have few spontaneous movements.
  - They are unable to lift their heads.
  - They have trouble sucking and swallowing.
  - They exhibit a loss of deep tendon reflexes.
  - Fasciculations, or constant, wormlike movements of the tongue, are noted.
  - Fasciculations can sometimes also be seen in the deltoid, biceps, and quadriceps muscles.
  - The respiratory muscles are weak, and death occurs by age 3 years because of respiratory compromise.
  - Infants who display symptoms at birth usually have a shorter life span and die before they are 12 months old.
- SMA type 2 is noted later in infancy.
  - It usually manifests between the ages of 6 and 24 months.
  - Deep tendon reflexes are absent.
  - Muscle fasciculations may or may not be present.
  - Life span for those with SMA type 2 is 20 to 30 years.
- SMA type 3 is a juvenile form of the disease.
  - It is also known as Kugelberg-Welander disease.
  - Onset of the disease is between ages 3 and 17 years.
  - Early symptoms are nonspecific and include delayed motor milestones.
  - Atrophy of proximal muscles may be present.
  - SMA type 3 is a milder form of the disease and children live into adulthood.

Assessment

- Thorough physical examination
- Thorough history of the child's illness

Diagnosis

- Diagnosis is derived from symptoms.
- Blood can be tested for genetic markers.
- EMG is performed to document muscle responses.
- A muscle biopsy is performed if blood tests are negative and the EMG is suggestive of SMA.

Treatment

- Treatment is aimed at supportive care.
- The family of a child with SMA requires additional support because of stress, typically in the areas of time, emotions, grief, and finances.

NEUROPATHY SYNDROMES

Neuropathy is a condition in which peripheral nerves are damaged (Fig. 13–9). Neuropathy can be an inherited disorder or result from a metabolic or endocrine disorder such as diabetes, exposure to toxins or chemotherapy, inflammation, vitamin deficiencies, and trauma. Sometimes the cause cannot be determined and the syndrome is termed *idiopathic.* Symptoms can include:

- Decreased sensation
- Pain
- Tingling
- Problems with balance
- Weakness in the extremities
    - Weakness can also occur in any other location in which autonomic nerves exist in the body.
        - This leads to conditions such as abnormalities in the heart rate and respiratory rate, inability to perspire, problems with food absorption, constipation, and bladder dysfunction.

Guillain–Barré Syndrome

Guillain–Barré syndrome is an acute, inflammatory, demyelinating polyneuropathy that affects the peripheral nervous system (Ward, 2014; World Health Organization, 2016). Demyelinating means that the protective myelin covering on nerve cells is being eroded, interrupting the smooth flow of impulses. The hallmark of Guillain–Barré is ascending paralysis, in which weakness occurs distally in the lower limbs and spreads to the upper extremities and torso.

- A complete loss of deep tendon reflexes occurs in patients affected by Guillain–Barré syndrome.
- This condition can be severe and affect the child's ability to breathe.
- Death may occur if the pulmonary system is severely compromised.
- Most patients recover fully, but the course of the disease is slow, showing improvement after 4 weeks and often taking up to a year to achieve full recovery.
- About 20% of those affected have lingering affects after 1 year if the disease course was severe or treatment was delayed.

Assessment

- Thorough physical examination
- Thorough history of the child's illness
- Deep tendon reflexes may indicate a loss of reflexes along with the ascending paralysis.

Diagnosis

- Diagnosis is made based on symptoms and diagnostic test results.
- EMG is done to test the electrical activity in the muscles.
- Nerve conduction velocity (NCV) testing is done to measure the speed of electrical signals traveling through a nerve.
- Lumbar puncture is done to assess protein and white blood cell count. In Guillain–Barré, the protein count is elevated and the white blood cell count is normal.

Treatment

- Treatment is aimed at supportive care.
- Plasmapheresis is a procedure in which plasma is removed from blood cells; then the blood cells are returned to the patient. This is thought to remove autoantibodies from the blood, and thus reduce the severity and duration of the syndrome.
- IV gamma globulins are substances that the body uses to help naturally fight the syndrome; they are given IV on a schedule until the patient shows normalization.
    - Immunizations should be delayed for 8 months after administration of IVIG. If the immunizations were given within 14 days before the IVIG, they should be repeated 8 months after the IVIG administration.
- Most patients recover fully, but the course of the disease is slow, showing improvement after 4 weeks and often taking up to a year to achieve full recovery.
- About 20% of those affected have lingering affects after 1 year if the disease course was severe or treatment was delayed.

Nursing care of the child with a neurological disorder requires critical thinking and physical assessment skills, as well as knowledge of developmental milestones of all ages of infants and children. The nurse must use the observations to provide safe and effective care for both acutely and chronically ill children and their families.

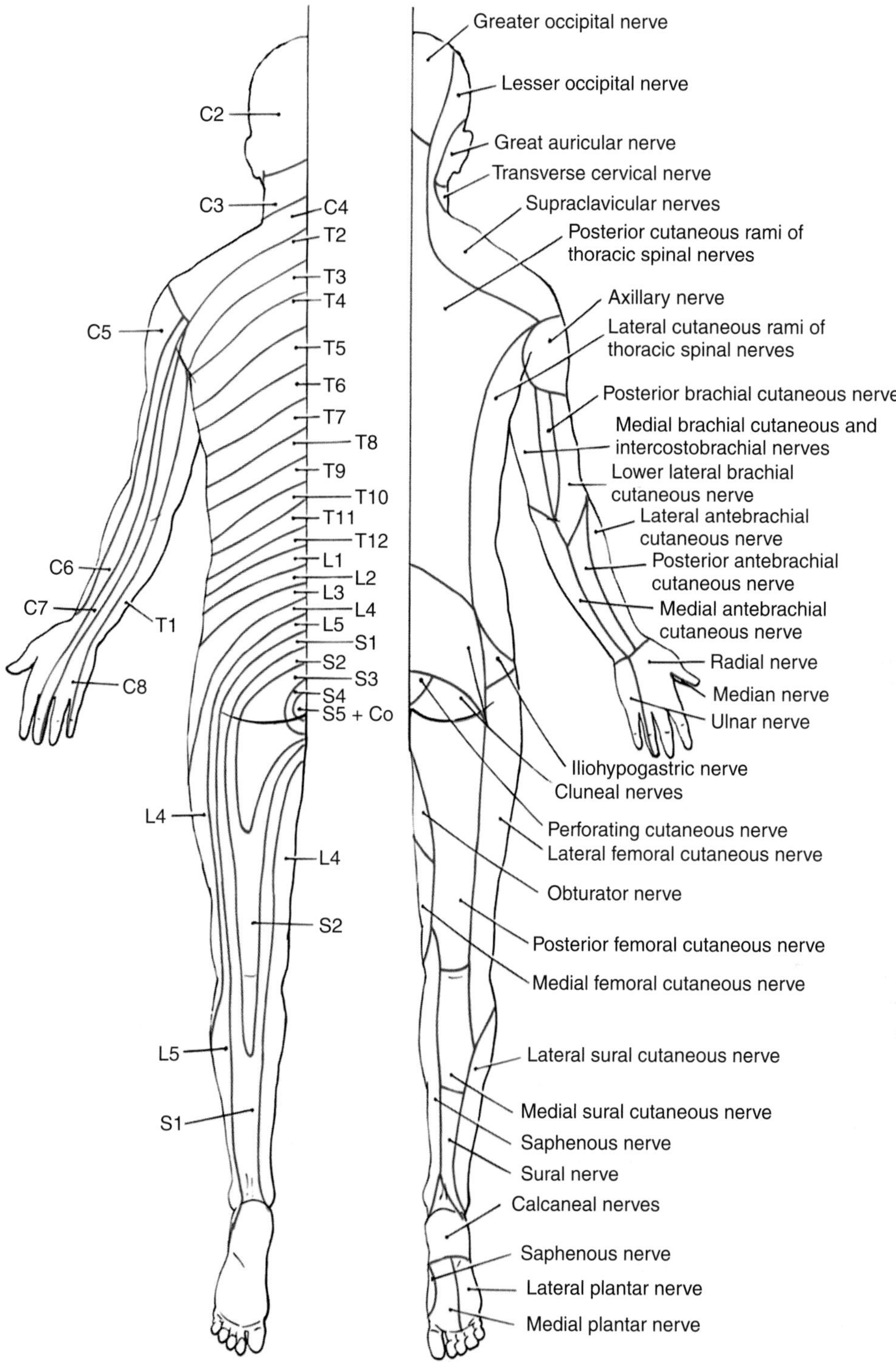

FIGURE 13–9 Pattern of innervations of the body by dorsal roots and peripheral nerves.

Case Study

Febrile Seizures

Isaac Hernandez is a 15-month-old boy who was brought to the emergency department with a seizure associated with fever. He has been in good health until today when he developed a fever of 104.8°F taken rectally. His mother gave him 1 teaspoon of acetaminophen 100 mg/5 mL. About 15 minutes after she gave the acetaminophen, she noticed shaking of his arms and legs, his eyes had a blank stare, and he would not respond when she called his name. His mother called 911 and an ambulance arrived in 5 minutes. When the ambulance arrived, the seizure movements had stopped, but Isaac was not fully awake. He was transported to the emergency department by ambulance and on arrival there was awake and somewhat irritable. His temperature on arrival was 100.2°F rectally, his heart rate was 100, respiratory rate was 26, blood pressure was 76/50 mm Hg, and oxygen saturation was 100%. He weighs 22 pounds, and his height is 31 inches. His physical examination was normal. He calmed considerably and was easily soothed by his parents. Isaac became playful and interactive with his family and the nursing staff in the emergency department.

1. What would you look for on examination of this baby?
2. What tests might be performed?
3. What information would you give his parents regarding his condition?

REFERENCES

American Academy of Pediatrics. (2017). *Acute flaccid myelitis in children.* Retrieved from https://www.aap.org/en-us/advocacy-and-policy/aap-health-initiatives/Children-and-Disasters/Pages/Acute-Flaccid-Myelitis-in-Children.aspx

American Stroke Association (ASA). (2017). *Stroke in children.* Retrieved from http://www.strokeassociation.org/STROKEORG/AboutStroke/StrokeInChildren/Stroke-In-Children_UCM_308543_SubHomePage.jsp

Association for Children's Mental Health. (2017). *Common mental health diagnosis in children and youth.* Retrieved from http://www.acmh-mi.org/get-information/childrens-mental-health-101/common-diagnosis/

Bird, S.J. (2016). Treatment of myasthenia gravis. *UptoDate.* Retrieved from https://www.uptodate.com/contents/treatment-of-myasthenia-gravis

Bodamer, O. A., & Miller, G. (2016). Neuromuscular junction disorders in newborns and infants. *UptoDate.* Retrieved from http://www.uptodate.com/contents/neuromuscular-junction-disorders-in-newborns-and-infants

Caserta, M.T. (2015). *Neonatal bacterial meningitis.* Retrieved from https://www.merckmanuals.com/professional/pediatrics/infections-in-neonates/neonatal-bacterial-meningitis

Centers for Disease Control and Prevention (CDC). (2017a). *Acute flaccid myelitis.* Retrieved from https://www.cdc.gov/acute-flaccid-myelitis/

Centers for Disease Control and Prevention (CDC). (2017b). *Child development—developmental screening.* Retrieved from http://www.cdc.gov/ncbddd/child/devtool.htm

Centers for Disease Control and Prevention (CDC). (2017c). *Congenital Zika syndrome and other birth defects.* Retrieved from https://www.cdc.gov/zika/hc-providers/infants-children/zika-syndrome-birth-defects.html

Centers for Disease Control and Prevention (CDC). (2017d). *Facts about anencephaly.* Retrieved from https://www.cdc.gov/ncbddd/birthdefects/anencephaly.html

Centers for Disease Control and Prevention (CDC). (2017e). *Meningitis.* Retrieved from https://www.cdc.gov/meningitis/

Centers for Disease Control and Prevention (CDC). (2017f). *Zika virus.* Retrieved from https://www.cdc.gov/zika/index.html

Chiu, S. (2016). Pediatric sleep disorders. *Medscape.* Retrieved from http://emedicine.medscape.com/article/916611-overview

Close, K. R., & Smirniotopoulos, J.G. (2015). Schizencephaly imaging. *Medscape.* Retrieved from http://emedicine.medscape.com/article/413051-overview

Dillon, P.M. (2016). *Nursing health assessment: the foundation of clinical practice* (3rd ed.). Philadelphia: F.A. Davis.

EBMedicine (2014). *Syncope: An ED approach to risk stratification.* Retrieved from http://www.ebmedicine.net/topics.php?paction=showTopic&topic_id=403&utm_source=TrendMD&utm_medium=cpc&utm_campaign=Ebmed_TrendMD_0

Ellenbrogen, R. G., & Roberts, T. S. (2015). Neural tube defects in the neonatal period. *Medscape.* Retrieved from http://emedicine.medscape.com/article/1825866-overview

Epilepsy Foundation. (2013). *Landau-Kleffner syndrome.* Retrieved from http://www.epilepsy.com/learn/types-epilepsy-syndromes/landau-kleffner-syndrome

Epilepsy Foundation. (2014). *Dravet syndrome.* Retrieved from http://www.epilepsy.com/learn/types-epilepsy-syndromes/dravet-syndrome

Epilepsy Foundation. (2015a). *Panayiotopoulos syndrome.* Retrieved from http://www.epilepsy.com/learn/types-epilepsy-syndromes/panayiotopoulos-syndrome

Epilepsy Foundation. (2015b). *Seizure action plan.* Retrieved from https://www.epilepsy.com/sites/core/files/atoms/files/seizure-action-plan-pdf_0.pdf

EpoMedicine (2016). *Gower's sign.* Retrieved from http://epomedicine.com/clinical-medicine/gowers-sign/

First Signs. (2014). *Recommended screening tools.* Retrieved from http://www.firstsigns.org/screening/tools/rec.htm

Hawley, J. S. (2015). Pediatric Tourette syndrome. *Medscape.* Retrieved from http://emedicine.medscape.com/article/289457-overview

Howard, J. F. (2015). *Clinical overview of myasthenia gravis.* Retrieved from http://www.myasthenia.org/HealthProfessionals/ClinicalOverviewofMG.aspx

Hsieh, D. T. (2016). Neurofibromatosis type 1. *Medscape.* Retrieved from http://emedicine.medscape.com/article/1177266-overview

Jallo, G. I., & Kao, A. (2015). Neural tube defects. *Medscape.* Retrieved from http://emedicine.medscape.com/article/1177162-overview

Ko, D. Y. (2014). Temporal lobe epilepsy. *Medscape.* Retrieved from http://emedicine.medscape.com/article/1184509-overview

Migraine Research Foundation. (2017). *Migraine in kids and teens.* Retrieved from http://migraineresearchfoundation.org/about-migraine/migraine-in-kids-and-teens/

Moeschler, J. B., Shevell, M., & Committee on Genetics. (2014). Comprehensive evaluation of the child with intellectual disability or global developmental delays. *Pediatrics,* 134, e903-18. doi: 10.1542/peds.2014-1839. Retrieved from http://pediatrics.aappublications.org/content/early/2014/08/19/peds.2014-1839

Muller, M. L. (2016). Pediatric bacterial meningitis. *Medscape.* Retrieved from http://emedicine.medscape.com/article/961497-overview

Muscular Dystrophy Association. (2017). *Spinal muscle atrophy.* Retrieved from https://www.mda.org/disease/spinal-muscular-atrophy

Myasthenia Foundation of America. (2014). *Myasthenia gravis: A nursing perspective and clinical guidelines.* Retrieved from http://www.myasthenia.org/LinkClick.aspx?fileticket=pQXk50m1RY0%3D&tabid=101

National Institutes of Health (NIH). (2017a). *Dandy-Walker malformation.* Retrieved from https://ghr.nlm.nih.gov/condition/dandy-walker-malformation

National Institutes of Health (NIH). (2017b). *Tethered cord syndrome.* Retrieved from https://rarediseases.info.nih.gov/diseases/4018/tethered-cord-syndrome

National Institutes of Health (NIH). (2017c). *Tuberous sclerosis complex.* Retrieved from https://ghr.nlm.nih.gov/condition/tuberous-sclerosis-complex

National Institute of Neurologic Disorders and Stroke (NINDS). (2017a). *Chiari malformation fact sheet.* Retrieved from https://www.ninds.nih.gov/Disorders/Patient-Caregiver-Education/Fact-Sheets/Chiari-Malformation-Fact-Sheet

National Institute of Neurological Disorders and Stroke (NINDS). (2017b). *Meningitis and encephalitis.* Retrieved from http://www.brainfacts.org/diseases-disorders/diseases-a-to-z-from-ninds/meningitis-and-encephalitis/

National Institute of Neurological Disorders and Stroke (NINDS). (2017c). *NINDS neurofibromatosis.* Retrieved from https://www.ninds.nih.gov/disorders/all-disorders/neurofibromatosis-information-page

National Institute of Neurological Disorders and Stroke (NINDS). (2017d). *Tethered cord syndrome.* Retrieved from https://www.ninds.nih.gov/Disorders/All-Disorders/Tethered-Spinal-Cord-Syndrome-Information-Page

National Organization for Rare Diseases (NORD). (2016). *Ataxia telangiectasia.* Retrieved from https://rarediseases.org/rare-diseases/ataxia-telangiectasia/

National Organization for Rare Diseases (NORD). (2017). *Agenesis of corpus callosum.* Retrieved from https://rarediseases.org/rare-diseases/agenesis-of-corpus-callosum/

National Stroke Association (NSA). (2017). *Pediatric stroke.* Retrieved from http://www.stroke.org/understand-stroke/impact-stroke/pediatric-stroke

Nelson, S.L. (2016). Hydrocephalus. *Medscape.* Retrieved from http://emedicine.medscape.com/article/1135286-overview

Ochoa, J. G., & Riche, W. (2016). Antiepileptic drugs. *Medscape.* Retrieved from http://emedicine.medscape.com/article/1187334-overview

Patel, M. (2017). Update on acute flaccid myelitis. *Medscape.* Retrieved from http://www.medscape.com/viewarticle/877314

Robertson, W. C. (2016). Migraine in children. *Medscape.* Retrieved from http://emedicine.medscape.com/article/1179268-overview

Selph, J. (2016). Juvenile myoclonic epilepsy. *Medscape.* Retrieved from http://emedicine.medscape.com/article/1185061-overview

Spratt, E.G. (2016). Sleep terrors. *Medscape.* Retrieved from http://emedicine.medscape.com/article/914360-overview

The Sturge-Weber Foundation. (2017). *Understanding Sturge-Weber.* Retrieved from http://sturge-weber.org/new-to-swf/understanding-sturge-weber.html

Vallerand, A. H., Sanoski, C. A., & Deglan, J. H. (2017). *Davis's drug guide for nurses* (15th ed.). Philadelphia: F.A. Davis.

Verklan, M. T., & Walden, M. (Eds). (2015). *Core curriculum for neonatal intensive care nursing* (5th ed.). St Louis, MO: Elsevier Saunders.

Ward, S. L. (2014). *Pediatric nursing care: Best evidence-based practices.* Philadelphia: F.A. Davis.

World Health Organization. (2016). *Guillain–Barré syndrome.* Retrieved from http://www.who.int/mediacentre/factsheets/guillain-barre-syndrome/en/

Wright, Z., Larrew, T. W., & Eskandari, R. (2016). Pediatric hydrocephalus: Current state of diagnosis and treatment. *Pediatrics in Review, 37*(11), 478–490. doi: 10.1542/pir.2015-0134. Retrieved from http://pedsinreview.aappublications.org/content/37/11/478

14 Mental Health Disorders

Andrea Warner Stidham, PhD, RN

LEARNING OUTCOMES

Upon completion of this chapter, the student will be able to:

1. Discuss three current trends in pediatric psychiatry.
2. Describe components of mental health assessment in children and adolescents.
3. Describe learning disabilities and recommended treatments.
4. Discuss reactive attachment disorder and its treatments.
5. Explain two mood disorders diagnosed in children and their recommended treatments.
6. Explain five anxiety disorders diagnosed in children and their recommended treatments.
7. Identify three disruptive disorders diagnosed in children and their recommended treatments.
8. Discuss impulse-control disorder and its recommended treatments.
9. Discuss schizophrenia in children.
10. Describe autism spectrum disorders.
11. Identify three eating disorders diagnosed in children and their recommended treatments.
12. Describe three current treatment modalities in pediatric substance abuse treatment.
13. Describe dual diagnosis in children.
14. Discuss child abuse assessment, diagnosis, and recommended treatments.

INTRODUCTION

Childhood and adolescence are periods of great transition and reorganization. Wide variation exists in normal developmental behavior. However, children can and do develop mental health disorders, and some of these disorders last a lifetime. As with any chronic illness, caregivers of children with mental illness need support and may grieve the loss of their "perfect" child and the ideal future that may have been planned. An estimated 20% of U.S. children have a mental disorder resulting in mild functional impairment (Avenevoli, Swendsen, He, Burstein, & Merikangas, 2015).

- Between 5% and 9% of the child population has a mental disorder resulting in extreme functional impairment (Olfson, Blanco, Wang, Laje, & Correll, 2014).

SAFE AND EFFECTIVE NURSING CARE: Cultural Competence

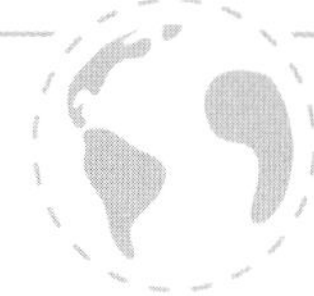

Incidence of Mental Illness

Incidence of mental illness is higher in subcultures of the population, such lesbian, gay, bisexual, and transgender youth (CDC, 2017).

- Of pediatric hospital admissions, 7% are for mental health reasons, with depression the primary diagnosis (Avenevoli et al., 2015).
- Approximately 80% of adolescents will experience at least one clinically significant depressive episode (Olfson et al., 2014).

- In the United States, the ratio of suicide attempt to suicide death in youths is approximately 25:1 (Centers for Disease Control and Prevention [CDC], 2015).
- Anna Freud, Sigmund Freud's youngest child, is considered the founder of pediatric psychiatry.

WHAT IS MENTAL ILLNESS?

Mental illness is a term that collectively refers to all mental disorders, health conditions characterized by alterations in thinking, mood, or behavior that are associated with distress and/or impaired functioning (American Psychological Association [APA], 2013). Individuals with mental illness may experience:

- A distorted view of self
- An inability to maintain personal relationships
- An inability to respond to the environment in ways that are in accord with oneself or society's expectations
- Thoughts or behavior patterns that impair functioning and cause the individual distress
- Impaired judgment
- Lack of insight regarding own abilities and consequences of actions

SAFE AND EFFECTIVE NURSING CARE: Clinical Pearl

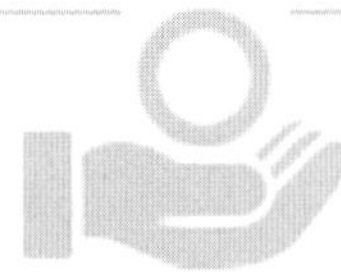

Mental Illness and Developmental Age

Developmental age must be considered when assessing behavior and thought patterns. Nurses working with youth should be knowledgeable about typical stages of growth and development. Understanding age-appropriate cognitive and behavioral abilities enables the clinician to distinguish between age-typical and abnormal functioning among youth.

Results of Mental Illness

- Cognitive distortions leading to lowered self-esteem
- Inability to form and/or maintain meaningful personal relationships
- Physical disability, morbidity, and/or death

Risk Factors for Mental Illness

Mental health disorders can occur across all social classes and families; however, there are risk factors for development of mental disorders in childhood. These include:

- Physical problems
- Intellectual disabilities
- Low birth weight
- Family history of mental illness or addictive disorders
- Multigenerational poverty
- Caregiver separation, abuse, or neglect

ETIOLOGY OF MENTAL ILLNESS IN CHILDREN

Research suggests that about half of all lifetime cases of mental illness manifest by age 14 years (Kessler, Chiu, Demler, Merikangas, & Walters, 2005). Genetic, psychological, environmental, and neurological factors all influence development of mental illness in children.

Genetic Influences

- Multiple genes, interacting with environmental factors, seem to confer risk for mental illness. Up to this point, no single gene has been pinpointed as causing mental illness.
- Major psychiatric disorders, such as depression, anxiety disorders, schizophrenia, and bipolar disorder, are found among family generations. Research indicates that autism, learning and language disorders, attention deficit-hyperactivity disorder (ADHD), and enuresis (bedwetting) seem to be genetically transmitted.
- Having a parent or sibling with a mental illness indicates increased risk for development of mental illnesses among other closely related family members.

Psychological Influences

- Stressful life events (e.g., caregiver illness, relocating, death of family member)
- Personality/temperament (e.g., how the child's temperament elicits reactions from parents or caregivers, accurate processing of social clues, sense of self-efficacy, ability to problem-solve)
- Gender (some psychiatric disorders affect males and females disproportionally, e.g., depression for girls and ADHD for boys)
- Age (children respond differently to events according to developmental maturity)

Social/Environmental Influences

- Parents (warm or supportive versus disregarding or neglectful)
- School adjustment (positive experiences versus negative experiences)
- Socioeconomic status (poverty and/or homelessness serve as barriers to normal developmental maturity and are risk factors for development of psychiatric disorders)
- Culture (view of diagnosis and treatment of mental illness can serve as barrier or protective factor in the development of mental illness)
- Religion (view of diagnosis and treatment of mental illness can serve as barrier or protective factor in the development of mental illness)
- Interpersonal relationships (positive, supportive relationships can serve as a protective factor in the development of mental illness)

Neurochemical Influences

- Norepinephrine deficiencies can cause:
  - Impaired attention
  - Problems concentrating
  - Problems with memory
  - Slow information processing
  - Depressed mood
  - Psychomotor developmental delay
  - Fatigue
- Serotonin deficiencies can cause:
  - Anxiety
  - Panic
  - Phobia
  - Obsessions
  - Compulsions
  - Food cravings
  - Bulimia
- Dopamine deficiencies can cause:
  - Decreased ability to experience pleasure
  - Increased irritability and aggression
  - Decreased cognitive functioning
  - Decreased motivation

SAFE AND EFFECTIVE NURSING CARE: Clinical Pearl

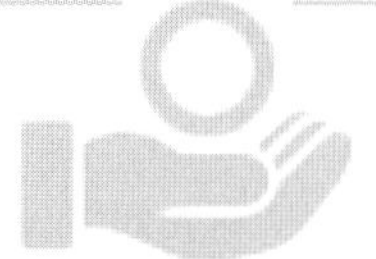

Emotional Intelligence

Emotional intelligence (EQ) stems from the prefrontal cortex and allows an individual to identify, analyze, understand, and regulate behavior. Children who have been abused or neglected, or who have a psychological disorder often lack EQ skills.

TRENDS IN PEDIATRIC MENTAL HEALTH

Child and adolescent mental health disorders are commonly influenced by familial, environmental, and economic factors (Collishaw, 2015). Although mental disorders and symptoms are relatively stable across time, factors that influence the development and treatment of such disorders are dependent on access to care, family structure and support, and appropriate diagnosis.

- One in five adolescents has a diagnosable disorder, yet many are undiagnosed and/or undertreated (Murphy, Barry, & Vaughn, 2013).
- Some estimates put the prevalence rate of ADHD as high as 10% among 12- to 17- year-olds (Murphy et al., 2013).
- Primary care providers may lack time and specific expertise to identify and manage mental illnesses (Murphy et al., 2013).
- Young people with mental illnesses, in general, are more likely than others to participate in risky activities that negatively affect their health (Murphy et al., 2013).
- A severe potential consequence of child/adolescent mental illness is suicide (Murphy et al., 2013).
- More clinical drug trials on pediatric participants are leading to more availability of appropriate psychotherapeutic treatments (Murphy et al., 2013).
- Parents, health-care providers, and friends can reduce stigma by encouraging youth experiencing emotional distress to seek help (Murphy et al., 2013).

CRITICAL COMPONENT

Adolescent Brain Development

New research shows that the adolescent brain is still in development until the early 20s, and it matures from back to front. In addition, at around age 11 or 12 years many brain connections are lost and the brain rewires itself to develop more adult patterns of thinking (Hayden & Mash, 2014).

ASSESSMENT

Mental health assessment must occur within family, social, and cultural contexts with the child's development taken into consideration. Assessment includes evaluation of the child's biological, social, and psychological factors. Mental health assessment generally takes place in schools and primary care offices. Families are essential partners in the provision of child mental health services.

CRITICAL COMPONENT

Puberty and Mental Health Illness

When taking a mental health history, the parents will often report that the child's symptoms started or got worse around the time of puberty.

Mental Status Examination

- The health-care provider will assess the child specifically for skills related to language, as well as cognitive, emotional, and social functioning. A mental status examination is conducted and includes the following:
  - Appearance, motor activity, self-concept, and behavior
  - Social interaction, general intelligence, memory, and orientation
  - Attention span and comprehension, speech, and language
  - Mood/feelings and insight and judgment
  - Thought processes and content
  - Auditory hallucinations (hearing voices that no one else hears)
  - Visual hallucinations (seeing things that no one else sees)
  - Delusional thoughts (such as thinking oneself to be a king)
  - Self-harm by banging head, cutting self, or by other means

- Substance use/abuse
- Sudden change in behavior
- Sudden change in school performance
- The health-care provider will ask several questions of both the child and caregiver to determine:
  - What caused the patient/family to seek help at this time
  - Psychiatric history (formal mental health services, family history of mental illness)
  - Current and past health status (symptoms child is experiencing and length of time they have been present)
  - Medications
  - Neurological history (handedness, dizziness, seizures, hyperactivity)
  - Responses to mental health problems (what helps or aggravates symptoms)
  - Developmental history (pregnancy, delivery, Apgar scores, developmental milestones)
  - Attachment, temperament, behavioral problems
  - Self-concept (identity, self-esteem)
  - Risk assessment (suicidal, homicidal ideation, substance use/abuse)
  - Risk of suicide, including history of suicidal thoughts/attempts, thoughts of and/or presence of a plan, lethality of the plan, and access to the means described in the plan
  - Risk of assaulting others and/or history of assaulting others
  - History of aggression toward animals
  - History of arson
  - History of running away
  - Family relationships (parents, deaths/losses, conflicts, siblings)
  - Relationships with peers and others in social settings (drug and alcohol use/abuse, dating, friends, participation in school-related activities)
  - School performance (adjustment, attendance, relationships with teachers)
  - Temper tantrums

SAFE AND EFFECTIVE NURSING CARE: Promoting Safety

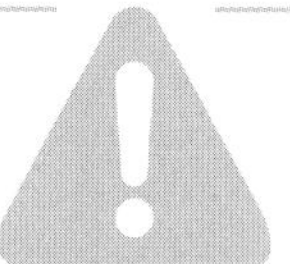

Assessing Risk for Suicide

When assessing suicidality, ask about a plan and whether the patient has means to carry out the plan. If the child does have access to a stash of pills or a weapon, it is the nurse's responsibility to work with the family and appropriate authorities to eliminate access.

- The three mental health conditions most common in children are:
  - Learning disabilities
  - ADHD
  - Behavioral conditions (for additional information, please see www.cdc.gov/nchs/hdi.htm)
- Common childhood problems include:
  - Death and grief
  - Parental separation and divorce
  - Sibling relationships
  - Physical illness
  - Adolescent risk-taking behaviors
  - Separation anxiety
  - Temper tantrums
  - School phobia
  - Bullying
  - Growth and development issues
  - Being abused or witnessing abuse, emotional, physical, or psychological

CRITICAL COMPONENT

The Effect of Certain Behaviors on Quality of Life

Behaviors that interfere with quality of life at home and school need to be evaluated by a professional. Examples of these behaviors include ongoing defiance, disruptive and frequent temper tantrums, excessive argumentativeness, and physical aggression toward self or others (APA, 2013).

- Nursing interventions to help a child through a common childhood problem include the following:
  - Provide support.
  - Encourage expression of feelings.
  - Provide information.
  - Answer questions honestly.
  - Assess for anger-related problems and suicidality.
  - Refer for individual and family therapy as needed.
- Before the child is diagnosed with a mental health disorder, a physical assessment, including laboratory tests, should be completed to rule out the following conditions that could produce symptoms similar to those of mental health problems:
  - Organic disorders
  - Sensory disorders
  - Medication-induced symptoms (e.g., weight loss, drug-induced psychosis)
  - Thyroid abnormalities
  - Intellectual disabilities
  - Brain tumors
  - Lead poisoning

Mental Illness Diagnosis

Mental health assessment occurs on many levels and in different settings to assess individual functioning. The *Diagnostic and Statistical Manual of Mental Disorders* (DSM) is a guide of all diagnosable mental illnesses (APA, 2013). This manual is updated periodically. The current version is DSM-5 (fifth edition). The DSM-5 offers guidelines for symptom assessment of various areas of individual functioning, taking into account age, gender, and cultural influences (APA, 2013). DSM-5 uses a single-axis system that assesses mental, medical, and other conditions with which individuals may present with in a clinical setting.

Limitations of the *DSM* with Children

- Of children currently diagnosed with a mental health disorder, 70% to 80% will not meet the criteria for the disorder a year from now because of childhood development, new coping behaviors, and/or factors related to assessment and diagnosis of childhood mental illness by clinicians (Ringoot et al., 2017).
- High comorbidity rates in children reflect a "general psychopathology" consistent with immature development and the consequent lack of ability to differentiate disorders into discrete categories (Stein et al., 2014).

SETTINGS OF CARE IN PEDIATRIC MENTAL HEALTH

Child and adolescent mental health care is available in a variety of settings. Depending on the diagnosis, severity of symptoms, and needs of youth and families, children or adolescents who are diagnosed with mental illness may receive care through one or more of the following:

- School counselor
- Home therapist
- Outpatient psychiatrist/psychologist
- Group home
- Residential treatment
- Partial hospitalization program
- Intensive outpatient program
- Inpatient psychiatric unit

SAFE AND EFFECTIVE NURSING CARE: Clinical Pearl

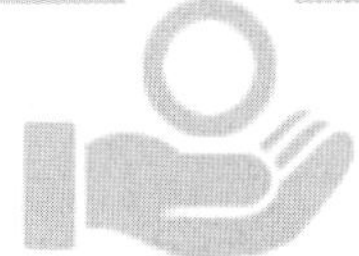

Residential Treatment

Residential treatment is expensive and often not covered under private insurance. Sometimes caregivers have to give up custody rights over the child for the county or state to fund residential treatment.

INPATIENT PSYCHIATRIC THERAPY

Inpatient psychiatric therapy is considered when the patient is at immediate risk of harming self or others. Admissions are either voluntary (guardian agrees to the admission) or involuntary (child is "pink-slipped" by a physician or police). Laws surrounding inpatient psychiatric treatment vary by state.

Therapeutic Milieu

- The environment of care is called the milieu in mental health care.
- The milieu itself is a treatment modality (Peplau, 1989) that provides structure and safety.
- All aspects of the milieu should contribute to care and recovery.
- Structured components of the milieu include group therapy, community meetings, and psychoeducation classes.
- Unstructured components of the milieu include interactions between patients, staff, and visitors.

Health-Care Providers in the Therapeutic Milieu

Inpatient hospitalization requires the coordination of many health-care disciplines to provide holistic care to children and adolescents. Health professionals in this setting work as a team to provide care to hospitalized youth in addition to support and information to parents and families of hospitalized children.

- Professionals who work in the therapeutic milieu include:
  - Psychiatric nurse
  - Psychiatric advanced practice nurse (adult, family, pediatric clinical nurse specialist or nurse practitioner)
  - Psychiatric social worker
  - Psychologist
  - Psychiatrist
  - Medical doctor
  - Occupational therapist
  - Certified addiction counselor
  - Milieu therapist
  - Mental health worker/technician
  - Activity therapist

Rules of the Milieu

- Refer to patients by first name only.
- Patients should not have shoelaces, belts, piercings, or anything else that could be used to hurt themselves or others.
- Pin numbers or a code word may be used to ensure patient confidentiality. Do not give information to someone who does not have the pin number/code word.
- No outside food is allowed in the milieu.
- Check all belongings/items that come in to ensure patient and staff safety.
- Check every patient at least every 15 minutes to ensure safety.
- Priority is personal safety. Do not wear necklaces/scarves that can be used as methods of choking.
- Be mindful of all items taken onto the milieu. Pencils, staples, and silverware can be used by patients to hurt self or others.
- Nurses should not give clients personal information like their phone number or e-mail address.

Admission Process

- Direct patient to change into a hospital gown.
- Check all belongings.
- Retain contraband items.
- Skin check: Document all rashes, cuts, and scars that a patient has on admission.
- Conduct psychological and risk assessment focusing on the child with input from parents and/or families.

- Obtain history and perform physical examination.
- Conduct laboratory tests (complete blood count with differential, comprehensive metabolic panel, thyroid-stimulating hormone, urine or blood toxicity, urinalysis, and pregnancy test for females).

Types of Restrictions With Interventions for Inpatient Psychiatric Patients

Children and adolescents who are hospitalized for mental illness require a structured environment that focuses on safety and health promotion. Specific interventions are needed to ensure that youth remain safe while hospitalized.

Suicide Precautions

- Frequently reassess for suicidal thoughts.
- Have child wear a cloth or paper gown.
- Monitor patient one on one.
- Assign room near nurse's station.
- Provide finger foods only.

Assault Precautions

- Frequently assess for signs of escalation.
- Do not assign a roommate.
- Do not allow patient off the unit.

Elopement Precautions

- Monitor exits and doors.
- Monitor patient's whereabouts frequently.
- Have child wear hospital gown and slippers.

Boundary Precautions

- Watch child for inappropriate verbal or physical interactions with others.
- Do not assign a roommate.

Restrict to Unit

- Child is not allowed to leave the unit because of psychological or medical condition.

Typical Day

Inpatient hospitalization provides a structured environment for youth being evaluated or treated for mental illness. Daily routines are implemented to reduce anxiety and promote well-being for hospitalized youth. A typical daily routine includes:

- Shower/clean room/breakfast
- Goal group
- Psychoeducational groups
- Art group
- Physical activity
- Visiting/phone calls
- Reflections

Discharge Process

- Distribute satisfaction surveys.
- Ensure that patient can contract for safety.
- Arrange follow-up appointments
- Make sure that patient/family has needed prescriptions.

Risks of Inpatient Psychiatric Admission

- Learning new (negative) behaviors from peers
- Hearing about subjects the child has not been exposed to previously, such as drugs and sex
- Physical/psychological violence from peers

Use of Restraints With Children

Restraints are used as an intervention when the child is hurting himself or herself or others and should always be a last resort. Policies surrounding the use of restraints vary by institution and state. Pediatric deaths have been associated with the use of restraints.

Application of Restraints

- When applying restraints:
  - Obtain a physician's order.
  - Check for contraindications to restraint, such as a physical health issue or history of prior abuse.
  - Do not restrain facedown.
  - Do not restrain with arms over head.
  - Make sure that two fingers can be placed in between the restraint and the limb. Recheck circulation of the extremities every 15 minutes.
  - Take vital signs every 15 minutes. Pay careful attention to respiratory status.
  - Offer fluids/toilet every 15 minutes.
  - Provide range of motion every 15 minutes.
  - Assign a staff member to provide one-to-one observation of the patient.
  - Discontinue as soon as the child is in control or has fallen asleep.
  - Debrief with the child and staff after the episode.

Use of Seclusion With Children

Seclusion should be used as a last resort when the child is at risk to harm or is actually harming others (Caldwell et al., 2014). If the child is harming himself or herself, do not seclude the patient. If the child starts to punch or kick the wall or head-bang, seclusion must be discontinued immediately.

- When implementing seclusion:
  - Obtain a physician's order.
  - Check for contraindications to restraint, such as a physical health issue or history of prior abuse.
  - Take vital signs every 15 minutes.
  - Offer fluids/toilet every 15 minutes.
  - Provide range of motion every 15 minutes.

- Assign a staff member to provide one-to-one observation of the patient.
- Discontinue as soon as the child is in control or has fallen asleep.
- Debrief with the child and staff after the episode.

SAFE AND EFFECTIVE NURSING CARE: Promoting Safety

Avoiding the Use of Seclusion and Restraints

Nurses can avoid the use of seclusion and restraints by using preventive measures, including awareness of the child's trauma history, forming and using plans to keep patients safe, using comfort rooms, maintaining communication with caregivers and families, and using de-escalation approaches (Caldwell et al., 2014).

PEDIATRIC THERAPEUTIC APPROACHES

Psychosocial therapies can be very effective alone as well as in conjunction with medication. Psychosocial therapy, sometimes called talk therapy, helps those with mental illness identify and change problematic thoughts and behaviors, and learn effective coping skills to manage mental illness (Evans, Owen, & Bunford, 2014). Therapy is generally an effective component of treatment for a variety of mental illnesses, and assists individuals and families to appropriately manage illness and lead healthy lives (Evans et al., 2014).

Key Influences

- Key factors that influence therapeutic approaches with children include the following:
  - Children need to be prepared for the future.
  - Children need to develop self-awareness.
  - Children use more nonverbal communication than verbal communication.

Goals of Therapy

- Improve communication skills.
- Build self-esteem.
- Stimulate development.
- Build an emotional repertoire.
- Improve emotional vocabulary.
- Encourage assimilation of traumatic events.
- Enable detachment from an emotional experience.

Approaches to Therapy With Children

Therapy is most effective when children are having fun. Allow the child to be in control of the therapy session provided he or she is following instructions and appropriately participating in the milieu.

Types of Therapy Used With Children

- Play therapy uses play as a tool to work within the developmental level of the child while not focusing on language abilities.
- Art therapy uses art to help identify and express thoughts and emotions.
- Music therapy uses music to help identify and express thoughts and emotions.
- Pet therapy uses animals to help identify and express thoughts and emotions.
- Cognitive behavioral therapy (CBT) links the relationships of distorted thoughts with moods and behaviors.
- Dialectical behavior therapy (DBT) is an intensive, highly structured therapy that addresses maladaptive learned behaviors as responses to problems. DBT focuses on extreme emotional instability, particularly regarding suicidal ideation and self-harm (Perepletchikova et al., 2011).

Tools Used in Therapy With Children

- Board games
- Group games
- Recreational equipment/approaches
- Arts and crafts
- Animals
- Worksheets
- Behavior charts
- Timers to teach patience/impulse control
- Videos
- Video games
- Relaxing music/sounds
- Weighted vests/body socks
- Visual supports

SCHOOL FOR CHILDREN WITH MENTAL ILLNESS

Teachers and other school staff need to be trained to recognize children with mental health disorders and help address these issues. Caregivers often feel frustrated by a lack of services and tired from being the child's advocate within the school system. Nurses should support caregivers and help them to be their children's best advocates.

Children with mental health disorders have certain rights under the Americans with Disabilities Act, such as nondiscrimination for selection into a school or program. Only children who are a direct threat to others may be excluded from school or certain programs within the school. Section 504 plans provide guidelines for the prevention of discrimination, including the use of accommodations, against children with disabilities (U.S. Department of Education, 2016). A Section 504 plan may be implemented to identify the accommodations needed by the child to be able to fully participate in a program/activity in school.

The Individuals with Disabilities Education Act ensures that children with mental illness have access to early intervention and special education services as needed. Children with mental illness may need an individualized education plan (IEP) at school to be successful. An IEP describes goals for the child and identifies the services needed to attain the goals. Periodic meetings between parents, teachers, the school counselor/psychologist, special education teacher, and others at the school ensure that services are modified as needed so that educational goals can be reached.

LEARNING DISABILITIES AND BEHAVIORAL CHALLENGES

Learning Disabilities

Learning disabilities are neurologically based processing problems that can interfere with learning basic skills such as reading, writing, and/or math. They can also interfere with higher level skills such as organization, time planning, abstract reasoning, long- or short-term memory, and attention (APA, 2013).

Learning disabilities may be caused by a number of factors, including:

- Intrauterine conditions such as maternal cigarette, alcohol, or drug use
- Genetics
- Environmental factors
- Comorbid ADHD or autism

CRITICAL COMPONENT

Learning Disabilities

Learning disabilities are more common in boys. Nearly one-third of individuals with learning disabilities also have ADHD (APA, 2013).

Nursing Interventions

- Be patient.
- Assess learning needs.
- Assess how child learns best.
- Design learning interventions accordingly.

Caregiver Education

Teaching for caregivers of a child with a suspected or diagnosed learning disability includes:

- Be patient with the child.
- Be an advocate for the child.
- Request testing through the school.
- Seek help as soon as a disability is suspected.
- Pursue an IEP as needed.

Behavioral Problems

Children with or without a mental illness may exhibit undesirable behaviors. These may include, but are not limited to:

- Failure to initiate behaviors requested by an adult in a reasonable time frame
- Failure to complete the directive
- Failure to follow previously learned rules of conduct in a situation
- Yelling
- Complaining
- Defiance
- Tantrums
- Throwing objects
- Insults
- Swearing
- Stealing
- Lying
- Arguing
- Annoying/teasing
- Engaging in physical fights
- Failing to complete schoolwork
- Refusing to go to school
- Ignoring self-care
- Talking back
- Disrupting others

Causes of Behavioral Problems

- Inconsistent discipline
- Inconsistent monitoring of the child's behavior
- Harsh or lax discipline methods
- Dysfunctional/inconsistent child–family member interactions
- Mental health diagnosis

Outcomes of Behavioral Problems

- Family conflict
- School problems
- Issues with peers
- Frustrated caregivers
- Frustrated child
- Caregivers feel hopeless, helpless
- Fewer family activities
- Fewer interactions between the caregivers and child
- Caregiver and child feel isolated

Help for Caregivers

Caregivers should seek help when:

- Behavior is developmentally inappropriate.
- Behavior is causing impairment at home, school, or with peer relationships.
- Behavior is causing a significant amount of emotional distress to self/parents.

Types of Help Available

- School counselor (counseling services available in the school setting)
- Individual/family counseling (counseling services available outside of school to address individual and/or family concerns)
- Inpatient treatment (focuses on acute crisis stabilization)
- Parent coaching (assisting parents to address child problems)

Nursing Interventions

Nursing interventions for the child who is behaviorally challenged include:

- Monitor behavior consistently.
- Praise the good.
- Be consistent (social predictability is key).
- Focus on giving positive attention.
- Defiance and aggressiveness produce the consistency the child craves, and therefore these behaviors increase.
- Use immediate and consistent punishments for noncompliance.
- Recognize and terminate escalating behaviors.
- Confront negative interactions.
- Provide incentives for compliance.
- Do not regress to name-calling/threats.
- Use joint problem-solving and negotiation techniques.
- Communicate in positive terms.
- Identify and reframe your expectations, especially if the child has a mental health diagnosis.

STRESS AND CHILDREN

Stress is a normal part of life. Children need to experience some stress to practice coping skills and gain confidence in handling future stressors.

Factors That Predispose Children to Stress

- Cognitive immaturity
- Lack of judgment/insight
- Home setting
- School setting
- Peers
- Events
- Family changes
- Emphasis on achievement
- Pace of life
- Media influences
- Lack of basic needs being met
- Anticipated events such as changing schools and starting menstruation

Manifestations of Stress

- Physical
  - Headaches
  - Abdominal pain
  - Cardiovascular disorders
  - GI upset
  - Enuresis (bedwetting/incontinence)
  - Encopresis (incontinence of stool)
  - Decreased immune functioning
- Behavioral
  - Acting inward, such as self-harming, isolating, abusing substances, or overeating
  - Acting outward, such as engaging in verbal/physical altercations with peers or adults
- Psychosocial
  - Anxiety
  - Depression
  - Irritability
  - Anger

Nursing Interventions

- Nursing strategies for stress management in children and adolescents include encouraging the following:
  - Exercise
  - Journaling/drawing
  - Deep breathing
  - Meditation
  - Hypnosis
  - Prayer
  - Talking with an adult or peer

SAFE AND EFFECTIVE NURSING CARE: Clinical Pearl

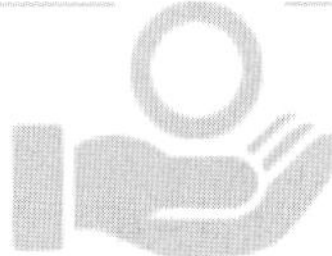

Capabilities Versus Expectations

When working with children with stress or anxiety, focus on the child's capabilities of dealing with stressful situations and not on the nurse's expectations of how he or she thinks the child should respond.

Caregiver Education

- Situations where the caregiver should seek additional help include:
  - Child is an immediate threat to self or others
  - Talk of suicide
  - Suicidal gestures
  - Symptoms interfere with relationships
  - Symptoms interfere with school/home/work

Crisis Intervention

A crisis is a time-limited, critical incident such as the death of a parent or the loss of a home due to fire. Crisis is personal; what is considered a crisis to one person may not be a crisis to another. The four main concepts of crisis intervention are:

- Safety: This includes safety of the patient and of the health-care professionals involved with the case.
- Catharsis: Patients in crisis have an overwhelming need to express feelings.
- Empathy-based listening: For example, "Help me to understand how you're feeling."
- Entropy: Do not add any more chaos to the situation. As the child escalates, the nurse should become even calmer by talking softer and controlling body language.

PERSONALITY DISORDERS

Personality influences everything that the person thinks, feels, and does—like a lens through which one views life. Personality is developed by age 2 years. Therefore, early childhood experiences influence whether the child will have a personality disorder (PD) as an adult. PDs are rarely diagnosed in childhood. However, pediatric nurses should be aware of them, because children may show features of a PD. The personality issues most often detected in childhood are MacDonald's triad and borderline PD.

Theories of Personality Disorders

- Psychodynamic/developmental—Someone with a PD is stuck in a developmental age of about 7 years old.
- Cognitive/behavioral—Behaviors are learned. Patients with a PD have learned maladaptive behaviors. These behaviors can be improved through self-awareness and behavior modification techniques.
- Biological/neurochemical—PDs are the result of atypical brain chemistry and can be treated with psychopharmacology, diet, and exercise (Lenzenweger & Clarkin, 2005).

MacDonald's Triad: The Precursor to Antisocial Personality Disorder

Young children who display bedwetting, cruelty to animals, and pyromania (MacDonald's triad) will likely have antisocial PD as an adult.

SAFE AND EFFECTIVE NURSING CARE: Clinical Pearl

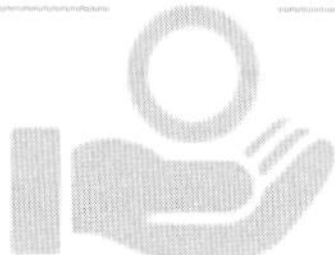

Risk Factors for MacDonald's Triad

When assessing enuresis, also ask about behavior toward animals and fire-setting.

Borderline Personality Disorder

- Adolescents can exhibit traits consistent with borderline PD. These can include:
  - Feeling as though bordering between sanity and psychosis
  - Staff splitting (attempting to manipulate staff to think that other staff members are not providing the best care)
  - Self-mutilating behaviors/suicidal gestures and attempts
  - Affective instability—shifts in moods
  - Identity disturbance
  - Role absorption—narrow definition of self
  - Painful incoherence—internal disharmony
  - Inconsistency in thoughts, feelings, and actions
  - Unstable interpersonal relationships
  - Fear of abandonment
  - Unstable, insecure attachments
  - Overidealized/intense relationships
  - Cognitive dysfunctions such as dissociation, disturbed thinking patterns, impaired problem solving, and impulsivity

Nursing Interventions

- Nursing management of a patient with borderline PD includes the following:
  - Monitor for suicidal ideation, gestures, and attempts.
  - Monitor for deliberate self-harm.
  - Establish a routine.
  - Be consistent.
  - Do not be manipulated.
  - Offer support.
  - Encourage individual and group therapy.
  - Administer antidepressants and other medications as ordered.

IMPAIRED EXECUTIVE FUNCTIONING

Executive functions are the cognitive processes that help manage an individual's resources to achieve a goal. It is an umbrella term for the neurologically based skills involving mental control and self-regulation. Impairments in executive functioning may exist with or without another clinical disorder. Many children with ADHD have issues with executive functioning (Diamond, 2013).

- Executive functioning is higher-order thinking that is necessary for:
  - Planning
  - Organizing
  - Sequencing
  - Using memory and information
  - Self-regulation of emotions and behavior
- The components of executive functioning include:
  - Working memory and recall
  - Activation, arousal, and effort
  - Controlling emotions
  - Internalizing language
  - Complex problem solving

Symptoms of Impaired Executive Functioning

A child with impaired executive functioning skills may exhibit:

- Forgetfulness
- Distorted sense of past events
- Altered sense of time
- Altered sense of self-awareness
- Altered sense of future

Impairments in executive functioning may exist with or without another clinical disorder. Many children with ADHD have issues with executive functioning.

Nursing Interventions

Nursing interventions for a child with impaired executive functioning include:

- Be concrete.
- Use visual aids.
- Reduce workload.
- Give extended time on tests.
- Increase support/supervision.

ATTACHMENT DISORDERS

The quality of the parent–child relationship is the cornerstone of future interpersonal relationships. Attachment is biologically driven and is manifested by the need to touch and be close to a parental figure (Blair-Gomez, 2013; Harlow, Harlow, & Suomi, 1971). Both mothers and fathers play a role in childhood attachment.

Disrupted attachments occur when the infant is unable to respond appropriately to a caregiver, when a caregiver does not respond appropriately to an infant, or a combination of the two. Infants need thousands of successful cycles of expressing a need and then having the need met to achieve attachment. Disrupted attachments can result in feeding disorders, failure to thrive, anxiety disorders, or reactive attachment disorder.

Reactive attachment disorder is characterized by the failure of a child younger than the age of 5 years to initiate or respond appropriately to caregivers and/or social situations. As a result, caregivers then disregard the child's physical and/or emotional needs.

A child may have diffuse attachments (inhibited type) or indiscriminate sociability (disinhibited type). Children at risk for attachment disorders include those who are abused, neglected, or adopted.

Primal Wound Theory of Attachment Disorders

- A child separated from his or her mother at birth loses his or her mother and a sense of self, because these are the same from the child's perspective (Verrier, 1993).
- The child will suffer from a sense of losing oneself.
- This is very hard to overcome, even years later.

Treatment

- Treatment of reactive attachment disorder of infancy or early childhood (Zeanah, Chesher, & Boris, 2016) includes:
  - Assessment related to demonstration of attachment behaviors to caregivers and appropriateness with strangers
  - Comprehensive safety assessment of child's current home or foster placement to avoid re-traumatization
  - Provision of an emotionally available attachment figure
  - Limiting contact with non-caregiving adults to avoid nondiscriminant behavior

MOOD DISORDERS

Mood disorders are disturbances in a person's emotional state that affect daily activities. Depression, characterized by persistent sadness and loss of interest in activities, and bipolar disorder, characterized by alternating periods of depression and mania (periods of euphoria, loss of rational thinking, and hyperactivity), are two types of mood disorders (APA, 2013). A mood disorder is an expression of depression in children and may manifest in the following ways:

- Infants
  - Sad expression or lack of expression
  - Look away when spoken to
  - Lack of interest in play
  - Problems sleeping or eating
  - Separation from primary caregiver, such as during prolonged hospitalizations where parent visits infrequently or foster care experience
  - Increased risk with babies of depressed mother
- Toddlers/preschoolers
  - Irritable
  - Act out
  - Suddenly begin getting in trouble at preschool or day care
  - Do not experience pleasure
  - Low self-esteem
  - Guilt
- School-age/adolescents
  - Act outward (physical or verbal aggression, temper tantrums)
  - Act inward (withdrawing from others)
  - Hopeless about the future
  - Angry
  - Defiant
  - Depressed adolescents are likely to use behaviors such as poor school performance, cutting, and suicidal gestures as attempts to communicate depression (American Academy of Child & Adolescent Psychiatry [AACAP], 2013)

Depression

Depression is diagnosed in approximately 5% of U.S. children and adolescents when persistent sadness and loss of interest in typically fun activities interfere with daily life (AACAP, 2013). Youth who experience stress or loss, or who have attentional, learning, conduct, or anxiety disorders have a higher risk for development of the disorder than same-age peers who do not experience these issues (AACAP, 2013). Theories of depression include faulty mood regulation of the brain, genetic vulnerability, stressful life situation, medications, and medical problems (AACAP, 2013).

- Children are less likely than adults to experience psychosis with depression.
- Depressed children are more likely than adults to manifest symptoms of anxiety and somatic symptoms.
- Mood may be irritable rather than sad (acting out instead of acting in).

- Suicide is a real risk, which peaks during mid-adolescence.
- Mortality from suicide increases steadily throughout the teenage years.
- Patient may be diagnosed with major depression, dysthymic disorder (persistent symptoms of depression for 2 years without respite [APA, 2013]), or depressive episode NOS (not otherwise specified).
- Patients aged 10 to 21 years should be assessed for depression at every well child visit (Siu, 2016).

Risk Factors for Development of Depression

- Prior episode of depression
- Family history of depressive disorder
- Lack of social support
- Stressful life event
- Current substance use/abuse
- Medical comorbidity

SAFE AND EFFECTIVE NURSING CARE: Clinical Pearl

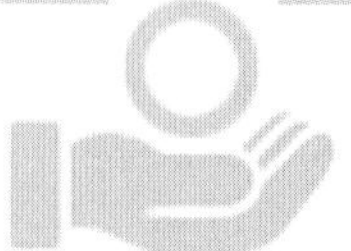

Assessing Depression Using SAD FACES

Assess for depression with the following tool:

S—sleep disturbances

A—anhedonia (inability to experience pleasure)

D—despair

F—fatigue

A—appetite changes

C—concentration

E—emotional sensitivity

S—suicidal ideation

Suicidality in Children

The number of children and adolescents admitted to inpatient psychiatric facilities has nearly doubled in the last decade (Plemmons, 2017). Older teens represent about 50% of hospitalizations, with younger teens and children comprising the other half of hospitalizations (Plemmons, 2017). U.S. youth are more likely to be hospitalized in the spring and fall versus summer months, suggesting a seasonal variation in symptoms (Plemmons, 2017).

Risk Factors for Suicide

Children who are experiencing depression are at risk for suicide. Even young children can have thoughts of suicide. Motivations behind suicidal thoughts/gestures/attempts include:

- A desire to die
- A desire to hurt others (i.e., to upset or get back at caregiver)
- A desire to escape a painful home or school situation, such as being bullied or abused
- A desire to punish oneself due to feeling guilty about something

Deterrents to Suicide

- Having family support
- Believing that suicide is wrong from a religious standpoint
- Having hope for future

CRITICAL COMPONENT

Bullycide

Bullycide is suicide due to becoming depressed and hopeless because of being bullied by peers (Wallace, 2011). Although bullying affects all victims, students who identify or are perceived by others as lesbian, gay, bisexual, or transgender are disproportionately targeted by bullies (Huebner, Thoma, & Neilands, 2015).

Indications for Medications

- Child is not responding to psychotherapy
- Severe symptoms that interfere with daily living
- History of recurrent depressive episodes
- Psychosis

Evidence-Based Practice: Treating Depression in Children

Ebert, E., Zarski, S., Christensen, D., Stikkelbroek, M., Cuijpers, P., Berking, M., & Riper, H. (2015). Internet and computer-based cognitive behavioral therapy for anxiety and depression in youth: A meta-analysis of randomized controlled outcome trials. *PLoS ONE 10*(3), e0119895. doi: 10.1371/journal.pone.0119895

CBT currently has the most research evidence for the treatment of depression in children, and CBT and interpersonal psychotherapy are preferred therapies for adolescent depression. Treatments can be administered in a variety of different formats, including individual and group therapy, in-person and online (Ebert et al., 2015). Computer-based CBT is useful when face-to-face options are not available (Ebert et al., 2015).

SAFE AND EFFECTIVE NURSING CARE: Understanding Medication

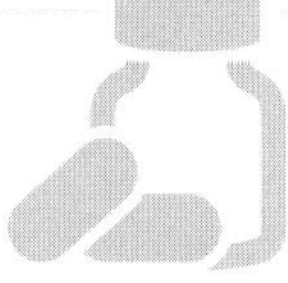

Treating Symptoms With Medication

Two rules of medicating children for psychiatric symptoms:

1. Skills before pills—try therapy first.
2. Start low, go slow—use low doses and titrate up slowly as needed.

Psychotropic Medication and Children

- The effects of most psychotropic medications are not well studied in children.
- Most psychiatric drugs are used off-label or for age groups not recommended by the U.S. Food and Drug Administration (FDA).
- Suicidal risks may increase in the initial days of treatment when first started on an antidepressant medication.
- In most cases, children need smaller doses of medication spaced throughout the day.

Antidepressants

- Antidepressants take 2 to 4 weeks to work.
- Goal of treatment is to restore normal levels of neurotransmitters.
- Act on serotonin, dopamine, or norepinephrine.
- Of patients, approximately 60% respond to treatment (defined as a 50% decrease in symptoms) (Walkup, 2017).
- Many have severe sexual side effects.
- These drugs do not cure depression; they reduce symptoms.
- They improve motivation and psychomotor retardation before they improve mood.
- Antidepressants are divided into the following classifications:
  - Tricyclic antidepressants
  - Monoamine oxidase inhibitors
  - Norepinephrine and dopamine reuptake inhibitors
  - Serotonin and norepinephrine reuptake inhibitors
  - Selective serotonin reuptake inhibitors (SSRIs)
  - Atypical antidepressants

Selective Serotonin Reuptake Inhibitors

SSRIs are the first-line agents used to treat depression in children. They have a lower risk of side effects than other classifications of antidepressants. These drugs work by blocking the reuptake of serotonin in the synaptic gap. Examples of SSRIs used in children include fluoxetine (Prozac), sertraline (Zoloft), and escitalopram (Lexapro). Side effects of SSRIs include gastrointestinal (GI) distress, sedation, anticholinergic effects such as dry mouth and constipation, sexual dysfunction, and orthostatic hypotension, as well as serotonin syndrome and serotonin discontinuation syndrome.

- Serotonin syndrome
  - Serotonin syndrome is an iatrogenic toxidrome that is the result of taking too many agents that block the reuptake of serotonin. These agents could be prescribed medications, over-the-counter medications, and herbal supplements such as St. John's wort.
  - Serotonin syndrome is usually mild, but can cause death.
  - Symptoms include thermal dysregulation, confusion, agitation, fever, shivering, diaphoresis, tremor, and diarrhea.
  - Treatment includes discontinuing one or more of the offending drugs and providing supportive care.
- Serotonin discontinuation syndrome
  - Serotonin discontinuation syndrome can occur when the patient suddenly stops taking an SSRI.
  - Symptoms include dizziness, feeling confused, flu-like symptoms, tremor, insomnia, agitation, anxiety, lability, and crying spells.

Predictors of Medication Noncompliance

- Poor insight into symptoms/disease
- Negative attitude toward medications by child and/or family members
- Substance use/abuse by the child or caregiver
- Acute illness of the child or caregiver
- Inadequate discharge plan/lack of follow-up care
- Poor therapeutic relationship with the child and/or caregiver

Nursing Interventions

- Nursing interventions for the child who is taking antidepressant medications include:
  - Provide patient and family medication education.
  - Monitor for compliance with medication regimen.
  - Monitor blood pressure.
  - Assess for suicidality, especially in the first month of medication administration.

Other Treatments for Depression in Children

Besides psychopharmacology, children who are experiencing depression may attend individual or group therapy and may even receive electroconvulsive therapy (ECT).

- ECT is the last-resort treatment for a pediatric psychiatric patient and will usually be used only for adolescents. It is the delivery of electrical current through the brain.
- A grand mal seizure is induced, which enhances dopamine sensitivity in the brain and reduces the reuptake of serotonin. Patients usually undergo a series of treatments, such as three times per week for 6 weeks.
- Nursing considerations for the patient undergoing ECT include:
  - Informed consent from caregiver
  - Assent from child if developmentally appropriate
  - Restriction of food/fluids for 6 to 8 hours before treatment to prevent aspiration
  - Completion of a preoperative checklist
  - Administration of a muscle relaxant
  - Assessment of vital signs during procedure
  - Assessment of patient for confusion and short-term memory loss after procedure
  - Placement of patient on falls precautions after procedure until patient physically and psychologically returns to baseline

Deliberate Self-Harm

Children who are depressed may exhibit self-harming behaviors such as head banging or cutting. This usually occurs as the result of a high level of psychological pain, especially when the patient feels like he or she is unable or unwilling to communicate feelings (alexithymia = "I have no words for my feelings").

Nursing Interventions

- Nursing interventions for the child who self-harms include:
  - Assess patient frequently for signs of psychological pain.
  - Assess skin frequently for signs of self-harm.

- Encourage expression of feelings.
- Maintain a safe environment free of objects that can be used for self-harm.

Bipolar Disorder

Bipolar disorder is a mood disorder characterized by unusual shifts in mood, energy, activity levels, and the ability to think clearly (APA, 2013). Youth with bipolar disorder experience fluctuating high (mania) and low moods (depression) that interfere with daily functioning (APA, 2013).

Types of Bipolar Disorder

- Bipolar type 1: alternating between major depression and mania
- Bipolar type 2: alternating between major depression and hypomania
- Mixed episodes: alternating between depressive and manic states in the same episode

Manic Episode

- Feeling unusually "high," euphoric, or irritable for at least 1 week
- Needing little sleep; great amount of energy
- Talking fast; others cannot follow
- Racing thoughts
- Easily distracted
- Inflated feeling of power, greatness, or importance
- Reckless behavior (e.g., with money, sex, drugs)

SAFE AND EFFECTIVE NURSING CARE: Clinical Pearl

Rage and Bipolar Disorder

Children with bipolar disorder mania often exhibit rage instead of or along with the symptoms just listed.

Nursing Interventions

- Frequently assess child for symptoms of depression or mania.
- Encourage participation in individual and group therapy as tolerated/appropriate.
- Keep child safe.
- Watch for boundary violations.
- Aid patient in the performance of activities of daily living (ADLs).
- Administer sleep aids as needed.
- Administer mood-stabilizing medications, such as lithium, aripiprazole (Abilify), and lamotrigine (Lamictal), as needed.
- Administer antipsychotic medications such as ziprasidone (Geodon), risperidone (Risperdal), quetiapine (Seroquel), and olanzapine (Zyprexa) during manic periods as needed.

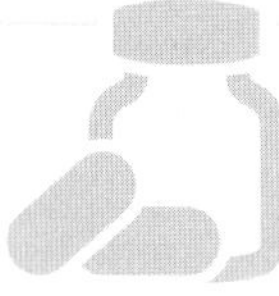

SAFE AND EFFECTIVE NURSING CARE: Understanding Medication

XR and ER Medications

Be cautious with medication orders containing "XR or ER." These medications are extended release and are *not* the same as medications without those labels.

Lithium

- The primary mood stabilizer used for bipolar disorder
- Mechanism of action: unknown
- Body cannot distinguish between lithium and salt
- Increased salt intake = decreased lithium uptake
- Facilitates reuptake of norepinephrine and serotonin (leaving less in the synapses)
- Blood levels: 0.5 to 1.2 mEq/L
- Side effects: GI upset, weight gain, polyuria, polydipsia
- Contraindicated in those with cardiac disease
- Caution in those taking diuretics
- Signs of lithium toxicity:
  - Runny nose
  - Coughing
  - Chest congestion
  - Fever
  - GI upset
  - Blurred vision
  - Ringing in the ears

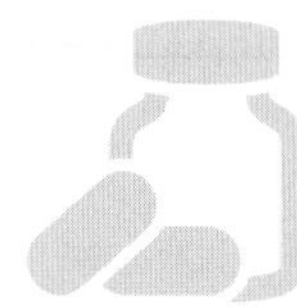

SAFE AND EFFECTIVE NURSING CARE: Understanding Medication

Medications for Pediatric Bipolar Disorder and Behavior Disorders

Divalproex sodium (Depakote) and clonidine (Catapres) are used off-label for pediatric bipolar disorder and behavior disorders. Depakote is an anticonvulsant medication that has mood-stabilizing effects on youth with bipolar. Catapres was first developed as a medication for hypertension but has been found to be an effective mood stabilizer in youth (Wagner, 2016).

Nursing Interventions

- Nursing interventions for the child who is taking mood stabilizers include:
  - Provide patient and family medication education.
  - Emphasize compliance.
  - Draw blood levels as ordered.

- Assess for symptoms of depression and mania.
- Assess suicidality.

ANXIETY DISORDERS

Anxiety disorders are characterized by persistent and excessive worry that interferes with daily activities. The feelings of worry may be accompanied by physical symptoms such as restlessness, irritability, fatigue, concentration problems, and/or insomnia (APA, 2013).

- The most common psychiatric disorder in children
- Separation anxiety is common in young children
- Test- or school-related anxiety is common in older children

SAFE AND EFFECTIVE NURSING CARE: Clinical Pearl

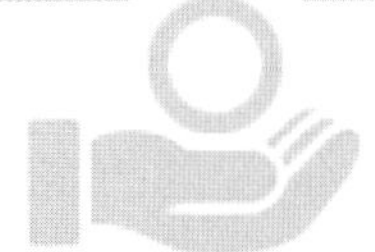

Expressions of Anxiety

Young children may not be able to verbally express anxiety. Instead, they may complain of physical symptoms such as headache or stomachache, nausea, or flatulence.

Health Consequences of Chronic Anxiety

Chronic anxiety is associated with:

- Decreased immune functioning
- Cardiovascular disease
- Diabetes
- GI issues
- Depression
- Forgetfulness
- Decreased attention span

Nursing Interventions

- Nursing interventions for the child with an anxiety-based disorder include:
  - Stay with patient during extreme anxiety.
  - Consult with key school personnel such as teachers and administrators.
  - Maintain a calm, relaxed approach.
  - Decrease environmental stimuli.
  - Encourage verbalization of feelings.
  - Encourage physical activity.
  - Teach relaxation techniques.
  - Teach problem-solving strategies.
  - Give positive feedback and support.
  - Provide psychoeducation.
  - Provide cognitive behavioral interventions.
  - Hypnosis is an option.
  - Administer anxiolytic medications as ordered.
- Nursing interventions for the child who is taking anxiolytic medications:
  - Provide patient and family medication education.
  - Monitor for compliance.
  - Assess for sedation, addiction, and suicidality.

SAFE AND EFFECTIVE NURSING CARE: Understanding Medication

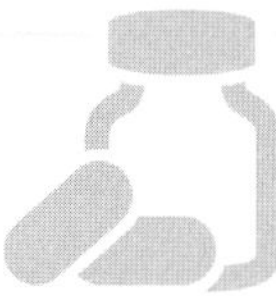

Anxiolytic Medications

Most anxiolytic medications are addicting, including benzodiazepines. These medications may be used in a crisis with children but not for long-term management of an anxiety-based disorder. Hydroxyzine (Vistaril) and diphenhydramine (Benadryl) are commonly used for acute anxiety in children. Buspirone (Buspar) is a long-acting anxiolytic medication that is nonaddicting and nonsedating, and is a better choice for treating an anxiety-based disorder. In addition, SSRIs have helped relieve chronic anxiety in children.

Obsessive-Compulsive Disorder

Obsessive-compulsive disorder (OCD) is characterized by severe obsessions (unwanted, reoccurring thoughts) and/or compulsions (repetitive behaviors) that interfere with quality of life. Obsessions create anxiety, and compulsions are performed to reduce anxiety.

- A common obsession is fear of contamination from contact with germs, which may result in compulsive hand washing.
- Common compulsions include washing self or objects, cleaning, checking, counting, repeating actions, ordering, making confessions, and requesting assurances.
- OCD affects about 2% of the child and adolescent population (APA, 2013).
- There seems to be a genetic component.
- Children with OCD are highly somatic (distress caused by placing significant focus on physical symptoms).
- OCD is often comorbid with PDs, autism, and Tourette's syndrome.
- The child may experience dissociation (a breakdown in integrated functions of memory, consciousness, perception of self, environment, or sensory and motor behavior) or depersonalization (loss of sense of personality).

Nursing Interventions

- Do not interrupt the ritual, as this will make the child more anxious
- Instruct child how to complete thought stopping—child becomes aware of the thoughts and tries to stop them
- Relaxation techniques
- Cue cards

Phobia

Phobia is characterized by excessive anxiety brought on by exposure to a specific feared object or situation, often leading to avoidance behavior.

- It involves a sense of dread so intense that the individual will do everything necessary to avoid the source of the fear.
- Common phobias in children include fear of the dark, spiders, enclosed places, heights, and social situations.

Nursing Interventions

- Provide support (e.g., anxiety management strategies such as deep breathing or distraction).
- Refer for CBT or exposure therapy as needed if the phobia is interfering with home/school.

Panic Disorder

Panic disorder is characterized by episodes of an overwhelming sense of dread/doom. These episodes are called panic attacks. Children often report a feeling of dizziness and faintness, as well as rapid heart rate and sweating during these episodes. Attacks may occur frequently or a child may experience an isolated attack during a period of extreme stress.

Nursing Interventions

- Nursing interventions for the child who is experiencing a panic attack include:
  - Staying with the child.
  - Reassuring him or her that you will not leave.
  - Giving clear directions.
  - Assisting patient to an environment with minimal stimulation.
  - Walking with the patient.
  - Administering prn anxiolytic medications.

Post-Traumatic Stress Disorder

Children may develop post-traumatic stress disorder (PTSD) after a traumatic event, including hospitalization for a medical condition.

- Experiencing any element that was present during the initial trauma (e.g., the time of day, an article of clothing, a smell or sound) can trigger a flashback.
- The flashback is the limbic system of the brain reminding the prefrontal cortex not to allow a repeat of the initial trauma.
- Research shows that administering a dose of propranolol (Inderal) right after a trauma decreases the risk for PTSD.

Nursing Interventions

- Nursing interventions for the child with PTSD include:
  - Provide support.
  - Encourage the patient to express feelings.
  - Refer the patient for psychotherapy.
  - Provide an anxiolytic medication after a flashback or on a long-term basis.

SAFE AND EFFECTIVE NURSING CARE: Clinical Pearl

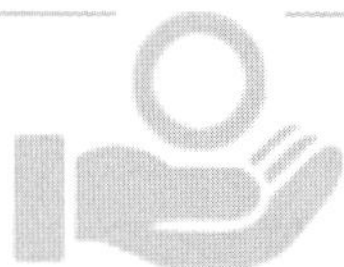

Flashbacks

Do not attempt to interact with a patient who is experiencing a flashback. If you touch or talk to the patient, you could become a part of the flashback and could be in physical danger.

DISSOCIATIVE DISORDERS

Dissociative disorders are characterized by a failure to integrate identity, memory, and consciousness, and are usually found in children with a history of horrific abuse. It is sometimes described as overuse of a defense mechanism. Patients report periods of loss of consciousness during which they have no memory; this is a means of escaping their current reality. Dissociating is easy for children between ages 2 and 7 years, who developmentally use magical thinking and have an ability to create and implement made-up friends and situations.

Types of Dissociative Disorders

- Dissociative amnesia—inability to recall
- Dissociative fugue—unexpected travel away from home
- Depersonalization disorder—being detached from one's body
- Dissociative identity disorder (formerly known as multiple PD)—having more than one personality
- Dissociative disorder NOS—does not fit the diagnostic criteria for any of the disorders, as described by the DSM

DISRUPTIVE DISORDERS IN CHILDREN

ADHD, oppositional defiant disorder (ODD), and conduct disorder (CD) belong in the group of disruptive behavior disorders characterized by significant and persistent behavior problems.

- They are also referred to as externalizing disorders due to the characteristic "acting out" behaviors associated with the disorders.
- These disorders are most common in school-age males, but can present in females as well.
- Children with these disorders are at high risk for physical injury as a result of fighting and impulsive behaviors. Adolescents are at high risk for sexually transmitted infections and/or pregnancy resulting from promiscuity.

Attention-Deficit Hyperactivity Disorder

ADHD is characterized by three core symptoms—inattention, hyperactivity, and impulsivity—that are pervasive and inappropriate for the child's developmental level (APA, 2013). Symptoms present both at school and at home. Children can present as predominantly hyperactive, predominantly inattentive, or combined.

- The inattentive subtype is very difficult to diagnose because the child does not display the hyperactivity most often attributed to the disorder.
- Children who are predominantly inattentive appear to not listen when spoken to, have difficulty following through and completing tasks that require sustained mental effort, frequently lose items necessary for task completion, and are easily distractible and appear forgetful.
- Children who are predominantly hyperactive may be squirmy or fidgety, run or climb inappropriately, talk excessively, interrupt, or have difficulty waiting.
- Discipline is frequently an issue because parents have difficulty managing their child's disruptive behaviors.
- These children often show a narrow range of emotions.
- They have difficulty sequencing information.
- They may have slow information processing.
- Symptoms often interfere with the ability to complete tasks at home and school.

Nursing Interventions

- Nursing interventions for the child with ADHD include:
- Individual and family therapy
- Behavior management
- Providing emotional support
- Promoting self-esteem
- Pharmacology (see later for further information)

SAFE AND EFFECTIVE NURSING CARE: Clinical Pearl

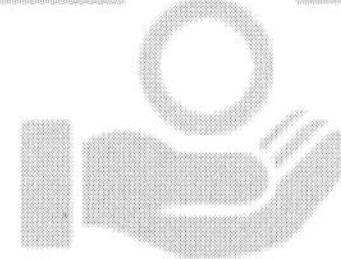

Medication for Attention-Deficit Hyperactivity Disorder

Medications used to reduce the symptoms of ADHD have a street value. Children who are not responding to treatment may not be taking the pills. Instead, the child or caregiver may be selling the medication.

Medications

- The most common medications used to treat ADHD are:
  - Methylphenidate (Ritalin)
  - Amphetamines mixed with salts (Adderall XR)
  - Methylphenidate (Concerta)
  - Lisdexamfetamine dimesylate (Vyvanse)
  - Daytrana transdermal patch
  - Atomoxetine HCl (Strattera)
  - Guanfacine (Tenex or Intuniv)—nonstimulant

Nursing Considerations

Nursing considerations when administering medications for ADHD include:

- Children may experience a decreased appetite and rapid weight loss.
- Other side effects include insomnia, increase in tics and/or compulsive behaviors, and/or psychotic reactions.
- ADHD medications should be given every day regardless of whether school is in session.

School-Based Interventions

School-based interventions for the child with ADHD include:

- Having child sit near teacher.
- Assigning a peer helper.
- Creating a daily schedule.
- Reviewing previously taught material.
- Allowing extra time for assignments or tests.
- Breaking assignments into shorter pieces.
- Giving shorter assignments.
- Giving directions one at a time.
- Decreasing environmental distractions.
- Giving the child periodic "errands" to run, such as picking up mail in the office or taking a book to the library.
- Allowing the child to keep a set of books at school and a second set at home.
- Color coding folders per subject.
- Helping the child organize his or her locker and desk.

Oppositional Defiant Disorder

ODD is characterized by a persistent pattern of disobedience, argumentativeness, angry outbursts, low tolerance for frustration, and tendency to blame others for misfortunes (APA, 2013).

- Of children with ADHD, 40% to 60% also have symptoms of ODD (Cuffe et al., 2015).
- Children have trouble with peer and social relationships and are often in conflict with adults.

Nursing Interventions

Nursing interventions for the child with ODD include:

- Consistent consequences
- Target a few behaviors at a time
- Positive reinforcement with activities
- Do not show emotional reactions to behavior
- Social skills training
- Caregiver training to manage behaviors

Conduct Disorder

- Childhood-onset type: at least one symptom before age 10 years
- Adolescent-onset type: at least three symptoms after age 10 years
- Characterized by *serious* violations of social norms, including aggressive behaviors, destruction of property, and cruelty to animals

- Children often engage in lying, larceny, theft, assault, and truancy from school
- More prevalent in boys than girls
- Most frequent disorder found among children residing in mental health facilities
- Anxiety disorders and substance use/abuse are common in children with CD
- Children generally present with a history of developmental delays, ADHD, and ODD
- Adolescents are often hostile, sarcastic, defensive, and provocative toward others

Nursing Interventions

Nursing interventions for the child with CD include:

- Give positive, specific feedback for desirable behavior
- Allow for natural consequences of actions
- Academic support
- Social skills training
- Limit the use of group therapy, as the group often reinforces negative behaviors
- Individual therapy
- Caregiver support
- Medications such as antipsychotics (e.g., haloperidol and low-dose risperidone), mood stabilizers (e.g., lithium carbonate), and Depakote

CRITICAL COMPONENT

Difference Between Oppositional Defiant Disorder and Conduct Disorder

The key difference between ODD and CD is that children with ODD feel remorseful when they break the rules or hurt someone, and children with CD do not because they lack empathy (APA, 2013).

IMPULSE-CONTROL DISORDERS

Impulse-control disorders are characterized by the inability to resist or control urges to do something that might harm themselves or others (APA, 2013). These disorders tend to develop around age 11 years in U.S. youth (APA, 2013).

Kleptomania

- Failure to resist the urge to steal things
- Feeling of tension before theft
- Pleasure and relief after the theft
- Unknown/unrecognized motives

Nursing Interventions

Nursing interventions for the child with kleptomania include:

- Psychotherapy
- Aversion therapy
- SSRIs

Pyromania

- Intentional fire-setting on more than one occasion
- Tension before the act
- Excessive interest in or attraction to fire
- Pleasure/gratification after the fire is set and while watching the fire
- Unknown/unrecognized motives

Nursing Interventions

Nursing care for the child who is experiencing pyromania includes:

- Behavior modification
- Psychotherapy

Intermittent Explosive Disorder

- Several occurrences of a failure to resist aggressive impulses that result in assaults or destruction of property
- The aggression is considered out of proportion to the perceived precipitants

Nursing Interventions

- Nursing interventions for the child who is experiencing intermittent explosive disorder include:
  - CBT
  - SSRIs
  - Antipsychotic medications such as olanzapine (Zyprexa) and risperidone (Risperdal)

Schizophrenia

- Childhood (or early-onset) schizophrenia is characterized by delusions or hallucinations, disorganized speech or behavior, and marked impairment in social and/or school functioning.
- Childhood schizophrenia is much rarer than later-onset, or adult, schizophrenia. It is a chronic illness with periods of exacerbation and remission.
- Patients with this disorder often need lifelong medication management.

Causes of Childhood Schizophrenia

- Genetic
- Biochemical differences in the brain, particularly with increased dopamine and/or cortisol reuptake
- Increased stress levels
- Youth who smoke marijuana laced with "wet" (formaldehyde)
- FOAD hypothesis—*f*etal *o*rigins of *a*dult *d*iseases. Child may develop schizophrenia because of intrauterine conditions.

Related Disorders

- Schizoaffective disorder
- Depression with psychotic features
- Mania with psychotic features
- Psychosis NOS

Risk Factors for Other Disorders

Patients with schizophrenia have an increased risk for:

- Cardiovascular disorders
- Depression and other dementias
- Substance abuse
- Cigarette smoking

Symptoms of Schizophrenia in Children

- Symptoms appear as inappropriate affect, loss of interest or pleasure, disturbances in sleep and concentration, and loss of appetite.
- Delays are common in social and cognitive functioning, linguistic and motor skills, and attentional and perceptual behaviors.
- These symptoms can be summarized with the acronym SLEPT; the patient with schizophrenia may experience alterations in:
  - S—social behavior
  - L—language
  - E—emotions
  - P—perceptions
  - T—thinking

Effects of Schizophrenia on Thought Processes and Content

- Loose association: thoughts are poorly related; thoughts are disorganized
- Autism: patient develops and retreats into a private world
- Slow or inhibited flow of thought: patient has difficulty expressing feelings
- Rapid thinking
- Perseveration: getting stuck on something
- Circumstantial: excessive or irrelevant detail
- Tangential: patient digresses in the conversation and never reaches the goal

Sensory and Perceptual Disturbances

- Hallucinations—sensory disturbances
- Delusions—perceptual disturbances rather than impairment in brain function
- Fixed false beliefs
- Cannot be validated in reality
- Exaggerated defense mechanisms
- Compensation for feelings of little worth
- The three phases to hearing voices are startling (person is disturbed by the voices), organization (coping), and stabilization (acceptance and integration of the voice into the life experience).

CRITICAL COMPONENT

Hallucinations

The more elaborate the description of a hallucination is, the less likely it is that the hallucination is real/truthful. Patients with schizophrenia see shadows and lights. They hear noises and muffled voices. Children sometimes have difficulty distinguishing between reality and imagination. Children who have been abused often imagine that they see or hear the abuser.

- Children with schizophrenia may be hospitalized for:
  - Initial diagnosis
  - Stabilization on medications
  - Patient safety
  - Inappropriate behavior
  - Inability to take care of basis needs

Nursing Interventions

Nursing interventions for the child with schizophrenia include:

- Maintain a safe environment (removal of sharp objects, locked windows, adequate supervision) with minimal stimulation
- Help with ADLs
- Encouragement to eat/drink
- Medications for sleep
- Psychotherapy
- Reality testing
- Social skills training
- Behavior modification
- Family education
- Referral to an outpatient provider for ongoing therapy and medication evaluation
- Medication education

Antipsychotic Medications

- Work by blocking dopamine receptors to prohibit uptake in the synapses
- Have a risk of weight gain; administering metformin (Glucophage) along with the medication will decrease this risk
- Can have severe side effects, such as extrapyramidal symptoms (EPS). EPS can occur after a one-time use of an antipsychotic medication or after prolonged use, depending on the medication. Types of EPS include:
  - Akathisia—motor restlessness
  - Dystonia—muscle tone impairment
  - Akinesia—muscular paralysis
  - Pseudoparkinsonism-like symptoms—tremors
  - Tardive dyskinesia—involuntary muscle movements

SAFE AND EFFECTIVE NURSING CARE: Understanding Medication

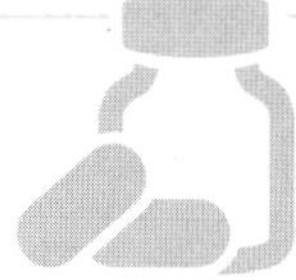

Extrapyramidal Symptoms

Children who are experiencing EPS often complain that the tongue feels thick, the neck is stiff, or the eyes keep looking up to the ceiling. EPS can also cause the throat to swell, causing shortness of breath.

- Medications to relieve EPS include benztropine (Cogentin) and diphenhydramine (Benadryl). The first is used for issues of increased motor movement such as akathisia, parkinsonism, and tardive dyskinesia. The latter is used for decreased motor issues such as dystonia and akinesia.

Haloperidol (Haldol)

- By mouth or intramuscularly (IM)
- IM version is given Z-track
- Haloperidol decanoate—long-acting; given monthly as an injection
- High risk for EPS
- Used across the life span
- Used to relieve symptoms that may lead to aggression
- Often given with Ativan (syringe compatible)

Olanzapine (Zyprexa)

- By mouth or IM
- Zyprexa Zydis is a sublingual (SL) form of Zyprexa
- Low risk for EPS
- Watch for orthostatic hypotension

Risperidone (Risperdal)

- By mouth
- Risperdal Consta: long-acting version; give every 2 weeks
- Few side effects
- No risk for EPS
- Watch for orthostatic hypotension

Quetiapine (Seroquel)

- By mouth
- May prolong the QT interval (get a baseline electrocardiogram [EKG] and follow-up EKGs)
- May cause sedation
- Useful for sleep or anxiety in low doses
- Little risk for EPS

Ziprasidone (Geodon)

- By mouth or IM
- May prolong the QT interval (get a baseline EKG and follow-up EKGs)
- Also helps with depression and anxiety (blocks reuptake of dopamine, serotonin, and norepinephrine)
- Few side effects
- Little risk for EPS
- Titrate up to a therapeutic range

Clozapine (Clozaril)

- Blocks reuptake of dopamine and serotonin
- Gold standard for treatment of schizophrenia, yet used as a last resort
- Risk for seizures
- May cause sialorrhea (excessive salivation)
- Serious side effect: agranulocytosis (low absolute neutrophil count)
- Regular blood draws are required
- Clozaril protocols:
  - If baseline white blood cell count (WBC) <3500, don't start medication.
  - Monitor WBC weekly for first 6 months, then biweekly.
  - Discontinue medication if WBC <3000 *or* absolute neutrophil count is <1500

Other Side Effects of Antipsychotic Medications

Although antipsychotic drugs are very effective in controlling psychotic symptoms, severe adverse side effects related to use of antipsychotic medications need to be closely assessed and monitored. Patient and family education regarding side effects is important to drug safety and effective maintenance by the patient and health-care provider.

Neuroleptic Malignant Syndrome

- Life-threatening neurological disorder most often caused by an adverse reaction to antipsychotic medications
- Can be summarized with the acronym FEVER:
  - F—fever
  - E—encephalopathy
  - V—vitals unstable
  - E—elevated creatinine phosphokinase (CPK) enzyme level
  - R—rigidity of muscles

NURSING INTERVENTIONS FOR NEUROLEPTIC MALIGNANT SYNDROME

Nursing interventions for the patient who is experiencing neuroleptic malignant syndrome include:

- Stop use of the drug.
- Provide supportive care to relieve symptoms (controlling rigidity and hyperthermia, and preventing major organ failure).

Metabolic Syndrome

- Onset of insulin resistance
- Lipid abnormalities
- Hypertension
- Abdominal obesity

NURSING INTERVENTIONS FOR METABOLIC SYNDROME

- Monitor blood pressure.
- Monitor blood glucose level.
- Monitor weight.
- Monitor lipid levels.

Nursing Interventions for the Child Who Is Taking an Antipsychotic Medication

- Provide patient and family education regarding effects and side effects.
- Emphasize importance of continuing medications.
- Monitor vital signs, weight, and EKG.
- Monitor for symptoms of EPS, neuroleptic malignant syndrome, and metabolic syndrome.

AUTISM SPECTRUM DISORDER

- Autism spectrum disorder (ASD) combines what the DSM-IV-TR called pervasive developmental disorders and combined autism and Asperger's syndrome. ASD is thought to have multiple causes, including genetic, biochemical, and environmental factors (APA, 2013).

- Characterized by severe and pervasive developmental impairment in social skills, communication, emotional attachment, or the presence of stereotyped behaviors or activities (APA, 2013).
- ASD is increasing at rates of 10% to 17% per year and is the fastest-growing pediatric disability (Christensen et al., 2016).
- Assessments for this disorder include examining the physical, psychological, and social contexts of the child.
- Diagnosed using DSM criteria. Children with ASD are more likely to be born to women 35 years and older and born breech.
- Deficits are usually apparent by age 18 months, with the disorder diagnosed before age 3 years.
- Genetic mutations relating to ASD have been discovered.
- Parents report concerns about child's interactions with others, language, or play.
- Examples of issues include: does not talk or babble by age 1 years, does not respond to name, does not seem to be able to hear, has violent tantrums, makes odd movements, does not smile, has poor eye contact, prefers to be alone, lines objects up, displays obsessions/compulsions, or shows unusual attachment to an object. For a complete list, see https://www.nichd.nih.gov/health/topics/autism/Pages/default.aspx.
- Essential features include abnormal and impaired social interaction and communication, and restricted behaviors and interests.
- Screening tools include:
  - The Checklist of Autism in Toddlers (CHAT)
  - The Modified Checklist of Autism in Toddlers (M-CHAT)
  - The Screening Tool for Autism in Two-Year-Olds (STAT)
  - The Social Communication Questionnaire (SCQ) for children age 4 and above

Nursing Interventions

- Early intervention
- Familial involvement in interventions
- Individual and family therapy
- Highly structured settings
- Social skills training
- Enhance communication skills
- Behavior modification
- Enhance cognitive skills
- Support and enhance academic and vocational readiness skills
- May need medication for OCD

Sensory Processing Disorder

- Children with an ASD often have a sensory processing disorder.
- These children are highly sensitive to sensory stimuli. Lights seem extra bright, noises seem extra loud, and even mild tactile stimulation seems like a big push or shove.

Nursing Interventions

- Early intervention
- Individual and family therapy
- Short periods of exposure to increased stimuli to build tolerance, such as using:
  - Massagers
  - Vibrating toothbrush
  - Aromatherapy
  - Weighted vests
  - Crafts involving clay, seeds, sand, soft pom-poms, or any other materials that are stimulating to touch
  - Lava lamp
  - Toys that encourage motion, such as a rocking horse or trampoline

EATING DISORDERS

Eating disorders are serious and often fatal illnesses that cause disturbances to an individual's eating behaviors. Common eating disorders are anorexia nervosa and bulimia nervosa (APA, 2013). Eating disorders are caused by a complex interaction of genetic, biological, behavioral, psychological, and social factors (APA, 2013). Adolescent females tend to develop eating disorders more often than males (APA, 2013).

Signs and Symptoms

- Focus on dieting
- Skipping meals
- Going to bathroom after eating
- Diet pills
- Laxatives
- Excessive exercise
- Extreme calorie counting
- Negative comments about self-body image

SAFE AND EFFECTIVE NURSING CARE: Clinical Pearl

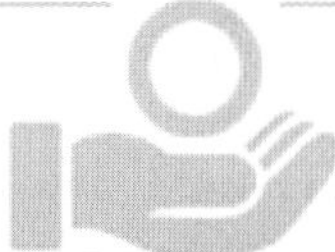

Screening for Eating Disorders

Screen for eating disorders using the SCOFF tool (Hill, Reid, Morgan, & Lacey, 2010):

1. Do you make yourself sick because you feel uncomfortably full?
2. Do you worry that you've lost control over what you eat?
3. Have you lost over 10 lb in the last 3 months?
4. Do you believe that you're fat?
5. Would you say that food dominates your life?

Anorexia Nervosa

- Self-starvation
- Person relentlessly pursues thinness
- Preoccupation with body and body image

- Despite extreme thinness, person thinks he or she is fat due to a distorted body image
- Diagnosed when a person drops to less than 85% of ideal body weight (Harrington, Jimerson, Haxton, & Jimerson, 2015)
- Onset is usually in early adolescence but can occur at any age
- Often found in females more than males
- Chronic condition with relapses characterized by significant weight loss
- Often continue to be preoccupied with food
- Of those affected, 10% to 25% go on to develop bulimia nervosa (Harrington et al., 2015)
- Poor outcome is related to initial lower minimum weight, presence of purging, and later age of onset

Complications

- Malnutrition
- Muscle wasting
- Dehydration
- Electrolyte imbalances
- Cardiac dysrhythmia
- Increased risk for infection

Nursing Interventions

- Monitor eating.
- Administer nutrition via nasogastric tube if ordered.
- Correct malnutrition.
- Resolve underlying psychological dysfunction.
- Encourage participation in psychotherapy.
- Restore weight within 10% of normal.
- Monitor bathroom behavior.
- Administer SSRIs as prescribed.
- Administer modafinil (Provigil) as ordered off-label to stimulate the appetite; however, it may prolong the QT interval, so a baseline EKG and follow-up EKGs are recommended

Bulimia Nervosa

- Bulimia nervosa is characterized by recurrent episodes of binge eating with or without purging
- Generally not life-threatening
- Usually child is of normal weight
- There are few outward signs; behavior usually occurs in secret and thus may go undetected for years

Signs and Symptoms

- Sneaking food
- Making excuses to use the bathroom after meals
- Eating large amounts of food on the spur of the moment
- Taking laxatives, vomiting, and/or overexercising to "purge" food
- Extreme concern with body weight and image
- Enamel on teeth begins to wear away, causing cavities
- May see Russell's sign—teeth marks on the knuckles from self-inducing vomiting

Nursing Interventions

- Stabilize and normalize eating patterns through nutrition counseling.
- Restructure dysfunctional thoughts and attitudes through individual therapy.
- Assess for comorbid depression, suicide, deliberate self-harm, and other impulsive behaviors such as shoplifting, overspending, or engaging in casual sexual encounters.
- Administer SSRIs as ordered.

Compulsive Overeating

- Binge-eating disorder
- Characterized by an addiction to food
- May have episodes of uncontrolled eating or binging
- Continues to eat even after becoming uncomfortably full
- Usually feels guilt/depressed afterward
- Does not purge

SUBSTANCE-RELATED DISORDERS

Substance-related disorders are characterized by recurrent use of one or more substances that cause clinical and functional impairments such as health problems, disability, and inability to meet school, home, or work responsibilities (APA, 2013). Approximately 9.4% of U.S. youth age 12–17 experience a substance use disorder (Center for Behavioral Health Statistics and Quality, 2015). Drug overdose is the leading cause of accidental death in the United States (National Institute on Drug Abuse [NIDA], 2015a).

Definitions of Substance Use

- Use—drinks alcohol; swallows, smokes, sniffs, or injects substance(s)
- Dependence—use despite adverse consequences; person feels "normal" only when on the drug
- Tolerance—the need for increasing amounts of a substance to achieve the same effects
- Abuse—use for purposes of intoxication or for treatment beyond intended use
- Addiction—psychological and behavioral dependence (Fig. 14–1)
- Withdrawal—physical signs/symptoms that occur when the addictive substance is reduced/withheld
- Codependency—stress-related preoccupation with an addicted person's life, leading to extreme dependence on that person

Signs and Symptoms

- Frequent absenteeism from school, work, or extracurricular activities
- Frequent injuries/accidents

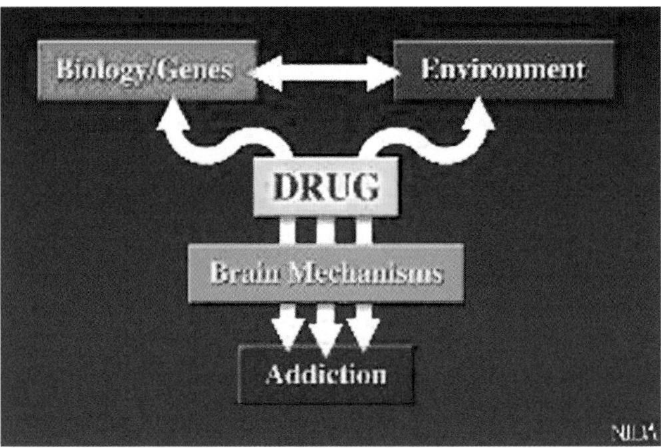

FIGURE 14–1 Addiction—psychological and behavioral dependence.

- Drowsiness
- Slurred speech
- Inattention to appearance
- Isolation
- Frequent "secretive" disappearances
- Tremors
- Flushed face
- Watery/red eyes
- Odor related to alcohol and/or marijuana use
- High number of physical complaints
- Missing medications/alcohol

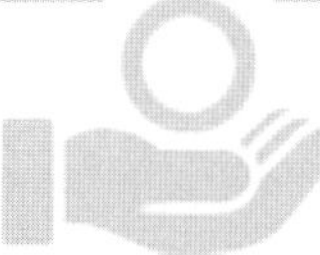

SAFE AND EFFECTIVE NURSING CARE: Clinical Pearl

CAGE Questionnaire

Assessing alcohol or substance use/abuse using the CAGE questionnaire:

1. Have you ever felt that you should cut down on your drinking/substance use?
2. Have people annoyed you by criticizing your drinking/substance use?
3. Have you ever felt bad or guilty about your drinking/substance use?
4. Have you ever had an eye-opener in the morning to steady your nerves or to get rid of a hangover?

Answers:

- Two yes responses are suggestive of a disorder.
- Three or more yes responses are diagnostic of a disorder (Ewing, 1984).

Assessment

- Interview tips
  - Be aware of risk of denial/minimizing.
  - Ask about peer and family use.

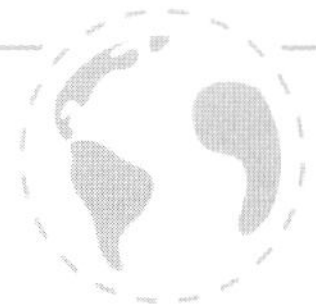

SAFE AND EFFECTIVE NURSING CARE: Critical Component

Peer and Family Substance Use/Abuse

If a peer or family member uses/abuses alcohol or drugs, a child is more likely to do so as well, so always ask about peer and family use/abuse.

- Be nonjudgmental.
- Do not be manipulated.
- Confront when necessary.
- Set and maintain limits.
- Provide option to verify interview data by urine, blood, or hair testing (Box 14–1).
- Drug withdrawal symptoms and severity depend on:
  - Type of drug used
  - Amount of drug used
  - Duration of drug use
  - Preexisting psychopathology

Nursing Interventions

- Discuss natural consequences of substance use.
- Provide substance/medication education.
- Offer hope for long-term recovery.

BOX 14–1 | Time After Ingestion That Drug Can Be Detected in Urine

Drug Detection Period

Heroin: 2–4 days

Morphine: 2–4 days

Demerol: 2–4 days

Methadone: 2–4 days

Fentanyl: Less than 1 hour

Barbiturates: 12 hours to 3 weeks

Benzodiazepines: up to 1 week

Amphetamines: 2–4 days

Cocaine: 2–4 days

Marijuana: 3 days to less than 1 month

PCP: 1 day to 1 month

- Encourage Alcoholics Anonymous (AA)/Narcotics Anonymous (NA) attendance.
- Encourage family therapy.
- Develop a nonuse contract with the patient.
- Encourage independence in ADLs.
- Administer medications and monitor side effects.
- Provide quiet environment.
- Assess vital signs, especially heart rate and blood pressure.
- Offer group therapy.

Alcoholism

- Alcohol is metabolized rapidly.
- Withdrawal is short term but can be severe.
- Symptoms begin hours after cessation of drinking.
- Symptoms peak in 2 to 3 days.
- Symptoms subside in 4 to 5 days.
- Delirium tremens is the most severe type of alcohol withdrawal.
  - Occurs within 1 week of cessation or severe reduction in alcohol use.
  - May lead to visual and/or tactile hallucinations.
  - Disorientation may occur.
  - Delusions and agitated behavior common.
  - Patient may be frightened and anxious.
  - High risk for grand mal seizures.

Nursing Interventions

- Individual and group therapy
- Assessment for the use of other substances
- Encourage attendance at AA meetings.
- Maintain a quiet environment.
- Monitor vital signs. Watch especially for increased heart rate and blood pressure.
- Monitor for seizures; put seizure precautions in place.
- Monitor for confusion and reports/signs of hallucinations/delusions.
- Administer long-acting sedative hypnotics such as chlordiazepoxide (Librium), diazepam (Valium), phenobarbitone (Phenobarbital), or lorazepam (Ativan) as ordered. These medications will be prescribed by a protocol using the Clinical Institute Withdrawal Assessment (CIWA) score:
  - CIWA for Alcohol (CIWA-Ar)
  - Validated 10-item assessment tool that can be used to quantify the severity of alcohol withdrawal syndrome, and to monitor and medicate patients going through withdrawal
  - Scores of 8 points or fewer correspond to mild withdrawal
  - Scores of 9 to 15 points correspond to moderate withdrawal
  - Scores of greater than 15 points correspond to severe withdrawal and an increased risk for delirium tremens and seizures
  - Medication decisions are based on CIWA score

Marijuana (Cannabis)

Marijuana refers to the dried leaves, flowers, stems, and seeds from the hemp plant, *Cannabis sativa*. The plant contains the mind-altering chemical delta-9-tetrahydrocannabinol (THC) and other related compounds. Extracts can also be made from the cannabis plant (NIDA, 2017). Marijuana remains the most used illegal substance among youth. By the time they graduate from high school, about 45% of U.S. teens have tried marijuana at least once (NIDA, 2017).

- Marijuana stimulates dopamine pathways.
- It causes euphoria, perception of slowed time, dry mouth, increased appetite, anxiety, and suspiciousness.
- All senses are enhanced with use.
- Patient may have red eyes.
- Patient may develop "amotivational syndrome," a lack of motivation to complete ADLs/tasks because of the THC found in marijuana.
- Marijuana may be laced with another substance, such as formaldehyde ("wet") or cocaine.
- Withdrawal is not as intense as that of alcohol or cocaine but can last 1 to 3 weeks.
- Medical marijuana is legally recognized in several U.S. states for adults, but its use is not yet recommended for children and adolescents (American Academy of Pediatrics, 2015).

Nursing Interventions

- Individual and group therapy
- Assessment for the use of other substances
- Maintain a quiet environment
- Administer anxiolytics for anxiety, as needed

Hallucinogens (LSD, PCP)

- Hallucinogens block reuptake of serotonin.
- These are considered psychedelic drugs that may cause hallucinations, suicidal and homicidal thoughts, and the experience of all of the senses "running together."
- Use of these substances can cause respiratory arrest, coma, seizure, and death.
- Patient may experience flashbacks of "bad trips" at unpredictable times years later.
- These substances are usually used sporadically in children and they do not necessarily become addicted to them or need to go through withdrawal. Instead, care is focused on the child who has used the substance and is actively having problems.
- Nursing interventions for the child under the influence of LSD or PCP include:
  - Maintain a safe environment.
  - Assess for the use of other substances.
  - Perform a reality test.
  - Administer a sedative.
  - Provide education on the effects of the drug once the patient is no longer under the influence.
  - Encourage individual and group therapy once the patient is no longer under the influence.

Cocaine/Crack Cocaine

Cocaine is a naturally occurring alkaloid extracted from the leaves of the coca shrub, which was originally found in the Andes Mountains of Peru and Bolivia. Cocaine can be used orally (rubbing on gums), intranasally (snorted), intravenously (dissolved in water), or by inhalation (pipe smoking) (NIDA, 2016). Common street names for cocaine include blow, snow, and powder. Crack cocaine, also known as candy, ball, and/or nuggets, is a mixture of baking soda and cocaine that is compressed into rock form. Even though adolescent cocaine use has declined in recent years, abuse of this substance is still an issue in this age group (NIDA, 2016).

- Cocaine decreases the reuptake of dopamine.
- Use of the drug causes hunger suppression, euphoria, relief of fatigue, decreased anxiety, and increased self-esteem.
- Use may lead to personality changes, irritability, disturbed concentration, compulsive behavior, and insomnia.
- Withdrawal from cocaine is rarely life-threatening.
- Symptoms of acute withdrawal include intense craving, agitation, depression, poor appetite, and insomnia; symptoms last 4 to 10 days.
- Symptoms of chronic withdrawal include fatigue, depression, anhedonia (lack of pleasure), mood disturbance, and cravings.

Nursing Interventions

Nursing interventions for the child or adolescent who is withdrawing from cocaine include:

- Encourage individual and group therapy.
- Assess for the use of other substances.
- Monitor vital signs, especially heart rate and blood pressure.
- Administer anxiolytics, antidepressants, antipsychotics, and dopamine agonists (amantadine, bromocriptine) as ordered.

Prescription Drug Abuse

Prescription drug abuse among youth is the most common form of drug abuse after marijuana and alcohol (NIDA, 2015b). Most youth who abuse prescription drugs are given them cost-free by a friend or family member (NIDA, 2015b). Children often view these drugs as safer than street drugs (NIDA, 2015b). Classes of drugs most commonly abused are opioid pain relievers, stimulants, and benzodiazepines.

Nursing Interventions

- Nursing interventions for the child who is abusing prescription drugs include:
  - Individual and family therapy
  - Group therapy specifically for prescription drug abusers
  - Assess for the use of other substances
  - Refer for inpatient or outpatient withdrawal management

Opiates

Opioids produce pleasurable feelings and reduce pain by interacting with opioid receptors in the central and peripheral nervous systems. Opioid substances can be licit (e.g., morphine) or illicit (heroin). Nearly 25% of individuals who try heroin will become addicted. Adolescent heroin use has more than tripled since 2014 (NIDA, 2015). Opioid addiction tends to start when individuals are prescribed opioids for an illness or injury. Eventually, they begin using heroin instead (NIDA, 2015a) because it is more accessible and costs less than prescription opioids (NIDA, 2015a).

- Examples include opium, heroin, morphine, codeine, and OxyContin
- Increases the release of dopamine
- Effects resemble those of alcohol
- Patient experiences decreased sex drive and decreased hunger, thirst, and pain
- Highly addictive
- Can be taken as by mouth or crushed into powder and inhaled or injected

Opioid Withdrawal

- Rarely life-threatening
- Symptoms vary based on last use of the substance:
  - 8 to 12 hours after last use: tearing, yawning, runny nose
  - 12 to 24 hours after last use: insomnia, poor appetite, abdominal cramping, tremors
  - 48 to 72 hours after last use: all of the above plus depression, diarrhea, goose pimples, bone pain, muscle spasm
- Clinical Institute Narcotic Assessment Scale (CINA) is used to make medication decisions.
  - 11 symptoms
  - The higher the score, the more severe the symptoms

Nursing Interventions

Nursing interventions for the child withdrawing from opioids include:

- Encourage individual and group therapy.
- Refer to NA.
- Assess for the use of other substances.
- Monitor vital signs, especially heart rate and blood pressure.
- Use CINA tool as needed.
- Administer an opiate substitute as ordered, such as methadone, tramadol, or buprenorphine (Suboxone), to suppress withdrawal symptoms and decrease cravings.
- Administer clonidine for increased heart rate, dicyclomine (Bentyl) for stomach cramps, anxiolytics for anxiety, and analgesics for pain, as needed.

Benzodiazepines

- Examples include lorazepam (Ativan), alprazolam (Xanax), temazepam (Restoril), chlordiazepoxide (Librium), and clonazepam (Klonopin).
- Symptoms of withdrawal include anxiety, restlessness, insomnia, and palpitations.
- Symptoms are assessed using the CIWA-B.
- Medication decisions are based on CIWA-B score.

Nursing Interventions

Nursing interventions for the child withdrawing from benzodiazepines include:

- Encourage individual and family therapy.
- Assess for use of other substances.

- Refer to NA.
- Monitor vital signs, especially heart rate.
- Administer phenobarbital as ordered based on CIWA-B score.

Tobacco/Nicotine

Tobacco plants are grown for the leaves, which are dried and fermented before being added to cigarettes and other tobacco products. Nicotine, an addictive substance, is found in tobacco products (NIDA, 2018). Nearly 20% of U.S. youth use tobacco products, and youth with mental illness use tobacco at higher rates than youth without mental illness (NIDA, 2018).

- Toxic and addictive
- Toxicity: 60 mg is fatal; 1 cigarette = 1/2 mg.
- Use can lead to cerebrovascular disease, cancer, and respiratory diseases.
- Dependence develops quickly.
- Increases blood pressure and peristalsis.
- Constricts blood vessels; decreases appetite.
- Stimulates the pleasure center (hypothalamus).
- Acute symptoms of withdrawal include anxiety, irritability, increased appetite, restlessness, increased blood pressure and heart rate, headaches, and fluid retention.
- Chronic symptoms of withdrawal include cravings, mood swings, agitation, inability to concentrate, and poor attention span.

Nursing Interventions

- Nursing interventions for the child who is withdrawing from nicotine include:
  - Assess for the use of other substances.
  - Administer nicotine replacements as ordered, such as gum or a patch.
  - Administer anticraving agents such as bupropion (Zyban, Wellbutrin).
  - May suggest alternative therapies such as hypnosis, acupuncture, or aversion therapy.

Caffeine

- Found in coffee, tea, cola, chocolate, and caffeine drinks/shots/pills
- Often not seen as harmful by children
- Increased alertness and verbal and physical performance
- Stimulates cardiac muscle
- Can lead to diuresis, ulcers, and psychological dependence
- Withdrawal symptoms include anxiety, agitation, restlessness, irritability, muscle twitching, rambling thoughts and speech, headache, irritability, and depression

Nursing Interventions

Nursing interventions for the child withdrawing from caffeine include:

- Provide support and encouragement.
- Educate about the ill effects of caffeine.
- Assess for the use of other substances.

Inhalants

- Examples include glue, gasoline, and anything in a can with a propellant, such as compressed air used to clean off computer keyboards.
- Slang terms include sniffing, huffing, and bagging.
- These substances quickly cross the blood–brain barrier.
- Children may develop mouth ulcers, confusion, headaches, and GI issues.

Nursing Interventions

Nursing interventions for the child using inhalants include:

- Encourage individual and family therapy.
- Assess for the use of other substances.
- Educate about the ill effects of inhalants (Fig. 14–2).
- Address any acute medical conditions caused by the inhalant.

SAFE AND EFFECTIVE NURSING CARE: Clinical Pearl

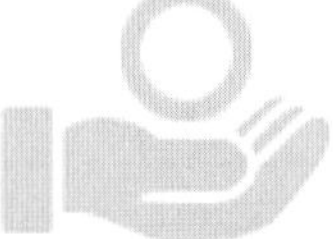

Dual Diagnosis

Dual diagnosis is having a primary mental health disorder with a co-occurring substance issue. These cases often require initial inpatient treatment with ongoing outpatient support. Interventions are aimed at addressing both mental health and addiction. Common dual diagnoses are mood disorders, psychotic disorders, and anxiety disorders (APA, 2013).

Warning Signs of Relapse

- Being around other users
- Severe craving
- Stop attending AA/NA
- Not expressing feelings
- Major emotional crisis

CHILDHOOD ABUSE

Risk factors for abuse and neglect include substance abuse, high levels of stress, unstable interpersonal relationships, and/or lack of social support. The experience of child abuse and neglect places a child at greater risk for development of psychiatric disorders later in life. Nurses are required by law to report any suspected abuse or neglect to child protective agencies. According to the CDC, child sexual abuse is "any completed or attempted (non-completed) sexual act, sexual contact with, or exploitation (ie, noncontact sexual interaction) of a child by a caregiver" (Leeb, Paulozzi, Melanson, Simon, & Arias, 2008).

- Evaluation should be done in a safe, supportive environment.
- Assessment includes questions about unwanted physical or sexual contact, photography, and/or secrecy surrounding the incident(s).

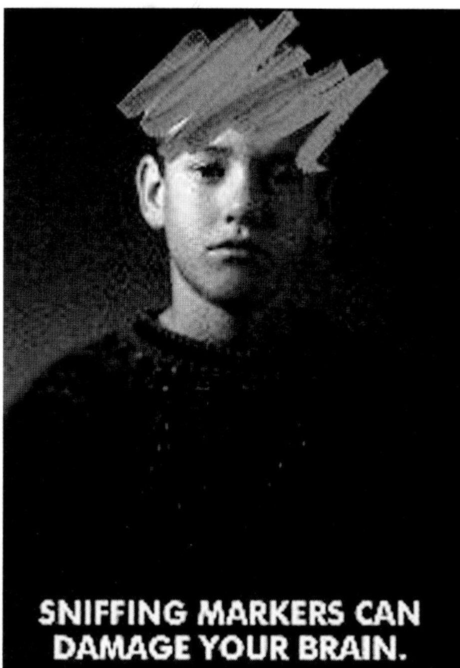

FIGURE 14–2 Educate children and families about the ill effects of inhalants.

- Signs of sexual abuse include bruises, bleeding of genitals and/or rectum, sexually transmitted infections, enuresis or encopresis, sexual acting out with peers, re-traumatizing self by putting objects into body orifices, somatic complaints, sleep difficulties, and/or withdrawal.
- Signs of physical abuse include bruises or lacerations, especially on areas that are not exposed by clothing; marks from objects such as belts, ropes, hands, or cords; bite marks from adults; bald spots on hair; aggression and/or fear toward, or withdrawal from, adults; indiscriminant seeking of affection; and defensive reactions when questioned about injuries.
- Abuse can also be verbal, such as calling the child names or demeaning him or her in front of others.
- Munchausen syndrome by proxy (also known as factitious disorder imposed on another, DSM-5) is when the caregiver, usually the mother, attempts to make the child appear ill. The caregiver may put blood in the child's urine, stool, or vomitus, or report made-up symptoms to health-care providers. The child may be admitted to the hospital for diagnostic tests. If so, the child should be put in a room with a camera so that the caregiver's actions can be monitored.
- Recommended treatments for abuse victims include stabilization of the physical condition, individual and family therapies, removal from the home and/or offender, and assessment for future psychiatric disorders related to the abuse (e.g., depression, anxiety, and PTSD).

Case Study

Alex is a 12-year-old boy who presents to the hospital with his mother and twin brother, Luke, with complaints of feeling "down" most of the time and "nervous" at school. Alex states he attends school regularly and achieves As and Bs, but that he becomes very nervous when interacting with other students, teachers, and school staff members. He states he often feels sad at home and sometimes thinks his mother and brother would be "better off" without him. Alex denies past suicidal ideation or attempts, but states that in the past 2 weeks he has had thoughts of wishing he was dead. Alex has a history of hypothyroidism, but that is controlled with medication. Alex's mother and brother express concern over Alex's sadness and occasional irritability at home. They state Alex has stopped participating in usual family activities such as family game and movie nights. Alex states he has little desire to participate in activities he used to enjoy, such as socializing with his twin, skateboarding, and playing video games. Instead, he spends most nights doing homework, reading, or sleeping. Alex used to enjoy attending school, but that has become difficult now that he has trouble interacting with others.

1. What assessment(s) would be appropriate for Alex based on his presenting complaints?
2. How would you assess for suicide risk for Alex?
3. What other information would you need to gather about Alex? How would you gather this information?

REFERENCES

American Academy of Child & Adolescent Psychiatry (AACAP). (2013). Depression in children and teens No. 4. Retrieved from http://www.aacap.org/AACAP/Families_and_Youth/Facts_for_Families/FFF-Guide/The-Depressed-Child-004.aspx

American Academy of Pediatrics. (2015). Committee on Substance Abuse and Committee on Adolescence. Technical report: the impact of marijuana policies on youth: clinical, research, and legal update. *Pediatrics, 135*, 1825.

American Psychological Association (APA). (2013). *The diagnostic and statistical manual of mental disorders* (5th ed.). Washington, DC: Author.

Avenevoli, S., Swendsen, J., He, J., Burstein, M., & Merikangas, K. (2015). Major depression in the national comorbidity survey–adolescent supplement: prevalence, correlates, and treatment. *Journal of the American Academy of Child & Adolescent Psychiatry, 54*(1), 37–44.e2. doi: 10.1016/j.jaac.2014.10.010

Blair-Gomez, C. (2013). The biological basis of parent-infant attachment: Foundations and implications for further development. *Informes Psicológicos, 13*, 23–40.

Caldwell, B., Albert, C., Azeem, M., Beck, S., Cocoros, D., Cocoros, T., Montes, R., & Reddy, B. (2014). Successful seclusion and restraint prevention efforts in child and adolescent programs. *Journal of Psychosocial Nursing and Mental Health Services, 52*(11), 30–38. doi: 10.3928/02793695-20140922-01

Center for Behavioral Health Statistics and Quality. (2015). Behavioral health trends in the United States: Results from the 2014 National Survey on Drug Use and Health (HHS Publication No. SMA 15-4927, NSDUH Series H-50). Retrieved from http://www.samhsa.gov/data/

Centers for Disease Control and Prevention (CDC). (2015). *WISQARS data and statistics fatal injury report.* Atlanta, GA: CDC.

Centers for Disease Control and Prevention (CDC). (2017). *Lesbian, gay, bisexual and transgender health: LGBT youth.* Atlanta, GA: CDC.

Christensen, D., Baio, J., Braun, K., et al. (2016). Prevalence and characteristics of autism spectrum disorder among children aged 8 years—autism and developmental disabilities monitoring network, 11 sites, United States, 2012. *Morbidity and Mortality Weekly Report 65*(SS-3), 1–23. doi: 10.15585/mmwr.ss6503a1

Collishaw, S. (2015). Annual Research Review: Secular trends in child and adolescent mental health. *Journal of Child Psychology and Psychiatry, 56,* 370–393. doi: 10.1111/jcpp.12372

Cuffe, S., Visser, S., Holbrook, J., Danielson, M, Geryk, L., Wolraich, M., & McKeown, R. E. (2015). ADHD and psychiatric comorbidity: Functional outcomes in a school-based sample of children. *Journal of Attention Disorders.* doi: 10.1177/1087054715613437

Diamond, A. (2013). Executive functions. *Annual Review of Psychology, 64,* 135–168. doi: 10.1146/annurev-psych-113011-143750

Ebert, E., Zarski, S., Christensen, D., Stikkelbroek, M., Cuijpers, V., Berking, M., & Riper, H. (2015). Internet and computer-based cognitive behavioral therapy for anxiety and depression in youth: A meta-analysis of randomized controlled outcome trials. *PLoS ONE, 10*(3), e0119895. doi: 10.1371/journal.pone.0119895

Evans, S. W., Owens, J., & Bunford, M. N. (2014). Evidence-based psychosocial treatments for children and adolescents with attention-deficit/hyperactivity disorder. *Journal of Clinical Child & Adolescent Psychology, 43*(4), 527–551. doi: 10.1080/15374416.2013.850700

Ewing, J. A. (1984). Detecting alcoholism: The CAGE questionnaire. *Journal of the American Medical Association, 252,* 1905–1907. doi: 10.1001/jama.252.14.1905

Harlow, H., Harlow, M., & Suomi, S. (1971). From thought to therapy: Lessons from a private laboratory. *American Scientist, 59,* 538–549.

Harrington, B. C., Jimerson, M., Haxton, C., & Jimerson, D. C. (2015). Initial evaluation, diagnosis, and treatment of anorexia nervosa and bulimia nervosa. *American Family Physician, 91*(1), 46–52.

Hayden, E., & Mash, E. (2014). Child psychopathology: A developmental-systems perspective. In E. Mash & R. Barkley (Eds.), *Child Psychopathology* (3rd ed.). New York: Guilford Press.

Hill, L.S., Reid, F., Morgan, J. F., & Lacey, J. H. (2010). SCOFF, the development of an eating disorder screening questionnaire. *International Journal of Eating Disorders, 43,* 344–351. doi: 10.1002/eat.20679/full

Huebner, D., Thoma B., & Neilands, T. (2015). School victimization and substance use among lesbian, gay, bisexual, and transgender adolescents. *Prevention Science, 16*(5), 734–743.

Kessler, R. C., Chiu, W. T., Demler, O., Merikangas, K. R., & Walters, E. E. (2005). Prevalence, severity, and comorbidity of 12-month DSM-IV disorders in the National Comorbidity Survey Replication. *Archives of General Psychiatry, 62,* 17–27.

Leeb, R. T., Paulozzi, L., Melanson, C., Simon, T. R., & Arias, I. (2008). Child maltreatment surveillance: Uniform definitions for public health and recommended data elements, version 1.0. Atlanta, GA: Centers for Disease Control and Prevention, National Center for Injury Prevention and Control. Retrieved from http://www.cdc.gov/violenceprevention/pdf/cm_surveillance-a.pdf

Lenzenweger, M., & Clarkin, J. (2005). *Major theories of personality disorders* (2nd ed.). New York: Guilford.

Murphy, D., Barry, M., & Vaughn, B. (2013). Mental health disorders. *Child Trends, 1,* 1–10. Retrieved from https://www.childtrends.org/wp-content/uploads/2013/03/Child_Trends-2013_01_01_AHH_MentalDisordersl.pdf

National Institute on Drug Abuse (NIDA). (2015a). *Drugs of abuse: Opioids.* Bethesda, MD: NIDA. Retrieved from http://www.drugabuse.gov/drugs-abuse/opioids

National Institute on Drug Abuse (NIDA). (2015b). *Drug facts: Prescription and over-the-counter medications.* Bethesda, MD: NIDA. Retrieved from http://www.drugabuse.gov/publications/drugfacts/prescription-over-counter-medications.

National Institute on Drug Abuse (NIDA). (2016, May 6). *Cocaine.* Retrieved from https://www.drugabuse.gov/publications/research-reports/cocaine

National Institute on Drug Abuse (NIDA). (2017, December 12). *Marijuana.* Retrieved from https://www.drugabuse.gov/publications/research-reports/marijuana

National Institute on Drug Abuse (NIDA). (2018, January 5). *Tobacco/nicotine and e-cigs.* Retrieved from https://www.drugabuse.gov/drugs-abuse/tobacconicotine-e-cigs

Olfson, M., Blanco, C., Wang, S., Laje, G., & Correll, C. (2014). National trends in the mental health care of children, adolescents, and adults by office-based physicians. *JAMA Psychiatry, 71*(1), 81–90. doi: 10.1001/jamapsychiatry.2013.3074

Peplau, H. (1989). Therapeutic nurse-patient interaction. In A. O'Toole & S. Welt (Eds.), *Interpersonal theory in nursing practice: Selected works of Hildegard E. Peplau* (pp. 192–204). New York: Sage.

Perepletchikova, F., Axelrod, S. R., Kaufman, J., Rounsaville, B. J., Douglas-Palumberi, H., & Miller, A. L. (2011). Adapting dialectical behaviour therapy for children: Towards a new research agenda for paediatric suicidal and non-suicidal self-injurious behaviours. *Child and Adolescent Mental Health, 16*(2), 116–121. doi: 10.1111/j.1475-3588.2010.00583.x

Plemmons, G. (2017, May 7). Trends in suicidality and serious self-harm for children 5-17 years at 32 U.S. children's hospitals, 2008-2015. Abstract presented at the meeting of Pediatric Academic Societies, San Francisco, CA.

Ringoot, A., Jansen, P., Rijlaarsdam, J., So, P., Jaddoe, V., Verhulst, F., & Tiemeier, H. (2017). Self-reported problem behavior in young children with and without a DSM-disorder in the general population. *European Psychiatry, 40,* 110–115. doi: 10.1016/j.eurpsy.2016.08.009

Siu, A. L., on behalf of the U.S. Preventive Services Task Force. (2016). Screening for depression in children and adolescents: U.S. Preventive Services Task Force Recommendation Statement. *Annals of Internal Medicine, 164,* 360–366. doi: 10.7326/M15-2957

Stein, D. J., McLaughlin, K. A., Koenen, K. C., Atwoli, L., Friedman, M. J., Hill, E. D., & Kessler, R. C. (2014). DSM-5 and ICD-11 definitions of post-traumatic stress disorder: Investigating "narrow" and "broad" approaches. *Depression and Anxiety, 31*(6), 494–505.

U.S. Department of Education. (2016). *Parent and educator resource guide to Section 504 in public elementary and secondary schools.* Washington, DC: USDOE.

Verrier, N. (1993). *The primal wound: Understanding the adopted child.* Baltimore, MD: Gateway Press.

Wagner, K. (2016). Update on treatment of pediatric bipolar disorder. *Psychiatric Times, 33*(4). Retrieved from http://www.psychiatrictimes.com/child-adolescent-psychiatry/update-treatment-pediatric-bipolar-disorder/page/0/2

Walkup, J. (2017). Antidepressant efficacy in children and adolescents: Industry and NIMH-funded studies. *American Journal of Psychiatry, 174,* 430–437.

Wallace, J. A. (2011). Bullycide in American schools: Forging a comprehensive legislative solution. *Indiana Law Journal,* 86(2), Article 8. Retrieved from http://www.repository.law.indiana.edu/ilj/vol86/iss2/8

Zeanah, C., Chesher, T., & Boris, N. (2016). Practice parameter for the assessment and treatment of children and adolescents with reactive attachment disorder and disinhibited social engagement disorder. *Journal of the American Academy of Child and Adolescent Psychiatry, 55,* 990–1001.

RESOURCES FOR THE NURSE

American Academy of Child & Adolescent Psychiatry (http://www.aacap.org for practice guidelines and resource centers)

American Psychiatric Nurses Association
https://www.apna.org/i4a/pages/index.cfm?pageid=1

American Psychological Association
http://www.apa.org/

FDA information for pediatrics (http://www.fda.gov/cder/pediatric)

Journal of Child and Adolescent Psychiatric Nursing

National Alliance of Mental Illness
https://www.nami.org/

National Guideline Clearinghouse (http://www.guideline.gov)

National Institute on Drug Abuse
https://www.drugabuse.gov/

National Institute of Mental Health
https://www.nimh.nih.gov/index.shtml

Gastrointestinal Disorders

15

Judith D. McLeod, DNP, RN, CPNP

LEARNING OBJECTIVES

Upon completion of this chapter, the student will be able to:

1. Identify the components of an abdominal examination.
2. Identify the important questions to ask when taking a history about gastrointestinal (GI) problems.
3. Identify and describe GI disease that is associated with the esophagus:
   - Tracheoesophageal fistula/atresia
4. Identify and describe GI diseases that present with abdominal pain:
   - Celiac disease
   - Appendicitis
   - Inguinal hernia
   - Inflammatory bowel disease, including Crohn's disease and ulcerative colitis
   - Irritable bowel syndrome (IBS)
   - Peptic ulcer disease
5. Identify and describe GI disorders associated with regurgitation or vomiting:
   - Gastroesophageal reflux
   - Pyloric stenosis
   - Intestinal obstruction, including volvulus and intussusception
   - Gastroenteritis
6. Identify and describe GI disorders associated with constipation:
   - Functional constipation
   - Hirschsprung's disease
7. Identify and describe GI problems manifested by an anterior abdominal wall defect:
   - Omphalocele
   - Gastroschisis
8. Identify and describe GI disorders associated with the liver, pancreas, or gallbladder:
   - Neonatal jaundice
   - Biliary atresia
   - Hepatitis
   - Fatty liver disease
   - Gallbladder disease
9. Identify and describe gastrointestinal disorders associated with nutrition problems:
   - Obesity
   - Failure to thrive (FTT)

ANATOMY AND PHYSIOLOGY

The gastrointestinal (GI) system encompasses the area from the mouth to the anus and includes the organs responsible for digestion and elimination. The organs in this system include (Fig. 15–1):

- Esophagus
- Stomach
- Small and large intestines
- Liver, gallbladder, and associated bile ducts
- Pancreas

Disruption of functions or disorders in the GI system may cause problems with the child's nutritional status. Children with disordered nutrition may be seen by a gastroenterologist for treatment.

ASSESSMENT

- This section will cover examination of the patient who presents with a GI problem, including the history and physical examination with pertinent findings.

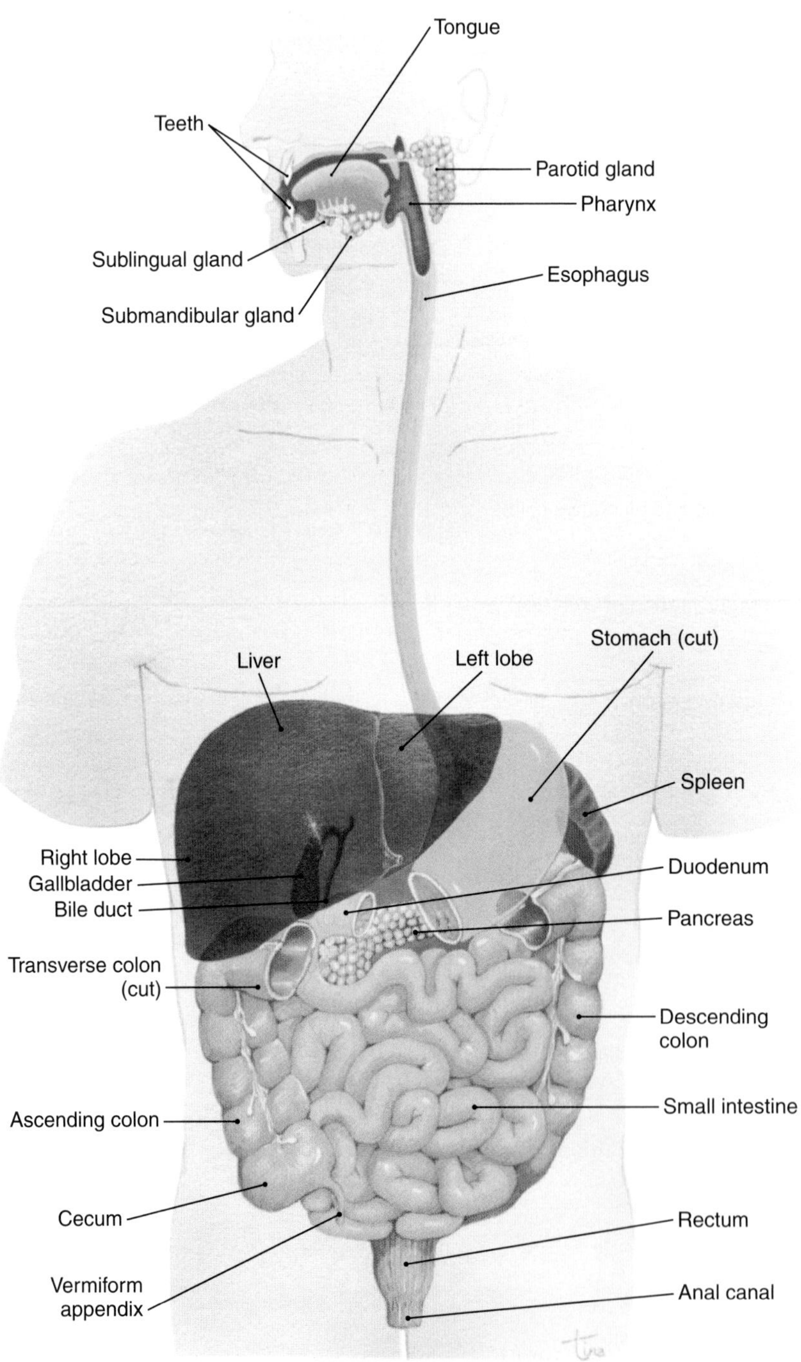

FIGURE 15–1 Digestive system.

History

- Important initial questions:
  - What is the problem?
  - How long has the child had this problem?
  - Has there been weight loss?
  - Is there a history of any previous illness?
  - Has the child recently traveled outside of the country?
- Symptoms:
  - Is the child having abdominal pain?
    - How often does the pain occur?
    - Where is the pain located?
    - Does anything help the pain?
    - Does the pain improve with eating?
    - Does the pain improve with defecating?
    - Does anything make it worse?
  - What is the normal stool pattern?
    - Does the child defecate every day?
    - Is the stool large? Small? Hard? Watery?
    - Does the child have a ritual before stooling?
    - Does the child go to the toilet willingly?
    - Does the child hide before stooling?
    - Does the stool block the toilet after the child defecates?
  - Does the child have diarrhea?
    - How frequent is the diarrhea?
    - Is it very watery?
    - Is it bloody or with mucus?
    - Is there pain associated with the diarrhea?
    - Does it exit the body explosively?
    - Does the patient have cramping or bloating?
    - What has been done to treat the diarrhea?
  - Does the patient have vomiting?
    - How often is the vomiting?
    - Are there symptoms associated with the vomiting?
    - Nausea? Cramping? Abdominal pain? Headache? Fever?
    - Does the child feel better after vomiting?
    - What has been done for the vomiting?
  - What does the child normally eat?
    - Is there a change in the eating pattern?
    - Is an infant refusing the breast or bottle?
- Review the family history, especially for history of GI problems. Complete a genogram with at least three generations to show patterns of illness, if possible.
- Review the social history:
  - Any problems at home
  - Any new stressors

Abdominal Examination

The abdominal examination of a child with GI issues should include the following elements.

Inspection

- Interaction of child with family
- Body positions and movements
  - Can the child climb up and down from the table?
  - Can the child jump down from the table?
  - Does the infant keep their legs drawn up toward the chest?
- Abdomen changes in size and shape with growth
  - Prominent in newborns
  - Flatter in older children
  - Abnormal findings include:
    - Marked distension with shiny appearance caused by air, fluid, or solid tissue enlargement
    - Scaphoid or very flat in newborn
    - "Missing" portions of GI tract may change appearance (Bickley, 2016)
- Children may need distraction during the examination.
  - Allow them to stay on the parent's lap as much as possible during the examination.
  - Infants can breastfeed or use pacifier.
  - Toddlers may be reluctant to leave parent—distraction with light, toy, or other means may be effective.
  - Preschoolers may want to know what is happening and ask questions; they want to know how their bodies work.
  - School-aged children and adolescents may be more cooperative, but they need an explanation of what will happen next.

Auscultation

- Bowel sounds are sounds of normal peristalsis.
- In newborns, air enters the stomach with first cry and reaches the rectum in 3 to 4 hours.
- Bowel sounds are recorded as present or absent.
- Assess bowel sounds in all four quadrants.
- There is an increase in sounds (frequency and volume) with eating.
- No diagnosis can be made on bowel sounds alone.
- Abnormal bowel sounds include:
  - Hyperactive—may indicate gastroenteritis or lactose intolerance
  - High-pitched, loud, tinkling rushes with obstructive process
  - Absence after 5 minutes indicates a paralytic ileus (Bickley, 2016)
- Auscultation of the infant's abdomen is easier if the baby is sucking and is quiet.
- Preschoolers and school-age children may want to listen with the stethoscope after the assessment; this will increase their cooperation.

SAFE AND EFFECTIVE NURSING CARE: Clinical Pearl

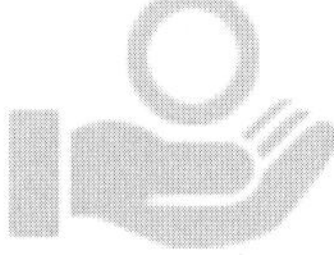

Auscultation Before Palpation

Always perform auscultation of the abdomen before you do palpation. Palpation will change the quality of the bowel sounds and, therefore, may change the assessment (Bickley, 2016).

Percussion

- Assesses distension, liver, and spleen size.
- Tympanic sound shows gaseous area, dull sound with fluid.

Palpation

- Child should be relaxed, supine, arms at side, knees flexed.
- Warm palm if possible; rest entire palm on abdomen.
- Gentle flexion of hand; avoid tickling and poking.
- Use light palpation to decrease pain.
- Having the child place his or her hand on top of the examiner's will allow the child to feel some control during the examination.
- The abdomen is divided into four quadrants; check each quadrant.
- Check for hernia.
- Examine perianal region for fissures, fistula, or skin tags.
- Digital examination may be done to assess anal sphincter tone.
- Note any of the following:
  - Site and severity of pain with any muscle guarding
  - Localized tenderness with involuntary guarding, a sign of peritoneal irritation
  - Check flank on each side for pain.

CLEFT LIP AND PALATE

Cleft lip is an opening in the formation of the lip that can vary in size from a slit to a large opening that extends into the nose. See Chapter 7 for a detailed description of this disorder.

TRACHEOESOPHAGEAL FISTULA

A tracheoesophageal fistula (TEF) is an abnormal connection (fistula) between the esophagus and the trachea. In most cases, the esophagus is discontinuous (atresia), causing immediate feeding difficulties (Wyllie, Hyams, & Kay, 2016).

Clinical Presentation

- History of polyhydramnios while in utero
- Inability to handle secretions—baby may have an overabundance of secretions
- Cyanosis with feeding
- Resistance with passage of a feeding tube
- Associated with syndromes that may have skeletal, anorectal, or limb abnormalities
- Continual choking with feedings after passage of a feeding tube will need further investigation for possible H-type fistula (Wyllie et al., 2016)
- Five types of TEFs:
  - Most common configuration (86%) is esophageal atresia with distal TEF: Proximal esophagus ends blindly in upper mediastinum; distal esophagus is connected to the tracheobronchial tree.
  - Second most common type (8%) is isolated esophageal atresia with no TEF: Has small stomach, gasless abdomen.
  - The third most common type (4%) is H- or N-type TEF with no esophageal atresia.
  - The fourth type (1%) is esophageal atresia with both a proximal and distal TEF.
  - The fifth type (1%) is esophageal atresia with a proximal TEF (Wyllie et al., 2016) (Fig. 15–2).

Diagnostic Tests

- Coiling of feeding tube is noted on x-ray.
- Bowel gas pattern may be abnormal.
- Ultrasound of renal system
- Echocardiogram
- A contrast evaluation for fistula may be performed.

Nursing Interventions

Nursing interventions for patients with TEF include emergency care, acute hospital care, and chronic care.

Emergency Care

- Prevention of aspiration is important
- Tube should be placed in proximal pouch until surgery
- IV access with fluids and antibiotics
- Supine position with head elevated
- Oxygen if needed

Acute Hospital Care

- Surgical repair is indicated
- Prepare caregiver/patient for surgery
- Witness informed consent
- IV support after surgery (Box 15–1)

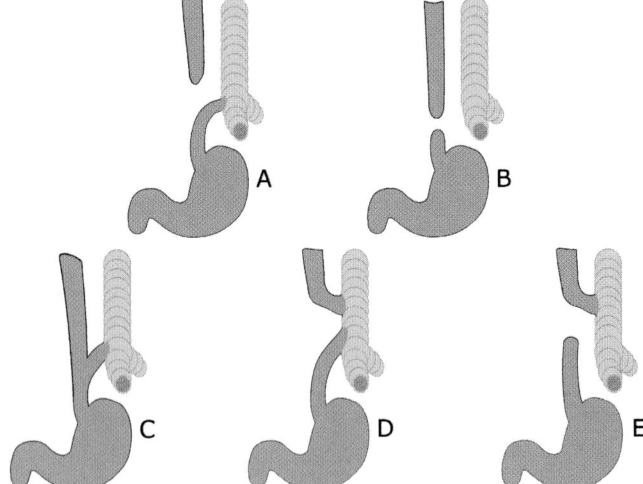

FIGURE 15–2 Tracheoesophageal fistulas. **A,** Esophageal atresia with distal tracheoesophageal fistula, **B,** isolated esophageal atresia with no tracheoesophageal fistula, **C,** H- or N-type tracheoesophageal fistula with no esophageal atresia, and **D,** esophageal atresia with a proximal tracheoesophageal fistula. **E,** Esophageal atresia with a blind pouch.

BOX 15–1 | Intravenous Therapy and Antibiotics in the Pediatric Gastrointestinal Patient

IV therapy in the GI patient may be administered because the pediatric patient is unable to maintain daily fluid requirements, or to restore or replace ongoing losses in fluid because of gastrointestinal disease. An example would be severe diarrhea or vomiting caused by acute gastroenteritis or diarrhea in IBD. Electrolytes may be administered in IV fluids to maintain and correct fluid and electrolyte imbalance.

Common IV Solutions

- Sodium chloride 0.9% (normal saline)
- Lactated Ringer's (LR)
- Sodium chloride 0.45% (0.45 NaCl)
- Dextrose 5%/sodium chloride 0.9% (D5 0.9 NaCl)
- Dextrose 5%/sodium chloride 0.45% (D5 0.45 NaCl)
- Dextrose 5%/sodium chloride 0.2% (D5 0.2 NaCl)
- Dextrose 5%/lactated Ringer's (D5LR)

Normal saline and lactated Ringer's are considered isotonic solutions. Normal saline is usually the solution of choice to begin treatment in the pediatric patient. A careful history and physical examination, as well as monitoring of laboratory values, such as electrolytes, glucose, bicarbonate, blood urea nitrogen, and creatinine, will help the provider determine the correct IV solution to use for each patient and whether a solution needs to be changed, such as changing to a solution containing dextrose because of low glucose levels.

Severe dehydration requires immediate treatment with IV or intraosseous (if an IV cannot be started) access. A patient who needs this therapy may have lethargy, tenting of the skin when pinched, depressed fontanels in infants, dry mucous membranes, decreased urine output, and/or lack of tears when crying. Normal saline is usually used for fluid resuscitation of the child with a bolus of fluid given at 20 mL/kg over 20 to 30 minutes. Careful monitoring of vital signs and level of consciousness, as well as laboratory values (electrolytes and glucose especially), is required. Several boluses of fluid may be required. Once the child is stable, the fluid may be infused at 10 mL/kg and the child started on oral rehydration as tolerated.

IV access also allows for the following:

- Administration of blood and its components
- Administration of parenteral medication (e.g., antibiotics, chemotherapy, analgesics)
- Administration of TPN
- Provides IV access in case of an emergency
- Provision of access for diagnostic purposes (e.g., dye injection before a procedure)

Antibiotics

The choice of antibiotics for each pediatric patient is determined by the provider caring for the patient and cultures that may have been drawn, which will show susceptibility of bacteria to the antibiotic.

Some common antibiotics used in pediatric GI care may include:

- Ampicillin (25 to 200 mg/kg/day) divided every 6 to 8 hours and gentamicin (2.5 mg/kg/day) every 8 hours commonly used in newborns and infants
- Cefazolin: 25mg/kg every 12 hours; may be used preoperatively and postoperatively
- Metronidazole: 30 mg/kg/day PO/IV divided every 6 hours; not to exceed 4 g/day
- Clindamycin: 20 to 40 mg/kg via IV infusion or IM injection per day, in 3 to 4 equally divided doses

Other antibiotics may be used if indicated.

(Burns et al., 2016; Wyllie et al., 2016)

- Chest tube care
- Continued antibiotics
- Frequent suctioning with a premeasured catheter
- Elevate head of bed 30 to 45 degrees
- Tube feedings start 2 to 3 days after surgery
- Acid suppression therapy with PPI such as lansoprazole, omeprazole, or pantoprazole after surgery to promote healing
- If no leak 5 to 7 days after surgery, start oral feedings
- Chest tube out with start of oral feedings
- Most babies respond well and do not experience complications

Chronic Care

- Leak of the surgical site requires continued IV therapy and chest tube.
- Leaks usually close spontaneously.
- Stricture may occur, which may require dilation of the stricture over 3 to 6 months.
- Reoccurrence of fistula formation may require more surgery for repair.

Caregiver Education

The nurse should educate caregivers in the following aspects of emergency, acute, and chronic care.

Emergency Care

- Explain need for IV fluids.
- Provide information about the diagnostic tests.
- Preoperative teaching for the caregiver is essential.
- Provide reassurance to caregivers as needed.

Acute Hospital Care

- Explain postoperative procedures.
- Provide emotional support.
- Nonnutritive sucking with a pacifier should be encouraged before oral feeding begins.
- Caregiver may assist with oral feeding once child has improved.
- Encourage caregiver to hold infant if stable; if unable to hold baby, then touching and stroking should be encouraged.
- Teach about signs to observe for at home on discharge.

Chronic Care

- Caregiver will need instruction on observing for and treating gastroesophageal reflux (see Gastroesophageal Reflux for treatment information).
- Caregiver should be taught baby feeding cues and signs of desire for interaction, as well as disengagement cues.
- Caregiver will need to keep all follow-up appointments.
- Caregiver will need to observe for and report any pulmonary difficulties.

GASTROINTESTINAL PROBLEMS MANIFESTED BY ABDOMINAL PAIN

GI conditions may be manifested by a description of either specific or vague symptoms of abdominal pain by the child.

Celiac Disease

Celiac disease is an immune-mediated systemic disease caused by the ingestion of wheat gliadin and related prolamines in genetically susceptible individuals. When people with celiac disease eat gluten (a protein found in wheat, rye, and barley), the body mounts an immune response that attacks the small intestine. These attacks lead to damage on the villi, small finger-like projections that line the small intestine that promote nutrient absorption. When the villi get damaged, nutrients cannot be absorbed properly into the body. Celiac disease is hereditary (Wyllie et al., 2016).

Assessment

See Figure 15–3 for the clinical presentation of celiac disease. Manifestations typically begin after food has been introduced into the diet at approximately 6 months of age and include:

- Abdominal bloating
- Diarrhea
- Vomiting
- Weight loss—may appear very skinny in the extremities but normal weight in the face
- Flatulence
- Foul-smelling stools
- Delayed growth and development, including short stature, delayed puberty
- Dental enamel defects in the teeth
- Dermatitis herpetiformis—blistering, pruritic skin rash on elbows, buttocks, or knees
  - More common in adults
  - Does not occur in all cases

In its most severe form, celiac disease can cause:

- Iron deficiency anemia
- B_{12} deficiency
- Osteopenia or osteoporosis due to calcium malabsorption (Palance, 2014)

> **CRITICAL COMPONENT**
>
> **Celiac Disease**
>
> Celiac disease is recognized as a genetic disorder, occurring in 1 in 141 people. In patients with a first-degree relative—parent, sibling, or child—the rate is 1 in 22 people (Rubio-Tapia, Ludvigsson, Brantner, Murray, & Everhart, 2012).
>
> Celiac disease may also occur in conjunction with other diseases, including diabetes, autoimmune thyroid disease, autoimmune liver disease, rheumatoid arthritis, systemic lupus erythematosus, and Sjögren's disease. It is recommended that any patient diagnosed with these diseases also be tested for celiac disease. A gluten-free diet used by a diabetic with concurrent celiac disease will result in a decrease in insulin needs (Palance, 2014).

Diagnostic Studies

- Complete blood cell count (CBC) with differential
- Anti-tissue transglutaminase antibodies
- Total immunoglobulin A (IgA)
- IgA antiendomysial antibodies
- Vitamin B_{12} level, ferritin, total iron-binding capacity, folate
- Stool for occult blood, fat, *Helicobacter pylori* antigen (Palance, 2014)
- Endoscopy and tissue biopsy for definitive diagnosis

Nursing Interventions

The nurse caring for a patient with celiac disease must perform the following interventions.

Emergency Care

- May require IV hydration for vomiting or diarrhea

Acute Hospital Care

- Prepare patient for endoscopy examination.
- Patient should not start gluten-free diet before endoscopy examination.
- Explain procedure to patient and family.
- Work with dietitian to teach patient and family about gluten-free diet before discharge.

Discharge

- Teach patient and family about gluten-free diet.
  - Refer family to http://celiac.org for information on disease and diet.
- Refer patient and caregivers to a support group for the disease.
- Alternative therapies:
  - Gluten-free diet is the definitive therapy and does not require medication.

Caregiver Education

Nurses must educate caregivers about the following aspects of caring for a child who has celiac disease.

Emergency Care

- Recognize celiac crisis, manifested by extreme vomiting, diarrhea, and dehydration. This may occur in susceptible children

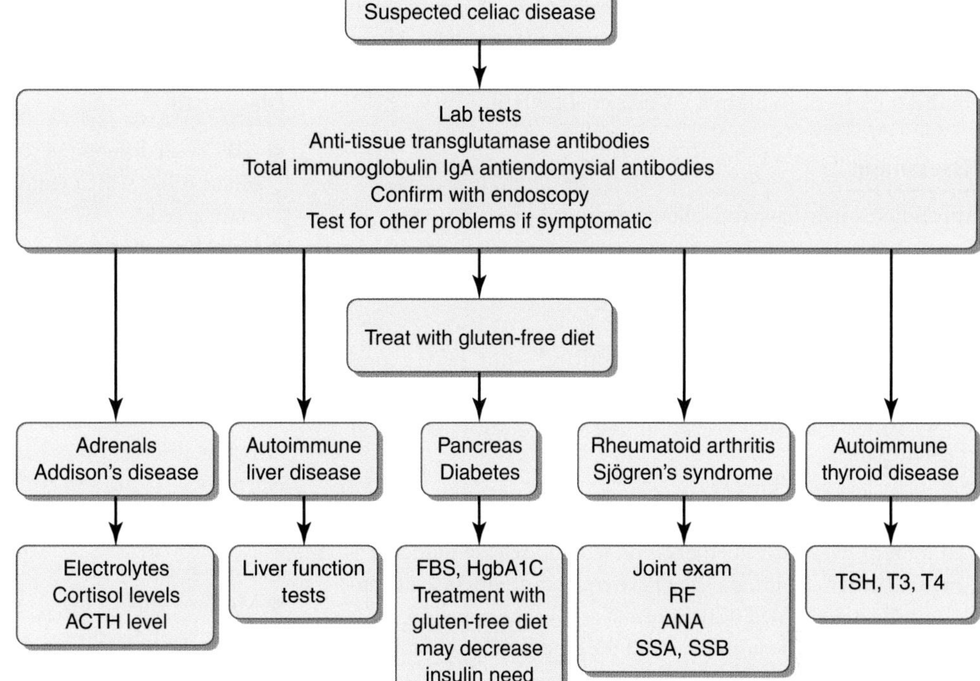

FIGURE 15–3 Diseases that can be associated with a diagnosis of celiac disease. ACTH, adrenocorticotropic hormone; ANA, antinuclear antibodies; FBS, fasting blood sugar; HgBA1C, hemoglobin A1C; RF, rheumatoid factor; SSA, Sjögren's syndrome antigen; SSB, Sjögren's syndrome B; TSH, thyroid stimulating hormone.

who received gluten-containing foods early and have increasingly severe reactions to gluten.

- Require IV therapy and electrolyte replacement, usually normal saline with potassium.
- Once on a gluten-free diet, most patients will not require emergency care.
- Failure to respond to the diet may indicate another underlying disease or failure to avoid gluten.

Acute Hospital Care

- Caregivers and patient will need to learn components of a gluten-free diet
- Referral to a dietitian
- Discuss food likes and dislikes, and teach family how to read labels for gluten
- Retrieve information from http://celiac.org about diet and support groups

Chronic Care

- Monitor adherence to the gluten-free diet by the patient.
- Many gluten-free products are available, so it is important to read labels.
- Provide a list of area stores/restaurants that carry gluten-free products if available.
- Regular follow-up with the gastroenterologist is essential.
- Participation in a support group either in person or online is helpful.
- Encourage child's participation in camps and outings with other children with celiac disease.
- Have caregivers and other family members screened also.

SAFE AND EFFECTIVE NURSING CARE: Cultural Competence

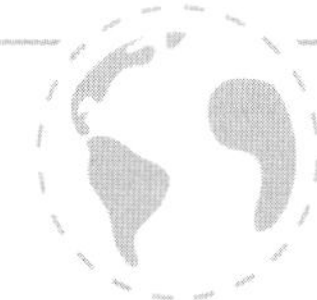

The Impact of Cultural Dietary Traditions on Illness

Food plays a part in many cultural traditions, including the dishes served during holiday meals. When a child is diagnosed with a GI problem that affects food intake, it is important to talk with the family members about how this will affect them in their food preparation, as well as their daily lives. The child may not be able to eat some traditional dishes because of gluten intolerance or intestinal pain, and the family and care providers both need to be sensitive to this issue.

For instance, the holiday turkey with traditional stuffing may not be appropriate for the child with gluten intolerance, and this diet restriction needs to be explained to all family members so they are not offended when the child does not eat this food. Many cultures use wheat in food products such as tortillas or noodles, and families need to be aware of the problems these foods could cause a child. Celiac disease may make it more difficult to participate in religious ceremonies such as communion, because communion wafers contain wheat. Discussing this problem with church leaders may help to find solutions, such as low-gluten wafers or communion with just wine (Palance, 2014). Nurses must be aware of cultural impact while teaching families about necessary changes in the child's diet (see Chapter 4 for further details).

Appendicitis

Appendicitis is inflammation of the appendix, a finger-shaped pouch that projects from your colon on the lower right side of your abdomen. Appendicitis is one of the most common surgical conditions affecting children (Wyllie et al., 2016).

Assessment

Appendicitis may have the following clinical presentation.

- Initial pain in the periumbilical area that moves to the right lower quadrant of the abdomen (Fig. 15–4)
- Low-grade fever
- May be nauseated and have vomiting—not taking oral intake
- Usually does not have stool, but may present with diarrhea or pelvic pain
- Usually lays with knees bent
- Rebound pain with examination in right lower quadrant
  - Pain in right side when press on left and release suddenly
  - McBurney's point is a site of extreme sensitivity in acute appendicitis, situated in the normal area of the appendix midway between the umbilicus and the anterior iliac crest in the right lower quadrant of the abdomen
  - Pain after internal rotation of flexed thigh
  - Pain on passive extension of right hip

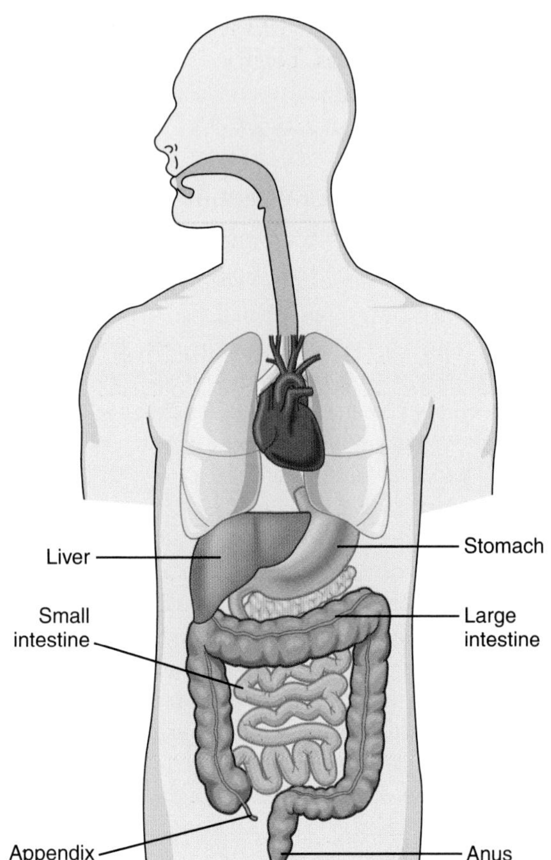

FIGURE 15–4 The appendix is a finger-like pouch attached to the large intestine in the lower right area of the abdomen.

  - Pain in right lower quadrant when jumping and landing on the heels (Bickley, 2016)
- Pain for several days with sudden resolution; an ill-looking child may indicate perforation of the appendix

Diagnostic Testing

- CBC with differential sometimes shows elevation of the white blood cells (WBCs) and a left shift of the WBCs toward less mature cells
- Urinalysis
- Ultrasound
- Computerized tomography (CT) scan usually ordered after consultation with a surgeon

Nursing Interventions

Nursing interventions for patients with appendicitis include emergency, acute, and chronic care.

Emergency Care

- Patient will be NPO.
- Monitor vital signs.
- Assist with diagnostic tests, including ultrasound and CT.
- Assist with positioning patient in position of comfort.
- Administer IV fluids as ordered.
- Explain tests to patient and family.
- Prepare patient for surgery, including required preoperative teaching.

Acute Hospital Care

- Monitor vital signs.
- Maintain IV therapy and then advance diet as tolerated.
- Assess pain with appropriate pain scale (FACES for young child, scale of 1–10 for older child) and administer pain medication as ordered.
- Encourage use of incentive spirometer.
- Encourage ambulation.
- Monitor incisional sites: three if done laparoscopically or right lower quadrant incision site if surgery is done using the traditional method.
- Provide discharge instructions to patient and caregiver.

Chronic Hospital Care

- If the appendix is ruptured, the patient may have a prolonged hospital stay because of possible peritonitis from contents of the appendix leaking into the abdomen.
- Administer IV therapy as ordered.
- Monitor nasogastric (NG) drainage if ordered.
- Monitor vital signs.
- Monitor laboratory tests, such as CBC and cultures.
- Monitor drainage and change dressings as needed.
- Assess for pain and administer medication as needed.
- Most acute appendicitis is now treated by laparoscopic removal.
- Nonsurgical treatment
  - Used occasionally if patient is not well enough to undergo surgery
  - Includes IV antibiotics
  - Liquid or soft diet until the infection subsides

Caregiver Education

Nurses must educate parents and caregivers of children with appendicitis on the following aspects of the condition.

Emergency Care

- Provide information about the diagnostic tests.
- Preoperative teaching for the caregiver and patient is essential.

Acute Hospital

- Instruct caregiver about medication administration for pain and antibiotics.
- Encourage caregiver to assist patient with ambulation as needed and stress its importance.
- Encourage child and caregiver to report pain and assist with medication or nonpharmacological methods of relief, such as massage, distraction, music, and aromatherapy.
- Teach caregiver and patient signs of infection—redness in incision, fever, unrelieved pain.
- Provide discharge instructions and follow-up care.

Discharge Instructions

- Instruct patient and caregivers to limit lifting and physical activity for several weeks.
- Teach patient and caregiver importance of medication administration after ruptured appendix.
- Teach caregiver and patient signs of infection—redness in incision, fever, unrelieved pain.
- Teach patient and caregiver importance of keeping follow-up appointments.

Inguinal Hernia

A hernia is a protrusion of contents through a defect or opening. The type of hernia is defined by its location. An inguinal hernia is a protrusion of the intra-abdominal contents through the external or internal inguinal rings (Wyllie et al., 2016).

Assessment

Inguinal hernia typically has the following clinical presentation:

- Lump in the groin, commonly on the right side
- History of intermittent pain and swelling in the groin
- Feeling of weakness or pressure in the groin
- A burning, gurgling feeling at the bulge
- Patient with a hydrocele should be checked for inguinal hernia
- With incarceration—increase in pain, fever, tachycardia, bilious vomiting due to obstruction and no stooling
- With strangulation—erythema and edema over a tender groin mass

Diagnostic Testing

- Palpation of the hernia on examination
  - Patient will be upright and cough or bear down, which causes the hernia to extrude and be felt during manual examination
  - Reduction of the hernia during examination
  - Transillumination of the hydrocele to rule out hernia—no intervention needed if only hydrocele
  - Report of caregiver of lump seen in groin area

Nursing Interventions

Nursing interventions with pediatric patients with inguinal hernia include emergency care, acute care, and discharge instructions.

Emergency Care

- Start IV fluids.
- Prepare patient for surgery.
- Witness informed consent.
- Provide support to caregivers as needed.

Acute Care

- May be performed on an outpatient basis if no incarceration.
- Start IV fluids if not emergent.
- Answer questions and provide support for caregivers.
- Provide appropriate pain medication postoperatively.
- Encourage nonnutritive sucking for infants.
- Keep suture line clean and dry.
  - In infants and toddlers who are not toilet trained, frequent diaper change is necessary.
  - Assess circulation on the side of the surgical incision.

Discharge Instructions

- Once repaired, the patient should not have additional problems with that side.
- The opposite side, if not repaired, will need periodic examination.
- Umbilical hernias may also occur, but are not repaired in newborns. They usually spontaneously close at 1 year.
- Older children may later need repair.

Caregiver Education

The nurse must educate the caregiver of a child with inguinal hernia on the following measures.

Emergency Care

- Provide information about the diagnostic tests.
- Preoperative teaching for the caregiver and patient is essential.

Discharge Teaching

- Teach caregiver care of surgical site.
- Encourage feeding of patient as tolerated.
- Administer pain medication as needed.
- Note importance of keeping scheduled appointments.
- Caregivers should observe opposite side for hernia.
- Report any problems to health-care provider.

INFLAMMATORY BOWEL DISEASE

A group of chronic intestinal diseases characterized by inflammation of the bowel (the large or small intestine). The most common types of inflammatory bowel disease (IBD) are ulcerative colitis and Crohn's disease (Wyllie et al., 2016).

Crohn's Disease

Crohn's disease is a chronic IBD characterized by immune response to injured tissue that causes redness, swelling, and pain of the GI tract. Crohn's disease can affect any part of the GI tract from the mouth to the anus, but it is more commonly found at the end of the small intestine and may extend through the entire thickness of the bowel wall (Wyllie et al., 2016).

Assessment

Crohn's disease may have the following clinical presentation.

- Abdominal pain
  - Often presents in the right lower quadrant (Fig. 15–5)
  - May mimic appendicitis
- Fever
- Diarrhea (possibly bloody)
- Nausea and vomiting
- Anorexia
- Weight loss and fatigue
- Anemia
- Delayed growth and development
- Oral aphthous ulcers: Canker sores are small, shallow lesions that develop on the soft tissues in the mouth or at the base of the gums. Unlike cold sores, canker sores do not occur on the surface of the lips and are not contagious.
- Intestinal blockage
- Fistula formation
- Periods of exacerbation and remission
- May be mild with minimal symptoms to severe with fulminant disease (Tanida et al., 2015; Wyllie et al., 2016)

Diagnostic Testing

- CBC, electrolytes, liver enzymes, sedimentation rate, C-reactive protein (CRP)
- Serum calcium and phosphorus, zinc, magnesium
- Total protein and albumin
- Urinalysis
- Stool for occult blood and WBCs, ova, and parasites
- Stool culture
- IBD laboratory panel
- Upper GI series with small bowel follow-up
- Ultrasound
- CT scan
- Colonoscopy with tissue biopsy
- Ophthalmic examination

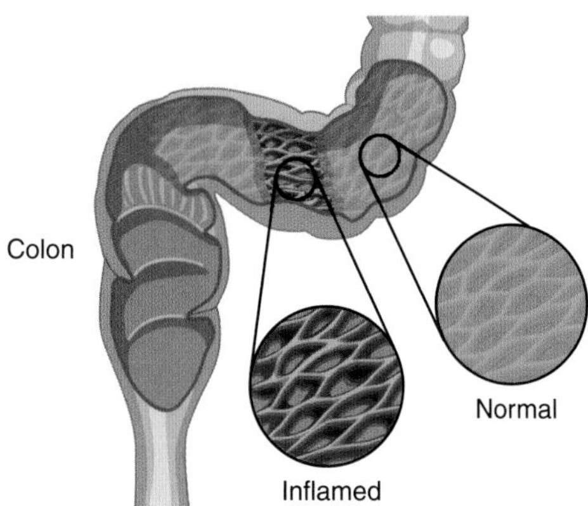

FIGURE 15–5 In Crohn's disease, portions of the digestive tract become inflamed. The diseased lining of the digestive tract becomes swollen and scarred.

Nursing Interventions

Nursing interventions for pediatric patients who have Crohn's disease include emergency, acute, and chronic care.

Emergency Care

- Periods of abdominal pain with bleeding require immediate treatment
- IV therapy
- High-dose corticosteroids, such as prednisone or prednisolone: for moderate flares of IBD, typical recommendation is prednisone at 10 to 40 mg/day; for more severe flares, dosages up to 60 mg/day may be used, tapered once patient improves

Acute Care

- May require IV therapy for hydration
- Corticosteroid therapy to induce remission
- Antibiotics may be used, such as ciprofloxacin (Cipro) and metronidazole (Flagyl)
- Tacrolimus or cyclosporine
- Start infliximab therapy
- May require surgery

Chronic Care

- Drug therapy
  - Mesalamine
  - Antibiotics such as ciprofloxacin or metronidazole
  - Immunosuppressives such as azathioprine, 6-mercaptopurine, or methotrexate
  - Infliximab therapy (tumor necrosis factor [TNF] blocker)—maintenance dosing every 6 to 8 weeks
- Nutritional supplementation may be necessary
- Surgery if medication does not control the symptoms and to correct potential complications of Crohn's disease—such as clearing an intestinal blockage or repairing damage to the intestines; damage to the intestines can include a perforation or abscess (Tanida et al., 2015; Wyllie et al., 2016)

Caregiver Education

Educate the parents and/or caregivers of Crohn's disease patients of the following measures.

Emergency Care

- Caregivers need to bring patient in for treatment with signs of bleeding or pain.

Acute Care

- Caregivers and patient need education about medications.
- Discuss concerns with caregiver and patient.

- Discuss feelings with child or adolescent about having a chronic disease.
- Work with child and adolescent on diet; discuss dietary likes and dislikes.
- Strive for some normalcy in diet between exacerbations.
- Teach patient and caregivers about stress-reduction techniques such as visualization and relaxation techniques.

Chronic Care

- Review use and side effects of medications with patient and caregivers.
- Review importance of regular follow-up examinations.
- Encourage patient to report if side effects of medications occur.
- Caregivers should report any illness to the gastroenterologist for possible medication adjustment.
- Refer caregiver and child to camps or other activities so that child can experience normal activities with other children with similar diseases.
- Discuss diet and how to maintain good nutrition, and incorporate dietary preferences.
- Refer patient and caregivers to a support group.

Ulcerative Colitis

Ulcerative colitis causes inflammation and ulcers in the lining of the large intestine. It usually affects the lower section (sigmoid colon) and the rectum, but can affect the entire colon. The more of the colon affected, the worse the symptoms will be (Wyllie et al., 2016).

Assessment

Ulcerative colitis may have the following clinical presentation:

- Abdominal pain (Fig. 15–6)
- Bloody diarrhea—watery with streaks of blood
- Urgency to defecate
- Anemia
- Fatigue
- Weight loss
- Loss of appetite
- Rectal bleeding
- Skin lesions
- Joint pain
- Growth failure
- Symptoms may be mild or with frequent bouts of bloody diarrhea, fever, and abdominal cramping.

Diagnostic Testing

- CBC, electrolytes, liver enzymes, sedimentation rate, CRP
- Total protein, albumin
- Serum iron, total iron-binding capacity, ferritin
- Stool for occult blood and WBCs, ova, and parasites; stool culture
- Stool for *Clostridium difficile*
- IBD laboratory panel
- Colonoscopy with tissue biopsy

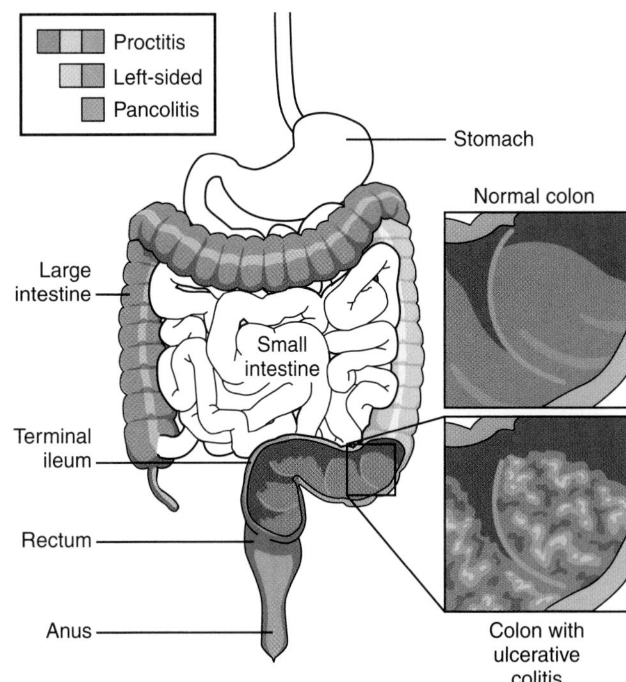

FIGURE 15–6 Ulcerative colitis is an inflammatory bowel disease (IBD), the general name for diseases that cause inflammation in the small intestine and colon.

Nursing Interventions

Nursing interventions for patients with ulcerative colitis may include emergency, acute, and chronic care.

Emergency Care

- Periods of abdominal pain with bleeding require immediate treatment:
  - IV therapy
  - Antibiotics such as ciprofloxacin or metronidazole

Acute Care

- May require IV therapy for hydration
- Corticosteroid therapy to induce remission
- Metronidazole, ciprofloxacin, and other antibiotics may be used when infections occur or to treat complications of ulcerative colitis
- Pain medication
- Antidiarrheals
- May require surgery

Chronic Care

- Drug therapy
  - Aminosalicylates such as sulfasalazine or mesalamine may be given orally, as a suppository, or as an enema
  - Corticosteroids—prednisone orally, IV, enema, or suppository; best suited for short-term control of IBD symptoms and disease activity
  - Immunosuppressives such as azathioprine, 6-mercaptopurine
  - Cyclosporine A may be given for severe disease (Wyllie et al., 2016)

- Nutritional supplementation may be necessary
- Surgery if medication does not control the symptoms
- If severe, surgical resection of the colon will be performed with creation of an ileostomy

Caregiver Education

Educate parents and caregivers about the following measures.

Emergency Care

- Caregivers need to bring patient in for treatment with signs of bleeding or pain.

Acute Care

- Caregivers and patient need education about medications.
- Discuss concerns with caregiver and patient.
- Discuss feelings about having a chronic disease with the child or adolescent.
- Teach patient and caregivers about stress-reduction techniques such as visualization and relaxation techniques.

Chronic Care

- Review use and side effects of medications with patient and caregivers.
- Review importance of regular follow-up examinations.
- Encourage patient to report if side effects of medications occur.
- Report any illness to the gastroenterologist for possible medication adjustment.
- If surgical intervention, answer patient and caregiver concerns about surgery.
- Refer patient and caregivers to a support group.
- Refer caregiver and child to camps or other activities so that child can experience normal activities with other children with similar diseases.

Peptic Ulcer Disease

Peptic ulcers are open sores that develop on the inside lining of the stomach or the upper portion of the small intestine. The most common symptom of a peptic ulcer is stomach pain. Peptic ulcers include:

- Gastric ulcers that occur on the inside of the stomach
- Duodenal ulcers that occur on the inside of the upper portion of the small intestine

The most common causes of peptic ulcers are infection with the bacterium *H. pylori* and long-term use of aspirin and certain other painkillers, such as ibuprofen (Advil, Motrin, others) and naproxen sodium (Aleve, Anaprox, others). Stress and spicy foods do not cause peptic ulcers. However, they can make the symptoms worse (Fashner & Gitu, 2015).

Assessment

Early clinical presentation includes the following symptoms with gastritis; however, some patients are asymptomatic (Fig. 15–7):

- Recurrent abdominal pain
- Nausea, vomiting, anorexia
- Decrease in growth

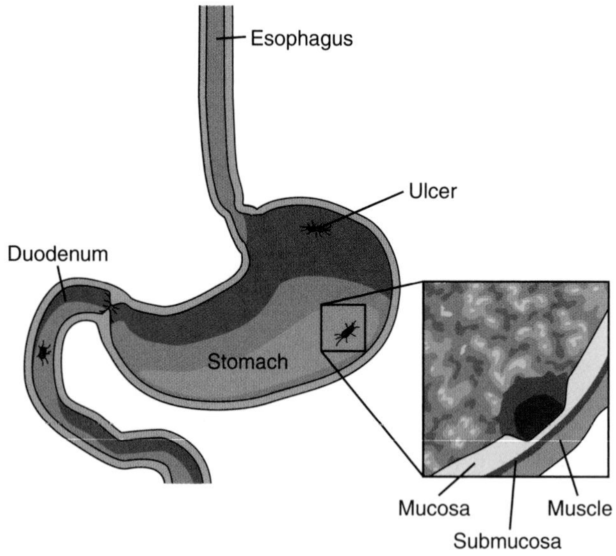

FIGURE 15–7 Peptic ulcers occur in the wall of the stomach and duodenum.

- Proceeds to crampy epigastric pain
- Change in eating habits

These symptoms proceed to:

- Chronic, recurrent abdominal pain
- Episodic epigastric pain
- Vomiting that is recurrent
- Nocturnal awakening
- Anemia
- May have life-threatening GI bleeding
- Perforation of the stomach or duodenum
- Shock

SAFE AND EFFECTIVE NURSING CARE: Clinical Pearl

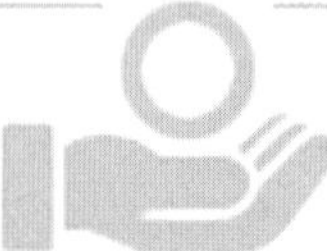

Symptoms of Peptic Ulcer

Infants may display hematemesis, melena, distention, and respiratory distress with an ulcer. Toddlers may have anorexia or vomiting. Bleeding follows within several weeks. Preschool children have pain as the presenting symptom, which occurs on arising and is not relieved by food. Older school-age children and adolescents will have symptoms similar to adult patients with ulcer (Wyllie et al., 2016).

Diagnostic Testing

- CBC, erythrocyte sedimentation rate (ESR)
- *H. pylori* antibody blood test
- *H. pylori* antigen in stool
- Stool for occult blood, WBC count
- Upper GI series
- Endoscopy with biopsy and *H. pylori* culture

Nursing Interventions

Nursing interventions for peptic ulcer disease include emergency, acute, and chronic care.

Emergency Care

- Patient should be seen immediately for:
  - Sudden, persistent stomach pain
  - Bloody or black stools
  - Bloody vomit or coffee-grounds vomit
- NPO
- IV therapy

Acute Care

- Maintain IV therapy if needed.
- Provide explanation of treatment to patient and caregiver.
- Start treatment using triple therapy.

SAFE AND EFFECTIVE NURSING CARE: Understanding Medication

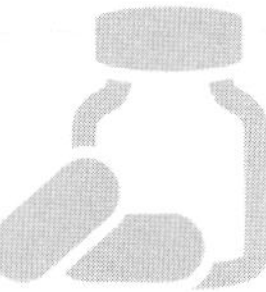

Triple Therapy

Ulcers are typically treated with a medication regimen known as triple therapy. Triple therapy usually consists of two antibiotics, often amoxicillin and Flagyl, tetracycline (for those older than 8 years), or clarithromycin, along with a proton pump inhibitor such as omeprazole, lansoprazole, or pantoprazole (Fashner & Gitu, 2015).

Chronic Care

- Monitor medication and patient compliance.

Complementary and Alternative Therapies

- A vaccine for *H. pylori* is currently under investigation; it has shown some success in animal models, but no active vaccine exists yet
- Avoidance of NSAIDs
- Good hand hygiene

Caregiver Education

Nurse education for caregivers of those with peptic ulcer disease should include the following measures.

Emergency Care

- Caregivers should be taught to recognize signs of serious disease, including bloody vomit or stools and severe pain.
- Instruct caregivers about therapy and diagnostic tests to be performed.

Acute Care

- Assist caregiver and patient with therapy.
- Explain importance of medication compliance (Table 15–1).
- Teach caregiver possible medication side effects.
- Reassure caregiver and patient when stress occurs.
- Teach stress-reduction techniques to child and caregiver.

Chronic Care

- Teach importance of completing therapy.
- Teach importance of follow-up care.
- Teach side effects of medication to report if they occur.

TABLE 15–1 Common Medications Used in Gastrointestinal Disease

DRUG	USES	DOSAGE	POSSIBLE SIDE EFFECTS OR WARNINGS
Omeprazole	GERD, acid-related stomach and esophageal problems, stomach and intestinal ulcers	1 mg/kg/day divided doses twice a day If >20 kg, give 20 mg daily	Long-term exposure may increase risk for gastric tumors Can cause palpitations, change in heart rate, nausea, flatulence, discolored stools, fever, or upper respiratory infection symptoms Elevated liver function tests, fatigue, dizziness, headaches and myalgias, leg pain, hematuria or glycosuria Do not crush or chew if enteric coated Can open and sprinkle in applesauce; do not chew when taking; should be administered immediately
Lansoprazole	GERD, acid-related stomach and esophageal problems, stomach and intestinal ulcers	0.5–1.5 mg/kg <10 kg: 7.5 mg once daily 10–20 kg: 15 mg once daily >20 kg: 30 mg once daily For GERD, 15 mg once daily up to 8 weeks	Can cause nausea, flatulence, discolored stools, elevated serum transaminase, fatigue, dizziness, headaches, and some cardiovascular symptoms, including hypotension Can be opened and sprinkled in applesauce, pudding, cottage cheese, or strained pears to administer to small children

Continued

TABLE 15-1 Common Medications Used in Gastrointestinal Disease—cont'd

DRUG	USES	DOSAGE	POSSIBLE SIDE EFFECTS OR WARNINGS
Pantoprazole	GERD, acid-related stomach and esophageal problems, stomach and intestinal ulcers	40 mg once daily	Nausea, vomiting, diarrhea, headache May cause vitamin B_{12} deficiency, weakness, sore tongue, tingling of hands and feet with longer-term use (over 3 years) Tablets should not be split or crushed May not be appropriate for children who cannot swallow tablets
Ranitidine	Histamine H2 antagonist, treatment of ulcers	Newborns: 2 mg/kg/day divided doses every 12 hours 1 month to 16 years ulcer treatment: 2–4 mg/kg day divided twice daily with maximum of 300 mg/day Maintenance: 1 month to 16 years, ulcer treatment: 2–4 mg/kg day divided twice daily with maximum of 150 mg/day GERD: 4–10 mg/kg/day divided into twice daily dose, maximum 300 mg/day Over age 16 years: 300 mg at bedtime for ulcers, for GERD 150 mg twice daily	The 150-mg effervescent tablet can be dissolved in 6–8 oz of water for administration The 25-mg effervescent tablet must be dissolved in at least 1 teaspoon of water If administering to a child, use a dose-measuring device Peppermint-flavored oral syrup for young children Can cause dizziness and sedation, constipation, nausea and vomiting, hepatitis, myalgia, tachycardia or bradycardia, gynecomastia
Metoclopramide (Reglan)	Prokinetic for gastroesophageal reflux—accelerates gastric emptying and intestinal transit without increasing secretions	<6 years: 0.1 mg/kg 6–14 years: 2.5–5 mg Children >14 years: 10 mg For GERD, neonates, infants and children: 0.4/0.8 mg/kg/day in 4 divided doses 30 minutes before meals	Can cause tardive dyskinesia with chronic use (lip smacking, impaired movement of the fingers, rapid eye movements, and tongue protrusion—not usually reversible) Can cause drowsiness and restlessness, constipation, diarrhea, gynecomastia, urinary frequency Use with caution with newborn because of possibility of increasing hyperbilirubinemia
Cimetidine	Histamine of H2 blocker used for ulcer treatment and GERD	Neonates: 5–10 mg/kg/day every 8–12 hours Infants: 10–20 mg/kg/day every 6–12 hours Children: 20–40 mg/kg/day every 6 hours	Bradycardia, tachycardia, dizziness, headache, drowsiness, rash, gynecomastia, diarrhea, nausea, vomiting, ALT, AST elevation, myalgias, elevated serum creatinine, possible relationship with pneumonia May interfere with metabolism of other medications
Famotidine	Histamine of H2 blocker used for ulcer treatment and GERD	Neonates and infants <3 months, GERD: 0.5 mg/kg once daily Infants >3 months to 1 year, GERD: 0.5 mg/kg twice daily Children 1–12 years, ulcer: 0.5 mg/kg/day at bedtime or twice daily (maximum 40 mg/day) Children 1–12 years, GERD: 1 mg/kg/day twice daily (maximum 80 mg/day) Children >12 years, ulcer: 20 mg twice daily Children >12 years, GERD: 20 mg twice daily for 6 weeks	Contains phenylalanine—use with caution with phenylketonuria Can cause bradycardia, tachycardia, dizziness, headache, seizures (patients with renal impairment), drowsiness, acne, rash, dry skin, diarrhea, nausea, vomiting, flatulence, dry mouth, thrombocytopenia ALT, AST elevation, cholestatic jaundice, arthralgias, muscle cramps, elevated serum creatinine and blood urea nitrogen, bronchospasm

TABLE 15-1 Common Medications Used in Gastrointestinal Disease—cont'd

DRUG	USES	DOSAGE	POSSIBLE SIDE EFFECTS OR WARNINGS
Polyethylene glycol 3350 without electrolytes	Treatment of chronic constipation	Children >6 months: 0.5–1.5 g/kg daily (initial dose 0.5 g/kg and titrate to effect) Fecal impaction, >3 years: 1–1.5 g/kg daily for 3 days (maximum 100 g/day) Administer in 4–8 oz of fluid	Patient needs to be evaluated for bowel obstruction before use Can cause urticaria, abdominal bloating, cramping, diarrhea, flatulence
Lactulose	Treatment of chronic constipation	1 mL/kg bid qd-bid (maximum 60 mL/day) May take up to 48 hours to see effect	Can cause flatulence, abdominal discomfort, diarrhea, nausea Oral antibiotics and antacids that are not absorbed may interfere with action of drug Should not be used with children on special diet low in galactose Use special dosing device for administration of smaller doses May be given in 4 oz of water, fruit juice, or milk
Mineral oil	Laxative, lubricant—decreases water absorption and softens stool	Children 5–11 years: 5–15 mL once daily for 1 week Children >12 years: 15–45 mL; may give in divided doses Can be given rectally as an enema	Nausea, vomiting, abdominal cramps, anal seepage Lipid pneumonitis if aspirated Can decrease the absorption of fat-soluble vitamins, carotene, calcium, and phosphorus May administer with meals if emulsified (better tasting)
Docusate sodium: Senokot or Senna preparation	Laxative, stimulant; short-term treatment of constipation May be combined with a stool softener	Infant 1 month to 2 years: 1.25–2.5 mL (syrup) at bedtime not to exceed 5 mL Children 2–5 years: 2.5–3.75 mL at bedtime or 1/2 to 1 tablet PO at bedtime Children 6–12 years: 5–7.5 mL at bedtime Tablets: 2 tablets at bedtime	Syrup can be mixed with juice, milk, or ice cream Can cause abdominal cramping, diarrhea, nausea and vomiting, and diarrhea; can have bitter taste Discolors feces and urine
Bisacodyl	Laxative, stimulant	Children 3–12 years: 5–10 mg in a single dose, oral Children >12 years: 5–15 mg/day in a single dose Rectal: Children <2 years: 5 mg/day as a single dose Children 2–11 years: 5–10 mg/day in a single dose Children >12 years: 10 mg/day	Long-term use may be habit forming and cause laxative dependence and possible electrolyte imbalance Can cause abdominal cramping, diarrhea, nausea and vomiting, sensation of rectal burning, and diarrhea May interact with antacids to cause delayed-release tablets to release sooner than in the small intestine, causing gastric irritation Do not take within 1 hour of dairy products

ALT, alanine transaminase; AST, aspartate transaminase; GERD, gastroesophageal reflux disease.

Adapted from Taketomo, C. K. (2016). Pediatric and neonatal dosage handbook *(23rd ed.). Hudson, OH: Lexi-Comp; Wyllie, R., & Hyams, J. (2016).* Pediatric gastrointestinal and liver disease *(3rd ed.). Philadelphia: Saunders Elsevier; Pediatric Lexi-Drugs Online. (2009).* Lexicomp online. *Retrieved from http://www.lexi.com/institutions/online.jsp?id=databases; and Epocrates Online. (2011). Retrieved from http://www.epocrates.com.*

- Teach stress-reduction techniques such as relaxation.
- Teach avoidance of food that may aggravate condition.
- Encourage normal activity and sleep habits.

Irritable Bowel Syndrome

Irritable bowel syndrome (IBS) is a common disorder that affects the large intestine (colon) and commonly causes cramping, abdominal pain, bloating, gas, diarrhea, or constipation. IBS is a chronic condition that needs to be managed long term. Even though symptoms are uncomfortable, IBS—unlike ulcerative colitis and Crohn's disease, which are forms of IBD—does not cause changes in bowel tissue or increase the risk for colorectal cancer.

Assessment

IBS may have the following clinical presentation:

- Cramping
- Bloating
- Diarrhea
- Constipation
- Change in appearance of the stool:
  - Loose or hard
  - Thin or like pellets
  - Mucus in the stool
- Urgency to have a bowel movement
- More common in women than men (Fig. 15–8)
- May be associated with other functional pain syndromes (e.g., chronic fatigue, fibromyalgia)

Diagnostic Testing

- In most cases, the diagnosis is established by history
- CBC, stool studies for ova and parasites, occult blood, WBC, stool culture
- Endoscopy if any bleeding occurs to rule out IBD

Nursing Interventions

Nursing interventions for patients with IBS include emergency, acute, and chronic care.

Emergency Care

- Patient may be evaluated for pain, but pain is usually relieved with a bowel movement.

Acute Care

- Stress the need to eat small meals and avoid trigger foods.
- Monitor medication administration and effects.

Chronic Care

- Dietary changes—removing trigger foods such as fatty foods, dairy, carbonated beverages, and caffeine
- Diary of symptoms, bowel habits, and diet
- Increase in high-fiber foods
- Eat several small meals
- Drink plenty of fluid
- Fiber supplements
- Laxatives such as MiraLAX (polyethylene glycol 3350) to relieve constipation
- Imodium to relieve diarrhea

Complementary and Alternative Therapies

- Probiotics may be helpful for some patients but are not well studied.

CRITICAL COMPONENT

Probiotic Use

Probiotics are being studied for a variety of uses, including acute infectious diarrhea, antibiotic-associated diarrhea, IBS, and IBD.

- Probiotics have demonstrated a decrease in the amount and duration of diarrhea in acute infectious diarrhea from bacterial infection or rotavirus. A short course of probiotics is beneficial for patients with diarrhea of more than 2 days and younger than 12 months. Probiotics are also beneficial for patients who had diarrhea previously with antibiotics. Co-administration with probiotics can reduce diarrhea.
- In patients with IBS, probiotics demonstrated a decrease in the frequency of pain and pain intensity. Patients may use *Lactobacillus rhamnosus* GG (LGG) for this therapy.
- Probiotics have shown promise for adjunct treatment in Crohn's disease and ulcerative colitis, but should not be used as a primary treatment for these conditions. Because there are not current recommendations for use in pediatrics and studies are ongoing, any use of probiotics for these conditions should be discussed with the pediatric gastroenterologist (May & So, 2014).

Caregiver Education

Caregiver education should include emergency, acute, and chronic care.

Emergency Care

- Emergency care may not be needed. Caregiver should know to have patient evaluated for unusual symptoms.

Acute Care

- Teach caregiver and patient importance of using medication for symptom management.
- Teach caregiver and patient use of diet and foods to avoid.

Chronic Care

- Review food diary with patient and caregiver to identify triggers.
- Review use of medication for symptoms.
- Teach use of diet—have child or adolescent help with planning meals and food selection (Table 15–2).
- Teach patient and caregiver stress-reduction techniques.

Complementary and Alternative Therapies

- Some use of probiotics
- Fish oil capsules

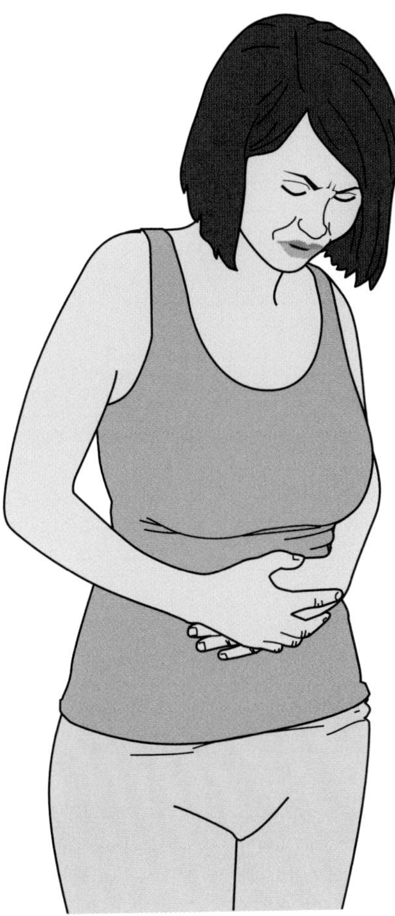

FIGURE 15–8 Girls with irritable bowel syndrome (IBS) often have more symptoms during their menstrual periods. Stress does not cause IBS, but it can make the symptoms worse.

GASTROINTESTINAL PROBLEMS MANIFESTED BY VOMITING

All babies spit up, some more than others. Approximately 40% of 4-month-olds regurgitate, approximately 20% to the extent that caregivers seek assistance (Orenstein, 2013). This section describes some of the GI problems that may be indicated by substantial vomiting in pediatric patients.

CRITICAL COMPONENT

Describing Regurgitation

Caregivers should be taught to describe the regurgitation by how much is on a cloth or blanket—dime-sized, quarter-sized, or covering the entire diaper. The vomiting may also be described as dribbling out of the nose, down the caregiver's leg or through the patient's nose, or forceful enough to travel several feet. The color of the emesis may be useful. An accurate description will help identify the problem causing the regurgitation or vomiting.

Gastroesophageal Reflux

In pediatric gastroesophageal reflux disease (GERD), immaturity of the lower esophageal sphincter function is manifested by frequent transient lower esophageal relaxations, which result in retrograde flow of gastric contents into the esophagus (Wyllie et al., 2016).

TABLE 15–2 Gastrointestinal or Other Problems That May Require a Special Diet

Celiac disease	Gluten-free diet (avoid wheat, barley, and rye and spelt) Can eat oats but need to be careful of cross-contamination from gluten-containing products Important to teach caregiver and child to read labels Child can learn to help plan meals with gluten-free foods Need to be on diet for life
Irritable bowel syndrome	Avoid trigger foods—caffeine, citrus, nuts, carbonated beverages, fatty foods, dairy Have child keep diet diary Discuss and teach diet choices Increase fiber in diet Increase fluid intake Encourage use of daily probiotics, either in capsule or by eating yogurt with probiotics
Crohn's disease	Nutritional therapy—inclusion of probiotics and fish oil; may need enteral therapy if severe Avoid irritating foods—fried foods, carbonated beverages Decrease intake of high-fiber food during inflammation Use small, frequent meals

Continued

TABLE 15–2 Gastrointestinal or Other Problems That May Require a Special Diet—cont'd

	Low-fat intake—may need emulsified fat Need vitamin supplements Increased caloric and protein needs
Lactose or milk intolerance	Avoid milk and milk products, including cheese and ice cream, and products that contain whey and casein
Constipation	Avoid constipating food such as bananas, excessive milk, pasta Needs increase in fresh fruit, vegetables, whole grains, and fiber
Glycogen storage disease	May need continuous feeding through a gastrostomy tube Frequent feedings in the daytime Cornstarch slurry at bedtime Monitoring of glucose
Gallbladder disease	Avoid foods that contain fat and cream-based soups
Short bowel syndrome	Will usually require parenteral nutrition at first with move to enteral nutrition and will need vitamin supplementation With very short colon: • No lipid restriction • High-dose antimotility agent • Soluble fiber to slow gastric emptying • Oral hydration solution with high sodium Small-bowel remnant: • Lipid restriction • Low-dose antimotility agent • Soluble fiber • Oral rehydration solution with low sodium
Failure to thrive (organic type)	Use a high-calorie formula such as Neocate or PediaSure Regular meals and frequent snacks Fortify milk by adding 1 cup of nonfat dry milk powder to a quart of milk; use in cooking as well as for drinking Add additional margarine or cheese to food Use instant breakfast in whole milk Watch infant or child for satiety cues

Adapted from Burns, C. E., Dunn, A. M., Brady, M. A., Starr, N. B., & Blosser, C. G. (2013). Pediatric primary care *(5th ed.). St. Louis, MO: Saunders; Celiac Disease Foundation. (2009).* Gluten free diet. *Retrieved from http://www.celiac.org; and Wyllie, R., Hyams, J., & Kay, M. (2016).* Pediatric gastrointestinal and liver disease *(5th ed.). Philadelphia: Saunders Elsevier.*

Assessment

- GERD may have the following clinical presentation:
  - With reflux, eating is unpleasant and hurts
  - A large amount of fluid may be present with recurrent vomiting
  - In silent GERD, milk enters the esophagus, causing burning, coughing, and choking
  - Slow weight gain or no weight gain due to association of eating with pain
  - Excessive irritability and crying, especially after meals
  - Arching during or after meals
  - Newborns or young infants may present with apnea
  - Children may have a chronic cough
  - May develop chronic episodes of pneumonia
  - Older children may have pain in the epigastric area
    - Mid-sternal discomfort
    - Sleep interruption
    - Persistent throat soreness not associated with any infectious disease (Wyllie et al., 2016)

CRITICAL COMPONENT

Sandifer's Syndrome

Sandifer's syndrome is characterized by sudden arching of the head, neck, and upper trunk during feeding due to reflux. The head is twisted side to side continuously, and the upper trunk is bent to one side so the head points to the floor. The patient may be very irritable during this time. Improvement of the reflux may appear with this posturing. Successful treatment with medication, such as ranitidine or omeprazole, will cause this behavior to stop (Cazan, Doborta, & Neamtu, 2014).

Diagnostic Testing

- Weight, length, head circumference
- Stool for occult blood
- Chest x-ray for respiratory symptoms
- pH probe
- Esophagram
- Gastric emptying study in older child
- In some cases, endoscopy may be used

Nursing Interventions

Nursing interventions for pediatric patients with GERD may include emergency care, acute hospital care, and discharge instructions.

Emergency Care

- If baby chokes and stops breathing, initiate CPR.

Acute Hospital Care

- Monitor intake and output.
- Monitor weight.
- Prepare infant for pH probe or other diagnostic tests.
- Assess mother's feeding style if breastfeeding; rule out overactive letdown with excessive milk.
- Administer medication as ordered.
  - Ranitidine
  - Reglan may be indicated for infants.
  - Proton pump inhibitors—lansoprazole, omeprazole (may be opened and sprinkled on food)
- May be treated with Nissen fundoplication, if severe (Wyllie et al., 2016)
- If surgery is indicated, provide preoperative teaching to the caregivers.
- Give support postoperatively.
  - Monitor intake and output, including NG tube secretions.
  - Gradually increase feedings.
  - Monitor weight daily.
  - Administer pain medication as needed.

Discharge Instructions

- Upright positioning is important for infants; caregivers should elevate head of the bed.
- Stress avoidance of food that may trigger symptoms.
- Teach administration of medication.
- May continue to breastfeed. Help correct overactive letdown if present; baby may breastfeed in upright position.
- Teach caregivers positioning.
- Teach importance of medication administration.
- Teach caregivers how to thicken feedings if medically ordered.
- In older children, teach avoidance of food that may trigger symptoms—fatty foods, acidic foods (citrus juices, carbonated beverages, tomato products).
- Encourage reduction in weight in older children who are obese.

Caregiver Education

Nurse education for caregivers of pediatric patients with GERD should include the following topics.

Emergency Care

- Teach caregiver to recognize symptoms of reflux and intervene immediately.
- Initiate CPR if reflux causes baby to stop breathing.

Acute Hospital Care

- Caregivers need to learn to administer medication as required.
- Assist caregivers with feedings.
- Teach caregivers to recognize symptoms.

Discharge Home Care

- Small, frequent feedings
  - May continue to breastfeed. Help correct overactive letdown if present; baby may breastfeed in upright position.
  - Frequent burping
- Change formula to protein hydrolyzed formula if bottle feeding
- Frequent burping during feeding
- Upright positioning during and after feeding
- Avoid placing patient in car seat or carrier after feeding
- Folded blanket in the well of the car seat to extend hips
- Administration of medication 30 minutes before morning feeding
- For older children:
  - No eating or drinking 2 hours before bedtime
  - Avoidance of caffeine, chocolate, spicy foods, fatty foods, acidic foods, and carbonated beverages
  - Avoidance of exposure to cigarette smoke
  - Weight loss if the child is obese
  - Medication administration of PPI before breakfast by 30 minutes

Complementary and Alternative Therapies

- A low-fiber diet may help reduce reflux.

Pyloric Stenosis

Pyloric stenosis occurs in infants when the pylorus blocks food from entering the small intestine. Normally, the muscular valve (pylorus) between the stomach and small intestine holds food in the stomach until it is ready for the next stage in the digestive process. In pyloric stenosis, the pylorus muscles thicken and become abnormally large, blocking food from reaching the small intestine. Pyloric stenosis can lead to forceful vomiting, dehydration, and weight loss. Babies with pyloric stenosis may seem constantly hungry (Wyllie et al., 2016).

Assessment

Pyloric stenosis may have the following clinical presentation:

- Found more in boys than girls (4:1); higher incidence if mother had disease (Wyllie et al., 2016)
- Forceful, progressive, nonbilious vomiting after each feeding
- Onset of vomiting from the first week of life to as late as 5 months of age
- Vomiting becomes projectile over time
- Observation of peristaltic waves from left to right before vomiting occurs
- Eventual dehydration with decrease in serum chloride

- Poor weight gain
- Failure to thrive (FTT)
- Risk for metabolic alkalosis
- Jaundice in 2% to 5% of cases

Diagnostic Testing

- Palpation of pyloric mass in the mid-epigastrium (olive sign)
- Ultrasound visualization of pyloric thickening
- Upper GI series
- CBC with electrolytes
- Liver function tests, including bilirubin total and direct

Nursing Interventions

The following nursing interventions are used for pediatric patients with pyloric stenosis.

Emergency Care

- Patient will need to be NPO.
- Provide patient with pacifier for comfort.
- Provide IV therapy with isotonic solution and added electrolytes as needed.
- Teach caregivers about diagnostic tests to be performed.

Acute Hospital Care

- Prepare patient for surgical correction.
- Teach caregivers about surgery to be performed and answer questions.
- Provide emotional support to caregivers.
- Provide breastfeeding mother with electric pump for pumping and storage.
- Give appropriate pain medication postoperatively.
- Monitor incisional site for infection.
- Fold diapers low to avoid incisional area.
- Monitor intake and output.
- Record daily weight.
- Advance diet as ordered; small amounts of fluid frequently.
- It is important to burp patient after feeding to decrease air in stomach.

Chronic Hospital Care

- Patient may continue to vomit postoperatively because of edema.
- Monitor intake and output.
- Provide caregiver reassurance.
- Assist with diagnostic tests as needed.
- In most cases, the surgery alleviates the problem.

Caregiver Education

Nurses must educate caregivers of children who have pyloric stenosis on the following measures.

Emergency Care

- Bring patient to the hospital or clinic for evaluation of persistent vomiting or lethargy.

Acute Hospital Care

- Assist with feeding as needed.
- Reassure caregivers about their ability to care for the patient.

Chronic Home Care

- Report continuation of vomiting if present.
- Advance diet as advised.
- Remind caregivers about keeping regular appointments and starting or continuing immunizations.

INTESTINAL OBSTRUCTION

Intestinal obstruction is mechanical or functional blockage of the intestines that prevents the normal movement of the products of digestion. The small or the large intestine may be affected.

SAFE AND EFFECTIVE NURSING CARE: Clinical Pearl

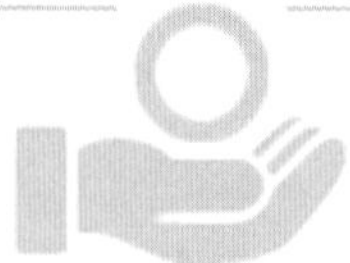

Bilious Vomiting

Bilious vomiting in an infant is a surgical emergency until proven otherwise (Wyllie et al., 2016). Malrotation (Fig. 15–9) occurs when the small or large intestine is not positioned in the abdominal cavity in the correct position. When either the small or large intestine is twisted or malpositioned, it carries with it the bands, vascular vessels, and ligaments that supply the organ. The symptom of bile in the emesis of an infant is therefore an ominous sign until proven otherwise.

Volvulus

A volvulus is an abnormal twisting of a portion of the GI tract, usually the intestine, which can impair blood flow. Volvulus can lead to gangrene and death of the involved segment of the GI tract, intestinal obstruction, perforation of the intestine, and peritonitis. The stomach, small intestine, cecum, and sigmoid colon are all subject to volvulus. Malrotation of the bowel during fetal development can predispose one to a volvulus, which often has a sudden onset (Wyllie et al., 2016).

Assessment

Volvulus may have the following clinical presentation:

- Most often occurs in the first 6 months (Fig. 15–10)
- Intense crying and pain
- Pulling up of the legs
- Abdominal distension
- Vomiting, usually bilious
- Tachycardia and tachypnea

Diagnostic Testing

- Upper GI series
- CBC with electrolytes

Nursing Interventions

Nursing interventions for patients with volvulus include emergency, acute, and chronic care.

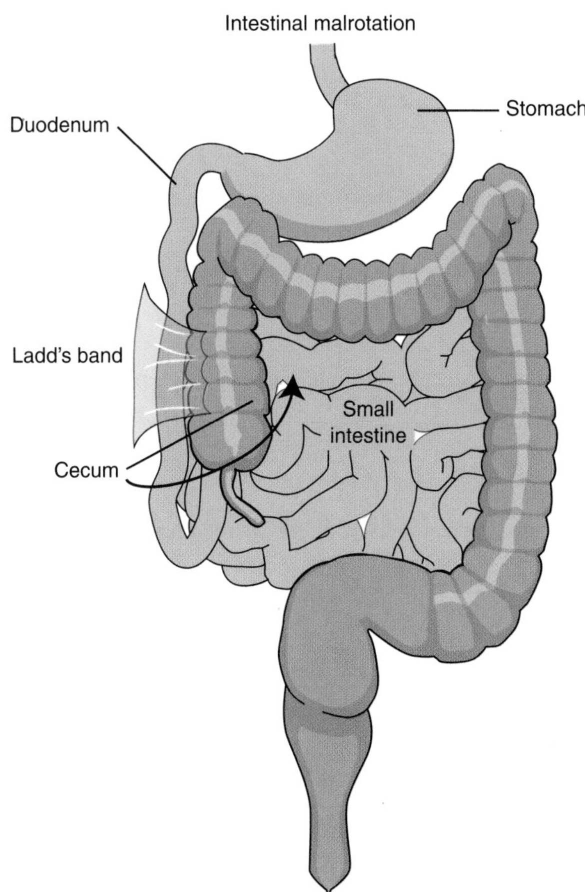

FIGURE 15–9 In malrotation, the cecum is not positioned correctly. The tissue that normally holds it in place may cross over and block part of the small bowel.

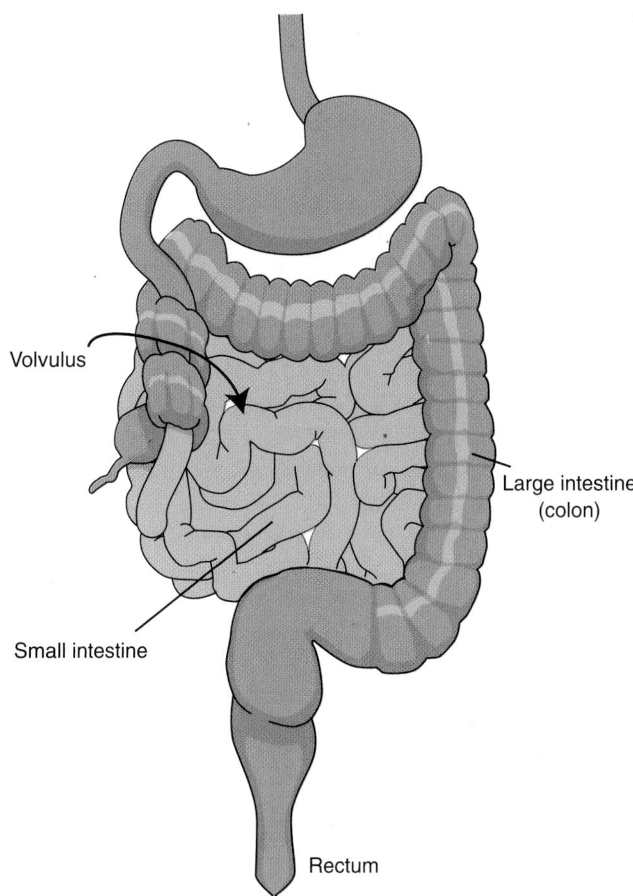

FIGURE 15–10 In volvulus, a portion of the intestine twists around itself.

Emergency Care

- Surgical emergency
- Patient needs counterclockwise rotation to restore normal perfusion
- With significant damage, may need resection

Acute Hospital Care

- Keep patient NPO.
- Establish IV therapy.
- Insert NG tube.
- Maintain record of intake and output.
- Prepare patient for surgery.
- Provide patient with pacifier.
- Provide emotional support for caregiver.
- Provide pain relief after surgery—use Neonatal Pain Scale for infants.
- Monitor incisional area.
- Monitor NG tube.
- With return of bowel sounds, start feedings.

Chronic Care

- Maintain record of intake and output.
- Once patient is maintaining good intake, he or she will be discharged.

Caregiver Education

Nurses must educate caregivers of pediatric patients who have volvulus on the following topics.

Emergency Care

- Explain procedures to caregivers.
- Answer caregiver questions as needed.
- Encourage caregiver to hold and rock patient.

Acute Care

- Explain procedures to caregiver.
- Encourage caregiver to hold patient, either postprocedure or postoperatively.
- Encourage caregiver to participate in oral feedings.
- Encourage nonnutritive sucking before oral feedings.

Chronic Care

- Teach caregivers signs of infection or complications.
- Teach caregivers importance of follow-up appointments.

Intussusception

Intussusception occurs when part of the intestine slides into an adjacent part of the intestine. This "telescoping" can block food or fluid from passing through. Intussusception also cuts off the blood supply to the affected portion of the intestine, which can lead to a perforation, infection, and death of bowel tissue. Intussusception is the most common cause of intestinal obstruction in children younger than age 3 years (Wyllie et al., 2016).

Assessment

Intussusception typically has the following cause and clinical presentation:

- May be caused by Meckel's diverticulum, polyp, or enlargement of lymph tissue
- Sudden drawing up of legs and crying with possible vomiting, then symptom free
- Pain will occur in regular intervals, every 15 to 20 minutes
- Vomiting will contain bile:
  - After 12 hours, develop currant-jelly stools (stool mixed with blood and mucus)
  - Increased abdominal distension
- As problem progresses:
  - Fever
  - Peritoneal irritation with tenderness and guarding
  - Tachycardia
  - Elevated WBC (Wyllie et al., 2016)

Diagnostic Testing

- Ultrasound
- CBC with differential
- Barium enema may correct the problem

Nursing Interventions

Nursing interventions for patients with this condition include emergency and acute care.

Emergency Care

- Begin IV therapy.

Acute Care

- Prepare patient for ultrasound.
- Keep patient NPO.
- Establish IV therapy.
- Maintain record of intake and output.
- Provide patient with pacifier.
- Reduction may be done with barium enema, air insufflation, or water-soluble solution.
  - Keep patient NPO.
  - Reintroduce to regular feeding gradually.
- Surgical reduction
  - Maintain NG tube.
  - Maintain IV therapy.
  - Provide pain medication as needed.
  - When bowel sounds return, start gradual oral feedings.
- Maintain record of intake and output.
- Once patient is maintaining good intake, he or she will be discharged.

Caregiver Education

Educate caregivers of pediatric patients with this condition on the following topics.

Emergency Care

- Explain procedures to caregivers.
- Answer caregiver questions as needed.

Acute Care

- Encourage caregiver to hold and rock patient.
- Explain procedures to caregiver.
- Encourage caregiver to hold patient, either postprocedure or postoperatively.
- Encourage caregiver to participate in oral feedings.

Chronic Care

- Teach caregivers signs of infection or complications.
- Teach caregivers importance of follow-up appointments.

SAFE AND EFFECTIVE NURSING CARE: Clinical Pearl

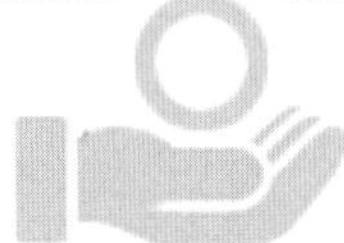

Atresia and Stenosis

Atresia, or complete obstruction of the lumen of the gut, and stenosis, which is an incomplete obstruction, can occur in the midgut, which is the duodenum, jejunum, and ileum. Atresia occurs more often than stenosis. These conditions present with bilious vomiting and abdominal distension, failure to pass meconium, and jaundice (Wyllie et al., 2016).

Necrotizing Enterocolitis

Necrotizing enterocolitis (NEC) is the death of tissue in the intestine. It occurs most often in premature or chronically ill infants (Wyllie et al., 2016).

Assessment

NEC may have the following clinical presentation:

- Happens in premature infants, especially after infection or ischemic incident
- Tense, distended abdomen
- Large gastric residual greater than 2 mL
- Stool positive for occult blood
- Increased periods of apnea
- Decreased blood pressure
- Poor temperature stability

Diagnostic Testing

- CBC, CRP
- Stool for occult blood

- Abdominal x-ray
- Increase in abdominal girth measurement

Nursing Interventions

Nursing interventions for pediatric patients with this condition may include the following measures.

Emergency Care

- Patient should be NPO to rest GI tract.
- Maintain IV therapy (see Box 15–1).

Acute Care

- Maintain and monitor IV therapy.
- Monitor total parenteral nutrition (TPN).
- Administer antibiotic therapy.
- If surgical intervention is required, prepare patient for surgery.
  - Monitor IV therapy postoperatively.
  - Maintain NG tube.
  - Monitor operative site.
- Surgical intervention may cause short bowel syndrome (SBS). SBS results from the alteration of intestinal digestion and absorption that occurs after extensive bowel resection. It is a complex disorder with nutritional, metabolic, and infectious consequences. Bowel obstruction is a potential complication of SBS.
- If patient develops SBS:
  - Start TPN.
  - Start enteral feedings early with continuous feedings.
  - Monitor stool output to advance feedings.
  - Monitor laboratory tests as appropriate, including electrolytes, albumin, alanine transaminase (ALT), and aspartate transaminase (AST).
  - If ostomy is present, consult with ostomy nurse.

Chronic Care

- After symptoms subside, restart feeding gradually, preferably with breast milk.
- Baby with SBS may require long-term parenteral nutrition.
- The goal of therapy for SBS is to advance to enteral feedings.
- If liver failure occurs, child may need liver transplant.

Caregiver Education

Nurse education for caregivers of these pediatric patients should discuss the following topics.

Emergency Care

- Explain procedures to caregivers.
- Answer caregiver questions as needed.

Acute Care

- Explain procedures to caregiver.
- Encourage caregiver to hold patient, either postprocedure or postoperatively.
- Encourage caregiver to participate in oral feedings.
- Encourage nonnutritive sucking with pacifier.
- Have caregiver provide breast milk if possible; provide breast pump for use as needed.

Chronic Care

- Teach caregivers signs of infection or complications.
- Teach caregivers importance of follow-up appointments.
- If patient has SBS:
  - Teach caregiver administration of enteral feedings.
  - Avoid hypertonic liquids (e.g., Kool-Aid, juices, soda).
  - Start patient on solids at normal developmental age, with meats first if possible.
  - Discuss long-term parenteral nutrition with caregiver if small bowel is less than 40 cm.
- Teach caregiver signs of infection and complications.

GASTROINTESTINAL PROBLEMS MANIFESTED BY DIARRHEA

GI conditions in this area are manifested by complaints of frequent loose or watery bowel movements and abdominal cramping.

Gastroenteritis

Acute gastroenteritis in children is often defined as the onset of diarrhea in the absence of chronic disease, with or without abdominal pain, fever, nausea, or vomiting. In the United States, the condition is a major source of morbidity and hospitalization in children younger than 5 years (Churgay & Aftab, 2012).

Assessment

Gastroenteritis may have the following clinical presentation:

- Watery diarrhea
- Abdominal cramping
- Vomiting
- Headache
- May have fever and chills—temperature above 102.5°F
- Stools with blood or pus
- Signs of dehydration—depressed fontanels, lack of tears, poor skin turgor, lethargy
- Symptoms last from 1 to 2 days up to 10 days

Diagnostic Testing

- Usually diagnosed by symptoms and examination
- May test stool for culture (bacterial and viral), ova and parasites, WBC count
- Blood work—CBC and electrolytes if patient appears dehydrated

Nursing Interventions

Nursing interventions for this condition include the following measures.

Emergency Care

- If the patient is dehydrated, IV therapy needs to be instituted. Initially an isotonic solution such as normal saline may be given followed by a hypertonic solution such as D5 1/2 normal saline.
- Patient may require additional electrolytes in the IV if there is an imbalance.
- There is a risk for metabolic acidosis.
- There is a risk for hypovolemic shock.

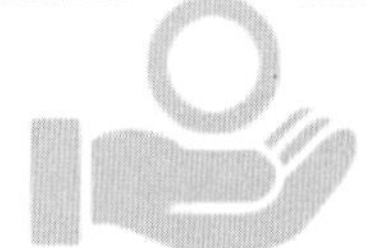

SAFE AND EFFECTIVE NURSING CARE: Clinical Pearl

Signs of Dehydration

Signs of dehydration include excessive thirst, dry mouth, little or no urine or dark urine, decreased tears, severe weakness or lethargy, and dizziness or lightheadedness. If children have any of these symptoms, caregivers should notify a health-care provider for further instructions about treatment (National Digestive Diseases Information Clearinghouse, 2017).

Acute Care

- If severe diarrhea or vomiting, may institute IV therapy.
- Antibiotics may be administered if stool culture is positive.
- If patient is not dehydrated, care may be given at home.
- Withhold fluids for 2 to 3 hours.
- Start with 1 tablespoon of fluid every 15 minutes for 1 hour, then 1 oz of fluid.
- Every half hour, give Pedialyte, water, popsicles, or oral rehydration solution.
- After several hours of retaining fluid, the patient may have clear broth and several saltines.
- If patient starts to vomit, then stop fluids and start over.
- If only diarrhea, provide brief period of rest from intake, then start fluids.
- Moisturize lips with Vaseline.
- Allow pacifier for infants for nonnutritive sucking.
- Keep perineal area clean and dry between diarrhea episodes.
- May continue to breastfeed.

Chronic Care

- Patient should return to a regular diet during the second 24 hours (Fig. 15–11).

Caregiver Education

Educate caregivers on emergency, acute, and chronic care.

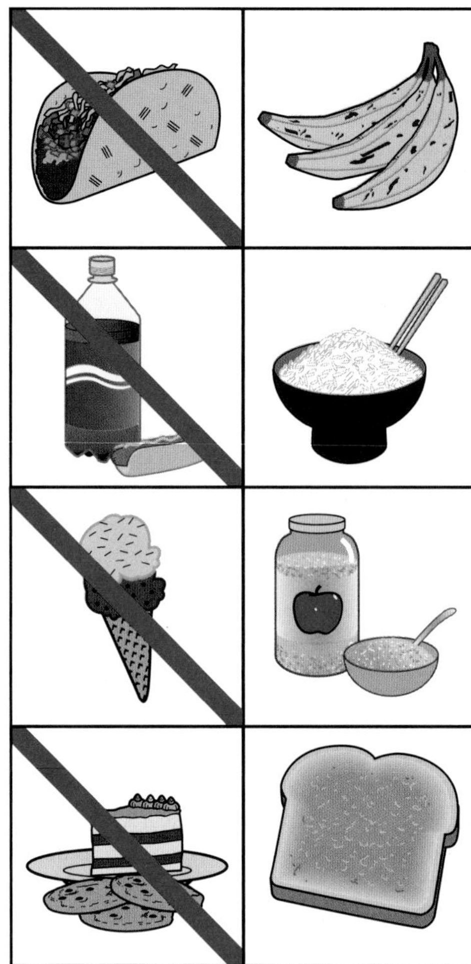

FIGURE 15–11 Treatment for diarrhea. As the patient feels better, he or she can begin eating soft, bland food, such as bananas, plain rice, boiled potatoes, toast, crackers, cooked carrots, and baked chicken without the skin or fat. Children can advance to a regular diet after 24 hours.

Emergency Care

- Caregiver should bring the patient to clinic or hospital if there are any of the following symptoms:
  - Prolonged vomiting
  - No urination for 8 to 12 hours or less than five to six wet diapers in an infant
  - Depressed fontanel
  - Dry mucous membranes
  - Lethargy

Acute Care

- Instruct caregivers on how to give fluids for recovery.
- Instruct caregivers not to give any antidiarrheals such as Imodium or Pepto-Bismol.

Chronic Care

- Teach caregivers not to give unlimited fluid.
- Remind caregivers to advance diet back to a regular diet after 48 hours.

SAFE AND EFFECTIVE NURSING CARE: Promoting Safety

Hand Hygiene

GI illness can be spread by handling items, especially food, after using the bathroom. Diarrheal illnesses can be especially contagious. Good hand hygiene is essential when caring for children with these illnesses or anytime stool needs to be collected for the laboratory. Practicing good hand hygiene is important, as well as teaching good hand hygiene to caregivers and children.

GASTROINTESTINAL PROBLEMS MANIFESTED BY CONSTIPATION

GI conditions in this area are manifested by complaints of infrequent or hard bowel movements and abdominal discomfort.

Functional Constipation

Constipation in infants and children is not typically caused by serious medical disease. The cause of most constipation is functional or idiopathic, meaning there is no sign of injury or infection, blood, or anatomic abnormality to explain the very real symptoms (Wyllie et al., 2016).

Assessment

Functional constipation may have the following clinical presentation:

- Infrequent stools (less than twice a week) that are usually hard and may be small and pebble-like or large
- Complaints of pain with stooling
- Leaking of stool between bowel movements (encopresis)
- Holding behaviors with stooling (hiding, dancing movements, squeezing buttocks together)
- Impaction—inability to stool with abdominal pain and sometimes vomiting
- History should cover general stooling habits
- On physical examination, stool may be palpated in the colon
- Assessment for anal wink and examination of anus for fissures on rectal examination

Diagnostic Testing

- Occult blood
- Flat plate of abdomen
- Barium enema (unprepped)—helps to rule out Hirschsprung's disease
- Colonic transport examination (done infrequently)
- Anorectal manometry

Nursing Interventions

Nursing interventions include emergency, acute, and chronic care.

Emergency Care

- Impaction accompanied by vomiting; may need admission for disimpaction.
- Child may need IV fluids.
- Enemas or oral electrolyte solutions may be used for disimpaction.

Acute Care

- If disimpaction is needed but child is not in acute distress, child may be treated at home with high-dose polyethylene glycol with close follow-up monitoring.
- Child may be admitted to the hospital if disimpaction does not work at home or child becomes worse with similar treatment as described earlier.
- Family must understand the importance of using medication as directed.

Chronic Home Care

- Medications, including:
  - Polyethylene glycol 3350 without electrolytes (MiraLAX or GlycoLax)
  - Mineral oil
  - Lactulose
  - Short-term therapy with Senna (Senokot)
  - Dulcolax also may be used for short-term therapy
  - Enemas may be helpful on a short-term basis
- Behavior modification
  - Regular times for stooling, usually after meals for 5 to 10 minutes
  - Daily record of stools and medication
  - Reward chart for success
- Increase in exercise
- Increase in fluid intake
- Dietary improvement, including increased fiber
- Elimination of cow's milk protein may help
- Biofeedback therapy
- Follow-up visits are important for weaning of medication

Caregiver Education

Parents and caregivers should be educated on emergency, acute, and chronic care.

Emergency Care

- If the child starts to vomit or has severe abdominal pain, caregiver should bring the child for immediate evaluation.

Acute Care

- Education of caregiver and child about procedures
- Education of caregiver and child about medication
- On discharge, caregiver and child need to know importance of continuing medication regularly

Chronic Care

- Regular use of medication

SAFE AND EFFECTIVE NURSING CARE: Understanding Medication

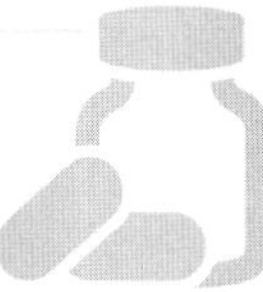

Treating Constipation

Regular medication administration is important in treating constipation. Oral laxatives have become the mainstay of treatment.

Polyethylene glycol 3350 without electrolytes (MiraLAX or GlycoLax) is the commonly used medication because it is well tolerated and easy to administer. The dose is adjusted according to the child's need, but may start at 17 g (1 capful) in 8 oz of water once or twice daily. Fluid volume may be adjusted for the child's age. Most children do not taste the medication.

Mineral oil is another alternative. Most caregivers do not like to administer mineral oil because the child complains of the taste and the mineral oil can leak from the rectum onto the underwear in high doses. Mineral oil is given as 1 to 4 mL/kg/day. Many health-care providers give mineral oil as 1 tablespoon per year of age.

Lactulose is usually administered to infants. One of the side effects is an increase in gassiness. It can be very effective in this population, especially with premature infants with constipation because of immaturity of the GI tract. The dosage is 1 to 2 mL/kg/day.

Occasional use of Senna or Bisacodyl may be necessary in those children with severe constipation and encopresis after disimpaction. These medications are considered short-term adjunct therapy only.

Caregivers need to understand the importance of complying with therapy and using the medication as prescribed, including during periods of weaning from the medication (Wyllie et al., 2016).

- Discuss behavior modification with caregiver and child.
  - Child should sit on toilet for set time and not get up until he or she has bowel movement or time is up (5–10 minutes at least, depending on child's age).
  - Child should sit on toilet after meals.
  - Record of stools and medication should be kept.
  - Use reward chart.
  - Participation of child is important for success in the therapy.
  - Reward should be a privilege such as extra TV or video game time; child should be part of selecting reward.
  - No food rewards should be given.
- Change in diet
  - Increase of fruits and vegetables
  - Increase of fluids
  - Increase fiber in diet—for age 1–3 years need 19 g; age 4–8 years, 25 g; age 9–13 years, 26 g for girls and 31 g for boys; age 14–18 years, 29 g for girls and 38 g for boys. Some health-care providers start with increased fiber in the diet because age in years +5 equals grams of fiber needed in the diet daily (Esmaeli, 2014; Koppen, Lammers, Benninga, & Tabbers, 2015). This can be used to start increase in fiber intake to work toward dietary recommendations.

Complementary and Alternative Therapies

- Dietary therapy alone may be helpful for mild constipation.
- Use of probiotics may be helpful. Study about their use is ongoing.

Hirschsprung's Disease

Hirschsprung's disease is a congenital condition that causes blockage of the intestine because of a lack of nerves in the bottom segment of the colon. These nerves normally allow the muscles in the wall of the bowel to contract and move digested material toward the anus to be eliminated.

Hirschsprung's disease occurs in 1 out of every 5,000 live births. The disease occurs more often in males than in females (Wyllie et al., 2016).

Assessment

Hirschsprung's disease may have the following clinical presentation:

- Failure to pass meconium in the first 24 hours of life with increased abdominal distension (Fig. 15–12)
- Constipation from birth
- No bowel movement more than once a week
- Ribbon-like or watery stools
- Thin child with protuberant abdomen
- Vomiting
- Poor weight gain

Diagnostic Testing

- Empty rectum on digital examination
- Abdominal x-ray (kidneys, ureter, bladder)
- Barium enema (unprepped)
- Rectal biopsy (definitive test for diagnosis)
- Anorectal manometry is more accurate for short or ultra-short segments and is not used in newborns

Nursing Interventions

Nursing interventions include the following measures.

Emergency Care for Dehydration

- Establish IV therapy for fluid and electrolyte balance.
- Antibiotic therapy as needed

Acute Care

- If not an emergency, caregiver may administer enemas before admission for surgery.
- Caregiver will need instruction in giving enema.
- Prepare child for surgery.
  - May need enema to evacuate colon.
  - Provide emotional support for caregiver.
- If surgical intervention is required, prepare patient for surgery.
  - Monitor IV therapy postoperatively.
  - Maintain NG tube.
  - Monitor operative site.
  - Administer antibiotics.

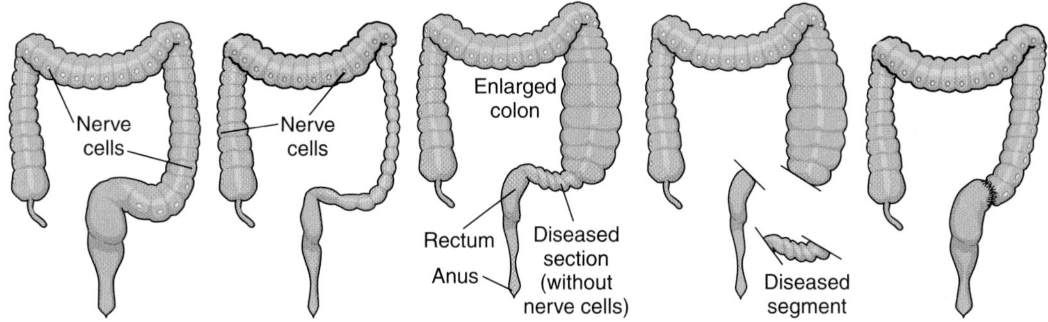

FIGURE 15–12 Hirschsprung's disease (HD) is a disease of the large intestine. The large intestine is also sometimes called the colon. The word *bowel* can refer to the large and small intestines. HD usually occurs in children. It causes constipation, which means that bowel movements are difficult. Some children with HD cannot have bowel movements at all. The stool creates a blockage in the rectosigmoid area of the colon.

- Observe for complications such as enterocolitis (watery diarrhea, abdominal distension, and fever).
  - Treat with IV fluids
  - Warm saline irrigation of rectum
  - Antibiotic therapy
- Advance feedings as tolerated if no complication.

Chronic Care

- Monitor for complications such as chronic constipation or impaction.
- Refer to gastroenterologist for follow-up.
- Observe stools for normal pattern and consistency.

Caregiver Education

Nurses should educate parents and caregivers on the following topics.

Emergency Care

- Explain procedures to caregivers.
- Answer caregiver questions as needed.
- Teach parent signs of enterocolitis and impaction that need immediate intervention.

Acute Care

- Explain procedures to caregiver.
- Encourage caregiver to hold patient, either postprocedure or postoperatively.
- Encourage caregiver to participate in oral feedings.
- Have caregiver provide breast milk if possible; provide breast pump for use.

Chronic Care

- Teach caregivers signs of infection or complications.
- Teach caregivers importance of keeping follow-up appointments.
- Child may be having difficulty with passing stools or leaking because of tight anus and pull-through surgery.
  - Caregiver needs to monitor stooling and be alert for problems.
- Teach caregiver that child may be a fussy eater at first; it is important to de-emphasize mealtime stress.
- Treatment for older child may be the same as for chronic constipation; child needs to be active participant in treatment.
- Genetic counseling may be recommended.

GASTROINTESTINAL PROBLEMS MANIFESTED BY ANTERIOR ABDOMINAL WALL DEFECT

GI conditions in this area are manifested by defects in the anterior abdominal wall.

Omphalocele and Gastroschisis

With omphalocele, the stomach and intestines are contained within a sac of amnio, peritoneum, and Wharton's jelly outside of the abdomen. A gastroschisis is an opening on the right side of the umbilical cord that affects the stomach, small and large intestines, and in rare cases, the liver.

Clinical Presentation

- Malrotation is present in both defects.

Omphalocele

- Defect varies from 4 to 12 cm.
- In large defects, the liver, spleen, gonads, and bladder may also be contained in the sac.
- Sac may rupture in utero.
- Commonly associated with anomalies (cardiac defects, neural tube defects, exstrophy of the bladder, or Beckman Wiedemann syndrome) (Wyllie et al., 2016)

Gastroschisis

- Intestine may be at risk for vascular compromise—matted with exudate
- Normally developed abdominal musculature
- Unusual to have other anomalies (Wyllie et al., 2016)

Diagnostic Testing

- Elevated maternal triple-screen alpha-fetoprotein (AFP)
- Usually diagnosed on prenatal ultrasound
  - Serial ultrasounds are recommended.
- Amniocentesis is recommended.

Nursing Interventions

Nursing interventions include the following measures.

Emergency Care

- Decision on type of delivery
  - Many babies delivered by cesarean section
- Immediate resuscitation after delivery
  - Orogastric insertion
  - IV insertion
  - Respiratory support if necessary
- Wrap and support defect to prevent fluid loss and hypothermia. Use sterile normal saline with nonadherent dressing. Newborn placed under warmer to prevent heat loss through the opening/exposed contents.

Acute Care

- Support fluid needs
- Closure of the defect by surgical means
  - May be done in stages.
- Orogastric tube to decompress intestines
- Parenteral nutrition
- IV antibiotics
- Support nonnutritive sucking needs—infant may need pacifier
- Observe surgical site for possible infection
- Observe for defecation
- Gradual resumption of feeding when ileus resolves, with breast milk or predigested formula

Chronic Care

- May have TPN for several months
- Slow increase in oral feedings
- Close monitoring of growth
- Teach importance of follow-up visits

Caregiver Education

Nurses must educate patients and caregivers on the following topics.

Emergency Care

- Explain procedures to caregivers.
- Answer caregiver questions as needed.

Acute Care

- Explain procedures to caregiver.
- Encourage caregiver to hold patient postoperatively, if possible.
- Encourage caregiver to participate in nonnutritive sucking.
- Have caregiver provide breast milk if possible; provide breast pump for use as needed.
- Have caregiver participate in oral feeding when feedings are started.

Chronic Care

- Teach caregivers signs of infection or complications.
- Teach caregivers importance of follow-up appointments.
- Teach caregivers that child may be a fussy eater at first; it is important to de-emphasize mealtime stress.

GASTROINTESTINAL PROBLEMS MANIFESTED BY LIVER, PANCREATIC, OR GALLBLADDER INVOLVEMENT

GI conditions in this area are manifested by conditions or abnormalities related to the liver, gallbladder, or pancreas.

Neonatal Jaundice

Neonatal jaundice is caused by the breakdown of red blood cells (which release bilirubin into the blood) and the immaturity of the newborn's liver (which cannot effectively metabolize the bilirubin and prepare it for excretion into the urine). Yellowish staining of the skin and whites of the newborn's eyes (sclerae) by pigment of bile (bilirubin) may occur. In newborns, a low level of jaundice is normal. Normal neonatal jaundice typically appears between the second and fifth days of life and clears with time. A high level of bilirubin or hyperbilirubinemia may cause the infant to be sleepy and eat poorly, causing the jaundice level to rise. Bilirubin lights may be necessary to help decrease the jaundice (Wyllie et al., 2016).

Assessment

Clinical presentation is as follows:

- Elevation of the bilirubin above normal
- Concern if jaundice develops before 24 hours
- Higher risk in preterm infants
- At higher levels of jaundice
  - Lethargy
  - Poor feeding
  - May have signs of infection
- Bilirubin encephalopathy (kernicterus)—may occur with severe jaundice; preventable
  - Opisthotonic posturing
  - Hypotonia or hypertonia
  - High-pitched cry
  - Seizures
  - Poor sucking (Ives, 2015; Muchowski, 2014)

Diagnostic Testing

- Transcutaneous bilimeter assessment—screening test
- Bilirubin total and direct
- CBC
- Reticulocyte count
- Urinalysis and urine culture if suspect infection
- Blood type and Rh, Coombs' test
- Test for glucose-6-phosphate dehydrogenase
- CRP and blood culture if signs of infection
- With elevated direct bilirubin, may need additional testing, including liver function tests, gamma-glutamyl transferase, alpha-1 antitrypsin, thyroid-stimulating hormone, and cortisol
- May also need ultrasound of gallbladder with elevated direct bilirubin

Nursing Interventions

Nursing interventions include the following measures.

Emergency Care

- Bilirubin results greater than 20 mg/dL may need admission to the neonatal intensive care unit or hospital if outpatient for phototherapy.
- Bilirubin results greater than 25 mg/dL may require exchange transfusion.

Acute Care

- Newborns should be assessed for jaundice before discharge.
  - Visual assessment is not always accurate.
  - Transcutaneous bilimeter reading
- Mothers should be encouraged to feed frequently; provide lactation support.
- Importance of early follow-up after discharge should be taught to caregivers.
- Jaundice in the first 24 hours requires intervention.
  - Close follow-up with repeat testing is necessary.
  - Phototherapy with biliblanket
- If level is high, may need additional interventions with fluids and phototherapy lights.
  - May require IV fluids.
  - Phototherapy—eyes will be patched.
  - Scrotal area should be covered in male infants.
  - Oral fluids—mother may continue to breastfeed if newborn is feeding well.
- Prepare for exchange transfusion if level is high.
  - Blood will be used, either typed or O negative.
  - Patient will need close monitoring during and after procedure.
- Patient may continue on biliblanket after discharge.

Chronic Care

- Patient may require follow-up appointment to follow bilirubin levels.
- If jaundice develops after first week, may interrupt breastfeeding for 12 to 24 hours to reduce level; done infrequently.
- Infant with elevated bilirubin that has a persistent direct component may need further testing to determine cause.

Complementary and Alternative Therapies

- Although once used as a therapy, indirect sunlight does not affect bilirubin levels.

Caregiver Education

Nurses must educate parents and caregivers on the following measures.

Emergency Care

- Caregiver should be taught to return to the hospital or clinic for blood tests if baby becomes jaundiced into the legs.
- Caregiver should also bring in patient if baby is feeding poorly or is very sleepy.

Acute Care

- Caregiver should feed patient frequently by breastfeeding or with formula.
- Time under the phototherapy lights or on the biliblanket should be maximized if possible; feeding without removing the biliblanket is essential.
- Monitor intake and output.
- Stress importance of follow-up visits and laboratory tests.

Chronic Care

- Patient may need frequent follow-up after discharge to follow bilirubin levels.
  - Caregivers must understand the need for and keep follow-up tests and appointments.
- Patients with problems that develop from bilirubin will need chronic care.
  - Although rare, bilirubin encephalopathy is a neurological problem that requires long-term care.

Biliary Atresia

A congenital absence or closure of the major bile ducts that drain bile from the liver, biliary atresia results in a progressive inflammatory process that may cause cirrhosis of the liver (Wyllie et al., 2016).

Assessment

Biliary atresia may have the following clinical presentation:

- Significant jaundice at 2 weeks of age (Fig. 15–13)
- Increase in the direct bilirubin (usually greater than 20% of the total value of bilirubin)
- Poor absorption of fat and the fat-soluble vitamins (A, D, E, and K)
- Dark urine
- Light-colored stools—after 2 months, may be pale, gray, or white
- Enlarged liver (Wyllie et al., 2016)

Diagnostic Testing

- Liver function tests—AST is normal early, then elevated
- Bilirubin, total and direct

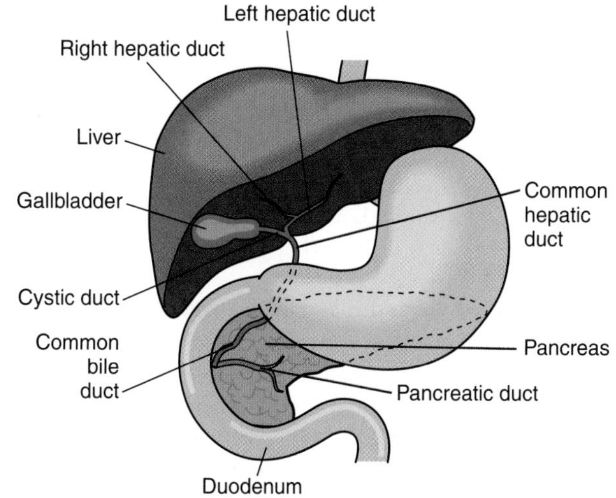

FIGURE 15–13 Biliary system.

- Alkaline phosphatase (elevated)
- Ultrasound of the abdomen and liver
- Liver scan
- Liver biopsy

Nursing Interventions

Nursing interventions include the following measures.

Emergency Care

- Stabilize patient with IV fluids.
- Prepare patient for diagnostic tests as needed.
- Explain tests to caregivers and provide reassurance as needed.

Acute Care

- IV fluids
- Low-fat, high-protein diet
- Administration of vitamins A, D, and K
- Surgery
  - After surgery, care of NG tube to suction for decompression
  - Daily weight input and output
  - Pain medication as needed
  - Administer antibiotics as ordered to prevent infection
  - Encourage nonnutritive sucking with pacifier
  - Care of the incisional site
  - Check abdominal girth size daily
  - With return of bowel function, diet to advance as tolerated from oral fluids
  - Description of stools, including color

Chronic Care

- Low-fat, high-protein diet
- Parenteral nutrition
- If initial surgery is not successful, then liver transplant may be indicated

Caregiver Education

Nurses must educate parents and caregivers about the following topics.

Emergency Care

- Bring child to hospital or clinic for care if he or she displays prolonged jaundice or pale, gray, or white stools.

Acute Care

- Teach caregiver importance of diet.
- Answer questions about NG tube.
- Teach caregiver dressing change as needed.
- Caregiver is to assist with nonnutritive sucking.

Discharge Teaching

- Teach caregiver about diet and maintenance of diet if needed.
- Stress with caregiver the importance of follow-up visits.
- Review possible signs of infection (redness or fever) or problems (increasing jaundice, vomiting, changes in stool color) to be reported.
- If liver transplant will occur, then refer to transplant team for teaching.
- Discuss caregiver concerns and provide emotional support.

Nonalcoholic Fatty Liver Disease

Two types of nonalcoholic fatty liver disease (NAFLD) are simple fatty liver and nonalcoholic steatohepatitis (NASH), which are considered two separate conditions. People typically experience development of one type of NAFLD or the other, although sometimes people with one form are later diagnosed with the other form of NAFLD.

Simple fatty liver, also called nonalcoholic fatty liver (NAFL), is a form of NAFLD in which the patient has fat in the liver but little or no inflammation or liver cell damage. Simple fatty liver typically does not progress to cause liver damage or complications.

NASH is a form of NAFLD in which fat in the liver is present along with inflammation and cell damage; this can cause fibrosis, or scarring of the liver. NASH may lead to cirrhosis or liver cancer (NIDDK, 2017).

Assessment

- NAFLD is becoming more prevalent in the adolescent population because of obesity; patients are usually (but not always) overweight
- May be diagnosed even earlier as prevalence of obesity continues to increase
- May be asymptomatic
- Fatigue
- Right upper quadrant pain
- Signs of insulin resistance include acanthosis nigricans, a usually benign skin condition characterized by hyperpigmentation (darkening of skin pigment), often accompanied by a velvety change in texture of the affected skin and/or menstrual irregularities
- Minimal to no alcohol consumption (less than two drinks daily/male or one drink or less/female) (Watanabe et al., 2015)
- Hepatomegaly (50%)
- May be associated with:
  - Diabetes
  - Familial lipodystrophies
  - Polycystic ovary syndrome
  - Celiac disease
  - Profound weight loss
  - TPN
  - Wilson disease is an autosomal recessive genetic disorder characterized by copper accumulation, leading to neurological or psychiatric symptoms and liver disease (Watanabe et al., 2015)

Diagnostic Testing

- Liver function tests
  - Hepatitis B and C testing
  - Fasting iron
  - Anti-nuclear antibody
  - Anti–smooth muscle antibody
  - Anti-mitochondrial antibody
  - Ceruloplasmin levels
  - Serum protein electrophoresis
  - Glucose
  - Triglycerides

- Ultrasound
- Liver biopsy in later stages (Watanabe et al., 2015)

Nursing Interventions

Nursing interventions should include the following measures.

Emergency Care

- Immediate care for acute liver failure is necessary.

Acute Care

- Assist with lifestyle modification.
  - Use group-based sessions
  - Increased physical activity
  - Dietary modification for weight loss (prevent rapid weight loss)

Chronic Care

- Lifestyle modification
- Pharmacological therapy
  - Vitamins A and E
  - Metformin (Watanabe et al., 2015)

Caregiver Education

Nurses must educate parents and caregivers on the following measures.

Emergency Care

- Caregiver must recognize signs of diabetic coma.
- Acute abdominal pain should be assessed immediately.

Acute Care

- Teach ways to modify lifestyle.
  - Discuss dieting and avoidance of fad diets.
  - Discuss exercise options, including increasing activity and decreasing screen time.
- Help family find an appropriate support group.
- Discuss feelings of child or adolescent about disease; provide emotional support.

Chronic Care

- Teach family importance of taking medications.
- Teach family importance of keeping follow-up appointments.
- Review lifestyle changes and diet modification with child or adolescent on a regular basis and modify as needed.

Cystic Fibrosis

Cystic fibrosis is a hereditary disorder that affects the exocrine glands. It causes the production of abnormally thick mucus, leading to the blockage of the pancreatic ducts, intestines, and bronchi, and often resulting in respiratory infection (Wyllie et al., 2016).

Assessment

- Pulmonary manifestations (discussed in Chapter 11)
- Effect on the pancreatic exocrine gland function—15% with normal gland function
  - FTT
  - Chronic diarrhea
  - Respiratory symptoms
- First manifestation may be meconium ileus (15%)
  - Lack of passage of meconium for 48 hours
  - Diagnosed by barium enema
- Rectal prolapse
- Steatorrhea
- Pancreatitis
- Diabetes mellitus
- May have slow or poor growth and nutrition (Wyllie et al., 2016)

Diagnostic Testing

- Sweat chloride test will be positive with elevated chloride.
- Chromosome analysis will indicate genes for cystic fibrosis.
- Seventy-two-hour fecal fat test result usually shows decreased fecal fat.

Nursing Interventions

Nursing interventions include emergency, acute, and chronic care.

Emergency Care

- Recognize signs of intestinal obstruction with meconium ileus.
- Recognize and treat signs of pancreatitis if they occur.
- Explain care and tests for diagnosis to caregivers.

Acute Care

- Assist with treatment as needed.
- Support nutrition; support breastfeeding if mother desires to breastfeed.
- Administer medication as needed.
  - Includes pancreatic enzymes and fat-soluble vitamins (A, D, E, K) (Table 15–3)
  - May take cystic fibrosis transmembrane conductance regulator (CFTR) modulator therapy (Table 15–3).
- Teach caregivers reason for medication and importance of use.

Chronic Care

- Measure and monitor growth.
- Teach family proper use of medications, including supplemental enzyme therapy.
  - Enzymes should be taken before eating and with all meals and snacks (unless a simple carbohydrate).
  - Enzymes should not be skipped.
  - Enzymes work for about 1 hour after eating. Higher dose may be needed for foods high in fat (e.g., fast food).
  - For infants and young children, enzymes should be mixed with a soft acidic food such as applesauce, not with milk-based food such as yogurt.
  - Enzymes should not be mixed in food ahead of time and should not be refrigerated.
  - If the child is on a tube feeding, the enzyme should be taken by mouth before the tube feeding.
- Encourage proper nutrition.
  - Teach child foods that may be eaten without taking enzymes, including fruits, juice, soft drinks or sports drinks, tea, lollipops, fruit snacks, jelly beans, gum, and popsicles or freezer pops.
  - Child may require gastrostomy tube if FTT occurs.
  - It has been shown that proper nutrition also supports respiratory status.
- Stress importance of regular immunizations.

TABLE 15–3 Pancreatic Enzymes and Other Medications Used to Treat Cystic Fibrosis

Pancreatic enzymes	Creon Pancrease, Pancrease MT, Pancrecarb (should not be given if allergic to pigs or pork), Ultrase, Ultrase MT, Viokase	Given before meals and snacks and may be opened for administration Young children can have it sprinkled in applesauce Helps to digest carbohydrate, protein, and fat and promote nutrient absorption, which will help increase weight
CFTR modulator therapies	Ivacaftor Adults and children ≥6 years: 150 mg every 12 hours with food containing fat Age 2–5 years: dosage by weight Lumacaftor/ivacaftor Age ≥6 years: 2 tablets every 12 hours with food containing fat	Given to children aged ≥2 years who have one of the following mutations in the CFTR gene: G551D, G1244E, G1349D, G178R, G 551S, R117H, S1251N, S549N, S549R Given to children aged ≥6 years with the F508del mutation (most common in CF) Medications work by regulating proper flow of fluids and sodium in and out of cells
Vitamin A	Age 0–1 years: 1,500 IU Age 1–3 years: 5,000 IU Age 4–8 years: 500 to 10,000 IU Age >8 years: 10,000 IU	Given as a supplement Also may be absorbed some from food such as orange-colored fruits and vegetables and dark green vegetables Take with pancreatic enzymes for better absorption
Probiotics	*Lactobacillus rhamnosus* GG capsules or in some yogurt	Reduces intestinal inflammation, reduces respiratory infection
Vitamin D	Infants: 400 IU Children with CF need 400–800 IU/day because of poor fat absorption	Will need supplement Some in foods—milk, salmon, tuna with oil, sardines, fortified cereal Take with pancreatic enzymes for better absorption
Vitamin E	Age 0–1 years: 40–450 IU Age 1–3 years: 80–150 IU Age 4–8 years: 100–200 IU Age >8 years: 200–400 IU	Is an antioxidant Used in the production of red blood cells Helps with intestinal health and protects against infection in lung lining Found in nuts, vegetable oil, wheat germ oil, olives, corn, leafy green vegetables, fortified cereal Take with pancreatic enzymes for better absorption
Dornase alfa/ Pulmozyme	Jet nebulizer or eRapid Nebulizer System: one 2.5-mg ampule inhaled daily May be used twice daily in some patients	Improves pulmonary function and reduces the risk for respiratory tract infections

CF, cystic fibrosis; CFTR, cystic fibrosis transmembrane conductance regulator.

Adapted from Cystic Fibrosis Foundation. (2016). Retrieved from http://www.cff.org; and National Institutes of Health, Office of Dietary GERD in Infants and Children Supplements. (2016). Fact sheets. *Retrieved from http://ods.od.nih.gov/factsheets/list-all/.*

Caregiver Education

Parents and caregivers must receive nurse education on emergency, acute, and chronic care.

Emergency Care

- Explain procedures and answer caregiver questions.

Acute Care

- Address caregiver concerns.
- Stress importance of maintaining medication regimen.
- Stress importance of nutrition.

Chronic Care

- Address caregiver concerns.
- Stress importance of maintaining medication regimen.
- Stress importance of nutrition.
- Review immunizations needed at each visit.
- Encourage caregiver to visit the Cystic Fibrosis Foundation Web site (https://www.cff.org) for more information about cystic fibrosis.
- Encourage caregivers to allow child to attend camp or other activities with other children with cystic fibrosis.
- Caregivers may need genetic counseling.

SAFE AND EFFECTIVE NURSING CARE: Clinical Pearl

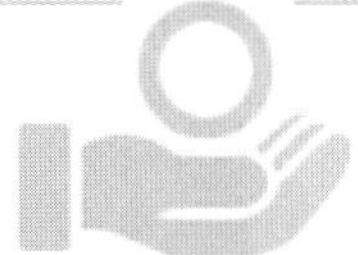

Symptoms of Cystic Fibrosis

Cystic fibrosis may be manifested by mainly respiratory or mainly GI symptoms, or a combination of both. Although it usually occurs in Caucasians, it may also be seen in African American and Native American populations (Wyllie et al., 2016).

Cholecystitis and Gallstones

Cholecystitis is the sudden inflammation of the gallbladder. If the condition persists for months, then it becomes chronic cholecystitis. Gallstones are small, hard crystalline masses formed abnormally in the gallbladder or bile ducts from bile pigments, cholesterol, and calcium salts. Gallstones can cause severe pain and blockage of the bile duct and cholecystitis (Wyllie et al., 2016).

Clinical Presentation

Cholecystitis and gallstones may have the following clinical presentation (Fig. 15–14):

- Jaundice in infants
- Fever
- Right upper quadrant pain with vomiting (older children and adolescents) and/or pain radiating to the right scapula region

Diagnostic Testing

- Localized tenderness to palpation
- CBC
- Bilirubin
- Alkaline phosphatase and gamma-glutamyl transferase

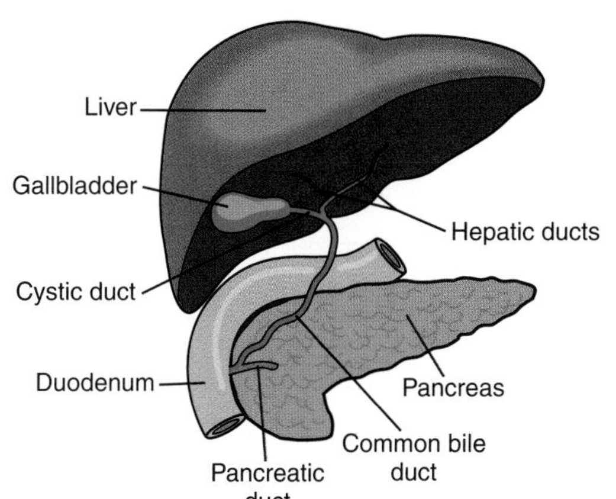

FIGURE 15–14 The gallbladder and the ducts that carry bile and other digestive enzymes from the liver, gallbladder, and pancreas to the small intestine are called the biliary system.

- Amylase
- Urinalysis
- Liver function tests
- Plain film radiograph
- Ultrasound

Nursing Interventions

Nursing interventions include the following measures.

Emergency Care

- Vomiting and pain may require immediate hospitalization.
- Start IV fluids.
- Patient should be NPO.
- Endoscopic retrograde cholangiopancreatography may be performed to remove gallstones from the bile duct.

Acute Care

- Continue IV therapy
- Analgesic medication as appropriate
- Administer antibiotics if ordered for persistent fever
- Prepare patient for surgery, which is usually laparoscopic
- Monitor patient postoperatively for any complications
  - Administer analgesics as appropriate.
  - Advance diet as tolerated; monitor intake and output.
  - Monitor incision sites.
  - Encourage coughing and deep breathing.
  - Encourage use of an incentive spirometer.
- Caregivers will need teaching about signs of infection, pain relief, and incision site care
- Surgery usually corrects problems
- Gallstones in infancy do not need removal unless symptomatic, because gallstones usually resolve spontaneously
- In patients with Crohn's disease who need a functioning gallbladder, gallstones may be removed from the bile duct without gallbladder removal
- Laser lithotripsy is currently an experimental therapy
- Enteral feedings for patients on TPN

Caregiver Education

Nurses should educate parents and caregivers on the following topics.

Emergency Care

- Bring patient to the hospital or clinic for evaluation for acute pain, vomiting, or signs of jaundice.

Acute Hospital Care

- Assist with feeding as needed.
- Reassure caregivers about their ability to care for the patient.
- Teach caregivers how to care for incision site.
- Teach caregivers about pain relief.

Chronic Home Care

- Advance diet as tolerated.
- Observe for signs of infection.
- Administer pain mediation as needed.
- Remind caregivers about keeping regular appointments and starting or continuing immunizations.

Hepatitis

Hepatitis is a disease that produces inflammation of the liver, usually resulting from a viral infection or liver damage (Wyllie et al., 2016).

Assessment

Hepatitis may have the following clinical presentation:

- Hepatitis A is caused by oral–fecal contamination, either through food or environmental contamination.
- Hepatitis B and C are caused by exposure to infected blood or blood products, or through sexual contact. Hepatitis B may be spread from mother to infant during delivery.
- Hepatitis A, B, and C may be asymptomatic.
- Symptoms may include:
  - Jaundice, including icteric sclera
  - Abdominal pain in right upper quadrant
  - Malaise
  - Loss of appetite
  - Low-grade fever
  - Dark urine and light-colored stools
  - Hepatosplenomegaly (HSM+)
  - Petechiae, ecchymosis, spider angiomas

Diagnostic Testing

- Liver function tests, including alanine aminotransferase
- Serological tests
  - Hepatitis A—anti-HAV-IgM: Confirms diagnosis of recent acute infection.
  - Hepatitis A—anti-HAV-total: Predominantly IgG, confirms previous exposure to hepatitis A, recovery, and immunity; does not distinguish recent from past infection.
  - Hepatitis B—hepatitis B surface antigen (HBsAg): If positive, earliest indicator of active infection. It is also present in chronic disease or carrier state. Does not become positive after immunization.
  - Hepatitis B surface antibody (anti-HBsAg): Presence without HBsAg indicates recovery from infection and immunity from previous exposure or vaccine.
  - Hepatitis B e antigen (HBeAg): In blood only when virus is present, and can be passed to others; monitors treatment. Useful to determine resolution of infection or presence of carrier state (persistence after 20 weeks indicates chronic or carrier state). Presence in HBsAg-positive mother indicates 90% chance of infant acquiring infection.
  - Anti–hepatitis B core antigen (HBc)-total: First antibody to appear after appearance of HBsAg. The presence with HBsAg and absence of anti-HBsAg indicate chronic infection.
  - Anti-HBc-IgM: This is the earliest specific antibody. It may be the only serological marker after HBsAg and HBeAg subside. Can differentiate acute from chronic infection.
  - Anti-HBe: This appears after HBeAg disappears; it is detectable for years. It indicates decreasing infectivity and good prognosis for recovery from acute infection. Presence with anti-HBc and absence of HBsAb and anti-HBs indicate recent acute infection.
  - HBV-DNA (polymerase chain reaction): It indicates active infection, is the most sensitive and specific assay for early diagnosis, and may be detected when all other markers are negative. It measures HBV replication.
  - Hepatitis C—anti-HCV test for antibody: It indicates infection, past or present, but does not differentiate. Confirmation of positive test with HCV RIBA. HCV RNA assay (viral load) now being used more because of better sensitivity. Viral genotyping may also be used (Williamson & Snyder, 2015).
- Ultrasound
- Liver biopsy

Nursing Interventions

Nursing interventions for hepatitis include the following measures.

Emergency Care

- Sudden onset of symptoms of liver failure may cause caregivers to bring patient for assessment.
- Development of ascites in a chronic patient may require hospitalization for supportive care.

Acute Care

- Hepatitis A is passed by the oral–fecal route, so good hand hygiene and standard precautions are essential
- Prevention of needle sticks
- Balanced diet that prevents dehydration
- Bedrest
- Antiviral therapy for hepatitis C: sofosbuvir (Sovaldi) and the combination product, ledipasvir/sofosbuvir (Harvoni), in children older than 12 years; peginterferon alfa-2b (PEG Intron) plus ribavirin (Rebetol) is approved for children 3 years or older; peginterferon alfa-2a (Pegasys) plus ribavirin (Copegus) is approved for children 5 years and older
- Supportive care, including monitoring for complications
- If patient remains in good health, no restrictions on activity
- With hepatitis A, child should not return to day care until virus has cleared
- Therapy will be related to the severity of disease; careful monitoring and follow-up are essential
- Family members should be vaccinated for hepatitis A and hepatitis B
- Children who are not infected should complete immunizations for hepatitis (Fig. 15–15)
- Infants should receive hepatitis B series of immunizations at birth and 2, 4, and 6 months
- All mothers should be tested for hepatitis B during pregnancy
- Infants of hepatitis B–positive mothers should receive the hepatitis B immunoglobulin vaccine at birth as well

Caregiver Education

Nurses must educate parents and caregivers on the following topics related to hepatitis.

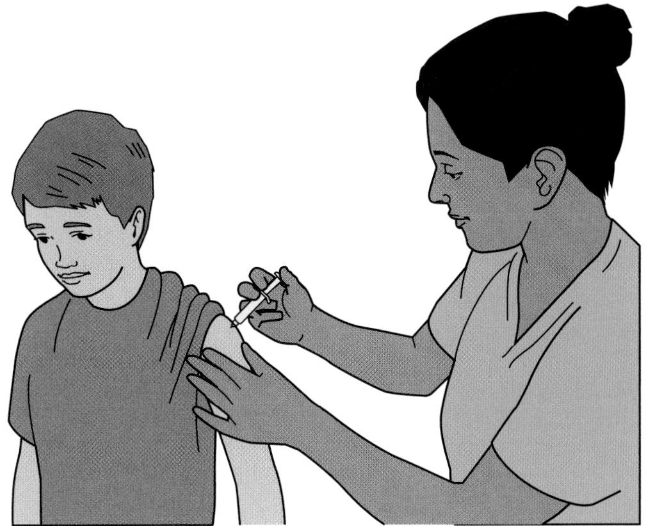

FIGURE 15-15 Vaccines protect you from getting hepatitis A.

Emergency Care

- Bring patient to hospital or clinic for evaluation if condition worsens.

Acute Care

- Help patient to maintain bedrest; encourage quiet activities for entertainment.
- Teach elements of proper nutrition to maintain calories and hydration.
- Teach importance of medication regimen if receiving antiviral therapy.

Discharge Teaching

- Teach importance of maintaining follow-up visits as scheduled.
- Teach importance of proper immunization for all family members.
- Teach caregivers to help child avoid medications that can cause liver damage.
- Always wash hands after using the toilet and before fixing food.
- Gloves are indicated for anyone handling another's stool.

Evidence-Based Practice: Decrease in Incidence of Hepatitis A With Immunization

Chugh, A., Maximus, M., Perlman, M., & Gonzalez-Peralta, R. (2016). Viral hepatitis in children: A through E. *Pediatric Annals, 45*(12), 420–426.

Hepatitis A has shown a decrease in incidence because of immunization strategies. Originally, vaccination was done in selected states with high rates of hepatitis A, but hepatitis A has now increased in states with lower risk, and universal immunization is now recommended for all children starting at age 1 year. It has been shown that children are a reservoir for hepatitis A, and immunization would reduce this risk to the elderly, as well as healthy adults. Immunization has helped reduce cases in the United States from 14,000 in 2000 to less than 2000 in 2012.

GASTROINTESTINAL PROBLEMS MANIFESTED BY NUTRITIONAL CHANGES

GI conditions in this area are manifested by changes in nutritional intake, either in excessive intake or deficit intake of calories.

Obesity

Whereas a body mass index (BMI) above the 85th percentile for the child's age and sex is defined as overweight, a BMI greater than or equal to the 95th percentile is defined as obesity by Centers for Disease Control and Prevention.

Assessment

- BMI greater than 95% is considered obese
- BMI of 85% to 94% is considered overweight
- Adiposity rebound at a young age
- Knee pain
- Abdominal pain
- Daytime somnolence
- Polycystic ovary disease
- Menstrual irregularities
- Acne
- Hirsutism
- Infertility
- May have associated problems
  - Diabetes
  - Fatty liver disease
  - Heart disease
  - Hypertension
  - Hyperlipidemia
  - Obstructive sleep apnea
  - Gallbladder disease
  - Slipped capital femoral epiphysis

Diagnostic Testing

- Height, weight, BMI at each visit
- CBC
- Lipid profile
- Fasting glucose
- Liver function tests
- Thyroid-stimulating hormone
- Cortisol a.m. (morning)
- Height and weight measurements
- BMI = weight in kilograms divided by the height in meters squared (kg/m^2)
  - Most commonly used measure
- Skinfold thickness—calipers measure subcutaneous fat from several areas and compare with controls
- Bioelectric impedance analysis
- Ultrasound
- Sleep study (Wyllie et al., 2016)

Nursing Interventions

Nursing interventions for obesity include emergency, acute, and chronic care.

Emergency Care

- Symptoms of heart disease, uncontrolled hypertension, or diabetes with blood sugar not well controlled may require hospitalization.
- Hip or leg pain should have immediate evaluation.

Acute Care

- Stabilize any health conditions.
- Encourage caregivers to not overfeed in infancy.

Chronic Care

- Patient needs individualized weight loss program
- Nutrition assessment
  - Referral to nutrition
  - Change in diet
  - Discuss speed of eating
  - Discuss caregiver effect on eating
  - Encourage patient to not skip meals
  - Encourage increase and change in physical activity
- Decrease screen time (television or video games) to 2 hours a day or less
- No eating in front of the TV
- Change daily routine to increase activity
- Behavior modification
  - Small, gradual changes over time
  - Positive reinforcement for changes
  - Provide some choice
- Family involvement
  - Family needs to be involved in plan and role-model healthy eating and physical activity.
  - Need education concerning short- and long-term consequences of obesity.
  - Promote positive parenting skills; consistent messages.
  - Provide healthy meals and snacks.
- Support groups
- Medication
  - Only for patient 16 years or older
  - Orlistat—needs close supervision if used
- Surgical intervention—bariatric surgery
  - It may be a consideration for late adolescent patient.
  - Patient must meet stringent criteria. The selection criteria for adolescents considered for a bariatric procedure should include a BMI ≥35 kg/m² with major comorbidities (i.e., type 2 diabetes mellitus, moderate-to-severe sleep apnea [apnea–hypopnea index >15], pseudotumor cerebri, or severe NAFLD) or a BMI ≥40 kg/m² with other comorbidities (e.g., hypertension, insulin resistance, glucose intolerance, substantially impaired quality of life or activities of daily living, dyslipidemia, sleep apnea with apnea–hypopnea index >5). The associated risk-benefit analysis should also include the consideration of the potential long-term health risks of untreated or inadequately treated obesity for the individual candidate (American Society for Metabolic and Bariatric Surgery, 2017).

SAFE AND EFFECTIVE NURSING CARE: Clinical Pearl

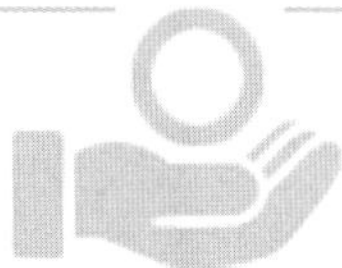

Smoking for Weight Control

Adolescents may use smoking as a weight-control strategy. Asking about this during history taking is important, as well as counseling the adolescent about risks of smoking (Wyllie et al., 2016).

Caregiver Education

Nurses must educate parents and caregivers on the following topics related to obesity.

Emergency Care

- Signs of complications such as uncontrolled diabetes and heart disease should be taught to the caregiver and patient.

Acute Care

- Caregiver should be taught short- and long-term consequences of obesity.
- Caregiver needs to know importance of not overfeeding.
- Importance of healthy diet and activity should be emphasized, with input from family.
- Discuss with caregiver and child feelings about food and mealtimes.

Chronic Care

- Obesity is a chronic condition that requires caregiver assistance for success with weight loss.
- Teach importance of diet—use resources such as *California Food Guide* (2016; see Box 15–2).
- Teach importance of regular exercise.
- Teach importance of reduction in sedentary behavior.
- Assist parent with learning positive parenting techniques.
- Encourage participation in support group.
- Reinforce importance of follow-up visits.

Failure to Thrive

FTT is defined as weight for age that is less than the 5th percentile on multiple occasions or weight deceleration that crosses two major percentile lines on a growth chart (Burns, Dunn, Brady, Starr, & Blosser, 2013).

Assessment

- The clinical presentation of FTT includes:
  - Poor weight gain of less than the 5th or 3rd percentile for age on graph
  - Vomiting
  - Food refusal
  - Food fixation
  - Abnormal feeding practices
  - Anticipatory gagging

BOX 15–2 | Resources for Digestive Disorders

This directory lists various organizations involved in digestive disease–related activities for patients.

American Celiac Disease Alliance (ACDA)

2504 Duxbury Place
Alexandria, VA 22308
Phone: 703–622–3331
E-mail: info@americanceliac.org
Internet: www.americanceliacsociety.org

Publications: *Celiac Disease: A Hidden Epidemic* and *Gluten-Free Diet: A Comprehensive Resource Guide* (books); *Gluten-Free Living* (magazine)

American Celiac Society—Dietary Support Coalition

Annette & James Bentley
P.O. Box 23455
New Orleans, LA 70183-0455
Phone: 504–737–3293
E-mail: info@americanceliacsociety.org
Internet: http://www.americanceliacsociety.org

Publications: Newsletter—*Whooo's Report. Call a Friend With Celiac Sprue*

American College of Gastroenterology (ACG)

P.O. Box 342260
Bethesda, MD 20827-2260
Phone: 301–263–9000
Internet: http://www.acg.gi.org

Publications: Journals—*American Journal of Gastroenterology* and *Nature Clinical Practice Gastroenterology & Hepatology*

American Gastroenterological Association (AGA)

National Office
4930 Del Ray Avenue
Bethesda, MD 20814
Phone: 301–654–2055
Fax: 301–654–5920
E-mail: member@gastro.org
Internet: https://www.gastro.org

Publications: Journals—*Gastroenterology* and *Clinical Perspectives in Gastroenterology*; weekly newsletter—*GI Practice Management News*; reports—*Legislative Report* and *Burden of Diseases Report*; membership magazine—*AGA Digest*

American Liver Foundation (ALF)

75 Maiden Lane, Suite 603
New York, NY 10038-4810
Phone: 1–800–GO–LIVER (465–4837),
1–888–4HEP–USA (443–7872), or 212–668–1000
Fax: 212–483–8179
E-mail: info@liverfoundation.org
Internet: https://www.liverfoundation.org

ARPKD/CHF Alliance

Autosomal Recessive Polycystic Kidney Disease & Congenital Hepatic Fibrosis Alliance
P.O. Box 70
Kirkwood, PA 17536
Phone: 717–529–5555
Fax: 1–800–807–9110
E-mail: info@arpkd.org
Internet: http://www.arpkd.org

Association of Gastrointestinal Motility Disorders, Inc. (AGMD) (formerly American Society of Adults with Pseudo-Obstruction, Inc.)

AGMD International Corporate Headquarters
12 Roberts Drive
Bedford, MA 01730
Phone: 781–275–1300
Fax: 781–275–1304
E-mail: digestive.motility@gmail.com
Internet: http://www.agmd-gimotility.org

Publications: Member publications—*AGMD Beacon* and *AGMD Search and Research*

Celiac Disease Foundation (CDF)

13251 Ventura Boulevard, #1
Studio City, CA 91604
Phone: 818–990–2354
Fax: 818–990–2379
E-mail: cdf@celiac.org
Internet: https://www.celiac.org

Publications: Quarterly newsletter—*Guidelines for a Gluten-Free Lifestyle;* brochures

Celiac Sprue Association/USA Inc.

P.O. Box 31700
Omaha, NE 68131-0700
Phone: 1–877–CSA–4CSA
Fax: 402–643–4108
E-mail: celiacs@csaceliacs.org
Internet: http://www.csaceliacs.org

Crohn's & Colitis Foundation of America (CCFA)

386 Park Avenue South, 17th floor
New York, NY 10016
Phone: 1–800–932–2423 or 212–685–3440
Fax: 212–779–4098
E-mail: info@ccfa.org
Internet: http://www.ccfa.org

Continued

BOX 15-2 | Resources for Digestive Disorders—cont'd

Cyclic Vomiting Syndrome Association (CVSA)

CVSA USA/Canada
3585 Cedar Hill Road, NW
Canal Winchester, OH 43110
Phone: 614-837-2586
Fax: 614-837-2586
E-mail: waitesd@cvsaonline.org
Internet: http://www.cvsaonline.org
Publication: Member newsletter—*Code V*

Digestive Disease National Coalition

507 Capitol Court NE, Suite 200
Washington, DC 20002
Phone: 202-544-7497
Fax: 202-546-7105
Internet: http://www.ddnc.org

Gastro-Intestinal Research Foundation

70 East Lake Street, Suite 1015
Chicago, IL 60601-5907
Phone: 312-332-1350
Fax: 312-332-4757
E-mail: girf@earthlink.net
Internet: http://www.girf.org
Publications: Several newsletters; patient education pamphlet—*Issues in Women's Gastrointestinal Health*

Gluten Intolerance Group of North America (GIG)

31214 124th Ave. SE
Auburn, WA 98092
Phone: 253-833-6655
Fax: 253-833-6675
E-mail: info@gluten.net
Internet: http://www.gluten.net
Publication: Member newsletter—*GIG Newsletter*

Hepatitis B Coalition

Immunization Action Coalition
1573 Selby Avenue, Suite 234
St. Paul, MN 55104
Phone: 651-647-9009
Fax: 651-647-9131
E-mail: admin@immunize.org
Internet: http://www.immunize.org and http://www.vaccineinformation.org
Publications: Semiannual publications—*NEEDLE TIPS, Vaccinate Adults,* and *Vaccinate Women*

Hepatitis B Foundation

3805 Old Easton Road
Doylestown, PA 18902
Phone: 215-489-4900
Fax: 215-489-4313
E-mail: info@hepb.org
Internet: http://www.hepb.org
Publications: Newsletters—*B Informed, B Connected,* and *B News You Can Use*; brochures—*The Hepatitis B Foundation Cause for a Cure, Someone You Know Has Hepatitis B, Protect Yourself and Those You Love Against HBV, What Hepatitis B Carriers Should Know,* and *The First Loving Act—Vaccination;* fact sheets—*Advice to Parents of Children With HBV* and *Hot Sheet*

Hepatitis Foundation International (HFI)

504 Blick Drive
Silver Spring, MD 20904-2901
Phone: 1-800-891-0707 or 301-622-4200
Fax: 301-622-4702
E-mail: hfi@comcast.net
Internet: www.hepatitisfoundation.org

International Foundation for Functional Gastrointestinal Disorders (IFFGD) Inc.

P.O. Box 170864
Milwaukee, WI 53217-8076
Phone: 1-888-964-2001 or 414-964-1799
Fax: 414-964-7176
E-mail: iffgd@iffgd.org
Internet: https://www.iffgd.org
Publications: Quarterly newsletters—*Participate, Digestive Health Matters,* and *Digestive Health in Children*

National Foundation for Celiac Awareness

P.O. Box 544
Ambler, PA 19002
Phone: 215-325-1306
Fax: 215-283-2335
E-mail: info@celiaccentral.org
Internet: http://www.celiaccentral.org
Publications: Books—*Celiac Sprue, A Guide Through the Medicine Cabinet; Gluten-Free Diet: A Comprehensive Resource Guide; Triumph Dining; NFCA Gluten-Free Resource Guide*

BOX 15-2 | Resources for Digestive Disorders—cont'd

Oley Foundation for Home Parenteral and Enteral Nutrition (HomePEN)

214 Hun Memorial, MC-28
Albany Medical Center
Albany, NY 12208–3478
Phone: 1–800–776–OLEY (6539) or 518–262–5079 (outside U.S.)
Fax: 518–262–5528
E-mail: info@oley.org
Internet: https://www.oley.org

Pediatric/Adolescent Gastroesophageal Reflux Association Inc. (PAGER)

P.O. Box 486
Buckeystown, MD 21717-0486
Phone: 301–601–9541
Fax: 630–982–6418
E-mail: gergroup@aol.com
Internet: http://www.reflux.org

Pull-thru Network

2312 Savoy Street
Hoover, AL 35226-1528
Phone: 205–978–2930
E-mail: info@pullthrunetwork.org
Internet: http://www.pullthrunetwork.org
Publications: Quarterly publication—*Pull-thru Network News;* free brochure—*Anorectal Malformations—A Parent's Guide*

Reach Out for Youth With Ileitis and Colitis Inc.

84 Northgate Circle
Melville, NY 11747
Phone: 631–293–3102
Fax: 631–293–3102
E-mail: reachoutforyouth@reachoutforyouth.org
Internet: http://www.reachoutforyouth.org

TEF-VATER International

15301 Grey Fox Road
Upper Marlboro, MD 20772
Phone: 301–952–6837
Fax: 301–952–9152
E-mail: info@tefvater.org
Internet: http://www.tefvater.org
Publication: Newsletter—*Inside Connections*

United Ostomy Associations of America, Inc.

P.O. Box 66
Fairview, TN 37062-0066
Phone: 1–800–826–0826 or 949–660–8624
Fax: 949–660–9262
E-mail: info@uoaa.org
Internet: http://www.ostomy.org
Publication: Journal—*Ostomy Quarterly*

Weight-control Information Network (WIN)

1 WIN Way
Bethesda, MD 20892–3665
Phone: 1–877–946–4627 or 202–828–1025
Fax: 202–828–1028
E-mail: win@info.niddk.nih.gov
Internet: http://www.win.niddk.nih.gov
Publication: Quarterly newsletter—*WIN Notes*

National Digestive Diseases Information Clearinghouse (NDDIC)

2 Information Way
Bethesda, MD 20892–3570
Phone: 1–800–891–5389
TTY: 1–866–569–1162
Fax: 703–738–4929
E-mail: nddic@info.niddk.nih.gov
Internet: http://www.digestive.niddk.nih.gov

The NDDIC is a service of the National Institute of Diabetes and Digestive and Kidney Diseases (NIDDK). The NIDDK is part of the National Institutes of Health of the U.S. Department of Health and Human Services. Established in 1980, the Clearinghouse provides information about digestive diseases to people with digestive disorders and to their families, health-care professionals, and the public. The NDDIC answers inquiries, develops and distributes publications, and works closely with professional and patient organizations and government agencies to coordinate resources about digestive diseases.

Its publications are not copyrighted. The Clearinghouse encourages users of its publications to duplicate and distribute as many copies as desired.

Adapted from Mullin, G. E. (2011). Integrative Gastroenterology. Directory of Digestive Diseases Organizations for Patients, Oxford, United Kingdom; and National Digestive Diseases Information Clearinghouse. *Directory of digestive diseases organization.* Retrieved from http://digestive.niddk.nih.gov/resources/Directory_Digestive_Diseases_Orgs_508.pdf

- Irritability
- Height, head circumference, and developmental skills may be affected
- Chronic physical problems
- Psychosocial problems in parent–child relationship can lead to nonorganic FTT
- May be caused by inborn error of metabolism with more severe symptoms
- Nonorganic: food restriction, food rituals, and poor appetite
- Organic: vomiting, diarrhea, and abdominal distension

Diagnostic Testing

- History: prenatal, perinatal, neonatal, postnatal health, developmental, family, psychosocial
- Height, weight, BMI, head circumference (<2 years), skinfold measurement
- Physical examination noting abnormalities
- Vital signs
- Feeding assessment
  - Quantity of food
  - Ability to suck, chew, swallow

- Meals and child feeding
- Feeding history including calorie intake, feeding behaviors, frequency, and intake
- Breastfeeding including frequency and length, formula preparation if bottle feeding
- Twenty-four-hour diet recall for infant, 3 days for older children

- Developmental assessment
- Basic metabolic profile
- Vitamin D, lead, zinc, iron screening
- Albumin with severe FTT
- CBC/ESR, serum electrolytes
- Urinalysis and urine culture
- Sweat chloride test
- Stool studies for fat, reducing substances, ova and parasites, and culture
- Thyroid-stimulating hormone
- Chest radiograph, renal ultrasound
- With growth failure: karyotype, bone age

Nursing Interventions

- Nursing interventions for FTT include the following measures.

Emergency Care

- Lack of intake or need for immediate intake may require hospitalization.
- Evaluate and intervene to protect the child from abuse if intentional abuse by withholding nutrition is suspected.
- Hospitalization may be necessary if outpatient management is not practical or feasible.

Acute Care

- Stabilize any conditions.
- Encourage caregivers to recognize feeding cues in infancy.
- Provide parent education about feeding and parental support.

Chronic Care

- Program for patient must be individualized
- Nutrition assessment (see Table 15–2)
  - Referral to nutrition
  - Feeding clinic
  - Discuss caregiver effect on eating
- Provide parent education and support
- Assist parent with learning positive parenting techniques
- Treat underlying chronic conditions
- Social work referral, especially if nonorganic FTT
- Evaluate for normal weight gain every 1 to 3 weeks
  - May take up to 2 weeks for growth to occur if the condition is severe.
  - Catch-up growth may occur rapidly.
  - Develop a goal weight within normal range for the child's age, sex, and height.
- Family involvement
  - Family needs to be involved in plan.
  - Need education concerning short- and long-term consequences of FTT.
  - Promote positive parenting skills; consistent messages.
  - Provide healthy meals and snacks, and recognize feeding patterns and behaviors.
- Reinforce importance of follow-up visits

SAFE AND EFFECTIVE NURSING CARE: Clinical Pearl

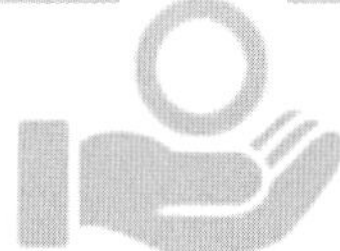

Definitions of Failure to Thrive

- Weight less than 80% of median weight for length
- Weight for length less than 80% of ideal weight
- Weight for length less than 10th percentile
- BMI for chronological age less than 5th percentile
- Weight for chronological age and sex less than 5th percentile or two standard deviations below the mean
- Length for chronological age less than 5th percentile
- Weight decrease crosses more than two major percentile lines on age and population appropriate growth chart
- Height, head circumference, and developmental skills may be affected
- Three basic causes: inadequate intake, inadequate caloric absorption, and excessive calorie expenditure with poor intake

Burns, C. E., Dunn, A. M., Brady, M. A., Starr, N. B., & Blosser, C. G. (2013). Pediatric primary care *(5th ed., p. 773). St. Louis, MO: Saunders.*

Caregiver Education

Caregivers must be educated on the following topics related to FTT.

Emergency Care

- Signs of complications should be taught to the caregiver and patient.

Acute Care

- Caregiver should be taught short- and long-term consequences of FTT.
- The importance of healthy diet and activity should be emphasized.
- Discuss with caregiver and child feelings about feeding, food, and mealtimes.

Chronic Care

- FTT can be a chronic condition that requires caregiver assistance for success with weight gain and maintenance.
- Teach importance of diet (see Table 15–2).
- Assist parent with learning positive parenting techniques.
- Reinforce importance of follow-up visits.

Case Study

Projectile Vomiting

Samuel Smith was born at 38 weeks' gestation by vaginal delivery and weighed 7 lb 14 oz at birth. Sammy had been breastfed since birth and has been spitting up breast milk since birth. His growth is slow but within the range of normal. Sammy comes to clinic with his caregivers. He is 5 weeks old today, and the caregivers are concerned because he has started to vomit his feeding. His weight is the same since the last visit. They state the "spitting up" became worse in the last week, and they state the vomiting is very forceful. The baby is fretful and acting hungry. They are wondering if they should be concerned.

1. What would you look for during an examination of this baby?
2. What tests might be performed?
3. What would you tell the caregivers about the treatment for this infant?

REFERENCES

American Society for Metabolic and Bariatric Surgery. (2017). *Pediatric best practice guidelines.* Retrieved from https://asmbs.org/resources/pediatric-best-practice-guidelines

Bickley, L. (2016). *Bates' guide to physical examination and history-taking.* Philadelphia: Lippincott Williams & Wilkins.

Burns, C. E., Dunn, A. M., Brady, M. A., Starr, N. B., & Blosser, C. G. (2013). *Pediatric primary care* (5th ed.). St. Louis, MO: Saunders.

Burns, C. E., Dunn, A. M., Brady, M. A., Starr, N. B., Blosser, C. G., & Garzon, D. L. (2016). *Pediatric primary care* (6th ed.). St. Louis, MO: Saunders.

California Food Guide. (2016). Sacramento, CA: California Department of Health Care Services and California Department of Public Health. Retrieved from http://www.dhcs.ca.gov/formsandpubs/publications/Pages/California FoodGuide.aspx

Cazan, C., Doborta, L., & Neamtu, M. L. (2014). Sandifer syndrome: A challenge for the pediatrician. *Archive of Disease in Children, 99*(Suppl. 2), A520.

Celiac Disease Foundation. (2009). *Gluten free diet.* Retrieved from http://www.celiac.org

Chugh, A., Maximus, M., Perlman, M., & Gonzalez-Peralta, R. (2016). Viral hepatitis in children: A through E. *Pediatric Annals, 45*(12), 420–426.

Churgay, C., & Aftab, Z. (2012). Gastroenteritis in children: Part I diagnosis. *American Family Physician, 85*(11), 1059–1062.

Cystic Fibrosis Foundation. (2016). Retrieved from http://www.cff.org

Epocrates Online. (2011). Retrieved from http://www.epocrates.com

Esmaeli, M. R. (2014). Distinguishing functional constipation from organic causes in children. *International Journal of Pediatrics, 2*(Suppl. 2), 12.

Fashner, J., & Gitu, A. (2015). Diagnosis and treatment of peptic ulcer disease and H. pylori infection. *American Family Physician, 91*(4), 236–242.

Ives, N. K. (2015). Management of neonatal jaundice. *Paediatrics and Child Health, 25*(6), 276–281.

Koppen, I., Lammers, L., Benninga, M., & Tabbers, M. (2015). Management of functional constipation in children: Therapy in practice, *Pediatric Drugs, 17,* 349–360. doi: 10.1007/s40272-015-0142-4

May, M. E., & So, T. (2014) Overview of probiotic use in the pediatric population. *Clinical Pediatrics, 53*(13), 1231–1238.

Muchowski, L. (2014). Evaluation and treatment of neonatal hyperbilirubinemia. *American Family Physician, 89*(11), 873–878.

National Digestive Diseases Information Clearinghouse. (2017). Viral gastroenteritis ("stomach flu") (NIH Publication No. 11–5103). Bethesda, MD: National Institutes of Health. Retrieved from http://digestive.niddk.nih.gov/ddiseases/pubs/viralgastroenteritis/index.aspx

National Institute of Diabetes & Digestive and Kidney Diseases. (2017). Non-alcoholic fatty liver diseasse & NASH. NIDDK. Retrieved from https://www.niddk.nih.gov/health-information/liver-disease/nafld-nash

National Institutes of Health, Office of Dietary GERD in infants and children Supplements. (2016). *Fact sheets.* Retrieved from http://ods.od.nih.gov/factsheets/list-all/

Orenstein, S. (2013). Infant GERD: Symptoms, reflux episodes & reflux disease, acid & non-acid reflux—Implications for treatment with PPIs. *Current Gastroenterology Reports, 15,* 353. doi: 10.1007/s11894-013-0353-1

Palance, I. (2014). Celiac disease and children. In L. Rodrigo & A. S. Pena (Eds.), *Celiac disease and non-gluten sensitivity* (pp. 221–233). Barcelona: OmniScience.

Pediatric Lexi-Drugs Online. (2009). *Lexicomp online.* Retrieved from http://www.lexi.com/institutions/online.jsp?id=databases

Pediatric Lexi-Drugs Online. (2016). *Lexicomp online.* Retrieved from http://www.lexi.com/institutions/online.jsp?id=databases

Rubio-Tapia, A., Ludvigsson, J. F., Brantner, T. L., Murray, J. A., & Everhart, J. E. (2012). Prevalence of celiac disease in the United States. *American Journal of Gastroenterology,* 107, 1538–1544.

Taketomo, C. K. (2016). *Pediatric and neonatal dosage handbook* (23rd ed.). Hudson, OH: Lexi-Comp.

Tanida, G., Ozeki, K., Mizoshita, T., Tzukamoto, H., Katano, T., Katanka, H., Kamiya, T., & Joh, T. (2015). Managing refractory Crohn's disease: Challenges and solutions. *Clinical and Experimental Gastroenterology, 8,* 131–140.

Watanabe, S., Hashimoto, E., Ikejima, K., Uto, H., Ono, M., Sumida, Y., ... Japanese Society of Gastroenterology; Japan Society of Hepatology. (2015). Evidence-based clinical practice guidelines for nonalcoholic fatty liver disease/nonalcoholic steatohepatitis. *Journal of Gastroenterology, 50,* 364–377.

Williamson, M. A., & Snyder, L. M. (2015). *Wallach's interpretation of diagnostic tests* (10th ed.). Philadelphia: Wolters Kluwer.

Wyllie, R., & Hyams, J. (2016). *Pediatric gastrointestinal and liver disease* (3rd ed.). Philadelphia: Saunders Elsevier.

Wyllie, R., Hyams, J., & Kay, M. (2016). *Pediatric gastrointestinal and liver disease* (5th ed.). Philadelphia: Saunders Elsevier.

16

Renal Disorders

Bonnie Kitchen, MNSc, APRN, PPCNB-BC

LEARNING OUTCOMES

Upon completion of this chapter, the student will be able to:

1. Review, comprehend, and apply the basic pathophysiology of selected renal disorders.
2. Understand and recognize normal and abnormal values of common laboratory findings in selected renal disorders.
3. Accurately distinguish between selected renal disorders based on clinical presentation.
4. Safely perform nursing interventions on selected renal disorders while in the acute hospital setting.
5. Educate family and patient regarding home therapies for selected renal disorders.

ANATOMY AND PHYSIOLOGY

- The two kidneys are located in the retroperitoneal space on each side of the vertebra, slightly above the umbilicus (Fig. 16–1).
- The renal arteries supply the kidney with blood flow.
- The right kidney is slightly lower than the left kidney.
- Each kidney contains 1 million nephrons.
  - The nephron contains a glomerulus, a tubule, and collecting duct.
  - Nephrons filter harmful products from the blood.
- Each renal pelvis extends to form a ureter.
- Each ureter drains into the urinary bladder.
- The urinary bladder collects urine, which is excreted via the urethra.
- The normal urethra has one-way valves allowing drainage and prevention of retrograde reflux of urine.
- Renal function is not completely mature until approximately 2 years of age (Kher, Schnaper, & Greenbaum, 2017) (Box 16–1).

CRITICAL COMPONENT

End-Stage Renal Disease and Pediatric Developmental Abnormalities

Congenital abnormalities account for 30% to 50% of all cases of end-stage renal disease in children (Kher et al., 2017).

ASSESSMENT

Nursing assessment of possible renal disorders for pediatric patients should include general, family, and dietary histories and physical examination.

General History

- Associated symptoms
- Alleviating factors
- Preceding illnesses
- Medical history

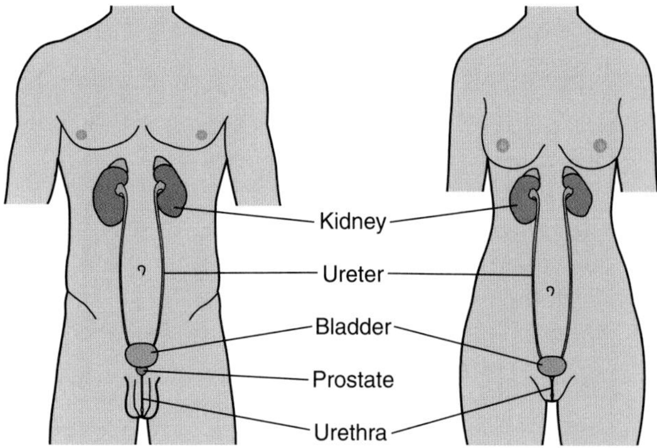

FIGURE 16–1 Urinary tract system.

BOX 16–1 | Fluid Needs

Fluid Needs Per Kilogram for 24-Hour Period (With Normally Functioning Kidneys)

WEIGHT	FLUID NEEDS
0–10 kg	100 mL/kg
11–20 kg	50 mL/kg
≥20 kg	20 mL/kg

Source: Engorn, B., & Flerlage, J. (2015). *The Harriet Lane handbook* (20th ed.). Philadelphia: Elsevier Mosby.

- Hospitalizations
- Use of indwelling catheters, which increases the risk for infection by contamination
- Recent or current medication usage
  - Nephrotoxic medications affect the kidney by altering renal blood flow, causing acute tubular necrosis, intratubular obstruction, or a hypersensitivity reaction.
  - Common nephrotoxic drugs include aminoglycosides, amphotericin B, vancomycin, nonsteroidal anti-inflammatories, heavy metals, and angiotensin-converting enzyme inhibitors.
- History of fractures with minimal trauma
  - Osteoporosis is a common finding in chronic renal diseases.
- History of growth retardation, frequent infections
- History of urological anomalies
- History of previous surgeries, sexual activity
  - Sexual activity is a risk factor, although the mechanism remains unclear.

Family History

- Recurrent urinary tract infections (UTIs)
- Chronic kidney disease (CKD), renal anomalies
- Deafness
- Metabolic disorders
- Immune disorders
- Renal calculi
- Thyroid disturbances
- Gout
- Family members needing dialysis
- Family members with growth retardation

Dietary History

- Protein intake
  - A high-protein diet may worsen kidney disease
- Fluid intake
  - Fluid restriction is an important component of many renal disorders.
  - Poor fluid intake or dehydration may lead to acute renal failure.
- Calories per kilogram per day
- Special dietary needs
  - A ketogenic diet increases the risk for nephrolithiasis.
  - High-oxalate foods may increase the risk for nephrolithiasis.
- History of failure to thrive
  - Many renal disorders manifest in infancy with failure to thrive.

Physical Examination

Aspects of physical examination for renal disorders include the following.

General Assessment

- Ill appearance—a child who has the appearance of not feeling well, but stable
- Toxic appearance—a child who has the appearance of not feeling well and not stable
- Well appearing—a child with a healthy appearance

Pulmonary System

- Alterations in breath sounds, cough, shortness of breath, and rapid respiratory rate should be investigated further, because these symptoms may indicate fluid overload of a renal origin.
- Pulse oximetry reading of less than 93% should be further investigated.

SAFE AND EFFECTIVE NURSING CARE: Clinical Pearl

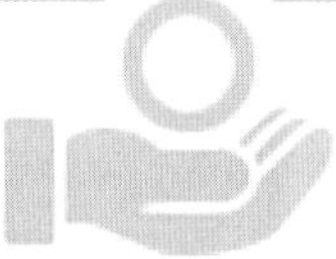

Fluid Balance

A major function of the renal system is to regulate fluid balance. Fluid accumulation from poor glomerular filtration and urinary excretion can lead to pulmonary edema.

Cardiovascular System

- Kidney function is crucial to the hemodynamic status of the human body because its major function is to maintain fluid

balance, maintain electrolyte balance, and excrete waste products (Kliegman, Behrman, Jenson, & Stanton, 2016)
  - Decreased pulses in lower extremities can indicate decreased blood pressure and poor perfusion from a renal origin.
  - A capillary refill of greater than 4 seconds indicates poor perfusion.
- Blood pressure
  - An elevated blood pressure can indicate glomerulonephritis, acute or chronic renal failure, renal artery stenosis, or dysplastic kidney (Bakris & Sorrentino, 2018).

SAFE AND EFFECTIVE NURSING CARE: Promoting Safety

Blood Pressure Cuff

Blood pressures must be taken with a cuff of the appropriate size for an accurate reading. The blood pressure cuff should encircle the arm without overlapping. A narrow cuff may give a false high reading, and a cuff that is too large may give a false low reading (Riley & Blulm, 2012).

- Pulses should be assessed for bounding, which can indicate fluid overload
- Heart sounds
- Extremity temperature (extremities should be the same temperature as the core to sensation)

Gastrointestinal System

- CKD is associated with anorexia, constipation, and failure to thrive.
  - Palpable stool in abdomen indicates constipation.
  - Diarrhea can indicate a UTI in infants (Kliegman et al., 2016).
  - Vomiting can indicate a UTI in children.
  - Weight loss or failure to thrive should be investigated for a UTI or renal disease.
  - Weight gain may reflect extracellular fluid collection and should be investigated for renal disease.
- Abdominal pain
  - Abdominal pain can be a hallmark symptom in UTIs in older children (Kliegman et al., 2016).
- Organomegaly, such as enlarged kidneys, can indicate a congenital anomaly or dysplastic kidneys.

Genitourinary System

- Anatomical abnormalities such as pulmonary hypoplasia, VATER/VACTERL syndrome, or Turner syndrome can be associated with renal disease (Kliegman et al., 2016).
  - Pulmonary hypoplasia is a congenital disorder that usually occurs in association with another intrauterine disorder that causes abnormal lung development.
  - VATER/VACTERL syndrome is a complex syndrome of multiple congenital anomalies, including vertebral, anorectal, cardiac, tracheal, esophageal, renal, and radial bone anomalies.
  - Turner syndrome is a genetic condition resulting from a complete or partial absence of the second X chromosome (see Chapter 17 for an in-depth review).
- Circumcision
  - Uncircumcised males have a higher incidence of UTIs (Kher et al., 2017).
- Suprapubic tenderness
  - Can be associated with a UTI or an enlarged bladder from posterior urethral valves.
- Frothy urine
  - Can be associated with proteinuria.
- Urine color
  - Hematuria causes urine to be tea colored, cola colored, or red.
  - Red urine can be caused by nephritis, medications, food dyes, or blood and should be further investigated (Kliegman et al., 2016).
- Urine flow
  - A poor or weak urine stream can be associated with the posterior urethral valves and secondary vesicoureteral reflux (VUR).
- Intake and output (Box 16–2)
  - Fluid maintenance requirements arise from the basal metabolism.
  - Based on the Holliday-Segar method, 100 mL of fluid will be needed for each 100 calories metabolized.
  - Approximately 50% to 65% of this fluid is needed for kidney filtration and subsequent urinary loss. The remaining 35% is required for skin, respiratory tract, stool losses, or insensible losses. These fluid needs are reduced in children with renal disease based on their renal function.

Dermatological System

- Rash
  - Palpable purpura on the posterior surface of the extremities is a sign of Henoch–Schönlein purpura (Stefek, Beck, Ionfreda, Gardner, & Stefanski, 2015). Palpable purpura can be described as a raised, port-wine-colored, nonblanching rash (Fig. 16–2).
- Sticky or dry mucosal moisture indicates dehydration.
  - Severe dehydration can lead to acute kidney injury (AKI).

Neurological System

- Hearing acuity/loss and/or physical ear anomalies
  - Embryonic development of the auditory and renal systems occurs at the same time, and the two systems may have associated anomalies.
- Pain is always pathological until proven otherwise
  - Can indicate infection, necrosis, or organomegaly.

Musculoskeletal System

- Appropriate linear growth and appropriate weight gain
  - Many renal disorders present with poor weight gain, growth retardation, and failure to thrive. Growth hormone is decreased in chronic renal diseases.

BOX 16–2 | Selected Normal Laboratory Values

Urinalysis

Specific gravity: 1.001–1.035

pH: 5.0–8.5

Protein: negative

Glucose: negative

Ketones: negative

Bilirubin: negative

Blood: negative

Nitrite: negative

Leukocyte esterase: negative

Serum Electrolytes

Sodium: 135–145 mEq/L

Potassium: 3.5–5.0 mEq/L

Chloride: 98–107 mEq/L

Carbon dioxide: 22–28 mEq/L

BUN: 8–20 mg/dL

Creatinine: 0.6–1.2

Complete Blood Cell Count

White blood cells: 5,000–10,000 cells/μL

Red blood cells: 4.6–4.8 million/μL

Hemoglobin: male 13.6–17.5 g/dL; female 12.0–15.5 g/dL

Hematocrit: male 39%–49%; female 35%–45%

Platelets: 150,000–350,000 (Custer & Rau, 2009)

Source: Adapted from Engorn, B., & Flerlage, J. (2015). *The Harriet Lane handbook* (20th ed.). Philadelphia: Elsevier Mosby.

- Muscle cramping may indicate electrolyte disturbances such as hypokalemia, hyponatremia, and hypocalcemia.
- Bone pain and fractures may be caused from osteodystrophy/osteopenia of chronic renal disease. Osteopenia is secondary to hypocalcemia, which arises from the inability of the kidney to convert vitamin D into the active form (Kliegman et al., 2016).
- Costovertebral tenderness is associated with UTIs in older children.
- Weakness and malaise may be secondary from anemia of chronic kidney failure and poor nutrition intake.

Lymphatic System

Edema can be caused by decreased circulating protein (hypoalbuminemia). Nephrotic syndrome is characterized by proteinuria and hypoalbuminemia resulting in edema (Kliegman et al., 2016).

- Periorbital edema
- Facial edema
- Ascites (excessive buildup of fluid in the abdominal cavity)
- Scrotal edema

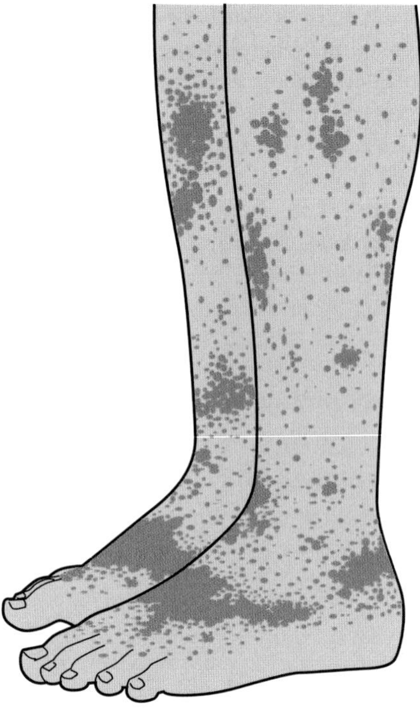

FIGURE 16–2 Palpable purpura in the lower extremities.

CRITICAL COMPONENT

Socioeconomic Factors in Growth and Development

Many chronic and acute illnesses can compromise the growth and development of children. However, most cases of poor growth and development are primarily caused by socioeconomic issues. Nursing should ask about household income, inquire about child's enrolment in government agencies for food assistance, ask family to demonstrate mixing formula, obtain an accurate daily dietary history, obtain household history (number of members in the house), family history of growth problems, and family medical and psychiatric history, and obtain the growth chart if possible. Red flags that indicate pathological conditions of poor growth are weight loss, retarded height velocity and head circumference growth, PICA, dermatological lesions, and regression of milestones attained.

- Sacral edema
- Dependent edema

Endocrine System

- A palpable thyroid may indicate hyperthyroidism, which is associated with CKD.

Renal System

- Large, dysplastic kidneys may be felt on physical examination.
- Urine output
  - Alterations in urine output can be associated with various renal diseases.

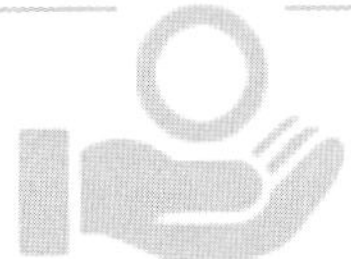

SAFE AND EFFECTIVE NURSING CARE: Clinical Pearl

Edema

Edema is associated with poor renal function and is often found in areas of dependence and large, hollow cavities. Assess edema by palpating dependent areas such as sacral process, labia, and scrotum. Assess for fluid wave in abdomen. Assess for pitting/nonpitting edema of the pretibial area. Weight is the most sensitive indicator of fluid changes. Every kilogram equals 1,000 mL of fluid.

- Normal urine output in children is 2 mL/kg/hr; 0.5 to 1.0 mL/kg/hr is acceptable in teenagers.

DISORDERS OF THE RENAL SYSTEM

Disorders or dysfunction of the renal system are common in children. Renal dysfunction may be primary, due to diseases originating in the kidney, or secondary, dysfunction due to systemic processes that alter the renal function. The kidney may be injured directly or from a systemic illness. The kidneys are both excretory and regulatory organs. The excretory function rids the body of excess fluids or substances that could be harmful. As a regulatory organ, the kidney maintains a constant fluid and electrolyte composition (Costanzo, 2018).

Urinary Tract Infection

A UTI is an infectious process that involves the urethra, bladder, ureters, renal pelvis, renal calyces, and renal parenchyma. It can be isolated or compromise the entire urinary tract.

- UTIs are more commonly seen in children between 2 and 6 years old.
- UTIs are the most frequent site of an occult serious bacterial infection in febrile infants without a recognizable source of infection (American Academy of Pediatrics Clinical Practice Guideline, 2011).
- *Escherichia coli* is the most common bacterial cause of UTIs, with other gram-negative organisms secondary.
- Symptoms of a UTI in infants and young children do not mimic the typical urinary symptoms in adults and may be as subtle as fever alone.
- If left untreated, UTIs can lead to renal scarring and renal failure (Traisman, 2016).

Assessment

Assessment for pediatric UTI should include the following elements.

Clinical Presentation

- Fever (temperature above 38.3°C [100.9°F])
- Vomiting
- Abdominal pain
- Flank pain
- Back pain
- Dysuria (painful urination)
- Frequency (urinating at frequent intervals not associated with increased volume)
- Urgency (an unstoppable urge to urinate)
- Hematuria (blood in the urine)
- Jaundice (a yellow discoloration of the skin and sclera caused by increased bilirubin levels)
- Poor oral intake
- Hyperthermia
- Hypothermia
- Failure to thrive

SAFE AND EFFECTIVE NURSING CARE: Promoting Safety

Children With Spina Bifida

Children with spina bifida are at increased risk for UTIs due to a neurogenic bladder. A neurogenic bladder is characterized by incomplete emptying, causing urinary stasis. Clean intermittent urinary catheterization is a safe standard of care for treatment of a neurogenic bladder.

Diagnostic Tests

- Urinalysis: nitrites, leukocyte esterase
  - A urinalysis can be suspicious, but not diagnostic, of a UTI.
  - Urine nitrites are almost always diagnostic of UTIs (Engorn & Flerlage, 2015).
- Urine microscopy: bacteria, white blood cells
- Urine culture: detection of specific bacterium with a culture is necessary to accurately diagnose a UTI (Table 16–1).

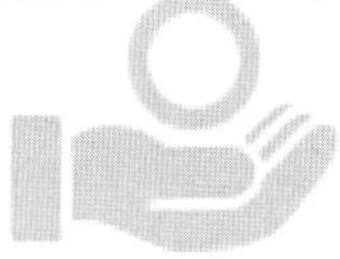

SAFE AND EFFECTIVE NURSING CARE: Clinical Pearl

Prevention of Contamination in Urine Cultures

A bag urine specimen is not an appropriate collection method for culture. Urine cultures should be obtained by catheterization, suprapubic tap, or clean catch if the patient is toilet trained. These methods decrease secondary contamination of the urine specimen.

TABLE 16–1 Urine Culture and Diagnostic Criteria for a Urinary Tract Infection

COLLECTION METHOD	Clean Catch	Urethral Catheterization	Suprapubic Aspiration
COLONY COUNT	>100,000 colony count of a colony-forming organism	>50,000 colony count of a colony-forming organism	>50,000 colony count of any colony-forming units

Adapted from Engorn, B., & Flerlage, J. (2015). The Harriet Lane handbook *(20th ed.). Philadelphia: Elsevier Mosby.*

CRITICAL COMPONENT

Urinalysis Evaluation Guidelines

The guidelines from the American Academy of Pediatrics report that a urinalysis suggestive of infection (pyuria and/or bacteriuria) and the presence of at least a colony count of 50,000/mL in febrile infants and children younger than 3 years is considered positive (American Academy of Pediatrics, 2011).

- Renal ultrasonography: structural anomalies or vascular compromise
- Voiding cystourethrogram (VCUG): VUR, hydroureter
  - During this procedure, the bladder is catheterized and a radioiodinated contrast is instilled into the bladder until the bladder is full. Radiographic images are taken of the full bladder, the ureterovesical junction, the kidneys, and the urethra. The contrast is eliminated by spontaneous voiding or catheter drainage.

SAFE AND EFFECTIVE NURSING CARE: Clinical Pearl

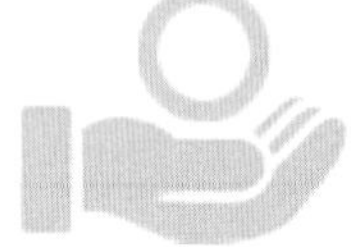

Voiding Cystourethrogram

A VCUG is no longer recommended to be performed routinely after the first febrile UTI. A VCUG is indicated if the renal ultrasound reveals hydronephrosis, renal scarring, or other abnormalities that would suggest VUR. It is also recommended for recurrent febrile UTIs (Traisman, 2016).

- DTc-dimercaptosuccinic acid (DMSA) scan: renal scarring
  - A radiopharmaceutical agent is infused IV, filtered by the glomeruli, and excreted in the urine. During the filtration phase, imaging is done to evaluate the renal parenchyma, as well as the anatomic structures of the urinary system.

Nursing Interventions

When a pediatric patient has a UTI, nursing interventions include the following measures.

Emergency Care

- Stabilization of circulatory status by delivering a 20-mL/kg IV fluid bolus of normal saline or lactated Ringer's

SAFE AND EFFECTIVE NURSING CARE: Clinical Pearl

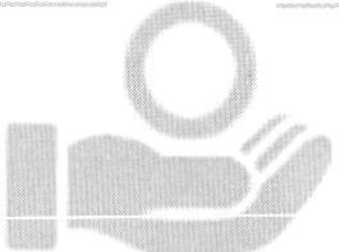

DTc-Dimercaptosuccinic Acid Scan

A DMSA scan should be obtained several months after the UTI has been treated. If a DMSA scan is obtained during the acute infection, the acute inflammatory changes can be misinterpreted as renal scarring, but can resolve after appropriate treatment (Traisman, 2016).

- Immediate administration of broad-spectrum IV antibiotics
  - Ceftriaxone 50 to 75 mg/kg/day IV
  - Cefotaxime 100 to 200 mg/kg/day divided every 6 to 8 hours daily IV (Engorn & Flerlage, 2015)

SAFE AND EFFECTIVE NURSING CARE: Promoting Safety

Guidelines for Infants Younger Than 2 Months

Any infant younger than 2 months who has a UTI needs a septic workup, hospitalization, and administration of IV antibiotics until cultures and sensitivities have been completed.

Acute Hospital Care

- Empiric broad-spectrum antibiotics should be started immediately after obtaining an appropriate urine specimen for culture.
- Antibiotics should be tailored to an appropriate IV or oral medication as soon as susceptibilities on culture are known.
  - Amoxicillin 25 to 50 mg/kg/day divided every 8 to 12 hours daily orally
  - Co-trimoxazole 8 to 12 mg/kg/day divided every 12 hours daily orally (Engorn & Flerlage, 2015)
- Ensure appropriate diagnostic testing is performed.
- Strictly monitor vital signs, with emphasis on temperature and blood pressure.
- Understand family values and cultural practices, and incorporate into the hospital plan of care, if possible.

Chronic Hospital Care

Urinary tract infections are the number one hospital-acquired infection. Prevention measures include:

- Good hand hygiene
- Aseptic technique
- Maintain a closed drainage system
- Remove Foley catheter when no longer needed (Children's Hospital Solution for Patient Safety, 2014)

Chronic Home Care

- Complete antibiotic course in its entirety (7 to 14 days).
- Educate family and patient on the importance of follow-up testing.
- Educate family and patient on prophylactic antibiotics if prescribed.
  - Co-trimoxazole 2 to 4 mg/kg/day as a single dose
  - Amoxicillin 10 mg/kg/day as a single dose orally
  - Nitrofurantoin 1 to 2 mg/kg/day as a single dose daily orally
  - Cephalexin 10 mg/kg/day as a single dose orally
- Encourage liquid intake appropriate for age and weight.
- Promote regular voiding.
- Avoid perineal irritants.
- Correct constipation.
  - High-fiber diet
  - Adequate water intake daily
  - Postprandial stooling attempts

Complementary and Alternative Therapies

- Cranberry juice has been effective in the prevention of UTI in healthy pediatric patients; however, there is no recommended dosing and frequency (Durham, Stamm, & Eiland, 2015).

Caregiver Education

Educate parents and caregivers of a child with a UTI on the following measures.

Emergency Care

- Seek medical attention immediately for fever in infants younger than 3 months.

Acute Hospital Care

- Include family's participation in daily care of the hospitalized child.
- Educate family and patient on medication administration, route, reason, and side effects.
- Use aseptic technique to prevent hospital-acquired infections.

Chronic Home Care

- Educate family and patient on home medication administration and side effects.
- Educate family and patient on importance of follow-up studies.
- Educate family and patient on any home procedures (in and out catheterization).

Complementary and Alternative Therapies

- Educate families and patients on reliable sources of information when researching alternative therapies.
- High-fiber diet and ample water intake may help constipation.
- Avoid tight clothing and diapers to prevent local irritation.
- Avoid the use of bubble baths or essential oils in baths to prevent local irritation.
- Encourage adults to practice postcoital urination to decrease chance of UTIs.

SAFE AND EFFECTIVE NURSING CARE: Promoting Safety

Chronic Urinary Tract Infections

Repetitive UTIs can cause permanent renal damage. Febrile illnesses without a recognizable source of infection should be investigated with a urinalysis and culture in a child with a previous UTI. Any prepubescent child with repetitive UTIs without a known etiology should be considered for sexual abuse.

Vesicoureteral Reflux

VUR is a congenital anatomical abnormality that allows the retrograde flow of urine from the bladder into the ureters and renal collecting system (Table 16–2).

- VUR is the most common congenital anomaly affecting the urinary tract in children.
- VUR and urinary stasis increase children's risk for UTIs and renal scarring, which could lead to end-stage renal disease.
- VUR is the most common pathological finding in children with UTIs.

Assessment

Assessment for possible VUR must include the following measures.

Clinical Presentation

- Frequent UTIs
- Suprapubic pain
- Urinary incontinence
- Family history of VUR
- Enlarged bladder

Diagnostic Tests

- Urinalysis
- Urine culture
- Postvoiding catheterization: residual urine present
- Renal ultrasound: evidence of hydronephrosis
- VCUG: gradation of VUR
- DMSA scan: detection of renal scarring

Nursing Interventions

The following nursing interventions are used in children who have VUR.

Emergency Care

- Prepare for dialysis if renal failure is present.

TABLE 16–2 Different Stages of Vesicoureteral Reflux

GRADE I	GRADE II	GRADE III	GRADE IV	GRADE V
Ureter only	Ureter, pelvis, calyces; no dilation, normal calyceal fornices	Mild or moderate dilation and/or tortuosity of ureter; mild or moderate dilation of the pelvis, but no or slight blunting of the fornices	Moderate dilation and/or tortuosity of the renal pelvis and calyces; complete obliteration of sharp angle of fornices, but maintenance of papillary impressions in the majority of calyces	Gross dilation and tortuosity of ureter; gross dilation of renal pelvis and calyces; papillary impressions are no longer visible in the majority of calyces

Reproduced with permission by Elsevier Mosby from Custer, J., & Rau, R. (2009). The Harriet Lane handbook *(18th ed.). Philadelphia: Elsevier Mosby.*

Acute Hospital Care

- Appropriate administration of empiric antimicrobials if UTI is suspected
- Ensure appropriate diagnostic testing is performed
- Postoperative care if surgical correction is performed
- Strict monitoring of vital signs, with emphasis on blood pressure
- Strict monitoring of intake and output
- Understand family values and cultural practices, and incorporate into the hospital plan of care, if possible

Chronic Hospital Care

- Accurate administration of medications if a UTI is present
  - Ceftriaxone 50 to 75 mg/kg daily IV
  - Cefotaxime 100 to 200 mg/kg/day divided every 6 to 8 hours IV daily
  - Co-trimoxazole 8 to 12 mg/kg/day divided every 12 hours daily orally
  - Amoxicillin 25 to 50 mg/kg/day divided every 8 to 12 hours daily orally (Engorn & Flerlage, 2015)
- Postoperative care if surgical correction is performed

Evidence-Based Practice

Continuous Prophylactic Antibiotics

Lee, T., & Park, J. (2017). Vesicoureteral reflux and continuous prophylactic antibiotics. *Investigative and Clinical Urology, 58*(Suppl 1), S32–S37.

Garcia-Roig, M., & Kirsch, A. (2016). Urinary tract infection in the setting of vesicoureteral reflux. *F1000 Research, 5*, 1552.

Several randomized controlled studies from 2006 to 2008 have failed to demonstrate UTI prevention by using continuous prophylactic antibiotics. Current studies challenge the long-standing practice of using prophylactic antibiotics to reduce the number of episodes of pyelonephritis and subsequent renal scarring in children with VUR. Continuous antibiotic prophylaxis may be beneficial for children with higher grade VUR.

The Randomized Intervention for Children with Vesicoureteral Reflux trial (RIVUR) demonstrated continuous prophylactic antibiotics does decrease the risk for recurrent UTI in patients with febrile UTIs and bowel/bladder dysfunction. It was also noted that there was an increase in the risk for antibiotic resistance and no decrease in renal scarring.

Caregiver Education

Nurses should educate caregivers of a child with VUR on the following topics.

Acute Hospital Care

- Educate family and patient on diagnostic tests.
- Educate family and patient on medication (reason, route, length of therapy, side effects).

Chronic Home Care

- Educate family and patient on medical therapy and compliance.
- Educate family and patient on medication (reason, route, length of therapy, side effects).
- Educate family and patient on need for follow-up diagnostic testing.

- Educate family that siblings are at higher risk for VUR and may need screening.
- Educate family on the need for aggressive treatment of constipation.

SAFE AND EFFECTIVE NURSING CARE: Clinical Pearl

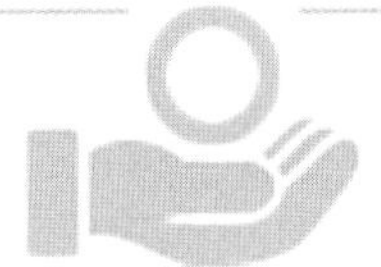

Surgical Intervention and Vesicoureteral Reflux

Most cases of VUR resolve with time; however, some forms may require surgical intervention (Kliegman et al., 2016). Medical management is generally safe and effective. In grades III and IV there was no advantage over surgical versus medical treatment. Surgical management is usually reserved for those children for whom medical management is ineffective (Okawada et al., 2016).

Nephrolithiasis (Renal Calculi)

Nephrolithiasis, or kidney stones, is a clinical condition in which urinary crystals coalesce and form growing renal calculi. There has been a steady rise in the incidence of nephrolithiasis in children and adolescents.

- Obesity, increased sodium consumption, decreased water intake, and decreased calcium consumption have been proposed but never proved to be contributing factors to the increased number of pediatric cases of nephrolithiasis (Hernandez, Ellison, & Lendvay, 2015).
- Other metabolic diseases, the use of loop diuretics, UTIs, or congenital anomalies of the urinary tract may increase the chance of stone formation.
- Vitamin D, calcium supplements, vitamin C, diuretics, steroids, ceftriaxone, and some antiepileptic medications are associated with nephrolithiasis.
- Children with metabolic disease or genetic or urinary tract abnormalities are at greater risk for recurrent kidney stones.
- Most recently, females are at greater risk than boys for development of renal calculi (Van Batavia & Tasian, 2016).

Assessment

Assessment for kidney stones in pediatric patients includes the following measures.

Clinical Presentation

- Colic-type abdominal, flank, or back pain
- Hematuria
- Urinary tract infection
- Poor feeding
- Acute renal failure if single kidney is present and obstructed
- Nausea and vomiting

Diagnostic Testing

- Urinalysis: hematuria or casts
- Abdominal radiograph: calcium calculi
- Ultrasonography: calculi, obstruction, or hydronephrosis
- Computed tomography: calculus
- Laboratory analysis of renal calculus
- 24-hour urine collection

Nursing Interventions

Nursing interventions for kidney stones in pediatric patients include the following measures.

Emergency Care

- Adequate fluid intake; IV fluids should be at 1.5 to 2 times the maintenance rate
- Tamsulosin for medical expulsive therapy (Henandez et al., 2015)
- Pain control with narcotic and non-narcotic medication
  - Morphine 0.1 to 0.2 mg/kg/dose every 2 to 4 hours IV
  - Oxycodone 0.05 to 0.15 mg/kg/dose every 4 to 6 hours orally
  - Acetaminophen 10 to 15 mg/kg/dose every 4 to 6 hours orally (Engorn & Flerlage, 2015)
- Accurate urinary output recording
- Monitor for urinary obstruction
  - Assist in percutaneous nephrostomy placement.
- Monitor for renal failure

SAFE AND EFFECTIVE NURSING CARE: Promoting Safety

Children With Renal Calculi and One Kidney

Children with a single kidney who have symptoms consistent with calculi (colicky flank pain, hematuria, vomiting, abdominal pain) and have signs of acute renal failure (oliguria, azotemia, hypertension, hyperkalemia) are to be treated as a surgical emergency.

Acute Hospital Care

- Provide adequate fluid intake (IV and oral).
- Strain urine for stone collection.
- Obtain laboratory studies appropriately and accurately.
- Provide pain control with narcotic and non-narcotic medication.
- Strictly monitor vital signs.
- Prepare family and patient for possible stone removal by open or closed surgical intervention.
- Prepare family and patient for possible extracorporeal shock-wave lithotripsy.
- Understand family values and cultural practices, and incorporate into the hospital plan of care, if possible.

Caregiver Education

Educate parents and caregivers on the following topics related to kidney stones.

Emergency Care

- Educate family and patient on presenting signs of nephrolithiasis, obstruction, and renal failure.

Acute Hospital Care

- Educate family and patient on diagnostic studies, medications, invasive treatment, and pain-control measures.
- Educate family and patient on how to strain urine.
- Educate family and patient on surgical procedures.

Chronic Hospital Care

- Educate family and patient on ongoing management.
- Educate family and patient on how to strain urine.
- Educate family and patient on medication administration (Table 16–3).
  - Furosemide 1 to 6 mg/kg/dose every 12 to 24 hours orally
  - Spironolactone 1 to 3.3 mg/kg/day divided every 1 to 4 times daily orally
  - Oxycodone 0.05 to 0.15 mg/kg/dose every 4 to 6 hours orally
- Educate family and patient on fluid intake and dietary modifications.

Chronic Home Care

- Educate family and patient on how to strain urine.
- Educate family and patient on appropriate nutrition requirements based on age.
- Educate family and patient on appropriate nutrition restrictions.
- Educate family and patient on appropriate fluid requirements based on age.
- Educate family and patient on home medications if ordered.
  - Thiazide diuretics may be beneficial in the treatment of certain types of kidney stones.
- Complete the course of antimicrobial therapy if UTI is present.
  - Amoxicillin 25 to 50 mg/kg/day divided every 8 to 12 hours daily orally
  - Co-trimoxazole 8 to 12 mg/kg/day divided every 12 hours daily orally (Engorn & Flerlage, 2015)
- Educate family and patient on importance of metabolic testing.

SAFE AND EFFECTIVE NURSING CARE: Understanding Medication

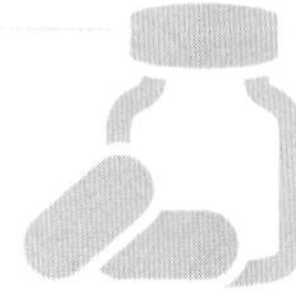

Potassium Citrate to Prevent Kidney Stones

Children on a ketogenic diet (high fat, low carbohydrate, adequate protein) for seizure control are at higher risk for development of kidney stones. Taking daily doses of potassium citrate can decrease the occurrence (Hallbook, Sjolander, Amark, Miranda, Bjurulf, & Dahlin, 2015).

TABLE 16–3 Commonly Used Diuretics

DRUG	DOSAGE	SIDE EFFECTS	ADMINISTRATION OPTIONS
Furosemide	Start at 2 mg/kg/dose and increase by 1–2 mg/kg/dose every 6–8 hours; maximum dose: 6 mg/kg/dose	Orthostatic hypotension, vertigo, photo sensitivity, electrolyte disturbances, nephrocalcinosis	Oral tablets or liquid
Furosemide	1–2 mg/kg/dose every 6–12 hours	Orthostatic hypotension, vertigo, photo sensitivity, electrolyte disturbances, nephrocalcinosis	IV injection
Metolazone	0.2–0.4 mg/kg/24 hr ÷ daily to twice daily	Orthostatic hypotension, syncope, vertigo, muscle cramps, electrolyte imbalances	Oral tablets; compounded liquid suspension
Bumetanide	0.015–0.1 mg/kg/dose once daily to twice daily; maximum dose: 10 mg/24 hr	Orthostatic hypotension, syncope, vertigo, muscle cramps, electrolyte imbalances	Oral tablets; IV injection
Spironolactone	1–3.3 mg/kg/24 hr ÷ twice daily to four times daily; maximum dose: 10 mg/24 hr	Lethargy, confusion, electrolyte disturbances, weakness, decreased renal function	Oral tablets; compounded liquid suspension

Adapted from Engorn, B., & Flerlage, J. (2015). The Harriet Lane handbook *(20th ed.). Philadelphia: Elsevier Mosby.*

Complementary and Alternative Therapies

- Low-oxalate diet
  - Oxalates are chemicals found in plant food that can increase stone formation in some people.
- Avoidance of high-protein intake
- Avoidance of fast foods and artificially flavored/sweetened drinks

Nephrotic Syndrome

Nephrotic syndrome, the most common kidney disease in children, is characterized by a combination of clinical manifestations, including massive proteinuria, hypoalbuminemia, edema, and hyperlipidemia of unknown etiology (Fig. 16–3). Macromolecules are filtered in the glomeruli, allowing albumin to cross the capillary wall. The loss of protein in the urine changes the oncotic pressure within the intravascular space, causing intravascular depletion of volume and extracellular edema (Bierzynska, 2017).

- The peak incidence is seen in children between 2 and 5 years of age.
- The types of nephrotic syndrome are minimal change disease (most common), focal segmental glomerulosclerosis, membranoproliferative glomerulonephritis, and mesangial proliferative glomerulonephritis.

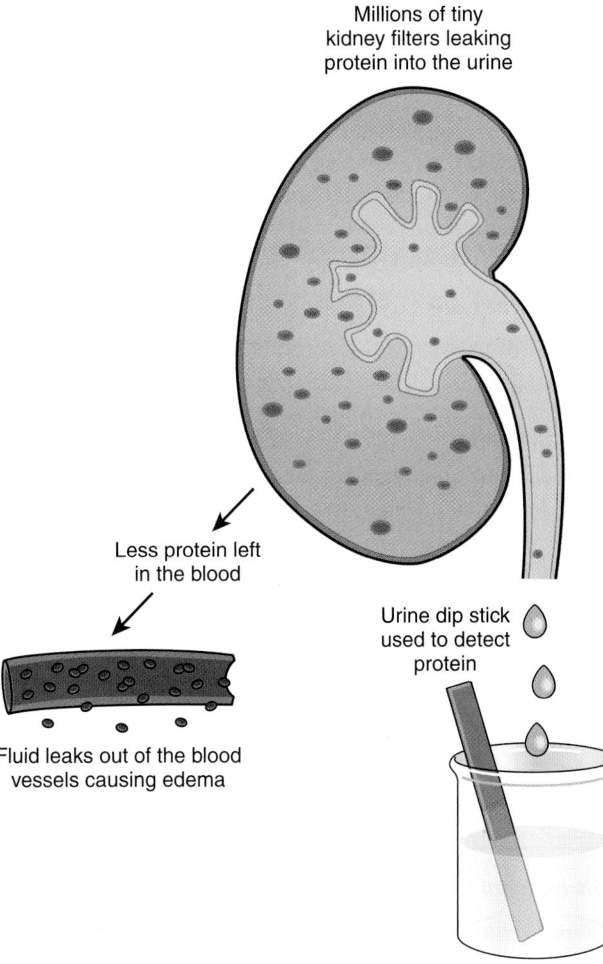
Millions of tiny kidney filters leaking protein into the urine
Less protein left in the blood
Urine dip stick used to detect protein
Fluid leaks out of the blood vessels causing edema

FIGURE 16–3 Nephrotic syndrome.

- Nephrotic syndrome often occurs after an upper respiratory tract infection.
- Edema is gravity dependent and occurs gradually.
- Decreased circulating volume is often present despite increased extracellular fluid volume, causing tachycardia, oliguria, and orthostatic hypotension.
- Complications of nephrotic syndrome include peritonitis, thromboembolism, AKI, and malnutrition.
  - Infection is the most common complication, followed by thromboembolism.

SAFE AND EFFECTIVE NURSING CARE: Understanding Medication

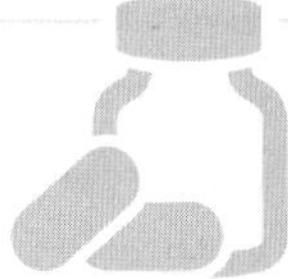

Antibiotic Use for Nephrotic Syndrome

Broad-spectrum antibiotics should be initiated when an infection is suspected. Antibiotics can be tailored later based on culture and susceptibilities (McCaffrey, Lennon, & Webb, 2016).

Assessment

The following areas are assessed for pediatric patients with nephrotic syndrome.

Clinical Presentation

- Edema (most notable around eyes, scrotal/sacral, ascites, and pretibial)
- Weight gain (tight clothing, umbilical hernia, protruding abdomen)
- Decreased urine output
- Anorexia
- Easily fatigued
- Hypertension

Diagnostic Testing

- Urinalysis: heavy proteinuria (greater than 50 mg/kg/day), +/– microscopic hematuria
- Serum protein: less than 2.5 g/dL
- Electrolytes: hyponatremia is occasionally seen
- Complements: +/– decreased C3 and C4
- Urea, creatinine: usually normal at presentation
- Serum cholesterol, low-density lipoproteins: grossly increased
- Serum calcium: reduced
- Ionized calcium: normal
- Renal ultrasound to detect possible structural anomalies
- Chest radiograph to detect possible pleural effusion

Nursing Interventions

Nurses perform the following interventions for pediatric patients with nephrotic disease.

Emergency Care

- Oxygen delivery for respiratory distress
- Computerized tomography to evaluate for pulmonary emboli

- Ultrasonography Doppler studies to evaluate for venous thrombosis in an extremity
- Preparation for drainage of pleural effusion
- Administration of IV fluids at 20-mL/kg bolus of normal saline for hemodynamic instability
- Administration of IV diuretics for fluid overload
  - Furosemide 1 to 2 mg/kg/dose every 6 to 12 hours IV (Engorn & Flerlage, 2015)
- Administration of IV antibiotics for suspected infection
  - Cefotaxime 100 to 200 mg/kg/day divided every 6 to 8 hours daily (Engorn & Flerlage, 2015)

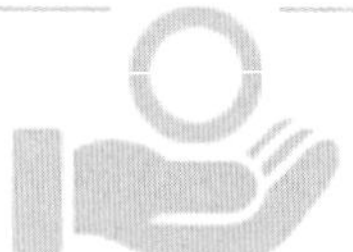

SAFE AND EFFECTIVE NURSING CARE: Clinical Pearl

Thrombus Formation

Children with nephrotic syndrome are at high risk for spontaneous peritonitis and thrombus formation (Kher et al., 2017), caused by the combination of immunosuppression from the high-dose steroids and the lowered function of the innate immune system. A combination of increased platelet aggregation, increased procoagulant factors, and increased loss of coagulation inhibitors in the urine are all thought to increase the risk for thrombus formation.

Acute Hospital Care

- Initiate corticosteroid therapy.
  - Prednisone 2 mg/kg/day with a maximum of 60 mg daily (Engorn & Flerlage, 2015)

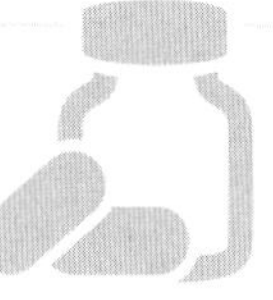

SAFE AND EFFECTIVE NURSING CARE: Understanding Medication

Comorbidities and Corticosteroid Therapy

The child with comorbidities such as diabetes still requires high-dose corticosteroids. Secondary complications such as hyperglycemia are individually managed.

- Initiate diuretic therapy
  - Furosemide 1 to 6 mg/kg/dose every 12 to 24 hours orally
  - Furosemide 1 to 4 mg/kg/dose every 12 to 24 hours orally (infants) (Engorn & Flerlage, 2015)
- IV albumin infusion
  - 25% albumin 0.5 to 1 g/kg/dose over 30 to 120 minutes IV every 1 to 2 days for symptomatic edema (hypertension, respiratory distress) (Engorn & Flerlage, 2015)
- Ensure nutrition consult to correct malnutrition and maintain appropriate fluid restriction
- Strict monitoring of daily weight
  - Weight should be taken at the same time each day, on the same scale, unclothed
- Strict monitoring of intake and output
- Monitoring of abdominal girth
- Monitoring of vital signs, with emphasis on heart rate and blood pressure
- Encourage ambulation and physical activity to prevent stasis complications
- Understand family values and cultural practices, and incorporate into the hospital plan of care, if possible

CRITICAL COMPONENT

Shortness of Breath

If a child with nephrotic syndrome is suddenly reporting shortness of breath and cannot speak in complete sentences, he or she has tachypnea, tracheal tug, and subcostal retractions. A pulmonary embolism must be considered until proven otherwise.

Chronic Hospital Care

- Monitor daily laboratory studies.
- Administer vaccinations appropriately.
  - Prevnar annually (pneumococcal vaccination)
- Prevent skin breakdown.
- Prevent infection with good hand washing and limitation of sick contacts.
- Provide patient/family emotional support.
- Administer purified protein derivative (PPD) before immunosuppressive treatment.

Chronic Home Care

- Provide instructions on medication administration and side effects.
- Provide appropriate supplies for home blood pressure monitoring.
- Provide appropriate supplies for urine chemistry checks.
- Provide written material regarding diet and fluid restriction.

Caregiver Education

Nurses should educate parents and caregivers on the following topics related to nephrotic syndrome.

Emergency Care

- Educate family and patient on signs of pulmonary emboli and respiratory distress.
- Educate family and patient on signs of peritonitis.

Acute Hospital Care

- Educate family and patient on medication administration and side effects.
- Educate family and patient on therapeutic treatments.

Chronic Hospital Care

- Educate family and patient on disease process and side effects.
- Educate family and patient on adherence to nutrition needs and fluid restriction.
- Educate family and patient on daily blood pressure monitoring and parameters.
- Educate family and patient on monitoring daily weight.
- Educate family and patient on activities to prevent venous stasis.

Chronic Home Care

- Daily monitoring of blood pressure and weight
- Daily monitoring of urine for proteinuria
- Compliance with nutrition requirements and fluid restriction
- Compliance with daily medication administration
- Knowledge of disease pathology and possible emergencies
- Knowledge of patient's immunosuppressive state and ways to minimize infection
- Knowledge of yearly vaccinations
- Provide information on local psychosocial support systems or agencies

SAFE AND EFFECTIVE NURSING CARE: Understanding Medication

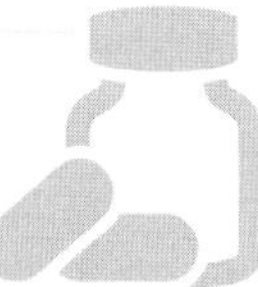

Vaccination Safety

Live vaccinations should be withheld if a child is receiving high doses of steroids or is taking cytotoxic agents.

Acute Postinfectious Glomerulonephritis

Acute postinfectious glomerulonephritis (APIGN) is an inflammation of the glomeruli in response to a preceding illness, most commonly a streptococcal upper respiratory or skin infection. APIGN is clinically apparent 10 to 14 days after the acute infection (Fig. 16–4).

- APIGN usually affects early school-age children, 95% of whom recover completely (Dagan et al., 2016).
- The peak ages of APIGN are 3 to 12 years.
- The most common and most studied form is poststreptococcal glomerulonephritis.
- Up to 6% of individuals with APIGN have sustained hypertension.

Assessment

Assessment of the pediatric patient with APIGN includes the following.

Clinical Presentation

- Painless hematuria; may be tea-colored, cola-colored, or bright red
- Proteinuria
- Oliguria
- Hypertension
- Edema
- Anorexia
- Antecedent upper respiratory or skin infection
- Arthralgias
- Pulmonary edema

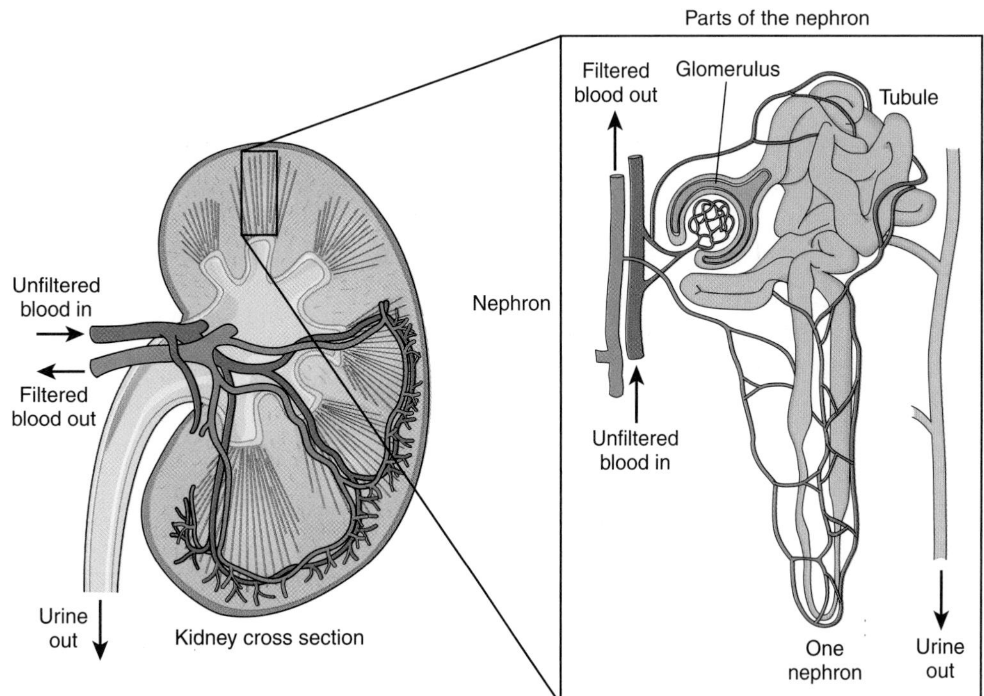

FIGURE 16–4 Nephron and glomeruli.

- Abdominal pain
- Malaise
- Impaired renal function

Diagnostic Testing

- Serum urea and creatinine: elevated
- Serum protein: decreased
- Serum white blood cell count: elevated
- Erythrocyte sedimentation rate: elevated
  - Reflective of systemic inflammatory process
- Serum complement (C3): decreased
- Serum complement (C4): normal to low
- Urinalysis: hematuria, proteinuria, red blood cell casts, hyaline casts
- Antistreptolysin O, anti-DNase B, monitor for a positive or negative streptozyme result
  - Reflective of previous streptococcal infection
- Anemia
- Hyperkalemia
- Renal biopsy may be necessary in some cases
- Throat culture: +/– beta-hemolytic *Streptococcus*

Nursing Interventions

Nurses perform the following interventions for patients with APIGN.

Emergency Care

- Hemodialysis for renal failure
- Antihypertensive management
  - Nifedipine 0.25 to 0.5 mg/kg/dose every 4 to 6 hours orally or sublingually (Engorn & Flerlage, 2015)
  - Administration of sodium polystyrene sulfonate for hyperkalemia
  - Seizure control for hypertensive encephalopathy
  - Lorazepam 0.05 to 0.1 mg/kg/dose every 15 minutes IV (Engorn & Flerlage, 2015)

Acute Hospital Care

- Antibiotics to eradicate the offending organism if present
  - Cefotaxime 100 to 200 mg/kg/day divided every 6 to 8 hours daily
  - Ceftriaxone 50 to 75 mg/kg/day divided twice daily IV (Engorn & Flerlage, 2015)
- Strict monitoring of vital signs, with emphasis on blood pressure
- Strict monitoring of intake and output
- Strict monitoring of daily weight
- Administration of diuretics
  - Furosemide 1 to 6 mg/kg/dose every 12 to 24 hours orally (Engorn & Flerlage, 2015)
- Monitoring and correction of electrolyte imbalances
- Understanding family values and cultural practices, and incorporating them into the hospital plan of care, if possible

Chronic Hospital Care

- Nutrition consult for no-added-salt diet and fluid requirements
- Assess neurological status for cerebral complications
- Renal replacement therapy if required
- Activities as tolerated

Chronic Home Care

- Provide appropriate home blood pressure monitoring equipment.
- Provide written dietary instructions.
- Provide psychosocial support.

Caregiver Education

Nurses should educate parents and caregivers of children who have APIGN on the following topics.

Emergency Care

- Educate family and patient on blood pressure elevations and appropriate intervention.
- Educate family and patient on seizure precautions.
- Educate family and patient on signs of hyperkalemia.

SAFE AND EFFECTIVE NURSING CARE: Promoting Safety

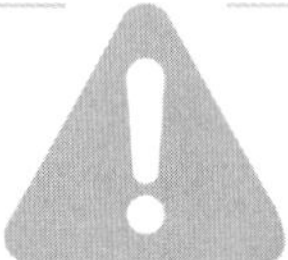

The Role of Electrocardiograms

Any child with hyperkalemia should have an emergent electrocardiogram to evaluate for life-threatening rhythm changes. EKG changes may include peaked T waves, prolonged PR segments, prolonged QRS complex, ST elevation, ectopic beats, and ventricular fibrillation.

Acute Hospital Care

- Educate family and patient on medication administration and side effects.
- Educate family and patient on pathology of disease.
- Educate family and patient on reason and necessity for testing.
- Educate family and patient about dialysis.

Chronic Hospital Care

- Educate family and patient on dietary restrictions and fluid restrictions.
- Educate family and patient on home medication administration and side effects.
- Educate family and patient on accurate intake and output monitoring.
- Educate family and patient on accurate daily weights.

Chronic Home Care

- Educate family and patient on daily monitoring of weight.
- Educate family and patient on daily blood pressure monitoring.
- Educate family and patient on importance of follow-up appointments.
- Educate family and patient on infection prevention.
- Provide family and patient information on local psychosocial support groups.

Henoch-Schönlein Purpura

Henoch-Schönlein purpura (HSP) is a common multisystem vasculitic disorder of children, classified by a tetrad of symptoms—rash, arthralgias, abdominal pain, and hematuria (Stefek et al., 2015).

- HSP is a self-limiting disorder, and most children have a full recovery.
- HSP frequently follows an antecedent upper respiratory tract infection.
- HSP is most common in children between 2 and 6 years of age but can affect all age groups.
- Intussusception is a common emergent condition seen in children with HSP that is thought to be caused by intestinal edema and hemorrhage (Fatima & Gibson, 2014).

Assessment

HSP is assessed using the following measures.

Clinical Presentation

- Colicky abdominal pain may represent intussusception
- Palpable purpura is most prominent in dependent areas (may not be the presenting complaint)
- Nonmigratory arthritis/arthralgia is located mostly in the lower extremities
- Edema of face, lips, dorsum of hands and feet, scrotum
- Occult or gastrointestinal bleeding
- Microscopic hematuria
- Proteinuria (+/–)
- Anorexia
- Malaise
- Erythema nodosum (red or purple subcutaneous nodules found in the pretibial area)

Diagnostic Testing

- Complete blood cell count (CBC): anemia with evidence of hemolysis, thrombocytosis, leukocytosis
- Erythrocyte sedimentation rate: elevated
- C-reactive protein: elevated
- Coagulation studies: normal
- Elevated serum creatinine
- Urinalysis: proteinuria and hematuria
- Stool occult blood: positive
- Abdominal ultrasound to evaluate for intussusception
- Skin biopsy: IgA deposition
- Renal biopsy: IgA deposition
  - Increased IgA is a histological confirmation of HSP.

Nursing Interventions

The following nursing interventions are used for patients with HSP.

Emergency Care

- Intussusception is a surgical emergency. The patient should be prepared for immediate transport to the operating room.
- If renal failure is present, emergent hemodialysis may be necessary. The patient should be prepared for surgical placement of a hemodialysis catheter.
- Evaluate family support for emergent procedures.
- Obtain family consent for emergent procedures.

SAFE AND EFFECTIVE NURSING CARE: Clinical Pearl

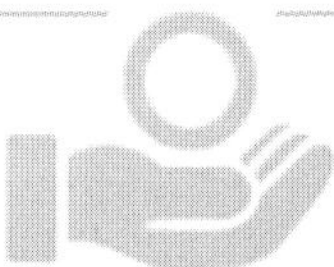

Colic and Intussusception

Any child with colicky abdominal pain and hematochezia should be evaluated for intussusception. An abdominal ultrasound is often the imaging modality to identify intussusception. If present, an air/contrast enema is performed for attempted reduction of the intussusception.

Acute Hospital Care

- IV fluid hydration with an isotonic fluid at 20-mL/kg bolus if hemodynamically unstable
- Fluid restriction to insensible losses if oliguric or anuric
- Strict monitoring of vital signs, with emphasis on blood pressure
- Accurate measuring of daily weights
- Pain control with pharmacological analgesics, avoiding NSAIDs
  - Acetaminophen 10 mg/kg/dose every 4 hours orally
  - Oxycodone 0.05 to 0.15 mg/kg/dose every 4 to 6 hours orally
  - Morphine 0.1 to 0.2 mg/kg/dose every 2 to 4 hours IV (Engorn & Flerlage, 2015)
- Pain control with nonpharmacological measures, such as positioning, distraction, therapeutic play
- Skin care to prevent breakdown from edema and rash
- Accurate monitoring for abdominal pain
- Accurate monitoring for occult blood in stool
- Understanding family values and cultural practices, and incorporating them into the hospital plan of care, if possible

Chronic Hospital Care

- Administer antihypertensive medications
  - Nifedipine 0.25 to 0.5 mg/kg/dose every 4 to 6 hours orally or sublingually
  - Enalapril 0.08 to 5 mg/kg/day divided 1 to 2 times daily orally (Engorn & Flerlage, 2015)
- Administer corticosteroids
  - Prednisone 1 mg/kg/day with a maximum of 60 mg daily orally (Engorn & Flerlage, 2015)
- Accurate blood pressure monitoring
- Accurate recording of daily weights
- Accurate recording of intake and output

Chronic Home Care

- Provide equipment for and educate family and patient about home blood pressure monitoring device and parameters.
- Provide family and patient with urine chemistry strips for hematuria and proteinuria.
- Educate family and patient on medication administration and side effects.
- Educate family and patient on possibility of relapse in condition.

SAFE AND EFFECTIVE NURSING CARE: Understanding Medication

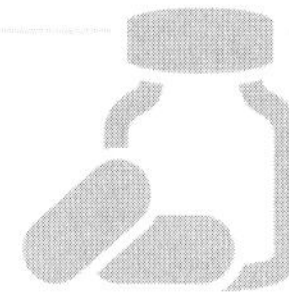

Henoch-Schönlein Purpura and Corticosteroid Use

Using steroids for HSP is not routinely recommended. However, if proteinuria is persistent, then a trial of systemic steroids may be beneficial (Kamat & Fischer, 2016).

Caregiver Education

Nurses must educate caregivers of patients who have VSP on the following topics.

Emergency Care

- Educate family and patient on need for surgical intervention.
- Educate family and patient on need for hemodialysis.
- Provide psychosocial support.

Acute Hospital Care

- Educate family and patient on medication administration and side effects.
- Incorporate family and patient in assessing need for analgesia.
- Educate family and patient on temporary status of rash.
- Educate family and patient on strict monitoring of vital signs, with emphasis on blood pressure.

Chronic Hospital Care

- Educate family and patient on medication administration and side effects.
- Educate family and patient on careful monitoring of intake and output.

Chronic Home Care

- Home blood pressure monitoring and parameters of acceptable blood pressures
- Monitoring for hematuria/proteinuria
- Importance of follow-up
- When to seek medical attention for HSP recurrences
- Medication administration and side effects

Hemolytic Uremic Syndrome

Hemolytic uremic syndrome (HUS) is a disease of unknown etiology, but consists of a triad of symptoms—microangiopathic hemolytic anemia, thrombocytopenia, and AKI after a recent illness (Kliegman, et al., 2016). HUS is diagnosed based on clinical findings and consistent laboratory studies.

- HUS is the most significant complication of infection by *Escherichia coli*, usually serotype O157:H7; however, *Streptococcus pneumoniae* and shigella have been implicated in HUS (Kher et al., 2017).
- HUS develops approximately 2 to 12 days after onset of hemorrhagic enterocolitis.
- HUS typically occurs in children younger than 5 years and seems to have a seasonal occurrence between summer and fall.

Assessment

Assessment for HUS includes the following measures.

Clinical Presentation

- Hematochezia (bloody diarrhea)
- Pallor
- Oliguria or anuria
- Hypertension
- Bruising, purpura, and/or petechiae
- Jaundice
- Edema
- Irritability
- Anorexia
- Seizures

Diagnostic Testing

- Urinalysis: hematuria, proteinuria, cellular casts
- CBC: anemia, thrombocytopenia, mild leukocytosis
- Peripheral smear: schistocytosis, helmet cells
- Reticulocyte count: elevated
- Lactate dehydrogenase: elevated due to increased hemolysis of blood cells
- Coombs' test: negative
- Prothrombin and partial thromboplastin: normal
- Blood urea nitrogen (BUN): elevated
- Creatinine: elevated
- Electrolytes: hyperkalemia, hyponatremia, hypocalcemia, hyperphosphatemia
- Anion gap: elevated with metabolic acidosis
- Total bilirubin: elevated

Nursing Interventions

Nursing interventions for patients who have HUS include the following measures.

Emergency Care

- Prepare family and patient for possible hemodialysis.
- Prepare family and patient for possible blood transfusion.
- Administer antiepileptic medications for seizure control.
  - Lorazepam 0.05 to 0.1 mg/kg/dose every 15 minutes IV
  - Fosphenytoin 15 to 20 mg PE/kg IV for loading dose
  - Fosphenytoin 5 mg/kg/day IV for maintenance (Engorn & Flerlage, 2015)
- Obtain appropriate consent for emergency procedures.

Acute Hospital Care

- Provide IV fluid hydration using isotonic fluid, paying careful attention to intake and output.
- Transfuse slowly with packed red blood cells as indicated.
- Monitor weight at least once daily.
- Accurately report intake and output.

- Assess meticulously for edema.
- Assess for mental status changes.
- Administer analgesics if necessary, avoiding nonsteroidal anti-inflammatory medications.
  - Acetaminophen 10 mg/kg/dose every 4 hours orally
  - Oxycodone 0.05 to 0.15 mg/kg/dose every 4 to 6 hours orally
  - Morphine 0.1 to 0.2 mg/kg/dose every 2 to 4 hours IV (Engorn & Flerlage, 2015)
- Administer antihypertensives as ordered.
  - Nifedipine 0.25 to 0.5 mg/kg/dose every 4 to 6 hours orally or sublingually
  - Enalapril 0.08 to 5 mg/kg/day divided 1 to 2 times daily orally (Engorn & Flerlage, 2015)
- Strictly monitor vital signs, with emphasis on blood pressure.
- Provide family and patient education regarding pathology and procedures.
- Provide family and patient psychosocial support.
- Understand family values and cultural practices, and incorporate into the hospital plan of care, if possible.

Chronic Hospital Care

- Monitor fluid and electrolyte status.
- Provide high-calorie, high-carbohydrate, no-added-salt, low-potassium diet.
- Provide enteral feeding if oral intake is inadequate.
- Monitor daily weight.
- Provide skin care for peritoneal or hemodialysis catheter site.
- Provide skin care for possible breakdown related to edema and decreased perfusion.

Chronic Home Care

- Provide home blood pressure monitoring device.
- Educate family and patient on appropriate medication administration and side effects.
- Educate family and patient on nutrition restrictions.
- Provide follow-up appointment dates and times.
- Educate family and patient on monitoring parameters

Caregiver Education

Nurses must educate parents and caregivers of patients with HUS on the following topics.

Emergency Care

- Educate family and patient on emergent procedures.

Acute Hospital Care

- Educate family and patient on possible complications of HUS.
- Educate family and patient on medication administration and side effects.
- Educate family and patient on need for accurate intake and output recording.
- Educate family and patient on dietary restrictions.
- Instruct family and patient on appropriate skin care.

Chronic Hospital Care

- Provide information regarding dietary restrictions.
- Educate family and patient on signs of fluid overload.
- Provide instructions on enteral or parenteral nutrition, if needed.
- Educate family and patient on how to provide skin care.

Chronic Home Care

- Educate family and patient on blood pressure monitoring and parameters.
- Instruct family and patient on importance of follow-up care.
- Instruct family and patient on dietary restrictions.
- Instruct family and patient on nonsteroidal medications and avoiding their use.
- Educate family and patient on avoiding the use of antidiarrheal medications and antibiotics with gastroenteritis-type illnesses.

Acute Kidney Injury

AKI, previously known as acute renal failure, is a decrease in the glomerular filtration rate (GFR) occurring over hours to days. This decreased renal function leads to an inability of the kidney to clear the blood of urea and regulate fluid and electrolyte balance (Shah et al., 2016).

- AKI is the result of poor renal perfusion or injury; in children, this is caused by ischemia, toxicity, nephropathy, or sepsis.
- Volume depletion is still the most common cause of AKI in pediatrics.
- The prognosis of AKI is dependent on the causative factor
- Renal replacement therapy (dialysis) is the mainstay of treatment.
  - Hemodialysis is effective in the acute setting for critically ill patients with fluid overload, intoxication/ingestion, and hyperkalemia. Hemodialysis uses a machine in which the blood flows through a series of components that act as a filter. This removes toxins and waste products.
  - Hemodialysis requires extensive specialized nursing training.

Assessment

Assessment for AKI includes the following measures.

Clinical Presentation

- History of fluid loss (vomiting, diarrhea, blood loss, burns)
- History of taking nephrotoxic agents (aminoglycosides, IV contrast, and NSAIDs are common nephrotoxic agents)
- Oliguria/anuria
- Hypertension
- Changes in level of consciousness
- Anemia
- Seizures
- Edema

Diagnostic Testing

- BUN: markedly elevated
- Creatinine: markedly elevated
- Electrolyte: hyperkalemia, hyponatremia, metabolic acidosis
- CBC: anemia
- Urinalysis: may be normal; proteinuria, hematuria
- Stool and blood cultures: identification of an organism for cause and appropriate treatment

- Renal ultrasound: normal or large kidneys
- Electrocardiogram: possible arrhythmias from electrolyte imbalance

Nursing Interventions

The following nursing interventions are used for patients with AKI.

Emergency Care

- IV fluid resuscitation with an isotonic fluid if hemodynamically unstable

SAFE AND EFFECTIVE NURSING CARE: Clinical Pearl

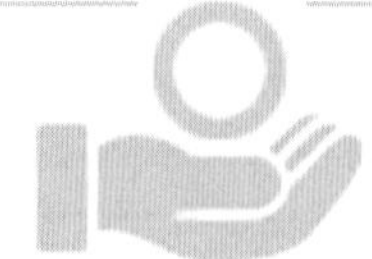

Renal Failure and IV Fluids

All children need concurrent IV fluids to combat ongoing losses of an acute illness or compensate for their insensible losses. Depending on the child's underlying condition, fluid needs vary. Regardless of the degree of renal failure, severe dehydration and/or shock need rapid correction of fluid balance to restore/preserve tissue perfusion (Kliegman, et al., 2016).

- Fluid removal with dialysis (hemodialysis) if fluid overload is present
- Prepare family and patient for possible hemodialysis
- Assist with obtaining appropriate consent for emergency procedures
- Seizure control
  - Lorazepam 0.05 to 0.1 mg/kg/dose every 15 minutes IV
  - Fosphenytoin 15 to 20 mg PE/kg IV for loading dose
  - Fosphenytoin 5 mg/kg/day IV for maintenance (Engorn & Flerlage, 2015)

CRITICAL COMPONENT

Seizures and Renal Failure

A child presents with tonic-clonic generalized seizure activity. The patient has a medical history of AKI. In addition to giving antiepileptic medications, laboratory studies are obtained. Specific abnormalities that can cause seizure activity are hyponatremia, hypoglycemia, and hypocalcemia. Accurate measurement of blood pressure is important because seizure activity can be from hypertensive encephalopathy.

Acute Hospital Care

- Preparation for renal replacement therapy
  - Hemodialysis
- Accurate fluid replacement of insensible losses (400 mL/m^2/24 hr)
- Accurate replacement of fluid losses from diarrhea, vomiting, urine production
- Recognition and correction of life-threatening electrolyte imbalances
- Obtaining electrocardiography with electrolyte imbalances
- Accurate administration of antihypertensive medications
  - Nifedipine 0.25 to 0.5 mg/kg/dose every 4 to 6 hours orally or sublingually (Engorn & Flerlage, 2015)
- Accurate monitoring of vital signs, with emphasis on blood pressure
- Accurate monitoring of intake, output, and weight daily
- Monitoring proper nutrition intake
- Understanding family values and cultural practices, and incorporating them into the hospital plan of care, if possible

Chronic Hospital Care

- Monitor fluid and electrolyte status.
- Provide adequate calories through no-added-salt, low-potassium, low-phosphate diet, without fluid excess.
- Provide enteral or parenteral feeding if oral intake is inadequate.
- Monitor daily weight.
- Provide skin care for peritoneal or hemodialysis catheter site.
- Provide skin care for possible breakdown related to edema and decreased perfusion.

Chronic Home Care

- Educate family and patient on home dialysis, if needed.
- Provide home blood pressure monitoring device.
- Educate family and patient on appropriate medication administration and side effects.
- Educate family and patient on nutrition restrictions.
  - Avoid high-protein diet
  - Appropriate fluid restriction
  - Low-potassium diet
  - Low-phosphorus diet
  - Avoid medications with phosphates (e.g., Fleet enema)
- Provide follow-up appointment dates and times.
- Educate family and patient on monitoring parameters.

Caregiver Education

Nurse education on the following topics is required for parents and caregivers of patients who have AKI.

Emergency Care

- Educate family and patient on emergent procedures.

Acute Hospital Care

- Educate family and patient on possible complications of AKI.
- Educate family and patient on medication administration and side effects.
- Educate family and patient on need for accurate intake and output recording.
- Educate family and patient on dietary restrictions.
- Instruct family and patient on appropriate skin care.

Chronic Hospital Care

- Provide information regarding dietary restrictions.
- Educate family and patient on signs of fluid overload.

- Provide instructions on enteral or parenteral nutrition, if needed.
- Educate family and patient on how to provide skin care.

Chronic Home Care

- Educate family and patient on blood pressure monitoring and parameters.
- Instruct family and patient on importance of follow-up care.
- Instruct family and patient on dietary restrictions.
- Instruct family and patient on nonsteroidal medications and to avoid their use.

Chronic Kidney Disease

CKD, including end-stage renal disease, is the irreversible function of the kidneys. Specifically, CKD is used to describe impaired kidney function for longer than 3 months.

- The GFR may be normal in children with CKD (Kher et al., 2017).
- CKD is staged from 1 (least severe) to 5 (most severe) (Table 16–4).
- Most cases of CKD in children are caused by congenital anomalies of the kidneys and urinary tract.
- Hypertension is the most common complication of CKD (Kher et al., 2017).
- African American children have a higher prevalence of CKD in the United States.
- Renal replacement therapy (dialysis) is the mainstay of treatment.
  - Hemodialysis is effective in the acute setting for critically ill patients with fluid overload, intoxication/ingestion, and hyperkalemia. Peritoneal dialysis is used with chronic renal failure and is delivered intraperitoneally. The peritoneal cavity is filled with a dialysate fluid and retained for a specific length of time or cycled throughout a time frame. At the end of the time period, the fluid is removed via gravity drainage. The dialysate acts as a filter by osmosis, removing toxins and waste products from the body.
  - Both hemodialysis and peritoneal dialysis require extensive specialized nursing training.

TABLE 16–4 Stages of Chronic Kidney Disease

CKD stage 1	GFR >90% plus signs of kidney disease
CKD stage 2	GFR 60%–89% plus mild kidney disease
CKD stage 3	GFR 40%–59% plus moderate kidney disease
CKD stage 4	GFR 15%–29% plus severe kidney disease
CKD stage 5/ESRD	GFR <15% or on dialysis

CKD, chronic kidney disease; ESRD, end-stage renal disease.
Reproduced with permission by the National Kidney Center (NationalKidneyCenter.org).

Assessment

Assessment for CKD includes the following measures.

Clinical Presentation

- Hypertension
- Poor growth/height
- Abdominal pain
- Edema
- Oliguria/anuria
- Arthralgias
- Fatigue
- Anemia
- Electrolyte abnormalities
- Muscle cramps
- Bone pain
- Seizure
- Nausea/vomiting
- Pruritus
- Dyspnea

Diagnostic Testing

- BUN: markedly elevated
- Creatinine: markedly elevated
- Electrolyte: hyperkalemia, hyponatremia, metabolic acidosis
- CBC: anemia
- Urinalysis: may be normal; proteinuria, hematuria
- Renal ultrasound: normal or large kidneys
- Electrocardiogram: possible dysrhythmias from electrolyte imbalance

Nursing Interventions

When a pediatric patient has CKD, the following nursing interventions are indicated.

Emergency Care

- IV fluid resuscitation with an isotonic fluid if hemodynamically unstable
- Fluid removal with hemodialysis if fluid overload is present
- Prepare family and patient for possible hemodialysis
- Assist with obtaining appropriate consent for emergency procedures
- Seizure control
  - Lorazepam 0.05 to 0.1 mg/kg/dose every 15 minutes IV
  - Fosphenytoin 15 to 20 mg PE/kg IV for loading dose
  - Fosphenytoin 5 mg/kg/day IV for maintenance (Engorn & Flerlage, 2015)

Acute Hospital Care

- Preparation for renal replacement therapy
- Hemodialysis/peritoneal dialysis
- Accurate fluid replacement of insensible losses (400 mL/m^2/24 hr)
- Recognition and correction of life-threatening electrolyte imbalances
- Obtaining electrocardiography with electrolyte imbalances
- Accurate administration of antihypertensive medications
  - Nifedipine 0.25 to 0.5 mg/kg/dose every 4 to 6 hours orally or sublingually (Engorn & Flerlage, 2015)

- Accurate monitoring of vital signs, with emphasis on blood pressure
- Accurate monitoring of intake, output, and weight daily
- Monitoring of proper nutrition intake
- Understanding family values and cultural practices, and incorporating them into the hospital plan of care, if possible

SAFE AND EFFECTIVE CLINICAL NURSING: Clinical Pearl

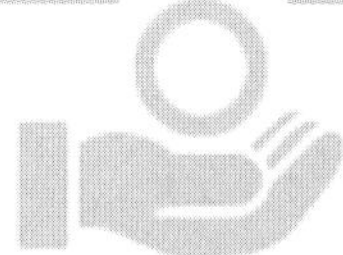

Hyperkalemia Prevention

Hyperkalemia is common in CKD and worsens as the GFR decreases (Kher et al., 2017). As the GFR worsens, the ability of the kidney to excrete potassium decreases. Metabolic acidosis also causes a cellular shift, thus increasing the serum potassium. Increased dietary intake of potassium-rich foods also causes hyperkalemia (Kliegman, et al., 2016).

Chronic Hospital Care

- Monitor fluid and electrolyte status.
- Provide adequate calories through no-added-salt, low-potassium, low-phosphate diet, without fluid excess.
- Provide enteral or parenteral feeding if oral intake is inadequate.
- Monitor daily weight.
- Provide skin care for peritoneal or hemodialysis catheter site.
- Provide skin care for possible breakdown related to edema and decreased perfusion.

Chronic Home Care

- Educate family and patient on home dialysis, if needed.
- Provide home blood pressure monitoring device.
- Educate family and patient on appropriate medication administration and side effects.
- Educate family and patient on nutrition restrictions.
    - Low-protein, low-potassium, low-phosphate diet
- Explain appropriate fluid restriction.

SAFE AND EFFECTIVE NURSING CARE: Clinical Pearl

Peritoneal Dialysis

Peritoneal dialysis involves the instilling of a hyperosmolar fluid into the peritoneal cavity via a surgically placed catheter. The fluid remains in the abdominal cavity for a prescribed length of time and then is drained out via gravity drainage. The goal is to remove excess fluid and help maintain electrolyte balance. Peritoneal dialysis education is taught by a specially trained nurse.

- Avoid medications with phosphates (e.g., Fleet enema).
- Provide follow-up appointment dates and times.
- Educate family and patient on monitoring parameters.

Caregiver Education

Nurse education for parents and caregivers of patients with CKD should cover the following topics.

Emergency Care

- Educate family and patient on emergent procedures.

Acute Hospital Care

- Educate family and patient on possible complications of CKD.
- Educate family and patient on medication administration and side effects.
- Educate family and patient on need for accurate intake and output recording.
- Educate family and patient on dietary restrictions.
- Instruct family and patient on appropriate skin care.

Chronic Hospital Care

- Provide information regarding dietary restrictions.
- Educate family and patient on signs of fluid overload.
- Provide instructions on enteral or parenteral nutrition, if needed.
- Educate family and patient on how to provide skin care.

Chronic Home Care

- Educate family and patient on blood pressure monitoring and parameters.
- Instruct family on importance of medication adherence.
- Instruct family and patient on importance of follow-up care.
- Instruct family and patient on dietary restrictions.
- Instruct family and patient on importance of monitoring weight consistently.
- Instruct family and patient to avoid nonsteroidal medications.
- Instruct family and patient to check with their nephrologist before starting any medications, supplements, or herbal therapies.

SAFE AND EFFECTIVE NURSING CARE: Understanding Medication

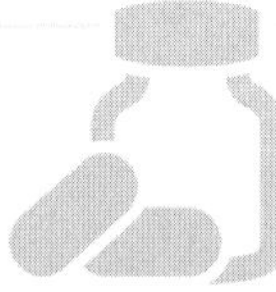

Vaccinations for Children With Chronic Kidney Disease

Children with CKD are at risk for development of illnesses that are preventable by vaccinations. Immunizations routinely administered to healthy children are provided to children with CKD. In addition, annual attenuated influenza vaccinations are recommended. Annual pneumococcal conjugate vaccinations are also encouraged. Live viral vaccinations such as varicella, MMR, and intranasal influenza vaccine are avoided in children with CKD.

GENITOURINARY ANOMALIES

Genitourinary disorders are conditions that occur when the organ is not functioning properly or has an incorrect anatomical location. These disorders are usually congenital.

Cryptorchidism

Undescended testis is the most common birth disorder of sexual differentiation in males (Kliegman et al., 2016). One percent of boys 1 year of age have cryptorchidism (Braga & Lorenzo, 2017).

Classification

- Abdominal: nonpalpable
- Peeping: abdominal but can be pushed into the upper part of the inguinal canal
- Gliding: can be pushed into the scrotum but immediately retracts
- Ectopic: perineal or superficial inguinal pouch

Assessment

Assessment for cryptorchidism includes the clinical presentation:

- Asymmetrical scrotum
- Small-appearing scrotum
- No palpable testis in scrotum

Nursing Interventions

Nurses conduct the following interventions for patients with cryptorchidism.

Acute Hospital Care

- If found in newborn care, refer to pediatrician or pediatric urologist.
- Consider the possibility of virilization from congenital adrenal hyperplasia in infants with bilateral undescended testes.

SAFE AND EFFECTIVE NURSING CARE: Promoting Safety

Cryptorchidism and Testicular Cancer

Men with a history of cryptorchidism are at increased risk for testicular cancer. Performing an orchiopexy prior to puberty seems to decrease this risk (Braga & Lorenzo, 2017).

- If outpatient admission for orchiopexy:
  - Pain control
  - Discharge education
  - Follow-up appointment arranged

Chronic Home Care

- Routine follow-up with pediatrician to track testis descent
- Surgical correction occurs between 6 and 18 months

Hypospadias

A hypospadias is a urethral opening on the ventral surface of the penis (Kliegman et al., 2016). One in 250 male newborns is born with this condition. It is usually an isolated anomaly.

Assessment

Assessment for hypospadias includes the following.

Clinical Presentation

- Urethral meatus on the glans penis (glanular), coronal, subcoronal, midpenile, penoscrotal, scrotal, or perianal area (Kliegman et al., 2016)
- Ventral curvature of the penis
- Hooded foreskin
- May have undescended testis
- May have inguinal hernia

CRITICAL COMPONENT

Hypospadias and Circumcision

Newborn males with hypospadias should not undergo a circumcision until evaluated by a pediatric urologist. Often the foreskin is used for the surgical repair of the hypospadias. The most common age for the surgical repair is between 6 and 12 months (Kliegman, et al., 2016).

Nursing Interventions

The following nursing interventions are used for patients with hypospadias.

Acute Hospital Care

- Avoid circumcision in the newborn period
- Surgical repair between 6 and 12 months of age
- Transfer to pediatric urologist

Chronic Home Care

- Routine follow-up with pediatric urologist

For additional resources, see Table 16–5.

TABLE 16–5 Kidney Disease Resources

American Association of Kidney Patients (AAKP) 14440 Bruce B. Downs Blvd. Tampa, FL 33613 Internet: https://aakp.org/	**National Kidney Foundation** Phone: 1.855.NKF.CARES (1.855.653.2273) E-mail: nkfcares@kidney.org Internet: https://www.kidney.org/patients
American Kidney Fund Internet: http://www.kidneyfund.org/	**National Kidney Registry** Internet: http://www.kidneyregistry.org
National Institute of Diabetes and Digestive and Kidney Diseases Phone: +1-800-860-8747 E-mail: healthinfo@niddk.nih.gov Internet: https://www.niddk.nih.gov	**Office of Disease Prevention and Health Promotion, U.S. Department of Health and Human Service** Internet: https://healthfinder.gov
National Kidney Center Phone: 703-662-1253 Internet: http://www.nationalkidneycenter.org	

Case Study

Demarcus S. is a 4-year-old boy who has a medical history of CKD. He was diagnosed with posterior urethral valves at 7 months of age. Since that time, he has had slow worsening of his CKD and is now stage 4. He has had increased blood pressure during his office visits for the past 3 months. He has not required dialysis. His mother reports that Demarcus has no restrictions to his diet that she adheres to, and she occasionally misses his evening medications because she has a part-time second job and is not home to administer the medications. He was admitted after a clinic visit where his blood pressure was greater than the 95th percentile for his age and height, with increased weight gain in the past 2 weeks and occasional vomiting.

The nurse taking care of Demarcus ensures that the blood pressure cuff is of the appropriate size. The nurse also ensures that his blood pressure is taken in the upper extremities. Demarcus's activities during and surrounding his blood pressure measurement should also be documented. Vomiting, pain, and agitation are examples of activities that may cause an elevated blood pressure reading. Conversely, if Demarcus is sedated or sleeping, his blood pressure readings may be lower.

In educating his mother about diet and hypertension, it is important to reinforce a low-sodium diet. Sodium requirements are based on age, but typically no more than 1,500 mg of sodium is allowed in the diet. Foods such as potato chips, soy sauce, ham, sausage, bacon, cured meats, and fast foods are high in sodium.

Children with CKD are also on a fluid restriction. Ensuring the family is aware of the fluid restriction is important because excess fluid will elevate the blood pressure.

In discussing medication administration with the family, it is important to stress that the medications need to be taken close to the same time each day. It is also important to avoid missing doses of medication. Often, medication charts and daily medication carriers are used to ensure appropriate administration of medications.

1. What are the stages of CKD and how are they defined?
2. What are some reasons that Demarcus's weight has increased recently?
3. What are some activities that may cause a decreased blood pressure reading?
4. Which foods are high in sodium?
5. How could you help the mother be more compliant with medication administration?

REFERENCES

American Academy of Pediatrics. (2004). The Fourth Report on the Diagnosis, Evaluation, and Treatment of High Blood Pressure in Children and Adolescents. *Pediatrics, 114*(2), 555–576.

Bakris, G., & Sorrentino, M. (2018). *Hypertension: A companion to Braunwald's heart disease* (3rd ed.). Elsevier: St. Louis.

Bierzynska, A. (2017). Recent advances in understanding and treating nephrotic syndrome. *F1000 Research, 6*, 121.

Braga, L. H., & Lorenzo, A.J. (2017). Cryptorchidism: A practical review for all community healthcare providers. *Canadian Urological Association Journal, 11*(Suppl. 1–2), S26–S32.

Children's Hospital Solution for Patient Safety. (2014). *SPS prevention bundle: Catheter associated urinary tract infections.* Retrieved from http://www.solutionsforpatientsafety.org/wp-content/uploads/SPS-Prevention-Bundles.pdf

Costanzo, L. (2018). *Physyiology* (6th ed.). Philadelphia: Elsevier Mosby.

Custer, J., & Rau, R. (2009). *The Harriet Lane handbook* (18th ed.). Philadelphia: Elsevier Mosby.

Dagan, R., Cleper, R., Davidovitis, M., Sinai-Trieman, L., & Krause, I. (2016). Post-infectious glomerulonephritis in pediatric patients over two decades: Severity-associated features. *Israel Medical Association Journal, 18*(6), 336–339.

Durham, S. H., Stamm, P. L., & Eiland, L. S. (2015). Cranberry products for the prophylaxis of urinary tract infections in pediatric patients. *Annals of Pharmacotherapy, 49*(12), 1349–1356.

Engorn, B., & Flerlage, J. (2015). *The Harriet Lane handbook* (20th ed.). Philadelphia: Elsevier Mosby.

Fatima, A., & Gibson, D. P. (2014). Pneumatosis intestinalis associated with Henoch-Schönlein Purpura. *Pediatrics, 134,* e880–e883.

Garcia-Roig, M., & Kirsch, A. (2016). Urinary tract infection in the setting of vesicoureteral reflux. *F1000 Research, 5*, 1552.

Hallbook, T., Sjolander, A., Amark, P., Miranda, M., Bjurulf, B., & Dahlin, M. (2015). Effectiveness of the ketogenic diet used to treat resistant epilepsy in Scandinavia. *European Journal of Paediatric Neurology, 19*(1), 29–36.

Hernandez, J., Ellison, J. S., & Lendvay, T. S. (2015). Current trends, evaluation and management of pediatric nephrolithiasis. *JAMA Pediatrics, 169*(10), 964–970.

Kamat, D. & Fischer, P. (2016). *Textbook of global health* (2nd ed.). Washington, DC: American Academy of Pediatrics.

Kher, K. K., Schnaper, H. W., & Greenbaum, L.A. (Eds.). (2017). *Clinical pediatric nephrology* (3rd ed.). Boca Raton, FL: Taylor & Francis Group.

Kliegman, R. M., Stanton, B. F., St. Geme, J. W., & Schor, N. F. (2016). *Nelson textbook of pediatrics* (20th ed.). Philadelphia: Elsevier.

Lee, T., & Park, J. (2017). Vesicoureteral reflux and continuous prophylactic antibiotics. *Investigative and Clinical Urology, 58*(Suppl. 1), S32–S37.

McCaffrey, J., Lennon, R., & Webb, N. (2016). The non-immunosuppressive management of childhood nephrotic syndrome. *Pediatric Nephrology, 31*, 1383–1402.

Okawada, M., Esposito, C., Esconlino, M., Farina, A., Cerulo, M., Turra, F., & Yamataka, A. (2016). Treatment of vesico-ureteral reflux in infants and children using endoscopic approaches. *Translational Pediatrics, 5*(4), 282–290.

Riley, M., & Blulm, B. (2012). High blood pressure in children and adolescents. *American Family Physician, 85*(7), 693–700.

Shah, S. R., Tunio, S. A., Arshad, M. H., Moazzam, Z., Noorani, K., Feroze, A. M., … Jeoffrey, S. A. H. (2016). Acute kidney injury recognition and management: A review of the literature and current evidence. *Global Journal of Health Science, 8*(5), 120–124.

Stefek, B., Beck, M., Ioffreda, M., Gardner, L., & Stefanski, M. (2015). Henoch-Schönlein purpura with posterior reversible encephalopathy syndrome. *Journal of Pediatrics, 167*(5), 1152–1154.

Traisman, E. (2016). Clinical management of urinary tract infections. *Pediatric Annals, 45*(4), e109–e111.

Van Batavia, J. P., & Tasian, G. E. (2016). Clinical effectiveness in the diagnosis and acute management of pediatric nephrolithiasis. *International Journal of Surgery, 36,* 698–704.

17

Endocrine Disorders

Kelly J. Betts, EdD, RN, CNE

LEARNING OUTCOMES

Upon completion of this chapter, the student will be able to:

1. Identify the anatomy and physiology of the endocrine system.
2. Identify areas of focus for performing an age-appropriate endocrine assessment.
3. Identify clinical manifestations of various endocrine disorders.
4. Recognize diagnostic and laboratory findings of patients with endocrine disorders.
5. Describe nursing interventions for the emergency care of patients with endocrine disorders.
6. Describe nursing interventions for the acute and chronic care of the patient with endocrine disorders.
7. Integrate home-care concepts into nursing interventions for the patient with an endocrine disorder.
8. Identify possible alternative therapy interventions for patients with endocrine disorders.
9. Develop a family teaching plan that will optimize therapy outcomes for patients with endocrine disorders.
10. Use critical thinking concepts to evaluate care of the patient with an endocrine disorder.

ANATOMY AND PHYSIOLOGY

The endocrine system regulates growth and development; energy use and storage; levels of glucose, fluid, and sodium in the bloodstream; sexual development; and the child's response to stress (Ward & Hisley, 2015). The endocrine system consists of organs that produce and secrete hormones (Fig. 17–1).

Hormones are chemicals produced by the endocrine glands and circulated in the bloodstream to another part of the body. They activate or inhibit cells in the target organs and act as messengers. There are two types of hormones: protein hormones from amino acids and steroid hormones from fat. The endocrine system communicates using positive and negative feedback systems of communication. Positive feedback occurs when hormone levels start to decline, causing the hypothalamus to secrete hormones that stimulate the pituitary gland to release hormones that then affect the target organ (Fig. 17–2).

Negative feedback occurs when hormone levels are too high. The hypothalamus secretes inhibitory hormones that stimulate the pituitary gland to release inhibitory factors.

Glands of the Endocrine System

The endocrine system releases hormones from glands located throughout the body; these hormones act on body tissues to perform an extensive range of function. Endocrine glands include the pituitary, thyroid, parathyroid, pineal body, thymus, pancreas, sex glands, and adrenal glands (Porth, 2015).

Hypothalamus

Located at the base of the brain, the hypothalamus sends messages from the autonomic nervous system to the target organs (Ward & Hisley, 2015) by secreting releasing or

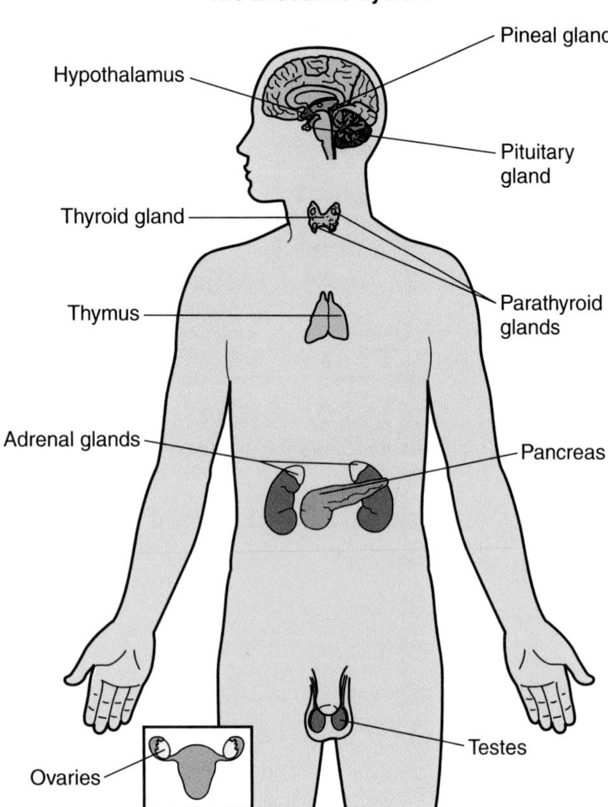

FIGURE 17–1 The endocrine system.

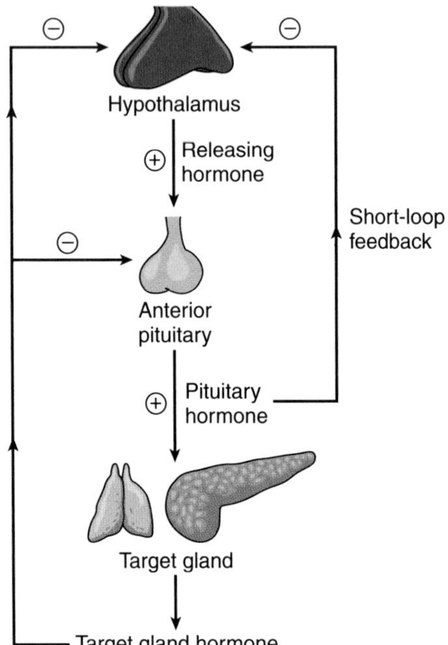

FIGURE 17–2 Feedback system from the pituitary to the target glands.

inhibitory hormones to the master gland (pituitary gland). These include:

- Thyroid-releasing hormone
- Corticotropin-releasing hormone (CRH)
- Luteinizing hormone (LH)-releasing hormone
- Growth hormone (GH)-releasing hormone
- Somatostatin—stimulates the pituitary gland to stop the release of GH

Pituitary Gland (Hypophysis)

Also called the master gland, the pituitary gland is located beneath the hypothalamus in the base of the brain. This gland controls other glands through stimulating hormones or inhibitory factors that turn the target glands on or off. The pituitary gland has two main lobes:

- The anterior lobe (adenohypophysis) secretes the following:
  - GH—stimulates growth of cells; stimulates protein synthesis and prevents protein breakdown
  - Thyroid-stimulating hormone—stimulates the thyroid glands to make thyroid hormones
  - Adrenocorticotrophic hormone (ACTH)—stimulates the cortex of the adrenal glands to make cortisone
  - Prolactin—stimulates milk production in the mammary glands of females
  - Follicle-stimulating hormone (FSH)—stimulates the ovaries to develop eggs within the follicles of the ovaries
  - LH—stimulates the follicles in the ovaries to rupture and release the egg and corpus luteum production in females; stimulates testosterone production in males
  - Melanocyte-stimulating hormone—stimulates melanin synthesis and release from skin and hair
- The posterior lobe (neurohypophysis) secretes the following:
  - Antidiuretic hormone (ADH) (vasopressin)—stimulates the kidneys to absorb and conserve water, increasing blood volume
  - Oxytocin (Pitocin)—stimulates smooth muscle contraction, milk letdown reflex, and the expulsion of the fetus and placenta

Pineal Body

- Located in the middle of the brain
- Stimulated by light exposure through the optic nerve
- Secretes the hormone melatonin
- Regulates wake-sleep cycles, circadian rhythms

Thymus

- Located in the anterior ventral aspect of chest at the base of the heart
- Atrophies with age
- Responsible for cellular immunity

Thyroid Gland

- Two lobes in anterior neck region below the larynx
- Produce T3 and T4 in response to TSH from pituitary gland
  - T3—tri-iodothyronine active
  - T4—thyroxine

- Responsible for synthesis of protein and cholesterol, glucose metabolism, heat production, growth and development, and metabolism
- Calcitonin—stimulates bone construction, thereby inhibiting calcium release from the bones and decreasing calcium blood levels

Parathyroid Glands

These four glands, two on each side of thyroid gland, produce parathyroid hormone (PTH) that:

- Increases calcium concentration in the bloodstream by stimulating the osteoclasts in the bone to release calcium
- Increases serum calcium levels by increasing the absorption of calcium from the gastrointestinal (GI) tract; increases calcium reabsorption in the kidneys
- Increases phosphate release from bones increasing blood levels; inhibits phosphate reabsorption in kidneys so that more phosphate is excreted

Adrenal Glands

- Located on top of the kidneys
- Two parts: cortex and medulla
    - Cortex produces steroids, hormones made from cholesterol
        - Glucocorticoids—mainly cortisone, which increases blood sugar, decreases inflammation, and aids in stress reduction
        - Mineralocorticoids (Aldosterone)—secreted in response to renin-angiotensin to conserve water, as well as retain sodium
    - Medulla
        - Adrenaline (epinephrine)—fight-or-flight response; increases heart rate, respiratory rate; dilates pupils; increases utilization of glucose; suppresses digestion and immune system
        - Norepinephrine—fight-or-flight response (same as above)
        - Dopamine—increases blood pressure

Pancreas

- Has both exocrine (with ducts) and endocrine function
    - Exocrine—secretes amylase, lipase, and trypsin for small-intestine digestion
    - Endocrine—islet of Langerhans
        - Beta cells secrete insulin, which forces glucose into the cells and stimulates glycogen formation; independent of pituitary control; stimulated by the ingestion of glucose.
        - Alpha cells work in the opposite manner as insulin; they break down glycogen in liver to increase blood sugar.

Sex Glands (Gonads)

The sex glands include the testes and the ovaries. These glands are responsible for the regulation of puberty and fertility. The ovaries are located on each side of the uterus (females), and the testes are located in the scrotum (males). The ovaries induce female sexual characteristics such as breast development, body around the hips and thighs, and the growth spurt that occurs during puberty. The testes induce the male sexual characteristics such as the development of muscles, increase in facial and body hair, and the growth spurt that occurs during puberty. In girls, the ovaries secrete hormones that regulate the menstrual cycle.

Testes

The testes produce androgens, mainly testosterone, in interstitial cells when stimulated by FSH and LH. Testosterone produces secondary sex characteristics in males, sperm formation, and sex drive.

Ovaries and Uterus

The ovaries produce estrogen and follicle cells.

- Estrogen produces secondary sex characteristics in females and mammary development.
- Follicle cells produce corpus luteum (meaning "yellow body"), which makes the hormone progesterone after the egg leaves the follicle.
    - Progesterone maintains pregnancy by relaxing the uterus and stimulates milk production in the mammary glands.

When a woman is pregnant:

- The ovaries and uterus produce relaxin, which is a hormone that relaxes the cervix, vagina, and ligaments around the birth canal in preparation for the delivery of a fetus.
- Human chorionic gonadotropin hormone is produced by the developing embryo; it inhibits immune response to the developing fetus.

ASSESSMENT

A comprehensive endocrine-focused assessment includes a general history, review of systems, and a physical examination. This section provides a systematic review of a complete endocrine assessment.

General History

The nurse should gather and assess the following aspects of the client's history.

Prenatal/Birth History

- Prenatal care
- Type of delivery
- Estimate of gestational age
- Complications of pregnancy or delivery
- Substance abuse
- Neonatal complications

Hospitalizations

- Overnight stays
- Surgeries—type and recovery time
- Accidents or injuries

Current Medications

- Prescribed
- Over the counter
- Dietary supplements
- Alternative/natural remedies

Allergies

- Medications
- Seasonal
- Foods/other

Immunizations

- Current, missed doses, and/or due dates

Family History

- Endocrine disorders
- Extreme short stature
- Parental heights/sibling heights
- History of other chronic disease

Developmental History

- Age of developmental milestones
- School performance
- History of behavioral problems

Nutrition

- Type of infant feeding (breast or formula)
- Types of food preferred
- Diet history—2 to 3 days
- Eating patterns
- Type and frequency of fast-food consumption
- Amount of milk consumed per day
- Any eating-related vomiting/GI distress
- Problems with chewing, swallowing, eating, or drinking

Activities

- Daily activities—type, quantity, how often
- Physical activity in school/team sports
- Number of TV/computer/video game hours per day

Physical Examination

A physical examination for endocrine conditions should include the following aspects.

Review of Systems

- Basic head-to-toe physical assessment of normal versus abnormal findings

Weight

- Infant weight without diaper on infant scale
- Minimal clothing for other children
- Scales should be calibrated for accuracy before weighing

Height

- Supine measurement for infants until age 24 months
- Children older than 24 months should be measured using a stadiometer (scales with measuring arms not recommended).
  - While using a stadiometer, take the child's shoes off and make sure the child is standing with feet together, heels against the wall, and standing straight with the hands down to the side. Girls with ponytails should take their hair down (Lipman et al., 2009; Phillips & Shulman, 2016).

Head Circumference

- Obtained using a measuring tape until age 36 months unless otherwise indicated by physician
- Level of fontanels should be assessed in infants

Vital Signs

- See vital sign parameters in Chapter 7.

Tanner Stage of Puberty

- Refer to Tanner staging chart in Chapter 10.
- Assess for signs of ambiguous genitalia and abnormal advancement in puberty (Horner, 2007; Houk & Levitsky, 2017).

Height and Weight

- Careful and accurate plotting of height, weight, and head circumference on growth chart (Lipman et al., 2009; Richmond & Rogol, 2017)
- Body surface area (refer to Chapter 10)
- Mid-parental height/target height
  - The mid-parental height is:

    Mother's height (inches) × father's height (inches) divided by 2

  - To get the target height, add 2.5 inches for boys and subtract 2.5 inches for girls.
- Body mass index (BMI) (Ball, Bindler, & Cowen, 2010):

$$\frac{\text{(Weight in kg)}}{\text{(Height in cm divided by 100)}^2} \quad or \quad \frac{\text{(Weight in kg)}}{\text{(Height in meters)}^2}$$

- Height velocity
  - Number of centimeters (cm) or inches (in) growth per year

Skin

- Assess skin for any unusual areas of skin discoloration or areas of increased skin pigmentation.

Body Odor

- Assess for unusual smells (e.g., musty, cheesy, sweet).

Neck

- Assess neck for the presence of any enlarged areas, nodules, or glands.

Muscles

- Assess strength and muscle tone. Note excess fat accumulation or decrease in muscle mass.

Facial Characteristics

- Assess the face for any unusual facial features such as a protuberant tongue, bulging of the eyes, excessive hair growth, or excessive roundness of the face.

HYPOPITUITARISM/ PANHYPOPITUITARISM

Hypopituitarism/panhypopituitarism is a condition in which one or more hormones secreted by the pituitary gland is deficient. GH is the most delicate of all the six hormones produced by the pituitary gland and is the first to become insufficient when the gland is damaged. This can occur as a result of trauma to the head during delivery or later in life, tumors of the hypothalamus or pituitary, infectious disease in the central nervous system (CNS), chemotherapy, radiation, surgical resection, and congenital syndromes.

Growth Hormone Deficiency

Children with growth hormone deficiency (GHD) have a clinical presentation of delayed growth of less than 2 inches (3 to 4 cm) per year. This is monitored by plotting serial growth points on the growth chart for his or her age and sex. Children with GHD have a consistent declination of growth measurements on the growth chart over time and a high weight-to-height ration with increased abdominal fat. Infants may present with a delay in closure of the anterior fontanel.

Other characteristics of children with GHD may include delayed dental eruption, decreased muscle mass, cherubic-like appearance or appearing to be younger than actual age, delayed puberty during adolescent period, and a high-pitched voice.

SAFE AND EFFECTIVE NURSING CARE: Clinical Pearl

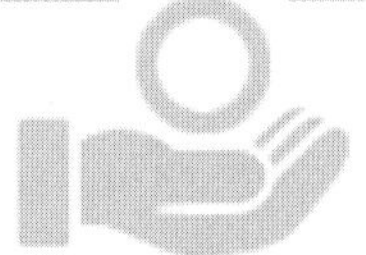

Congenital Hypopituitarism

Frequent or recurrent hypoglycemia, prolonged jaundice, small penis/testes, lethargy, feeding problems, and excretion of excessive amounts of urine in the neonatal period may indicate congenital hypopituitarism. Infants with this condition are prescribed GH replacement therapy immediately to help regulate blood sugar levels. This type of neonatal hypoglycemia can be fatal if not treated immediately upon diagnosis. These infants undergo further testing to detect other possible pituitary hormone deficiencies that need to be treated. Other common hormone deficiencies are hypothyroidism, ACTH deficiency, and ADH deficiency (Khardori & Kemp, 2015; Ward & Hisley, 2015).

Diagnostic Testing

- Thorough review of growth plots on a growth chart is done to determine the rate of growth per year; special attention is given to those children whose growth is less than the 3rd percentile.
- Biological parental heights are calculated to determine the mid-parental height of the parents or the average. This is used as an estimate only.
- Bone age x-ray of the left hand and wrist is used to determine the actual age of the bones in comparison with the child's actual (chronological) age. Bone age greater than 2 standard deviations (SD) below normal merits further evaluation (Alt et al., 2013).
- Magnetic resonance imaging (MRI) of the head, with a focus on the pituitary gland, is used to look for abnormalities or absence of the gland.
- Baseline blood tests include cortisol, complete blood cell count, and electrolytes.
- Provocative GH testing—this test uses certain medications that stimulate the pituitary gland to make GH (Ball et al., 2010).

CRITICAL COMPONENT

Growth Hormone Secretion

GH is secreted in pulsatile spurts during a 24-hour period, not constantly. A single laboratory measurement of GH is not indicative of GHD.

- Insulin-like growth factor 1 (IGF-1) and insulin-like growth factor binding protein 3 to test for GHD
- Karyotype in girls to rule out Turner syndrome
- Thyroid function test to detect hypothyroidism
- ACTH and cortisol levels to detect the presence of other hormone deficiencies
- Urine creatinine, pH, specific gravity, blood urea nitrogen (BUN), and electrolytes to detect the possibility of short stature being caused by chronic renal failure
- Complete blood cell count and sedimentation rate to rule out any inflammatory bowel disease
- Antigliadin antibodies to screen for celiac disease

Nursing Interventions

- Careful measurement and documentation of growth on the child's age- and sex-appropriate growth chart, noting any declining trends in the child's growth patterns over a 6-month to 1-year period
- Assess for psychosocial clues that the child or parents are having trouble dealing with the child's stature. Examples may include the following:
  - Child does not want to be involved in team activities for fear of being bullied or fear that he or she cannot physically play the games/sports.

- Parents won't allow the child to be involved in activities, because they believe the child is not capable or "too small" to be involved.
- Siblings or other children treat the child as if he or she is younger than his or her age. For example, the child's peers carry the child with a growth disorder around or treat him or her like a baby.

- Educate the patient and parents regarding the disease process of GHD, including the causes, diagnostic testing methods, and medical treatments available.
- Educate the family regarding the medications administered for the treatment of GHD and the potential side effects of the medication.
- GH replacement therapy is a medical regimen administered in the home setting. Follow-up with the endocrinologist every 3 to 4 months is crucial for assessing response to therapy.

Caregiver Education

- Provide detailed instructions regarding the administration of GH replacement therapy.
- Provide the parents with educational and online resources and support groups.
  - The Human Growth Foundation (http://www.hgfound.org)
  - The Magic Foundation (http://www.magicfoundation.org)
- Stress the importance of medication compliance and clinic follow-up appointments with the endocrinologist every 3 to 4 months to ensure the patient is responding to therapy.
- Educate the parent regarding the side effects of somatropin and when to contact the physician with concerns.

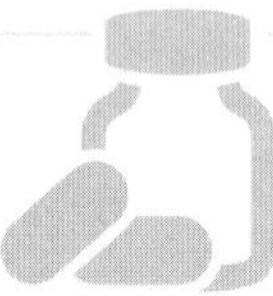

SAFE AND EFFECTIVE NURSING CARE: Understanding Medication

Growth Hormone Replacement Therapy

GH replacement therapy consists of the child receiving daily subcutaneous injections of manufactured GH called somatropin. As with many medications, several manufacturers have developed GH with different trade names, including Genotropin, Nutropin, Humatrope, Tev-Tropin, and Norditropin. These derivatives of GH lack one amino acid but are otherwise identical to human GH. Somatropin is dosed differently depending on the manufacturer, but recommended doses start at 0.24 to 0.3 mg/kg/week. As with insulin, GH is available in vials that must be reconstituted, pen devices that contain cartridges, and needleless injection devices. Some of the side effects include headache and achiness in the joints and muscles, particularly the knees, ankles, and wrists. If side effects occur, the physician may decrease the starting dose and then increase the dose slowly until the side effects resolve. It is recommended to start children on GH therapy as early as possible to achieve the maximum growth benefit (Rogol, 2017; Vallerand, Sanoski, & Deglin, 2017).

DIABETES INSIPIDUS

Diabetes insipidus (DI) is insufficient production of ADH, which is stored in the posterior pituitary gland and acts on the kidneys to restore water and control the amount of urine excreted. There are two forms of DI: central (or neurogenic) DI and nephrogenic DI. Central DI is caused by insufficient ADH production. Nephrogenic DI occurs when the kidneys fail to respond to appropriate levels of ADH. Both forms of DI can have an abrupt onset and similar manifestations.

Assessment

Assessment for DI includes the following measures.

Clinical Presentation

- Central (neurogenic) DI:
  - Polyuria, polydipsia, enuresis
  - Getting up to drink water throughout the night
  - Irritability in infants that can only be relieved by giving water instead of formula or breast milk
  - Constipation, fever, dehydration, and hypernatremia
- Nephrogenic DI:
  - Polyuria, polydipsia
  - Hypernatremia in the neonatal period
  - Dilute urine, vomiting, dehydration
  - Fever and possible changes in mental status

CRITICAL COMPONENT

Dehydration

Dehydration is a critical effect of DI in children. Severe dehydration can occur very quickly in infants and smaller children, so fluids must be increased as soon as possible during exacerbation. The nurse must be able to recognize signs and symptoms of dehydration, such as dry mucous membranes, sunken fontanel in infants, tachycardia, minimal or no tears when crying, and decreased skin turgor. Severe dehydration can lead to hypovolemic shock. The administration of IV fluids is essential to treat severe dehydration, especially when the child is unable to tolerate liquid intake (Mishra & Chandrashekhar, 2011; Suddaby & Mowery, 2007).

Diagnostic Testing

- Measure 24-hour urine collection for daily output.
- Serum sodium is elevated (greater than 150 to 170 mEq/L) (Ward & Hisley, 2015).
- Urine osmolality is decreased (less than 300 mOsm/L).
- Urine specific gravity is decreased (less than 1.005).
- Urine-to-serum osmolarity ratio is less than 1 (Ball et al., 2010).
- Water Deprivation Testing: Water deprivation testing is performed to diagnosis DI. The patient is under direct supervision by the nurse while the nurse carefully monitors vital signs and weight. Urine and blood are collected early in the day and

tested for osmolarity and electrolytes. Then the child is deprived of water intake until significant dehydration occurs. The child is weighed every 2 hours until 2% to 5% of body weight is lost. Urine-specific gravity is monitored every hour. This test is stopped once the urine-specific gravity reaches 1.014 or higher. The testing should never last more than 4 hours for an infant and 7 hours for a child. During the test, vital signs are carefully monitored for signs of hypotension and fever (Styne, 2016).

Evidence-Based Practice Research

Elder, C., & Demitri, P. J. (2017). Diabetes insipidus and the use of desmopressin in hospitalized children. *Archives of Disease in Childhood Education and Practice Edition, 102,* 100–104. doi: 10.1136/archdischild-2016-31076

In 2016, a group of researchers in England (United Kingdom) released a patient safety alert that highlighted the association between mortality and morbidity when desmopressin is omitted in individuals with DI. The UK National Reporting System reported 76 near misses, 56 dosing errors leading to harm, and 4 cases where the lack of administering desmopressin resulted in severe dehydration and even death. Key messages from this research article for health-care personnel taking care of patients with DI are as follows:

- The administration of desmopressin is highly individual, and patients should be monitored based on their clinical effect.
- Never restrict fluids to a patient with DI.
- The doses of the different formulations of desmopressin are not interchangeable. Seek advice from a pharmacist or endocrine specialist when converting a patient taking desmopressin to a different formulation.
- Strict monitoring of intake and output, as well as serum electrolytes, osmolality, and urine osmolality, is needed to ensure safe care of patients with DI.

(Elder & Dimitri, 2017)

Nursing Interventions

- Recognition of the differences between central (neurogenic) and nephrogenic DI is essential to assess and make decisions regarding the appropriate nursing care of the patient.
- Acute hospital care includes nursing responsibility related to the diagnostic water deprivation test, such as obtaining vital signs, weights, blood and urine samples, and then careful assessment for signs and symptoms of dehydration.
- The nurse is responsible for administration and education regarding the use of medications to treat the two types of DI.
- Accurate intake and output should be constantly monitored.

Caregiver Education

- Emergency care involves teaching the parents about the signs and symptoms of dehydration, and the need to take the child to the hospital for IV fluid replacement.
- During the initial states of exacerbation, it is important to teach the parents and child to increase fluids until the medication begins to take effect.
- Chronic home care involves teaching the parents of the child with DI the importance of medication compliance and the correct way to administer the medications, because DI is a lifelong condition that will require long-term use of medications for treatment.
- It is also important for the nurse to educate the parents regarding the importance of making the child's school aware of the condition so that appropriate care can be provided at school.
- The parents should provide the child with an emergency alert bracelet, and the bracelet should be worn at all times by the infant or child.

SAFE AND EFFECTIVE NURSING CARE: Understanding Medication

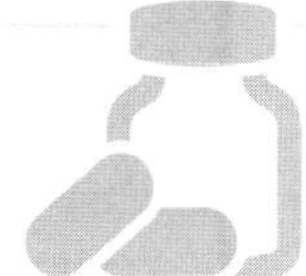

Types of Diabetes Insipidus Medications

Central DI medications include vasopressin analogs such as vasopressin or desmopressin (DDAVP). This medication is usually given intranasally, but it can be given orally or subcutaneously (SQ). Vasopressin analogs are usually the first line of treatment for patients with DI. Diuretics may also be used to treat central DI because they paradoxically decrease urine volume as much as 75% (Ward & Hisley, 2015). Midamor is an example of a potassium-sparing diuretic that may be used in patients with DI. Indomethacin (Indocin) is a cyclooxygenase inhibitor and may be taken to inhibit prostaglandin, which in turn reduces urine output.

CRITICAL COMPONENT

Vasopressin

Vasopressin (DDAVP) cannot effectively treat nephrogenic DI because the kidney is unresponsive to the mechanism of action of the drug, so it is critical to diagnose the correct type of DI.

SAFE AND EFFECTIVE NURSING CARE: Clinical Pearl

Intranasal Medications

Tips regarding the administration of intranasal medications include:

- Have the child blow his or her nose before the administration of the medication.
- In infants, clear the nose with a bulb syringe before administering the medication.
- Positioning can enhance the absorption of the medication.
- Infants and children with colds or severe congestion should receive an alternate route of the medication, because this interferes with its absorption.

HYPERPITUITARISM (GROWTH HORMONE EXCESS)

Hyperpituitarism is a rare condition characterized by excess GH secretion from the pituitary gland, causing children to experience uncontrolled growth. If the patient has precocious puberty in conjunction with hyperpituitarism, the condition may be caused by a tumor on or near the hypothalamus or pituitary gland. Once the closure of the epiphyseal plates occurs and hyperpituitarism continues, overgrowth of the bones occurs. This is referred to as acromegaly. Enlargement of the hands and feet, and coarseness of facial features, including the forehead, nose, lips, tongue, and jaw, are common. Other symptoms may include generalized muscle weakness and pain in the muscles and joints.

Diagnostic Testing

- Early identification is essential. Monitoring growth charts for excessive growth spurts or consistent growth greater than the 95th percentile is warranted. An estimated mid-parental height that is greater than 2 SD scores above normal should be monitored.
- IGF-1 levels will be elevated with hyperpituitarism.
- Radiological testing such as a bone age x-ray will depict advancement of bone growth.
- An MRI may be necessary to evaluate the hypothalamus and pituitary gland to rule out a GH-producing or other type of tumor.

Nursing Interventions

- Nursing care should focus on accurate assessment of growth trends by carefully documenting height and weight on the appropriate growth chart.
- Physical assessment is important to evaluate for early physical signs of excess bone growth characteristics and other features of gigantism.
- Evaluation of laboratory values indicative of hyperpituitary function is essential.
- If surgery is indicated, preoperative and postoperative nursing interventions such as neurological assessment, vital signs, wound assessment, and dressing care and assessment for potential complications are important.
- Follow-up home care may be indicated depending on the status of the patient after surgical intervention. The nurse should take responsibility to refer the patient/family to a home-care provider.

Caregiver Education

- Focus on educating patients and families about the disorder, treatment options, psychosocial support, and surgical preparation if indicated.
- Patient and family education regarding home medications such as somatostatin analogs, dopamine agonists, and GH receptor antagonist.
- Promote medication compliance.
- Focus on long-term complications of noncompliance, such as hypertension, cardiomegaly, subsequent cardiovascular disease, diabetes mellitus, osteoarthritis, sleep apnea, and early death.

SYNDROME OF INAPPROPRIATE ANTIDIURETIC HORMONE

Syndrome of inappropriate antidiuretic hormone (SIADH) occurs in the presence of excessive ADH production. The kidneys are unable to conserve appropriate amounts of water so the body retains water, leading to water intoxication, hyponatremia, and cellular edema. SIADH is very closely associated with children who have had CNS infections or intrathoracic disease, and may occur in postoperative patients as a complication. The signs and symptoms have varying degrees of seriousness. Excessive SIADH may include nausea, vomiting, seizures, and personality changes such as irritability, combativeness, hallucinations, and confusion leading to stupor of coma (Ward & Hisley, 2015). Other signs may include increased blood pressure, neck vein distention, crackles heard on lung examination, weight gain with no external visible edema, decreased urine output despite a high urine-specific gravity, and low sodium levels.

Diagnostic Testing

Serum laboratory levels are monitored and diagnosis is confirmed when the laboratory levels present the following results:

- High urine osmolarity (greater than 1,200 Osmol/kg)
- High urine-specific gravity (more than 1.030)
- Low serum osmolarity (greater than 275 mOsm/kg)
- Low serum sodium (greater than 125 mEq/L)
- Decreased BUN (more than 10 mg/dL)
- Decreased hematocrit

Nursing Interventions

- Fluid restriction is essential for a child with SIADH. The fluid restriction protocol may begin with restricting 75% of fluid maintenance and decreasing the fluids to half of maintenance if there is no improvement in 4 to 6 hours.
- Emergency management of severe SIADH may include the administration of a hypertonic sodium chloride solution, especially if hyponatremia is severe and neurological disease is present.
- If adrenal insufficiency is present, corticosteroids will be administered according to stress dosing protocols.
- Very detailed intake and output must be monitored by the nurse, including accounting for all routes of fluid administration. Careful attention must be paid to those children old enough to reach water fountains or toilets.
- Strict diaper weights must be obtained when caring for infants with SIADH.
- Medications should be given during the meal so that additional fluid intake is not needed when administering medications.
- Irrigate all feeding tubes with normal saline as opposed to water to prevent the pulling of sodium from the body.
- A diet high in sodium and protein should be encouraged.

- Neurological assessment is crucial for patients with SIADH, because decreased sodium levels can cause an altered level of consciousness that may lead to seizures.
- Seizure precautions at the bedside should be used and documented on the patient's chart.

Caregiver Education

- Emergency patient/family education should consist of teaching how to recognize the signs and symptoms of sodium depletion, such as weight gain, altered level of consciousness, confusion, complaints of headache, and irritability. The parents should be taught to take the child to the emergency department or call for emergency assistance.
- Education regarding the importance of fluid balance is essential. The child and parents/family should be taught to carefully assess intake and output, including fluid restrictions, obtaining diaper weights, and urinals or "toilet hats" to monitor output. Careful precautions must be taken to teach patients and family about hidden water in food sources such as popsicles and watermelon. Encouraging a diet high in sodium and protein is also indicated.
- Encourage the patient to wear a medical alert bracelet.

CRITICAL COMPONENT

Low Sodium and Risk for Seizure

Low sodium levels less than 125 mEq/L may cause seizure activity in children with SIADH. Keeping sodium levels as near to normal as possible is the primary goal of treatment. The pediatric nurse must be very thorough in keeping accurate track of the child's intake, output, and daily weights (Ward & Hisley, 2015).

PRECOCIOUS PUBERTY

Precocious puberty is defined as early pubertal development in girls younger than 8 years and boys younger than 9 years. It can be caused by premature release and secretion of gonadotropin hormones from the pituitary. There are three classes of precocious puberty (Table 17–1):

- Complete or true precocious puberty
- Incomplete precocious puberty
- Puberty caused by other conditions, such as injury to the CNS

TABLE 17–1 Classification of Sexual Precocity

TRUE PRECOCIOUS PUBERTY, COMPLETE	INCOMPLETE PRECOCIOUS PUBERTY	PRECOCIOUS PUBERTY CAUSED BY OTHER CONDITIONS
Caused by premature activation of gonadotrophic hormones from the hypothalamic–pituitary feedback system **Examples:** Familial or constitutional central precocious puberty CNS tumors such as craniopharyngiomas, hamartoma, and hypothalamic astrocytoma Idiopathic precocious puberty	Caused by ovarian or adrenal secretion of, or ingestion of, estrogen (Styne, 2016); in this case, the serum gonadotropins will be suppressed and serum estradiol levels will be elevated **Examples:** ***Boys*** Gonadotropin-releasing tumors Increased androgen secretion from the adrenal gland or testis, such as in congenital adrenal hyperplasia Leydig cell adenoma Familial testotoxicosis (sex-limited autosomal dominant disorder) ***Girls*** Ovarian cyst Estrogen-secreting ovarian or adrenal tumor Peutz-Jeghers syndrome ***Both sexes*** McCune-Albright syndrome Hypothyroidism Iatrogenic or exogenous exposure to estrogens in foods, drugs, or cosmetics	May be caused by condition that directly affects the CNS **Examples:** Encephalitis Static encephalopathy Brain abscess Hydrocephalus Head trauma Arachnoid cyst Myelomeningocele Vascular lesions Cranial irradiation

From Alt, P., Babler, E. K., Betts, K. J., Carney, P. H., Courtney, J. A., Flores, B. M., … Worley, D. D. (2013). Clinical handbook of pediatric endocrinology *(2nd ed.). St. Louis, MO: Quality Medical Publishing.*

Tanner staging is an assessment guide that should be used for every child's physical examination, and it is especially important for children and adolescents during pubertal age.

Assessment

Assessment for precocious puberty includes the following measures.

Clinical Presentation

- Presence of breast development (Tanner stage 2 or greater) for girls younger than 8 years
- Presence of testicular development (Tanner stage 2 or greater) for boys younger than 9 years
- Scrotum is reddened and thinner
- Tanner stage 2 pubic hair or greater
- Vaginal mucosa pink and thicker
- Sebaceous activity on face; acne
- Café au lait spots, presence of bone lesions on x-ray may indicate McCune-Albright syndrome
- Advanced bone age; bone age x-ray of the left hand and wrist to determine the actual age of the bones in comparison with the child's actual (chronological) age; bone age above normal merits further evaluation (Alt et al., 2013; Kaplowitz & Hoffman, 2017)
- Increased height velocity
- Gonadotropin-releasing hormone (GnRH) stimulation test results with increased LH response greater than 10 IU/L (Alt et al., 2013)
- Leuprolide acetate stimulation test results with LH levels greater than 8 IU/L (Alt et al., 2013)

Diagnostic Testing

- Serum studies include LHs, estradiol, FSH, and testosterone.
- Provocative stimulation testing: GnRH stimulation testing and leuprolide acetate stimulation testing
- Radiological studies such as bone age x-ray and MRI

Nursing Interventions

- Early identification and treatment are essential.
- Careful monitoring of height velocity is necessary to determine whether treatment methods are providing effective hormone suppression.
- Carefully assess sexual characteristics (Tanner staging) at each visit.
- Administer a gonadotropin-releasing hormone analogue (GnRHa) to stop the progression of pubertal development and suppress the release of gonadotropin hormones monthly.
- If GnRHa is given intramuscularly, assess injection sites for signs of sterile abscess.
- Perform psychological assessment of the child's response to the advanced pubertal development to determine whether psychological referral is indicated.

Caregiver Education

- Provide education about the condition and treatment options prescribed.
- Teach parents the importance of dressing the child age-appropriately despite development of sexual characteristics.
- Encourage the importance of medication compliance to avoid elevation of gonadotrophic hormones and advancement of sexual characteristics and height velocity.
- Discuss with the parents the need to talk about issues of sexuality at an earlier age than normal. Protective guidance measures should be offered, because children with precocious puberty may be at risk for sexual advances by older children, teens, or adults.
- Educate parents that medication should suppress the child's moodiness and emotional lability.
- Educate parents that use of GnRHa will not cause infertility problems later in life and that once the child is at an age where puberty is appropriate, the medication can be discontinued and spontaneous puberty will appear normally.

CRITICAL COMPONENT

Symptoms of Precocious Puberty

Variations in pubertal development may lead the health-care professional to suspect precocious puberty. These variations are usually benign and do not progress into full sexual pubertal development, but they must be evaluated frequently to make a definitive diagnosis. These variations include:

- Premature thelarche
  - Isolated breast development that occurs earlier than normal
  - Most common when younger than 2 years and older than 6 years
  - No increased growth velocity
  - May have unilateral/bilateral breast development with areolae maturation
  - No other signs of puberty are present
- Premature adrenarche
  - Early development of pubic hair in girls younger than 8 years and boys younger than 9 years
  - No increase in growth velocity
  - Tanner 2 or greater pubic hair
  - May also be accompanied by axillary hair, body odor, mild acne, and oily skin
  - May also be seen in girls born prematurely
  - Testis 3 mL or less by Tanner stage
- Adolescent gynecomastia of boys
  - Glandular enlargement greater than 0.5 cm of the male breast tissue
  - Most common between 13 and 14 years of age, but usually resolved by age 17 years
  - May be caused by high estrogen-to-testosterone ratio

HYPOTHYROIDISM

Hypothyroidism is caused by an underactive thyroid gland. The thyroid gland produces three types of hormones: T4 (thyroxine), T3 (tri-iodothyronine), and thyroid-stimulating hormone. Hypothyroidism can be congenital or acquired.

SAFE AND EFFECTIVE NURSING CARE: Understanding Medication

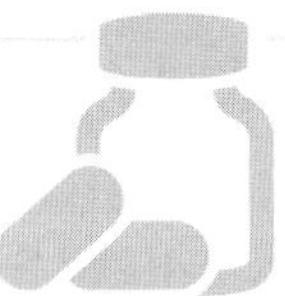

Lupron

Leuprolide acetate (Lupron Depot Pediatric) is the most common medication for treating true central precocious puberty in children. Because this medication is also used to treat adults for other causes, it is critical to ensure that the child receives the pediatric formulation. Beginning doses start at 3.75 mg and are increased based on weight to a maximum dose of 15 mg. This medication can be given intramuscularly (IM) or SQ. The medication should be given as directed or the child may experience increased hormone levels that cause signs of puberty to progress (Vallerand et al., 2017).

Congenital Hypothyroidism

Congenital hypothyroidism occurs at birth. State newborn screening programs identify infants born with congenital hypothyroidism and report the results immediately to the family and the infant's health-care provider. It is important that a newborn with congenital hypothyroidism get the appropriate treatment as soon as possible to avoid delays in cognitive development.

Assessment

Assessment for hypothyroidism must include the following elements.

Clinical Presentation

- Most infants are born asymptomatic.
- Ten percent of affected infants have symptoms that develop within weeks to months of birth.
- Symptoms may include hypotonia, lethargy, open posterior fontanel, open cranial sutures, umbilical hernia, prolonged jaundice, pallor, enlarged tongue, hoarse cry, constipation, dry skin, respiratory difficulties, poor weight gain, generalized edema, goiter, abdominal distention, and increased birth weight.

Diagnostic Testing

- Thyroid laboratory tests are part of the state mandatory newborn screening.
- In children with suspected acquired hypothyroidism, T4, TSH, and antithyroid antibodies are taken.
- Thyroid scan or ultrasound may be indicated to confirm the presence and position of the thyroid gland.
- Assessment of the infant's or child's growth velocity may also indicate hypothyroidism, especially if there are extreme differences between height and weight percentiles.

Nursing Interventions

- Immediate initiation of thyroid replacement hormone is essential to prevent cognitive damage in newborns and infants.
- Follow-up with newborn screening results prior to or at the first newborn visit within 1 week of birth.
- Carefully assess height and weight on the growth chart to determine growth delay.
- Obtain history of infant's activity level, feeding ability, frequency of feedings, and bowel habits during follow-up visits.
- Provide patient/family education regarding thyroid replacement therapy and medication administration.

Caregiver Education

- Teach parents how to administer thyroid medications by having them crush and mix the medication with a small amount of water, breast milk, formula, or baby food.
- Instruct parents to give thyroid medications at the same time each morning and not to skip or double doses.
- Instruct parents to administer medication via needleless syringe and not to put medication in bottle.
- Instruct parents that formula should be milk-based and not soy-based, because soy-based formulas can break down the effects of the medication.
- Reinforce the importance of medication compliance and the lifelong need for thyroid medications.
- Instruct parents on the potential side effects of thyroid replacement medications, and instruct them to notify their physician immediately if side effects are experienced.

Acquired Hypothyroidism

- Onset in childhood or teen years
- Cause may be related to an autoimmune condition known as Hashimoto's thyroiditis
- Medications such as lithium may interfere with thyroid synthesis

Assessment

Assessment for acquired hypothyroidism includes the following measures.

Clinical Presentation

- Decreased appetite, thinning of the hair or hair loss, dry and cool skin, depressed tendon reflexes, bradycardia, constipation, extreme fatigue, sensitivity to cold temperatures, abnormal menstrual cycles
- Manifestations unique to children include changes or deceleration in growth velocity, weight increase, delayed bone age, delayed dentition, muscle weakness, and delayed or precocious puberty
- School-age children may show a decline in school performance
- A goiter may be present

Diagnostic Testing

- In children with suspected acquired hypothyroidism, laboratory results of T4, TSH, and anti-thyroid antibodies are evaluated.
- Thyroid scan or ultrasound may be indicated to confirm the presence and position of the thyroid gland.
- Bone age x-ray is used to assess delayed growth.
- Assessment of infant's or child's growth velocity may also indicate hypothyroidism, especially if there are extreme differences between height and weight percentiles.

Nursing Interventions

- Assess height and weight on the growth chart to determine growth delay and/or excessive weight gain.
- Obtain history of the child's activity level, appetite, incidences of hair loss or thinning, constipation, or other symptoms of hypothyroidism.
- Obtain family history for autoimmune thyroid problems, especially in female family members.
- Provide patient education regarding thyroid replacement therapy and medication administration.

Caregiver Education

- Instruct parents to give thyroid medications at the same time each morning and not to skip or double doses.
- Instruct parents to administer medication via needleless syringe and not to put medication in bottle.
- Reinforce the importance of medication compliance and the lifelong need for thyroid medications.
- Instruct parents on the potential side effects of thyroid replacement medications, and instruct them to notify their physician immediately if side effects are experienced.
- Stress the importance of follow-up physician visits every 6 months so that thyroid blood levels can be assessed. The dosage of thyroid medications depends on body weight, and the dose may need to be adjusted frequently as the child grows.
- Teach parents to modify child's diet with fruit and bulk if the child is experiencing constipation.
- Teach parents about the complications related to lack of thyroid treatment, such as myxedema.

SAFE AND EFFECTIVE NURSING CARE: Promoting Safety

Myxedema

A severe complication of hypothyroidism is a condition known as myxedema. This life-threatening crisis occurs when thyroid levels are extremely low. TSH levels are critically high, and T4 levels are usually undetectable. The clinical manifestations of myxedema include nonpitting edema, severe edema of the face (face will appear round), edema of the tongue, metabolic disturbances, and hypothermia. If this condition is not treated immediately, the child or infant will progress to hypoglycemia, hypotension, cardiovascular arrest, and coma (myxedema coma). This condition is rare in children but does exist in children who are untreated for hypothyroidism.

SAFE AND EFFECTIVE NURSING CARE: Clinical Pearl

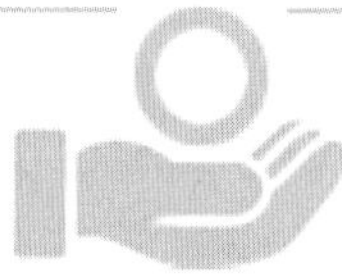

Laboratory Indicators for Hypothyroidism

When evaluating laboratory results for hypothyroidism, the nurse will see the following laboratory indicators:

Serum T4 ↓

Serum T3 normal

Serum TSH ↑

SAFE AND EFFECTIVE NURSING CARE: Understanding Medication

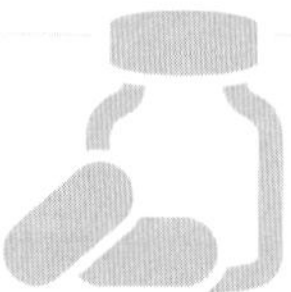

Thyroid Hormone Replacement Therapy

DRUG: levothyroxine sodium (Synthroid, Levoxyl, Levothroid, and others)

PREPARATIONS:

- Tabs—25, 50, 75, 88, 100, 112,125, 137, 150, 175, 200, or 300 mcg
- IV, IM—50% to 75% of oral dose
- Injection—0.2 mg/vial, 0.5 mg/vial

DOSING RECOMMENDATIONS:

Age Range	Daily Dose (mcg/kg)	Daily Dose (mcg/day)	Weight Range (kg)
<6 months	6–10	25–50	3–9
6–12 months	6–8	37.5–75	6–12
1–5 years	4–5	75–100	9–23
6–12 years	5–6	75–100	15–55
12–18 years	2–3	75–175	30–90

Adapted from Vallerand, A. H., Sanoski, C. A. & Deglin, J.H. (2017). Davis's drug guide for nurses *(15th ed.). Philadelphia: F.A. Davis.*

HYPERTHYROIDISM

Hyperthyroidism is an overproduction of thyroid hormone often referred to as Graves' disease. It occurs most frequently in teens between 12 and 14 years old. It tends to be familial, and the manifestation period is between 6 and 12 months. If untreated, hyperthyroidism can cause lifelong complications to the body systems, especially the eyes, CNS, and GI tract. Thyroid storm is a life-threatening condition that requires medical intervention and hospitalization. This can occur if the symptoms go untreated for a long period and become severe.

Assessment

Assessment for hyperthyroidism in pediatric patients includes the following measures.

Clinical Presentation

- Elevated serum levels of T4 and T3 with low or undetectable levels of TSH
- A goiter may be present, along with exophthalmus (bulging of the eyes)
- Other symptoms may include physical restlessness, fatigue, tachycardia, high blood pressure, increased perspiration, increased appetite, weight loss, difficulty sleeping, tremor, heat intolerance, fine hair, systolic murmurs, absence of menses, and mood changes or irritability

SAFE AND EFFECTIVE NURSING CARE: Clinical Pearl

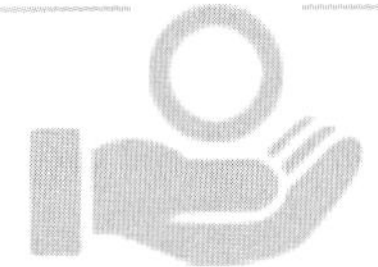

Laboratory Indicators for Hyperthyroidism

When evaluating laboratory results for hyperthyroidism, the nurse will see the following laboratory indicators:

Serum T4 ↑

Serum T3 ↑

Serum TSH ↓ (may be undetectable)

Diagnostic Testing

- Serum T4, T4, TSH, and thyroid antibodies
- Thyroid ultrasound

Nursing Interventions

- Complete physical assessment, especially for children who are referred for symptoms of attention deficit-hyperactivity disorder (LaFranchi, 2016)
- A complete school history of performance and behavioral problems; history of sleep patterns and changes in mood
- Menstruation cycle history in girls
- Outpatient follow-up is recommended every 4 to 6 months until stabilized
- The nurse must understand the administration, dosage, side effects, and nursing interventions of medications administered for hyperthyroidism
- Radioactive iodine therapy may be indicated to decrease the production of thyroid hormone; in this case, the nurse must be familiar with patient education and outcomes related to the therapy
- If surgery is indicated to remove an overactive nodule of the thyroid gland, the nurse must take precautions postoperatively to make sure the patient's respiratory status is stable and the environment is quiet and calm, and assess the operative site for excessive edema or excessive bleeding
- Patients who have a thyroidectomy will require lifelong thyroid hormone replacement therapy to treat hypothyroidism
- Emotional support should be provided to patients with hyperthyroidism and their families

Caregiver Education

- Patient/family education regarding the importance of medication compliance, adverse reactions to medications, and follow-up care is essential.
- For patients who have had a thyroidectomy, teaching the importance of lifelong hormone replacement therapy is crucial.
- Parents should be encouraged to educate teachers and school personnel about the child's physical and emotional instability during the treatment period.
- Emergency care involves teaching the patient/family signs and symptoms of thyroid storm and instructing them to bring the child to the hospital immediately if these symptoms occur.
- Stress the importance of a low-stress, low-pressure environment during and after hospitalization, and until the child's symptoms of hyperthyroidism are decreasing.

SAFE AND EFFECTIVE NURSING CARE: Understanding Medication

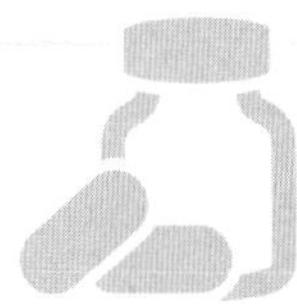

Medications for Hyperthyroidism

The most common medications used to treat hyperthyroidism are antithyroid medications and beta blocking agents. The antithyroid agents help to lower the level of T4 by blocking the synthesis of T4 and T3. Beta blocking agents do not decrease the amount of thyroid hormone, but provide comfort for the patient who is experiencing tachycardia, restlessness, and tremors.

Side Effects of Antithyroid Medications

Mild effects: skin rash, mild leucopenia, loss of taste, arthralgia, and loss of hair or abnormal hair pigmentation

Severe effects that can be fatal: agranulocytosis (as evidenced by sore throat and high fever), symptoms similar to lupus, hepatitis, hepatic failure, and glomerulonephritis

HYPOPARATHYROIDISM

Hypoparathyroidism is rare in children. This condition is caused by inadequate production of PTH. In some cases, PTH is released from the parathyroid gland, but the kidneys or bones do not respond to it. PTH mediates the parathyroid glands to regulate the homeostasis of calcium and phosphate concentrations in the extracellular fluid through regulation of their absorption from the intestines, mobilization from the skeleton, and reabsorption from the kidneys. A delay in the diagnosis of hypoparathyroidism may result in permanent brain dysfunction or death.

Assessment

Pediatric assessment for hypoparathyroidism should include the following measures.

Clinical Presentation

- Vomiting, poor tooth development, headaches, confusion, seizures, and spasms of the face, hands, arms, and feet
- Infants may experience increased irritability, muscle rigidity, abdominal distention, and episodes of apnea or cyanosis

Diagnostic Testing

- Serum calcium levels are low, phosphate levels are high, magnesium levels are low, and PTH levels are low
- Decreased bone mineral density
- Bone or soft tissue abnormalities as confirmed by x-ray or computed tomography (CT) scans
- Evidence of prolonged QT interval confirmed by 12-lead electrocardiogram (EKG)

Nursing Interventions

- A thorough physical assessment and history should be taken to determine whether the patient has experienced muscle spasms, muscle twitching, seizure activity, vomiting, or headaches.
- Thorough knowledge of medications used to treat hypoparathyroidism, such as calcium and vitamin D, is necessary.
- In the beginning phase of diagnosis, the patient may require IV calcium infusions. The nurse must frequently check the IV site for symptoms of infiltration or extravasations. Carefully check and recheck the calcium dose and dilution order, and follow facility IV calcium infusion protocols.
- Once the patient's calcium has normalized, the nurse must evaluate the oral tolerance of vitamin D and calcium for 24 hours to make sure the patient is able to tolerate the medication before discharge.
- Vital signs are assessed frequently.
- Seizure precautions are exercised until calcium levels normalize.
- Cardiac telemetry may be indicated, and the nurse should carefully monitor cardiovascular status.
- Assessment for hyperreflexia of the muscles should be performed frequently while calcium levels are unstable.
- The nurse must provide dietary recommendations to the patient/family.

SAFE AND EFFECTIVE NURSING CARE: Clinical Pearl

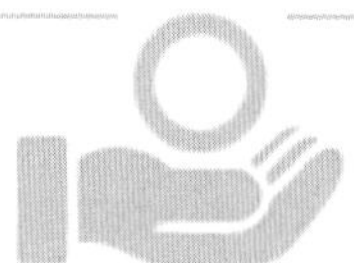

Chvostek Sign

Assessment of hyperreflexia of the muscles can be performed by tapping on the facial nerve. If a spasm occurs in the facial muscles, then a positive Chvostek sign has occurred. This confirms that the child has muscle spasms, pain, cramping, and twitches. This is an important test for infants and small children, because they are unable to communicate pain or muscle spasms.

Caregiver Education

- Encourage dietary compliance, such as avoiding caffeine and limiting the intake of carbonated beverages.
- Encourage foods high in calcium and vitamin K.
- Instruct parents to give calcium and vitamin D with acidic substances such as orange juice or with salads that contain lemon juice in the dressing.
- Provide dietary instruction regarding alternative dietary supplements in addition to calcium and vitamin D, such as magnesium, boron, and vitamin K.
- Encourage follow-up appointment with physician to have calcium levels checked.
- Instruct family and patient regarding the need for lifelong medication therapy.

HYPERPARATHYROIDISM

Hyperparathyroidism is rare in children. This condition is a result of overproduction of PTH from the parathyroid gland. It is most common in females during adolescence. The classic symptoms are severe malaise, constipation, dehydration, headache, and vomiting. Cardiac abnormalities such as heart block and shortening of the ST segment may be present on EKG. Approximately 50% of patients with hyperparathyroidism do not have any symptoms, and approximately 1% of patients are undiagnosed (Ward & Hisley, 2015).

Assessment

Hyperparathyroidism assessment includes the following measures.

Clinical Presentation

- Signs and symptoms may include bone and joint pain, bone loss or evidence of osteoporosis, bone fractures, muscle weakness, abdominal pain, heartburn, nausea, vomiting, constipation, lack of appetite, kidney stones, excessive thirst, excessive urination, depression, anxiety, memory loss, and drowsiness or fatigue.

Diagnostic Testing

- Serum calcium is elevated along with elevated PTH levels.
- X-ray or bone densitometry reveals signs of bone loss.
- Renal calculi may be present in the kidneys.

Nursing Interventions

- Postoperative care of the child with a parathyroidectomy focuses on maintaining the airway and breathing.
- The nurse should assess the surgical site for edema that may lead to altered respiratory status.
- Frequently assess for sign and symptoms of infection and hematoma.
- The nurse should administer IV fluids as ordered and keep track of intake and output.
- Careful monitoring of electrolytes is also important.

Caregiver Education

- Instruct parents to monitor for the signs and symptoms of infection at the operative site.
- Nutrition guidance should include food and liquids high in calcium and vitamin D, because removal of the parathyroid glands can cause the patient to be deficient in both.
- Parents should be taught the signs and symptoms of hypocalcaemia and when to alert their physician.
- Remind parents and patient that calcium and vitamin D supplements are a lifelong therapy.

CUSHING SYNDROME

Cushing syndrome is a metabolic disorder caused by an overproduction of cortisol by the adrenal glands. The most common causes of Cushing syndrome are cortisol-producing tumors, adrenal hyperplasia, and benign adrenal tumors. Children who are prescribed chronic steroids may be at risk for Cushing disease. It can be very difficult to diagnose and may take up to 5 years to manifest. Cushing disease is unusual in infancy and childhood. Clinical manifestations tend to develop slowly. Psychologically, the child may experience mood changes such as depression, anxiety, irritability, and euphoria. Growth delay may also be found on physical examination. Excessive cortisol levels may lead to hyperglycemia, causing diabetes, high blood pressure, or arteriosclerosis.

Assessment

Assessment for Cushing disease includes the following measures.

Clinical Presentation

- Clinical manifestations develop slowly
- Alkalosis related to hypokalemia and hypercalcemia
- Excessive urinary calcium excretion
- Other symptoms include weight gain, pendulous abdomen, fatigue, muscle wasting, weakness of the extremities, round "moon-shaped" face, facial flushing, fat pad located between the shoulder blades known as a buffalo hump, and pink or purple stretch marks on the abdomen, thighs, and arms
- Females may experience irregular or absent menstrual cycles

Diagnostic Testing

- Referral to a pediatric endocrinologist is warranted
- 24-hour urine collection for urinary free cortisol and 17-hydroxycorticosteriod
- Dexamethasone suppression test: a test used to assess the status of the hypothalamic–pituitary–adrenal axis for the differential diagnosis of adrenal overproduction
- Saliva swabs to test cortisol levels
- Serum blood levels of glucose, cortisol, and electrolytes
- Bone scan to rule out osteoporosis
- MRI of the pituitary gland
- CT scan of the adrenal glands

Nursing Interventions

- Nursing care is dependent on the cause of the overproduction of cortisol.
- The nurse must be knowledgeable regarding the pharmaceutical treatments that inhibit the production of cortisol.
- If surgery is not possible, the nurse may have to educate the patient/family regarding the use of radiation therapy.
- Surgical intervention may be necessary to excise or remove a tumor. The nurse must provide preoperative and postoperative education.
- Postoperative nursing care involves maintaining IV fluids, monitoring hydration status, providing pain control, and postoperative assessment and initiation of medications.
- The nurse must monitor serum electrolytes.

Caregiver Education

- Emergency care involves educating the patient regarding lifelong cortisol replacement therapy daily and in emergency situations.
- The patient will need to be taught stress dosing with hydrocortisone injections during times when the child is extremely ill, has a fever, is vomiting, experiences trauma, or is having surgery.
- The parents should be reassured that the child's symptomatic appearance will improve over time with treatment.
- Offer nutritional guidance for healthy food selections that will help the child maintain a healthy weight.
- Instruct the parents on the signs and symptoms of adrenal insufficiency, such as increased irritability, headache, confusion, restlessness, nausea and vomiting, diarrhea, abdominal pain, dehydration, fever, loss of appetite, and lethargy. These symptoms can be life-threatening, and the parents should take the child to the emergency department as soon as symptoms are identified.

CONGENITAL ADRENAL HYPERPLASIA

Congenital adrenal hyperplasia (CAH) is the inability to produce cortisol in the adrenal glands, caused by excessive amounts of CRH and adrenocorticotropic hormone production (ACTH). Because of the surplus of CRH and ACTH, the adrenal gland begins to develop hyperplasia, leading to excessive androgen hormone production from the adrenal glands. Defective conversion of 17-hydroxyprogesterone (17-OHP) to 11-deoxycorticol accounts for more than 95% of the cases of CAH. The defective conversion is caused by mutations in the CYP21A2 gene, hence making 21-hydroxylase deficiency one of the more common inherited disorders (Merke, 2015). CAH can present in two clinical syndromes: (1) salt losing or (2) non–salt losing.

Assessment

Assessment for CAH includes the following measures.

Clinical Presentation

- Males typically do not experience manifestations until later in childhood. These symptoms include early development of pubic hair, enlargement of the penis, or both; advancement in growth velocity; and advanced bone age compared with the child's chronological age.
- In females, CAH manifests at birth with abnormal development of the genitalia called ambiguous genitalia. The clitoris may be enlarged and labial folds may be fused. These manifestations give the appearance that the female may be male; however, the internal sex organs will be normal.
- Virilization (development of secondary sexual characteristics) occurs in females.

Diagnostic Testing

- Genetic paternal screening is available; however, the screening may show "false positive" results. In this case, the health-care provider will need to evaluate for symptoms at birth.
- Serum 17-OHP will be elevated. If the levels continue to be elevated after birth, CAH is expected, because normal growth and development will decrease 17-OHP as the infant matures.
- Chromosomal analysis will be performed to determine the infant's gender in the case of ambiguous genitalia.
- In some cases, surgery of the genitalia is performed to meet the needs of the determined sex of the child.

Nursing Interventions

- Early diagnosis is the key to successful treatment. The nurse must be able to carefully assess for prenatal and postnatal risk factors.
- Referral to a genetics clinic may be indicated.
- Dehydration is a complication of CAH, and the nurse must assess for signs and symptoms of dehydration, electrolyte imbalance, and hypovolemic shock when the child is salt wasting.
- Careful monitoring of cardiopulmonary status is necessary.
- Frequently assess vital signs.
- Assess the parents' emotional status related to the ambiguity of the infant's genitalia. Understanding cultural and spiritual beliefs when counseling parents is important.
- Provide detailed education regarding the cause of the diagnosis, symptoms, and available treatment options.
- If the infant's gender is questionable at birth, refer to the infant as "your baby" and not "your son" or "your daughter."

Caregiver Education

- Emergency care involves teaching the parents and family how to administer medications.
- Teaching the family the signs and symptoms of adrenal crisis and the performance of stress dosing is crucial.
- Instruct the parents regarding the signs and symptoms of dehydration.
- Encourage the parents to seek emotional support from CAH support groups in their area or through a national organization.

CRITICAL COMPONENT

Administering Corticosteroids and Mineralocorticoids

Emergency care involves education regarding the administration of lifelong medications such as corticosteroids and mineralocorticoids. Emergency administration of corticosteroids given via injection should be taught to the parents for use when the child is in a crisis, such as febrile illness, surgery, trauma, or severe stress. The doses will need to be doubled or tripled during the period of crisis. This is referred to as "stress dosing." The most common medications administered are hydrocortisone and fludrocortisone (Florinef) (Alt et al., 2013).

- Educate the parents regarding future pregnancies and the importance of prenatal screening for CAH, and refer them to a genetics clinic.
- Allow parents and family members to discuss their concerns, feelings, and beliefs regarding their infant's condition. Refer them to the appropriate center for psychological support; involve the social work team and offer spiritual support such as the clergy or designated chaplain for their faith.
- If surgery is indicated, provide education regarding preoperative and postoperative care, and let the parents know that there may be more than one surgery to correct the genitalia.

ADRENAL INSUFFICIENCY (ADDISON'S DISEASE)

Insufficient cortisol and aldosterone production from adrenal glands leads to adrenal insufficiency. Usually the cause is unknown. Thirty percent of cases occur from a direct attack on the adrenal gland (e.g., cancer, infections, autoimmune diseases, or chronic steroid use). Children with CAH may experience hypoglycemia, especially during stressful times such as surgery or febrile illness. The symptoms may be mild unless the child gets sick. Symptoms are very individualized.

Assessment

Assessment for Addison's disease should include the following measures.

Clinical Presentation

- Manifestations include but are not limited to weakness, fatigue, dizziness, and rapid pulse; dark skin that appears as if the child is very tanned; black freckles; bluish-black discoloration around the nipples, scrotum, and vagina; and weight loss, dehydration, loss of appetite, intense salt cravings, nausea and vomiting, and cold intolerance.

Diagnostic Testing

- Low serum sodium, high potassium, and low blood sugar
- Diagnosed by assessing manifestations

CRITICAL COMPONENT

Adrenal Insufficiency, Congenital Adrenal Hyperplasia, and Hormone Replacement

It is important to remember that children with adrenal insufficiency and/or CAH require lifelong hormone replacement. Children with adrenal insufficiency tend to grow poorly in height and weight, but puberty will present at a normal age despite the growth delay. These children may require GH replacement therapy along with corticosteroid and mineralocorticoid replacement therapy.

- Low blood pressure
- Serum cortisol level drawn around 8 a.m. because the levels are the highest upon arising in the morning
- Cortisol levels less than 3 mg/dL indicate Addison's disease; levels between 3 and 19 mg/dL are considered suspicious, and further testing is needed to confirm diagnosis

SAFE AND EFFECTIVE NURSING CARE: Promoting Safety

Addisonian Crisis

Addisonian crisis is a life-threatening event that requires the child to receive immediate medical attention. If ignored, the child may die. The symptoms of an Addisonian crisis are sudden, penetrating pain in the lower back or legs, severe vomiting and diarrhea, dehydration, low blood pressure, and loss of consciousness (Smans, Van der Valk, Hermus, & Zelissen, 2016). This type of crisis is very overwhelming for parents, and a detailed plan of care and patient education can help the parents be ready for an emergency if it occurs.

Nursing Interventions

- Frequent laboratory assessment
- Administration of corticosteroids such as Solu-Cortef; this medication is given two to three times per day (Merke, 2015)
- Administer IM Solu-Cortef if the child is vomiting, nauseated, or has diarrhea and is unable to tolerate oral intake (Table 17–2)
- Assessment of hydration status
- Strict intake and output to avoid dehydration
- Teach the parents how to administer IM Solu-Cortef for home emergencies
- Careful assessment for signs and symptoms of hypovolemic shock in the severely dehydrated patient (Riepe & Sippell, 2007)
- Make sure that the child has been referred to a pediatric endocrinologist to diagnose and treat this condition

Caregiver Education

- Emergency care involves teaching parents the signs and symptoms of adrenal crisis and how to administer IM Solu-Cortef if the child develops crises outside of the hospital (Riepe & Sippell, 2007).
- Chronic home care involves teaching the parents the importance of medication compliance and avoidance of skipping doses, because this can lead to adrenal crisis.
- The child should wear a medical alert bracelet at all times.
- Teach the parents how to "stress dose" in times when the child has fever, vomiting, diarrhea, emotional stress, trauma, or surgery.
- Teach the parents to make sure the child is well-hydrated before being involved in a physical activity or sports.
- Educate school teachers and staff regarding the potential for dehydration and hypovolemic shock so that measures can be taken to provide the child with extra fluids before and during physical activity.
- Encourage the child and parents to increase salt intake during the warmer months of the year to maintain adequate mineralocorticoid levels.

PHEOCHROMOCYTOMA

Pheochromocytoma rarely occurs in children; when it does occur, it is usually caused by a childhood tumor that can originate in any chromaffin tissue in the body. The most common location is in the right adrenal gland. The peak incidence is between 9 and 12 years of age. When the tumor occurs, excessive amounts of catecholamines are produced. Hypertension can be present with a systolic blood pressure as high as 250 mm Hg. Pheochromocytoma may mimic the symptoms of hyperthyroidism and diabetes mellitus.

Assessment

Assessment for pheochromocytoma includes the following measures.

Clinical Presentation

- Typical symptoms include increased heart rate (tachycardia), headache, palpitations, dizziness, poor weight gain, nausea and vomiting, and growth failure.
- Other symptoms may include abdominal pain, profuse sweating, cool extremities, polydipsia, and polyuria.

Diagnostic Testing

- 24-hour urine to assess the presence of catecholamines
- MRI or CT scan to determine the location of the tumor

Nursing Interventions

- Removal of the tumor is usually indicated.
- Preoperative administration of medications to inhibit the release of catecholamines may begin 1 to 3 weeks before surgery.
- If surgery is not an option, administration of medications such as alpha-adrenergic blocking agents is used to provide

TABLE 17–2 Medications Used to Treat Adrenal Disorders

	FLUDROCORTISON ACETATE (FLORINEF)	HYDROCORTISONE (SOLU-CORTEF, HYDROCORTONE, CORTEF)
How supplied	0.1-mg tablets	Tablets—5, 10, 20 mg Injection—100, 250, 500, 1,000 mg/vial Acetate (Hydrocortone)—25, 20 mg/mL
Dose/route	*Addison's disease:* 2.1 mg/daily (dose may vary from 0.1 mg three times/week to 0.2 mg/daily) *Salt-losing congenital adrenal hyperplasia:* 0.1–0.2 mg/daily PO	*Physiological dosing:* *PO:* 0.5–0.75 mg/kg/day or 20–25 mg/m²/day divided every 8 hours *IM:* 0.25–0.35 mg/kg/dose or 12–15 mg/m²/day every day *Stress dosing:* Two to three times the normal physiological dose, depending on the severity of the illness or stress
Potential side effects	Hypertension, edema, cardiac enlargement, congestive heart failure, potassium loss, hypokalemia alkalosis	Hypertension, euphoria, insomnia, acne, hyperglycemia, growth suppression, immunosuppression, and adrenal suppression

From Vallerand, A. H., Sanoski, C. A. & Deglin, J.H. (2017). Davis's drug guide for nurses *(15th ed.). Philadelphia: F.A. Davis.*

medical management. This medication may be combined with beta-adrenergic blocking agents to maximize the efficacy of treatment.

- Careful assessment of vital signs, especially blood pressure, is crucial.
- Blood glucose levels should be taken and assessed daily preoperatively and postoperatively, because blood sugar levels may be higher than normal.
- Postoperatively, the patient should be placed in a minimally stimulating environment.

CRITICAL COMPONENT

Avoid Palpating the Adrenal Glands

During the physical assessment of the patient, the nurse should avoid palpating the area of the adrenal glands where the tumor is located because it can cause an elevated release of catecholamines, which will increase metabolism and produce a potential hypertensive crisis or tachydysrhythmias.

Caregiver Education

- Preoperative education begins with providing information regarding the cause, symptoms, and treatment options for the condition.
- If surgery is not an option, the nurse must provide thorough education regarding medications used for the treatment of the condition.
- Parents should provide a low-stress environment for the child during the preoperative and postoperative periods.

TYPE 1 DIABETES MELLITUS (INSULIN-DEPENDENT DIABETES)

Type 1 diabetes mellitus (T1DM) is caused by destruction of the beta cells in the pancreas. The pancreas is the organ that produces insulin that regulates blood sugar levels in the body. When the beta cells are destroyed, the pancreas can no longer produce insulin, so glucose levels in the bloodstream are too high. Children with T1DM must have exogenous insulin to survive. The clinical syndrome of diabetes mellitus results from a variety of causes, including genetic influence, autoimmune mechanisms that negatively affect the pancreatic islet cells, and viral illnesses that attach and destroy pancreatic function (Hockenberry, Wilson, & Rodgers, 2016).

Assessment

Assessments for T1DM include the following.

Clinical Presentation

- Polyuria, polydipsia, and polyphagia
- Unintentional weight loss over several days or weeks
- High-glucose levels in the blood and urine
- Nausea and vomiting, excessive fatigue, abdominal pain, increased susceptibility to infections, dehydration, blurred vision, irritability, and restlessness (Hockenberry et al., 2016)

Diagnostic Testing

- Elevated blood glucose levels greater than 200 mg/dL
- Elevated hemoglobin A1C levels greater than 7.0
- Decreased serum insulin levels

- Presence of serum and urine ketones
- Of affected individuals, 85% to 90% may have one or more of the following positive autoantibodies:
  - ICA
  - IAA
  - GAD_{65}
  - IA-2β (Halvorson, Yasuda, Carpenter, & Kaiserman, 2005)

Nursing Interventions

Nursing interventions should focus on the following major areas:

- Physical assessment
- Administration of insulin (Table 17–3)
  - Always double-check insulin orders to make sure orders are clear and concise. When drawing up insulin, another registered nurse (RN) must verify that the correct dosage is drawn up in the syringe.
  - Make sure that the correct strength of insulin has been ordered because multiple strengths and types are available.
  - Only use insulin syringes to draw up insulin doses.
  - When using insulin pen devices, replace the pen needle with each dose and store the insulin pen in the refrigerator. Some insulin may be stored at room temperature for up to 28 days after opening. Always check the manufacturer's recommendations in the prescribing information that comes with the insulin vial or pen cartridge.
  - Only regular insulin may be used IV during the management of diabetic ketoacidosis (DKA).
  - Verify dose with a second RN and document the dose of insulin administration in the chart.
  - Rotate insulin injection sites with each dose (abdomen, arms, legs, buttocks).
  - Assess for injection-site reactions.
  - Monitor body weight daily, because weight loss or gain will indicate a possible increase or decrease in insulin dose.
  - If a sliding-scale insulin regimen is ordered, the nurse must be diligent with obtaining blood glucose levels before meals and at bedtime to adjust insulin dose. Sliding scales are individualized per patient.
- Diet and nutrition education
  - Once the diagnosis of T1DM has been made, the nurse needs to take a thorough dietary history of the patient's eating habits. The patient and parents should have a dietary consult so that the patient can be placed on a diabetic diet or be taught to count carbohydrate exchanges and adjust insulin requirements based on dietary intake.
- Education regarding physical exercise
  - Assessment of the child's exercise ability and regimen should be considered to determine the possibility for hypoglycemia during exercise and the need for pre-exercise snacks.
  - The child must eat an extra complex carbohydrate and protein serving at least 30 minutes to 1 hour before engaging in exercise or sports.
- Education regarding differences between hypoglycemia and hyperglycemia (Table 17–4)
- Stress management or "sick day rules" should be established and taught to the patient, parents, family members, and teachers to have basic guidelines for how to manage diabetes in times of stress such as sickness, emotional stress, minor accidents, surgery, or dehydration
- Blood glucose and urine ketone monitoring
  - Monitor blood glucose every 4 to 6 hours or as ordered by physician.
  - Test urine for the presence of ketones using urine ketosticks.
  - On follow-up clinic visits to the endocrinologist, it is important to evaluate the patient's blood sugar log for daily blood sugar trends, doses of insulin, the presence of ketones in the urine, and the presence of hypoglycemia.
  - Many blood glucose monitors now have the capability to download blood sugar data into software at the endocrinologist's office so that trends in data can be evaluated and the health-care provider can use the data to adjust insulin or other medications.
- Assessment of laboratory values
  - Assess laboratory values such as phosphorus, magnesium, and potassium, because insulin may decrease serum levels.
  - Frequently monitor hemoglobin A1C levels to assess average blood glucose levels over a 90-day period. This will also help to identify whether the insulin regimen is appropriate or requires adjustment.
- Psychosocial support
  - Provide psychosocial support to patient, parents, and family, taking into consideration the age-appropriate developmental needs of the patient.
  - Refer the patients to diabetes support organizations:
    - American Diabetes Association (ADA): http://www.diabetes.org
    - Juvenile Diabetes Foundation: http://www.jdrf.org
  - Encourage participation in diabetes education classes and diabetes support groups provided by the institution.
  - Make referral to social services or psychosocial counselor if indicated.

Caregiver Education

- Patient and family education regarding the administration of insulin (Fig. 17–3; Box 17–1)

SAFE AND EFFECTIVE NURSING CARE: Clinical Pearl

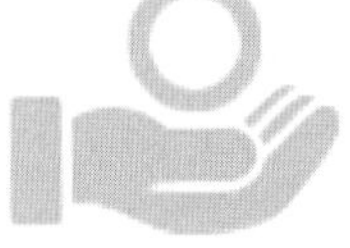

Important Things to Teach Regarding Sick Day Rules

M—Monitor blood sugar levels more frequently.

D—Do not stop taking insulin.

C—Check urine for ketones.

B—Be careful with over-the-counter medicines.

H—Have a game plan and don't hesitate to ask for help.

F—Force fluids.

TABLE 17–3 Types of Insulin Used to Treat Diabetes Mellitus

INSULIN TYPE	ONSET	PEAK	DURATION	AVAILABILITY	DOSE	ROUTE	CONSIDERATIONS
Short-Acting Insulin							
Humulin R, Humulin R U-500, Novolin R	30–60 minutes	2–4 hours	5–7 hours	100 units/mL in 10-mL vials, 3-mL disposable delivery devices, 500 units/mL in 20-mL vials	SQ doses individualized per patient IV; doses start at 0.5–1.0 unit/kg/day	SQ	May be given IV to treat diabetic ketoacidosis (DKA)
Intermediate-Acting Insulin							
NPH Insulin, Humulin N, Novolin NPH, Novolin N	1–2 hours	4–12 hours	18–24 hours	100 units/mL in 10-mL vials, 3-mL disposable delivery devices	0.1 unit/kg/day	SQ	Only given SQ
Long-Acting Insulin							
Insulin detemir (Levemir) **Insulin glargine** (Lantus)	**Insulin detemir:** 3–4 hours **Insulin glargine:** 3–4 hours	**Insulin detemir:** 3–14 hours **Insulin glargine:** No peak	**Insulin detemir:** 24 hours **Insulin glargine:** 24 hours	**Detemir:** 100 units/mL in 10-mL vials, 3-mL cartridges, or prefilled syringes **Glargine:** 100 units/mL in 10-mL vials, 3-mL cartridges, or prefilled disposable pens	**Detemir:** 0.1–0.2 units/kg once daily in the a.m. or 10 units once or twice daily **Glargine:** 50%–75% of daily insulin requirements once daily	SQ	Only administered SQ Only indicated for children >6 years old Glargine cannot be given in the same site as other insulin
Insulin Mixtures							
Insulin lispro protamine suspension/insulin lispro solution mixtures, rDNA origin (Humalog 75/25, Humalog Mix 50/50)	15–30 minutes	2.8 hours	24 hours	100 units/mL in 10-mL vials, 3-mL disposable delivery devices	0.5–1.0 unit/kg/day	SQ	Only administered SQ
Insulin aspart protamine suspension/insulin aspart	15 minutes	1–4 hours	18–24 hours	100 units/mL in 10-mL vials, 3-mL disposable delivery devices	0.5–1.0 unit/kg/day	SQ	Only administered SQ

TABLE 17-3 Types of Insulin Used to Treat Diabetes Mellitus—cont'd

INSULIN TYPE	ONSET	PEAK	DURATION	AVAILABILITY	DOSE	ROUTE	CONSIDERATIONS
				Insulin Mixtures			
solution mixtures, rDNA origin (NovoLog Mix 70/30)							
NPH/ regular insulin mixtures (Humulin 50/50, Humulin 70/30, Novolin 70/30)	30 minutes	4–8 hours	24 hours	100 units/mL in 10-mL vials, 3-mL disposable delivery devices	0.5–1.0 unit/kg/day	SQ	Only administered SQ

SQ, subcutaneously.
From Vallerand, A. H., Sanoski, C. A. Deglin, J.H (2017). Davis's drug guide for nurses *(15th ed.). Philadelphia: F.A. Davis.*

TABLE 17-4 Clinical Comparison of Hypoglycemia and Hyperglycemia

CLINICAL CONDITION	MANIFESTATIONS	CRITICAL NURSING ACTIONS
	Hypoglycemia	
Too much insulin for amount of food eaten	Rapid onset Irritable Nervous	• Give 15 grams of carbohydrates
Injected insulin into muscle	Shaky feeling, tremors	• Recheck blood glucose in 15 minutes
Too much activity for insulin dose	Difficult to concentrate Difficult to speak	• If blood glucose is <70 mg/dL, give another 15 grams of carbohydrates
Too much time between meals	Behavior change Confused Repeats over and over	• Recheck again in another 15 minutes
Too few carbohydrates eaten	Unconscious Seizure	• If unconscious, give IM glucagon
Illness or stress	Tachycardia Shallow breathing Pale, sweaty Hungry Headache Dizzy Vision blurry or double	

Continued

TABLE 17–4 Clinical Comparison of Hypoglycemia and Hyperglycemia—cont'd

CLINICAL CONDITION	MANIFESTATIONS	CRITICAL NURSING ACTIONS
	Hypoglycemia	
	Photophobic Numbness or mouth or lips	
	Hyperglycemia	
Too little insulin for the food eaten	Gradual onset Lethargic Sleepy	• Give additional insulin at usual injection time
Illness or stress	Slow response Confused	• Use sliding-scale doses for specific level of blood glucose
Too many carbohydrates eaten	Breathes deeply and rapidly Skin flushed and dry	• Increase fluids
Meals too close together	Mucous membranes dry	• If ketones are elevated, give an extra insulin injection
Too many snacks	Thirsty Hungry Dehydrated	
Insulin given just under the skin	Weak Tired Headache	
Too little activity	Abdomen hurts Nausea and vomiting Vision blurry Shock	

Source: Ward, S. L., & Hisley, S. M. (2015). Maternal-child nursing care: Optimizing outcomes for mothers, children, & families *(2nd ed.). Philadelphia: F.A. Davis.*

BOX 17–1 | Teaching Parents How to Inject Insulin

Purpose

To teach parents how to inject insulin

Equipment

Insulin bottle from refrigerator (remove up to 1 hour before injection to allow it to warm to room temperature)

Appropriate syringe (U-30, U-50, or U-100)

Alcohol wipes

Container for the dirty, used syringe

Steps

1. Check the expiration date on the insulin bottle.
   RATIONALE: *Ensures that the insulin has not expired.*
2. Wash hands.
   RATIONALE: *Prevents the spread of bacteria.*
3. Clean rubber stopper on insulin bottle with alcohol wipe.
   RATIONALE: *Promotes asepsis.*
4. Remove syringe cap and pull air into the syringe; line up the end of the black plunger to the exact amount the insulin dose will be.
   RATIONALE: *Ensures accurate dosage of insulin to be drawn up.*
5. Put the syringe needle through the bottle rubber top and push syringe plunger so that all the air goes from the syringe into the bottle.
6. Turn the insulin bottle upside down and pull the syringe plunger so that the insulin enters the syringe until the top of the black plunger exactly lines up with the dose of insulin to be given.
7. Remove every air bubble, always checking that the dose is exact.
   RATIONALE: *Exact dosing is essential in managing the child's condition.*

BOX 17–1 | Teaching Parents How to Inject Insulin—cont'd

8. Choose (or let the child choose) the site of the injection.
RATIONALE: *Allowing the child to participate may help the child feel more in control of the condition.*
9. Clean the injection site with an alcohol swab.
RATIONALE: *Alcohol will decrease the presence of microorganisms.*
10. Pinch up the skin slightly and gently, with the syringe at a 90-degree angle (perpendicular) to the skin; with a dart-like motion, insert the needle into the skin; release the skin.
RATIONALE: *Ensures proper medication administration.*
11. Slowly inject the dose of insulin.
12. Discard the used syringe in a hard, rigid container with a tight-fitting lid.

Clinical Alert

The nurse teaches the parents to evaluate the child for the signs and symptoms of either hypoglycemia or hyperglycemia. In understandable terms, explain these signs and symptoms to the parents so they can watch for them at home.

HYPOGLYCEMIA (LOW BLOOD SUGAR)	HYPERGLYCEMIA (HIGH BLOOD SUGAR)
Cold, pale skin (cold sweat)	Increased thirst, even if consuming a large amount of liquids
Shakiness/hand tremors	Loss of appetite, nausea/vomiting
Sudden hunger (crave salt/sweet)	Weakness, stomach pains/aches
Emotional outbursts (personality changes)	Heavy, labored breathing
Drowsiness/extremely tired	Fatigue, tired, often sleepy
Pounding heartbeat/palpitations	Large amounts of sugar in urine
Nervousness/dizziness	Ketones in urine
Anxiety/irritability	Frequent urination
Headache, mental confusion, difficulty concentrating	Blurred/double vision
Numbness or tingling of lips/mouth	
Poor coordination/staggering unable to walk	
Slurred or slow speech	
Dilated, enlarged pupils	
Fainting (needs emergency treatment *NOW*)	

Teach Parents

If the child expresses that the injection is painful, the following measures can be taken to decrease the pain:

- Inject room-temperature insulin.
- Clear even the tiniest air bubbles from the syringe.
- Let the alcohol dry completely before injection.
- Tell the child to relax the muscles in the area of injection (the tenser the muscles during injection, the more painful the procedure).
- Use syringe-like dart to pierce the skin quickly.
- Do not change the needle direction during insertion or withdrawal.
- Never reuse syringes.
- Rotate sites with *each* injection (giving the insulin in the *same* place twice in one day can cause unnecessary discomfort for the child and undue stress on the tissue).

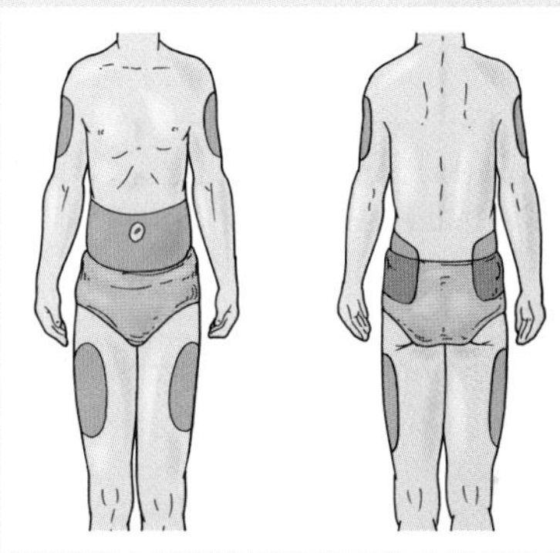

- Document exactly where each injection was given to avoid using the same place more than once a day.
- Create and keep a Diabetes Management Notebook with the plan and a place to record daily blood sugar values as well as doses of insulin administered, including injection site. *For example:*

DATE	BLOOD GLUCOSE A.M.	BLOOD GLUCOSE P.M.	INSULIN DOSE GIVEN AND TIME	INJECTION SITE	GIVEN BY
8/9/07	124		4 units regular at 0700	Right mid-arm	Mom
8/9/07		144	4 units regular 4 units NPH 1230	Left mid-thigh	Dad

Documentation

Mother gave 4 units of Regular at 0700 in right mid-arm

—noted by R. Such, RN

Father gave 4 units of Regular and 4 units NPH at 1230 in left mid-thigh

—noted by R. Such, RN

Source: Adapted from Ward, S. L., & Hisley, S. M. (2015). *Maternal-child nursing care: Optimizing outcomes for mothers, children, & families* (2nd ed.). Philadelphia: F.A. Davis.

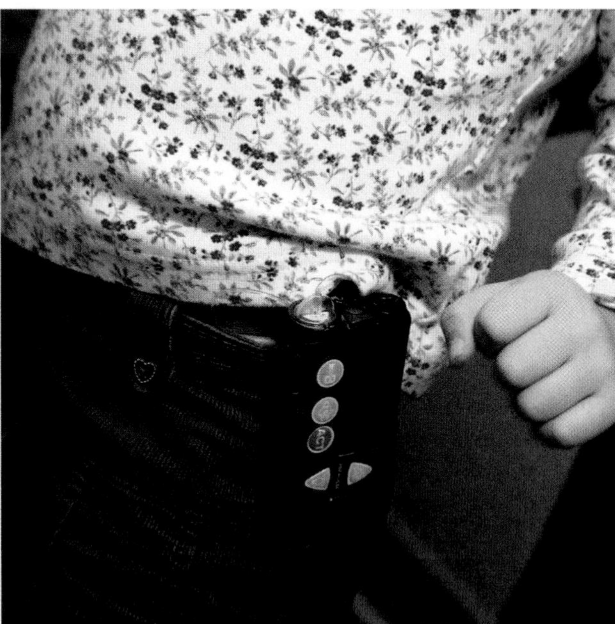

FIGURE 17–3 Wearing an insulin pump allows children to control the release of insulin throughout the day, more closely resembling the body's natural response.

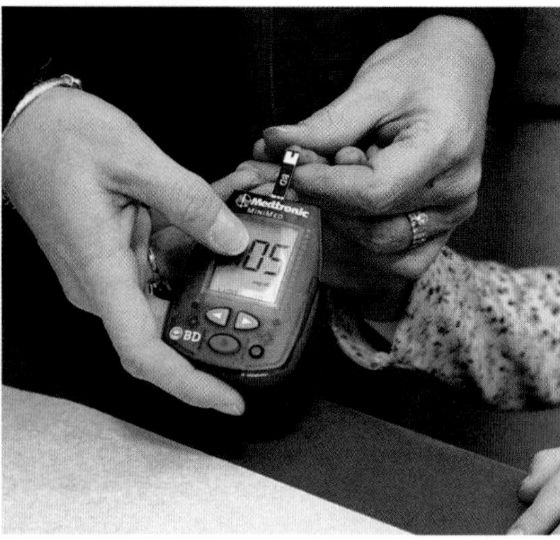

FIGURE 17–4 Home monitoring requires parents to perform glucose checks on the child with diabetes.

- Patient and family education regarding stress management or "sick day rules" (Hockenberry et al., 2016)
- Patient and family education regarding blood glucose monitoring (Fig. 17–4)
  - Patient and family should demonstrate proficiency with glucometer.
  - Discuss importance of monitoring blood sugar three to four times daily and keeping a blood sugar log with readings.
- Patient and family education regarding assessment of urine for urine ketones, especially when sick or under stress
- Patient and family education regarding how to manage hypoglycemia
- Preparing the patient and family for school guidance
- Preparing teachers and school administrators regarding insulin regimen of the child, sick day rules, monitoring of blood glucose levels, signs and symptoms of hypoglycemia, and the administration of glucagon
  - Emergency doses of glucagon and Gluco-Gel should be kept at home and at school if severe hypoglycemia occurs.
- Management of DKA
  - Administer IV fluids and IV insulin as ordered.
  - Correct acidosis and restore acid-base balance.
  - Correct electrolyte imbalance by administering IV fluids with electrolytes.
  - Monitor laboratory values.
  - Frequently check blood sugar and vital signs.
  - Frequently assess for signs of further complications.
  - Assess respiratory status for signs of complications, such as Kussmaul breathing. This type of breathing is very deep and laborious, and means that the patient is trying to correct the metabolic acidosis and "blow off" excess carbon dioxide (CO_2).
  - Frequently assess IV site, because multiple infusions of fluids, electrolytes, and insulin will increase chances of infiltration. The nurse must use an IV Y-Port to allow for multiple infusions at the same time. The nurse must also check drug compatibility before infusing multiple infusions through the same IV tubing.
  - Patients in DKA may have a "fruity" or "sweet" odor to their breath, which smells similar to Juicy Fruit gum.

CRITICAL COMPONENT

Diabetic Ketoacidosis

In 2014, the International Society for Pediatric and Adolescent Diabetes (Wolfsdorf et al., 2014) defined DKA according to the following parameters:

- Hyperglycemia—blood glucose of more than 200 mg/dL (11 mm/L)
- Metabolic acidosis—venous pH less than 7.3 or a plasma bicarbonate less than 15 mEq/L (15 mmol/L) *and*
- Ketosis—determined by the presence of ketones in the blood or urine

There are three levels of acidosis to consider:

0—mild DKA: venous blood pH is 7.2 to 7.3

1—moderate DKA: venous blood pH is 7.10 to 7.19

2—severe DKA: venous blood pH is less than 7.0

DKA is a complex, emergent condition that combines hyperglycemia, acidosis, and ketosis, resulting in severely deficient insulin levels that alter metabolism of carbohydrates, protein, and fat. Some of the precipitating factors that the nurse must assess are:

- Poor compliance with insulin regimens
- Patients entering puberty and beginning of the menstrual cycle
- Caregiver lack of competence regarding insulin management
- Insulin pump failure
- Insulin that is out of date
- Underlying illness, surgery, or trauma

CRITICAL COMPONENT

Family Teaching Guidelines: Dealing With a Hypoglycemic Crisis

How to: Recognize the signs of hypoglycemia—child is pale, sweaty, dizzy, "shaky" (tremors), confused, irritable, numb on lips or mouth, and can have an altered mental status.

Essential Information:

- Check blood glucose level.
- If blood glucose is below 70 mg/dL, rapidly give one of the following sources of carbohydrates (about 10–15 grams each), in the right amount to treat hypoglycemia:
  - ½ to ¾ cup of orange or grape juice (a juice box is good when one is away from home)
  - 2 glucose tablets or 2 doses of glucose gel
  - 2–4 pieces of hard candy
  - Gumdrops
  - 1–2 tablespoons of honey
  - 1 small box of raisins
  - 6 oz regular (not diet) soda (about half a can)
  - 2 tablespoons of cake icing
- Recheck blood glucose in 15 minutes. If reading is still below 70 mg/dL, then:
  - Give another glass of juice, etc.
  - Recheck blood glucose again after another 15 minutes.
- When blood glucose returns to at least 80 mg/dL, a more substantial snack (non-concentrated sugar) may be given (i.e., cheese and crackers, bread and peanut butter, etc.) if the next meal is more than 30 minutes away or if a physical activity/exercise is planned.
- If the child is unconscious, glucagon should be given either subcutaneously or intramuscularly (ADA, 2017a,b).

Safety Note:

If the child is conscious, a 4-oz glass of orange juice will help increase blood sugar levels. When a child is severely hypoglycemic and unable to take glucose tablets by mouth due to confusion or loss of consciousness, a dose of glucagon must be given IM or IV. In most cases the drug is administered IM in the home or school setting to reverse the effects of severe hypoglycemia. The recommended dose to administer for children <20 kg is 0.5 mg and for children >20 kg is 1.0 mg. Doses may be repeated in 15 minutes if needed.

Source: Ward, S. L., & Hisley, S. M. (2015). Maternal-child nursing care: Optimizing outcomes for mothers, children, & families *(2nd ed.). Philadelphia: F.A. Davis.*

TYPE 2 DIABETES MELLITUS

Type 2 diabetes mellitus (T2DM) occurs when the body becomes resistant to insulin production from the pancreas. T2DM is also termed "adult-onset" diabetes; however, pediatric obesity has led to a sharp increase in type 2 diabetes among children and adolescents. Risk factors for the development of T2DM are obesity, sedentary lifestyle, family history of diabetes, and poor dietary intake (especially high-carbohydrate, simple-sugar foods). Children with T2DM usually have no symptoms, and the condition is diagnosed with routine well-check visits. Any child with a BMI more than the 85th percentile for weight and age should be monitored for early signs of T2DM, because obesity is a key predisposing factor, followed by hypertension and high cholesterol levels.

Assessment

The following measures are used to assess for T2DM among pediatric patients.

Clinical Presentation

- The initial symptom will be an elevated blood glucose level or complications such as DKA.
- Acanthosis nigricans (dark pigmented areas of the skin on the back of the neck, axilla, and arms) is evidence of insulin resistance.
- Other symptoms that might occur are gradual and may consist of a burning sensation of the feet, ankles, and legs; poor wound healing; changes in vision; and fatigue.

Diagnostic Testing

- Elevated fasting blood glucose levels greater than 125 mg/dL
- Random blood glucose levels greater than 200 mg/dL
- Elevated hemoglobin A1C level greater than 7 percent
- Oral glucose tolerance testing

Nursing Interventions

- Early assessment for risks, detection, and diagnosis is crucial.
- Obtain dietary history and refer to dietitian for dietary counseling.
- Encourage exercise and refer the parents to a physical therapist if indicated.
- Administer oral anti-hyperglycemic medications as ordered to help decrease high blood glucose levels.
- Assess for symptoms of psychosocial problems, such as altered body image, depression, and ineffective individual coping, and refer to a psychologist if needed.

CRITICAL COMPONENT

Risk Factors for Type 2 Diabetes Mellitus

Obesity in children and adolescents has led to an increased incidence of insulin resistance and T2DM. As a result of the increased incidence of T2DM, established guidelines have identified certain risk factors that may appear while obtaining the history and physical information. These risk factors include but are not limited to:

- BMI greater than 85th percentile for age and weight
- Family history of T2DM
- Certain race/ethnicity groups: African American, Latino, Asian American, American Indians, and Pacific Islanders
- Signs of insulin resistance as evidenced by acanthosis nigricans
- Maternal history of gestational diabetes or diabetes

Diagnosis is confirmed when the child has a fasting glucose greater than 126 mg/dL or two random blood glucose readings greater than 200 mg/dL. The child's hemoglobin A1C level must also be ≥6.5% on two laboratory confirmed tests (Laffel & Svoren, 2017; Ward & Hisley, 2015).

Caregiver Education

- Explain to the family that treatment options include dietary compliance and exercise to help lose weight and lower glucose levels.
- Involve the entire family in the dietary and exercise education, because many patients have obese parents and siblings with prediabetes or T2DM. The concept of working as a team is very important because the child will not be compliant with treatment unless the family is involved and supportive of the child.
- Educate the child and family regarding the long-term effects of T2DM, such as permanent vision loss, cardiovascular disease, hypertension, high cholesterol, and orthopedic problems.
- Teach the parents how to limit sedentary playtime such as playing video games and watching TV, and encourage team sports and daily exercise.
- If oral anti-hyperglycemics are ordered, the nurse must teach the parents and patient regarding reasons for the medication, dose, route, and frequency. Potential side effects should also be discussed.
- The patient should be taught the signs and symptoms of hypoglycemia, hyperglycemia, and DKA.

Case Study

Mallory S. is a 15-year-old who has been diagnosed with hyperthyroidism since age 13 years. Mallory's hyperthyroidism has been well controlled with antithyroid medications. However, she has been missing doses of her medication due to being "too busy and forgetting" to take her medication as prescribed. Over the last 2 weeks, she has had an increased appetite, increased perspiration, and extreme fatigue, and has become very irritable and restless. She tells her mother that she is having trouble concentrating in school. She begins to have severe diarrhea and tells her mother that she feels like her heart "is racing." Mallory's mother takes her to the emergency department, where she is diagnosed with thyroid storm and hospitalized. During the hospitalization, she is placed on a beta-blocking agent.

1. As the nurse taking care of Mallory, what do you think has caused the thyroid storm to develop?
2. What nursing interventions would be appropriate in caring for Mallory?
3. What patient educational topics are warranted for Mallory and her parents?

REFERENCES

Alt, P., Babler, E. K., Betts, K. J., Carney, P. H., Courtney, J. A., Flores, B. M., … Worley, D. D. (2013). *Clinical handbook of pediatric endocrinology* (2nd ed.). St. Louis, MO: Quality Medical Publishing.

American Diabetes Association (ADA). (2017a). Glucagon training for standards for school personnel: Providing emergency medical assistance to pupils with diabetes. Retrieved from http://web.diabetes.org/Advocacy/school/glucagon.pdf

American Diabetes Association (ADA). (2017b). *Hypoglycemia (low blood glucose).* Retrieved from http://www.diabetes.org/living-with-diabetes/treatment-and-care/blood-glucose-control/hypoglycemia-low-blood.html?loc=lwd-slabnav

Ball, K., Bindler, K. J., & Cowen, R. C. (2010). *Child health nursing: Partnering with children and families* (2nd ed.). Upper Saddle River, NJ: Prentice Hall.

Elder, C., & Demitri, P. J. (2017). Diabetes insipidus and the use of desmopressin in hospitalized children. *Archives of Disease in Childhood Education and Practice Edition, 102*, 100–104. doi: 10.1136/archdischild-2016-31076

Halvorson, M., Yasuda, P., Carpenter, S., & Kaiserman, K. (2005). Unique challenges for pediatric patients with diabetes. *Diabetes Spectrum, 18*, 167–173. doi: 10.2337/diaspect.18.3.167

Hockenberry, M., Wilson, D., & Rodgers, C. (2016). *Wong's essentials of pediatric nursing* (10th ed.). St. Louis, MO: Mosby Publishers.

Horner, G. (2007). Genitourinary assessment: An integral part of a complete physical exam. *Journal Pediatric Health Care, 21*, 162–170. Retrieved from http://www.jpedhc.org/

Houk, C. P., & Levitsky, L. L. (2017). Evaluation of the infant with atypical genitalia (disorder of sex development). *UpToDate.* Retrieved from https://www.uptodate.com/contents/evaluation-of-the-infant-with-atypical-genitalia-disorder-of-sex-development?source=search_result&search=ambiguous%20genitalia%20children&selectedTitle=1~58

Kaplowitz, P., & Hoffman, R. (2017). Precocious puberty clinical presentation. *Medscape.* Retrieved from http://emedicine.medscape.com/article/924002-clinical

Khardori, R., & Kemp, S. F. (2015). Pediatric hypopituitarism. *Medscape.* Retrieved from http://emedicine.medscape.com/article/922410-overview

Laffel, L., & Svoren, B. (2017). Epidemiology, presentation, and diagnosis of type 2 diabetes mellitus in children and adolescents. *UpToDate.* Retrieved from https://www-uptodate-com.libproxy.uams.edu/contents/epidemiology-presentation-and-diagnosis-of-type-2-diabetes-mellitus-in-children-and-adolescents?source=search_result&search=type%202%20diabetes%20in%20children&selectedTitle=1~150

LaFranchi, S. (2016). Clinical manifestations and diagnosis of hyperthyroidism in children and adolescents. *UpToDate.* Retrieved from https://www-uptodate-com.libproxy.uams.edu/contents/clinical-manifestations-and-diagnosis-of-hyperthyroidism-in-children-and-adolescents?source=search_result&search=hyperthyroidism%20in%20children&selectedTitle=1~150

Lipman, T. H., Hench, K. D., Benyi, T., Delaune, J., Gilluly, K. A., Johnson, L., … Weber, C. (2004). A multicentre randomized controlled trial of an intervention to improve the accuracy of linear growth measurement. *Archives of Disease in Childhood, 89*, 342–346. doi: 10.1136/adc.2003.030072

Merke, D. P. (2015). Diagnosis of classic congenital adrenal hyperplasia due to 21-hydroxylase deficiency. *UpToDate.* Retrieved from https://www.uptodate.com/contents/diagnosis-of-classic-congenital-adrenal-hyperplasia-due-to-21-hydroxylase-deficiency?source=search_result&search=congenital%20adrenal%20hyperplasia%20children&selectedTitle=1~125

Mishra, G., & Chandrashekhar, S. R. (2011). Management of diabetes insipidus in children. *Indian Journal of Endocrinology and Metabolism, 15*(Suppl. 3), S180–S187. doi: 10.4103/2230-8210.84858

Phillips, S. M., & Shulman, R. J. (2016). Measurement of growth in children. *UpToDate.* Retrieved from https://www.uptodate.com/contents/measurement-of-growth-in-children?source=see_link

Porth, C. M. (2015). *Essentials of pathophysiology* (4th ed.). Philadelphia: Wolters Kluwer.

Richmond, E. J., & Rogol, A. D. (2017). Diagnosis of growth hormone deficiency in children. *UpToDate.* Retrieved from https://www.uptodate.com/contents/diagnosis-of-growth-hormone-deficiency-in-children/print?source=see_link

Riepe, F. G., & Sippell, W. G. (2007). Recent advances in diagnostic, treatment and outcome of congenital adrenal hyperplasia due to 21-hydroxylase deficiency. *Reviews in Endocrine & Metabolism Disorders, 8*, 349–363. doi: 10.1007/s11154-007-9053-1

Rogol, A. D. (2017). Treatment of growth hormone deficiency in children. *UpToDate.* Retrieved from https://www-uptodate-com.libproxy.uams.edu/contents/treatment-of-growth-hormone-deficiency-in-children?source=search_result&search=treatment%20for%20growth%20hormone%20deficiency%20in%20children&selectedTitle=1~115#H6

Smans, L. C., Van der Valk, E. S., Hermus, A. R., & Zelissen, P. M. (2016). Incidence of adrenal crisis in patients with adrenal insufficiency. *Clinical Endocrinology (Oxford). 84*(1), 17–22. doi: 10.1111/cen.12865

Styne, D. M. (2016). *Pediatric endocrinology: A clinical handbook.* Cham, Switzerland: Springer International Publishing.

Suddaby, B., & Mowery, B. (2007). Complications of diabetes insipidus: The significance headache. *Pediatric Nursing, 33*, 58–59.

Vallerand, A. H., Sanoski, C. A., & Deglin, J. H. (2017). *Davis's drug guide for nurses* (15th ed.). Philadelphia: F.A. Davis.

Ward, S. L., & Hisley, S. M. (2015). *Maternal-child nursing care: Optimizing outcomes for mothers, children, & families* (2nd ed.). Philadelphia: F.A. Davis.

Wolfsdorf, J. I., Allgrove, J., Craig, M. E., Edge, J., Glaser, N., Jain, V., … International Society for Pediatric and Adolescent Diabetes. (2014). ISPAD Clinical Practice Consensus Guidelines 2014. Diabetic ketoacidosis and hyperglycemic hyperosmolar state. *Pediatric Diabetes, 15*(Suppl. 20), 154–179.

Reproductive and Genetic Disorders

18

Irene Cihon Dietz, MD, FAAP

LEARNING OUTCOMES

Upon completion of this chapter, the student will be able to:

1. Identify the anatomy of the male and female reproductive systems.
2. Discuss common pediatric reproductive health concerns.
3. Describe the signs and symptoms and interventions for common sexually transmitted infections.
4. Explain the human genome and its function.
5. Describe errors in reproduction, including mitosis, meiosis, and their contribution to genetic disorders.
6. Explain differences and similarities among autosomal dominant, recessive, and X-linked disorders.
7. Describe a variety of common genetic syndromes.
8. Explain the recommended age-appropriate care and pediatric surveillance for common genetic syndromes.

FEMALE ANATOMY AND PHYSIOLOGY

The female anatomy contains organs that work together for reproduction (Fig. 18–1).

- Ovaries: the two walnut-sized female organs that produce the ova (eggs) and sex hormones
- Ovum: mature female reproductive cell, also known as the egg or oocyte
  - Ova are formed within the ovaries and released on a cyclic basis.
  - The development of the ovum is under hormonal control.
- Fallopian tube(s): also known as the oviducts, two 4-inch muscular tubes that extend from the uterus to each ovary
- Uterus (Fig. 18–2): Commonly called the womb, the pear-shaped organ in the female abdominal cavity that holds the developing fetus
- Endometrium: a layer of cells lining the uterus that sheds to produce the menstrual cycle
  - Responds to hormones (estrogen and progesterone)
- Clitoris: A small area of erectile tissue situated below the pelvic bone and partially covered by the labia minora
- Vagina: tubular area connecting the external female genital tract from the vulva to the cervix
- Hymen: thin fold of skin that lies between the labia minora
  - Disrupted by sexual intercourse or other means of rupture
- Urethra: muscular tube through which urine exits the bladder

Pubertal Changes in Girls

- Adrenarche occurs when the adrenal gland starts to produce sex hormones. These outward changes are characterized by the stages of puberty (Table 18–1).
- These staging events have been published by Marshall and Tanner (1969) and are referred to as Tanner stages (see Chapter 10).

SAFE AND EFFECTIVE NURSING CARE: Clinical Pearl

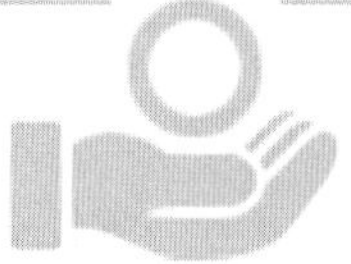

Age of Pubertal Onset

The age of pubertal onset varies with genetic and environmental influences, including physiological stress. In the United States, pubertal onset before age 8 years is considered precocious, and later than age 16 years is considered delayed and merits endocrine evaluation.

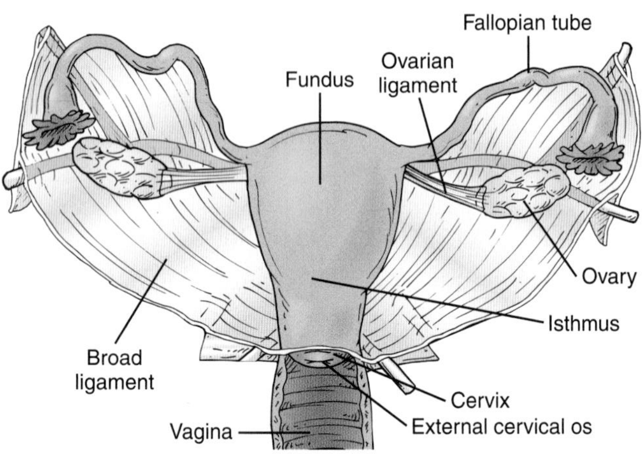

FIGURE 18–1 Female reproductive system.

TABLE 18–1 Stages of Puberty in Females

Pubarche	Appearance of pubic hair
Thelarche	Appearance of breast tissue maturation
Menarche	Onset of first menstrual period

COMMON PEDIATRIC PROBLEMS OF THE FEMALE GENITAL TRACT

Genital and urinary complaints are very common in pediatrics. Girls and young women often present with vague complaints of redness, itching, discharge, and sometimes bleeding and painful urination and/or vaginal burning. Urinary tract infection can present as vague abdominal pain. When evaluating girls with broad complaints, focus your inquiry based on age of presentation, activities, whether they are toilet trained, whether they tend to take baths or showers, and degree of sexual maturity. Careful consideration of possible sexual abuse when performing the history, examination, and laboratory tests is always necessary (Jenny, Crawford-Jakubiak, J., & Committee on Child Abuse and Neglect, 2013).

Straddle Injury

- Injury to genitals as the result of a fall over a blunt object in which tissues are compressed between bone and blunt object

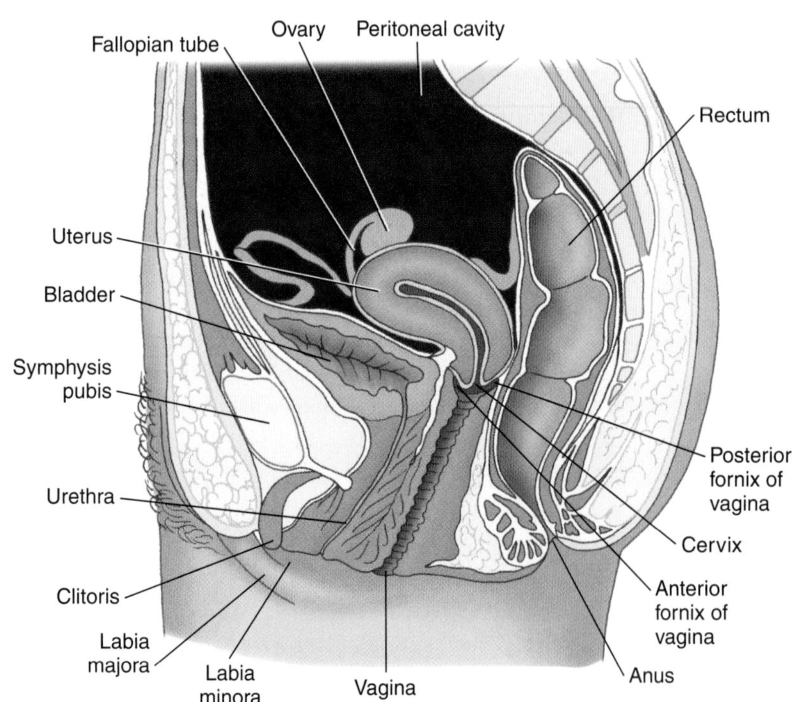

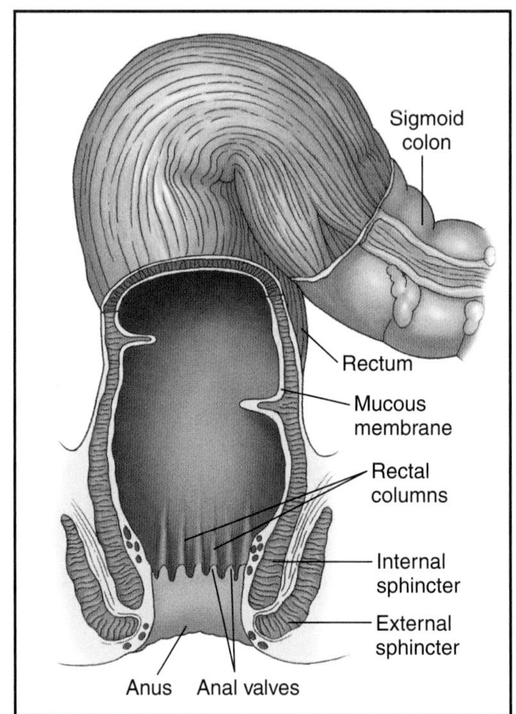

FIGURE 18–2 Internal female genitalia and cross-section of rectum.

- Common in school-age children
- Commonly caused from monkey bars or bicycle

Nursing Interventions

- May cause a hematoma (trapped blood between tissues): most do not need special treatment
- Avoid surgical drainage to prevent introduction of bacteria and abscess
  - Small (size of a hen's egg): bedrest, intermittent use of ice pack with pressure for 12 to 24 hours
  - Medium (size of an orange): as above, bedrest, ice for first 12 to 24 hours, then warm tub baths or Sitz-type soaking bath in addition
  - Large (size of a grapefruit or larger): must assess for urethral obstruction; may require suprapubic catheter

Lacerations or Skin Tears

- Lacerations or skin tears may require examination under anesthesia to identify the source of the bleeding.
  - Bleeding control is key with labial or vulvar tears.
  - Avoid treatment by suturing superficial injuries with controlled bleeding, and instead allow to heal by secondary intention if possible.
  - Large areas need repair and exploration under anesthesia for additional vaginal injury.
  - Puncture wounds need to be cleaned and assessed for foreign bodies (Laufner & Makai, 2017).
- Hymenal injuries occur most often from penetrating trauma.
  - Penetrating injury can cause vaginal and/or internal injury; treatment varies by degree of bleeding.

Nursing Interventions

- Evaluate for possible sexual abuse.
- Area and type of injury and placement of bruising should be examined by abuse expert.

Vulvovaginitis

- Vulvovaginitis is inflammation of the vulva and vaginal areas.
- It is the most common complaint involving the genital area of prepubescent girls (Laufner & Emans, 2016).
- Symptoms may include vaginal itching (pruritus), soreness, redness (erythema), thin vaginal discharge, or painful urination (dysuria).
- This condition can be caused by an infection or by nonspecific irritants such as tight nylon undergarments, bubble bath, or perfumed bath products.
- Prepubescent girls are more susceptible.
  - Labial tissue lacks estrogen.
  - Tissue is thinner and more susceptible to irritants.
  - Infection and chronic masturbatory activity in small children is irritating.
  - Vulvovaginitis may also indicate the presence of vaginal foreign body.
  - Of girls with a foreign body, 25% to 75% may present with odor or discharge (Laufner & Emans, 2016).

Nursing Interventions

- Teach hygiene with front-to-back wiping after bowel movements.
- Consider using moist wipes rather than dry paper to wipe.
- Allow air flow by wearing cotton underwear. Avoid wearing tight clothing on lower body.
- Daily warm bath for 10 to 15 minutes in clear water; minimal use of gentle soap, rinsed just before getting out of tub; pat dry, or may use hair dryer distant from skin on cool or low setting.

Specific Causes of Vulvovaginitis

Common causes of vulvovaginitis in the pediatric population are pinworm, vulvar ulcers, and imperforate hymen.

Pinworm

- Tiny worms with fecal–oral spread
- Adult female worms live in gastrointestinal (GI) tract, are not shed in stool, and come out to lay eggs in warm perineal areas, mostly at night
- Vulvar and perianal itching usually present (Laufner & Emans, 2016) (Fig. 18–3)
- "Tape test": use sticky side of tape to lift bean-shaped white eggs from area; may see white 5- to 13-mm adult worms

Nursing Interventions

- Teach proper hand hygiene after using the bathroom and after contact with feces.
- Administer medications as prescribed by physician.
- Avoid scratching perianal area.

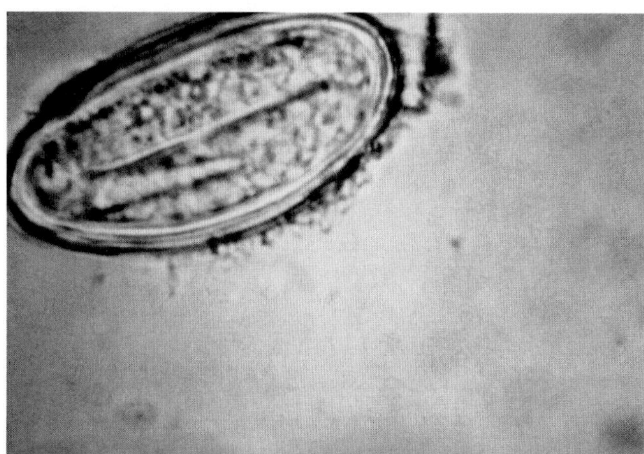

FIGURE 18–3 Pinworm.

Vulvar Ulcers

- Also known as Lipschütz ulcers, "virginal" ulcers, or "aphthous" ulcers
- Generally seen in girls aged 10 to 15 years
- Present as one or more painful ulcers more than 1 cm in diameter with purulent bases and raised red edges
- Nonsexually transmitted; associated with viral infections such as influenza A, Epstein–Barr virus, or cytomegalovirus, but should also test for herpes simplex virus types 1 and 2

Nursing Interventions

- May require a Foley catheter to urinate
- Topical antibiotic if secondary infection
- Usually heals in 1 to 3 weeks
- Pain management

Imperforate Hymen

- Congenital malformation
- May be seen at birth with white or mucoid material detained behind the area, but will reabsorb if missed
- More often presents as a bluish bulge in a teen with reports of amenorrhea
- Can be associated with chronic pain in abdomen or back from retained blood within the vagina

Nursing Interventions

- Provide anticipatory guidance for the surgical repair
- Pain management
- Reassure teen girl if body image issues are present

ADOLESCENT VAGINAL COMPLAINTS

Adolescent girls presenting with symptoms of vaginal discharge and bleeding require taking a careful history, including symptoms and timing around of first pubertal cycle, normal menstrual patterns, and degree of sexual maturity and contraceptive use.

Bacterial Vaginosis

- Bacterial vaginosis (BV) is the most common cause of vaginal discharge in postmenarchal adolescents and women of childbearing age.
- The absence of inflammation is the basis for the term "vaginosis" rather than "vaginitis" (Kenyon et al., 2013).
- Of affected women, 50% to 75% may have minimal symptoms, including fishy-smelling, thin, whitish-gray discharge (Kenyon et al., 2013).
- BV results not from one organism, but from a complex change in normal vaginal organisms and increase in other organisms (Fig. 18–4).

Nursing Interventions

- Up to one-third of cases will resolve spontaneously.
- May consider treatment in partners for women who have sex with other women.
- Presence of BV is associated with HIV acquisition, as well as increased risk for preterm labor in pregnant women.

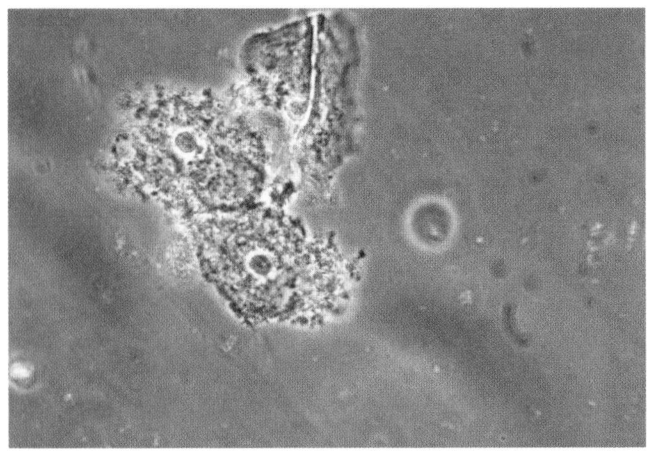

FIGURE 18–4 Vaginosis "clue cells" indicating a change in normal vaginal organisms.

> **CRITICAL COMPONENT**
>
> **Normal Menstrual Cycle**
>
> The normal menstrual cycle results from a complex feedback system involving the hypothalamus, pituitary, ovary, and uterus. The cyclic changes in the major pituitary and gonadal hormones are illustrated in Figure 18–5. Although the development of secondary sexual characteristics varies by race and geographic location, the average age of menarche in the United States is 12.3 years (Harrington & Palmert, 2016).

Abnormal Uterine Bleeding

- Menstruation is the active shedding of the endometrial lining of the uterus in a cyclic fashion in response to estrogen and progesterone hormone changes (Fig. 18–5)
- Menstrual cycles are often irregular in the first months to up to 3 years after menarche.
- The average adult menstrual cycle lasts 28 to 35 days with 4 to 6 days of menstrual bleeding.
- The median blood loss during each menstrual period is 30 mL; the upper limit of normal is 80 mL (DeSilva, 2017).
- The median length of the first cycle after menarche is 34 days, with 38% of cycles exceeding 40 days and 7% occurring less than 20 days apart (World Health Organization, Task Force on Adolescent Reproductive Health, 1986).
- Abnormal uterine bleeding is the cause of most frequent gynecological complaints.
- Most cases of abnormal uterine bleeding in adolescents are caused by anovulatory cycles, where no ovum (egg) is released. This is seen most often during the first 12 to 18 months after menarche.
- Other common causes are pregnancy, infection, the use of hormonal contraceptives, stress (psychogenic or exercise induced), bleeding disorders, and endocrine disorders (e.g., hypothyroidism, polycystic ovary syndrome).

Amenorrhea

Amenorrhea is the absence of monthly menses.

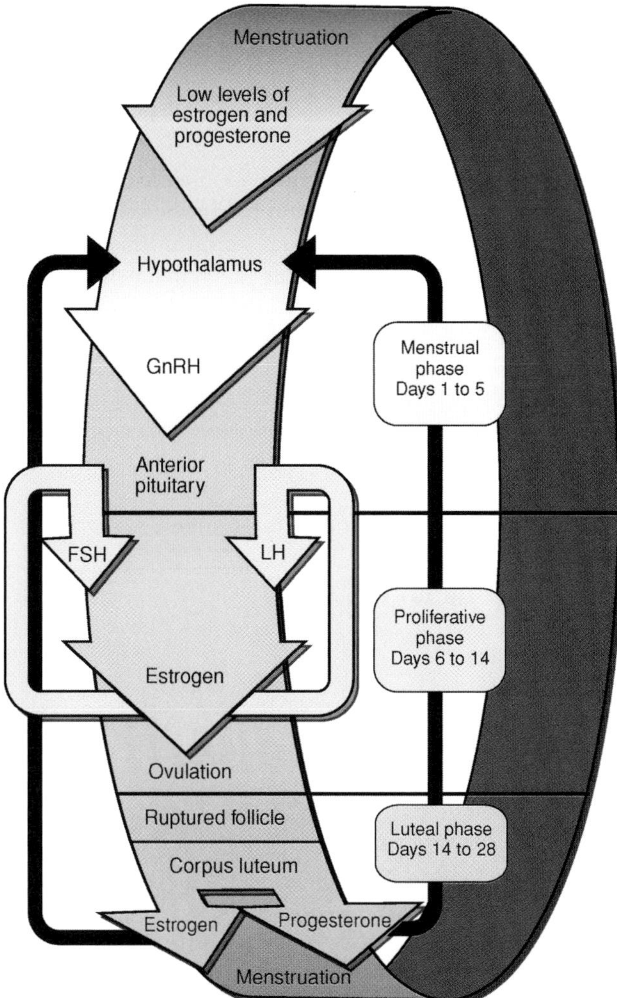

FIGURE 18–5 Menstrual cycle. FSH, follicle-stimulating hormone; GnRH, gonadotropin-releasing hormone; LH, luteinizing hormone.

Primary Amenorrhea

- Period has never been present
- The average age of menarche is 12.3 years, and 95% of females in the United States have onset of menses by 14.7 years
- Girls need endocrine evaluation if no menses by 16 years

Nursing Interventions

- Obtain detailed physical history.
- Obtain family history of reproductive problems.

Secondary Amenorrhea

- Absence of menses for more than three cycles or 6 months in women who previously had menses
  - Cause of secondary amenorrhea is most often pregnancy
  - Work up by excluding pregnancy through urine or blood pregnancy test

Nursing Interventions

- Hormone therapy as indicated by physician
- Assess for vaginal bleeding
- Document amount of vaginal bleeding as output

Caregiver Education

- Teach the importance of keeping track of when the period starts and when it ends.
- Teach that hormone therapy does not prevent sexually transmitted infections (STIs).

Menorrhagia

- Menorrhagia is characterized by menstrual flow of excessive duration, greater than 7 days, and/or heavy volume, greater than 80 mL/cycle (DeSilva, 2017).
- Typically occurs at irregular intervals, indicating anovulatory (lack of ova release) cycles.
- Need to also consider coagulation disorders, especially if present with very heavy first menses or among those with significant anemia after treatment.

Nursing Interventions and Caregiver Education

- Obtain complete blood cell count, platelets, and iron level as indicated by physician.
- Consider evaluation for von Willebrand disease.
  - The most common inherited cause of excessive bleeding
  - Individuals have missing or decreased function of von Willebrand factor (important for clotting and adherence of platelets)
- Provide education to evaluate amount of vaginal discharge.
- Encourage a well-balanced diet including food rich in iron during menses.

MALE ANATOMY AND PHYSIOLOGY

- Penis: male reproductive organ (Fig. 18–6)
  - Both urine and semen leave the body through the penis.
  - Contains the urethra and two tubular and honeycombed areas of erectile tissue.
- Glans: external bulbous area at the end of the penis; a particularly sensitive area
- Prepuce (foreskin): small area of skin that covers the glans; removed in male circumcision

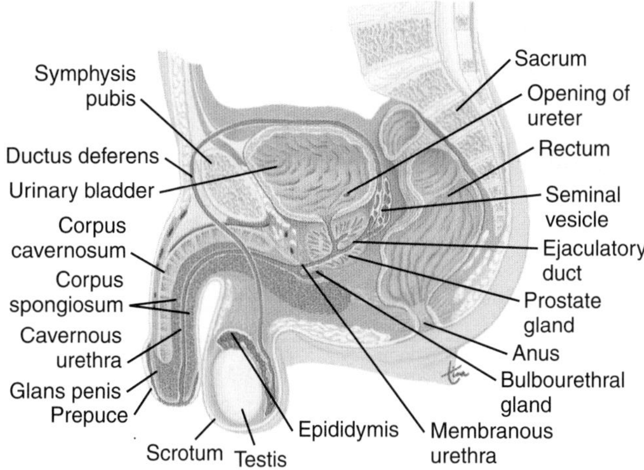

FIGURE 18–6 Male reproductive system.

- Testis (testicle): one of the male reproductive organs (gonads)
  - After puberty, the testes produce the male hormone testosterone and the reproductive cells (sperm).
  - Each is about 1.5 inches (4 cm) long in adults.
- Sperm: the male sex cell produced within the testicles and ejaculated in semen, also known as the spermatozoon
  - Each sperm (and ovum) contains half of the normal number of chromosomes required to form a single cell
- Semen: creamy discharge secreted through the penis during ejaculation
  - Consists of sperm and fluids secreted by the prostate gland and seminal vesicles, certain epithelial cells, and other gland secretions
- Spermatic cord: the cord that suspends the testicle within the scrotum and encloses the vas deferens, blood vessels, and testicular nerves
- Epididymis: long, coiled tube that rests on the backside of each testicle
  - Transports and stores sperm cells that are produced in the testes.
  - Brings the sperm to maturity, as the sperm that emerge from the testes are immature and incapable of fertilization.
  - Each male has two epididymides.
- Vas deferens (sperm duct): tube that carries mature sperm to the epididymis to the seminal vesicles where sperm is stored
- Prostate gland: a walnut-shaped organ that lies beneath the bladder and surrounds the urethra
  - Produces secretions that maintain the vitality of the sperm
- Scrotum: The baglike structure of skin that contains the testicles, epididymides, and parts of the spermatic cords
  - The skin of the scrotum contains muscles that can raise or lower the testicles, thereby keeping them at optimum temperature for sperm reproduction.

Puberty in Boys

Pubertal changes in boys include enlargement of the genitals, both in length of the penis and size of the testicles; pubic hair development and increased body hair; deepening of the voice; and rapid skeletal and muscle growth (Table 18–2).

TABLE 18–2 Stages of Puberty in Males

Adrenarche	Adrenal medulla area starts to produce androgens (testosterone and estrogen); typically occurs before the onset of puberty
Pubarche	Appearance of pubic hair
Gonadarche	Activation of the gonads by the pituitary hormones: follicle-stimulating hormone and luteinizing hormone

COMMON PEDIATRIC AND ADOLESCENT PROBLEMS OF THE MALE GENITAL TRACT

Concerns about the penis, scrotum, and testes in children and adolescents require careful attention to history including presence of pain, swelling, redness, and warmth. The age of the patient, as well as activities including prior circumcision, toilet training and diaper use, sexual maturity, and exposures must be considered.

Circumcision

- Surgical removal of the foreskin (Fig. 18–7)
- Often done in infancy
- May be done for religious or cultural purposes

CRITICAL COMPONENT

Circumcision

Circumcision in the United States is most often performed for social reasons, often as part of a religious rite of passage near birth or an initiation into adulthood. Frequently it is because it is the tradition in the family or because most boys in the neighborhood are circumcised. The most recent statement of the American Academy of Pediatrics (AAP), released in 2012, reports specific benefits of circumcision including prevention of urinary tract infections, penile cancer, and transmission of some STIs, including HIV (AAP, 2012). In the United States and worldwide, circumcision is still considered elective surgery (World Health Organization & Joint United Nations Programme on HIV/AIDS, 2010).

Nursing Interventions

- Provide pain management.
- Wash with soap and water.
- Dressing may not be necessary.
- Alert physician to excessive bleeding.

Caregiver Education

- Notify physician if oozing, swelling, or drainage noted around surgical site.
- Notify physician of fever.
- Wash with soap and water after diaper changes.
- Provide Tylenol as ordered by physician.

Uncircumcised Penis

- Phimosis is the inability to retract the foreskin.
- Not all male infants have a fully retractable foreskin, but the ability to fully retract increased with age.
- By seventh grade, only about 1% of uncircumcised boys cannot retract the foreskin (Hsieh, Chang, & Chang, 2006; Wilcox, 2017)

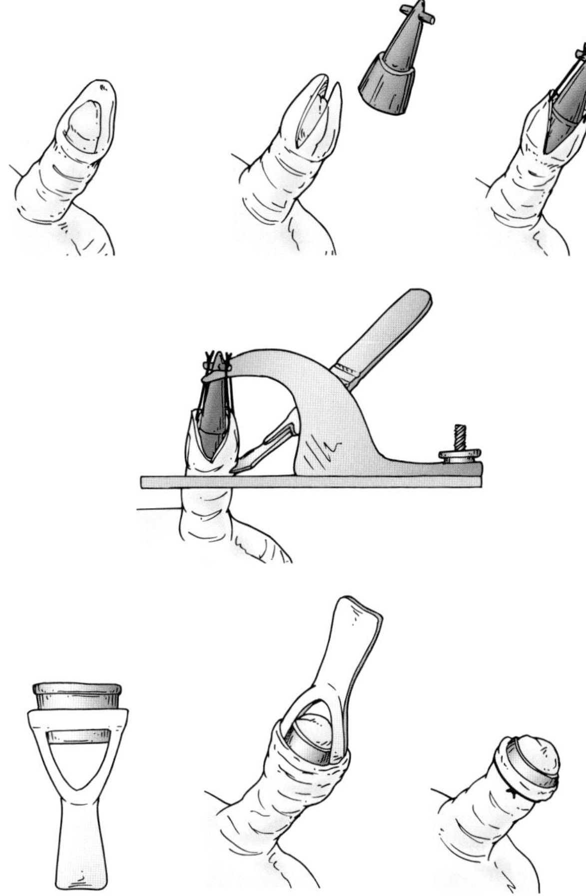

FIGURE 18–7 Circumcision.

Nursing Interventions

- Wash or cleanse the penis and glans as you would any other part of the body.
- The foreskin does not need to be retracted in infancy or toddler years.

Caregiver Education

- During this time, caregivers should leave the foreskin alone.
- Avoid forced retraction.
- As the foreskin naturally begins to retract, cleaning and then drying underneath the foreskin can be performed.
- Foreskin should always be pulled down to its normal position covering the glans after drying.

Physiological Phimosis

- Inability to retract the foreskin beyond the glans penis
- Physiological phimosis is present in almost all newborn males

Nursing Interventions

- School-age boys without a fully retractable foreskin and/or their parents should be counseled that there is normally a wide range of retractability.
- Reinforce proper hygiene.

Caregiver Education

- Patients and/or parents can be taught to perform gentle stretch exercises.
- As ordered by a physician, a 4- to 8-week course of topical corticosteroids may be prescribed.
- Counsel parents and child that nearly all men develop the ability to retract the foreskin by adulthood without specific treatment.

Pathological Phimosis

- Secondary nonretractability of the foreskin after retractability at an earlier age
- Irritation or bleeding from the preputial orifice
- Pain with urination (dysuria)
- Painful erection
- Chronic urinary retention with ballooning that is only resolved with manual compression

Nursing Interventions

- Pediatric urological consultation should be sought.

Paraphimosis

- Inability to return the foreskin to its natural position once retracted, resulting in swelling and pain in the glans penis
- Medical emergency to avoid vascular injury to the glans

Nursing Interventions and Caregiver Education

- Educate child and caregiver that anesthesia is generally required to return foreskin and may require possible circumcision.
- Steroid may also be used as noted earlier if circumcision is not desired.

Zipper Injuries

- Penile injuries related to zipper entrapment
- One of the more common genital injuries
- Usually entrapment of the foreskin or redundant skin, with localized edema and pain being the most common complications; skin loss or necrosis is rare

Nursing Interventions

- Treatment is release of the zipper.
- Most often recommend cutting the zipper's median bar with wire cutters, bone cutters, or small hacksaw.
- Sedation or local pain control is recommended.

Caregiver Education

- Teach child to carefully zip pants once underwear has been pulled up.
- Do not force zip-up if difficulty is noted.
- Encourage the child to ask for assistance when zipper is difficult to manage.

DEVELOPMENT OF THE TESTIS

Understanding of the development and movement of the testis into the scrotum is important to understand types of masses of the scrotum.

- The testicles develop in the abdomen of the male fetus in a position very close to that of the ovaries in the female.
- At around 10 weeks of gestational age, an outpouching through the abdominal cavity develops.
- By 12 weeks, the testicles start to migrate down through the abdominal wall to reside in the scrotum.
- The processus vaginalis forms from an outward protrusion of the peritoneum that lines the abdominal wall.
- Between the seventh and ninth months of gestation, the testes descend into the scrotum, pushing the processus vaginalis ahead, and then protrude into its cavity.
- Once this process is complete, the processus vaginalis obliterates spontaneously, usually by age 2 years.
- Many males are born with incomplete descent of the testis, and the process may be completed after birth.

Cryptorchidism (Undescended Testis)

- Cryptorchidism is a congenital condition in which the testis fails to descend into the scrotum.
- Most often, the testis remains in the inguinal canal or higher up in the groin.
- May be palpated on examination.

Nursing Interventions

- Refer to urology or surgery by age 2 years if undescended testicle is palpated in the groin or inguinal area.
- Anticipate ultrasound of the scrotum if the testicle is not palpated within the scrotum or canal.

Caregiver Education

- Encourage loose clothing worn on the lower body.
- Ultrasound or other tests may be needed to evaluate the current condition.

Scrotal Swelling

- Causes vary from benign incidental findings to medical emergencies, and by age and clinical symptoms (Brenner & Ojo, 2017)
- Generally divided into painless versus painful swelling or chronic versus acute changes

Hydrocele

- A painless collection of fluid between the layers of tissue or capsule covering the testis, the tunica vaginalis
- Fluid moves through the processus vaginalis to surround the testis
- Very common in newborns, generally resolves by 1 year of age
- Examination is of a cystic structure and can be transilluminated (light easily passes through the area)
- May occur in older children and adolescents, both spontaneously or related to infection or trauma

Nursing Interventions and Caregiver Education

- Monitor for resolution of fluid/swelling before 1 year of age.
- Refer for further evaluation after 1 year of age.

Varicocele

- A painless collection of dilated and tortuous veins in the plexus surrounding the spermatic cord in the scrotum
- Can be asymptomatic or present with a dull ache or fullness of the scrotum upon standing
- A palpable varicocele has the texture of a "bag of worms" and may become fuller with bearing down or in Valsalva maneuver
- May be associated with infertility

Nursing Interventions

- No clear guidelines have been established for treatment of a varicocele in childhood
- Observation until teen years

Child and Caregiver Education

- Provide anticipatory guidance when aggressive surgical treatment is necessary.

Testicular Torsion

- Testicular torsion, or twisting of the testicle, has the following characteristics:
  - Painful scrotal swelling
  - Abrupt, severe constant pain in the scrotum, lower abdomen, and groin area; 90% with nausea and vomiting (Brenner & Ojo, 2017)
  - Peak incidence in boys 12 to 18 years old; smaller group in neonatal period
  - Present with scrotal edema; the affected testis is tender, swollen, and slightly elevated; the testis may lie horizontally and may have a reactive hydrocele
  - Intermittent torsion can present with intermittent sharp pain and swelling, then rapid resolution
  - This is a surgical emergency in which action must be taken to preserve the testes; ultrasound or Doppler flow scan of scrotum may be indicated
  - Long-term viability of the testis relies on time to derotation (Brenner & Ojo, 2017)
- Torsion of the appendix testis
  - Twisting of a very small remnant in the upper pole of the testis, a residual appendage with no function after fetal development

Nursing Interventions

- Provide pain management.
- Prepare for possible surgery.
- Prepare child age-appropriately for diagnostic testing.

Epididymitis

- Inflammation of the epididymis related to infection
  - May have diffuse swelling; may also have increased urination (frequency), painful urination (dysuria), or discharge from the urethra; sometimes fever.
  - Testis is in normal vertical lie on examination, and scrotum may be red or edematous.
  - Chlamydia is the most common cause of epididymitis in sexually active adolescent males and is also associated with gonorrhea, but can be caused by *Escherichia coli* and even some viruses. Most often idiopathic in prepubertal males.

Nursing Interventions

- Can occur in young boys after infection with enteroviruses, adenovirus, and mycoplasma
- Associated with structural anomalies of the urinary tract in prepubertal boys
- Diagnosis is by clinical examination, but must rule out differential of testicular torsion
- Doppler or nuclear scan considered if testicular torsion needs immediate surgical referral

Child and Caregiver Education

- Review care and antibiotic use.
- Prepare for diagnostic Doppler ultrasound and the possible surgery if necessary.
- Preparation should be explained in a developmentally appropriate manner.

Orchitis

- Painful inflammation/infection of the testis
- Presents with scrotal swelling, pain, tenderness, and redness/shininess of the overlying skin

Nursing Interventions

- Associated with other systemic infections
- Anticipate treatment to be based on cause of infection (viral or bacterial)

Child and Caregiver Education

- Bedrest
- Ice packs as ordered
- NSAIDs (ibuprofen) as ordered by physician
- Support of the inflamed testis
- Appropriate antibiotics as ordered by physician

Primary Inguinal Hernia

- A hernia is a protrusion of any organ or tissue through an abnormal opening in the wall that should contain it.
- Passage of tissue into the groin area occurs in 1% to 5% of all newborns and 9% to 11% of those born prematurely (Ramsock, 2016).
- Inguinal hernias occur three to four times more often in males than females, and they occur bilaterally in about 10% (Brenner & Ojo, 2017) (Fig. 18–8).
- Inguinal hernia repair is the most commonly performed surgical procedure in children.
- Groin hernia may be caused by injury.
- Factors that increase the pressure in the abdomen may produce a groin hernia in susceptible adolescents, such as lifting heavy objects, obesity, constipation and resultant straining, and recurrent coughing or sneezing.
- Incarceration of hernia is the inability to push herniated tissue back through the opening; this is a surgical emergency that must be treated quickly.
- Strangulation of hernia is vascular compromise of the contents of an incarcerated hernia caused by progressive edema from venous and lymphatic obstruction.
  - Strangulation can occur within 2 hours of incarceration.
  - Children with hernias may present with a painless intermittent mass, a constant reducible mass, or pain with strangulation.

Nursing Interventions

- Assess for signs and symptoms of infection after surgery.
- Provide adequate pain control and offer nonpharmacological methods for pain relief.
- Assess for bleeding at surgical site.
- Brace lower abdomen with pillow when coughing or deep breathing to prevent dehiscence of wound.

Child and Caregiver Education

- Discourage heavy lifting after repair.
- Watch for bleeding or drainage from surgical site.
- Notify physician if fever is present.

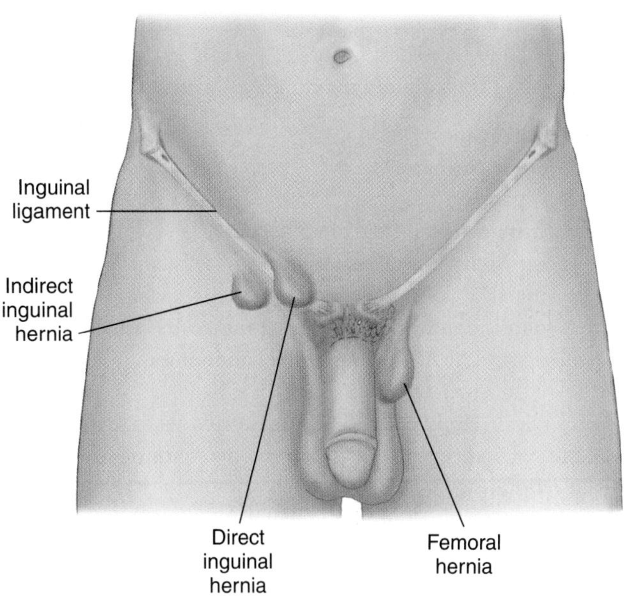

FIGURE 18–8 Hernia.

- Provide pain medications as ordered by physician.
- Brace lower abdomen with a pillow when coughing or deep breathing.

SEXUALLY TRANSMITTED INFECTIONS

The term STIs refers to a variety of clinical syndromes and infections caused by pathogens that can be acquired and transmitted through sexual activity. Health-care teams must be aware of the risks for STIs and changing practices, including screening special populations to decrease the worldwide incidence.

Evidence-Based Practice Research: Adolescents at Highest Risk for Sexually Transmitted Infection

Centers for Disease Control and Prevention (CDC). (2015). *2015 STD treatment guidelines.* Retrieved from http://www.cdc.gov/std/tg2015/default.htm

Prevalence rates for STIs (previously called sexually transmitted diseases) are highest among adolescents. Adolescents and young adults, aged 15 to 24 years, account for half of all new STD infections. STIs are among the highest of all racial/ethnic health disparities—71% of all gonorrhea, 48% of chlamydia, and 52% of syphilis infections occur in African Americans, according to the Centers for Disease Control and Prevention (CDC). Screening guidelines have been updated by the CDC for even asymptomatic persons in certain high-risk populations, including adolescent clinics, pregnant women, men who have sex with men, and teens in detention centers. Nurses involved in the care of youth and adolescents must be aware of these guidelines and knowledgeable about high-risk groups to assist with confidential questioning and screening of even asymptomatic patients when presenting for care. This may include pediatrics annual wellness visits even outside specialized adolescent clinics.

Risk Factors for Sexually Transmitted Infections

Behavioral and biological factors play a role in the increased incidence of STIs in adolescents compared with adults.

- Behavioral issues
  - Multiple partners
  - New partners
  - Partners with multiple other partners
  - Inconsistent use of condoms, especially with established partners
  - Alcohol and other drug consumption, often associated with inappropriate birth control and condom use
- Biological issues
  - Cervical ectopy or cervical immaturity, which refers to the area of ectocervix that is covered by columnar epithelium after puberty
  - Columnar epithelium is thought to be more susceptible than is squamous epithelium to sexually transmitted organisms: *Neisseria gonorrhoeae*, *Chlamydia trachomatis*, and human papillomavirus

Screening for Sexually Transmitted Infections

- Follow CDC and American College of Gynecology recommendations (CDC, 2015).
- Annual *C. trachomatis* screen is recommended for all sexually active females younger than 25 years.
- Annual *N. gonorrhoeae* screen is recommended for all sexually active females at risk for infection.
- Females younger than 25 years are at highest risk for gonorrhea infection.
- All teens or young adults should have at least one HIV screen.
- Routinely screen sexually active adolescents who are asymptomatic for certain STIs (e.g., syphilis, trichomoniasis, BV, herpes simplex virus).
- Young men who have sex with men and pregnant adolescent females might require more thorough evaluation and testing.
- Pap screens should be done on younger teens who engage in high-risk behavior, such as having multiple sexual partners.

Pelvic Inflammatory Disease

- Acute infection of the upper genital tract structures in women
- Can involve the uterus, oviducts, and ovaries, or all three
- Often accompanied by involvement of the neighboring pelvic organs
- Involvement of these structures may result in:
  - Endometritis—infection of uterine lining
  - Salpingitis—infection of the fallopian tubes
  - Oophoritis—infection of the ovaries
  - Peritonitis—infection of the abdominal lining or peritoneum
  - Perihepatitis—inflammation of the hepatic area, and tubo-ovarian abscess
- Caused most often by genital gonorrhea and the effect of other infections
- Douching may increase the risk for development of pelvic inflammatory disease (PID), especially when performed frequently
- Health-care providers should maintain a low threshold for the diagnosis of PID
- Sexually active young women with the combination of lower abdominal, ovarian, or fallopian structures (adnexa), and cervical motion tenderness should receive empiric treatment (CDC, 2015)

Nursing Interventions

- Complete antibiotic regimen as ordered.
- Educate child or adolescent to take medication as directed.
- Provide pain management.
- Teach signs and symptoms of infection.
- Educate about the prevention of STIs.
- Educate about condom use.
- Educate about abstinence.

Child and Caregiver Education

- Complete antibiotics as prescribed.
- Educate about the prevention of STIs.
- Educate about the use of condoms.
- Educate about abstinence.

Trichomoniasis

- The responsible organism is the flagellated protozoan *Trichomonas vaginalis*, a single-celled organism with a tail (Fig. 18–9).
- Humans are the only natural host; it is rarely cultured from surfaces.
- Transmission is nearly always through sexual contact.

Classic Signs and Symptoms in Females

- Purulent, malodorous, thin discharge (70% of cases)
- Burning, pruritus (itching)
- Dysuria (painful urination), frequency
- Dyspareunia (pain with intercourse)
- Postcoital bleeding can occur
- Urethra is also infected in the majority of women
- Symptoms may be worse during menstruation
- Discharge classically described as green, frothy, and foul-smelling is found in fewer than 10% of symptomatic women

Classic Signs and Symptoms in Males

- Symptoms in men are generally less severe; often affected men remain asymptomatic, and spontaneous resolution may occur.
- Less than 10% of men experience any symptoms.
- Symptoms are the same as those for urethritis from any cause and consist of a clear or mucoid, purulent urethral discharge and/or pain with urination.
- Potential complications include prostatitis, balanoposthitis, epididymitis, and infertility.

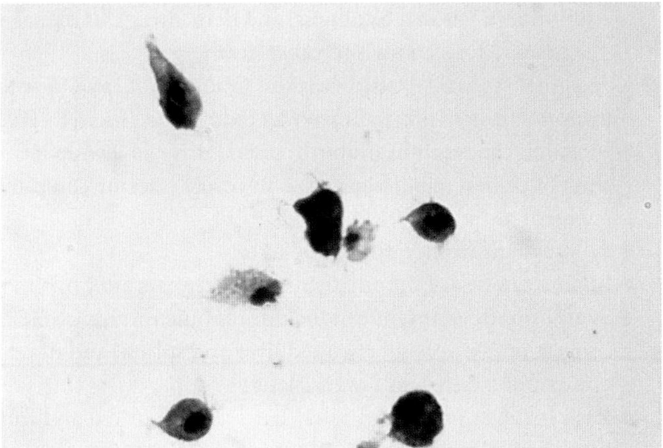

FIGURE 18–9 Trichomonas vaginalis.

- The only reliable test to diagnose trichomonas in the male is polymerase chain reaction testing of urine, which is not widely available; other tests, such as saline microscopy of urethral swabs, have low sensitivity.

Nursing Interventions

- Complete antibiotic regimen as ordered.
- Should avoid any alcohol consumption for at least 72 hours after treatment completion to avoid severe vomiting (medication interaction).

Child and Caregiver Education

- Teach all nonpregnant females to be treated.
- Teach to abstain from sexual contact with partner until treatment is complete and symptoms are gone, generally 1 week.
- Follow-up clinical examination or testing is usually not necessary for women who are then asymptomatic, because the drugs are very effective.
- Treatment is the same for men and nonpregnant women.

Gonorrhea

- Gonorrhea is caused by *N. gonorrhoeae*.
- Infection can occur in the cervix, vagina, and fallopian tubes in women, but also the eyes, throat, urethra, and anus of males and females.
- Gonorrhea may also spread to the blood or the joints, causing painful arthritis with red, swollen joints.
- Is spread by contact with infected sites, most often through sexual contact in adolescents, and can signal sexual abuse in children.
- Can be spread from mother to infant during delivery.
- Severe eye infection in infants can lead to blindness.
- Often associated with co-infection of *C. trachomatis.*

SAFE AND EFFECTIVE NURSING CARE: Understanding Medication

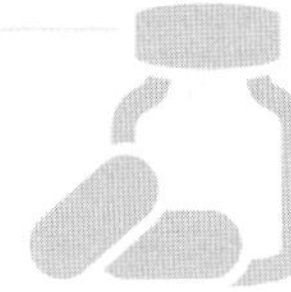

Preventing Gonorrhea Eye Infections in Infants

Ophthalmia neonatorum refers to neonatal conjunctivitis as the result of infection transmitted from the mother to the child during delivery. This is typically caused by gonorrhea but can also result from chlamydia. Eyedrops or ointment should be administered after birth if infection is suspected. Erythromycin ointment is used in most countries. As these pathogens become more resistant, good prenatal care, with screening and treatment of infected mothers during pregnancy, is key (Moore, MacDonald, & Canadian Paediatric Society, Infectious Diseases and Immunization Committee, 2015).

Signs and Symptoms

- Pain with urination
- Yellow, white, or green urethral discharge, more often in men
- May be asymptomatic or mimic signs of urinary tract infection
- Symptoms of rectal infection in both men and women may include discharge, anal itching, soreness, bleeding, or painful bowel movements
- Rectal infection also may cause no symptoms
- Infections in the throat may cause a sore throat, but usually cause no symptoms

Nursing Interventions

- Obtain cultures before the start of antibiotics.
- Administer antibiotics as prescribed.

Child and Caregiver Education

- Educate about the use of condoms.
- Educate about abstinence.
- Complete antibiotics as prescribed.

Chlamydia

- Caused by the bacterium *C. trachomatis*
- Most common bacterial agent of sexually transmitted genital infections
- Significant numbers of patients are asymptomatic, providing an ongoing reservoir for infection; this includes men and women
- Conjunctivitis and pneumonia can occur in infants born to mothers through an infected birth canal

Nursing Interventions

- Complete antibiotic regimen as ordered.
- Educate about the prevention of STIs.
- Educate about condom use.
- Educate about abstinence.

Child and Caregiver Education

- All females should be tested for pregnancy, and a test of cured status is necessary in about 3 weeks for pregnant women only.
- Notify physician if infection is not appearing to improve.
- Test of cured status is not recommended for others, even HIV-positive persons.

Syphilis

- Syphilis is an STI caused by the bacterium *Treponema pallidum,* is a very long, thin, and coiled bacterium, a spirochete.
- It has often been called "the great imitator" because so many of the signs and symptoms are indistinguishable from those of other diseases.
- Syphilis is a chronic infection that occurs in several stages.
  - Primary stage
    - Marked by the appearance of a single sore (called a chancre), but there may be multiple sores.
    - The time between infection with syphilis and the start of the first symptom can range from 10 to 90 days (average 21 days).
    - The chancre is usually firm, round, small, and painless. It appears at the spot where syphilis entered the body.
    - The chancre lasts 3 to 6 weeks, and it heals without treatment. However, if adequate treatment is not administered, the infection progresses to the secondary stage.
  - Secondary stage
    - Skin rash and mucous membrane lesions characterize the secondary stage; starts with the development of a rash on one or more areas of the body.
    - Rashes associated with secondary syphilis can appear as the chancre is healing or several weeks after the chancre has healed.
    - Characteristic rash of secondary syphilis may appear as rough, red, or reddish-brown spots both on the palms of the hands and the bottoms of the feet.
    - Rashes with a different appearance may occur on other parts of the body, sometimes resembling rashes caused by other diseases.
    - Other symptoms of secondary syphilis may include fever, swollen lymph glands, sore throat, patchy hair loss, headaches, weight loss, muscle aches, and fatigue.
    - The signs and symptoms will resolve with or without treatment.
    - Without treatment, the infection will progress to the latent and possibly late stages of disease.
  - Late and latent stages
    - The latent (hidden) stage of syphilis begins when primary and secondary symptoms disappear.
    - Without treatment, the infected person will continue to have and be contagious, even without active symptoms.
    - The late stages develop in about 15% of people who have not been treated for syphilis.
    - It can appear 10 to 20 years after infection was first acquired and last for years, even decades.
    - The disease may subsequently damage the internal organs, including the brain, nerves, eyes, heart, blood vessels, liver, bones, and joints.
    - Signs and symptoms of the late stage of syphilis include difficulty coordinating muscle movements, paralysis, numbness, gradual blindness, and dementia. This damage may be serious enough to cause death.
- Congenital syphilis occurs when the spirochete *T. pallidum* is transmitted from a pregnant woman to her fetus (Fig. 18–10):
  - Infection can result in stillbirth, prematurity, or a wide spectrum of clinical manifestations; only severe cases are clinically apparent at birth.
  - All pregnant women should be tested.
  - Infants can be asymptomatic for up to 2 years after birth.
  - Symptoms in an infant can include chronic rhinitis or nasal congestion, "snuffles," enlarged liver and spleen, and development of a rash 1 to 2 weeks later.
  - Rash involves palms and soles; starts as pink or red and can turn dark or even coppery.

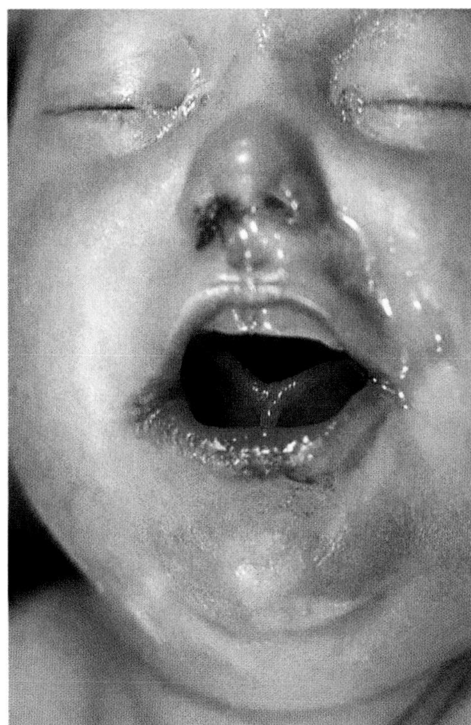

FIGURE 18–10 Infant with congenital syphilis.

- Long-bone abnormalities may occur, with possible fractures or pain, and may limit movement of the involved extremity, giving the appearance of paralysis ("pseudoparalysis of Parrot").
- Central nervous system (CNS) involvement can occur, and long term may cause seizures, hydrocephalus, developmental delay, or loss of developmental milestones.

Nursing Interventions

- Assess for localized and systemic infection.
- Infants need to have long-term follow-up care to evaluate for chronic infections.
- A lumbar puncture is needed to evaluate cerebral spinal fluid.

Child and Caregiver Education

- Give antibiotics as ordered.
- Assess for penicillin allergy, because this is the typical drug of choice.

GENETICS AND GENETIC DISORDERS

Humans are composed of almost a trillion cells of different types, each of which derives from a single cell. This single cell then differentiates, or develops, into highly specific cell types. The cell is composed of a central enclosed core, or nucleus, and the outer area, or cytoplasm, which contains fluid and other cell organelles. The nucleus houses the chromosomes, the highly organized structures that contain the genetic code, DNA. The DNA is then organized into hundreds of units of heredity, or genes. The genes are responsible for determining our physical attributes and biological functions. Under the direction of genes, the cell cytoplasm then produces products necessary for the organism's functions, such as growth, release of energy, and elimination of waste products at the cellular level.

Genetic Inheritance

- Human cells have a total of 46 chromosomes, organized into 23 complementary pairs. Each pair contains two copies, or two alleles.
- There are 22 pairs of autosomes, which both males and females have.
- There is one pair of sex chromosomes, one from each parent.
  - These are called X and Y; females have XX and males have XY.
  - The Y chromosome is only about one-third as large as the X and contains many fewer genes.
  - The presence of the Y chromosome determines "maleness."

Genetic Errors

- Defects can occur with the ongoing processes of cell reproduction
- Mitosis—cell division into identical sister cells, each with 46 chromosomes, or 23 pairs of alleles.
  - Ongoing cell mitosis is essential throughout the life span to maintain proper body function; it takes place in nearly all cells of the body.
  - Different types of cells reproduce by mitosis at different rates.
  - Skin cells divide about every 10 hours, liver cells about once a year.
  - More highly differentiated cells, such as muscle and nerve cells, may take many years to reproduce, and brain cells do not appear to reproduce or undergo mitosis after birth.
  - This accounts for the different rates in healing from injury.
  - As organisms age, the rate and ability for cells to divide decrease, limiting the body's capacity to recover.
  - Errors or changes in the process of mitosis account for diseases such as cancers, but do not contribute to inherited disorders.

Meiosis

- Meiosis is reproductive division, that is, creating four daughter cells, each one containing only 23 single alleles.
- Meiosis can only take place in the germ cell to create the reproductive gametes, the egg and sperm.
- There are two meiotic divisions, and unique to meiosis, both copies of the chromosomes match up and then are intertwined.
- The intertwined chromosomes may wrap around and then break and recombine so that portions of each are exchanged, a process called recombination.
- In the second meiotic division, the pairs are separated into the reproductive cells, or gametes, each with just 23 alleles.

- This process may result in disorders by some loss or gain of material—the reason for genetic variance.
- Nondisjunction occurs when chromosome pairs divide unequally, for example, one daughter cell with 24 chromosomes and another with 22.

Oocyte

- Oocyte is the result of meiosis in females.
- It is commonly called the egg, the female reproductive cell.
- All immature oocytes are produced during the fetal stage; the first meiotic division takes place at birth.
- Baby girls are born with a certain number of "pre-egg" cells that are arrested at an early stage of meiosis.
- In fact, the pre-egg cell does not complete meiosis until after fertilization has occurred.
- Fertilization itself triggers the culmination of the process.
- This means that meiosis in women typically takes decades and can take as long as 40 to 50 years.
- Increased maternal age can result in increased gene errors, because these oocytes have been present for the life span of the mother.

Spermatocyte

- The result of meiosis in males
- Spermatocytes are the immature sperm cells that contain 23 single chromosomes in the male
- Produced throughout the life span of the male
- The average life span of a single sperm is about 1 week to maturation within the epididymis

Reproduction

- Egg and sperm unite, forming a zygote with 46 chromosomes.
- The zygote undergoes rapid cell division to form the embryo and ultimately the fetus.
- Errors may occur during this rapid time of cell proliferation.
- Rarely, some of the cell's chromosomes are normal and others abnormal, a condition called mosaicism.

Alterations in Chromosomes and Development

- In reproduction, the 23-chromosome, or haploid, egg and sperm unite to form a diploid cell with the full 46 chromosomes; this then rapidly divides by mitosis to form the embryo and ultimately the fetus.
- Additional errors or abnormalities can occur at any time during the process, from meiosis, to mitotic division after fertilization, to cell differentiation, and organ formation and development.

Trisomy 21 (Down Syndrome)

- In about 95% of those with Down syndrome, each cell has three copies of chromosome 21, or 47 chromosomes.
- Associated with advanced maternal age (older than 35 years) with alteration in oocyte before reproduction.
- Rarely, pieces of the long arm of chromosome 21 are attached to another chromosome, usually chromosome 14, 21, or 22; this is known as translocation Down syndrome and affects about 4% of those with Down syndrome (Mai et al., 2013) (Fig. 18–11).
- Mosaicism (see earlier) is a condition where nondisjunction occurs in mitosis of the fertilized egg, resulting in a different makeup from cell to cell—some are normal and some are not—and affects about 1% of persons with Down syndrome.

Signs and Symptoms

Features of Down syndrome include (Fig. 18–12):

- Small head (microcephaly)
- Flattened, broad head with flat posterior areas
- Underdeveloped, flattened middle of face (midface hypoplasia)
- Almond-shaped, up-slanting eyes, with redundant tissue along inside
- Prominent epicanthal folds, with small, downturned mouth
- Small oral opening with protruding tongue
- Small, low-set ears that may be cupped (Fig. 18–13)
- Chest may be broad, with heart murmurs related to defects
- Short hands that may have a single crease (Fig. 18–14)
- Congenital heart defects—very high incidence rate of about 44%
- Endocardial cushion effect (atrioventricular canal)—connection between the atria, upper chambers, and ventricle, lower chambers, most common
- Low tone; can be floppy, with breathing and feeding problems at birth

Nursing Interventions

- Health-care providers are a vital link in helping parents and families to adapt to the initial shock and disappointment in learning their child has Down syndrome.
- Diagnosis is usually suspected based on physical appearance, and specific testing should take place as soon as possible to

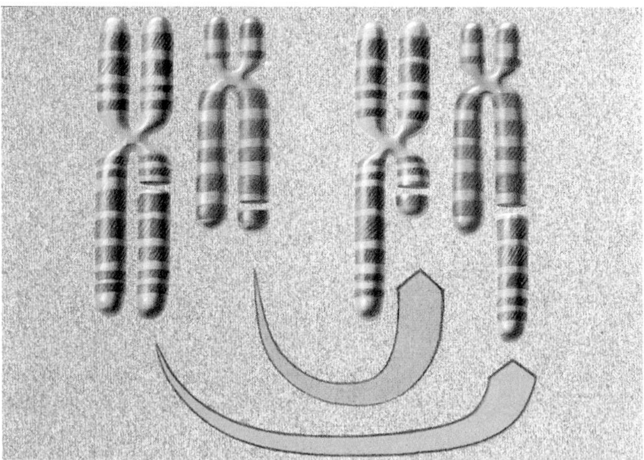

FIGURE 18–11 Translocation.

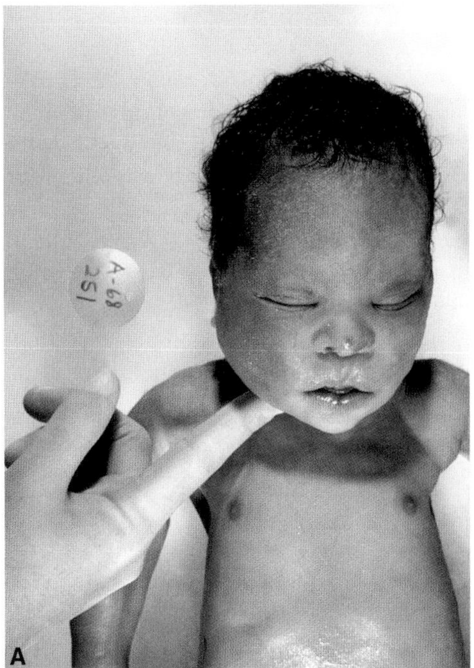

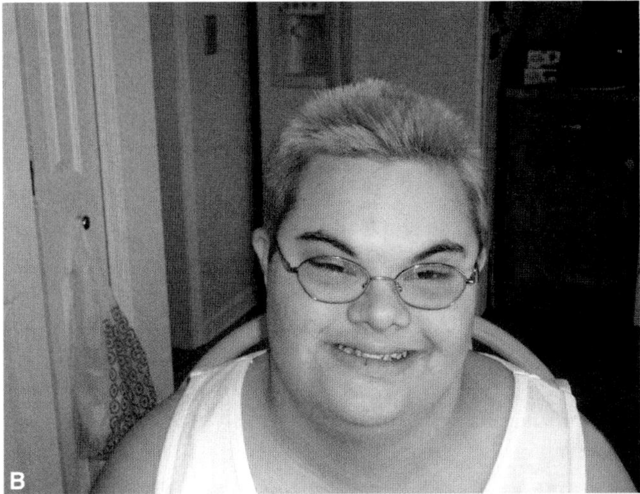

FIGURE 18–12 **A**, Infant with Down syndrome. **B**, Adolescent with Down syndrome.

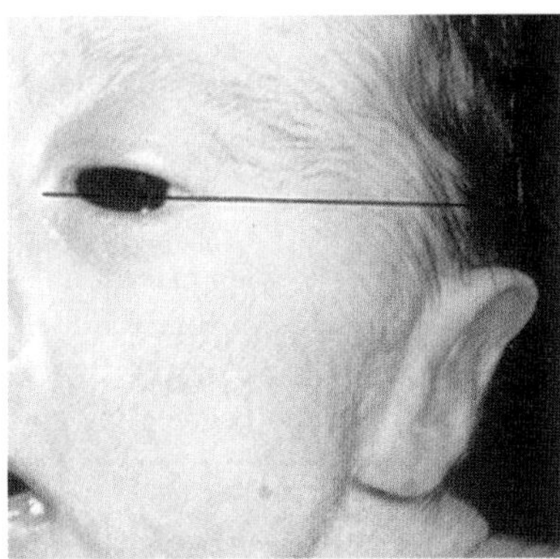

FIGURE 18–13 Low-set ears in Down syndrome.

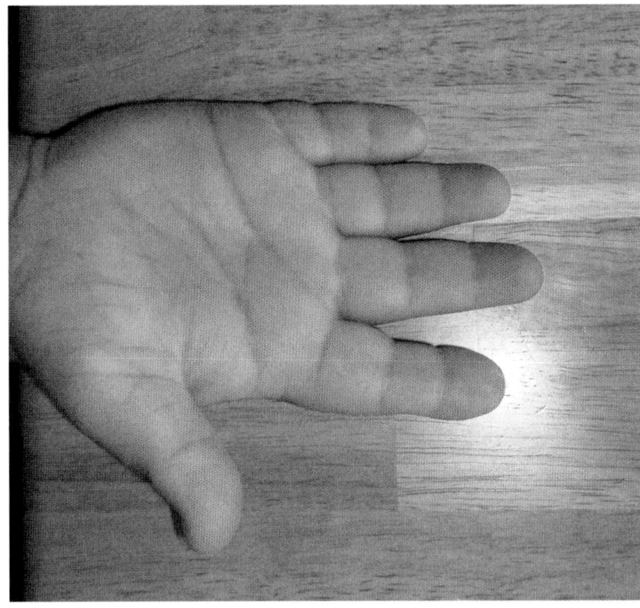

FIGURE 18–14 Hand of an adolescent with Down syndrome.

avoid diagnostic error and instances of translocation or partial duplication of trisomy 21.

- Parents should ideally be informed as soon as possible of the definitive diagnosis, by someone known to the couple, and literature about Down syndrome, as well as support groups and community supports, should be made available before discharge.
- Newborn can by hypotonic and hyperextensible, with poor feeding; the large, protruding tongue produces tendency for mouth breathing.

SAFE AND EFFECTIVE NURSING CARE: Promoting Safety

Aspects of Feeding With Down Syndrome

When feeding an infant with Down syndrome, take the following steps to assess respiration:

- Make sure the infant is well awake, and mouth and nares are cleared of mucus.
- Position correctly and steady the chin.
- May need to be burped more frequently and offered smaller, more frequent feedings.
- Monitor color and respiratory patterns, because these may be clues for congenital heart defects.
- Infants with heart defects also tire easily at feeding.

- Need strict attention to feeding and elimination related to high association of malformations of the gut.
  - Atresia of the duodenum—may have a blind pouch, so feeding may result in immediate emesis
  - Annular pancreas—wraps around the gut to cause obstruction

- Hirschsprung's disease—lack of ganglia that affects motility in the colon; can present as severe constipation or frank obstruction
- Specific growth curves for children with Down syndrome need to be used to plot weight, height, and head circumference; overall, these children are smaller, shorter, and have smaller heads, as well as increased obesity in the teen years

- Motor development takes about twice as long as in the usual child; about 90% can walk by age 3 years.
- All children with suspected delay and or known syndromes need to be referred to local early intervention services.
- Developmental delay, including intellectual disabilities, is common; IQs typically range from very low to near normal, and average around 55.
- Thyroid disease, especially hypothyroidism, is very common and needs to be monitored across the life span.
  - Newborn screens are required in all 50 states for congenital hypothyroidism.
  - Thyroid studies need to be done several times in the first years of life and then at a minimum of yearly; they are considered related to poor growth velocity.
- Immune dysfunction is common, such as abnormalities in immunoglobulin levels and other cellular types of immunity.
- The risk for pneumonia is high, although mortality is less frequent with modern antibiotics.
- Ear infections are more common, in part due to anatomy and known immune dysfunction, and the risk for both conductive and sensorineural hearing loss is higher as well.
- Musculoskeletal concerns related to joint laxity are common.
  - Instability of the neck, specifically at the area between the first and second cervical vertebrae or atlanto-axial joint, is also possible.
  - Routine films for this condition are believed to have poor sensitivity; regular and careful assessment of young children with Down syndrome and monitoring for signs and symptoms of cervical cord changes—such as in gait, flexion, and bladder or bowel function—are more sensitive.
  - Protection of the spinal cord through avoidance of high-risk sports and neutral neck positioning, including during surgery and dental procedures, should be implemented for all children with Down syndrome.
- Malignancies are also more common with Down syndrome, and incidence of leukemia is about 18 times greater than in the general population (see Chapter 19).
- Skin problems, such as dry skin and allergic dermatitis, are also very common.
- Hair loss and thin hair may be evident.
- Sleep problems, including obstructive sleep apnea, are associated with a narrow posterior throat (hypopharynx) and hypotonia, even with a relatively normal size of the tonsils and adenoids. Even children presumed to be asymptomatic should be referred to a sleep center for a polysomnogram (sleep study) by 4 years old (AAP, 2011; Bull & Committee on Genetics, 2011; Santor, Yin, & Hopkin, 2017).
- Suspicion should be raised if parents or caregivers note snoring or unusual sleeping positions, such as with the head hyperextended, looking up and back, or on the stomach with the knees drawn up, as well as restless, disturbed sleep.

Trisomy 18 (Edward's Syndrome)

- Each chromosome has three copies of chromosome 18; this is the second most common trisomy after Down syndrome.
- Characterized by prenatal growth deficiency, craniofacial features, characteristic hand gestures with overriding fingers, nail hypoplasia, and short sternum.
- Internal anomalies and severe heart defects are common.
- A bedside scoring system has been developed to help clinicians without specialized training make the diagnosis of trisomy 18 in the newborn period.

Trisomy 13 (Patau Syndrome)

- Trisomy 13 is the least common and most severe of the viable autosomal trisomies.
- Average survival is fewer than 3 days.

Nursing Interventions (Trisomy 18 and Trisomy 13)

- A plan for minimal intervention can be initiated from the time of delivery.
- Provide support and end-of-life care as necessary.

Caregiver Education (Trisomy 18 and Trisomy 13)

- Central apnea and its presence with other congenital malformations may result in death within a few weeks (see Chapter 5 for end-of-life issues).
- Although severe heart defects are noted, these alone do not account for early death, and some may be amenable to surgeries.
- At 1 year of age, 5% to 10% of children may be alive without any extraordinary means of support, and may exhibit very slow developmental gains in milestones (Carey, 2005; Weremowicz, 2017).
- Some children do live to later childhood years, but this is rare.
- It is impossible to predict whether an infant with Trisomy 13 or 18 will live beyond the first year of life, even if the infant does not require a ventilator.

Turner Syndrome

- Result of chromosomal loss of entire X chromosome (45, X)
- Only known disorder where a fetus can survive despite loss of an entire chromosome
- Affects only girls; no known living males with 45, Y
- Usually the result of abnormal meiotic error in the sperm
- Girls receive no sex chromosome from the sperm of the father and receive the X from the mother

Signs and Symptoms

- Prematurity
- Feeding difficulties, with spitting, emesis, and difficulty latching on
- Frank gastroesophageal reflux and failure to thrive

Physical Assessment Findings

- Often webbed, thick, short neck or nuchal folds
- Short stature
- Broad "shieldlike" chest with wide-spaced nipples
- Nonfunctional ovaries
- Common to have thyroid dysfunction
- Common to find heart defects
  - Obstruction of the left side of the heart
  - Coarctation or narrowing of the aorta
- Most affected girls have normal intelligence, but many have visual-perceptual impairments that predispose them to nonverbal learning disabilities.
- Endocrine disorders result in short stature that can be improved with growth hormone injections.
- Absence of a single kidney (renal agenesis), horseshoe kidney, duplication of the collecting system, and aberrant renal arteries can occur.
- Approximately one-fifth to one-third of affected girls are identified at birth because of the presence of lymphedema, a notable swelling or puffiness of the hands and feet (Gravholt et al., 2017; Sybert, 2005).

Nursing Interventions

- Anticipate feeding difficulties and be patient when feeding.
- Lack of secondary sexual characteristics by mid-teens may be the first symptom noted.
- Assess for hypothyroidism.
- Assess for cardiovascular disorders.
- Baseline electrocardiograms and then monitoring on a regular basis are recommended.

Child and Caregiver Education

- Lack of pubertal development can be treated with estrogen supplementation so that girls can develop secondary sexual characteristics; however, they will remain infertile.
- Endocrine referral is recommended so that growth hormone treatment can be started early.
- Provide anticipatory guidance on obesity, which can become a problem in later childhood and adult life.
- Height and weight are usually within normal parameters at birth, and then deceleration of height velocity continues.

Cri Du Chat Syndrome

- "Cat cry" syndrome—the result of a deletion or loss of a portion of chromosome 5 (Fig. 18–15)

Assessment

- Distinctive high-pitched, catlike cry
- Profound microcephaly, round face with widely spaced eyes, epicanthal folds, and low-set ears; significant intellectual disability

Nursing Interventions

- Supportive care—feeding issues and poor growth
- All children with this diagnosis need early referral to genetics and neurology

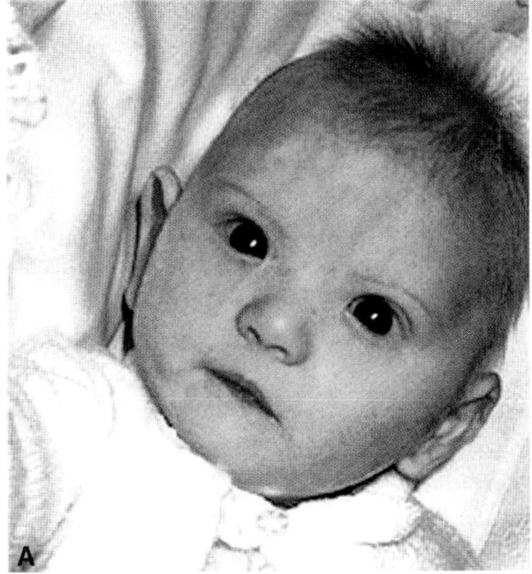

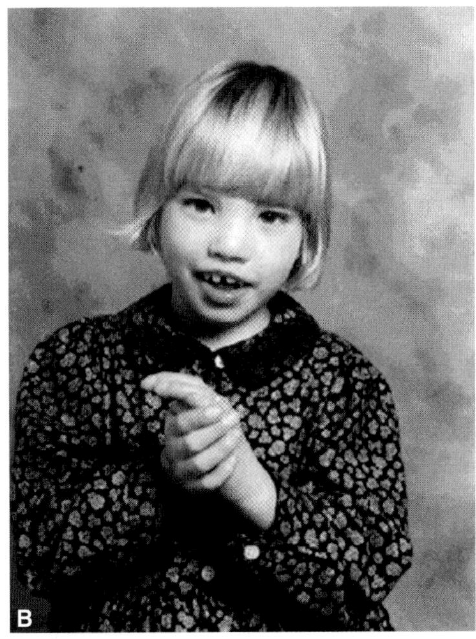

FIGURE 18–15 **A,** Infant with cri du chat. **B,** School-age child with cri du chat. *(© Genetic Diseases, http://www.genetic-diseases.net, with permission)*

Caregiver Education

- Severe CNS irritability and minimal developmental progress of the child put family members at very high risk for depression.
- Provide education and information regarding family support groups.

Williams Syndrome

- Result of a microdeletion in the long arm of chromosome 7 (7q11.23)

Assessment

- Characteristic pattern of dysmorphic facial features:
  - Broad forehead
  - Bitemporal narrowing
  - Low nasal root
  - Periorbital fullness

- Stellate/lacy iris pattern
- Bulbous nasal tip
- Strabismus (crossed or wandering eyes)
- Long philtrum, full lips, wide mouth
- Full cheeks, small jaw
- Prominent earlobes
- Malocclusion of the teeth and a long neck in older children

- Developmental delay
  - IQ scores on standard tests range from severe intellectual delay to low normal
  - Highly verbal and overly sociable, "cocktail personality"
- Connective tissue abnormalities, including cardiovascular disease
  - Hoarse and deep voice, hernias, soft and loose skin, joint laxity or limitation
  - Supravalvular aortic stenosis

Nursing Interventions

- Affected children often have severe feeding difficulties and short stature; growth and height should be plotted on Williams syndrome growth curve chart.
- Idiopathic infantile hypercalcemia is a distinctive feature of children with Williams syndrome, contributing to the presence of extreme irritability, vomiting, constipation, and muscle cramps associated with this condition.
- Excess calcium and vitamin D should be avoided because persistent elevated calcium in the urine (hypercalciuria) contributes to renal stones (nephrocalcinosis) (Sindhar, 2016).
- Difficulty with gross motor function and depth perception; very difficult to negotiate uneven surfaces and stairs.
- Attention deficit-hyperactivity disorder (ADHD) is present in about 70%. Children are overly friendly to others, especially adults, and may have generalized anxiety (Mervis & John, 2010).
- Elastin problems cause arterial defects, including supravalvular aortic stenosis, but can involve any artery and lead to morbidity and mortality.

Child and Caregiver Education

- Puberty commonly occurs early (anticipatory guidance needed)
- Difficulty with handwriting, drawing, buttoning, and pattern construction; poor math skills; strong memory for auditory information, such as instructions read out loud

Velocardial Facial Syndrome

- Results from a microdeletion in the q, or long arm, of chromosome 22 at the 11th position (22q11 deletion)

Assessment

- Variable physical presentations: congenital heart disease, palate abnormalities, immune system dysfunction including autoimmune disease, low calcium (hypocalcemia) and other endocrine abnormalities such as thyroid problems and growth hormone deficiency, GI problems, feeding difficulties, kidney abnormalities, hearing loss, seizures, skeletal abnormalities, minor facial differences, and learning and behavioral differences
- The symptoms of this condition are extremely variable, even among members of the same family who are affected
- Because of the variability in the severity of defects, this deletion in the same gene has been described under many different names, for example, VCF syndrome, DiGeorge syndrome, CATCH 22, Sphrintzen syndrome, Cayler syndrome, deletion 22q11 syndrome, and conotruncal anomaly face syndrome (McDonald-McGinn et al., 2015)
- No specific criteria for diagnosis are noted because of variability, but presence of cleft palate and heart defects should indicate need for chromosomal testing
- Right-sided heart defects or defects of the aortic arch, including:
  - Right-sided, double or interrupted, ventriculoseptal defect
  - Pulmonary atresia
  - Tetralogy of Fallot
  - Aberrant subclavian arteries
  - Tracheal ring
- Characteristic but subtle facial appearance
  - Increased vertical length
  - Long cylindrical or tubular nose
  - Small posterior jaw (retrognathia)
  - Hooded upper eyelids
- Mild developmental delays
  - Learning disabilities
  - Social immaturity
  - Hypernasal speech
  - Impulsivity
  - Anxiety or phobias
- Classic DiGeorge sequence includes absent thymus, hypocalcemia, and immune deficiency with characteristic facial features
- Cayler syndrome, also known as asymmetric crying face syndrome, with unusual "crying" mouth and face asymmetry with movement, as well as heart defects

Nursing Interventions

- Vascular anomalies and heart defects can be noted in the newborn nursery as murmurs, feeding difficulties, color change, and stridor or breathing difficulty related to vascular rings.
- Seizures can occur related to hypocalcemia.
- Aspiration pneumonias may occur in relation to immune dysfunction and cleft palate.
- Hypotonia can lead to breathing problems.
- Low gut motility is also seen with constipation.
- Immune disorders can lead to chronic upper and lower respiratory infections.
- Sensorineural hearing loss is present in up to 15% of cases (McDonald-McGinn, 2015; Shprintzen, 2005).

Caregiver Education

- Provide education on prevention of constipation.
- Provide education on prevention of chronic respiratory infections.
- Promote good hand hygiene.

Phenylketonuria

- Phenylketonuria (PKU) is caused by a single mutation at a single site or base pair mutation.
- PKU results in abnormality in the production of phenylalanine hydroxylase (PAH), the enzyme that breaks down the protein phenylalanine.
- More than 950 PAH gene variants have been identified in people with PKU (Blau, 2016).
- The result is accumulation of phenylalanine in the blood and brain, causing brain damage with progressive intellectual disability.
- Testing for PKU is performed during the newborn period (Fig. 18–16).

Assessment

- Affected children appear completely asymptomatic at birth, although commonly fair, blonde, and blue-eyed, then progressive intellectual disability occurs.

Nursing Interventions

- All 50 states now screen for PKU as part of standard newborn screening. Ensure the screening is performed when child has been fed full-strength formula or breast milk, ideally for 48 hours.

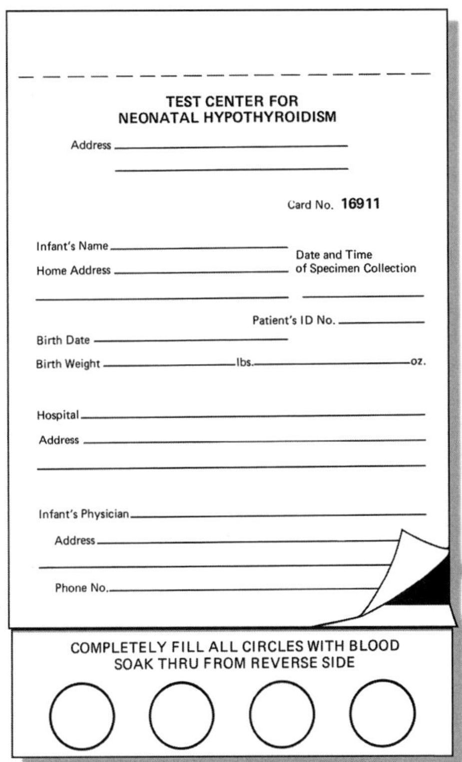

TEST CENTER FOR
NEONATAL HYPOTHYROIDISM
Address

Card No. 16911

Infant's Name
Home Address
Date and Time of Specimen Collection
Patient's ID No.
Birth Date
Birth Weight lbs. oz.
Hospital
Address
Infant's Physician
Address
Phone No.

COMPLETELY FILL ALL CIRCLES WITH BLOOD
SOAK THRU FROM REVERSE SIDE

Example of Specimen Card
with Essential Information Requested

FIGURE 18–16 Specimen card to test for phenylketonuria.

- During development, must regularly measure phenylalanine level because some individuals have a residual amount of the enzyme.
- Phenylalanine is an essential protein; it cannot be removed completely from the human diet, but caregivers need to provide a phenylalanine-free formula and low-protein diet with very close monitoring by a nutrition specialist.
- The fetus needs to have phenylalanine to develop.

Child and Caregiver Education

- Women with PKU can become pregnant.
- Teens often want to disregard the diet; encourage compliance and measuring serum levels.
- Once brain injury occurs, it is irreversible, so the restrictive diet is recommended for life.
- Once screened as abnormal, individuals require immediate referral to a geneticist and a metabolic nutritionist for information on protein restriction and replacement formula.
- Can continue to breastfeed without risk for brain injury.
- Pregnant women with PKU need referral to a high-risk center with nutrition and genetics support, and ideally pregnancies should be planned.

Neurofibromatosis, Type 1 (Von Recklinghausen's Disease)

- Also known as peripheral neurofibromatosis; the result of a single "non-sense" mutation on the long arm of chromosome 17, locus 11.2 (17q11.2) (North, 2000)
- Autosomal dominant inheritance pattern—presence of just one copy of the abnormal 17q11.2 mutation plus one normal allele results in the disease syndrome
- There is a 50% chance with each pregnancy that the newborn will inherit the disease syndrome from an affected parent

Assessment

- Wide range of variability
- Neurofibromin is a tumor-suppressor protein; absence of neurofibromin results in multiple tumors that form on the body and in the brain
- Instead of neurofibromin, a useless protein is produced
- Variable expression in different individuals; various physical presentations
- Age-related abnormal tissue proliferation caused by lack of neurofibromin
- Seven recognized cutaneous manifestations (change based on age; develop over time)
- Diagnosis is usually clinical, and the presence of just two of seven characteristics is considered enough to make a clinical diagnosis
- The presence or number of these physical characteristics does not, however, indicate the ultimate severity of the disease or long-term prognosis

Seven Criteria for Diagnosing Neurofibromatosis Type 1 (Viskochil, 2005)

1. Six or more café au lait macules, patches, or spots; pigmented birthmarks, more than 5 mm in greatest diameter

in prepubertal children, or more than 15 mm in greatest diameter after puberty
- The name café au lait is French for "milky coffee" and refers to their light-brown color (Fig. 18–17).
- These can be present from birth, but others may develop later.

2. Two or more neurofibromas of any type, or one or more plexiform neurofibroma
   - Neurofibromas are benign nerve sheath tumors. They arise from the supportive tissue within the nerve itself.
   - As these neurofibroma tumors grow, they displace and compress important nerve fascicles within the nerve. This causes pain, weakness, and numbness.
   - Although neurofibromas are frequently solitary and occur at random, they can also occur in multiple locations in patients with neurofibromatosis.
3. "Freckling" in the axillary or inguinal regions—minute irregular and sometimes raised areas
4. Optic glioma—enlargements of the optic nerve; symptomatic lesions usually seen after age 3 years as progressive visual loss (National Institute of Neurological Disorders and Stroke [NINDS], 2017)
   - Optic pathway gliomas occur in 15% of children younger than 6 years with neurofibromatosis type 1 (NF-1); they may rarely occur in older children and adults.
   - Presence of optic gliomas is usually asymptomatic but can cause progressive visual loss, loss of color sensitivity, and possible bulging of the eyes as tumors become enlarged.
   - They are low-grade tumors; injury results from location along the optic pathways.
   - Incidence is enough to recommend serial eye examinations by a pediatric ophthalmologist on a regular basis for children with known NF-1 up to age 6 years.
   - Annual magnetic resonance imaging (MRI) may be recommended until age 6 years for detection, and more frequently if present.
   - Screening MRI is not currently recommended unless presence is suspected by eye examination. Still, many clinicians often opt for a screening MRI of the brain and orbits at 1 to 2 and 2 to 3 years of age to detect optic pathway tumors before they become symptomatic, primarily because of the difficulty assessing vision in this age group.
   - Eye examinations should be performed every 3 to 6 months until age 6 years and then yearly after that time.
5. Two or more Lisch nodules (iris hamartomas)
   - Lisch nodules characteristically are raised, often pigmented hamartomas of the iris and represent a relatively specific finding for NF-1.
   - These do not affect vision in any manner.
   - These are present in only about 10% of children with NF-1 at age 6 years, but in nearly 90% of adults (Lewis & Riccardi, 1981; NINDS, 2017).
   - A slit-lamp examination by an ophthalmologist is recommended but may be seen without this examination in persons with light or blue iris color.
6. A distinctive bony lesion such as sphenoid dysplasia or thinning of the long bone cortex with or without pseudoarthrosis
   - A pseudoarthrosis, or false joint, is formed by nonunion of bone fragments. Pseudoarthrosis in NF-1 results from impaired healing caused by bone dysplasia and may severely compromise the function of the limb.
   - Sphenoid dysplasia describes abnormalities of the sphenoid bone, commonly seen by computed tomography (CT) scan, and can result in asymmetry of the face.
   - Scoliosis, sideways curving, and kyphosis, anterior curvature, can be seen in 10% to 25% of children with NF-1, often presenting around 6 to 10 years of age or early adolescence.
7. A first-degree relative (parent, sibling, or offspring) with NF-1 based on the previous six criteria
   - Genetic testing is increasingly being used in the diagnosis of NF-1 for patients who meet only the two criteria of café au lait spots and axillary freckling, because these can be seen in other conditions as well (see Fig. 18–17).
   - If the child is the first identified case in the family, a clinician with experience with NF-1 needs to examine the parents; however, the criteria of a first-degree relative cannot be used for diagnosis in that parent, two of the other criteria must be met.

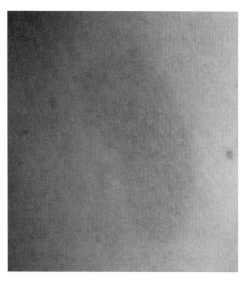

FIGURE 18–17 Café au lait spot on left arm.

Nursing Interventions

- Obtaining and plotting accurate growth parameters, including height, weight, and head circumference, at every visit is recommended. Children with NF-1 are almost always macrocephalic, with larger head circumference than typical peers.
- Blood pressure should also be checked yearly at minimum because of high incidence of hypertension.
- Infants can present with a single or a few café au lait spots in early childhood; then other changes develop over time. Careful skin examinations during bathing and diaper changing are always necessary.
- Initially children with NF-1 can grow normally, but there is a higher incidence of short stature related to less growth throughout the pubertal growth spurt.
- Scoliosis is also seen and should be screened for at every examination starting in early childhood.
- Growth curves specific for NF-1 have been published.
- Complications of NF-1 result from direct involvement of multiple organ systems by plexiform neurofibromas.

- The lifelong risk for malignancy in affected individuals is increased.
- Malignant peripheral nerve sheath tumors represent the most common neoplasm, occurring in approximately 5% to 10% of individuals with NF-1 (NINDS, 2017).

Health Supervision for Children With Neurofibromatosis

- NF-1 is associated with an increased incidence of intellectual disability (4% to 8%) compared with 3% risk for all persons.
- Usually, overall intellectual abilities are in the average to low-average range.
- In contrast, specific learning disabilities are observed in as many as 40% to 60% of affected children, and impaired performance on at least one test of academic achievement is present in 65% of children with NF-1.
- ADHD also occurs more frequently in children with NF-1.
- Children with NF-1 have a higher likelihood of being hypotonic and having subtle neurological abnormalities that affect balance and gait.
- Speech problems also may occur.
- Because of these issues, and autosomal dominant inheritance, parents may have multiple children with learning and physical problems, and may also be affected themselves.
- Child psychology and referral for early intervention and then special education evaluation are recommended if there are any developmental delays or concerns.

Neurofibromatosis, Type 2

- Neurofibromatosis type 2 (NF-2) is less common than NF-1.
- Symptoms usually appear in the teens or young adulthood.
- Tumors frequently occur on the auditory nerve, causing:
  - Hearing loss
  - Ringing in the ears
  - Problems with balance
- Problems with hearing and balance worsen over time, causing greater disability than children experience with NF-1 (NINDS, 2017).

Assessment

- General physical examination
- Thorough skin examination
- Hearing evaluation

SAFE AND EFFECTIVE NURSING CARE: Clinical Pearl

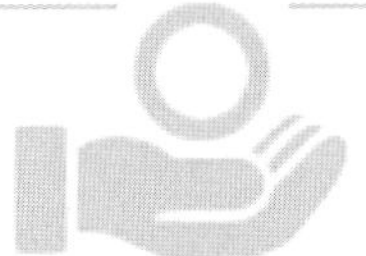

Comparing Neurofibromatosis Types 1 and 2

Children with NF-2 do not have the café au lait spots or axillary freckling that is seen in NF-1, but they do exhibit similar tumors on the skin. There are different risks then for optic glioma with NF-1 or hearing loss caused by tumors in the auditory canal with NF-2.

Diagnosis

- Diagnosis is based on clinical findings.
- MRI of the brain and auditory nerve should be performed.
- An electroencephalogram (EEG) should be performed if seizures occur.
- A blood test can be performed to evaluate for a genetic marker.

Nursing Interventions

- Treatment focuses on managing the symptoms.
- Sometimes the neurofibromas are removed by surgery.
- Referral to an audiologist is necessary because of the problems with hearing.
- Physical therapy can be helpful in treating the problems with balance.
- Seizures can usually be controlled with medication.
- A child may need specialized educational plans because learning problems are common.
- Psychological therapy may be needed for children and adolescents with self-esteem problems because of the visible tumors.

Tuberous Sclerosis

- Tuberous sclerosis (TSC) causes benign growths called "tubers" to form on different body organs, including the brain, eyes, kidneys, heart, skin, and lungs (Behrman, Kliegman, Jenson, & Stanton, 2007; TS Assic, 2017).
- It occurs in approximately 1 in 6,000 births.
- A child of a parent with TSC has a 50% chance of inheriting the disorder.
- Skin lesions are called ash leaf lesions, which are patches of skin with less color or pigment than other skin.
- Symptoms of TSC include:
  - Mild skin abnormalities
  - Lung tumors
  - Heart tumors
  - Tumors in the retina or along the optic nerve
  - Kidney failure
  - Seizures
  - Intellectual disability

Assessment

- General physical examination
- Thorough skin examination
- Measurement and documentation of skin lesions

Diagnosis

- Diagnosis is based on clinical findings.
- A baseline MRI of the brain should be performed and then repeated as the child grows to monitor for tumors.
- Screening studies of the heart, lungs, kidneys, and eyes should be performed at regular intervals.
- An EEG should be performed if seizures occur.

Nursing Interventions

- The treatment focuses on managing the symptoms.
- Sometimes surgery is required to remove tumors from vital organs.

- Medication may be needed to treat seizures.
- A child may need specialized educational plans if learning is a problem.
- Genetic counseling is recommended.

SAFE AND EFFECTIVE NURSING CARE: Clinical Pearl

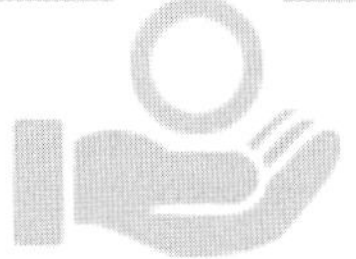

Diagnosing Tuberous Sclerosis

The specific tests that are performed depend on the age of the individual who is suspected of having TSC and may include:

- MRI scan of the brain
- CT scan of the lungs, liver, and kidneys
- Ultrasound scan of the kidneys
- Echocardiogram ultrasound to examine the structures of the heart
- Eye examination to look for abnormalities of the retina
- Skin examination under ultraviolet light
- Genetic testing to diagnose and/or confirm a diagnosis of TSC

Sturge-Weber Syndrome

- Sturge-Weber syndrome is a rare condition caused by a spontaneous genetic mutation in the GNAC gene that affects the skin and the brain.
- This mutation cannot be transmitted from parent to child (Shirley et al., 2013).
- The symptoms vary widely, and some patients are undiagnosed for many years.
- The most common symptom is a skin lesion called a port-wine stain that is present at birth (DeSai & Glasier, 2017).
    - This is so named for its distinctive purple-red color that gives the appearance of "spilled wine"; it usually covers at least one eyelid and a portion of the forehead.
- Blood vessel growths called angiomas can occur on the brain.
    - These lesions can cause seizures, usually occurring before the first birthday.
    - The seizures tend to worsen with age and may be convulsions on the opposite side of the body from the skin discoloration.
    - These angiomas may or may not be surgically repairable, depending on their size and location.
- Glaucoma is also common, usually in the eye affected by the port-wine stain. The eye may sometimes become enlarged.
- Children with Sturge-Weber syndrome are also at higher risk for strokes.

Assessment

- General physical examination
- Careful skin examination

Diagnosis

- Diagnosis is based on physical findings.
- An MRI of the brain and the brain blood vessels should be performed to evaluate for angiomas.
- An EEG may be performed if the child experiences seizures.

Nursing Interventions

- Treatment is aimed at symptom management.
- In some cases, laser surgery can be done for infants as young as 1 month to reduce the size (and therefore the long-term effects) of the port-wine stain lesion.
- Seizures and glaucoma can be managed with medications.
- Screening should be done for angiomas.
- Measures to prevent stroke should be instituted, such as weight management and control of blood pressure, blood glucose levels, and blood lipids.

Charcot-Marie-Tooth Disease

- Charcot-Marie-Tooth (CMT) disease is an inherited neurological disease characterized by a slowly progressive degeneration of the muscles in the foot, lower leg, hand, and forearm, and a mild loss of sensation in the limbs, fingers, and toes.
- The first sign of CMT is generally a high-arched foot or gait disturbances.
- Symptoms usually manifest in late childhood or adolescence and usually begin with foot drop, in which the child cannot dorsiflex the foot.
- Some children experience development of hammer toes, where the toes remain curled.
- Later wasting of the lower leg gives the appearance of an inverted champagne bottle or a stork's leg.
    - The leg exhibits hypertrophy of the proximal muscles.
    - The peroneal muscles show marked atrophy.
    - The distal portion of the extremities is thin due to the atrophied muscles.
- As the condition progresses, other weaknesses can occur in the pelvis and trunk (NINDS, 2012).
- CMT disease can be divided into two classes, depending on where the dysfunction occurs in the peripheral nerves:
    - In CMT type 1, the peripheral nerves' axons, the part of the nerve cell that transmits electrical signals to the muscles, lose their protective outer coverings (myelin sheaths). This disrupts the axons' function.
    - In CMT type 2, the axons' responses are diminished because of a defect within the axons themselves. CMT type 2, the less common of the two classes, can be further separated into at least six subtypes, caused by defects in different genes.

Assessment

- Thorough physical examination
- Thorough history of the child's illness

Diagnosis

- Diagnosis is made based on symptoms.
- Blood can be tested for genetic markers for this disorder.
- Electromyography is done to determine the extent of the disease.
- Nerve conduction velocity studies are done to determine the speed of the electrical signal through the nerves. Delayed or weakened responses indicate a neuropathy such as CMT.
- Nerve biopsy is done to confirm the disease. A small piece of a peripheral nerve is taken from the calf of the leg.

Nursing Interventions

- Treatment is supportive care for the child and prevention of further disability.

Achondroplasia

- Achondroplasia is one of a group of disorders called chondrodystrophies or osteochondrodysplasias.
- It is a bone growth disorder that causes the most common type of dwarfism.
- It is the most common form of disproportionate short stature.
- Occurs once in every 15,000 to 40,000 live births (National Organization for Rare Disorders, 2017).
- Achondroplasia is caused by a gene alteration (mutation) in the *FGFR3* gene on chromosome 4, short arm (4p16.3).
- The *FGFR3* gene makes a protein called fibroblast growth factor receptor 3 that is involved in converting cartilage to bone.
- *FGFR3* is the only gene known to be associated with achondroplasia.
- It may be inherited as an autosomal dominant trait, so there is a 50% chance for affected parent to pass to his or her child.
- Most cases appear as spontaneous mutations. More than 80% of individuals who have achondroplasia have parents with normal stature and are born with achondroplasia as a result of a new (de novo) mutation of parental gamete (Bacino, 2017; Pauli, 2005).
- Infants born to two parents with achondroplasia have a 50% chance of having achondroplasia, but a 25% chance of inheriting the abnormal gene from both parents, resulting in "double dominant dwarfism"; these infants may be stillborn or live only a few months.

Assessment

- The typical appearance of achondroplastic dwarfism can be seen at birth
- Some cases are now identified in utero by routine prenatal ultrasound
- Prenatal ultrasound may show excessive amniotic fluid surrounding the unborn infant (polyhydramnios)
- There may be signs of hydrocephalus
- X-ray films of the long bones can reveal achondroplasia in the newborn
- Disproportionately large head-to-body-size difference (macrocephaly) with specific facial features, such as a prominent forehead (frontal bossing) and mid-face hypoplasia (flattening)
- Shortened arms and legs (especially the upper arm and thigh)
- Short stature
  - Significantly below the average height for a person of the same age and sex
  - Adult height is generally 4 feet for men and women
  - Individuals rarely reach 5 feet in height
- Decreased muscle tone (hypotonia)
- Spinal stenosis
  - Narrowing of the spinal column that causes pressure on the spinal cord
  - Narrowing of the openings (called neural foramina) where spinal nerves leave the spinal column
- Abnormal hand appearance with persistent space between the long and ring fingers—a trident-shaped hand
- Bowed legs (see Chapter 20)
- Defects of the joints at the knee that may later cause premature joint degeneration and pain
- Clubbed feet can also occur (see Chapter 20)

Nursing Interventions

- There is no specific treatment for achondroplasia
- Intelligence and life span are normal for most persons with this condition
- Prenatal diagnosis
  - Close, high-risk monitoring of a mother carrying a child with achondroplasia
  - Close monitoring for mothers with achondroplasia themselves
- Children affected with achondroplasia commonly have delayed motor milestones related to tone
- Should be referred for early intervention
- Growth curves
  - Track appropriate head circumference, weight, and height with close attention to weight-for-height curves specific to achondroplasia.
- Sudden death may occur
  - In the first year of life, central apnea related to abnormalities or narrowing of the foramen magnum and cord compression may occur.
  - Careful neurological examination, noting for any changes or loss of function, sleep study (polysomnogram), and CT/MRI of the craniocervical junction are recommended.
- Great care needs to be taken with any neck manipulation, such as preparing for intubation
- Upper airway obstruction can occur
  - Related to tone and relatively small posterior airway, the hypopharynx
  - About 5% of persons with achondroplasia may require tracheostomy
- Related abnormalities
  - Spinal stenosis and spinal cord compression, which should be treated by neurosurgery when they cause problems such as pain or change in gait

- Obstructive sleep apnea due to decreased tone and obesity
- Increased incidence of otitis media

Caregiver Education

- Parents need to be instructed to use caution and care when lifting the infant and to only use infant carriers with firm backs that provide good neck support.
- Child should be placed in rear-facing car seat for as long as possible.
- Unsupported sitting should not be encouraged until the child has adequate trunk muscle strength, including discouraging the use of infant walkers or "excer-saucer"-type seating and infant swings that can cause excessive head movement and have poor trunk support.

X-Linked Hydrocephalus

- X-linked recessive disorder (Haridas & Tomita, 2017) caused by mutation mapped to Xq28, L1CAM protein
- Because girls have one typical and one atypical X, they do not present with symptoms, but males are affected
- The most common genetic form of congenital hydrocephalus
- Stenosis of the aqueduct of Sylvius causing obstruction (Haridas & Tomita, 2017; Schrander-Stumpel & Fryns, 1998)
- This disorder is due to mutations in the gene encoding L1, a neuronal cell adhesion molecule that belongs to the immunoglobulin "superfamily" and is essential in neurological development

Assessment

- Approximately 50% of affected boys have adducted thumbs (held inward toward the palms), which is helpful in making the diagnosis.
- Some have other CNS abnormalities:
  - Malformation of the corpus callosum
  - Small brainstem
  - Absence of the pyramidal tract
- Mutations in L1 also result in other conditions, known as the L1 spectrum, which is characterized by neurological abnormalities and mental retardation.
  - These include MASA spectrum (mental retardation, aphasia, shuffling gait, adducted thumbs), X-linked spastic paraplegia type 1, and X-linked agenesis of the corpus callosum.

Nursing Interventions

- Close monitoring of head circumference and then management of a CNS shunt if placed
- Assessment for age-appropriate developmental milestones

Caregiver Education

- Prenatal diagnosis may be made based on ultrasound and then amniocentesis.
- Referral to early intervention and neurosurgery, neurology, and developmental specialists is necessary.

Fragile X Syndrome

- Fragile X syndrome (FXS) is formerly known as fragile X mental retardation syndrome.
- It is a result of decreased or absent levels of fragile X mental retardation protein (FMRP) due to a mutation in the fragile X mental retardation (*FMR1*) gene located at Xq27.3.
- Males inherit a single X chromosome from their mother and, therefore, show many more symptoms if there is a mutation present.
- Females have two copies of the X chromosome; they may inherit an abnormal X from one parent, but a typical X from the other. Only one X per cell is active; the other is said to be inactivated. Therefore, females can show varying symptoms, from only a few to very severe (Hagerman & McCandless, 2005; Van Esch, 2017).
- Fragile X is caused by an expansion, a series of repeats, in the DNA at Xq27.3. This number of repeats generally accounts for the severity of symptoms.
- Most individuals have between 5 and 40 repeats; 41 to 58 repeats is called an intermediate or gray-zone; 59 to 200 is called premutation; and more than 200 is referred to as full mutation.
- Repeats of more than 200 essentially turn off production of FMRP.
- Typically, mutated genes are passed on in a relatively stable fashion.
- In fragile X, when passed on from mother to children, the number of repeats tends to "expand," with more repeats at each generation. The greater the number of premutation repeats a mother may have, the more likely the child will inherit a full mutation.
- An affected father will pass the mutation to his daughters, but they tend to contract, or have less repeats. Daughters do not inherit the full mutation from an affected father, but become carriers.
- Males that possess the full FMR1 mutation of more than 200 repeats are considered fully affected and have FXS.

SAFE AND EFFECTIVE NURSING CARE: Clinical Pearl

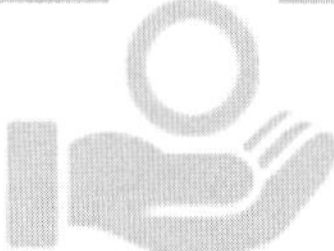

Diagnosing Fragile X

Males and females may have FXS, and not all males are severely affected. All children diagnosed with global developmental delay or autism should have specific fragile X testing. FXS cannot be detected with a standard chromosome test or microarray. A specific test, the FMR1 DNA Test for Fragile X, must be ordered.

Assessment

- Males with more than 200 repeats tend to have physical features such as:
  - Long, narrow face
  - Prominent jaw and forehead
  - Large, protruding ears

- High, arched palate
- Loose connective tissue
- Loose connective tissue can cause:
  - Hyperextensible joints
  - Flat feet
  - Mitral valve dysfunction
- After puberty, men have remarkably enlarged testicles (macro-orchidism)
- Males with FXS often have intellectual disabilities, including:
  - Issues with communication, generally speech and language delays
  - IQ in mild-to-moderate intellectual disability range
  - Hyperactivity
- Stereotypic behaviors may also be displayed, such as the following:
  - Hand flapping
  - Lack of eye contact and inattention
  - Aggression and anxiety
  - Higher incidence of meeting criteria of autistic spectrum disorder
- Females with the full mutation often have the following characteristics:
  - Subtler facial features
  - Less severe degrees of developmental delay and speech and language issues
  - Higher IQ than males with FXS
- Females who are direct carriers occur more frequently, although significant shyness and anxiety may be evident (Hagerman & McCandless, 2005; Van Esch, 2017).

Nursing Interventions

- Routine well-child care and immunizations should be performed.
- Seizures occur in about 20% of those affected.
- Newborns can have feeding issues, and mild motor delays are common.
- Language delays tend to appear between 2 and 3 years of age, and autistic features such as hand flapping and hand biting, poor eye contact, and social anxiety and shyness may appear as well.
- Stimulants and parental guidance are necessary to address behaviors and hyperactivity.
- Complications include eye issues such as alignment errors (strabismus) and orthopedic issues with joint laxity and flat feet related to the connective tissue defects.
- Heart murmurs require echocardiograms and monitoring of the mitral valve.

Caregiver Education

- Daughters do not inherit the full mutation from an affected father, but become carriers.
- Genetic counseling concerning pregnancy for females affected by FXS is necessary.
- Girls with the full mutation may display early puberty, and women with direct effects may have early menopause (Hagerman & McCandless, 2005).
- Tantrum behavior and hyperactivity may begin by age 2 years.

Prader-Willi Syndrome

- Prader-Willi syndrome is another unique inheritance pattern genetic syndrome, caused by several different genetic alterations on chromosome 15's long arm (15q) (Cassidy & McCandless, 2005; Schiemann, 2017).
- In about 75% of individuals with Prader-Willi syndrome, there is a small deletion on chromosome 15 between q11 and q13.
- Additional cases can result from inheriting two maternal alleles of chromosome 15 and no paternal alleles, known as uniparental disomy.
- Inheritance of two paternal alleles results in Angelman syndrome, a completely different syndrome.
- A third cause, in less than 5% of cases, is the result of a defect in the imprinting process. These individuals do not have a notable deletion and have inherited alleles from each parent, but only the maternal allele is active.

Assessment

- Result of hypothalamic/pituitary gland dysfunction when the gland itself is structurally normal
- Infants born with hypotonia often have feeding difficulty and display early failure to thrive
- Rapid onset of weight gain and large appetite presenting between 1 and 6 years of age (hyperphagia)
  - May consume nonfood items
- Characteristic facial features:
  - Almond-shaped eyes
  - Narrow nasal bridge
  - Down-turned mouth
  - Thin upper lip
- Small genitals (hypoplasia) and pubertal deficiency
- Developmental delay and intellectual disabilities:
  - IQ median range is 60 to low 70s
  - May have mild intellectual delay within normal limits
- Behavioral profile:
  - Stubbornness
  - Can be manipulative
  - Obsessive-compulsive qualities
  - Great difficulties without routines
- Physical traits:
  - Hypopigmentation, fair hair and skin compared with family members (Schiemann, 2017)
  - Small hands and feet for height, tapered fingers
  - Overall short stature, genu varum (knock-knees; see Chapter 20)
  - Near-sighted (myopia) and cross-eyed
  - Thick, viscous saliva
  - Speech articulation defects
  - Skin picking
  - High pain threshold
  - Temperature-control problems
  - Scoliosis and kyphosis
  - Osteoporosis

Nursing Interventions

- Feeding support and possible supplements in newborn period; rarely can breastfeed
- May see hyperphagia and lack of emesis with severe gastric distention in older children and teens (Schiemann, 2017)
- Endocrine involvement; improvement with growth hormone supplementation
- Early adrenarche but overall pubertal delay; many are not sexually active as adults
- Infertility also common

Caregiver Education

- Feeding support and possible supplements in newborn period; rarely can breastfeed
- Early intervention for developmental delay
- Need to establish clear health routines early, with limited oral intake, daily exercise, and skin examination daily; treatment of picked skin areas with antibiotics
- Strict attention to feeding recommendations and dietary restriction; may eat to point of severe gastric distention without emesis
- Need to restrict access to items such as garbage, pet food, paste, and glue

Angelman Syndrome

- Deletion on maternal chromosome 15
- Characteristic features:
  - Developmental delay
  - Intellectual disabilities
  - Severe speech and language impairment
  - Problems with movement, coordination, and balance
  - Happy, laughing demeanor
  - Hand-flapping behaviors
  - Hyperactivity with short attention span
  - Short sleep cycles
  - Epilepsy
  - Scoliosis is common

Assessment

- General physical assessment
- Documentation of dysmorphic features or obvious abnormalities
- Assess presence or absence of developmental milestones
- Screening for other associated conditions

Diagnosis

- Children with chromosomal abnormalities are diagnosed by examination and documentation of characteristics seen with specific disorders.
- A blood test is necessary to evaluate the chromosomes and genetic codes.
- Because some chromosomal disorders may cause multiple malformations, such as heart defects or kidney defects, as well as dysmorphic features, evaluations for other malformations should be performed.

Nursing Interventions

- Treatment is aimed at supportive care.
- Medications to treat medical disorders may be necessary, such as to control seizures.
- Physical, occupational, and speech therapies are often needed to help children progress in developmental milestones.
- Families require support because of added stressors, such as:
  - Time to care for the child with special needs
  - Education of medical procedures that may be needed at home, such as tube feedings
  - Emotions
  - Grief
  - Finances

Fetal Alcohol Spectrum Disorder

- Fetal alcohol spectrum disorder (FASD) is an umbrella term to describe the broad range of disorders caused by exposure to excessive maternal alcohol use. This is not a genetic syndrome, but the result of the toxic effect of alcohol on a developing fetus.
- At one end of the spectrum are persons with typical FASD facial features and neurocognitive disorders, and at the other end are children with no physical features but behavioral and cognitive deficits.
- The exact amount of alcohol necessary to cause the full spectrum is unknown, so no alcohol should be consumed during pregnancy.
- Some persons appear to be at higher risk for FASD related to variance in the three different types of alleles for alcohol dehydrogenase that result in different levels of enzyme activity.

Fetal Alcohol Spectrum Disorder Subtypes

The spectrum can be divided into four subtypes (CDC, 2017; Hoyme et al., 2005):

1. Fetal alcohol syndrome (FAS): This is the most severe form of FASD and is defined by abnormalities in three domains: poor growth, abnormal brain growth or structure, and specific dysmorphic facial features. Prenatal alcohol exposure may or may not be confirmed.
2. Partial FAS: These children display the typical facial dysmorphic features associated with FAS, have abnormalities in only one of the other domains, and prenatal alcohol exposure is confirmed.
3. Alcohol-related birth defects: These children have the typical facial features associated with FAS, normal growth, and normal brain function and structure, but have structural congenital anomalies in other organs (such as cardiac or renal abnormalities). Confirmation of prenatal alcohol exposure is required.
4. Alcohol-related neurodevelopmental disorder: These children have normal growth and lack the facial features of FASD but display a pattern of behavioral or cognitive abnormalities typical of prenatal alcohol exposure. These children are at risk for significant cognitive impairment, abnormalities on testing

of verbal learning and memory skills, and low IQ scores (CDC, 2017; Mattson et al., 1997). Confirmation of prenatal alcohol exposure is required.

Assessment

- Typical facial features at birth:
  - Flat midface
  - Thin upper lip
  - Small chin (micrognathia)
  - Short, upturned nose
  - Short palpebral fissures
  - Prominent epicanthal fold at inner portion of eyes
- Growth deficiency, starting at infancy and lasting throughout life
  - Brain anomalies/defects can include abnormalities of the corpus callosum, cerebellum, and frank microcephaly.
  - Sensory, motor, and regulatory behaviors are also affected at the cellular level.
  - Communication and language can be affected.
  - Organ damage, including congenital heart defects, can occur.

Nursing Interventions

- There may be difficulties with suck/swallow/breath coordination or aspiration.
- Gastrostomy feeding may be necessary.
- Sensory overreactivity to textures is often present.
- Behavioral management and environmental changes are necessary to address inattention.
- Comorbidities must be recognized.

Caregiver Education

- No alcohol is to be consumed during pregnancy.
- Impulsivity, attention issues, and frank ADHD are common.
- Executive dysfunction is common.

Case Study

Snoring and Down Syndrome

Timmy is a 5-year-old with Down syndrome, born to a mother who was 37 years old at the time of his delivery. His genetic studies have confirmed Trisomy 21. He has missed a number of well-child visits because his mother does not like to see him "hurt" with shots, and she has not followed routine recommendations for blood and medical studies. His last laboratory studies were at age 12 months with a lead and complete blood cell count, but his shots are up to date. His newborn screen showed normal thyroid function. Timmy is pale and often very sleepy during the day, but restless when he naps or overnight, and often snores very loudly. His mother is concerned that something is wrong. At the 5-year well-child visit, she confides in you that she does not want to attend the many follow-up visits ordered for her special needs son, because her three other children never needed more than yearly visits after age 2 years. She is also upset that the doctor keeps telling her that he is too heavy, but he is smaller than her other children at this same age and loves to eat. He had trouble growing in infancy and she had to work on getting him to eat, and now she likes to reward him with snacks as he works very hard in preschool to keep up with his peers.

1. How can the office nurse counsel the mother about testing and follow-up needs for Timmy?
2. Is Timmy at risk for abnormal laboratory studies? When should these be performed?
3. Should his mother be concerned about his sleep pattern snoring at this young age?
4. Should Timmy's mother be concerned now about his feeding and weight?

REFERENCES

Alasdair, G. W. H. (2005). Down syndrome. In S. Cassidy & T. Allanson (Eds.), *Down syndrome in management of genetic syndromes* (2nd ed., pp. 191–210). Hoboken, NJ: John S. Wiley & Sons.

American Academy of Pediatrics (AAP) & Committee on Genetics. (2001). Health supervision for children with Down syndrome. *Pediatrics, 107*, 442–449. Retrieved from pediatrics.aappublications.org/content/pediatrics/107/2/442.full.pdf?download=true

American Academy of Pediatrics, Committee on Substance Abuse and Committee on Children with Disabilities. (2000). Fetal alcohol syndrome and alcohol related neurodevelopmental disorders. *Pediatrics, 106*, 358–361. Retrieved from http://aappolicy.aappublications.org/cgi/content/full/pediatrics;106/2/358

American Academy of Pediatrics. Health supervision for children with Down Syndrome. *Pediatrics*, 2011;128(2):393–406. doi: 10.1542/peds.2011-3113

Anderson, S. E., & Must, A. (2005). Interpreting the continued decline in the average age at menarche: results from two nationally representative surveys of U.S. girls studied 10 years apart. *Journal of Pediatrics, 147*, 753–760. doi: 10.1016/j.jpeds.2005.07.016

Bacino, C. (2017) Achondroplasia. In E. TePas (Ed.), *UpToDate*. Retrieved from http://www.uptodate.com/contents/achondroplasia

Behrman, R. E., Kliegman, R. M., Jenson, H. B., & Stanton, B. F. (2007). *Nelson textbook of pediatrics* (18th ed.). St. Louis, MO: W.B. Saunders.

Berry-Kravis, E. (2002). Epilepsy in fragile X syndrome. *Developmental Medicine and Child Neurology, 44*, 724–728. doi: 10.1017/S0012162201002833

Blau, N. (2016). Genetics of phenylketonuria: Then and now. *Human Mutation, 37*, 508–515. doi: 10.1002/humu.22980

Brenner, J., & Ojo, A. (2017). Causes of painless scrotal swelling in children and adolescents. In J. Wiley (Ed.), *UpToDate*. Retrieved from https://www.uptodate.com/contens/cause-of-painless-scotal-swelling-in-children-and-adolescents

Bull, M., & Committee on Genetics. (2011). Health supervision for children with Down syndrome. *Pediatrics, 128*(2), 393–406. doi: 10.1542/peds.2011.1605

Butler, M. G. (1989). Hypopigmentation: A common feature of Prader-Labhart-Willi syndrome. *American Journal of Human Genetics, 45*, 140–146. Retrieved from http://www.ncbi.nlm.nih.gov/pmc/articles/PMC1683374/

Carey, J. (2005). Trisomy 18 and trisomy 13 syndromes. In S. Cassidy & T. Allanson (Eds.), *Management of genetic syndromes* (2nd ed., pp. 555–568). Hoboken, NJ: John S. Wiley & Sons.

Cassidy, S. B., & McCandless, S. E. (2005). Prader-Willi syndrome. In S. B. Cassidy & J. E. Allanson (Eds.), *Management of genetic syndromes* (pp. 429–448). Hoboken, NJ: Wiley-Liss.

Centers for Disease Control and Prevention (CDC). (2010). *2010 STD treatment guidelines*. Retrieved from http://www.cdc.gov/std/treatment/2010/default.htm

Centers for Disease Control and Prevention (CDC). (2012). *Male circumcision.* Retrieved from http://www.cdc.gov/hiv/malecircumcision/

Centers for Disease Control and Prevention (CDC). (2015). *2015 STD treatment guidelines.* Retrieved from http://www.cdc.gov/std/tg2015/default.htm

DeSai, S., & Glasier, C. (2017). Sturge-Weber syndrome. *New England Journal of Medicine, 377*(9), e11. doi: 10.1056/NEJMicm1700538

DeSilva, L. (2017). Abnormal uterine bleeding in adolescents: Evaluation and approach to diagnosis. In M. Torchia (Ed.), *UpToDate.* Retrieved from http://www.uptodate.com/contents/abnormal-uterine-bleeding-in-adolescents

Gravholt, C. H., Anderson, N. H., & Conway, G. S., Dekkers, O. M., Geffner, M. E., Klein, K. O., ... International Turner Syndrome Consensus Group. (2017). Clinical practice guidelines for the care of girls and women with Turner syndrome: Proceedings form the 2016 Cincinnati International Turner Syndrome Meeting. *European Journal of Endocrinology, 177*(3), G1–G170. Retrieved from http://www.eje-online.org/content/177/3/G1

Hagerman, R., & McCandless, S. (2005). Fragile X syndrome. In S. Cassidy & T. Allanson (Eds.), *Management of genetic syndromes* (2nd ed., pp. 251–264). Hoboken, NJ: John S. Wiley & Sons.

Haridas, A., & Tomita, T. (2017). Hydrocephalus in children: Physiology, pathogenesis, and etiology. In C. Armsby (Ed.), *UpToDate.* Retrieved from http://www.uptodate.com.contents/hydrocpehalus-in-children-pathyphysiology-pathogenesis-and-etiology

Hicks, C., & Sparling, P. F. (2011). *Pathogenesis, clinical manifestations, and treatment of early syphilis.* Retrieved from https://www.uptodate.com/contents/definition-etiology-and-evaluation-of-precocious-puberty

Hoyme, H. E., May, P. A., Kalberg, W. O., Kodituwakku, P., Gossage, J. P., Trujillo, P. M., ... Robinson, L. K. (2005). A practical clinical approach to diagnosis of fetal alcohol spectrum disorders: Clarification of the 1996 institute of medicine criteria. *Pediatrics, 115,* 39–47. doi: 10.1542/peds.2005-0702

Hsieh, T. F., Chang, C. H., & Chang, S. S. (2006). Foreskin development before adolescence in 2149 schoolboys. *International Journal of Urology, 13,* 968–970. doi: 10.1111/j.1442-2042.2006.01449.x

Jenny, C., Crawford-Jakubiak, J., & Committee on Child Abuse and Neglect. (2013). The evaluation in the primary care setting when sexual abuse is suspected. *Pediatrics, 132,* e558. doi: 10.1542/peds.2013-1741

Kenyon, C., Colebunders, R., & Crucitti, T. (2013). The global epidemiology of bacterial vaginosis: a systematic review. *American Journal of Obstetrics and Gynecology, 209*(6), 505–523. doi: 10.1016/j.ajog.2013.05.006

Laufner, M., & Makai, G. (2017). Evaluation and management of female lower genital tract trauma. In S. Falik (Ed.), *UpToDate.* Retrieved from http://www.uptodate.com/contents/evaluation-and-management-of-female-lower-genital-tract-trauma

Lewis, R. A., Gerson, L. P., Axelson, K. A., Riccardi, V. M., & Whitford, R. P. (1984). Von Recklinghausen neurofibromatosis. II. Incidence of optic gliomata. *Ophthalmology, 91,* 929–935.

Lewis, R. A., & Riccardi, V. M. (1981). Von Recklinghausen neurofibromatosis. Incidence of iris hamartomata. *Ophthalmology, 88,* 348–354. Retrieved from http://www.ncbi.nlm.nih.gov/pubmed/6789269

Mai, C. T., Kucik, J. E., Isenburg, J., Feldkamp, M. L., Marengo L.K., Bugenske, E. M., Kirby, R. S., & National Birth Defects Prevention Network. (2013). Selected birth defects data from population-based birth defects surveillance programs in the United States, 2006 to 2010: Featuring trisomy conditions. *Birth Defects Research Part A: Clinical Molecular Teratology, 97,* 709–725.

Marshall, W. A., & Tanner, J. M. (1969). Variations in pattern of pubertal changes in girls. *Archives of Disease in Childhood, 44,* 291–303. doi: 10.1136/adc.44.235.291

Mattson, S. N., Riley, E. P., Gramling, L., Delis, D. C., & Jones, K. L. (1997). Heavy prenatal alcohol exposure with or without physical features of fetal alcohol syndrome leads to IQ deficits. *Journal of Pediatrics, 131,* 718–721.

McDonald-McGinn, D., Sullivan, K, Marino, B., Philip, N., Swillen, A., Vorstman, J., & Bassett, A. (2015). 22q11.2 deletion syndrome. *National Review in Disease Primer, 1,* 15071. doi: 10.1038/nrdp.2015.71

Mervis, C., & John, A. (2010). Cognitive and behavioral characteristics of children with Williams syndrome: Implications for intervention approaches. *American Journal Genetics Clinical Seminars in Medical Genetics, 154C*(2), 229–248. doi: 10.1002.ajmg.c.30263

Moore, D. L., MacDonald, N. E., & Canadian Paediatric Society, Infectious Diseases and Immunization Committee. (2015). Preventing ophthalmia neonatorum. *Paediatric Child Health, 20,* 93–96. Retrieved from https://www.ncbi.nlm.nih.gov/pmc/articles/PMC4507834/

Morris, C. (2005). Williams syndrome. In S. Cassidy & T. Allanson (Eds.), *Management of genetic syndromes* (2nd ed., pp. 665–665). Hoboken, NJ: John S. Wiley & Sons.

National Institute of Neurological Disorders and Stroke (NINDS). (2012a). *Charcot Marie Tooth fact sheet.* Retrieved from http://www.ninds.nih.gov/disorders/charcot_marie_tooth/detail_charcot_marie_tooth.htm#102833092

National Institute of Neurological Disorders and Stroke (NINDS). (2012b). *NINDS neurofibromatosis information page.* Retrieved from http://www.ninds.nih.gov/disorders/neurofibromatosis/neurofibromatosis.htm

National Institute of Neurological Disorders and Stroke (NINDS). (2017). *Neurofibromatosis fact page.* Retrieved from https://www.ninds.nih.gov/Disorders/Patient-Caregiver-Education/Fact-Sheets/Neurofibromatosis-Fact-Sheet

National Organization for Rare Disorders (NORDS). (2017). *Achondroplasia.* Retrieved from https://rarediseases.org/rare-diseases/achondroplasia/

North, K. (2000). Neurofibromatosis type 1. *American Journal of Medical Genetics, 97,* 119–127. doi: 10.1002/1096-8628(200022)97:2{119:AID-AJMG3>3.0.CO;2-3

Pauli, R. (2005). Achondroplasia. In S. Cassidy & T. Allanson (Eds.), *Management of genetic syndromes* (2nd ed., pp. 13–30). Hoboken, NJ: John S. Wiley & Sons.

Ramsock, C. (2017). Inguinal hernia in children. In J. Wiley (Ed.), *UpToDate.* Retrieved from https://www.uptodate.com/contents/inguinal-hernia-in-children?search=17,%20inguinal%20hernias%20in%20children&source=search_result&selectedTitle=1-150&usage_type=default&display_rank=1/aa/

Reyes Mendez, D. (2017). Straddle injuries in children: Evaluation and management. In J. Wiley (Ed.), *UpToDate.* Retrieved http://www.uptodate.com/contents/straddle-injuries-in-children-evaluation-and-management

Santor, S. L., Yin, H., & Hopkin, R. (2017) Adherence to symptom-based care guidelines for Down syndrome. *Clinical Pediatrics, 56,* 150. doi: 10.1177/0009922816653416

Schiemann, A. (2017). Clinical features, diagnosis, and treatment of Prader-Willi syndrome. In A. Hoppin (Ed.), *UpToDate.* Retrieved from http://www.uptodate.com/clinical-features-diagnosis-and-treatment-of-prader-willi-syndrome

Schrander-Stumpel C., & Fryns, J. P. (1998). Congenital hydrocephalus: Nosology and guidelines for clinical approach and genetic counseling. *European Journal of Pediatrics, 157,* 355–362. doi: 10.1007/s004310050830

Shirley, M. D., Tang, H., Gallione, C. J., Baugher, J. D., Frelin, L. P., Cohen, B., ... Pevsner, J. (2013). Sturge-Weber syndrome and port-wine stains caused by somatic mutation in GNAQ. *New England Journal of Medicine, 368*(21), 1971–1975. doi: 10.1056/NEJMoa1213507

Shprintzen, R. (2005). Velo-cardio-facial syndrome. In S. Cassidy & T. Allanson (Eds.), *Management of genetic syndromes* (2nd ed.). Hoboken, NJ: John S. Wiley & Sons.

Sindhar, S., Lugo, M., Levin, M., Danback, B., Brink, B., Yu, E., ... Kozel, B. (2016) Hypercalcemia in patients with Williams-Beuren syndrome. *Journal of Pediatrics 178,* 254–260.e4. doi: 10.10167jped.08.027

Sybert, V. (2005). Turner syndrome. In S. Cassidy & T. Allanson (Eds.), *Management of genetic syndromes* (2nd ed.). Hoboken, NJ: John S. Wiley & Sons.

Tuberous Sclerosis Complex. (2017). *The genetics of TSC.* Retrieved from http://www.tuberous-sclerosis.com/adult-patients/tuberous-sclerosis-gene.jsp?site=43700022043234060&source=01030&usertrack.filter_applied=true&NovaId=4029462223569761294

Van Esch, H. (2017). Fragile X syndrome: Management in children and adolescents. In E. TePas (Ed.), *UpToDate.* Retrieved from https://www.uptodate.com/contents/fragile-x-syndrome-management-in-children-and-adolescents

Viskochil, D. (2005). Neurofibromatosis type 1. In S. Cassidy and T. Allanson (Eds.), *Management of genetic syndromes* (2nd ed.). Hoboken, NJ: John S. Wiley & Sons.

Weremowicz, S. (2017). Congenital cytogenetic abnormalities. In E. TePas (Ed.), *UpToDate*. Retrieved from http://www.uptodate.com/contents/congenital-cytogenic-abnormalities

Wilcox, D. (2017). Care of the uncircumcised penis in infants and children. In M. Kim (Ed.), *UpToDate*. Retrieved from https://www.uptodate.com/contents/care-of-the-uncircumcised-penis-in-infants-and-children

World Health Organization, Task Force on Adolescent Reproductive Health. (1986). Longitudinal study of menstrual patterns in the early postmenarcheal period, duration of bleeding episodes and menstrual cycles. *Journal of Adolescent Health Care, 7*, 236–244. Retrieved from http://www.ncbi.nlm.nih.gov/pubmed/3721946

World Health Organization & Joint United Nations Programme on HIV/AIDS. (2010). Neonatal and child male circumcision: a global review. Retrieved from http://www.who.int/hiv/pub/malecircumcision/neonatal_child_MC_UNAIDS.pdf

Hematological, Immunological, and Neoplastic Disorders

19

Sheryl Stuck, MSN, RN, CNS, CDP

LEARNING OUTCOMES

Upon completion of this chapter, the student will be able to:

1. Identify the classifications of anemia.
2. Compare iron deficiency and sickle cell anemia.
3. Identify the major pathophysiology associated with the care of the child with cancer.
4. Identify nursing assessments and interventions that promote health during the care of children with cancer and their families.
5. Develop a nursing care plan for the child with cancer who is experiencing pain.
6. Develop a caregiver education plan for high-risk oncology clients.
7. Demonstrate an understanding of the pathophysiology of and nursing interventions for the child with immunodeficiency disorders.
8. Identify the categories of hematopoietic stem cell transplant.

HEMATOLOGICAL DISORDERS

Hematopoiesis is the process through which the bone marrow produces blood cells and platelets, whereas erythropoiesis is the production of the red blood cells (RBCs) with erythropoietin and iron. RBCs increase a patient's hemoglobin and oxygen capacity. The life span of RBCs is 120 days, after which they are destroyed by phagocytes in the spleen and liver through a process called hemolysis. Hematological disorders occur when disruptions occur in these processes.

Iron Deficiency Anemia

The most common type of anemia, iron deficiency anemia occurs when there are not enough healthy RBCs to carry oxygen to the body's tissues. This condition is a dietary deficiency and is more common among infants who are given cow's milk. Iron deficiency anemia is the most common microcytic anemia characterized by small, pale RBCs and depleted iron stores, with subsequent decrease in bone marrow erythropoiesis.

Assessment

- Screening hemoglobin concentration at 12-month health supervision visits is recommended by the American Academy of Pediatrics (Kleinman & Greer, 2014).
- Children with this condition may have the following characteristics:
  - Irritability, anorexia, tachycardia, systolic murmur, brittle and concave nails
  - Poor muscle tone
  - Prone to infection
  - Skin may be described as porcelain-like
  - Edematous
  - Retarded growth
  - Decreased serum concentration of the proteins albumin, gamma globulin, and transferrin
  - Delayed learning

Diagnostic Testing

- Complete blood cell count (CBC) with RBC indexes normal, borderline, or moderately reduced
- RBCs small in size
- Low serum iron (serum iron concentration circulating; reference values: newborn 100 to 250 mcg/dL, infants 20 to 105 mcg/dL, and 20 to 145 mcg/dL for 10 to 14 years old) (Van Leeuwen & Bladh, 2015)
- Serum ferritin (reference values 6 months to 15 years is 7 to 140 ng/mL) (Van Leeuwen & Bladh, 2015)
- Total iron-binding capacity (reference values 250 to 350 mg/dL) (Van Leeuwen & Bladh, 2015)
- Erythropoietin level of reference values: 0 to 3 years, 1.7 to 17.9 mIU; 4 to 6 years, 3.5 to 21.9 mIU; 7 to 9 years, 1.1 to 13.5 mIU; 10 to 12 years, 1.1 to 14.1 mIU, and 13 to 15 years, 2.2 to 14.4 mIU (Van Leeuwen & Bladh, 2015)
- Reticulocyte hemoglobin content

Nursing Interventions

- Dietary therapeutics with oral elemental iron preparations (Table 19–1)
- Liquid dosage of iron sipped through a plastic straw to avoid discoloring tooth enamel
- Iron supplementation may be necessary in adolescence
- Use Z-track injection method for iron dextran (Imferon)

Caregiver Education

- Use commercial iron-fortified formula; if bottle feeding, iron supplements are not needed.
- Avoid consumption of cow's milk in infants until age 12 months. Whole milk is recommended from 12 months to 2 years.
- For breastfed infants, provide an iron supplement (1 mg/kg of body weight/day) if the infant does not consume sufficient iron-rich foods (Hagan, Shaw, & Duncan, 2017).
- Teach parents to add iron-rich foods to the child's diet (Table 19–2).

Acquired Thrombocytopenia

With acquired thrombocytopenia, platelet counts decrease because of an infection such as Rocky Mountain spotted fever, Colorado tick fever, malaria, or other bacteria. Drug or chemical exposure may also be a factor. With removal of the causative agent, platelet count recovers.

Assessment

- Recent spontaneous bleeding such as epistaxis, blood in feces, blood in mucous membranes or gums, scabbed areas, hematemesis
- Assess for petechiae, often over bony prominences
- Recent exposure to chemicals, insecticides, paint, gasoline, kerosene, and lawn care supplies may be the causative agent
- Recent exposure to Rocky Mountain spotted fever, malaria, bacteremia, viral infection, measles, mumps, rubella, and chickenpox
- Petechiae, purpura on face, thorax, and extremities

TABLE 19–1 Iron and Folic Acid Preparations

DRUG (PREGNANCY CATEGORY)	PHARMACOLOGICAL CLASS	USUAL DOSAGE RANGE	INDICATIONS/USES
Ferric gluconate (B)	Parenteral iron salt	>6 years: 1.5 mg/kg/dose for 8 doses	Iron deficiency associated with hemodialysis
Ferrous fumarate (A)	Oral iron salt	4–6 mg/kg/day	Severe iron deficiency anemia Iron deficiency anemia
Folic acid (A)	Water-soluble B-complex vitamin	PO/IV/IM/subcutaneous: 0.1–0.4 mg/day	Folate deficiency tropical sprue, nutritional and pregnancy-related supplementation
Iron dextran (C)	Parenteral iron salt	IM/IV: 5–10 kg: 25 mg/day; >10 kg: 50 mg/day Epinephrine available in case of anaphylaxis	Iron deficiency when oral iron therapy is unsatisfactory
Iron sucrose	Parenteral iron salt	Adult IM/IV: 100 mg/day (2 mL/day) Give with epinephrine in case of anaphylaxis	Iron deficiency in adult with chronic renal failure

Adapted from Skidmore-Roth, L. (2017). Mosby's drug guide for nursing students e-book *(12th ed.). St. Louis, MO: Mosby.*

TABLE 19–2 Recommendations for Foods Rich in Iron and Folate

Iron	Organ meats, shellfish, poultry, legumes, molasses, fortified cereals
Folate (folic acid)	Legumes, liver, dark green or leafy vegetables, lean beef, potatoes

Adapted from Baker, R. D., Greer, F. R., & Committee on Nutrition American Academy of Pediatrics. (2010). Diagnosis and prevention of iron deficiency and iron-deficiency anemia in infants and young children (0–3 years of age). Pediatrics, 126, *1040–1050.*

Diagnostic Testing

- Platelet countdecreased (normal: 2- to 6-year-old boys and girls, 205 to 405 × 10^3/αL, 7- to 12-year-old boys, 195 to 365 × 10^3 /αL; 7- to 12-year-old girls, 185 to 370 × 10^3 /αL) (Van Leeuwen & Bladh, 2015)

Nursing Interventions

- Provide mouth care with soft toothettes.
- Monitor stools for occult or frank blood.
- Avoid intramuscular injections and suctioning.
- Avoid use of salicylates (aspirin), which interfere with platelet aggregation.
- Administer steroids to increase platelet production and decrease vascular fragility.
- Modify age-appropriate activities to avoid injuries.
- Collaborate with physical therapist when needed. The child may have had prolonged time in bed without activity.
- Encourage a positive self-image and self-care.

Caregiver Education

- Teach about side effects of steroid therapy including possible fluid retention and weight gain.
- Give steroids with food and limit sodium intake.
- Provide range of activity based on platelet count.
- Avoid exposure to causative agent.
- Encourage parent to support positive self-concept of child.
- Support appropriate activities for child.

Sickle Cell Disease

Sickle cell disease is the most common genetic condition, characterized by partial or complete replacement of abnormal hemoglobin S for normal hemoglobin A. The deformed cell changes from round to sickle (crescent) shape (Fig. 19–1). Tissue damage can occur all over the body, and complications relate to delayed growth and sexual maturation, acute and chronic pulmonary dysfunction, stroke, aseptic necrosis of the hip and shoulders, retinopathy, dermal ulcers, severe and chronic pain, and psychosocial dysfunction. When both parents have the sickle cell trait, there is a one in four chance with each pregnancy that the child will have sickle cell disease (SCD).

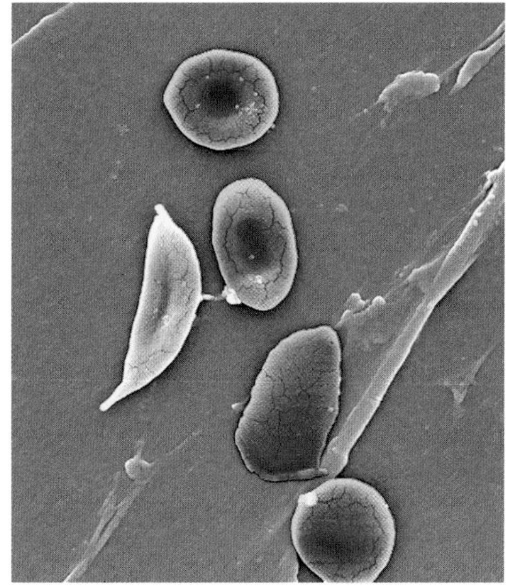

FIGURE 19–1 Example of a sickle cell.

About 1 in 13 African-American babies are born with this sickle cell trait (Centers for Disease Control and Prevention, 2016).

Assessment

- Asymptomatic until 4 to 6 months due to presence of fetal hemoglobin, which resists sickling and suppresses symptoms. Sickle hemoglobin and sickle-shaped cells replace the fetal hemoglobin at 5 months old.
- The sickled RBCs die early. There are not enough healthy RBCs to carry oxygen in the body. As the disease worsens over time, sickle cells do not flow smoothly through the vessels.
- Vaso-occlusive crisis (obstruction of blood flow causing tissue hypoxia and necrosis) is a painful episode with hand-foot syndrome (dactylitis), causing symmetrical infarct in the bones of the hands and feet, and very painful swelling of soft tissue.
- Acute chest syndrome occurs as a new pulmonary infiltrate with chest pain, fever, cough, tachypnea, wheezing, and hypoxia.
- Sequestration crisis is the loss of spleen function from frequent infarcts and the pooling of a large amount of blood, causing spleen enlargement.
- A cerebrovascular accident is a blocking of the blood vessels in the brain with impaired neurological function; severe headache; twitching of the face, legs, or arms; seizures; change in speech; weakness in the hands, feet, or legs; or abnormal behavior.
- Assess for psychological adjustment, including emotional and behavioral problems related to long periods of hospitalization.

Diagnostic Testing

- Sickle turbidity test (Sickledex) with fingerstick blood yields results in 3 minutes to determine whether hemoglobin S is present.
- Hemoglobin electrophoresis is accurate and rapid; quantifies the percentages of various types of hemoglobin S and hemoglobin A.

Nursing Interventions

- Analgesics for the pain of vasoocclusion
- Pain distraction techniques, including self-hypnosis
- Activity and rest cycling for periods of activity intolerance
- Hydration with IV therapy and oral fluids
- Antibiotics for infection treatment
- Penicillin prophylaxis significantly reduces the risk for pneumococcal infection starting at 2 months of age
- Hydroxyurea is cytoxic and is used to reduce the frequency of painful crises and reduce the need for blood transfusions in patients with recurrent, moderate-to-severe crisis (Skidmore-Roth, 2017).
- Metabolic acidosis treatment with IV electrolyte replacement
- Physical therapy
- Complementary therapy, including cognitive-behavioral therapy approaches, controlled breathing, positive self-talk, behavioral rehearsal, transcutaneous electrical nerve stimulation, hand holding, humor, music, and memory reframing
- Splenectomy as a lifesaving measure
- Hematopoietic stem cell transplantation (HSCT) may be an option
- Monitor for acute chest syndrome for possible severe chest, back, or abdominal pain; fever; congested cough; dyspnea; tachypnea; retractions; decreased oxygen saturation (less than 92%)
- Administer blood transfusions for treatment of anemia

SAFE AND EFFECTIVE NURSING CARE: Cultural Competence

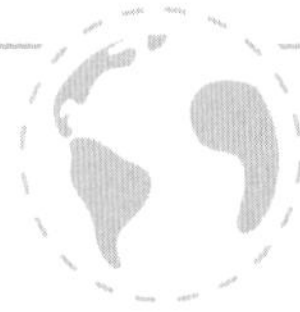

Health-Care Practices Involving Blood Transfusions

Children with cancer or recurrent sickle cell crises frequently need blood transfusions. Children who have Jehovah's Witness beliefs and their caregivers may not accept blood products because of their beliefs, so caregivers may therefore refuse the administration of blood to the child. During the preparation of the patient treatment plan, the interprofessional team, including the oncologist, surgeon, nurse, and hematology members, may arrange for alternative treatment modalities as possible (Campbell, Machan, & Fisher, 2016).

Caregiver Education

- Provide resources for the family, including genetic counseling.
- Teach caregivers signs of infection.
- Seek medical care with temperature of 38.0°C (100.4°F) as directed by prescribing physician.
- May need prophylactic penicillin before dental procedures.
- Advise immunizations against haemophilus influenzae type B (HIB), pneumococcal, and meningococcal organisms.
- Discuss feelings of altered self-concept manifested as poor academic performance, low social and interpersonal functioning, and withdrawal.
- Resulting pain contributes to depression, anxiety, and other psychiatric disturbances.
- Develop a relationship with the child and caregiver to work together to find the safest medical solution.
- Take the time to get to know the child and answer any questions.

Aplastic Anemia

Pathophysiology of aplastic anemia is a deficiency of the formation of blood elements; pancytopenia is decreased leukocytes, platelets, and erythrocytes. Damage to the three blood cell types produced within the bone marrow causes anemia.

Assessment

- Fatigue
- History of illness or injury that does not heal

Diagnostic Testing

- CBC with differential and platelet count to diagnose the specific type of anemia
- Reticulocytes are less mature RBCs, and an increase in the percentage of reticulocytes indicates that a release of RBCs is occurring more rapidly than usual to compensate for deficiency (reference value of 0.8% to 2.1% of the total RBC count for 3 months to 18 years) (Van Leeuwen & Bladh, 2015).
- Bone marrow aspiration confirms red bone marrow conversion to yellow, fatty bone marrow.

Nursing Interventions

- Monitor immunosuppressive therapy to remove functions that prolong aplasia.
- Monitor blood transfusions and IV infusion access care to decrease infection.
- Prevent infection with hand hygiene.

SAFE AND EFFECTIVE NURSING CARE: Clinical Pearl

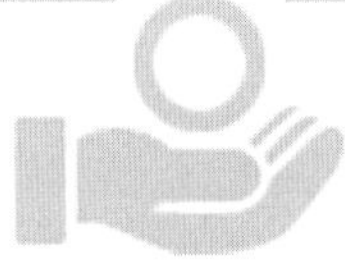

Blood Transfusion Preparation

In preparation for a blood transfusion, the patient and family need information before providing informed consent. Involve family with the results of the blood counts and plan of care. Monitor blood infusion for reactions during the first 15 minutes. Obtain vital signs and assess for temperature changes. Stop the infusion and notify the physician immediately if a blood transfusion reaction is identified (Williams, Estrada, Gary-Bryan, & MacKeil-White, 2012).

Caregiver Education

- Describe the possibility of bone marrow transplant before multiple transfusions; transfusions increase the child's sensitivity to human leukocyte antigens (HLAs), which decreases the likelihood of a successful transplant.
- Encourage caregiver participation in daily care.
- Support the balanced diet of the child, including meat and meat substitutes.

Hemophilia

Hemophilia is commonly a deficiency of factor VIII, a substance produced by the liver that assists with thromboplastin formation in blood coagulation. The clotting factors are present, but in a diminished capacity. The defective factor is unable to do its job in the clotting cascade, so the cascade is halted and the fibrin clot is unable to form, leading to uncontrolled bleeding when injury occurs. Both hemophilia A and B are inherited as X-linked recessive traits, which affect males. Females are carriers and do not have the disease.

Assessment

- History of bleeding, nosebleeds, and bruising
- Hemarthrosis into the joint cavities of the knees, ankles, elbows
- Hematoma with pain, swelling, and limited motion
- Spontaneous hematuria

Diagnostic Testing

- Partial thromboplastin time (PTT) prolonged, indicating ineffective clotting factors except factor VII (reference value 25 to 35 seconds for activated PTT) (Van Leeuwen & Bladh, 2015)
- Low level of factor VII or IX coagulant
- Often no bleeding in first year of life, until child starts to walk and fall; common first injury is oral mucosal membrane bleeding

Nursing Interventions

- Administration of factor VIII concentrate from pooled plasma as prescribed by physician
- Administration of DDAVP (1-deamino-8D-arginine vasopressin), a synthetic form of vasopressin to increase plasma factor VIII in mild cases as prescribed by physician
- Corticosteroids for child with hematuria, hemarthrosis, and synovitis as prescribed by physician
- NSAIDs for relieving pain; may interfere with platelet formation (Skidmore-Roth, 2017)
- Avoid aspirin, which interferes with platelet function
- Avoid chronic use of codeine
- Supportive care with exercise and physical therapy

Caregiver Education

- Prevent injury in the environment with supervision, helmet use, and activity restrictions. Avoid contact sports. Provide soft toothbrushes and venipuncture in place of fingersticks to decrease bleeding.
- Medical alert tag is important.
- Prophylaxis by administrating periodic factor replacement of factor VIII, including self-administration as child is capable (Table 19–3).
- Provide resources from the National Hemophilia Foundation publications.
- Anticipate altered family dynamics and how illness may impact financial resources

SAFE AND EFFECTIVE NURSING CARE: Promoting Safety

Development of Independent Functioning

A child's recreational activities should include other children for socialization whenever possible. Alternatives should be fun and build self-esteem and positive body image. An adolescent focuses on egocentrism, and has a feeling that "nothing will happen to me" and is unable to see consequences of actions. Encourage the adolescent's involvement in care, allowing as much control as possible over aspects of care. Isolation from school, work, and community may cause a loss of independent functioning.

Lead Poisoning

Lead poisoning is a condition caused by chronic ingestion or inhalation of materials that contain lead, characterized by physical and mental dysfunction. Children with iron deficiency absorb lead more readily than those with sufficient iron stores, making them more susceptible to lead poisoning.

Assessment

- Screening no later than 12 months; selective screening at ages 3, 4, 5, and 6 years (American Academy of Pediatrics Council on Environmental Health, 2016)
- Inquire about sources of lead: interior and exterior paint, plaster, caulking on playgrounds, soil, foods or liquids, water from leaded or copper pipes, cigarette butts and ashes, colored newsprint, unglazed pottery, painted lead crib rails, and window ledges
- Inhalation sources: sanding and scraping of lead-based painted surfaces, burning of automobile batteries, burning of colored newspaper, automobile exhaust, sniffing leaded gasoline, cigarette smoke, dust (Fig. 19–2)
- Health-care professionals should work with local health authorities to develop culturally competent questions appropriate to housing hazards and public utility usage
- Signs of anemia: abdominal pain, vomiting, constipation, anorexia, headache, fever, lethargy
- Central nervous system signs: hyperactivity, impulsiveness, lethargy, irritability, loss of developmental progress, hearing impairment, learning difficulties

TABLE 19–3 Blood Transfusion Products

TRANSFUSION PRODUCTS	INDICATIONS	CRITICAL NURSING ACTIONS
Red blood cells	Hemoglobin <8 grams in a stable patient with chronic anemia Hypovolemia due to acute blood loss Evidence of impending heart failure secondary to severe anemia Patients on hypertransfusion regimen for sickle cell disease and history of: Cerebral vascular accident Splenic sequestration Acute chest syndrome Recurrent priapism Preoperative preparation for surgery with general anesthesia Hypoxia Children requiring increased oxygen-carrying capacity (i.e., complex congenital heart, intracardiac shunting, severe pulmonary disease—ARDS): Shock states (decreased BP, increased peripheral vasoconstriction, pallor, cyanosis, diaphoresis, clamminess, mottled skin, increased oxygen requirement, decreased urinary output) Cardiac failure Respiratory failure requiring significant ventilatory support Postoperative anemia	Observe for clinical signs and symptoms of anemia: • Fatigue • Syncope • Pallor • Tachycardia • Diaphoretic • Shortness of breath • Inability to perform activities of daily living Don appropriate personal protective equipment (PPE) for all blood product transfusions Monitor vital signs per hospital policy and procedure Monitor hemoglobin and hematocrit During blood product infusions, observe for adverse reactions Blood can be stored only in a designated blood refrigerator Generally 10–15 mL/kg of packed red blood cells are transfused (Khilnani, 2005)
Autologous blood (self-donated blood product)	For general scheduled surgical procedures in which there are clinical indications that a blood transfusion may be necessary during the intraoperative or postoperative period, the patient may elect to self-donate; check with blood bank facilities for time criteria for this type of donation For general surgical procedures, the recommended hemoglobin is 10 grams or greater and for orthopedic surgery the recommendation is hemoglobin of 11.5 or greater	Verify with parents that self-donation has occurred Patient identification and administration process is the same as for all other blood products
Whole blood or packed red blood cells (PRBCS) reconstituted with fresh frozen plasma (FFP)	Hypovolemia due to acute blood loss nonresponsive to crystalloids Hct <35% Hypovolemia due to acute massive blood loss (i.e., major trauma) History of blood loss at delivery or large amount of blood drawn for lab studies (10% blood volume) Cardiac patients Hct <40% (structural heart disease, cyanosis, or congestive heart failure) Drop in Hgb to below 10 gm intraoperatively Exchange transfusion	Same nursing actions applicable to red blood cell infusions In major trauma situations, patient may be transfused with O-negative blood, the universal donor Use blood warmer and rapid infuser if available

TABLE 19-3 Blood Transfusion Products—cont'd

TRANSFUSION PRODUCTS	INDICATIONS	CRITICAL NURSING ACTIONS
Platelets	Platelet count <20,000 Active bleeding with symptoms of DIC or other significant coagulopathies Platelet count <50,000 with planned invasive procedure (i.e., surgical procedure, central line insertion, does not include drawing blood or intramuscular injection of intravenous catheter insertion) Prevention or treatment of bleeding due to thrombocytopenia (secondary to chemotherapy, radiation, or bone marrow failure) Treatment of patients with severe thrombocytopenia secondary to increased platelet destruction or immune thrombocytopenia associated with complication of severe trauma Massive transfusion with platelet dilution	Know normal platelet count (150,000–400,000) Obtain CBC Assess bruising, petechiae, and bleeding
Fresh frozen plasma (FFP)	Replacement for deficiency of factors II, V, VII, IX, X, XII; protein C or protein S Bleeding, invasive procedure, or surgery with documented plasma clotting protein deficiency (i.e., liver failure, DIC, or septic shock) Prolonged PT and/or PTT without bleeding Significant intraoperative bleeding (10% blood volume/hr) in excess of normally anticipated blood loss that is at high risk of clotting-factor deficiency Massive transfusion Therapeutic plasma exchanges Warfarin anticoagulant overdose	Notify blood bank to thaw FFP; product must be used within 6 hours of thawing Don appropriate PPE for all blood product transfusions Monitor vital signs per hospital policy and procedure Monitor coagulation studies During FFP infusions, observe for adverse reactions
Cryoprecipitate (CRYO)	Fibrinogen levels below 150 mg/dL with active bleeding Bleeding or prophylaxis in von Willebrand's disease or in factor VIII (hemophilia A) deficiency unresponsive to or unsuitable for DDAVP or factor VII concentrates Replacement therapy, bleeding, or invasive procedure in patients with factor XIII deficiency Patients with active intraoperative hemorrhage in excess of normally anticipated blood loss who are at risk of clotting factor deficiency	Assess for signs and symptoms of bleeding Don appropriate PPE for all blood product transfusions Monitor vital signs per hospital policy and procedure Monitor coagulation studies During cryoprecipitate infusions, observe for adverse reactions
Granulocytes (white blood cell transfusion)	Bacterial or fungal sepsis (proven or strongly suspected) unresponsive to antimicrobial therapy Infection (proven or strongly suspected) unresponsive to antimicrobial therapy	Type and crossmatch required for all WBC transfusions Pre-medications may be ordered, such as antihistamines or acetaminophen

Continued

TABLE 19–3 Blood Transfusion Products—cont'd

TRANSFUSION PRODUCTS	INDICATIONS	CRITICAL NURSING ACTIONS
Factor VII	Treatment of factor VII deficiency Treatment of factor VIII inhibitors Treatment of factor IX inhibitors Idiopathic uncontrolled bleeding	Assess for signs and symptoms of bleeding Don appropriate PPE for all blood products, even recombinant Monitor coagulation studies If undiluted, dilute vial with indicated amount of sterile water and administer intravenously as per manufacturer's guidelines
Factor VIII concentrate	Hemophilia A (factor VIII deficiency) Patients with factor VIII inhibitors Patients with von Willebrand's disease	Assess for signs and symptoms of bleeding Don appropriate PPE for all blood products Monitor coagulation studies Check product to see if refrigeration necessary Record expiration date and lot number of product
Factor IX concentrate (prothrombin complex)	Treatment of hemophilia B Hemophilia A with factor VIII inhibitors Patients with congenital deficiency of prothrombin, factors II, VII, IX, and factor X	Assess for signs and symptoms of bleeding Don appropriate PPE for all blood products Monitor coagulation studies Record expiration date and lot number of product
Intravenous immunoglobulin (IVIG)	Congenital or acquired antibody deficiency Immunological disorders such as idiopathic thrombocytopenia (ITP), Kawasaki disease Posttransplant patients used prophylactically, newborns with severe bacterial infections	Don appropriate PPE for all IVIG infusions Monitor vital signs per hospital policy and procedure Start infusion slowly and increase rate/titrate per physician orders During IVIG infusion, observe for adverse reactions such as fever, chills, and headache Product is obtained from pharmacy Record expiration date and lot number of product

ARDS, acute respiratory distress syndrome; BP, blood pressure; CBC, complete blood cell count; DDAVP, 1-deamino-8D-arginine vasopressin; DIC, disseminated intravascular coagulation; Hct, hematocrit; Hgb, hemoglobin; IVIG, intravenous immunoglobulin; PT, prothrombin time; PTT, partial thromboplastin time; WBC, white blood cell.

From Skidmore-Roth, L. (2017). Mosby's Drug Guide for Nursing Students e-book *(12th ed.). St. Louis, MO: Mosby.*

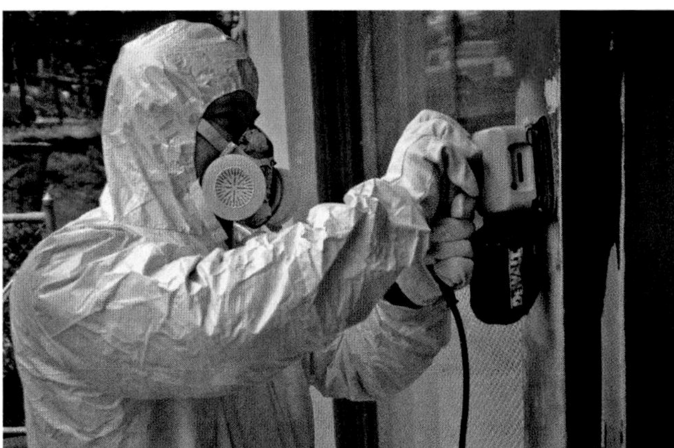

FIGURE 19–2 Man wearing protective clothing and mask to protect against lead-based paint dust.

Diagnostic Testing

- Blood lead level
- Free erythrocyte protoporphyrin level is less than 30 mcg/dL in males and less than 40 mcg/dL in females (Van Leeuwen & Bladh, 2015)
- Bone radiography
- Urinalysis
- Hemoglobin and CBC

Nursing Interventions

- Prevent further exposure to lead
- Chelation therapy with injections of calcium disodium edetate and succimer into a large muscle mass after administration of local anesthetic procaine

Caregiver Education

- Instruct about safety from lead hazards
- Remove paint chips or dust; remove with a damp paper towel and discard in the trash. Use a wet paper towel to clean the surface and discard (U.S. Environmental Protection Agency, 2017)
- Possible relocation of child until removal of lead
- Speech and child developmental specialist to evaluate child as needed

IMMUNOLOGICAL DISORDERS

Immunology is the mechanism with which the body defends itself against infectious agents and foreign substances. Without a strong immune system, the body is unable to defend against the HIV. Development of an antibody to HIV is the first step in determining HIV infection.

Acquired Immunodeficiency Syndrome

Acquired immunodeficiency syndrome (AIDS) develops from HIV infection, which most commonly affects children when transmitted in utero from a mother who has HIV. Using preventive medicine during pregnancy can reduce risk for HIV transmission (U.S. Department of Health and Human Services, 2017). Youth aged 13 to 24 years accounted for 22% of new HIV cases in the United States during 2015. Most new cases were among gay and bisexual males (Centers for Disease Control and Prevention, 2017).

The HIV virus infects specific T lymphocytes found in blood, semen, vaginal secretions, and breast milk. Acute infection increases the viral load, which decreases slowly in infected children. It has an incubation period of months to years. Hematological deficiencies including neutropenia increase the risk for complications.

Assessment

- Lymphadenopathy
- Mucocutaneous eruptions
- Failure to thrive and delayed development
- Hepatosplenomegaly
- Oral candidiasis
- Parotitis
- Chronic or recurrent diarrhea

Diagnostic Testing

- Testing includes HIV enzyme-linked immunosorbent assay and Western blot immunoassay for children 18 months and older.
- HIV polymerase chain reaction (PCR) is used for detection in infants born to HIV-infected mothers because of the presence of maternal antibodies transferred transplacentally; preferred virological assays include HIV DNA PCR and HIV RNA assays (Fig. 19–3).
- Virological diagnostic testing is recommended at birth in infants at high risk for HIV infection (e.g., infants born to HIV-infected mothers who did not receive prenatal care or prenatal antiretroviral therapy).

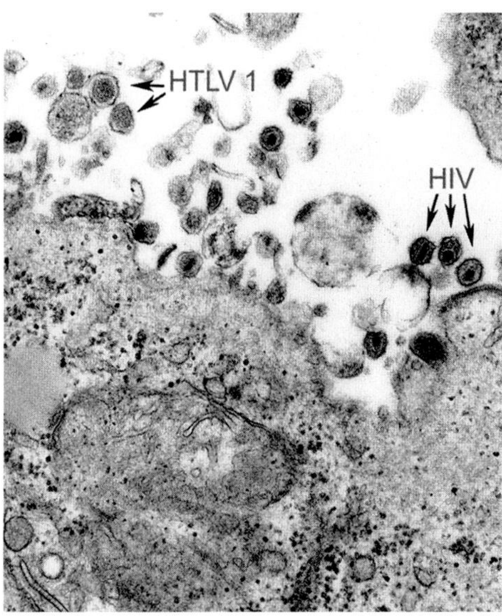

FIGURE 19–3 HIV cell.

- In children 18 months or older, HIV antibody assays are ordered.
- Rapid HIV testing may include oral specimen collection.

Nursing Interventions

- Administration of highly active antiretroviral therapy drugs combination therapy (a strategy analogous to the treatment of infectious diseases) has improved efficacy, minimized toxicity, and delayed drug resistance (Fig. 19–4).
- Immunization against common childhood illnesses is recommended if exposed to HIV.
- Nutritional management includes high-calorie, nutrient-dense foods.
- Maintain confidentiality.
- Follow standard precautions when providing care.
- Prevent and manage opportunistic infections (OPs) of children with severe immune suppressions. OPs include *Pneumocystis jiroveci* pneumonia and tuberculosis.

Caregiver Education

- Teach pain management techniques.
- Tolerance to opioids may require increased dosing.
- Encourage use of nonpharmacological pain interventions.
- Emphasize time of administration of highly active antiviral therapy and its importance to maintain drug efficacy.
- Support caregivers with complex day-care arrangements or social/family problems.
- Educate day-care and school staff on current HIV information.
- Encourage positive self-concept and avoid the HIV-related stigma.
- Support the child with a life-threatening illness.

ONCOLOGICAL DISORDERS

Oncological (cancer) disorders are a group of complex diseases with uncontrolled growth and spread of abnormal cells. Treatment for cancer varies according to the pathophysiology and subsequent diagnosis but may include chemotherapy, surgery, radiation, and/or bone marrow transplant.

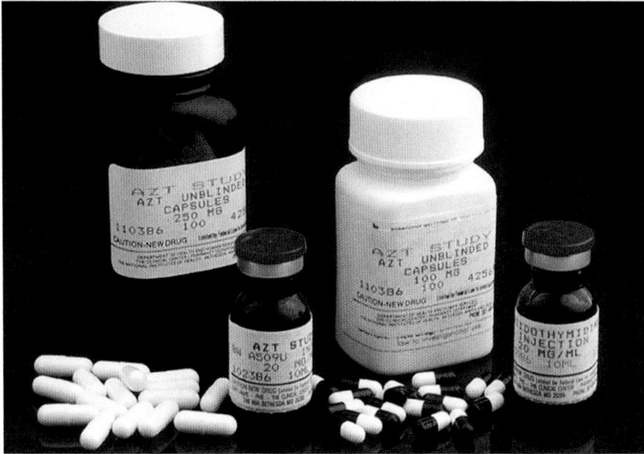

FIGURE 19–4 AZT is a common antiviral medication.

Neoplasm

- Pathophysiology: Uncontrolled abnormal cell growth forms a tumor. Tumors are classified as benign (noncancer) or malignant (cancer cells with uncontrolled growth). Metastasis is the ability of cancer cells to invade surrounding tissue or spread to other areas of the body.
- Causes of most cancers are unknown. Possible causes are chemical carcinogens, radiation, and viruses.
- Genetic and hereditary conditions with oncogenes allow unregulated genetic activity and tumor growth (Wilms' tumor).
- Patterns of onset of tumor include the developmental stages of infancy and adolescence.
  - Infancy/early childhood (neuroblastoma, retinoblastoma) (Fig. 19–5)
    - Wilms' tumor of the kidney is typically discovered by caregivers noticing a lump in the abdominal area while dressing or bathing a child.
  - Adolescence (Hodgkin's lymphoma, osteosarcoma)
    - This is a treatable disease with cure as a realistic goal.

Assessment

- Pain with neoplasm directly or indirectly affecting nerve receptors
- Cachexia with anorexia, weight loss, weakness
- Anemia due to chronic bleeding, iron deficiency, and limited RBCs in bone marrow
- Infection prevention due to an altered immune system from side effects of cancer treatment
- Bruising from uncontrolled bleeding with decreased platelets
- Hematuria

CRITICAL COMPONENT

Absolute Neutrophil Count and Calculation

A nursing priority is the high risk for infection for the child with an oncological disorder. Calculating the absolute neutrophil count (ANC) requires three numbers from the CBC and differential. The following formula calculates the ANC:

(% Bands + % segmented cells) × total WBC count = ANC

Example:

(3% Bands + 50% segmented cells) × 1,500 = 795

When the ANC is less than 500, the client is at high risk for infection.

(Pagana, 2009)

Diagnostic Testing

Genomics, personalized, and precision medicine approaches to care are rapidly advancing. Nurses need to provide information to enhance patient genetic risk testing and caregiver understanding.

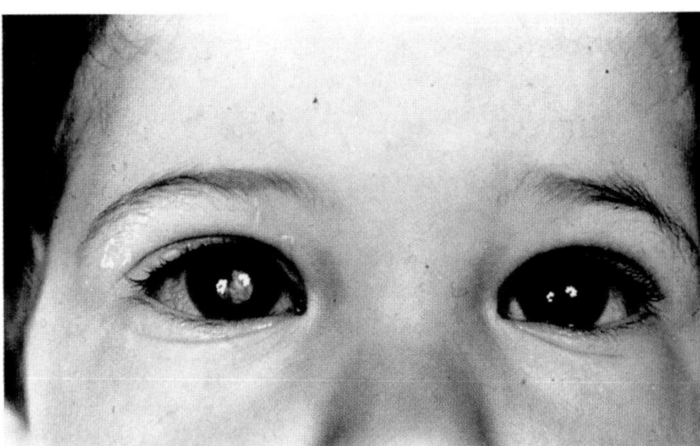

FIGURE 19–5 Young child with retinoblastoma.

Care coordination is key (Vorderstrasse, Hammer, & Dungan, 2014). Diagnostic measures include:

- CBC, including ANC
- Lumbar puncture (Fig. 19–6)
- Computed tomography (CT), magnetic resonance imaging (MRI), ultrasound
- Biopsy to determine the type of benign or malignant tumor
- Bone marrow aspiration
- Surgery
- Chemotherapy following protocols based on research findings for type of cancer, staging of disease process, and cell type
- Radiation therapy as specific treatment protocol
- Bone marrow transplantation
- Biological response modifiers stimulate the body's immune system to destroy cancerous cells

SAFE AND EFFECTIVE NURSING CARE: Understanding Medication

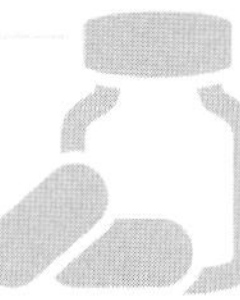

Types of Antioncological Medications

Classifications of medications include but are not limited to monoclonal antibodies, interleukins, interferon, tumor necrosis factors, and colony-stimulating factors to increase the production of blood cells using filgrastim and erythropoietin.

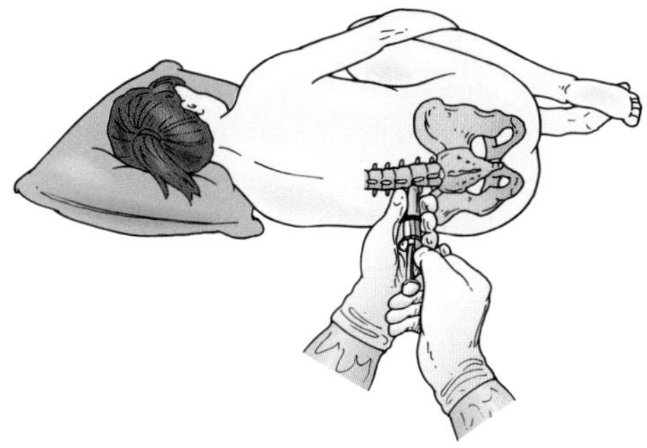

FIGURE 19–6 Lumbar puncture.

SAFE AND EFFECTIVE NURSING CARE: Promoting Safety

Nursing Care Priorities for Complex Pediatric Hematology and Oncology Patients

- Triage patients quickly and place in a treatment room as soon as possible.
- Begin neutropenic precautions (protective isolation).
- Use strict hand hygiene. To prevent infection, dedicate stethoscopes and equipment to the room.
- Initiate cardiopulmonary monitoring. Add oxygenation as necessary. Obtain and monitor frequent vital signs for trends. Hypotension is a sign of sepsis.
- Avoid invasive procedures.
- Access central lines and use only 10-mL syringes to flush the line.
- Obtain laboratory values including blood cultures, basic metabolic panel (BMP), CBC, type and screen, and prothrombin time (PT)/PTT.
- Start antibiotics if febrile within 60 minutes of assessment. Monitor for adverse reactions.
- If febrile (temperature greater than 38.0°C or 100.4°F), give acetaminophen 15 mg/kg every 4 to 6 hours. Avoid ibuprofen to reduce risk for platelet dysfunction (Hymes & Steele, 2016; Williams et al., 2012).

Nursing Interventions

- Complementary and alternative medicine therapies: aromatherapy is the therapeutic use of essential oils from plants (flowers, herbs, or trees) for the improvement of physical, emotional, and spiritual well-being; it can be used by cancer patients for general well-being (National Cancer Institute at the National Institute of Health, 2017)
- Administration of medications to prevent nausea and vomiting
- Hydration with IV fluid and replacement according to emesis loss
- Nutrition and calorie intake
- Prevent infection in peripheral IV central catheter or implanted central venous access port (Fig. 19–7)
- Appropriate age and developmental stage nursing care for hospitalized child
- Listen, debrief, and offer support for daily care

Nonpharmacological pain management includes role-play with the child, "acting out" the procedure on dolls; adolescents can observe a visual demonstration, video, or computer simulation. Answer questions as age appropriate and clarify medical language unfamiliar to caregivers.

Oncology Emergencies

- Tumor lysis syndrome: destruction of tumor cells releases uric acid, potassium, phosphates, calcium

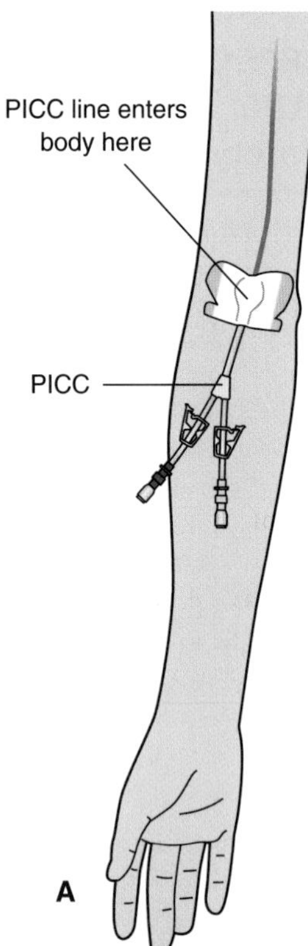

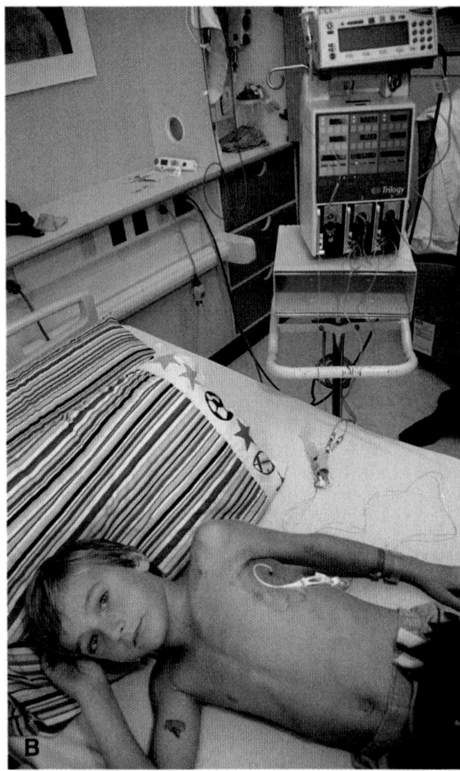

FIGURE 19–7 A, B Peripheral intravenous central catheters (PICCs) in children.

- Septic shock from overwhelming infection
- Hyperleukocytosis is the infiltration of brain and lung tissue with blast cells
- Increased intracranial pressure (ICP) due to space-occupying lesions in brain

Caregiver Education

- Support a sense of control for child, family, and others.
- Encourage support system and coping with uncertainty of future.
- Acknowledge potential loss of future of the child and future generations, including grieving the loss of their dreams and aspirations for the child (see Chapter 5).
- Grief and sadness may fade as hope grows.
- Hope gives strength to endure treatments and renewed appreciation for life.
- Identify financial support as needed.

Side Effects of Radiation Therapy

Rapidly dividing cells are more radiosensitive. The cancer cells are susceptible to destruction from the inability of the skin cells to keep up with the accelerated cell loss caused by radiation. Caregivers should be made aware of the various possible side effects of radiation therapy, such as:

- Integumentary system: skin erythema, ulceration, alopecia (Yarbro, Wujcik, & Gobel, 2018)
- Nervous system: learning disabilities, attention difficulties, headache, edema
- Ophthalmological: dry eyes, cataracts, retinopathy, sclera melting
- Cardiac: pericarditis, valve dysfunction, cardiomyopathy
- Pulmonary: radiation pneumonitis, fibrosis
- Gastrointestinal: mucositis, esophagitis, nausea, vomiting, diarrhea, abdominal cramping, rectal ulceration, proctitis, anorexia, dysphagia, obstruction of small bowel
- Genitourinary: radiation nephritis, bladder radiation cystitis, amenorrhea, decrease in sperm production, sterility
- Hematological: myelosuppression
- Skeletal: slow bone growth at epiphyseal plates, growth arrest with high doses
- Miscellaneous: lethargy, headache, increased need for sleep, fatigue

Leukemia

Leukemia is a group of malignant diseases of the bone marrow and lymphatic system. White blood cell (WBC) overproduction occurs, although the count is actually low. Immature cells do not deliberately attack and destroy normal cells but are in competition for metabolic elements. Leukemia represents 29% of all childhood cancers, 76% of which are lymphoid leukemias. It is the most common form of pediatric cancer (Siegel, Miller, & Jemal, 2017). With the use of targeted therapies, dramatic improvements in survival rates in recent years have occurred (Table 19–4). The survival rates for leukemia may fluctuate from irradiation, prior x-rays, or exposure to chemicals.

Assessment

- Anemia with weakness, fatigue, pallor, dyspnea, cardiac dilation, and anorexia

CRITICAL COMPONENT

Radiation Types and Side Effects

The treatment goal of radiation therapy is to destroy tumor cells and allow normal cells to regrow and repopulate surrounding tissues. Radiation is dependent on cell cycle for cell death. The principles of radiation exposure include duration of time of exposure and distance from the radiation to minimize exposure. Wear a lead shield and radiation film badge.

Types of Radiation Therapy

1. According to target theory, cells with a direct radiation hit are most effective.
2. Three-dimensional conformal radiotherapy is a computerized delivery of a high dose of radiation while maintaining a tight margin to deliver only a low dose of radiation to the surrounding nontargeted tissues.
3. Hyperfractionated radiation therapy delivers two radiation treatments per day to treat aggressive, fast-growing tumors.
4. Proton-heavy particle therapy is used to deliver maximum radiation energy to the treatment site and minimize the dose to surrounding tissue. Protons are used in patients with medulloblastoma, rhabdomyosarcoma, retinoblastoma, and glioma.
5. Brachytherapy is the implantation of radioactive sources directly into the tumor bed under CT guidance. The goal is to deliver optimizing doses of radiation in higher doses over several weeks.
6. Image-guided CyberKnife radiosurgery uses a stereotactic frame, radiation delivery, computer planning, a robotic arm, and x-ray cameras to deliver highly focused beams of radiation. Used for the brain and spine tumors (Yarbro et al., 2018).

- Cough, wheezing, tracheal/bronchial compression, and respiratory distress/arrest related to mediastinal mass and compression of great vessels
- Neutropenia with infection of skin and lungs, fever, decreased wound healing
- Thrombocytopenia (low platelet count) with bruises, petechiae, purpura, large ecchymosis, epistaxis, gums and sclera hemorrhages
- Hematuria and melena occasionally
- Bone and joint pain due to infarction, bone destruction, and pressure caused by hyperplastic neoplastic tissue in medullary spaces; gait problems
- Liver and enlarged spleen with pain, gastrointestinal symptoms, urinary symptoms
- Enlarged lymph nodes greater than 1 cm and firm but not painful in regional areas, elbow, and supraclavicular nodes
- Necrotic, ulcerative rectal lesions
- Painless testicular enlargement
- Central nervous system signs: nausea, vomiting, lethargy, morning headache, irritability, convulsions, cranial nerve palsies, papilledema, pain upon neck flexion, hyperphagia, blindness, decreased coordination, growth deceleration, and precocious puberty

Diagnostic Testing

- Bone marrow test for a positive diagnosis of abnormal cells
- CBC screen for abnormal cells
- Low reticulocyte count
- Thrombocytopenia with platelet count less than 140×10^3 /αL (reference values: 2- to 6-year-old boys and girls, 205 to 405×10^3/αL; 7- to 12-year-old boys, 195 to 365×10^3/αL; and 7- to 12-year-old girls, 185 to 370×10^3/αL) (Van Leeuwen & Bladh, 2015)
- WBC with differential

TABLE 19–4 Types of Leukemia (Acute and Chronic)

TYPE OF LEUKEMIA	POSSIBLE CAUSE	SYMPTOMS	TREATMENT
Acute lymphocytic leukemia: most common type in children	Chromosome problems, radiation, previous chemotherapy	Bone and joint pain, bruising, bleeding, fatigue, swollen glands, weight loss	Chemotherapy, transfusion of blood products, antibiotics, stem cell transplant, immunotherapy
Acute myeloblastic leukemia	Certain chemicals, chemotherapy drugs, radiation	Bleeding from nose and/or gums, fever, shortness of breath, skin rash	Antibiotics, chemotherapy, stem cell transplant, blood and platelet transfusion
Chronic myelogenous also known as chronic myeloid leukemia	Philadelphia chromosome abnormality, radiation exposure	Fever without infection, bone pain, swollen spleen with pain, night sweats, fatigue, rash	Imatinib (Gleevec) oral pill associated with remission in Philadelphia chromosome-positive patient, bone marrow transplant
Chronic lymphocytic	Cause unknown, common in adults aged ≥70 years	Bruising, enlarged lymph nodes, night sweats, fatigue, fever, infections that recur, weight loss	In early stages, no treatment; later stages, chemotherapy, radiation, stem cell transplants

Adapted from Penn State Hershey (2011).

- Lumbar puncture to determine central nervous system infiltration and increased pressure, leukemia cells, blast cells, negative cultures, increased protein, decreased sugar
- CT, MRI

Nursing Interventions

- Blood transfusion
- Chemotherapy to suppress production of abnormal cells
- Prevention of infection

See Table 19–5 for information on two common childhood cancers and the nursing care for each.

Caregiver Education

- Teach hand hygiene.
- Avoid plants to prevent exposure to fungus.

Lymphomas

Lymphoma is a type of cancer that affects the immune system. The pathophysiology may be cellular proliferation of the lymphoid tissue. Malignancy develops as apoptosis (programmed cell death) and uncontrolled cell growth occurs.

Two major types of lymphomas are Hodgkin's lymphoma and non-Hodgkin's lymphoma (NHL; Table 19–6). The main difference is the abnormal lymphocyte cell. Hodgkin's disease develops in a single lymph node and contains Reed-Sternberg cells. This cancer is more curable. NHL occurs in the peripheral lymph nodes and spreads to tissues throughout the body (Fig. 19–8). The NHL cell type may be poorly differentiated and spread early. The chest mediastinum may be involved.

TABLE 19–5 Two Common Childhood Cancers and Their Nursing Care

TYPE OF CANCER	MEDICAL TREATMENT	BASIC NURSING CARE OF THE CHILD
Acute lymphocytic leukemia	Remission reduction postinduction with one of the following: consolidation/intensification *or* maintenance/continuation therapy	Prevent infection, including hand hygiene; reduction of environmental molds and organisms from plants and fresh fruits. Prevent bleeding from mouth with use of a soft toothbrush, offer mouth care, and provide a safe environment.
Acute myeloblastic leukemia	Induction (initial aggressive treatment) to attain remission with combination chemotherapy Second phase of treatment is postremission consolidation/intensification therapy	Use personal protective equipment to reduce child exposure to infection. Promote nutrition and monitor elimination patterns.

TABLE 19–6 Characteristics of Hodgkin's and Non-Hodgkin's Lymphoma

	PATHOPHYSIOLOGY	STAGING	NURSING ASSESSMENT	NURSING INTERVENTIONS
Hodgkin's	Reed-Sternberg cells Metastasis (spleen, liver, lungs)	Stages I–IV using the Cotswold Modified Ann Arbor system	Enlarged cervical or supraclavicular nodes	Administer chemotherapy Monitor for effects of irradiation
Non-Hodgkin's	Group of malignancies of lymphoid cells Undifferentiated or poorly differentiated cells, mediastinal and meninges involved Waldeyer's ring has lymphoid tissue encircling the tonsils	Revised European-American lymphoma system	Enlargement of lymph nodes causes airway and intestinal obstruction, cranial nerve palsies, spinal paralysis	Administer chemotherapy and prepare child for radiation Prevent infection

Data from Yabro, Wujcik, and Gobel (2018).

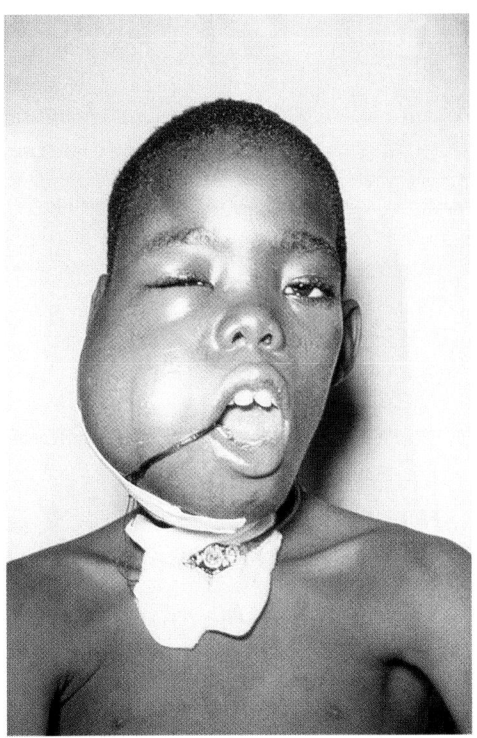

FIGURE 19–8 Child with non-Hodgkin's lymphoma.

Both diseases involve a staging system to inform treatment options. A stage of lymphoma is assigned based on number of lymph nodes, presence of extranodal disease, and history of any symptom. Other lymphoid types of cancers include:

- Mature B cell, identified as Burkitt lymphoma
- Lymphoblastic lymphoma of precursor T cell and precursor B cell
- Anaplastic large-cell lymphoma

Assessment

- Enlarged cervical lymph node or supraclavicular lymphadenopathy
- Monitor for symptoms related to pressure for enlargement of adjacent lymph nodes, including airway obstruction, intestinal instruction, cranial nerve palsies, and spinal paralysis
- Fever, weight loss, night sweats, cough, abdominal discomfort, anorexia, nausea, pruritus

Diagnostic Testing

- CBC and coagulation studies
- Erythrocyte sedimentation rate
- Presence of uric acid, liver function test, T-cell function studies, urinalysis
- CT scans of neck, chest, abdomen, pelvis
- Gallium scan to identify metastatic or recurrent disease
- Chest x-ray
- Bone scan
- Lumbar puncture and bone marrow aspiration to identify metastatic disease

See Table 19–7 for more information about diagnostic tests for lymphomas (Yarbro et al., 2018).

Nursing Interventions

- Administer chemotherapy.
- Prepare child for radiation and decrease activity intolerance.
- Patient treatment may include immunotherapy directed to specific lymphoma subtype that will target antibodies on the surface of the lymphoma cells (Yarbro et al., 2018).
- Allow for medical play when age appropriate (Fig. 19–9).
- Administer pneumococcal and meningococcal immunizations.
- Prevent infection using standard precautions and isolation as required (Fig. 19–10).

TABLE 19–7 Diagnostic Tests for Hematological, Immunological, and Oncological Disorders

TEST	PREPARATION	TIME TO COMPLETE	DATA GIVEN	RISKS INVOLVED
Complete blood cell count	EMLA cream on skin surface to anesthetize Visual imagery	Time varies from time of collection from peripheral or central venous catheter Laboratory reports may be ordered STAT	Differential for rapid treatment of antibiotics or need for further diagnostic tests	Low due to blood loss and prevention of infection
Tissue sample from an excisional lymph node biopsy	Preprocedure informed consent and patient safety precautions per agency protocol	Surgical asepsis of patient before physician intervention Duration of 1–4 hours in postanesthesia area	Type of cancer and staging of disease to determine treatment protocol	Moderate due to risk for infection and risk for cancer cell dissemination

Continued

TABLE 19–7 Diagnostic Tests for Hematological, Immunological, and Oncological Disorders—cont'd

TEST	PREPARATION	TIME TO COMPLETE	DATA GIVEN	RISKS INVOLVED
Bone marrow aspiration	Informed consent before procedure and note laboratory values at risk for patient bleeding	Patient preparation for procedure	Removal of bone marrow demonstrates initial disease and progression of treatment protocol	Low due to care of needle insertion and prevention of bleeding

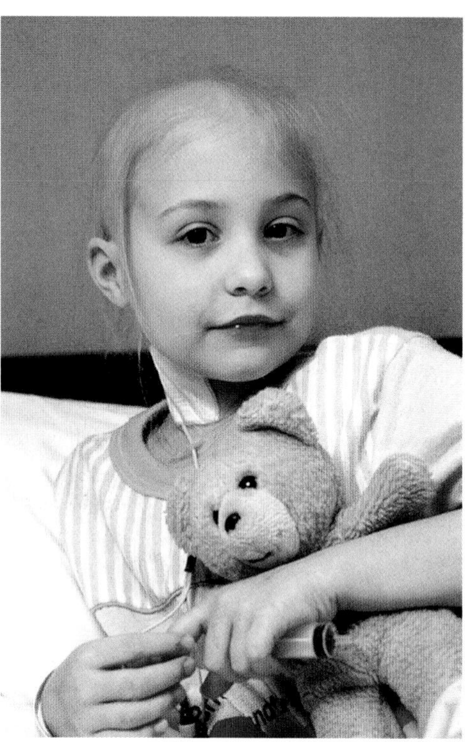

FIGURE 19–9 Girl with cancer using a syringe during medical play.

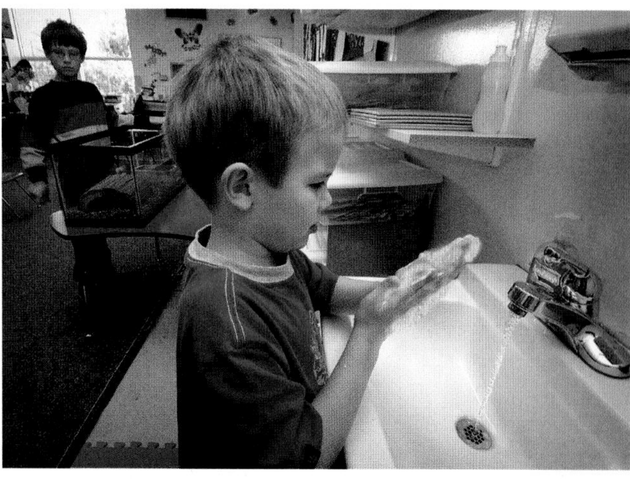

FIGURE 19–10 Encourage good hand hygiene to prevent infection.

SAFE AND EFFECTIVE NURSING CARE: Understanding Medication

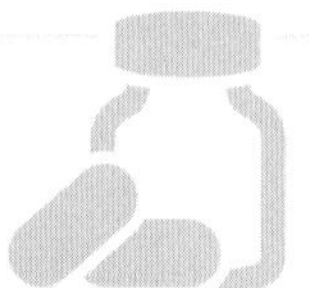

Special Considerations in Chemotherapy and Biotherapy Administration

The nursing priority is to assess child and caregiver understanding of the disease and treatment.

- Anticipate need for anti-emetic medication and hydration.
- Provide child safety by using two forms of patient identifiers.
- Verify drug order and dosage calculation by body surface area and/or weight calculation. Double-check with another nurse for the correct dosage.
- Intervene with education, explain protective precautions as needed, and use aseptic technique for venous access.
- Monitor medication administration, collect data, document treatment, and evaluate patient-centered outcomes.
- Prompt identification of adverse effects of medication is critical (Yarbro et al., 2018).

Caregiver Education

- Monitor activity level to provide for rest.
- Explain high risk for sterilization; sperm banking may be possible.
- Teach about disease; explain all procedures, expected side effects, and toxicities.
- Drug reactions may be complications of treatment.

SAFE AND EFFECTIVE NURSING CARE: Promoting Safety

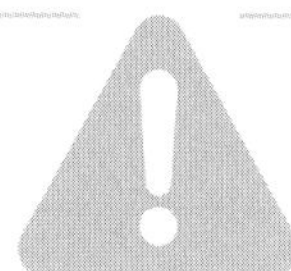

Chemotherapy Precautions

- Assure that the written policies and procedures are followed regarding protective equipment required, restricted access to hazardous drug spills, and posted signs.
- Cleanup of a large spill is handled by workers trained in handling hazardous materials.
- Locate spill kits in the immediate area where exposures may occur (Connor, et al., 2016).

- Describe what to do when side effects occur.
- Encourage discussion of feelings regarding disease.

Brain Tumors

A brain tumor begins when healthy cells in the brain grow spontaneously due to random cell mutations. Medulloblastoma is a type of solid brain tumor originating in the cerebellum. The cerebellum controls body movement and coordination. Neuroblastoma is a type of peripheral nervous system cancer common in children younger than 5 years of age.

Brain tumors can arise from any cell within the cranium and are classified by their location of origin. Neuroblastoma, the most common type of brain tumor, originates from embryonic neural crest cells. In 70% of neuroblastoma cases, the cancer is discovered after it has metastasized to the head, neck, chest, or pelvis.

Assessment

- Increased head size in infants is a sign of increased ICP, frequently a complication from the presence of a brain tumor
- Headache on awakening
- Nausea and vomiting is a sign of ICP
- Monitor pulse pressure (difference between systolic and diastolic pressure)
- Pupils sluggish, dilated, or unequal and weak hand grasp

Diagnostic Testing

- MRI to determine extent of tumor and location
- CT, angiography, electroencephalography
- Lumbar puncture without increased ICP to prevent herniation
- Brain tissue removal during surgery to diagnose tumor type
- Single-photon emission tomography scan to differentiate between brain cells, tumor cells, and scars
- Positron emission tomography scans used to study the biochemical and physiological effects of tumor

SAFE AND EFFECTIVE NURSING CARE: Clinical Pearl

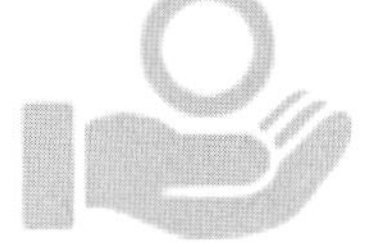

Preparing Children for Diagnostic Testing

The upcoming procedure should be explained to the child by the nurse and/or the child life specialist.

- Consider the developmental level of the child and use words he or she can understand.
- State what the child will hear, see, feel, touch, and smell.
- Tell the child it is okay to cry.
- Give the child any equipment or pictures of equipment to play with before the procedure.
- Tell the child what can be done to encourage cooperation during the procedure.
- Distract with songs, listening to music, or counting aloud.
- Explain how caregiver will be present before, during, and after the procedure. Anesthesia may put the child to sleep with a mask or IV medication. Administer medication for any pain, including headache, as needed.
- Share with the child the procedure is complete and acknowledge his or her feelings.
- Provide a special box of toys to have a treat to look forward to after the procedure.

Nursing Interventions

- Provide care of child during radiotherapy to shrink tumor.
- Assess response of child to targeted therapy (Yarbro et al., 2018).
- Assess postsurgical wound, including estimate of dressing drainage.
- Chemotherapy administration should be according to protocol.
- Assess mouth for soreness and open areas of stomatitis.
- Monitor for seizures and changes in posturing.
- Monitor temperature increases, pulse, respirations, blood pressure, and visual disturbances.
- Monitor blood pressure and pulse pressure, which is the difference between systolic and diastolic pressures, and report variations immediately.
- Assess pupil equality, size, reactivity, accommodation, reaction to light, extraocular eye movements, and cranial nerve function.
- Monitor level of consciousness and sleep patterns.
- Monitor movement of all extremities, gag reflex, and blink or swallowing reflex.
- Elevate head of bed 30 degrees in a supratentorial craniotomy; avoid Trendelenburg position because of increases in ICP.
- Align the body with pillows so neck and head are in midline.
- With infratentorial craniotomy, give fluids with return of gag and swallowing reflex.
- Prevent vomiting to prevent aspiration and avoid increased ICP (Yarbro et al., 2018).
- Monitor IV fluid to prevent cerebral edema, increased ICP, and hydrocephalus.
- Provide pain management measures.

CRITICAL COMPONENT

Nursing Interventions for Promoting Nutrition and Hydration in Children With Cancer

- Frequently offer any tolerated food and drink.
- Allow child to be involved in food and drink selection.
- Families can bring favorite foods from home or foods with appealing packaging.
- Culture-specific foods commonly served at home may comfort child.
- Fortify food with nutritious supplements, including liquids.
- Monitor child's weight.

Caregiver Education

- Encourage discussion of feelings of guilt caused by parents ignoring initial complaints (Aukema, Last, Schouten-van Meeteren, & Grootenhuis, 2011).

- Explain plan of care and survival rates (Table 19–8).
- Encourage emotional support of the child with a life-threatening illness (Fig. 19–11).

Wilms' Tumor

Wilms' tumor originates in fetal development, with a tumor typically found on the child's kidneys at age 3 or 4 years (American Cancer Society, 2017). Parents usually report finding a bump around the waistband or diaper area of the child, often during bath time. Wilms' tumors may affect one or both kidneys.

Assessment

- Lump is evident in the abdomen/waistband area
- May have pain in the area associated with the lump
- May have increased blood pressure due to changes in the renin-angiotensin system
- May have a fever for no identified reason

Diagnostic Testing

- May be associated with congenital anomalies; chromosomal testing may be ordered
- Abdominal CT scan
- MRI
- Laboratory work to include:
  - CBC
  - Liver function test
  - Urinalysis
  - Renal function test

Nursing Interventions

- Do not palpate the tumor site because it can cause metastasis.
- Provide caregiver with information regarding treatment and current clinical trials.
- Ensure that blood pressure is obtained as ordered; manual pressures are indicated with the changes in the renin-angiotensin system.
- Assess input and output to ensure that the child is urinating.
- Chemotherapy will likely be ordered before surgery.
- Provide strict aseptic technique with central venous line care.
- Monitor nutritional intake.
- The child should wear clothing that is loose around the waistband.

Caregiver Education

- Do not palpate the tumor because this can cause the proliferation or spread of cancer cells.
- Avoid pushing or lifting in tumor area when handling and bathing the child.
- Instruct parents that it is important to arrange care at a facility with a multidisciplinary team that is experienced with caring for many types of childhood cancers (National Cancer Institute, 2014).
- Side effects of the cancer treatments can be seen years after the treatment (National Cancer Institute, 2014).

TABLE 19–8 Common Childhood Cancers and Survival Rates

COMMON CHILDHOOD CANCERS AND USUAL AGE AT DIAGNOSIS	COMMON PERCENTAGE OF OCCURRENCE	5-YEAR SURVIVAL RATES (1999–2005)
Leukemia	30%	82%
Brain cancer and other nervous system cancers	26%	72%
Neuroblastoma, <1 year of age	7%	78%
Wilms' tumor, 3–6 years of age	5%	92%
Lymphoma		
Hodgkin's cancer, 15–40 years of age	4%	98%
Non-Hodgkin's	4%	86%
Soft tissue sarcoma	7%	74%
Rhabdomyosarcoma	3%	69%
Eye cancer, <4 years of age	3%	97%
Bone cancer		69%
Osteosarcoma	3%	
Ewing sarcoma	2%	

Data from American Cancer Society. (2016). Cancer treatment & survivorship facts & figures 2016–2017. *Atlanta, GA: American Cancer Society. Retrieved from https://www.cancer.org/content/dam/cancer-org/research/cancer-facts-and-statistics/cancer-treatment-and-survivorship-facts-and-figures/cancer-treatment-and-survivorship-facts-and-figures-2016-2017.pdf*

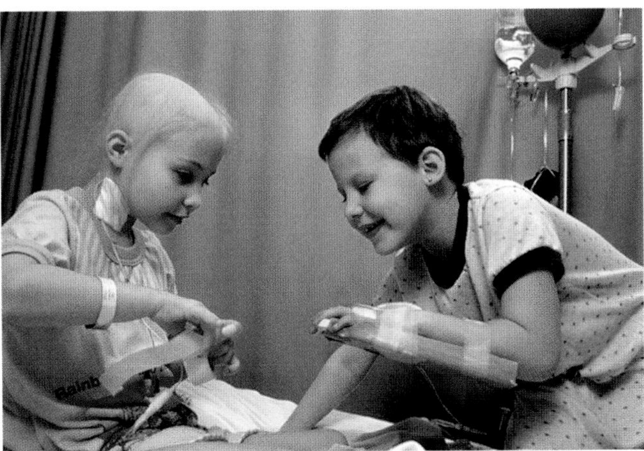

FIGURE 19–11 Children with cancer playing in the hospital.

- Genetic counseling may be ordered. Provide information and support to parents who may feel guilt that they passed this disease on to their child.
- Educate about the side effects of chemotherapy.
- Surgery will be needed to remove the tumor. Parents should be aware of the risks involved with this surgery.

HEMATOPOIETIC STEM CELL TRANSPLANTATION

With HSCT, a lethal dose of chemotherapy is administered to kill the cancer cells and suppress bone marrow production.

- Conditions considered for treatment using the process of HSCT are aplastic anemia, malignant disorders, nonmalignant hematological disorders (sickle cell anemia), and immunodeficiency disorders.
- The body is resupplied with stem cells (autologous, allogeneic, umbilical cord blood).
- Disease-free marrow replaces cancerous marrow.
- Peripheral stem cell transplant: Autologous collection of stem cells from the blood with an apheresis machine; frozen until needed (Yarbro et al., 2018).

Assessment

- Malignancy is life-threatening, and family is supported in the decision to agree to HSCT.
- Prepare child for isolation to undergo intensive ablative therapy.

Diagnostic Testing

- HLA system complex matching is completed to prevent graft versus host disease (GVHD).
  - GVHD is incompatibility of the donor bone marrow with the intended recipient related to the immunological response of the recipient.
  - Histocompatibility testing for allogeneic transplantation decreases risk for rejection.
  - The most common complication of a transplant is when the donor is mismatched with two to three antigens using HLA tissue matching.
  - Signs and symptoms of acute GVHD occur 7 to 30 days after transplant and affect the gut, liver, lungs, and skin.
  - Signs and symptoms of chronic GVHD occur about 100 days after transplant and affect the liver, gastrointestinal system, oral mucosa, and lungs. The skin has scleroderma-like skin, and the oral mucosa is abnormally dry.
  - Therapy for GVHD includes high doses of methylprednisolone, antithymocyte globulin, antilymphocyte globulin, cyclosporine, and anti-T-cell immunotoxins as ordered by the physician.

Nursing Interventions

- Administer high-dose chemotherapy with or without total body irradiation to suppress rejection of the transplanted marrow
- IV transfusion of stem cells harvested from bone marrow, peripheral blood, or umbilical vein of the placenta
- Strict asepsis with central venous catheter care
- Monitor intake and output of fluids
- Monitor nutritional intake

Caregiver Education

- Inform caregivers about medications and the use of nonpharmacological techniques.
- Teach the procedure for care of the venous access device.
- Caregiver should continue to participate in the child's care as much as possible to empower the caregiver and maintain a sense of control.
- Encourage siblings to be involved by bringing toys or food items if condition of patient is stable without danger of bacterial exposure.
- Normalize caregiver processes.
- Access the injection cap with the syringe or IV tubing (opening the clamp, if necessary).
- Perform hand hygiene when done.

SAFE AND EFFECTIVE NURSING CARE: Clinical Pearl

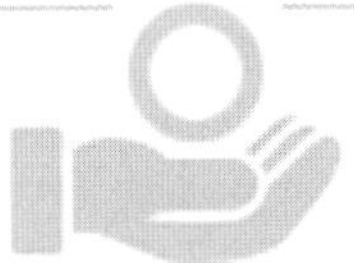

Palliative Care

The World Health Organization defines palliative care as "an approach that improves the quality of life of patients and their families facing the problem associated with life-threatening illness, through the prevention and relief of suffering by means of early identification and impeccable assessment and treatment of pain and other problems, physical, psychosocial and spiritual" (World Health Organization, 2017). Seek out individual preferences of patients and their families facing life-limiting illnesses. For more information on end-of-life care, see Chapter 5.

Case Study

Adolescence and Adherence to Medications

A 14-year-old male adolescent is receiving medications according to the HIV research protocol in a regional medical center several miles from home. He has had HIV all of his life and the prognosis is currently poor. The adolescent and family decided to enroll in a drug trial in an effort to increase life expectance and quality of life. The treatment protocol requires accuracy for time of medication administration. After weeks of hospitalization, the adolescent is experiencing the complications of fatigue and social isolation. Family members describe how the present changes of the body, progression to a new school building, and an additional group of friends have influenced his behavior. Goals agreed on with the adolescent are to maximize immune function and maintain normal development.

1. What priority nursing assessment information does the nurse identify?
2. What nursing interventions would support the nursing goals?
3. When the adolescent develops boredom with the initial nursing interventions, what other activities are suggested?
4. How will the nurse evaluate these goals?

REFERENCES

American Academy of Pediatrics Council on Environmental Health. (2016). Prevention of childhood lead toxicity. *Pediatrics, 138*(1), e20161493.

American Cancer Society. (2016). *Cancer treatment & survivorship facts & figures 2016–2017.* Atlanta, GA: American Cancer Society. Retrieved from https://www.cancer.org/content/dam/cancer-org/research/cancer-facts-and-statistics/cancer-treatment-and-survivorship-facts-and-figures/cancer-treatment-and-survivorship-facts-and-figures-2016-2017.pdf

American Cancer Society. (2017). *What are the key statistics about Wilms tumors?* Retrieved from https://www.cancer.org/cancer/wilms-tumor/about/key-statistics.html

Aukema, E., Last, B., Schouten-van Meeteren, A., & Grootenhuis, M. (2011). Explorative study on the aftercare of pediatric brain tumor survivors: A parents' perspective. *Supportive Care in Cancer, 19*, 1637–1646. doi:10.1007/s00520-010-0995-6

Baker, R. D., Greer, F. R., & Committee on Nutrition American Academy of Pediatrics. (2010). Diagnosis and prevention of iron deficiency and iron-deficiency anemia in infants and young children (0–3 years of age). *Pediatrics, 126*, 1040–1050.

Campbell, Y. N., Machan, M. D., & Fisher, M. D. (2016). The Jehovah's witness population: Considerations for preoperative optimization of hemoglobin. *American Association of Nurses Anesthetists Journal, 84* (3), 173–178.

Centers for Disease Control and Prevention. (2016). *Sickle cell disease (SCD).* Retrieved from https://www.cdc.gov/ncbddd/sicklecell/data.html

Centers for Disease Control and Prevention. (2017). *HIV among youth.* Retrieved from https://www.cdc.gov/hiv/group/age/youth/index.html

Connor, T. H., MacKenzie, B. A., DeBord, D. G., Trout, D. B., & O'Callaghan, J. P. (2016). Preventing Occupational Exposure to Antineoplastic and Other Hazardous Drugs in Health Care Settings [U.S. Department of Health and Human Services, Centers for Disease Control and Prevention, National Institute for Occupational Safety and Health, DHHS (NIOSH) Publication Number 2016-161 (Supersedes 2014-138)]. Retrieved from https://www.cdc.gov/niosh/docs/2004-165/default.html

Hagan, J. F., Shaw, J. S., & Duncan, P. M. (2017). *Bright futures: Nutrition* (4th ed.). American Academy of Pediatrics. Retrieved from https://brightfutures.aap.org/Bright%20Futures%20Documents/BF4_Introduction.pdf

Hymes, S. R., & Steele, R. W. (2016). Fever without a focus. *Medscape.* Retrieved from http://emedicine.medscape.com/article/970788-overview

Khilnani, P. (2005). *Practical approach to pediatric intensive care.* New York: Oxford Press.

Kleinman R. E., & Greer F.R. (Eds.). (2014). *Pediatric nutrition: Policy of the American Academy of Pediatrics* (7th ed.). Elk Grove Village, IL: American Academy of Pediatrics; 2014:449-466.

National Cancer Institute at the National Institutes for Health. (2014). *Wilms tumor and other childhood kidney tumors.* Retrieved from http://www.cancer.gov/cancertopics/pdq/treatment/wilms/HealthProfessional

National Cancer Institute at the National Institutes for Health. (2017). *Aromatherapy and essential oils (PDQ®)—Health professional version.* Retrieved from https://www.cancer.gov/about-cancer/treatment/cam/hp/aromatherapy-pdq

Pagana, K. (2009). What does the absolute neutrophil count tell you? *American Nurse Today, 4*, 12–13. Retrieved from http://www.americannursetoday.com/article.aspx?id=4332&fid=4302

Siegel, R. L., Miller, K. D., & Jemal, A. (2017). Cancer statistics, 2017. *CA A Cancer J Clin, 67*, 7–30. doi: 10.3322/caac.21387

Skidmore-Roth, L. (2017). *Mosby's drug guide for nursing students e-book* (12th ed.). St. Louis, MO: Mosby.

U.S. Department of Health and Human Services. (2017). *Preventing mother-to-child transmission of HIV.* Retrieved from https://aidsinfo.nih.gov/understanding-hiv-aids/fact-sheets/20/50/preventing-mother-to-child-transmission-of-hiv/

U.S. Environmental Protection Agency. (2017). *Protect your family from exposures to lead.* Retrieved from https://www.epa.gov/lead/protect-your-family-exposures-lead

Van Leeuwen, A. M., & Bladh, M. L. (2015). *Davis's comprehensive handbook of laboratory & diagnostic tests with nursing implications* (6th ed.). Philadelphia: F.A. Davis.

Vorderstrasse, A. A., Hammer, M. J., & Dungan, J. R. (2014). Nursing implications of personalized and precision medicine. *Seminars in Oncology Nursing, 30* (2), 130–136.

Ward, S. L., & Hisley, S. M. (2009). *Maternal-child nursing care: Optimizing outcomes for mothers, children, and families.* Philadelphia: F.A. Davis.

Williams, A. M., Estrada, C., Gary-Bryan, H., & MacKeil-White, K. (2012). The hematology and oncology pediatric patient: A review of fever and neutropenia, blood transfusions, and other complex problems. *Clinical Pediatric Emergency Medicine, 13*(2), 91–98.

World Health Organization. (2017). *WHO definition of palliative care.* Retrieved from http://who.int/cancer/palliative/definition/en/

Yarbro, C. H., Wujcik, D., & Gobel, B. H. (Eds.). (2018). *Cancer nursing: Principles and practice* (8th ed.). Burlington, MA: Jones & Bartlett Learning.

Musculoskeletal Disorders

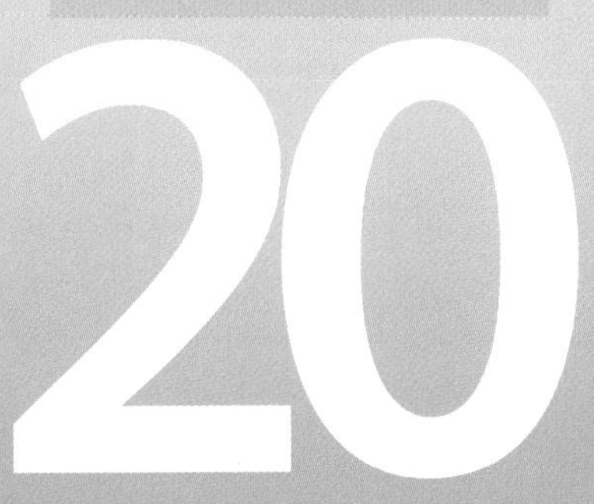

Suzanne Fortuna, DNP, APRN-BC, CNS, FNP

LEARNING OUTCOMES

Upon completion of this chapter, the student will be able to:

1. Describe the anatomy and physiology of the musculoskeletal system.
2. Describe the common disorders of the musculoskeletal system.
3. Identify specific physical assessment skills for evaluation of the musculoskeletal system.
4. Describe the diagnostic tests and laboratory values typically monitored in musculoskeletal disorders.
5. Explain the applicable nursing interventions for musculoskeletal disorders.
6. Integrate acute hospital care concepts for musculoskeletal disorders.
7. Integrate chronic hospital care concepts for musculoskeletal disorders.
8. Integrate emergency care or trauma concepts for musculoskeletal disorders.
9. Describe strategies to support patient/caregiver education about musculoskeletal disorders.

ANATOMY AND PHYSIOLOGY

The musculoskeletal system is composed of bones, muscles, joints, tendons, and ligaments that interconnect. Muscle contraction is innervated by the somatic nervous system. Fetal development of the musculoskeletal system begins with the formation of pure cartilage, which is then transformed by osteoclasts and osteoblast formation. The rapid formation of the skeletal structures makes abnormalities somewhat common (Fig. 20–1). Considerations in abnormalities include:

- Environment
- Genetics
- Trauma

Bones are cartilaginous structures while children are growing and developing. Growth plates are open in children, making certain diagnoses more difficult at times due to age-specific qualities of bone and joint structures. Once maturation occurs, bones are characteristically dense osseous structures typical of the description of a skeleton framework. As a rule of thumb with children, skin, muscles, and ligaments protect the maturing bones; therefore, if these parts are weakened or not developed properly, the bones suffer.

Anatomy of Growing Bone

- Epiphysis: ends of long bones
- Physis: segment of bone responsible for lengthening during growth
- Metaphysis: wide part of long bones where diaphysis and epiphysis meet
- Diaphysis: formed from primary center of ossification; sometimes referred to as the shaft
- Periosteum: sheath covering the bones

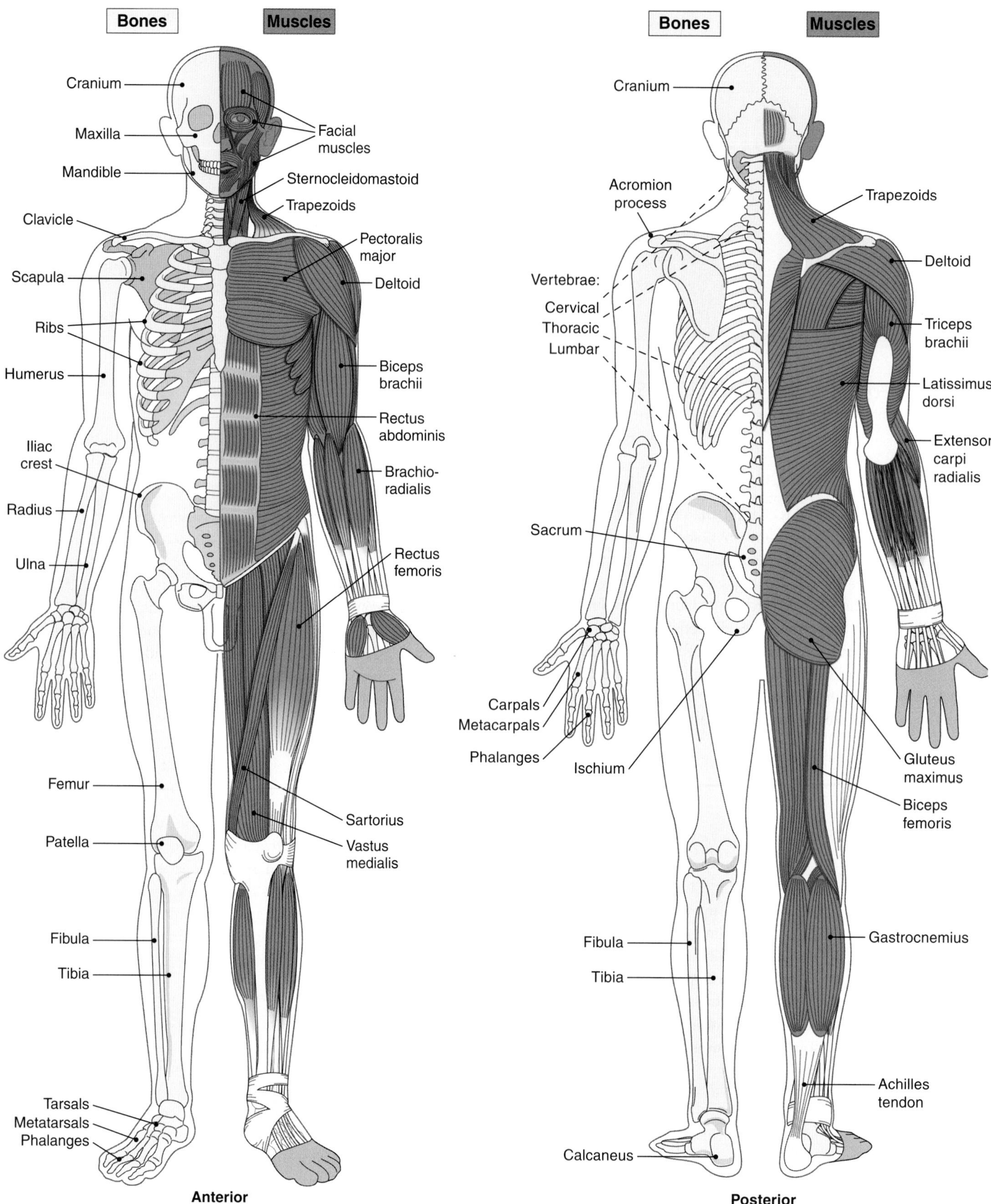

FIGURE 20–1 Cross-section of the musculoskeletal system.

CRITICAL COMPONENT

Physis

Injury to the physis can cause long-term impact of a child's physical development.

- Children's bones are different from adult bones.
- Adult fractures must be aligned perfectly.
- Children with open growth plates will remodel, or form new bone to repair the fractured area. The younger the child, the better remodeling will occur depending on the extent of deformity. Injuries that occur after age 16 years may not have enough time to remodel completely. Risk for physeal arrest with subsequent growth disturbance is present.

Skeleton

Children have an immature skeleton, characterized by:

- Increased resiliency to stress
- Thicker periosteum
- Increased potential to remodel
- Shorter healing times
- Presence of a physis

Injury Pattern in Growing Bones

- Bones tend to bow rather than break.
- Compressive force = torus fracture/buckle fracture.
- Ligaments and tendons are stronger than young bone.
  - Bone is more likely to be injured than soft tissue.
  - Periosteum, a sheath covering the bones, is biologically active in children. This means that the periosteum is developing new bone and also supplying blood.
    - Stabilizes fracture
    - Promotes healing

Unique Properties of the Immature Skeleton

- Children tend to heal fractures faster than adults (Sofu et al., 2015).
- Advantage: The immobilization times are shorter.
- Disadvantage: Misaligned fragments become "solid" sooner.
- Anticipate bone remodeling, the absorption of bone tissue while new bone is simultaneously deposited, if child has more than 2 years of expected growth left.
- Mild angulation deformities (less than 2 mm) often correct themselves.
- Rotational deformities, those that are twisted, require reduction, or placement of correct alignment, will not remodel.
- Fractures in children may stimulate longitudinal bone growth.
- Some degree of bone overlap is acceptable and may even be helpful.
- Children do not tend to get as stiff as adults after immobilization, yet still need to regain strength after immobilization in 1 to 3 weeks of slow return to full activities once pain, swelling, and stiffness have resolved.
- After casting, a callus is formed but still may be fibrous. A provisional callus is temporary and is still developing new bone. A definitive callus forms permanent osseous or bone tissue after several weeks.
- Children should avoid contact activities for 2 to 4 weeks once out of cast.

ASSESSMENT

Many clinical tools are used for the evaluation of musculoskeletal system abnormalities, and all require an understanding of musculoskeletal system anatomy. The overall assessment of the musculoskeletal system involves simple to complex physical tests to evaluate changes or deficits. Mainly, the evaluation involves:

- Inspection
- Palpation
- Range-of-motion (ROM) maneuvers
- Laboratory tests if indicated (Table 20–1)
- Radiographic tests: X-rays, computed tomography (CT) scans, magnetic resonance imaging (MRI), arthrograms (Table 20–2)

Understanding normal motor development and screening tools also helps the health-care provider determine problems or potential delays. Motor development is the child's increasing ability to move and interact with the environment. Although the rate of motor development varies among individuals, it follows a predictable pattern (Noritz, Murphy, & Neuromotor Screening Expert Panel, 2013). The common goal for children is mastery of certain skills and improvement in efficiency, precision, and speed along the way. When musculoskeletal abnormalities exist, motor skills may be delayed or nonexistent. Taking a thorough history, including birth history and the degree of prenatal and postnatal care, is important to understanding the child's development and predicting potential delays that may occur.

General Assessment

Screening for appropriate growth and development includes the following:

- Physical examination
- History taking
- Height and weight
- Diagnostic imaging if applicable
- Laboratory testing if applicable
- Motor development evaluation
- Family expectations

EMERGENT AND INITIAL NURSING CARE OF THE MUSCULOSKELETAL SYSTEM

The usual nursing care and positioning of the affected extremity involve:

- PRICE (protect, rest, ice, compression, and elevation)
- Neurovascular checks

TABLE 20–1 Blood and Body Fluid Analysis for the Child With Alterations in Musculoskeletal Conditions

DIAGNOSTIC TEST	FUNCTION OF THE TEST	INDICATIONS	NORMAL VALUES
Complete blood count (CBC)	Blood sample evaluates many aspects	Platelets indicate a bleeding disorder >WBC indicates a bacterial infection or septic arthritis	Platelets: 150,000–400,000/μL WBC: 4500–10,000/μL
CBC differential	Breaks down WBC into various types (five total) Numbers indicate a percentage of total WBC Indicates the type of infection	Monocytes indicate a long-term infectious process Lymphocytes indicate an increase in viral illness Eosinophils indicate an allergic or parasitic condition Basophils indicate a chronic inflammatory condition Neutrophils (polys) Bands are immature neutrophils Segs are mature neutrophils (left-shift describes an increase in the band neutrophils) Suggests a severe bacterial infection such as sepsis	Monocytes normal = 2%-10% Lymphocytes normal = 20%–40% Eosinophils normal = 1%-6% Basophils normal = 1-2% 0% for bands and 31%–57% for segs Presence of bands is highly indicative of a bacterial infection
C-reactive protein (CRP)	Measures a protein in blood that is released when an infection is present Normal=less than 1	>0.9 indicates an infection or septic arthritis	<1.0 mg/dL
Calcium and phosphate	Measures the amount of these minerals	Low levels may indicate rickets	Calcium: 8.5–11 mg Phosphorus: 3.0–4.5 mg/dL
Rheumatoid factor (Rh factor)	Measures the body's autoimmune response to an antigen	If positive, may indicate juvenile arthritis Not all children with juvenile arthritis have a positive Rh factor	Negative
Erythrocyte sedimentation rate (ESR)	Measures the speed at which RBCs settle out in solution	Elevated indicates septic arthritis May also indicate infection	0–10 mm/hr
Blood cultures	Measures whether microorganisms grow in the laboratory	Can identify an organism causing infection Forty percent of children with septic arthritis have a positive blood culture	No growth
Bone biopsies	Diagnose tumor or infection of the bone	Osteomyelitis Bone tumor	Normal bone cells
Fluid aspiration from joints	Diagnose an infection of the joint or drain fluid from joint to relieve pressure	Drainage is purulent Culture of fluid is positive	Clear fluid No growth from culture

RBC, red blood cell; Segs, segmented cells; WBC, white blood cell.

From Ward, S. L., & Hisley, S. M. (2015). Maternal-child nursing care: Optimizing outcomes for mothers, children, & families, *2nd edition (p. 1164). Philadelphia: F.A. Davis.*

TABLE 20–2 Orthopedic Diagnostic Tests

DIAGNOSTIC IMAGING TEST	BENEFITS	LIMITATIONS
Radiograph	Easily available Visualizes fractures well No sedation needed Inexpensive	Two-dimensional Does not visualize soft tissue such as cartilage Patient must be positioned properly Radiation exposure
Fluoroscopy	Guides many orthopedic procedures Can be used with contrast Real-time radiography Inexpensive	Radiation exposure
Arthrography	Provides visualization of joints Three-dimensional view	Risk of reaction to contrast Depends on the skill of the radiographer Radiation exposure
Computed tomography (CT) scan	Cross-sectional view of anatomy Clearer than radiographs Software programs can show reconstruction Can use contrast	Expensive May require sedation Risk of reaction to contrast
Bone scan (nuclear medicine)	Excellent at finding changes in bone as a result of infection, trauma, or tumor	Takes 4 hours Not always available on emergency basis Cannot distinguish benign from malignant tumors Radiation exposure to entire body IV access required
Ultrasound	Easily available No radiation No sedation needed Good for visualizing soft tissue masses and cysts Painless Inexpensive	Limited use Depends on the skill of the radiographer
Magnetic resonance imaging (MRI)	Visualizes hard and soft tissue and bone marrow No radiation	Not readily available No metal can be present in the vicinity Sedation may be needed Need experienced radiologist to read MRI

From Ward, S. L., & Hisley, S. M. (2015). Maternal-child nursing care: Optimizing outcomes for mothers, children, & families, 2nd edition *(p. 1164). Philadelphia: F.A. Davis.*

- Natural alignment is best to prevent deformity, improve function
- Keep splint/cast/brace application intact
- Reinforcement of bandage or splint as needed
- Maintenance of weight-bearing status
- Teach/monitor use of assistive aids as needed
- Activity-level precautions can be age specific.
- Pain medication usage, side effects, discontinuation
- Nonpharmacological methods, especially distraction
- Problems or concerns that require immediate medical attention include slipped bandage or splint, high fever, and/or foul odor from the bandage or splint
- Postoperative coping and family support or community resources
- Interdisciplinary team involvement, such as social work or rehabilitation services
- School and gym class participation restrictions
- Toileting and other activities of daily living
- Follow-up visits

FRACTURES

Fractures in children are more complicated than in adults due to the nature of maturing bones, cartilaginous features, and open growth plates. Torus (buckle) fractures are some of the most common among children. The mechanism of injury is usually a direct fall onto an outstretched arm/hand or a fall from some height with a landing that compresses the bones either at or away from the growth plate. The acronym FOOSH (fall onto outstretched hand) is used to describe this type of injury.

Occult fractures are also common due to the maturation process. An occult fracture of the tibia commonly is called a toddler's fracture. An occult fracture is rarely seen on emergent x-rays, but the child may cry or refuse to bear weight on the affected extremity.

The softness of developing bone in children means that simple stressors, such as jumping from a height or twisting unnaturally, can cause injury to the bone.

- Placing the child in either a walking boot or cast relieves the pressure and pain. Upper extremities use a brace or sling to immobilize and elevate pain.
- Repeat films after 3 to 4 weeks note healing callous formation along the seam of the bone, proving occult fracture validity.
- Sometimes just symptom relief is the treatment for fractures.
- Advise families that new bone formation may or may not be visible, but clinical examination and immobilization are still recommended.

SAFE AND EFFECTIVE NURSING CARE: Promoting Safety

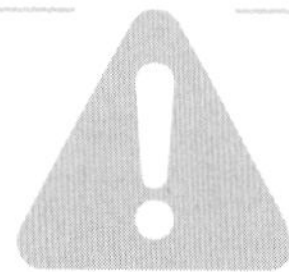

General Fracture Care

Typically, instruct patients and families about the following activity limitations (if applicable):

- Keep two feet on the ground; no running, jumping, or climbing with splints or casts unless otherwise indicated.
- No activities with balls or bicycles.
- Do not insert food, toys, or other objects into casts/splints.
- Upper arms: Use sling/brace if instructed. No slings around the neck to bed. Slings should be at heart level.
- Lower extremities: Use brace, crutches (for children older than 8 years), wheelchair (older than 4 years), or stroller (younger than 3 years) as instructed.

Physeal Injuries

- Many childhood fractures involve the physis (Arora, Fichadia, Hartwig, & Kannikeswaran, 2014; Eastwood & de Gheldere, 2011).
- Account for 27% of all skeletal injuries in children (Kunes, 2011); 15% to 25% of pediatric fractures (Arora et al., 2014). Many fractures occur during adolescence.
- Can disrupt growth of bone.
- Injury near but not at the physis can stimulate bone growth.

Incidence of Pediatric Fractures

- Approximately 10% to 25% of children who seek attention for injury have a fracture (Arora et al., 2014; Kunes, 2011; Naranje, Erali, Warner Jr., Sawyer, & Kelly, 2016)
- From birth to 16 years, chance of fracture:
  - Boys: 42% (Jawetz et al., 2015; Kunes, 2011)
  - Girls: 27% (Jawetz et al., 2015; Kunes, 2011)
- Peak incidence of fractures: age 14 years for boys and age 11 years for girls (Arora et al., 2014)
- Most commonly involved sites:
  - Distal radius (most frequently fractured along with metacarpal and phalanges) accounts for 50% of injuries (Arora et al., 2014)
  - Clavicle (second most common)
  - Hand
  - Elbow
  - Radius
  - Tibia

Classification of Fractures

Fractures in general can be classified in several different categories (Fig. 20–2):

- Greenstick, buckle or torus, and plastic deformation fractures
- Simple fractures
- Comminuted fractures
- Complex fractures

Physeal fractures are classified as Salter Harris I through IV based on the level of growth plate involvement (Arora et al., 2014). This system delineates risk for growth disturbance from fracture. While higher-grade fractures are more likely to cause growth disturbance, it can happen with any physeal injury.

- Type I
  - Fracture passes transversely through physis, separating epiphysis from metaphysis

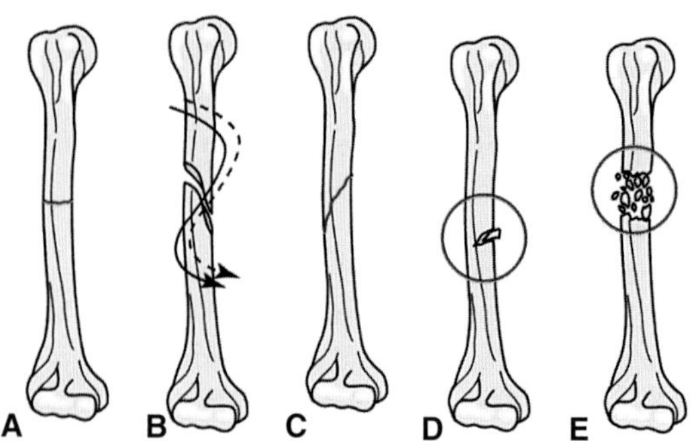

FIGURE 20–2 Different classes of fractures. **A,** Transverse. **B,** Spiral. **C,** Oblique. **D,** Greenstick. **E,** Comminuted.

- Type II
  - Fracture passes transversely through physis but exits through metaphysis
  - Triangular fragment
- Type III
  - Fracture crosses physis and exits through epiphysis at joint space
- Type IV
  - Fracture extends upward from the joint line, through the physis, and out the metaphysis
- Type V
  - Crush injury to growth plate

The level of severity and the child's age may direct treatment modalities and outcomes.

Torus Fractures

With this type of fracture, the bone bends and buckles but does not break; it occurs commonly in the radius or ulna, or both. This fracture occurs only in children because their bones are softer than those of adults. Many torus fractures are not diagnosed until days after the injury occurs. Treatment strives to alleviate pain and prevent further deformity. If the bones are anatomically aligned, no reduction is needed. Children with this injury typically wear a short arm cast for 3 to 4 weeks. If the injury is more than 24 hours old, it will be casted immediately; newer injuries are splinted for 5 to 7 days before casting.

Greenstick Fractures

Greenstick fractures are incomplete fractures of long bones that are commonly mid-diaphyseal. If nondisplaced, this injury is typically treated with a short arm cast for 4 weeks followed by a removable split for 2 weeks. If the fracture is displaced more than 15 degrees, it is reduced and immobilized in a long arm cast.

Distal Radius Fracture

Distal radius fracture is a common bone fracture that affects the radius in the forearm. Because of its proximity to the wrist joint, this injury is often called a wrist fracture. When displaced, this fracture should be reduced as soon as possible. Nondisplaced fractures are given a short arm cast for 3 to 6 weeks. The older the child is when the injury occurs, the longer the immobilization. If the x-rays do not initially show a fracture but the child has tenderness over the growth plate, the wrist should be immobilized for 2 weeks and then re-examined with a follow-up x-ray. Fracture is unlikely if no callus is present.

Elbow Fractures

Elbow fractures comprise 10% to 12% of pediatric fractures (Arora et al., 2014), most of which are supracondylar fractures. Elbow fractures in children are complex to diagnose and manage due to immature bones and involvement of many different bones at the joint. Early recognition and referral will provide the best outcomes.

Supracondylar Fractures

- A supracondylar fracture affects the weakest part of the elbow joint where humerus flattens and flares.
- Peak incidence is 5 to 7 years old, and it represents 60% to 80% of pediatric elbow fractures (Arora et al., 2014).
- Most commonly extension fracture is characterized by elbow pain and swelling.
- Potential for vascular compromise
  - Indicated by 5 Ps: pain, pulse, pallor, paresthesia, paralysis
  - Reduce fracture if pulse is compromised
- Check nerve function in hand.
- Most supracondylar fractures are displaced and need surgery.
- Nondisplaced fractures can be managed with long arm cast, forearm neutral, elbow at 90 degrees for 3 weeks.
- Follow-up x-rays are taken 3 to 7 days later to document alignment.
- X-rays are taken at 3 weeks to document callus.
- Once callus is noted at 3 weeks, discontinue cast, pull out pins in the office, and start active ROM slowly over the next 1 to 2 weeks.
- If no ROM improvement in 2 to 3 weeks, can recheck in office or send to occupational therapy as needed.

Lateral Condylar Fractures

- Second most common elbow fracture (Arora et al., 2014)
- Most common physeal elbow injury
- FOOSH (fall on outstretched hand) + varus force = lateral condyle avulsion
- Examination: focal swelling at lateral distal humerus
- Most are displaced and require surgical pinning
- If nondisplaced, treat with casting
- Posterior splint acutely, elbow at 90 degrees
- At follow-up (weekly), check for late displacement
- If stable for 2 weeks, long arm cast for another 4 weeks
- Complications: growth arrest, nonunion

Medial Condyle Fractures

- Third most common elbow fracture (Arora et al., 2014)
- Common injury of baseball pitchers between ages 9 and 14
- Overuse injury caused by repetitive motion and increased muscle fatigue
- Conservative treatment for nondisplaced and stress injuries
- Long arm splint or cast for 3 weeks
- Surgical intervention possible for displaced fractures in more than minimal displacement intra-articularly or presence of loose bodies
- Side effects include stiffening, ulnar nerve injury, and symptomatic non-union

Clavicle Fractures

Clavicle fracture is the most common birth injury. It can also result from FOOSH, a fall on the shoulder, or direct trauma. Eighty percent of clavicle fractures occur in the middle third of the bone, 15% in the distal third, and 5% in the proximal third (Arora et al., 2014; Kunes, 2011). Patients with a clavicle fracture typically hold their arm to the chest and experience pain with shoulder movement. Obvious deformity often occurs. This injury is occasionally missed in infants until callous formation causes a visible bump. Without trauma, this injury can indicate the presence of bone cysts. Abuse should be ruled out in infants and young children (Arora et al., 2014).

- Surgical intervention is required if open fracture is displaced more than 100% of width, tenting skin (bone is pushing the skin outward), comminution (fracture pieces), or neurological compromise (vascularity, pulselessness, or loss of sensation) (Arora et al., 2014).
- Although a figure-eight bandage was once the standard of care, this can redisplace the fracture, which complicates healing. Most pediatric fractures of this kind can be treated with a simple sling, which provides comfort and reminds others to proceed with caution.
- When fracture is fully healed, the shoulder's full ROM will be painless.
- Children can generally return to pain-free activity by 4 weeks, but should not play contact sports for at least 6 weeks.
- Children may have a bump in the injured area even after full healing; it will shrink but may not completely disappear.

Tibia Fractures

A tibia fracture typically occurs when the foot is twisted during a fall (Palmu et al., 2014).

- Because it takes a lot of force to injure the tibia shaft, this fracture is rarely displaced.
- Posterior lower leg split is required for an acute fracture because swelling occurs 24 to 48 hours postinjury.
- Nondisplaced fractures require a long leg cast for 6 to 8 weeks.
- Weekly radiographs may be required to monitor position.
- Surgery is required if the break angulates more than 15 degrees.

Toddler Fractures

- Toddler fractures occur with children younger than age 2 years who are learning to walk (Bauer & Lovejoy, 2017).
- No specific injury is notable most of the time.
- Child refuses to bear weight on leg.
- Examine hip, thigh, and knee to rule out other causes of limping.
- Consider and rule out abuse; spiral fractures are a common signifier.
- Examine for soft tissue injury to buttocks, back of legs, head, and neck.
- Transverse fractures of the midshaft are more suspicious for child abuse.
- Management: long leg cast for 3 to 4 weeks
- Weight-bearing as tolerated
- Heals completely in 6 to 8 weeks

CRITICAL COMPONENT

Radiograph Pearls

- Nearly 20% of children with injury have a fracture (Arora et al., 2014; Kunes, 2011).
- Consider bilateral x-rays in children if unsure of or difficulty visualizing fracture lines.
- Physeal injuries are common and may have no radiographic findings—treat as fracture!
- Remember to tell caregivers about possible future growth problems.

Femur Fractures

The femur is the most commonly fractured long bone, representing 1.4% to 1.7% of all pediatric fractures (American Academy of Orthopedic Surgeons, 2015; Kocher et al., 2009; Sela, Hershkovich, Sher-Lurie, Schindler, & Givon, 2013). This injury is usually a diaphyseal fracture and more commonly affects males and children older than age 3 years. Incidence of femur fracture is highest in summer months and is typically caused by trauma, including falls, recreational sports, and car accidents. When this injury occurs in toddlers, rule out potential abuse, particularly when a spiral or corner fracture is seen in a child who does not yet walk (Kocher et al., 2009; Sela et al., 2013).

Treatment

Treatment aims to restore length, alignment, and rotation of the femur while preventing disruption of blood supply to the femoral head (osteonecrosis) and physeal injury that will impact growth. Treatment options include the following:

- Traction presurgery if bone needs to be reduced, usually skin traction (Fig. 20–3)
    - Older child may need skeletal traction depending on fracture and amount of translation. Traction is often not required because of the increased ability to use femoral rods or sliding plates with minimally invasive surgery options.
- Casting: applying stabilizing forces to prevent further injury
- Plate and screw fixation: open reduction internal fixation
- External fixation: nails or pins to hold a fracture in place outside the skin
- Flexible nailing: thinner nails to hold fracture pieces in alignment with severe deformity
- Rigid nailing: firmer and can permanently realign bones with severe deformity
- Traction: application of splinting and bracing techniques to hold position or realignment until definitive treatment can occur

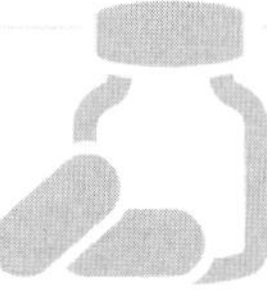

SAFE AND EFFECTIVE NURSING CARE: Understanding Medication

Medication for Muscle Spasms

With fractures surrounding large muscle groups such as femur fractures, children will have muscle spasms while in traction. The use of IV lorazepam (Ativan) every 4 to 6 hours as needed may be ordered. The child may need oral lorazepam at home for 1 to 3 days. Spasms typically subside once a Spica cast has been placed.

Care of Child in a Spica Cast

A Spica cast (Fig. 20–4) is used for treatment of femur fractures in toddlers and preschoolers. Care measures for this treatment include the following:

- Turn and reposition every 2 to 4 hours while awake to prevent pressure sores at heals or sacrum

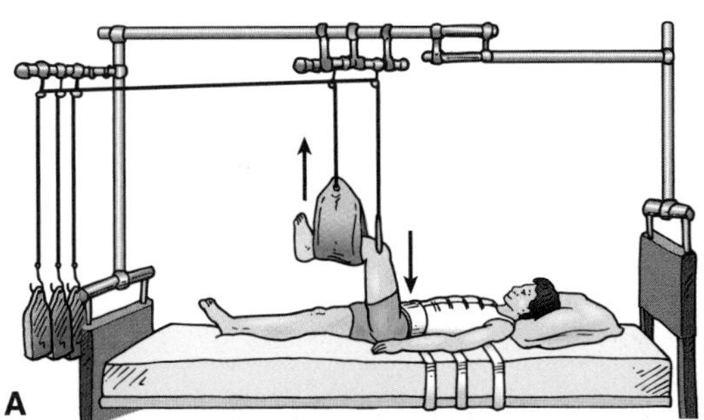

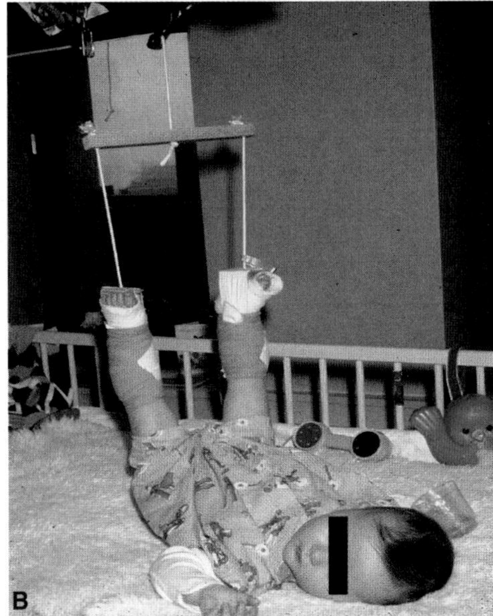

FIGURE 20–3 **A**, The 90/90 femoral traction is most commonly used to treat femur fractures and complicated femur fractures. **B**, Example of baby in traction.

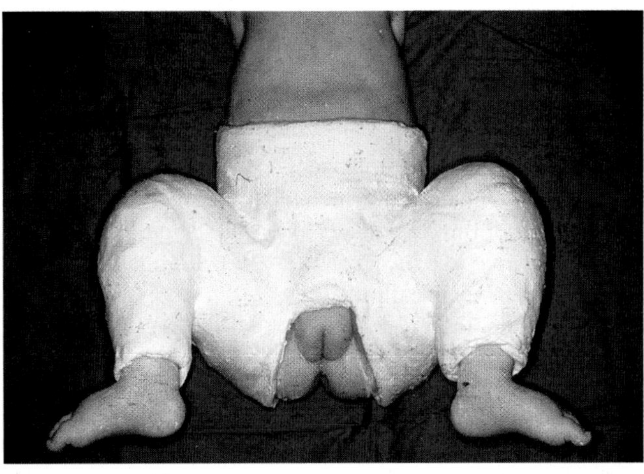

FIGURE 20–4 Child in Spica cast.

- Neurovascular checks every 2 hours for 24 hours postoperatively.
- Insert two fingers along abdomen of cast to verify it is not too tight, especially with position changes such as side lying or from side to back.
- Toileting: Use diapers in incontinent child, urinal or bedpan in continent child.
- Padding protects the cast from urine and feces; use chux pads with absorbent side placed next to skin.
- Oxycodone every 4 to 6 hours as needed, around the clock for initial 24 to 48 hours, then before bed for up to 1 week postoperatively; may encourage ibuprofen or acetaminophen during the day as needed.
- Constipation prevention includes:
  - Increase consumption of clear fluids.
  - Increase consumption of fresh fruits and veggies.
  - Decrease consumption of fried foods and constipation triggers such as cheese and milk until no longer taking narcotics.
  - Explain decreased physical activities are associated with gastric motility.
  - Regulate consumption of high-fat and high-carbohydrate foods, and encourage more lean and green types of foods.
  - Decrease intake of sweet, sugary food and drink until cast is off and normal activity is resumed.

CONGENITAL MUSCULOSKELETAL ABNORMALITIES

Congenital refers to a condition that a child is born with, develops in utero, or inherits. Many congenital abnormalities or birth defects are apparent either in utero or shortly after birth. Other disorders remain unrecognized until the child reaches a later stage of growth and development. Some abnormalities are caused by packaging, which refers to the size of and amount of amniotic fluid in the womb.

Clubfoot

Clubfoot is a congenital abnormality (Fig. 20–5); it may also be neurogenic or idiopathic (no known reason).

- Syndrome development includes deformity along with other physical or developmental defects.
- Teratological (myelodysplasia and arthrogryposis) causes include possible in utero exposures to environmental factors, chemicals, or genetic disorders.
- Positional (in utero malposition)

Risk Factors and Incidence

The incidence of clubfoot in infants occurs with the following considerations:

- Presentation may be unilateral or bilateral; bilateral presentation in 50% of cases (Kliegman, Stanton, St. Geme, Schor, & Behrman, 2011; Radler, 2013).
- Family history increases incidence.
- Males are more often affected (2:1) than females (Kliegman et al., 2011; Radler, 2013).
- Affects the entire lower extremity from the knee down
- The calf looks smaller and has less ability to develop muscle strength than a typical lower-extremity limb.
- The affected foot may be smaller in dorsal height and length.
- The foot itself is fixed and rigid in a plantar-flexed and pronated position that cannot be dorsiflexed or manually stretched into a neutral position.
- The Achilles tendon is extremely tight or shortened, with the inability to have the talus and calcaneus lowered into the neutral equinus position.

Treatment

Treatment options include both nonsurgical and surgical modalities.

Nonsurgical Modalities

The first approach is to start the Ponseti technique of serial casting within the first week of life. This is a very time-consuming but successful treatment option. The casts are changed weekly for up to 12 weeks, which allows for a gradual change in position. The goal is to first re-create the deformity, then slowly progress to full correction in an abducted fully dorsiflexed turned-outward presentation. See Ponseti method as above.

After casting is complete, the correction is maintained either with ankle-foot orthotics or the use of a Denis-Browne bar or Dobb's bar. This device is a bar with shoes attached that keeps the foot in external rotation to prevent recurrent deformity. It is used at least 23 hours a day for 3 months, then during naps and nighttime sleep until age 3 years. Without strict adherence to follow-up regimen, the failure rate for this treatment is high. It is essential to teach symptom monitoring so caregivers can recognize an acute need to return for further medical care.

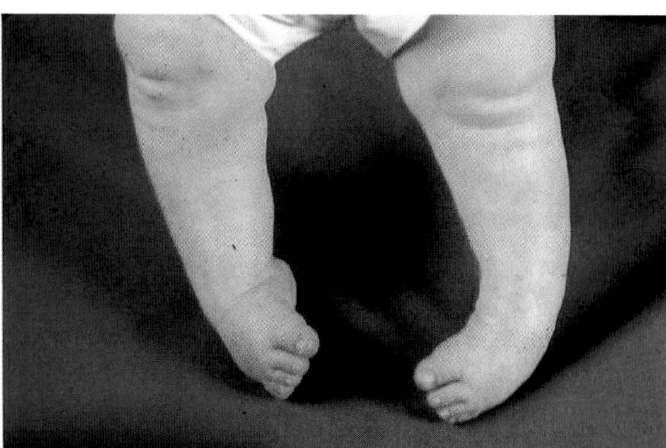

FIGURE 20–5 Clubfoot.

CRITICAL COMPONENT

Alerts for Caregivers

After clubfoot treatment, the caregiver should be instructed to return to the health-care provider if the child presents with any of the following symptoms:

- Feet appear to turn inward
- Walking on the lateral border of foot
- Tiptoe walking
- Rocker-bottom foot, in which the navicular bone at the neck of the talus is malpositioned, the ankle is in severe equinus, and the forefoot is in dorsiflexion

Other nonsurgical treatment options include:

- Physical therapy: manually stretching heel cords at home and/or kinesiology taping to hold the foot in place
- Serial splinting beginning at age 12 weeks
- Removable splits that hold the foot in a fixed position
- Molded or prefabricated orthotic bracing that holds the foot in proper positioning while child matures

SAFE AND EFFECTIVE NURSING CARE: Clinical Pearl

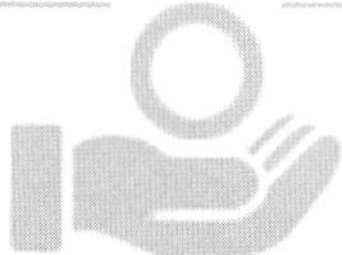

Casting Material

The casting material is always plaster because of its ability to be molded, whereas fiberglass is more rigid. A fiberglass cast overlay may be placed over plaster to maintain the mold that was created and provide stability so the plaster does not break down as easily and cause cracks or ripples in the material that may lead to skin breakdown. It is important to keep either type of cast dry.

Surgical Modalities

Indications for surgical treatment are:

- Failed serial casting
- Referral for treatment after first 10 days of life
- Failure to follow-up and/or early discontinuation of treatment options
- Recurrent deformity

Surgical treatment options include:

- Soft tissue releases: surgical procedure to release tight muscles or release scar tissue formation
- Tendon transfers: moving insertion of hypermobile tendons to work at a different point of fixation
- Bony surgical procedures, which align bone fragments to reposition a deformity, will improve shape and function of deformed bone structures

Metatarsus Adductus

Metatarsus adductus is a common foot deformity that involves the forefoot only in which the patient presents with the foot turned inward (Fig. 20–6).

Risk Factors and Incidence

- More common in males than in females (Williams, James, & Tran, 2013)
- Usually bilateral
- Inheritance factor minimal
- In utero molding—petite mother, prima gravida

Clinical Presentation

- Abducted forefoot
- Normal hind foot
- Prominent fifth metatarsus tuberosity
- Variable rigidity

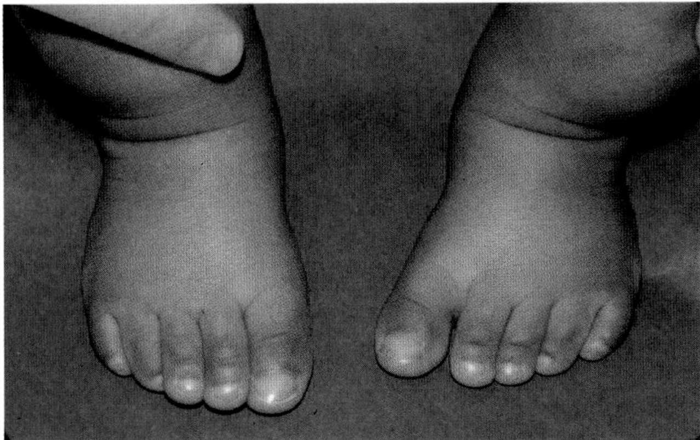

FIGURE 20–6 Metatarsus adductus.

Treatment

Treatment options are dependent on the flexibility of the forefoot:

- Flexible
  - No treatment required
  - Resolves spontaneously
- Moderately flexible
  - Passive stretching (with infants, apply gentle stretch at every diaper change)
  - Corrective shoes/splinting (reverse last shoes)
- Rigid
  - Serial casting (0–3 years of age)
  - Surgery (4 years of age and older)

Internal Tibial Torsion

Internal tibial torsion is the most common cause of in-toeing in children younger than 3 years (Harris, 2013; Lincoln & Suen, 2003; Sass & Hassan, 2003). In the orthopedic outpatient clinic, it is the most common cause for parental referral to a specialist (Fig. 20–7). Internal tibial torsion manifests with a twisted shin that makes the foot appear to turn inward.

The usual cause is in utero positioning or intrauterine molding. If unilateral, it is typically left-sided (Harris, 2013; Lincoln & Suen, 2003). Patients generally have ligament laxity and are very comfortable sitting on their feet. Parents often report stomach sleeping with the child's feet tucked underneath and excessive tripping and falling. Treatment for this condition is conservative; it often resolves spontaneously by age 4 years, sometimes after aggressive ambulation or running. Patients and other caregivers should be instructed to encourage the child to avoid sitting on the heels or feet.

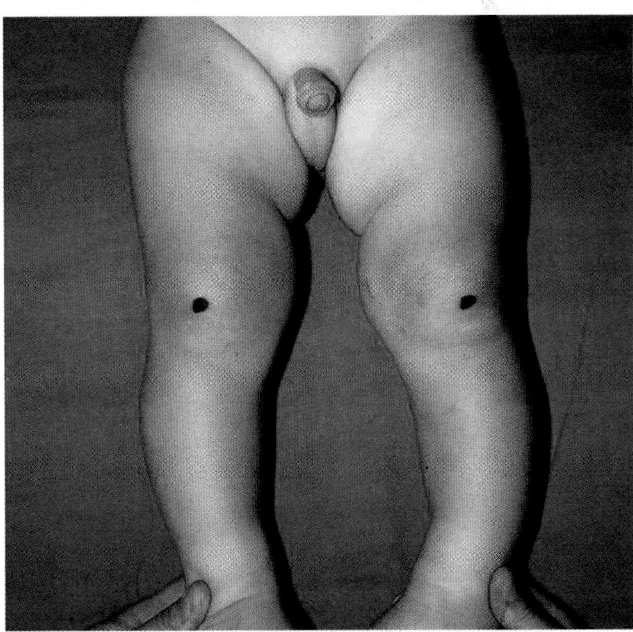

FIGURE 20–7 Internal tibial torsion.

Internal Femoral Torsion

Internal femoral torsion is the most common cause of in-toeing in children older than 2 years (Fig. 20–8) and is more common among females (Harris, 2013; Lincoln & Suen, 2003). This condition typically presents with generalized ligament laxity and abnormal seating preferences, commonly the "W" seating position (Fig. 20–9). Children with this condition have excessive medial rotation and limited lateral rotation. The deformity commonly corrects itself when the child corrects his or her sitting habits. If it is still present at age 9 years, surgical correction will be required.

- There are two types of internal femoral torsion:
  - Medial femoral torsion, characterized by extreme lateral or medial twisting rotation of the femur on its longitudinal axis that may be caused by the action of the gluteal or other muscles
  - Femoral anteversion, characterized by abnormal medial rotation of the thigh at the hip joint
- If the deformity is present and severe by 8 or 9 years of age, surgical intervention is required for correction.
- Most spontaneously resolve; of the few that do not, either a proximal femoral or tibial osteotomy is performed (Harris, 2013; Lincoln & Suen, 2003). This is a surgical procedure in which the bone is cut at the site of the deformity, then rotated to realign into better anatomical position to stop the rotation from occurring.
- Non-weight-bearing long leg casts for 6 to 8 weeks.
- This intervention is offered as a last resort and for very severe cases of deformity that do not spontaneously resolve.

Genu Varum (Bowlegs)

Genu varum (varus deformity), also called bowlegs or Blount's disease, is a lower leg deformity often seen in children between 18 months and 3 years of age, although it can also affect adolescents. The typical clinical presentation is in-toeing to the extent that a bowling ball could be placed between the legs (Fig. 20–10). Although some level of bowing is normal among this age group, certain features differentiate genu varum from typical development. The normal progression of limb development is physiological bowing, then the lower legs straighten out, then physiological knock-knees, then the legs again straighten out, and by the time a child is 7 years old or so, the limbs should be straight and not change throughout their remaining growth. Typical developmental bowing has these characteristics:

- Usually symmetrical
- Does not worsen with growth
- No lateral knee thrust
- No radiographic changes in severity
- Present in infancy but resolves by age 2

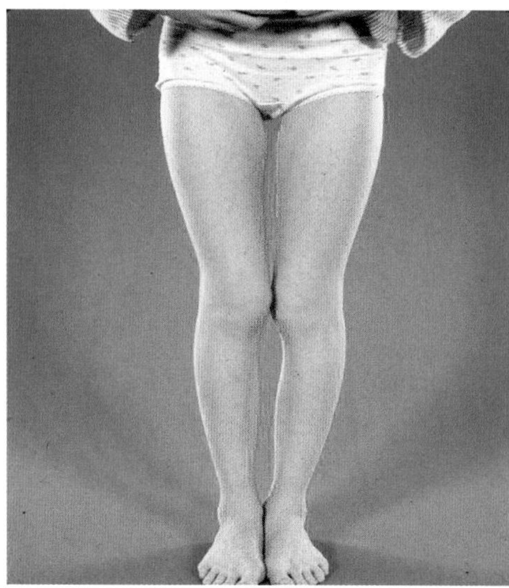

FIGURE 20–8 Internal femoral torsion.

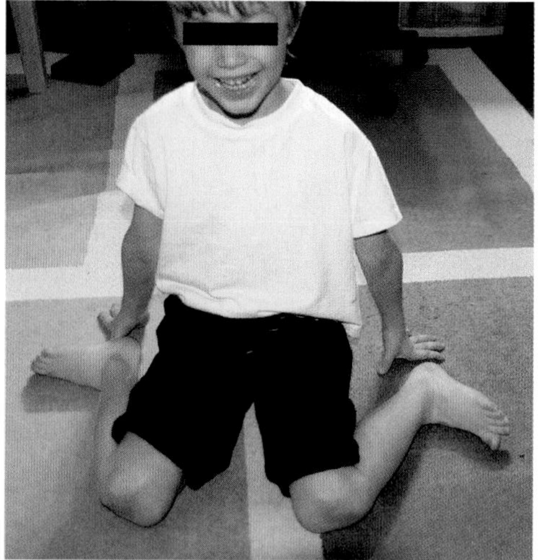

FIGURE 20–9 Ligament laxity and "W" sitting position.

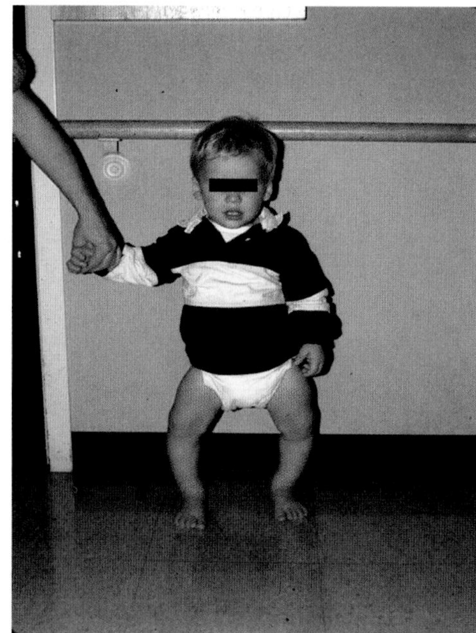

FIGURE 20–10 Genu varum.

In infantile Blount's disease, the deformity may be related to the following risk factors:

- Ambulation or full independent weight bearing before or between the ages of 9 and 12 months
- Heavy children (greater than 95th percentile in early years) with early ambulation

In adolescent Blount's disease, the deformity occurs during growth maturation. Those at risk include morbidly obese children at greater than 95th percentile for weight but average or below average height. Adolescent Blount's disease causes premature closure of the lateral epiphysis in unilateral or bilateral tibias. Causes of genu varum include:

- Physiological, with no known reason
- Tibial vara or Blount's disease
- Metabolic disorders: vitamin D–resistant rickets or hypophosphatemia
- Skeletal dysplasia: achondroplasia, or dwarfism
- Focal fibrocartilaginous dysplasia: benign dysplasia causing the upper leg to bow or unilateral varus of the tibia (most common location)
  - May also occur in humerus, forearm, phalanx, and femur
  - Epidemiology or demographics usually seen in infant or toddlers
  - Pathophysiology: etiology and the pathogenesis of the deformity are unknown
  - Associated conditions include infantile tibia vara; it is important to recognize this variation of infantile tibia vara because it can resolve without surgery
- Physeal abnormality such as tumor, infection, or trauma

Treatment

Genu varus must be observed and treated by age 4 years, after which it becomes more difficult to correct and carries an increased risk for damage to the growth plates of the knees.

- Bracing in cumbersome long leg orthoses is a treatment option, but compliance is often difficult.
- The bracing slows down the progression of the deformity, but it does not reverse it.
- The surgical correction for adolescent Blount's disease is tibial derotational osteotomies.
  - Patients are placed in either long leg casts for the first 4 to 6 weeks followed by short leg non-weight-bearing casts for 6 to 12 weeks total, or in short leg non-weight-bearing casts for 6 to 12 weeks total.
  - It is highly recommended to treat one leg at a time to allow for assisted ambulation and activities of daily living, with 6 to 8 weeks or more between procedures.
  - It is also customary to encourage lifestyle changes before the surgery to decrease the risk for complications such as bone nonunion or deep vein thrombosis postsurgery. Education about healthy weight loss and nutrition choices is vital.
  - Most present with a history of teasing because of obesity compounded by ridicule due to bowed legs—the condition is very visible or apparent.
  - Not only are patients emotionally scarred, but the families may be argumentative because they rarely feel that the obesity is due to family eating choices and habits. Many children who are overweight have overweight family members, so helping everyone improve nutrition habits can be beneficial. By getting the whole family involved the children do not feel isolated or that it is their fault.
  - Nutritionists, physical therapists, nursing staff, and social workers all need to meet with family members to discuss the rationales and expected outcomes for doing this complicated procedure; otherwise, recurrence and/or failure to return to correct the opposite side is more likely.

Genu Valgum (Knock-knees)

Genu valgum (valgus deformity), or knock-knees, is the opposite of genu varum (Fig. 20–11). Affected children present with "knees kissing" and often run with an abnormal gait.

Types of Genu Valgum

- Physiological: growth related
- Asymmetric growth, such as after trauma or infection causing premature growth arrest
- Metabolic disorders such as rickets or arthritis
- Skeletal dysplasia
- Neuromuscular deformity, such as with cerebral palsy

Treatment

The treatment modalities are both nonsurgical and surgical. Children aged 2 to 10 years are often treated with observation or orthosis, although the latter is controversial because children don't

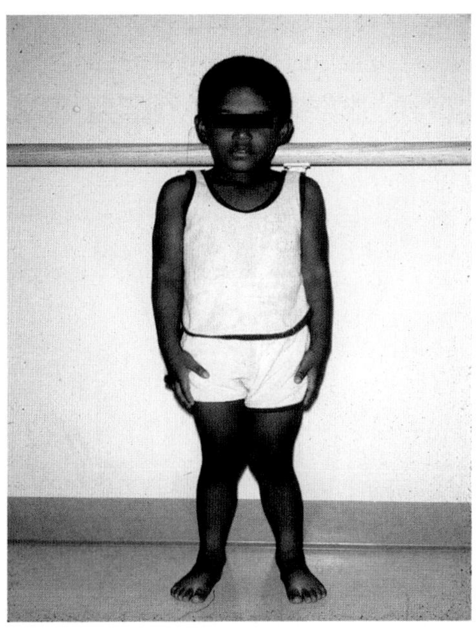

FIGURE 20–11 Genu valgum.

tend to like wearing braces. Surgery is indicated for children aged 11 to 13 years and may include:

- Medial physeal stapling, which prevents deformity by allowing the opposing side to catch up
- Medial physeal hemiepiphysiodesis, which stops the growth plate on the side of the deformity to allow the deformity to correct
- Osteotomy, in which a wedge of bone is removed to correct the deformity

Calcaneovalgus Foot

Calcaneovalgus foot is one of the most common causes of foot deformity due to packaging in utero. This condition is often confused with clubfoot. Clinically, this deformity is not classically considered as problematic in terms of growth and development, but children and families are often concerned because it may hinder sports performance and cause untoward attention from peers. However, this condition usually resolves spontaneously between 2 and 6 months of age, although stretching exercises are indicated in rare cases. Clubfoot is most often attributed to the following positions in utero:

- One foot against the wall of the uterus
- Dorsiflexed, everted foot
- Lateral tibial torsion (usually flexible) (see Fig. 20–12)
- Treatment: This condition usually resolves itself once the infant is out of the enclosed womb and relaxation of the tight positioning occurs.

Lateral Tibial Torsion

Lateral tibial torsion is often associated with calcaneovalgus foot deformity. It presents as out-toeing in infants but usually resolves around 18 to 24 months of age after walking begins and does not cause lifelong problems. In older children, tibial osteotomy is done to derotate the limb into its correct neutral alignment.

Hip Dysplasia

Hip dysplasia can be either congenital or caused by in utero positioning and is also called developmental dislocating hips

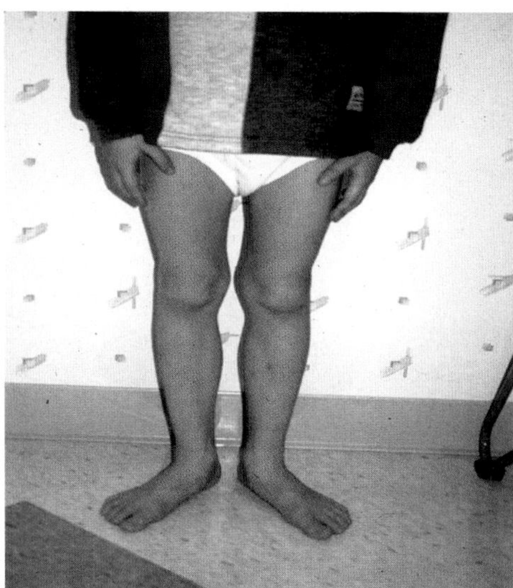

FIGURE 20–12 External tibial toeing.

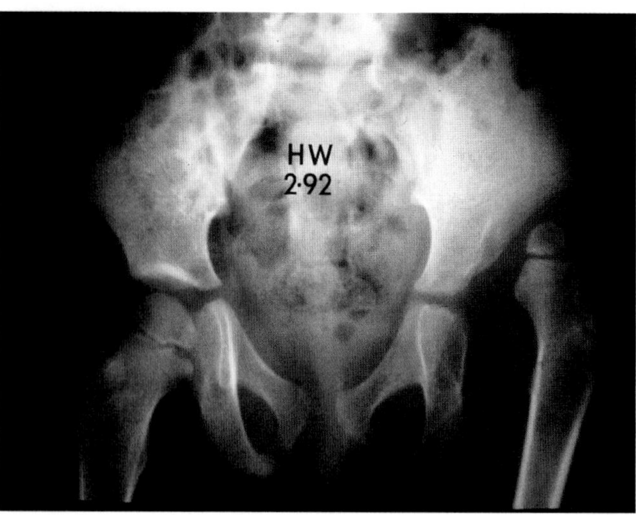

FIGURE 20–13 Radiograph of dislocated hip.

and congenital dislocating hips (Fig. 20–13). The cause of hip dysplasia development is multifactorial. Some features can result from a combination of mechanical factors, physiological factors, and postnatal positioning. Therefore, the condition can be subtle and is often missed or misdiagnosed because initially infants are symptom-free. Pelvic x-rays after age 6 weeks assist with diagnoses. Dynamic ultrasound is used for diagnosis before 6 weeks of age.

Risk Factors

Risk factors that may be related to the development of hip dysplasia include (Guille, Pizzutillo, & MacEwen, 1999; Harris, 2013):

- Firstborn child
- Female gender (ratio of 6:1 to 8:1); 80% of affected children are female
- Left side affected often associated with left occiput anterior positioning in utero
- Breech presentation
- Limited hip motion
- Petite mother with or without low amniotic fluid or gestation of multiples; maternal hormones and additional estrogen secretion of the female infant's uterus
- Family history
- Generalized ligament laxity
- Neuromuscular disorders, such as cerebral palsy, myelomeningocele, or spina bifida
- Extension/adduction cradle boards
- Occurs more often among children born in winter

Neuromuscular conditions can cause gradual development of hip dysplasia.

- Children with neurological conditions such as cerebral palsy or myelodysplasia could develop hip subluxation or dislocation.
- The spasticity in children with cerebral palsy overpowers the muscles that keep the femoral head located in the socket.
- Tone control is helpful, but patients may need more aggressive treatment options to slow down the progression.

- Some may develop hip pain in the future or higher incidences of arthritis without treatment.
- Surgical intervention is common before the hip dislocates in a growing child to prevent femoral head and acetabular deformities.
- Children with myelodysplasia may develop this disorder because of the inherent loss of muscle and nerve innervation caused by the condition.
- Children with certain spinal abnormalities such as spinal muscular atrophy are at higher risk.
- However, many live either sedentary or ambulatory lives without any problems or procedural treatment interventions.

Clinical Presentation

Clinical presentations most commonly observed in children with hip dysplasia include:

- Limited hip abduction
- Asymmetrical thigh skinfolds (number not size)
- Absence of knee flexion contractures (infants should have some contraction)
- Barlow test—measures hip stability along with Ortolani test
- Ortolani test—dislocated
- Galeazzi sign—uneven knee heights in bent-knee position
- Infants must be calm to elicit tests

Treatment

- Pavlik harness is a type of abduction brace (Fig. 20–14). Safety measures include ensuring proper fit and checking toes for vigorous capillary refill and movement after application.

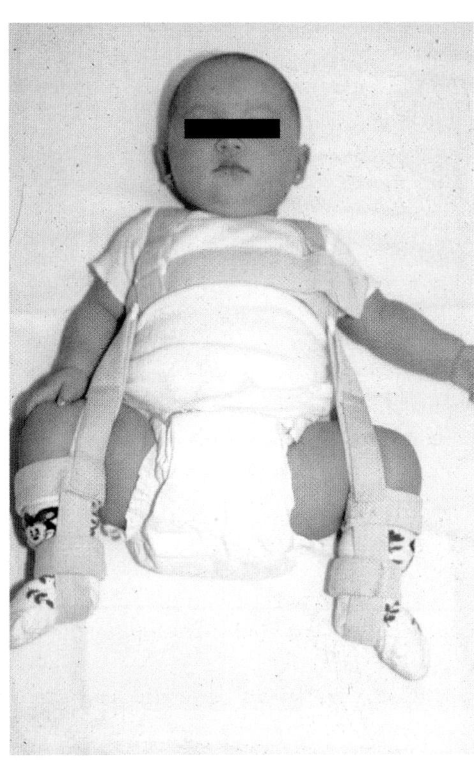

FIGURE 20–14 Example of the Pavlik harness.

- With Bryant's traction, an extremity is suspended. Keep weights free from bed frame, and monitor skin for breakdown and irritation. Prevent falls and maintain alignment with traction. Assist caregivers and family members with positioning to decrease friction to skin and bony prominences.
- Spica cast: Keep the cast clean and dry. Frequent position changes, especially by bony prominences, are necessary to prevent decubitus ulcer formation.
- Surgery may be required.

Legg-Calvé-Perthes Disease

Legg-Calvé-Perthes disease is a loss of blood supply to the femoral head with unknown cause (Fig. 20–15). It most often affects boys aged 2 to 9 years and is sometimes painful. The most common sign of this condition is limping or inability to bear weight on the affected leg.

Incidence

- Male-to-female ratio of 5:1 (Mazloumi, Ebrahimzadeh, & Kachooei, 2014; Mehlman & McCourt, 2010)
- Mean age: 7 years; often children 4 to 8 years of age affected due to standard deviation from mean
- Unilateral, 90%; bilateral, 10% to 15% (Mazloumi et al., 2014)
- Family history, 3%
- Most common among Caucasians, Asians, and Alaska Natives (Mazloumi et al., 2014; Rowe, Jung, Lee, Bai, & Kang, 2005)

SAFE AND EFFECTIVE NURSING CARE: Cultural Competence

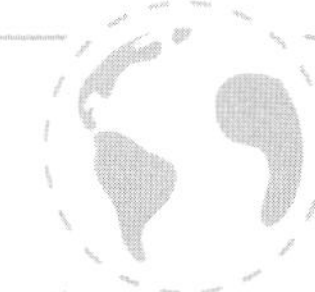

Causative Factors for Legg-Calvé-Perthes Disease

Multiple theories exist regarding causation of Legg-Calvé-Perthes disease. Incidence and geography are also widely varied. Some centers claim no causation; others note either thrombolytic components or trauma as causative factors. Geographical locations have noted higher and lower incidents of cases. According to Mehlman & McCourt (2010), "Rates that are four times higher than [in] Korea have consistently been noted in Great Britain" (Mazloumi et al., 2014; Mehlman & McCourt, 2010).

Clinical Presentation

- Pain
  - Sudden
  - Can be referred to groin, thigh, knee
  - Increases with movement
  - Decreases with rest
  - Not similar to pain of internal hip rotation
  - Limpness
- Decreased ROM
  - Hip abduction
  - Hip internal rotation

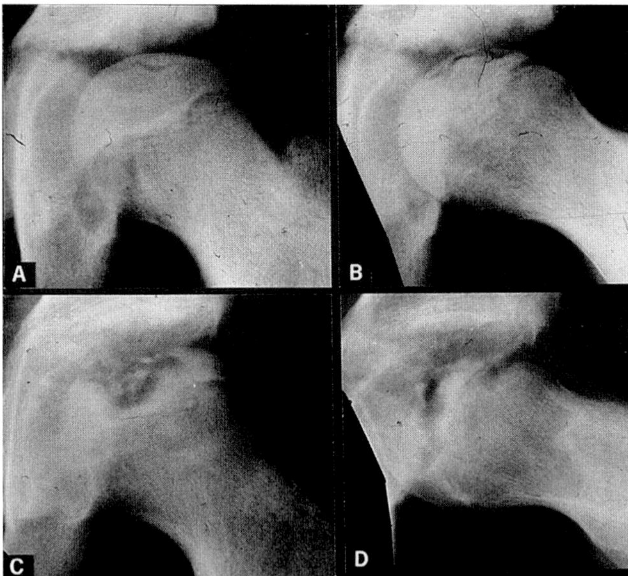

FIGURE 20–15 Legg-Calvé-Perthes disease.

Avascular Necrosis

Avascular necrosis (AVN) results in blood loss to the femoral head of the femur caused by fracture or dislocation. The blood flow to the bone is interrupted. Symptoms of AVN may not be evident for up to 2 years, meaning it may take 2 years for bone healing to complete (International Hip Dysplasia Institute, 2016).

- Severity depends on the child's age of development. The younger the child is at the time of diagnosis, the better the outcome.
- The femoral head is sometimes oddly shaped and ovoid, with a widened femur neck shaft.
- The AVN process occurs over approximately 1 to 4 years and has telltale stages of development and rebuilding (remodeling): prenecrosis, necrosis, and space revascularization.
  - Prenecrosis
    - Insult causing loss of blood supply
  - Necrosis
    - Femoral head without blood supply
    - Femoral head structurally intact
    - Asymptomatic
    - Radiographs may be normal
  - Revascularization (1- to 4-year process)
    - New bone deposition
    - Dead bone reabsorption
    - Femoral head weak and susceptible to pathological fracture
  - Bone healing
    - Reossification occurs gradually.
    - Reabsorption stops.
    - Bone returns to normal strength.
- Remodeling
  - The younger the age of development, the greater the potential for remodeling.
- The child usually presents with limping plus or minus hip, thigh, or knee pain.
- Patients have good days and bad days.
- The condition waxes and wanes for months to years.
- The goal is to keep the femoral head in the hip socket to maintain a good hip joint and decrease the risk for permanent deformity to the femoral head and acetabulum.
- Classification of Legg-Calvé-Perthes disease is categorized using Catterall and Salter/Thompson systems (Rampal et al., 2017; Salter & Thompson, 1984).

Treatment

Treatment aims to:

- Eliminate hip irritation (pain).
- Restore and maintain ROM.
- Prevent collapse of the capital femoral epiphysis (proximal femur growth plate).
- Attain a spherical femoral head.
- Contain the femoral head in the rim of the acetabulum.

Treatment modalities include:

- Traction—Bryant's or Buck's, either with hips off the bed or feet up over the head presentations using weights and pulleys to gently release pressure from the hip joint
- Casting—Petrie casts changed every 6 to 12 weeks; this cast extends from mid-chest to just above the knee; an opening is left for toileting
- Surgery—proximal femoral derotational (opposing deformity to be in better alignment) osteotomy

Bracing is controversial (Hardesty, Liu, & Thompson, 2011; Mazloumi et al., 2014).

Slipped Capital Femoral Epiphysis

Slipped capital femoral epiphysis is a hip deformity of childhood (Fig. 20–16) with widespread epidemiology due to both environmental and neurological factors.

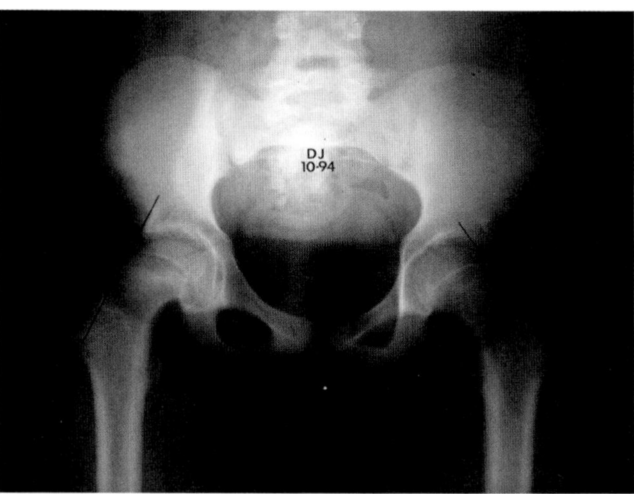

FIGURE 20–16 Slipped capital femoral epiphysis.

Risk Factors and Incidence

The following factors increase the incidence of slipped capital femoral epiphysis:

- Adolescent onset, usually at the time of a growth spurt
  - Males: 10 to 16 years old
  - Females: 10 to 14 years old
- More common among African Americans
- Incidence is bilateral in 25% to 30% of cases (Gettys, Jackson, & Frick, 2011; Millis, 2017).
- Manifests with obesity or tall, lanky physique
- Developmental delay

Causative factors for this condition are as follows:

- Idiopathic—most common
  - Obesity
  - Juvenile hormonal changes
- Endocrine problems such as diabetes
- Radiation exposure
- Chemotherapy

Clinical Presentation

- Anterior thigh and knee pain
- Antalgic gait: a limp adopted to avoid pain on weight-bearing structures, characterized by a very short stance phase
- Externally rotated lower leg
- Decreased ROM in hip(s)

Treatment

Slipped capital femoral epiphysis is treated with use of crutches or wheelchair for protected activities for 6 to 8 weeks. The treatment goals include:

- Stabilize the hip joint with open reduction internal fixation, a surgical technique in which a femoral screw is used to hold the joint in place and support healing.
- Promote epiphysiodesis.
- Avoid complications such as further injury to growth plate, deep vein thrombosis, and infection.
- Improve hip function.

Transient Monoarticular Synovitis

Transient monoarticular synovitis is the most common cause of acute-onset, short-duration limping in children (Naranje, Kelly, & Sawyer, 2015). This is due to intermittent inflammation of the hip joint.

- It is more common in males than females.
- The average age of onset is 6 years (can range from 2 to 12 years).
- The cause is nonspecific synovitis or hip irritation.
- Classified as the following types of synovitis:
  - Allergic or inflammatory reaction
  - Viral-like—following an upper respiratory infection or other minor ailment
  - Result of a minor trauma

Clinical Presentation

The following clinical presentations are indicative of typical toxic synovitis:

- Mild limp
- Low-grade fever (38°C/100.4°F)
- Anterior thigh or knee pain
- Irritable hip (positive roll test)
- Mild limb rotation (favored position is to hold the lower leg turned outward)

Other conditions that mimic limping and other characteristics of TMS include:

- Septic arthritis
- Osteomyelitis
- Legg-Calvé-Perthes disease

Diagnostic Testing

- Normal complete blood cell count (CBC) and differential
- Elevated erythrocyte sedimentation rate
- Negative arthrocentesis (negative cultures, no crystals)

Treatment

- Bedrest for 7 to 10 days
- Traction to hold the hip in a restful position to relieve fluid buildup
- Bone scan to determine location of other sites of irritation, inflammation, or infection, especially in young children who cannot describe the location of pain

Septic Arthritis and Osteomyelitis of the Hip

Staphylococcus aureus is the most common bacterial pathogen causing osteomyelitis in children of all ages. "Group A streptococcus (especially complicating varicella), *Streptococcus pneumoniae*, and the emerging pathogen *Kingella kingae* are the next most common organisms in infants and children. Group B streptococcus and gram-negative enterics are common causes of osteomyelitis in the neonatal period" (Kaplan, 2005; Simonsen, Anderson-Berry, Delair, & Davies, 2014).

Patients are managed closely after hospital discharge, usually by both pediatric orthopedics and infectious disease specialists, until laboratory levels have returned to normal and full restoration of pain-free ROM of the hip occurs. The length of antibiotic treatment both IV and then orally depends on the severity of the infection and the type of organisms involved. Most children need yearly follow-up after treatment to be sure the hip joint and bony anatomical features develop correctly.

Septic arthritis and osteomyelitis of the hip are acute orthopedic emergencies. Delay of treatment in either case can cause severe deformity and even death. Both are primarily seen in infants and can follow an antecedent illness by several weeks. Many patients initially present at the doctor's office with an ear infection or strep throat several weeks before onset of osteomyelitis symptoms. Ask about history of a fever, runny nose, cold, or cough several weeks ago.

Clinical Presentation

Infants typically present with the following symptoms:

- Irritable; refuses to eat
- Hip flexion contracture
- Abduction and externally rotated position of comfort
- Pain with hip ROM
- Erythema, edema
- Minimal fever but may progressively get worse
- Child may look septic
- Normal CBC

Clinical presentations in children include:

- Limp—may refuse to walk or bear weight
- History of trauma, surgery, or infection
- Hip abnormality
    - Flexed
    - Abducted
    - Externally rotated
- Pain with hip ROM, especially internal rotation
- Febrile, toxic
- Positive leukocytosis

Treatment

Treatment of choice is to admit urgently to the hospital for care:

- Emergency surgery for incision and drainage (I&D)
- Drainage or repeat I&D every 1 to 3 days
- Systemic antibiotics coverage, usually via peripherally inserted central catheter line for 3 to 12 weeks, depending on organism growth, followed by oral therapy depends on the type of organism but may be ciprofloxacin (Cipro, Ciloxan), linezolid (Zyvox), or trimethoprim/sulfamethoxazole (Bactrim)
- Maintenance of hip motion

Prognosis is determined by several factors:

- Age of onset
- Site of initial infection
- Delay of diagnosis
- Organisms present

Scoliosis

Scoliosis is a term for curvature of the spine that deviates from normal spinal alignment (Fig. 20–17). Scoliosis is predominantly idiopathic in origin, meaning it occurs for no known reason. Some experts think it may be related to intrauterine molding as with other musculoskeletal disorders that occur with spinal curves, such as torticollis and hip dysplasia.

Congenital Scoliosis

- Congenital or infantile scoliosis occurs before age 6 months.
- It can be genetic or caused by intrauterine or external uterine forces applied to infants during growth and development.
- Clinical evaluation at well-infant checkups by a health-care professional or parent observation usually detects deviation from normal infant anatomy.

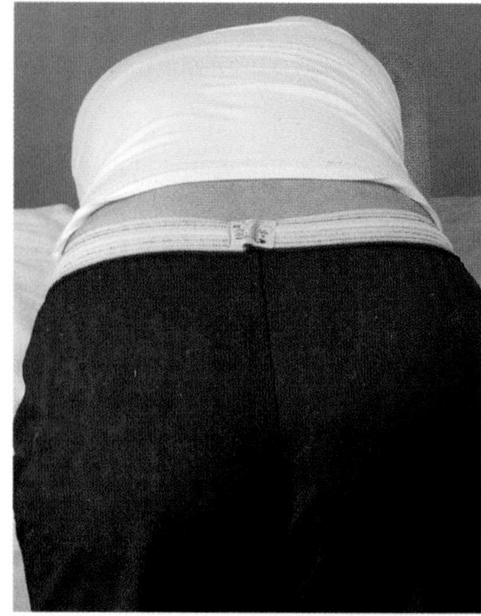

FIGURE 20–17 Adolescent with obvious scoliosis.

- X-rays determine the level of severity of the curvature.
- A complete neurological examination is crucial to rule out other deformities or conditions.
- Severe cases are evaluated with MRI scans, especially left-sided curves.
- The curvature is measured from the thoracic-to-lumbar curvature and lumbar-to-sacral curvature using the Cobb method of angles to the deformity, usually in an S-shaped curve.

Clinical Presentation

- Rare condition representing 1% of all idiopathic scoliosis cases (Yang, Andras, Redding, & Skaggs, 2016)
- More common in Europe than in United States
- Left-sided is more common in infants
- Girls with right-sided infantile scoliosis tend to have a worse prognosis (Larson, 2011; Yang et al., 2016)

Treatment

- Bracing—thoracolumbosacral orthosis (TLSO) bracing to hold positional curvature while child matures
- Casting—Risser cast holds the deformity from progressing chest high to thigh
- Surgical instrumentation—growing rods, changed every 6 months
- Definitive spinal fusion

Juvenile (Early-Onset) Scoliosis

Juvenile scoliosis is a spinal curvature diagnosed before age 10 years. It is more common than infantile scoliosis but less common than in adolescents.

Risk Factors and Incidence

- Accounts for 10% to 15% of all idiopathic cases (Colliard, Circo, & Rivard, 2010; Yang et al., 2016)
- Tends to be right sided, but children with left-sided curves fare better than those with right-sided ones because the latter tends to become more severe and require treatment
- Is not painful
- Follows a common progression

Clinical Presentation

- Forward bend test; characteristic rib hump (Figs. 20–18 and 20–19)
- Asymmetrical shoulder heights
- Asymmetrical pelvic obliquity: One side of the pelvis appears to be elevated, which can create a scoliosis misdiagnosis.
- Decreased ROM of upper trunk (e.g., leans forward and back and side to side or twists with difficulty)
- Radiographs reveal more than 10-degree curve, usually S- or C-shaped

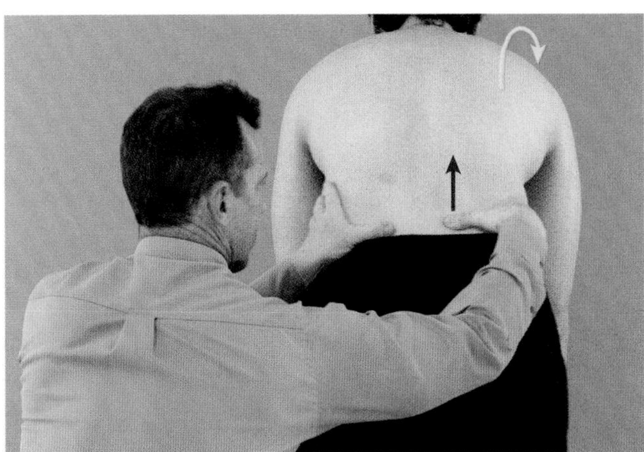

FIGURE 20–18 Forward bend.

Treatment

Treatment options are based on the time of diagnosis, age of child, and likelihood of progression.

- Observation for minor curves of 15 to 25 degrees
- Bracing for flexible moderate curves of 25 degrees plus, such as with TLSO bracing (Fig. 20–20)
- Riser cast for rigid curves, changed every 6 to 12 weeks and followed by bracing (Cincinnati Children's, 2016)
- Surgical intervention—instrumentation such as rods, or definitive fusion
- With correct diagnosis and treatment options for juvenile scoliosis, good outcomes are the norm
- Many children grow up without any limitations and participate in active lifestyles

Adolescent Idiopathic Scoliosis

Adolescent idiopathic scoliosis is a condition that affects children aged 9 years through young adulthood. This is the most common type of idiopathic scoliosis, accounting for 80% of cases and affecting between 2% and 4% of those aged 10 to 16 years (Arlet & Reddi, 2007; Maruyama, Kobayashi, Miura, & Nakao, 2015). It is more common among girls than boys. Adolescent idiopathic scoliosis is characterized by a C- or S-shaped lateral curve to either the left or right. It often goes undetected because it rarely causes pain or affects activity levels, but it may be found early in puberty or during a growth spurt.

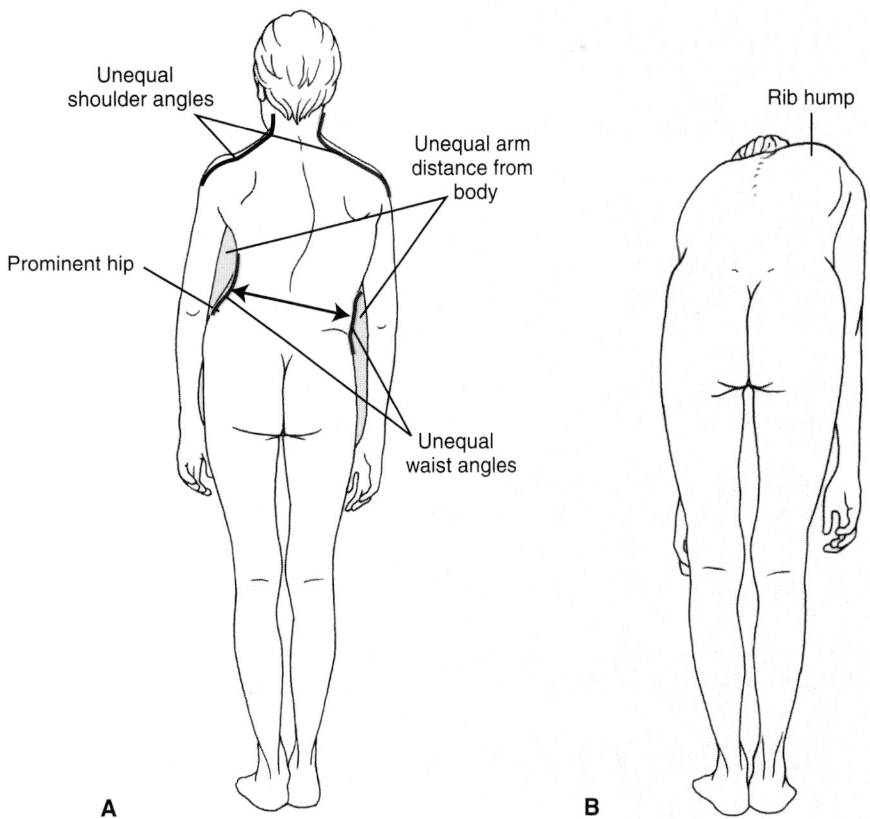

FIGURE 20–19 Rib hump.

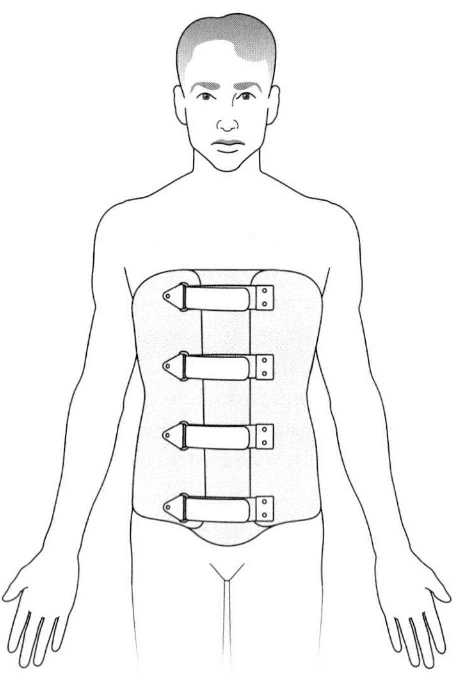

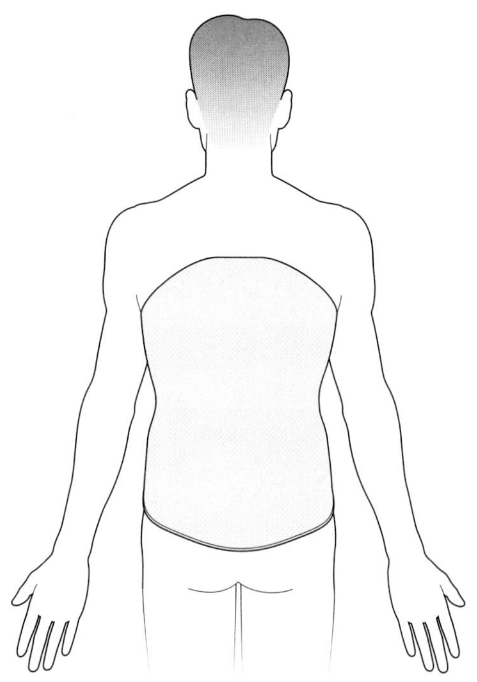

FIGURE 20–20 Thoracolumbosacral orthosis (TLSO) brace.

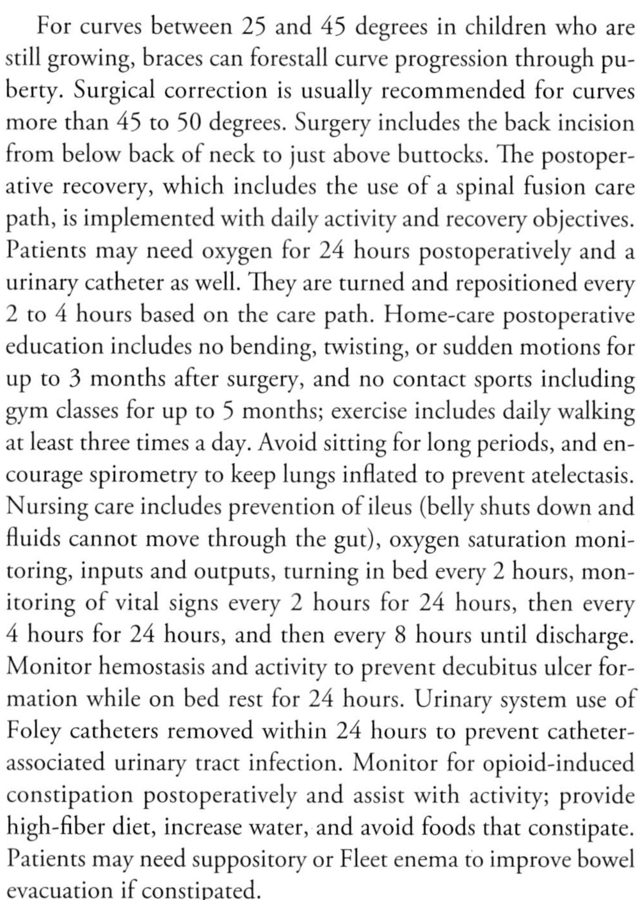

For curves between 25 and 45 degrees in children who are still growing, braces can forestall curve progression through puberty. Surgical correction is usually recommended for curves more than 45 to 50 degrees. Surgery includes the back incision from below back of neck to just above buttocks. The postoperative recovery, which includes the use of a spinal fusion care path, is implemented with daily activity and recovery objectives. Patients may need oxygen for 24 hours postoperatively and a urinary catheter as well. They are turned and repositioned every 2 to 4 hours based on the care path. Home-care postoperative education includes no bending, twisting, or sudden motions for up to 3 months after surgery, and no contact sports including gym classes for up to 5 months; exercise includes daily walking at least three times a day. Avoid sitting for long periods, and encourage spirometry to keep lungs inflated to prevent atelectasis. Nursing care includes prevention of ileus (belly shuts down and fluids cannot move through the gut), oxygen saturation monitoring, inputs and outputs, turning in bed every 2 hours, monitoring of vital signs every 2 hours for 24 hours, then every 4 hours for 24 hours, and then every 8 hours until discharge. Monitor hemostasis and activity to prevent decubitus ulcer formation while on bed rest for 24 hours. Urinary system use of Foley catheters removed within 24 hours to prevent catheter-associated urinary tract infection. Monitor for opioid-induced constipation postoperatively and assist with activity; provide high-fiber diet, increase water, and avoid foods that constipate. Patients may need suppository or Fleet enema to improve bowel evacuation if constipated.

Neuromuscular and Syndromic Scoliosis

Neuromuscular scoliosis can occur in children with neurological conditions at any age and at any stage of growth and development. It is common in children with cerebral palsy or myelodysplasia, or those born with syndromes like Costello or Klippel-Feil syndrome. With this type of scoliosis, the potential for curve progression is less accurately defined.

If surgical intervention or casting is required, then a similar course of care to previously mentioned should be followed.

JUVENILE IDIOPATHIC ARTHRITIS

Juvenile idiopathic arthritis (JIA; formerly JRA) is a common diagnosis for pain and inflammation in multiple joints that can occur as early as age 2 years. Caregivers typically seek medical help when children present with on-and-off joint pain in several different joints over a period of months, although some cases involve only one joint. JIA commonly first affects the knees, ankles, and hips, and is usually bilateral.

JIA is the most common chronic rheumatic illness in children that causes significant short- and long-term disability (Shenoi, 2017). It is regarded as a complex genetic trait, with multiple genes causing inflammation and immune response. Some literature has implied that certain people are more genetically prone to develop JIA by triggers of stress, abnormal hormone levels, trauma to a joint, or infections (Lang & Shore, 1990; Shenoi, 2017; Weiss & Ilowite, 2007).

Diagnostic Testing

Laboratory tests that are common in the evaluation of rheumatic conditions include:

- CBC with differential
- Anti-nuclear antibody titer
- Rheumatoid factor
- Human leukocyte antigen (HLA B27)
- Complement component 3 (C3) and C4

- Epstein-Barr virus titer
- Erythrocyte sedimentation rate, C-reactive protein

Children with JIA should be monitored for:

- Nutrition deficits
- Uveitis: inflammation of the iris of the eye
- Growth disturbances, including delayed puberty
- Psychological concerns due to the chronicity of the disease and active disease causing functional limitations

Treatment

Treatment goals include:

- Controlling pain and inflammation: naproxen (Naprosyn, Aleve) and methotrexate (Trexall, Rheumatrex)
  - Take medications with food; stop if causes nausea and vomiting, rash, or diarrhea
- Preserving function
- Promoting normal growth and development
- Promoting psychological well-being

Evidence-Based Practice: Treatment Options for Juvenile Idiopathic Arthritis

Weiss, J. E., & Ilowite, N. T. (2007). Juvenile idiopathic arthritis. *Rheumatic Disease Clinics of North America, 33,* 441–470. doi: 10.1016/j.rdc.2007.07.006

Shenoi, S. (2017). Juvenile idiopathic arthritis—changing times, changing terms, changing treatments. *Pediatrics in Review, 38*(5), 221–232.

Weiss and Ilowite (2007) categorized the following treatment options:

- Therapeutic modalities
  - Physical therapy and occupational therapy as vital adjuncts to all medical treatment options
  - Splints
  - Arthroplasty
- NSAIDs
- Glucocorticoids
- Disease-modifying antirheumatic agents
- Sulfasalazine
- Methotrexate
- Leflunomide
- Biological agents (treats polyarticular and systemic JIA manufactured in or extracted from biological sources): Different biologics tend to work better for different subgroups of the disease. In recent years, the U.S. Food and Drug Administration has approved several of these treatments. Following are their names, the type of JIA they treat, and approval dates:
  - Adalimumab (Humira) for polyarticular JIA, February 2008
  - Abatacept (Orencia) for polyarticular JIA, April 2008
  - Etanercept (Enbrel) for polyarticular JIA, May 1999
  - Tocilizumab (Actemra) for systemic JIA, April 2011, and polyarticular JIA, April 2013
  - Canakinumab (Ilaris) for systemic JIA, May 2013
- U.S. Food and Drug Consumer updates retrieved July 30, 2017
  - Etanercept (Infliximab)
  - Adalimumab (Humira)
  - Anakinra
  - Humanized anti-interleukin-6 receptor antibody
  - Autologous stem cell transplantation

OSTEOGENESIS IMPERFECTA

Osteogenesis imperfecta (OI), also called brittle bone disease, is an inherited disorder resulting from a collagen defect or dominant gene mutation. Some children diagnosed with OI have no known hereditary linkage. With this disorder, fractures of the shoulder, humerus, clavicle, or femur commonly occur at birth via the birth canal. Little external trauma is present; infants may be sent home and later present in the emergency department with inability to move the upper extremity or swollen and painful lower extremity.

The disorder is classified into types I through VI, denoting mild to severe in its symptomatology. Without a known family history, the diagnosis is sometimes made later in infancy or even at toddler age if the OI is a very mild case.

- Children with severe OI have multiple fractures of the long bones of the body multiple times, often in short time periods.
- These multiple fractures can lead to growth plate deformities or unusual bowing of the extremities, especially in all four extremities.
- The infant can also present with "blue sclera," a bluish tinge of the eyes.
- Laboratory tests can assist in the diagnosis of OI.
  - Sodium dodecyl sulfate–polyacrylamide gel electrophoresis (SDS-PAGE)
  - Two-dimensional SDS-PAGE
  - Cyanogen bromide (CNBr) mapping
  - Thermal stability studies
- Sometimes the diagnosis is detectable in utero by ultrasound, with identification of bowing or unusual shortness of the long bones.

SAFE AND EFFECTIVE NURSING CARE: Clinical Pearl

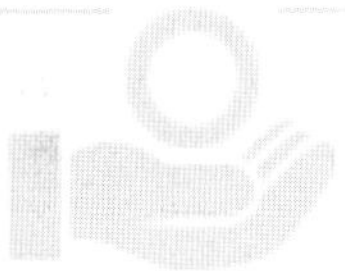

Osteogenesis Imperfecta or Abuse?

Often, infants are sent home and then present in the emergency department with the chief complaint of inability to move an upper extremity or a swollen and painful lower extremity. This often prompts social work to get involved and/or a child protection team to rule out physical child abuse before a diagnosis of OI. Many families are traumatized by the negative social implication and then are shocked by the diagnosis of a chronic genetic disorder. Nurses should be supportive and aware of this issue, and take the following measures:

- Refer affected families to resources that can help them navigate chronic disease.
- Ask families about previous fracture patterns.
- Assist with holding/feeding/changing to decrease incidence of trauma to the infant while in hospital care.
- Forego taking blood pressure if this has caused an upper arm fracture in the past.
- Place signs over the bed that remind staff to use caution and care while moving the patient.
- Ask nursing staff for assistance to caution ancillary departments about fragility of infant.

- Specific types can be diagnosed at certain gestational weeks.
- The more severe the type, the more identifiable is the clinical presentation.

Nursing Interventions

Nursing interventions to promote the safety of a child with OI include:

- Use noninvasive blood pressure measures when appropriate.
- Use caution when repositioning.
- Alert ancillary staff about precautions to prevent injury, such as during phlebotomy procedures.
- Fall-prevention education for all age groups.
- Nursing care in the hospital should be directed at demonstrating to the families gentle holding positions and, if severe OI, avoiding or limiting procedures that could "squeeze" extremities and induce fractures.
- Procedures can be minimally invasive, such as manual and automatic blood pressure readings, or more invasive, such as placing IVs or obtaining radiographs.
- The OI Foundation's website has detailed brochures for parents, health-care providers, and daycare centers/schools.

SPORTS-RELATED INJURIES

In the United States, about 30 million children and teens participate in some form of organized sports, and those aged 14 years and younger experience more than 3.5 million sports-related injuries each year. More children are getting involved in competitive sports at younger ages. Using data from the U.S. Consumer Product Safety Commission's *National Electronic Injury Surveillance System*, the report focused on pediatric sports injuries related to 14 common sports activities, including football, soccer, and basketball. The number of children involved in year-round sports has also increased because of the availability of indoor arenas such as those for soccer and baseball. Common orthopedic injuries in children include:

- Sprains and strains
- Dislocations and subluxations
- Tears
- Fractures
- Hematomas
- Overuse injuries—Little Leaguer's elbow, tendonitis, and growth plate fractures

Sports injuries in children may present with:

- Swelling
- Pain
- Ecchymosis skin discoloration caused by bruising

With the typical ankle sprain:

- Mechanism of injury is often rolled the ankle into inversion
- Treatment options include splint, cast, or boot; graduate to sports lace-up ankle brace
- Prevention with physical therapy

Dislocations and Subluxations

- Mechanism of injury—hyperextension or pulling, or varus/valgus stress
- Pain
- Swelling
- Nursemaid's elbow is the most common dislocation in the toddler population
- Ehlers-Danlos syndrome causes laxity due to collagen defects and may affect adolescents
- Treatment usually requires sedation in emergency department for true dislocation to be relocated
- Prevention—occupational therapy and physical therapy to strengthen and prevent recurrence
- Surgical intervention for repeated dislocation or subluxation—either bony or soft tissue procedures

Tears and Contusions

- Mechanism of injury—usually foot planted and body continues moving forward or some type of twisting injury
- Usually hear or feel "pop"
- Pain
- Swelling
- Diagnostic testing: x-rays and MRI
- Treatment typically includes use of crutches or braces to protect the extremity to rest and provide comfort; surgical intervention is reserved for conservative treatment failure or continues to have recurrent injury or more serious injury
- Prevention includes education on proper body mechanics and weight training before the sports season, as well as use of plyometrics to learn proper landing techniques
- Continued sports participation is dependent on injury and severity

Overuse Injuries

- Mechanism of injury—repetitive forces such as in pitching, tennis, diving, gymnastics
- Occurs when activity levels exceed the body's ability to recover
- Evaluate for intensity, duration, and magnitude of training
- Proper coaching
- Tips for prevention of overuse injuries in pediatric and adolescent athletes:
  - Always stretch before play or exercise.
  - Cool down after hard sports or workouts.
  - Wear shoes and equipment that fit properly, are stable, and have good shock absorption.
  - Learn to do your sport right; use proper form; if unsure, ask coach or trainer for help.

- Know your body's limits.
- Build up your exercise level gradually.
- Do a total-body workout consisting of cardiovascular, strength-training, and flexibility exercises.
- Get a physical examination before you start playing competitive sports.
- Follow the rules of the game.
- Don't play if you are tired or in pain.

Case Study

A 12-year-old boy presents to your office with his right leg turned out to the side. He is morbidly obese but says he used to play a lot of basketball outside. His mother reports less physical activity for the last several years and increased consumption of sweets and soft drinks. He likes to have a bag of chips each night after dinner while doing his homework. He denies fever and numbness or tingling in his right leg. He was in the pediatrician's office for a weight check and had gained more than 20 lb in the last 6 months. The doctor recommended a diet log and visit with the nutritionist.

1. What other questions do you need to ask the patient or family?
2. What could the diagnosis be for this boy?
3. What is the next diagnostic tool to help determine the medical condition?
4. What follow-up care is needed for this boy?

REFERENCES

American Academy of Orthopedic Surgeons. (2015). *Treatment of pediatric diaphyseal femur fractures evidence-based clinical practice guideline.* Retrieved from https://www.aaos.org/Research/guidelines/PDFF_ReIssue.pdf

Arlet, V., & Reddi, V. (2007). Adolescent idiopathic scoliosis. *Neurosurgery Clinics of North America, 18*, 255–259. doi: 10.1016/j.nec.2007.02.002

Arora, R., Fichadia, U., Hartwig, E., & Kannikeswaran, N. (2014). Pediatric upper-extremity fractures. *Pediatric Annals, 43*(5), 196–204. doi: 10.3928/00904481-20140417-12

Bauer, J. M., & Lovejoy, S. A. (2017). Toddler's fractures: Time to weight-bear with regard to immobilization type and radiographic monitoring. *Journal of Pediatric Orthopaedics*. 28141694. doi: 10.1097/BPO.0000000000000948

Cincinnati Children's. (2016). *Risser, mehta and pantaloon casts.* Retrieved from https://www.cincinnatichildrens.org/health/r/risser-pantaloon

Colliard, C., Circo, A., & Rivard, C. (2010). SpineCor treatment for juvenile idiopathic scoliosis: SOSORT award 2010 winner. *Scoliosis Journal, 5*, 25. doi: 10.1186/1748-7161-5-25

Eastwood, D., & de Gheldere, A. (2011). Physeal injuries in children. *Surgery, 29* (4), 146–152. doi: 10.1016/j.mpsur.2011.01.003

Gettys, F., Jackson, J., & Frick, S. (2011). Obesity in pediatric orthopaedics. *Orthopaedic Clinics of North America, 42*, 95–105. doi: 10.1016/j.ocl.2010.08.005

Guille, J., Pizzutillo, P., & MacEwen, D. (1999). Developmental dysplasia of the hip from birth to six months. *Journal of the American Academy of Orthopaedic Surgeons, 8*, 232–242. Retrieved from http://jaaos.org/content/8/4/232.abstract

Hardesty, C. K., Liu, R. W., & Thompson, G. H. (2011). The role of bracing in Legg-Calvé-Perthes disease. *Journal of Pediatric Orthopaedics, 31*, S178–S181. doi: 10.1097/BPO.0b013e318223b5b1

Harris, E. (2013). The intoeing child. *Clinics in Podiatric Medicine and Surgery, 30*(4), 531–565.

International Hip Dysplasia Institute. (2016). *Infant and child hip dysplasia.* Retrieved from http://hipdysplasia.org/developmental-dysplasia-of-the-hip/problems-after-treatment/avascular-necrosis/

Jawetz, S. T., Shah, P. H., & Potter, H. G. (2015). Imaging of physeal injury: Overuse. *Sports Health, 7*(2), 142–153.

Kaplan, S. L. (2005). Osteomyelitis in children. *Infectious Disease Clinics of North America, 19*, 787–797. doi: 10.1016/j.idc.2005.07.006

Kliegman, R. M., Stanton, B. M. D., St. Geme, J., Schor, N., & Behrman, R. E. (2011). *Nelson textbook of pediatrics* (19th ed.). Philadelphia: W. B. Saunders.

Kocher, M., Sink, E., Blasier, R., Luhmann, S. J., Mehlman, C. T., Scher, D. M., ... Hitchcock, K. (2009). Treatment of pediatric diaphyseal femur fractures. *Journal of the American Academy of Orthopaedic Surgeons, 17*, 718–725. Retrieved from http://www.jaaos.org/content/17/11/718.abstract

Kunes, J. (2011). Pitfalls in assessing common pediatric fractures. *Journal of Urgent Care Medicine, 1*. Retrieved from http://www.jucm.com/

Lang, B. A., & Shore, A. (1990). A review of current concepts on the pathogenesis of juvenile rheumatoid arthritis. *Journal of Rheumatology, 21*, 1–15.

Larson, N. (2011). Early onset scoliosis: What the primary care provider needs to know and implications for practice. *Journal of the American Academy of Nurse Practitioners, 23*, 392–403. doi: 10.1111/j.1745-7599.2011.00634.x

Lincoln, T. L., & Suen, P. W. (2003). Common rotational variations in children. *Journal of the American Academy of Orthopaedic Surgeons, 11*, 312–320. Retrieved from http://jaaos.org/content/11/5/312.abstract

Maruyama, T., Kobayashi, Y., Miura, M., & Nakao, Y. (2015). Effectiveness of brace treatment for adolescent idiopathic scoliosis. *Scoliosis, 10*(Suppl. 2): S12. http://www.scoliosisjournal.com/content/10/S2/S12

Mazloumi, S. M., Ebrahimzadeh, M. H., & Kachooei, A. R. (2014). Evolution in diagnosis and treatment of Legg-Calve-Perthes disease. *Archives of Bone and Joint Surgery, 2*(2), 86.

Mehlman, C., & McCourt, J. (2010). Legg-Calvé-Perthes disease: Where are we 100 years later? *The Orthopod, 18*, 30–35. Retrieved from http://www.jaaos.org/content/18/11/643.citation

Millis, M. B. (2017). SCFE: Clinical aspects, diagnosis, and classification. *Journal of Children's Orthopaedics, 11*(2), 93–98.

Naranje, S. M., Erali, R. A., Warner Jr., W. C., Sawyer, J. R., & Kelly, D. M. (2016). Epidemiology of pediatric fractures presenting to emergency departments in the United States. *Journal of Pediatric Orthopaedics, 36*(4), e45–e48.

Naranje, S., Kelly, D. M., & Sawyer, J. R. (2015). A systematic approach to the evaluation of a limping child. *American Family Physician, 92*(10), 908–918.

Noritz, G. H., Murphy, N. A., & Neuromotor Screening Expert Panel. (2013). Motor delays: Early identification and evaluation. *Pediatrics, 131*, e2016–e2027. doi: 10.1542/peds.2013-1056

Palmu, S. A., Auro, S., Lohman, M., Paukku, R. T., Peltonen, J. I., & Nietosvaara, Y. (2014). Tibial fractures in children: A retrospective 27-year follow-up study. *Acta Orthopaedica, 85*(5), 513–517.

Radler, C. (2013). The Ponseti method for the treatment of congenital club foot: Review of the current literature and treatment recommendations. *International Orthopaedics, 37*(9), 1747–1753.

Rampal, V., Clément, J.-L., & Solla, F. (2017). Legg-Calvé-Perthes disease: classifications and prognostic factors. *Clinical Cases in Mineral and Bone Metabolism,* 14(1), 74–82. http://doi.org/10.11138/ccmbm/2017.14.1.074

Rowe, S. M., Jung, S. T., Lee, K. B., Bai, B. H., & Kang, K. D. (2005). The incidence of Perthes' disease in Korea. A focus on differences among races. *Journal of Bone and Joint Surgery. British Volume, 87*, 1666–1668. doi: 10.1302/0301-620X.87B12.16808

Salter, R. B., & Thompson, G. H. (1984). Legg-Calvé-Perthes disease: The prognostic significance of the subchondral fracture and a two-group classification of the femoral head involvement. *Journal of Bone Joint Surgery, 66*, 479–489.

Sass, P., & Hassan, G. (2003). Lower extremity abnormalities in children. *American Family Physician, 68*, 461–468.

Sela, Y., Hershkovich, O., Sher-Lurie, N., Schindler, A., & Givon, U. (2013). Pediatric femoral shaft fractures: Treatment strategies according to age—13 years of experience in one medical center. *Journal of Orthopaedic Surgery and Research, 8*(1), 23.

Shenoi, S. (2017). Juvenile idiopathic arthritis—changing times, changing terms, changing treatments. *Pediatrics in Review, 38*(5), 221–232.

Simonsen, K. A., Anderson-Berry, A. L., Delair, S. F., & Davies, H. D. (2014). Early-onset neonatal sepsis. *Clinical Microbiology Reviews, 27*(1), 21–47. doi: 10.1128/CMR.00031-13

Sofu, H., Gursu, S., Kockara, N., Issin, A., Oner, A., & Camurcu, Y. (2015). Pediatric fractures through the eyes of parents: An observational study. *Medicine (Baltimore), 94*(2), e407.

U.S. Consumer Product Safety Commission, (2017). National electronic injury surveillance system. Retrieve from https://www.cpsc.gov/s3fs-public/2017-NEISS-data-highlights-age.pdf?pKuMH.4NqENxSLIyA9fVd1U0g0F5MGV.

Ward, S. L., & Hisley, S. M. (2009). *Maternal-child nursing care: Optimizing outcomes for mothers, children, & families.* Philadelphia: F.A. Davis.

Weiss, J. E., & Ilowite, N. T. (2007). Juvenile idiopathic arthritis. *Rheumatic Disease Clinics of North America, 33*, 441–470. doi: 10.1016/j.rdc.2007.07.006

Williams, C. M., James, A. M., & Tran, T. (2013). Metatarsus adductus: Development of a non_surgical treatment pathway. *Journal of Paediatrics and Child Health, 49*(9), E428–E433.

Yang, S., Andras, L. M., Redding, G. J., & Skaggs, D. L. (2016). Early-onset scoliosis: A review of history, current treatment, and future directions. *Pediatrics, 137*(1), e20150709.

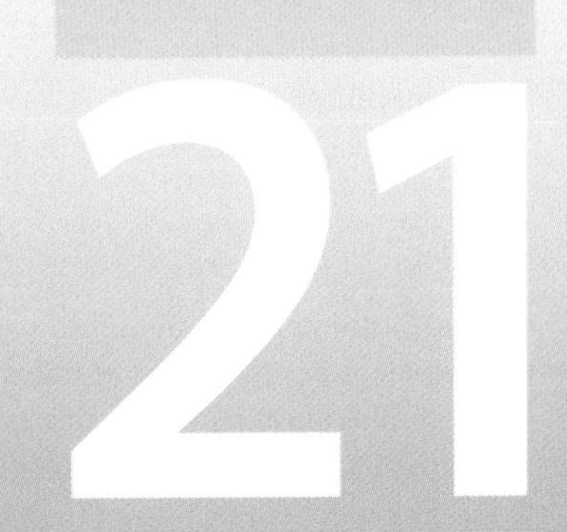

Dermatological Diseases

Teresa Whited, DNP, APRN, CPNP-PC

LEARNING OUTCOMES

Upon completion of this chapter, the student will be able to:

1. Identify causes and precipitating factors of skin conditions and skin injuries seen in children and adolescents.
2. Outline critical components of skin assessment in children and adolescents.
3. Describe the clinical presentation of acquired skin diseases, skin infections and infestations, and various injuries to the skin.
4. Explain diagnostic and laboratory studies used for skin conditions.
5. Describe emergency care given for acute infections, bites, and burns to the skin.
6. Describe care in the hospital for a child or adolescent with an acute or chronic skin condition or with an injury to the skin.
7. Develop a home-based plan of care for a child or adolescent with a chronic skin condition.
8. Discuss alternate therapies used for various skin conditions or injuries to the skin.
9. Develop a teaching plan for caregivers of children or adolescents with skin conditions or injuries to the skin.

ANATOMY AND PHYSIOLOGY

The skin is the largest organ of the body, with functions that include temperature regulation, barrier to environment, prevention of body fluid loss, vitamin D production, toxin excretion, and the sensation of touch. The epidermis, dermis, and subcutaneous layers of the skin are all critical in the function and integrity of the skin in children. Newborns and infants are especially at risk for skin issues because their skin is thinner and weaker. As the child ages, the skin takes on more adult characteristics with increase in hair, increase in sweat and sebaceous gland secretions, and thickened texture (Gehris, 2018).

ASSESSMENT

Skin assessment in pediatric patients consists of the elements described in the following subsections.

General History

Ask about the following issues:

- General health of the child
- Date or time of onset of symptoms
- Growth or changes in rash or lesions
- Presence of itching
- Recent immunizations or medications
- Allergies

- Recent illness
- Similar rash or lesions in family members

Physical Examination

- Distribution or pattern of rash over body
- Are lesions on flexural or extensor surfaces of the body?
- Are lesions clustered (herpetiform) or scattered (diffuse)?
- Do lesions follow a dermatomal (nerve) pattern?
- Are lesions in a straight line (linear), serpiginous (wavy), annular (ring-shaped), circular, or reticulated (lacy)?
- Is the epidermis involved? These lesions include scales, papules, vesicles, and pustules.
- Is the dermis involved? If markings on the epidermis are normal, but there is an elevated area, this indicates dermal involvement (examples: nodule, tumor).
- What color are the lesions?
- Primary lesions arise from the skin itself. These include macules, papules, plaques, vesicles, pustules, wheals, and nodules.
- Secondary lesions grow out of primary lesions or occur when a primary lesion becomes irritated or injured by scratching. Secondary lesions include crusts, ulcers, fissures, and scars.
- Check for any systemic signs and symptoms such as fever, headache, decreased responsiveness, and pain (Chiocca, 2015).

SAFE AND EFFECTIVE NURSING CARE: Clinical Pearl

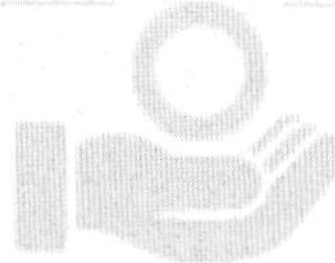

Purpura

Purple or blue lesions that do not blanch suggest purpura. Purpura is an ominous symptom in children that can be associated with critical conditions. The most notable conditions associated with purpura are bacterial meningitis and thrombocytopenia. If purpura is found, the nurse should notify the provider immediately.

SAFE AND EFFECTIVE NURSING CARE: Cultural Competence

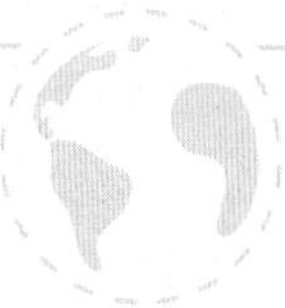

Assessing Pallor, Cyanosis, and Jaundice in Dark Skin

When assessing pallor, cyanosis, or jaundice in a child with dark skin, examine the palpebral conjunctivae (lower eyelids) and the oral mucosa. Jaundice may also be observed in the sclera.

CRITICAL COMPONENT

Skin Integrity and the Hospitalized Child

Skillful nursing care of a hospitalized infant or child includes constant skin assessment, prevention of skin breakdown, and management of impaired skin integrity. Several areas are key to the assessment of the skin in the hospitalized child, including:

- Care of surgical incisions
- Maintenance of IV catheters with careful monitoring for infiltration
- Maintenance of invasive tubes or probes that must be taped: Common equipment such as urinary catheters, pulse oximeter probes, and nasal tubes must be taped in place, and skin integrity is threatened when the tape is in place and when it is removed. Tape removal may damage the epithelium.
- Tracheostomies, gastrostomies, and colostomies all put the child at risk for skin breakdown due to leakage of fluids and body secretions
- Monitor for skin breakdown at the site of external medical equipment such as endotracheal tubes, traction, IV boards, casts, splints, cables, and sensors
- Children who are acutely or chronically ill are at risk for pressure ulcers (Kiss & Heiler, 2014; Schluer, Schols, & Halfens, 2014)

SAFE AND EFFECTIVE NURSING CARE: Clinical Pearl

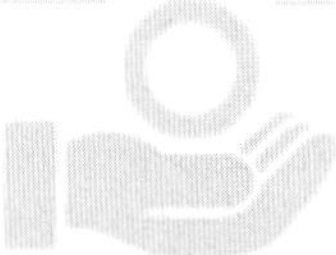

Braden Q Scale

The Braden Q Scale (published by Curley, Razmus, Roberts, & Wypij [2003] and further validated by Tume, Siner, Scott, & Lane [2014]) can be used for children older than 1 year. This tool outlines seven factors that predict the likelihood that a child will experience a pressure ulcer (Fig. 21–1):

- Mobility or the likelihood that a child can change his or her own body position
- The degree of activity
- The ability to respond in a developmentally appropriate way to uncomfortable sensations of pressure
- The degree of moisture on the skin
- The degree of friction or shear from moving across bed linens or other surfaces
- The child is well nourished
- Whether the child is well oxygenated and the tissues are well perfused

The Braden Q Scale					
Intensity and Duration of Pressure					**Score**
Mobility The ability to change and control body position	**1. Completely immobile:** Does not make even slight changes in body or extremity position without assistance.	**2. Very Limited:** Makes occasional slight changes in body or extremity position but unable to completely turn self independently.	**3. Slightly Limited:** Makes frequent though slight changes in body or extremity position independently.	**4. No Limitations:** Makes major and frequent changes in position without assistance.	
Activity The degree of physical activity	**1. Bedfast:** Confined to bed	**2. Chair fast:** Ability to walk severely limited or nonexistent. Cannot bear own weight and/or must be assisted in to chair or wheelchair.	**3. Walks Occasionally:** Walks occasionally during day, but for very short distances, with or without assistance. Spends majority of each shift in bed or chair.	**4. All patients too young to ambulate OR walks frequently:** Walks outside the room at least twice a day and inside room at least once every 2 hours during waking hours.	
Sensory Perception The ability to respond in a <u>developmentally</u> appropriate way to pressure-related discomfort	**1. Completely Limited:** Unresponsive (does not moan, flinch, or grasp) to painful stimuli, due to diminished level of consciousness or sedation **OR** limited ability to feel pain over most of body surface.	**2. Very Limited:** Responds only to painful stimuli. Cannot communicate discomfort except by moaning or restlessness **OR** has sensory impairment which limits the ability to feel pain or discomfort over half of body.	**3. Slightly Limited:** Responds to verbal commands, but cannot always communicate discomfort or need to be turned **OR** has some sensory impairment which limits ability to feel pain or discomfort in 1 or 2 extremities.	**4. No Impairment:** Responds to verbal commands. Has no sensory deficit, which limits ability to feel or communicate pain or discomfort.	
Tolerance of the Skin and Supporting Structure					
Moisture Degree to which skin is exposed to moisture	**1. Constantly Moist:** Skin is kept moist almost constantly by perspiration, urine, drainage, etc. Dampness is detected every time patient is moved or turned.	**2. Very Moist:** Skin is often, but not always moist. Linen must be changed at least every 8 hours.	**3. Occasionally Moist:** Skin is occasionally moist, requiring linen change every 12 hours.	**4. Rarely Moist:** Skin is usually dry, routine diaper changes, linen only requires changing every 24 hours.	
Friction - Shear ***Friction:*** occurs when skin moves against support surfaces ***Shear***: occurs when skin and adjacent bony surface slide across one another	**1. Significant Problem**: Spasticity, contracture, itching or agitation leads to almost constant thrashing and friction.	**2. Problem:** Requires moderate to maximum assistance in moving. Complete lifting without sliding against sheets is impossible. Frequently slides down in bed or chair, requiring frequent repositioning with maximum assistance.	**3. Potential Problem:** Moves feebly or requires minimum assistance. During a move skin probably slides to some extent against sheets, chair, restraints, or other devices. Maintains relative good position in chair or bed most of the time but occasionally slides down.	**4. No Apparent Problem:** Able to completely lift patient during a position change; Moves in bed and in chair independently and has sufficient muscle strength to lift up completely during move. Maintains good position in bed or chair at all times.	
Nutrition *Usual* food intake pattern	**1. Very Poor**: NPO and/or maintained on clear liquids, or IVs for more than 5 days **OR** Albumin <2.5 mg/dl **OR** Never eats a complete meal. Rarely eats more than half of any food offered. Protein intake includes only 2 servings of meat or dairy products per day. Takes fluids poorly. Does not take a liquid dietary supplement.	**2. Inadequate:** Is on liquid diet or tube feedings/TPN which provide inadequate calories and minerals for age **OR** Albumin <3 mg/dl **OR** rarely eats a complete meal and generally eats only about half of any food offered. Protein intake includes only 3 servings of meat or dairy products per day. Occasionally will take a dietary supplement.	**3. Adequate:** Is on tube feedings or TPN, which provide adequate calories and minerals for age **OR** eats over half of most meals. Eats a total of 4 servings of protein (meat, dairy products) each day. Occasionally will refuse a meal, but will usually take a supplement if offered.	**4. Excellent:** Is on a normal diet providing adequate calories for age. For example: eats/drinks most of every meal/feeding. Never refuses a meal. Usually eats a total of 4 or more servings of meat and dairy products. Occasionally eats between meals. Does not require supplementation.	
Tissue Perfusion and Oxygenation	**1. Extremely Compromised:** Hypotensive (MAP <50mmHg; <40 in a newborn) **OR** the patient does not physiologically tolerate position changes.	**2. Compromised:** Normotensive; Oxygen saturation may be <95 % **OR** hemoglobin may be < 10 mg/dl **OR** capillary refill may be > 2 seconds; Serum pH is < 7.40.	**3. Adequate:** Normotensive; Oxygen saturation may be <95 % **OR** hemoglobin may be < 10 mg/dl **OR** capillary refill may be > 2 seconds; Serum pH is normal.	**4. Excellent:** Normotensive, Oxygen saturation >95%; Normal Hemoglobin ; & Capillary refill < 2 seconds.	
				Total:	

FIGURE 21–1 Braden Q Pressure Ulcer Risk Assessment Scale.

CRITICAL COMPONENT

Skin Integrity in the Hospital

Nursing care to maintain skin integrity in the hospitalized infant or child includes the following measures:

- Change diapers and linens frequently to keep the skin dry.
- Use barrier creams containing zinc oxide as needed on the diaper area for diaper dermatitis. It is not necessary to completely remove all the barrier cream with each diaper change, as removing the cream may cause further skin breakdown. Remove soiled areas only.
- Use water-based hypoallergenic moisturizers for dry skin.
- Bathe the child with mild, nonalkaline, pH-balanced cleansing agents. Avoid vigorous cleaning or scrubbing.
- Pay special attention to skin around tracheostomies and other ostomies. Keep the skin clean and dry. Foam dressings may help absorb exudates around tracheostomies and gastrostomies.
- Keep the child well oxygenated and well nourished.
- If the child is confined to a bed or chair, turn or change position at least every 2 hours. Elevate the head of the bed no more than 30 degrees. Lower the head of the bed before repositioning the child. Keep the heels from rubbing on surfaces, and place the child on an egg crate or air flotation mattress as needed. Pay special attention to the back of the head and ears in children who are immobile. These areas are the most common sites of pressure ulcers in children.
- Place foam dressings over bony prominences that are at risk for breakdown.
- Minimize taping and use gauze or self-adherent wrap as an alternative when possible. Tape without tension. Use barriers such as skin preps under tape to protect the skin. Remove tape carefully to avoid stripping the epithelium.
- Monitor carefully all probes, tubes, and IV catheters for skin irritation or breakdown at the site. Change pulse oximeter probes every 2 to 6 hours.

ACQUIRED DISORDERS

Multiple skin lesions are a result of acquired disorders from external forces such as pressure, contacts with allergenic substances, or processes that affect skin integrity. Based on the disorder, treatment for these conditions varies significantly. Nurses must thoroughly assess the skin and implement practices that can help prevent disruption in the normal skin barrier. This section will cover the most common acquired disorders of the skin in childhood.

Pressure Ulcers

The child who is immobile or hospitalized is at risk for pressure ulcers, which most commonly affect the ears, occiput, sacrum, scapula, and feet. Nurses must minimize risk factors associated with pressure ulcers; in children, these include:

- Immobility
- Comorbid conditions, especially those affecting circulation
- Patients who are critically ill
- The use of mechanical ventilation with endotracheal tubes, IV lines that prevent movement of the head or other body parts, cables on the skin, or devices of immobility like traction, splints, and IV boards
- Poor sensory perception
- Immobility of the patient for long periods
- Poor nutrition
- Amount of friction/shear forces on the area (Manning, Gauvreau, & Curley, 2015; Schluer et al., 2014)

Clinical Presentation of Pressure Ulcers

Pressure ulcers can be in multiple areas on the body and should be staged appropriately. According to the National Pressure Ulcer Advisory Panel (2017), pressure ulcers can be staged by the following criteria:

- Stage 1: nonblanchable erythema of intact skin
- Stage 2: partial-thickness skin loss with exposed dermis
- Stage 3: full-thickness skin loss
- Stage 4: full-thickness skin and tissue loss
- Unstageable: obscured full-thickness skin and tissue loss
- Deep tissue: persistent nonblanchable deep red, maroon, or purple discoloration

Nursing Interventions

The most critical portion of nursing care for pressure ulcers is prevention of the occurrence of the ulcers by early identification of risk factors and prevention strategies. Treatment of ulcers is dependent on the stage of the ulcer, bacterial infection, and location of the ulcer. Common nursing interventions include:

- Assess skin regularly and assess risk factors using Braden Q or other scale appropriate for skin integrity.
- Use interventions that allow pressure redistribution and prevent further breakdown such as padding devices, egg crate, dressings, and frequent position changes when possible.
- Assess pain and treat with prescribed medications.
- Prevent and treat infection with dressings and prescribed topical or oral antibiotics.
- Debridement may be necessary for wounds with necrotic tissue present.
- Many adjunct therapies are used, such as hyperbaric oxygen, negative pressure wound therapy, ultrasound, and electrical stimulation; however, these require additional study (Berlowitz, 2017; National Pressure Ulcer Advisory Panel, 2017).

Caregiver Education

Nurses must educate parents and caregivers on the following measures to prevent pressure ulcers.

Home Care

- Monitor wound closely for healing or worsening.
- Call provider if signs of infection or necrosis develop.
- Continue medications and dressings as prescribed to promote healing.
- Keep area clean and dry when possible.

- If still immobile, use prevention measures to redistribute pressure and monitor for worsening or new breakdown of skin (Rodriguez, 2016).

DERMATITIS

The three main types of pediatric dermatitis are diaper, seborrheic, and contact.

Clinical Presentation of Diaper Dermatitis

- The skin around the diaper area becomes irritated from chemicals and enzymes in the urine or feces (Fig. 21–2). Skin becomes erythematous, with scaling and confinement to the convex surfaces of the diaper area.
- Infection with *Candida albicans*, a yeastlike fungus, results in candidiasis of the diaper area. Erythematous areas are well demarcated, and satellite lesions may be noted on the buttocks, legs, and abdomen. These characteristics differentiate candidiasis from milder forms of diaper dermatitis (Fig. 21–3).

Nursing Interventions

- Apply an ointment containing zinc oxide for irritants and nystatin (Mycostatin) as ordered for candidiasis in the diaper area.
- Hydrocortisone 1% cream may be ordered for severe diaper rash with short duration of therapy to prevent skin thinning.
- Monitor for signs of bacterial infection with severe diaper rash: pustules, purulent discharge, increasing ulcerations, and erythema. Refer for medical treatment as needed.

Caregiver Education

Caregivers should receive nurse education on the following topics related to diaper dermatitis.

Home Care

- For prevention and home care for diaper rash, keep diaper area dry; change diapers frequently.

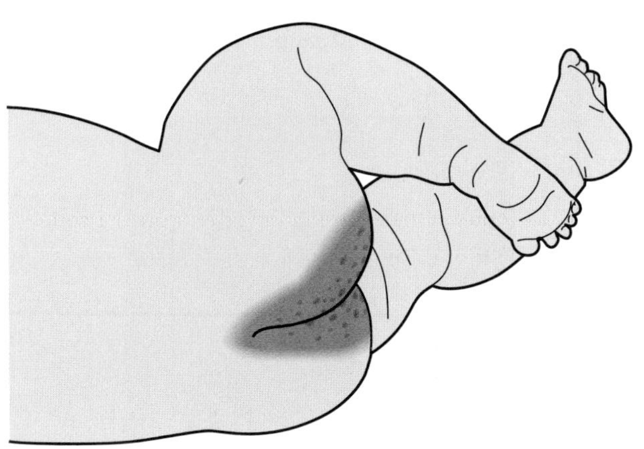

FIGURE 21–2 Diaper rash.

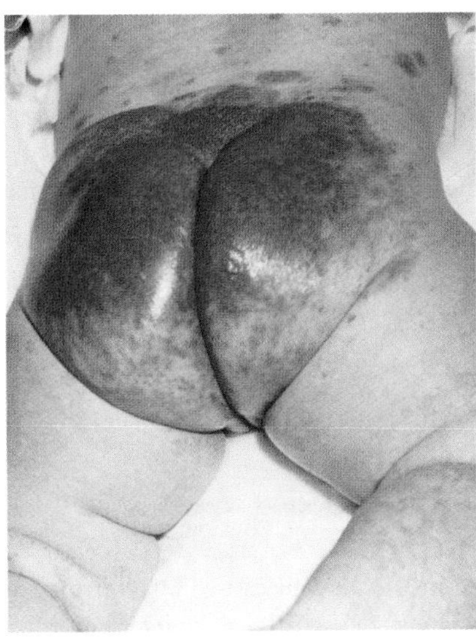

FIGURE 21–3 Candidiasis has a beefy-red appearance, different from the appearance of typical diaper rash.

- Clean diaper area with warm water each time diaper is changed. If soap is required, use a mild soap such as Cetaphil, Neutrogena, Dove, or Basic. Avoid vigorous scrubbing. Use caution with commercial wipes; some infants are sensitive to the chemicals in these wipes.
- Leave diaper area open to air when possible. Fifteen minutes four times daily is recommended.
- Do not use plastic diaper covers. These hold in heat and moisture.
- Barrier ointments containing zinc oxide may be used. Examples are A&D ointment and Desitin ointment.
- Do not use baby powder or cornstarch because it can get in the infant's lungs (Klunk, Domingues, & Wiss, 2014).

Clinical Presentation of Seborrheic Dermatitis

- Seborrheic dermatitis (called cradle cap when it appears on scalp) manifests with scaling and a greasy appearance on the scalp and in folds of the body. It may also appear on the face or behind the ears.
- It is nonpruritic, which helps to distinguish it from atopic dermatitis.

Diagnostic Studies

Most cases can be diagnosed based on the clinical picture described earlier. However, if the diagnosis is uncertain or not responsive to traditional therapies, a biopsy can be obtained. The cause of seborrheic dermatitis is often unknown, but it can be caused by *Pityrosporum* or *Candida.*

Caregiver Education

Caregivers should receive education on the following topics related to seborrheic dermatitis.

Home Care

- Daily shampoos with a mild pH-balanced infant shampoo will help to prevent seborrheic dermatitis (cradle cap) in infants.
- Avoid vigorous scrubbing of the scalp.
- An antiseborrheic shampoo or topical steroid may be recommended for cases of severe cradle cap.

Complementary and Alternative Therapies

- If cradle cap is present, apply warm olive oil or baby oil, wait 15 minutes, shampoo hair, and brush gently (Clark, Pope, & Jaboori, 2015).

Clinical Presentation of Contact Dermatitis

- Contact dermatitis may be caused by an irritant or allergy.
- Irritant contact dermatitis is characterized by erythema, papules, vesicles, hives, burning, and weeping. Causes include soaps and irritating chemicals.
- Allergic contact dermatitis is characterized by pruritus that is usually severe, erythema, papules, vesicles, and streaks or patches.
- Common causes of allergic contact dermatitis in children include poison oak, poison ivy, and poison sumac. Nickel found in buckles and jewelry can also be a problem.

Caregiver Education

Nurses should educate parents and caregivers on the following topics related to contact dermatitis.

Home Care

For prevention and home care of poison oak, ivy, or sumac:

- Wash area thoroughly with soap and water. This must be done within 15 minutes of exposure to remove the resin oils that cause the irritation.
- Apply cool, wet compresses four times daily. Burrow's solution or Domeboro solution may be helpful as a wet compress.
- Apply lotions or creams to help control itching. Examples include Calamine lotion and pramoxine (Prax) or Sama with menthol, camphor, and phenol. Low-dose over-the-counter (1%) corticosteroid creams may also be applied in a thin coat to relieve inflammation and itching.
- Refer for medical help if the rash is extensive or involves the face. Higher concentrations of topical corticosteroid creams or oral therapy may be prescribed.

Complementary and Alternative Therapies

- Bathe with oatmeal bath such as Aveeno.

ATOPIC DERMATITIS (ECZEMA)

Eczema is a chronic skin disorder with multifactorial causes including genetic, environmental (allergies or topical irritants), skin barrier dysfunction, and hyperimmune activation of T-helper cells that results in dry, pruritic skin lesions (Otsuka et al., 2017) (Fig. 21–4).

SAFE AND EFFECTIVE NURSING CARE: Clinical Pearl

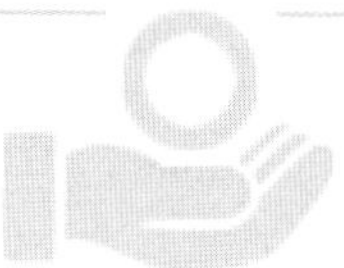

Latex and Contact Dermatitis

Latex allergies to gloves may produce contact dermatitis of the hands in health-care providers or patients with chronic conditions/prolonged hospitalizations. Nurses can prevent sensitization or allergic reactions by minimizing or eliminating the use of latex products. Prevention can be accomplished by using vinyl, nitrile, or polymer gloves in place of latex products, or using power-free gloves if latex gloves are required to be used.

(Centers for Disease Control and Prevention, 2014)

CRITICAL COMPONENT

Poison Oak, Poison Ivy, and Poison Sumac

Plant resins are responsible for the skin lesions and intense itching associated with poison ivy and similar plants. Allergic dermatitis resulting from contact with poison ivy is not contagious. However, resins can be spread not only by direct contact with the plants, but by indirect contact, causing typical signs and symptoms of poison ivy. The resins may be spread indirectly through contact with clothing and pets. Resins may also be spread through the air if these plants are burned.

Clinical Presentation

- Children from families with a history of asthma, allergies, or atopic dermatitis are at greater risk for development of atopic dermatitis or eczema.
- Eczema is characterized by skin scaling and intense itching. There may be patches of skin with erythema, papules, vesicles, crusting, and sometimes weeping. Patches of eczema may become infected. Scratching places the child at greater risk for infection.
- Infantile eczema involves mainly the extensor surfaces of the extremities and the face and scalp.

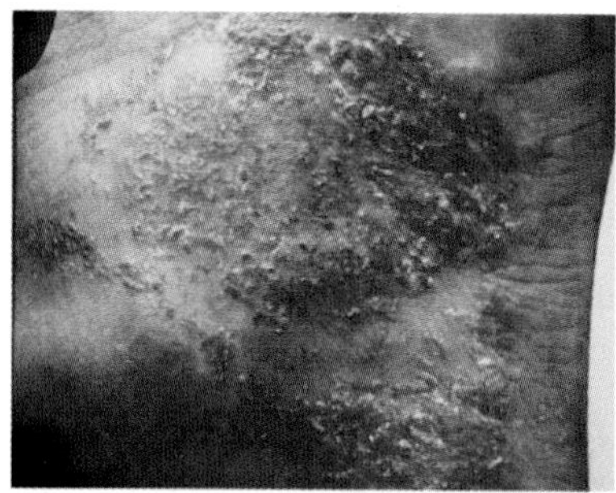

FIGURE 21–4 Child with atopic dermatitis (eczema).

- Childhood eczema involves mainly the flexural surfaces of the extremities, the wrists, the neck, areas behind the ears, and sometimes the hands.
- Adolescent eczema is more common on the hands and in skin creases (Eichenfield et al., 2015; Saeki et al., 2016).

SAFE AND EFFECTIVE NURSING CARE: Promoting Safety

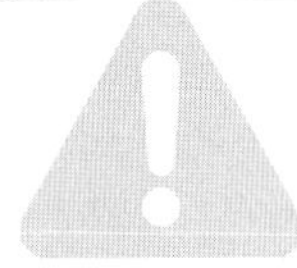

Preventing Infection

Children with atopic dermatitis (eczema) are at risk for skin infections due to the underlying defects in the skin and constant breakdown of the skin barrier. Skin should be assessed for infection, and patients should be encouraged to avoid exposure to people with warts, herpes simplex, and other infectious skin conditions.

Diagnostic Testing

- Cultures may be carried out if infection develops.

Caregiver Education

Caregivers and parents of pediatric patients who have eczema should be educated on the following topics.

Home Care

- Wear loose, cotton clothing. Avoid wool clothing or blankets. Use mild, fragrance-free laundry detergents and fabric softeners. Wash all new clothing before wearing.
- Apply moisturizers three times daily.
- Bath every other day in warm (not hot) water and use mild soaps such as Dove, Basic, Cetaphil, or Neutrogena. May bathe in diluted bleach baths.
- Keep the environment cool and humidified.
- Identify foods or irritants that trigger eczema or make it worse.
- Prevent scratching. Oral antihistamines may be given at night to promote sleep. Keep fingernails short.
- Apply topical steroids and immunomodulators as ordered.
- Carefully assess for signs of infection such as redness, swelling, pustules, and purulent drainage (Eichenfield et al., 2015; Saeki et al., 2016).

Complementary and Alternative Therapies

- Vitamin A (50,000 IU daily), vitamin E (400 IU daily), zinc (50 mg daily), omega 3 fatty acids, and evening primrose oil (3,000 mg daily) may be used by adolescents and adults to treat eczema (Arcangelo, 2017). However, it is important not to dose children with vitamins over and above their daily requirements.

CRITICAL COMPONENT

Dry Skin and Eczema

The key to successful treatment of atopic dermatitis (eczema) is hydration of the skin. Dry skin is a significant factor in the progression of eczema; therefore, moisturizers (emollients) are very effective in the management of this condition. Examples of moisturizers include Eucerin cream, Cetaphil cream, Aquaphor, and petroleum jelly. Moisturizers are applied to the skin two or three times daily and immediately after bathing while the skin is still moist. The skin is patted dry instead of rubbed.

Evidence-Based Practice: Diet and Atopic Disease

Fleisher, D., Sicherer, S., Greenhawt, M., Campbell, D., Chan, E., Muraro, A., . . . Rosenwasser, L. (2015). Consensus communication on early peanut introduction and the prevention of peanut allergy in high-risk infants. *Pediatrics, 136*(3), 600–604. doi: 10.1542/peds.2015-2394

Du Toit, G., Roberts, G., Sayre, P. H., Bahnson, H. T., Radulovic, S., Santos, A. F., . . . LEAP Study Team. (2015). Randomized trial of peanut consumption in infants at risk for peanut allergy. *New England Journal of Medicine, 372*(9), 803–813. doi: 10.1056/NEJMoa1414850

The Learning Early About Peanut Allergy (LEAP) randomized trial evaluated 640 high-risk infants aged 4 to 11 months who had severe eczema, egg allergy, or both. This study found that introduction of highly allergic foods such as peanuts should not be delayed past 4 to 11 months. It further found that exposing these infants to peanuts may reduce their risk for peanut allergy up to 80% (Du Toit et al., 2015).

The American Academy of Pediatrics with the National Institute of Allergy and Infectious Disease and American College of Allergy, Asthma & Immunology along with multiple other worldwide organizations have endorsed a statement recommending introduction of peanut-containing foods into the diets of high-risk infants by 4 to 11 months of age. Further, infants who have early-onset atopic disease or egg allergy in the first 4 to 6 months of life may benefit from evaluation by allergy specialist for food allergy testing and management including introduction of foods (Fleischer et al., 2015).

ACNE

Acne is a common condition in older children and adolescents. Although the condition is often self-limited to adolescence, significant lesions can result in long-term scarring and social distress in this age group. Acne is a very manageable condition with multiple treatments available in over-the-counter and prescription forms. Acne management prevents complications and promotes healthy skin in children and adolescents.

Clinical Presentation

- The primary lesions of acne are comedones or plugged sebaceous follicles (Fig. 21–5). The problem in mild acne is not inflammation but plugged sebaceous follicles in the skin that

SAFE AND EFFECTIVE NURSING CARE: Understanding Medication

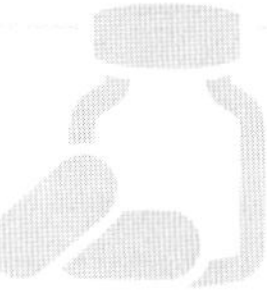

Medication to Treat Eczema

The two most effective medications for eczema are topical steroids and immunomodulators. Topical steroids may be applied at the same time as emollients. The steroid cream is applied in a thin layer first, and the emollient is applied over the steroid cream. Occlusive dressings such as a plastic wrap or damp towel may be placed over steroid creams for 10 minutes to promote absorption.

Topical immunomodulators such as tacrolimus (Protopic) or pimecrolimus (Elidel) may be used as alternates to topical steroid creams for children older than 2 years. However, occlusive dressings should never be placed over topical immunomodulators. If topical agents are ineffective, the patient may benefit from a short course of oral steroids.

Topical steroids come in multiple preparations including creams, ointments, lotions, and gels. Steroid creams are the preferred method. However, ointments and gels are the most potent and lubricating of the preparations. Steroid creams come in three strengths: low, medium, and high. Low-strength creams are available over the counter, but medium- and high-strength creams may be obtained by prescription only and are used for the more severe cases. Special care must be taken not to apply medium- or high-strength steroid creams to the face or neck where the skin is thin, because they may produce skin atrophy, ecchymosis, or acne. Steroid creams must be applied in a thin coat and should not be used for prolonged periods (usual course is 7 days).

produce open comedones (blackheads) and closed comedones (whiteheads).

- The bacterium *Propionibacterium acnes* may produce inflammation in individuals with more severe acne. The inflammation leads to pustules, cysts, and scarring (Fig. 21–6).
- Acne lesions generally start on the face but also appear on the chest and back.

Caregiver Education

Parents and caregivers should receive education on the following topics related to acne.

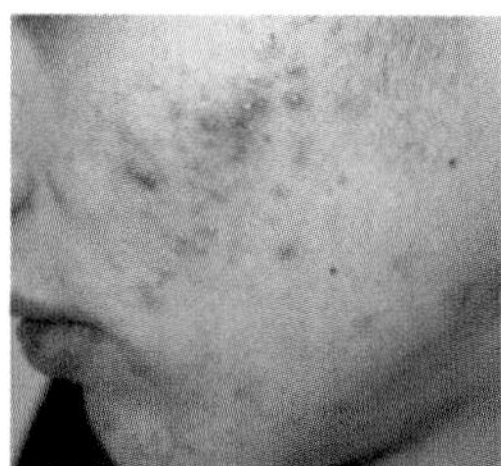

FIGURE 21–5 Adolescent acne (comedones).

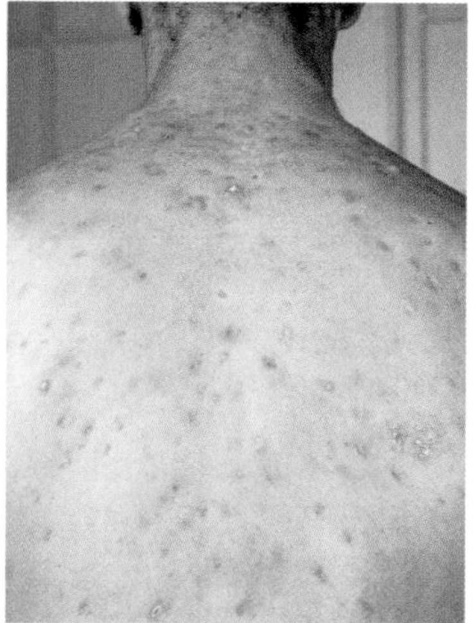

FIGURE 21–6 Adolescent with inflammatory acne (pustules, cysts).

Home Care

- Avoid touching the face or squeezing comedones.
- Avoid oil-based creams or cosmetics on the face. Makeup must be oil free. Teach adolescents to read labels.
- Clean the face gently two or three times daily with a mild soap or cleanser such as Cetaphil, Basis, or Neutrogena. Harsh soaps and astringents are damaging to the skin.
- Keep hair clean and off the face.
- Administer topical comedolytic agents as ordered for noninflammatory acne (examples: tretinoin, azelaic acid, adapalene).
- Administer topical antibiotics as ordered for mild inflammatory acne (examples: benzoyl peroxide, erythromycin, clindamycin ointments).
- Administer oral antibiotics as ordered for inflammatory acne (minocycline or doxycycline).

SAFE AND EFFECTIVE NURSING CARE: Clinical Pearl

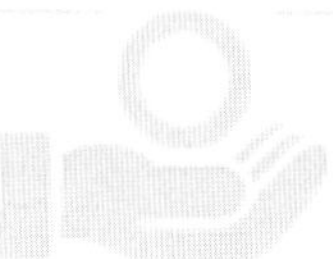

Management of Acne

The key to successful management of acne is skin care with gentle cleansing and avoidance of oil-based substances on the face. Dietary changes do not affect acne.

SAFE AND EFFECTIVE NURSING CARE: Understanding Medication

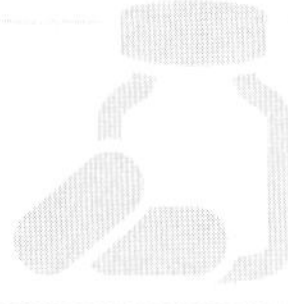

Skin Sensitivity With Comedolytic Creams

When comedolytic creams such as tretinoin, azelaic acid, or adapalene are ordered for the treatment of acne, it is important to teach patients to use sunscreen, because these creams make the skin more sensitive to the sun.

Evidence-Based Practice: Oral Contraception and Acne Reduction

Zaenglein, A. L., Pathy, A. L., Schlosser, B. J., Alikhan, A., Baldwin, H. E., Berson, D. S., . . . Bhushan, R. (2016). Guidelines of care for the management of acne vulgaris. *Journal of the American Academy of Dermatology, 74*(5), 945–973.e33. doi: 10.1016/j.jaad.2015.12.037

Combination oral contraceptives that contain both an estrogen and a progestin have been shown to be effective in reducing acne lesions in women. If first-line therapies are ineffective, oral contraceptives or spironolactone can be added to the treatment regimen in females.

BACTERIAL INFECTIONS

Bacterial infections of the skin occur when the normal skin barriers break down and allow overgrowth of bacteria. Skin breakdown can be caused either by an unintentional injury or a surgical incision. Most bacterial infections occur as a result of normal skin flora such as *Staphylococcus* or *Streptococcus*; however, any type of bacteria can be present. It is important to identify the type of infection present and treat appropriately to prevent worsening infection. Nurses need to identify and help manage these conditions to restore the normal skin integrity.

Impetigo

Impetigo is a bacterial infection characterized by vesicles with a honey-colored crust. Nonbullous impetigo, the most common form, usually presents on the face, extremities, or trunk. Bullous impetigo is less common and only caused by *Staphylococcus*. Bullous impetigo is more likely to occur in infants in the diaper area. Impetigo is extremely contagious and should be managed with topical or oral medications.

Clinical Presentation

- Papules turn into vesicles that crust over with a honey-colored crust (Fig. 21–7).
- Lesions around the nose and mouth are common.
- Infection may develop in areas where skin has been damaged or area around nose has been irritated from nasal secretions.
- Contagious until the child has been on antibiotics for 24 hours

Diagnostic Testing

- Caused by *Staphylococcus aureus* or group A beta-hemolytic streptococcus

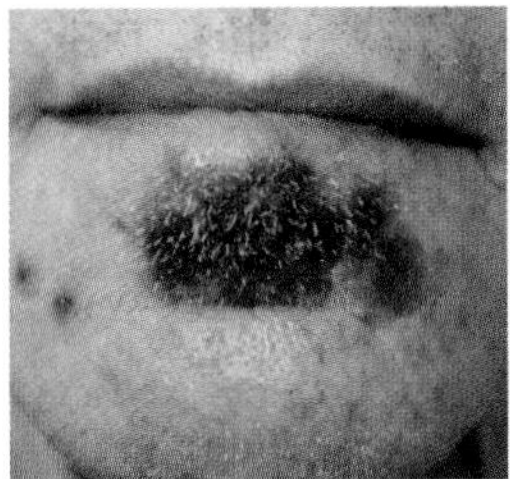

FIGURE 21–7 Child with impetigo.

Nursing Interventions

Nursing interventions during hospital care for patients with impetigo include the following measures.

- Careful hand hygiene and contact isolation
- Administration of topical antibiotics as ordered for mild cases with small, localized lesions
- Administration of oral antibiotics as ordered for more extensive infections

Caregiver Education

- Practice careful hand hygiene during and after child care.
- Teach hand hygiene to child.
- Keep fingernails clean and trimmed to prevent scratching.
- Disinfect surfaces such as sink, bathtub, and toys.
- Wash child's clothes and linens in contact with lesions daily.
- Cover impetigo lesions with loose, cotton clothing if possible.
- Administer of topical or oral antibiotics as ordered.
- Complete all antibiotics.
- If infection worsens or fails to resolve, seek medical care (Hartman-Adams, Banvard, & Juckett, 2014).

Methicillin-Resistant *Staphylococcus aureus*

Methicillin-resistant *Staphylococcus aureus* (MRSA) infection is caused by bacteria that has become resistant to common antibiotics used to treat staphylococcal infections. MRSA can be either hospital or community acquired and must be treated by specific antibiotics depending on sensitivity studies. MRSA tends to be a more significant and more difficult to treat infection than typical staphylococcal infections. MRSA can easily be spread from patient to patient, so preventive measures must to be used in a health-care setting. It is important for nurses to identify, care for, and prevent these types of infections.

Clinical Presentation

- A MRSA infection of the skin may begin as a small red bump that may be mistaken for an insect bite.
- Infections may develop where there has been a small break in the skin.
- The infection may begin as a red macule and progress to a warm, swollen, reddened area that is tender to touch. Purulent drainage may be present.
- The infection may present as a furuncle (boil), carbuncle (cluster of boils), or abscess.
- If the infection spreads to surrounding soft tissue, cellulitis will result (see later Cellulitis section).

Diagnostic Testing

- Culture drainage to identify the bacteria involved.
- Sensitivity tests should also be performed to determine whether the bacteria are resistant or susceptible to certain antibiotics.

Nursing Interventions

Nursing interventions for patients receiving outpatient care include:

- Incision and drainage procedures are performed on skin lesions to release purulent material and promote healing.
- Culture any drainage present.

- Cover the lesion with a gauze dressing and give instructions on dressing the lesion at home.
- Administer antibiotics as ordered.

Nursing interventions for MRSA in the hospital include:

- More severe infections that involve cellulitis may be treated in the hospital. Patient will require contact isolation protocols. Refer to the later Cellulitis section.
- MRSA infections may complicate the healing of surgical wounds in the hospital. Meticulous hand hygiene, gloving, and sterile technique when changing dressings is essential.
- Complications of severe infections may include pneumonia, meningitis, and osteomyelitis.

Caregiver Education

- Keep wound covered with sterile gauze and change as needed.
- Hand hygiene with soap for 30 seconds before and after changing dressing.
- Disinfect shower, bathtub, and other surfaces used by the child.
- Complete course of antibiotics as ordered.
- Seek medical help for signs of cellulitis such as increasing redness, streaks of red around lesion, increasing swelling or tenderness, or fever.
- Seek medical advice for repeated infections. Nasal mupirocin or chlorhexidine baths may help to prevent infections in a colonized person.

CRITICAL COMPONENT

Hospital-Acquired and Community-Acquired Methicillin-Resistant *Staphylococcus aureus*

MRSA infections may present as health hazards in the hospital (hospital-acquired MRSA) or in the community (community-acquired MRSA). Community-acquired MRSA infections develop in otherwise healthy people who have not been in the hospital or other health-care facility. Most community-acquired MRSA infections involve the skin or soft tissues. Hospital-based MRSA infections are more likely to affect people who are already ill, and they tend to be more serious and affect internal organs such as the lungs.

SAFE AND EFFECTIVE NURSING CARE: Clinical Pearl

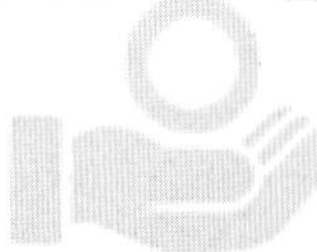

Colonization

An individual may be colonized with MRSA from an old infection. This person will not have any sign of infection, but carries the bacteria on his or her body. Persons colonized with MRSA are more likely to have surgical-site infections or pass the bacteria on to other close contacts. Careful hand hygiene is essential. Community-acquired MRSA may also be carried in the nose. Nasal mupirocin two or three times daily for 1 week, bathing in chlorohexidine, and bleach in the bath water may prevent recurrent infections (American Academy of Pediatrics, 2015).

SAFE AND EFFECTIVE NURSING CARE: Understanding Medication

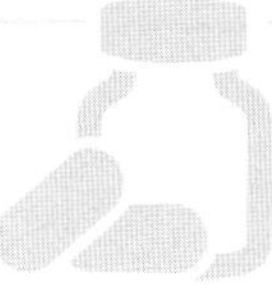

Resistance to Antibiotics

MRSA developed because some *S. aureus* bacteria became resistant to penicillin-based antibiotics. Three common practices may be contributing to the development of resistant bacteria: (1) taking antibiotics unnecessarily for viral infections, (2) failing to complete the entire dose of antibiotics as ordered, and (3) saving leftover antibiotics for later self-medication. Antibiotic stewardship is a national mandate for health care to reduce the number of antibiotic-resistant organisms. An important part of the nurse's role is to teach proper administration of antibiotics (Pollack et al., 2016).

Vancomycin, linezolid, clindamycin, sulfamethoxazole-trimethoprim, and rifampin are all used to treat community-acquired MRSA infections in children. However, health-care providers must be alert for development of resistance or adverse effects of the medications. Liquid clindamycin is foul tasting and may be difficult for children to take. Consider mixing this antibiotic with flavored syrup.

SAFE AND EFFECTIVE NURSING CARE: Promoting Safety

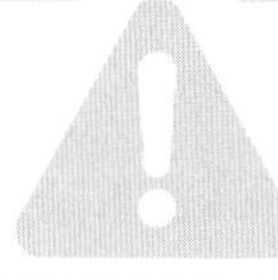

To prevent MRSA infections, follow these guidelines:

- Careful hand hygiene after touching infected skin or changing bandages: wash hands with soap, and rub hands for 30 seconds before rinsing thoroughly.
- Avoid touching the nose.
- Disinfect equipment and surfaces.
- Do not share towels and other personal equipment.
- Avoid line drying of clothes; use a clothes dryer.
- Keep any wound, boils, and draining sores covered.

(Salge, Vera, Antons, & Cimiotti, 2016)

SAFE AND EFFECTIVE NURSING CARE: Clinical Pearl

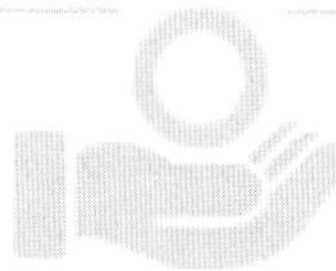

Disinfectants

Disinfectants are used to clean surfaces such as showers and locker-room benches that have been in contact with bare skin. When purchasing a disinfectant, check the label to ensure that it is effective against MRSA and that the label includes an Environmental Protection Agency (EPA) registration number.

Cellulitis

Cellulitis may develop where there has been a small break in the skin or recent trauma. It may also follow sinusitis or otitis media.

Clinical Presentation

- The organism may be *S. aureus*, MRSA, *Haemophilus influenzae*, or group A streptococcal (GAS) infection. Refer to the earlier section on MRSA for additional information on this common type of bacterium.
- GAS is responsible for common strep throat and impetigo. However, on rare occasions, GAS may spread to the blood and then to the muscles or lungs. If it spreads to the soft tissues and muscles, it causes necrotizing fasciitis.
- Local clinical manifestations include redness, warmth, swelling, and tenderness. There may also be lymphangitis and red streaking in the area.
- Systemic clinical manifestations include fever, chills, and malaise.

Diagnostic Testing

- Culture and sensitivity tests on any drainage present
- Blood cultures if fever and systemic signs and symptoms are present
- Complete blood cell count (CBC) with white blood count (WBC) differential to assess for bacterial infection

Nursing Interventions

- Assess temperature, heart and respiratory rate, and blood pressure at regular intervals (every 2–4 hours as needed).
- Assess local clinical manifestations and monitor site for increasing redness, swelling, warmth, tenderness, drainage, or streaking.
- Assess perfusion (color, warmth, capillary refill) of affected extremity or body part (every 2 to 4 hours as indicated).
- Assess hydration status and maintain intake and output records.
- Monitor child's behavior and level of consciousness.
- Apply warm, wet compresses to affected area as ordered.
- Elevate affected extremity or body part.
- Use contact isolation and meticulous hand hygiene.
- Administer acetaminophen or ibuprofen as ordered for pain and fever.
- Encourage oral fluids and administer IV fluids as ordered.
- Administer IV antibiotics as ordered.
- Provide for quiet play according to the child's activity level.

Caregiver Education

- Seek medical help for increased fever or for increasing redness, streaking, and pain and swelling at the infection site.
- Complete course of antibiotics as ordered.
- Administer acetaminophen or ibuprofen for pain or fever.
- Apply warm, wet compresses or dressings if indicated.
- Practice careful hand hygiene before and after dressing changes or touching infected area.
- Refer to home-care instructions for MRSA.

VIRAL INFECTIONS

Viral infections of the skin result from common viruses and are usually spread through close contact with others infected by the virus. Some viral infections are self-limiting, whereas others are lifelong infections that recur. Viral infections of the skin usually present in distinct patterns and should be treated appropriately based on the underlying disorder. Nurses play a crucial role in the identification and treatment of these infections.

Papillomavirus (Verruca or Warts)

Human papillomavirus (HPV) has multiple strains and can result in warts in multiple areas of the skin. The most common types of warts are caused by HPV-2 in children. Warts can be unsightly and concerning for families whose children are affected. Multiple modalities are available for management of these warts.

Clinical Presentation

- Is caused by HPV.
- Plantar warts on the soles of the feet or the palms of the hands are caused by HPV-1.
- Common warts or verruca vulgaris are caused by HPV-2. In children, these commonly appear on the hands and appear as rough, scaly papules.

Caregiver Education

- Warts may be mildly contagious. Perform hand hygiene after touching warts.
- Do not scratch or pick at warts. This may lead to a secondary bacterial infection and scarring.
- Do not share towels.
- Many warts heal spontaneously and disappear without treatment within 2 to 3 years.
- Treatments such as liquid nitrogen stimulate the body's immune system and help it to fight against the papillomavirus.
- Cryosurgery may be required for warts that are resistant to other therapy.
- Salicylic acid in the form of liquid, gel, or a patch (Duofilm) may be effective in removing warts.

SAFE AND EFFECTIVE NURSING CARE: Clinical Pearl

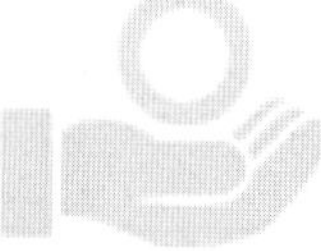

Nail Biting

Children who constantly bite fingernails or pick at cuticles are at higher risk for development of warts under the nails.

Herpes Simplex Virus 1 (Cold Sores or Fever Blisters)

Herpes simplex virus 1 (HSV1) can result in a skin infection, often affecting the mouth and gums, and also occurring in genital areas. Herpes simplex is endemic worldwide. Most HSV1 infections are known as cold sores or fever blisters because lesions tend to occur during periods of illness, fever, or high stress. The HSV1 infection is lifelong, with intermittent outbreaks of the lesions. Herpes simplex is most contagious during outbreaks but can be spread without obvious lesions. The most common transmission is through oral-to-oral exposure. In infants, this occurs through transmission from parents to the child with kissing or touching of the mouth. It is important for nurses to educate families on prevention and management of these conditions.

Clinical Presentation

- Present as small vesicles on the lips, in the mouth, and/or on the gums (Fig. 21–8). These vesicles are painful and may leak clear fluid or bleed slightly. Vesicles eventually crust over.
- The incubation period is 2 days to 2 weeks.
- The person is contagious for at least 1 week and sometimes longer after initial infections; most contagious 3 to 4 days after recurrent infections, although viral shedding may continue after lesions have cleared.
- Transmission is by direct contact or contact with toys that have been put in the mouth.
- Systemic signs and symptoms include fever, irritability, and enlarged, tender lymph nodes.

Nursing Interventions

- Contact isolation with gown and gloves
- Careful hand hygiene and sanitizing of surfaces
- Cool, bland liquids with careful attention to hydration status because mouth becomes very sore
- In severe cases, the child or adolescent may be unable to tolerate oral liquids and may require total parenteral nutrition or IV therapy to maintain nutrition and hydration status
- IV acyclovir is required for severe cases

Caregiver Education

- Practice careful hand hygiene.
- Do not share cups or utensils between family members.
- Sanitize toys between children.
- Avoid touching sores on the mouth.
- Prescription creams may provide relief and facilitate healing in small, localized lesions. Examples are docosanol cream 10% (Abreva) and penciclovir cream 1% (Denavir).
- Administer oral acyclovir as ordered for widespread or recurrent infections.

Complementary and Alternative Therapies

- Apply cool water compresses to lips.
- Use a lip balm with sun-blocking agents to prevent additional injury to lips.
- Over-the-counter creams such as those containing tetracaine cream 1% may be helpful.
- A mouthwash with 1 teaspoon diphenhydramine or 1/2 teaspoon sodium bicarbonate in a cup of slightly warm water may be soothing. The child must be taught to swish the medication in the mouth and then spit it out.

TINEA (FUNGAL) INFECTIONS

Tinea infections are caused by a fungal infection of the skin. These types of infections can occur in multiple sites throughout the body, including the scalp, groin, and feet. Based on the location of the infection, treatment will vary. Tinea infections commonly occur in warm, moist environments or with significant close contact with pets or other individuals affected by tinea, such as locker rooms. Tinea infections often have to be treated for long periods to eradicate the infection. Nurses need to be aware of these types of infections and how to treat the different presentations of tinea.

Clinical Presentation

- Tinea infections are spread by direct contact, contact with personal items, and in some cases by pets (cats and dogs).
- Tinea corporis: fungal infection (ringworm) on the body (Fig. 21–9). These infections appear as circular lesions with raised edges and central clearing. Itching is common.
- Tinea capitis: fungal infection (ringworm) on the scalp. There are circular patches with scaling and erythema. There may be patches with hair loss or broken hair.

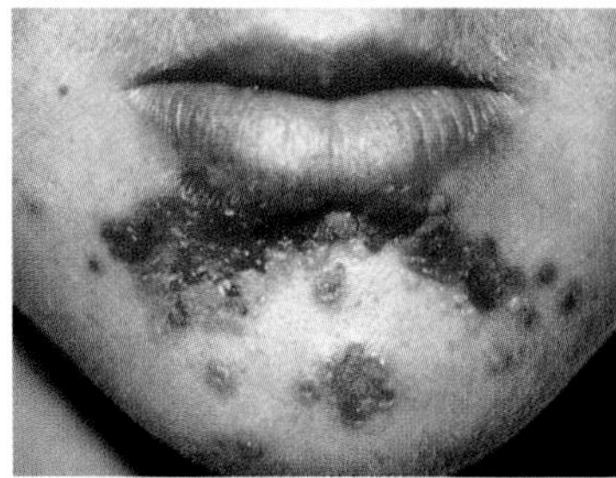

FIGURE 21–8 Child with herpes simplex (cold sore) on lips.

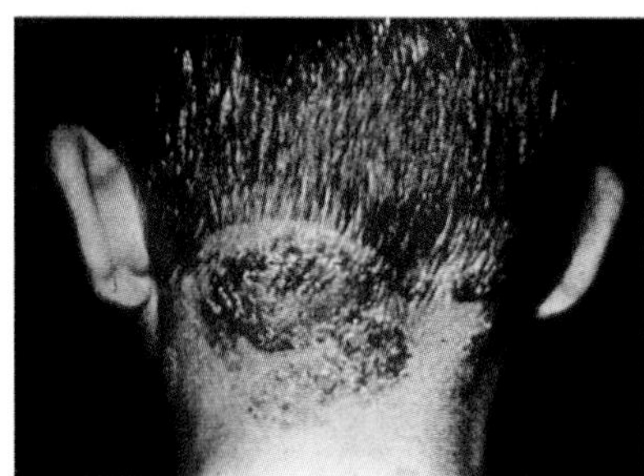

FIGURE 21–9 Child with ringworm (tinea capitis or tinea corporis).

- Tinea pedis: fungal infection of the foot (athlete's foot); more common in adolescents. Lesions may be scaly or made up of vesicles and pustules. Itching is common.
- Tinea cruris: fungal infection of the groin (jock itch); more common in adolescent males. There are scaling patches in the folds of the groin and upper thighs that are sharply demarcated. Itching can be intense.

Diagnostic Testing

- A Wood's lamp will cause some types of tinea to fluoresce and show as green. However, not all types of fungi will fluoresce under a Wood's lamp.
- The lesion can be scraped, and the tissue mixed with potassium hydroxide (KOH) before examining under a microscope. If fungi are present, branching strands (hyphae) may be seen under a microscope.

Caregiver Education

- Apply an antifungal cream such as miconazole to the lesion twice daily.
- If lesions are moist, such as in the groin area or between toes, apply wet compresses using Burrow's solution twice daily to dry the area.
- Do not share hats, combs, brushes, ribbons, scarves, clothing, or bedding.
- Cover skin lesions.
- For tinea pedis (athlete's foot), air the feet as much as possible. Sandals are recommended for airing the feet. Change socks daily and alternate shoes to give them a chance to air out.
- For tinea capitis (ringworm on the scalp), shampoo the hair twice daily for 2 weeks with shampoos such as selenium sulfide 2.5% or ketoconazole 2%. Shampoos are effective in mild cases and as adjunct therapy to oral medications. Systemic oral medications are also required.

SAFE AND EFFECTIVE NURSING CARE: Understanding Medication

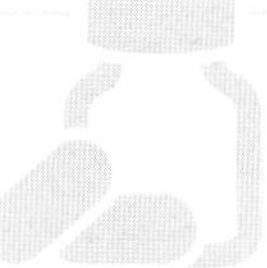

Medication for Tinea Capitis

Systemic oral medication is required for children with tinea capitis. Griseofulvin is given once or twice daily for 4 to 6 weeks or up to 8 to 12 weeks as needed. This medication must be given with high-fat foods such as ice cream or peanut butter to enhance absorption. Side effects of griseofulvin include nausea and sensitivity to the sun. Educate caregivers on the importance of using a sunscreen with an SPF of 15 or greater. Children must be reevaluated monthly, and the renal, hematological, and hepatic systems must be monitored during administration of this medication. Griseofulvin is approved in children 2 years of age and older (American Academy of Pediatrics, 2015; Zampella, Kwatra, Blanck, & Cohen, 2016).

DISORDERS RELATED TO CONTACT WITH INSECTS

Certain insects can cause infestations of the hair and skin that commonly affect children. Infections such as scabies or head lice are easily spread from one person to the next with sharing of items or direct contact, resulting in outbreaks in schools, healthcare facilities, shelters, and daycares. The reaction of the body to these types of infestations often causes distressing symptoms such as pruritus, erythema, edema, or skin breakdown. Nurses need to identify and prevent these types of infections in children and adolescents.

Pediculosis Capitis (Head Lice)

Pediculosis, commonly referred to as head lice, is an infestation of the hair by small insects called lice. Head lice are easily spread from one individual to the next through close proximity and can result in outbreaks in schools. Head lice are becoming more immune to common treatments and therefore need to be treated promptly and effectively. An important component of head lice management is education on prevention and management of the condition, which nurses are poised to provide.

Clinical Presentation

- Nits or lice eggs appear as very small white, translucent, or yellow dots that are firmly attached near the base of the hair shaft (Fig. 21–10). Nits hatch in 7 to 10 days.
- An adult louse is approximately the size and shape of a sesame seed. Lice feed on blood from the scalp and cannot live more than 48 hours away from the scalp.
- Lice may cause a tickling sensation as they move through the hair. They may also cause intense itching. Scratching the scalp may result in excoriation and bacterial infection.
- Lice move by crawling and do not fly or hop. They are usually spread by direct contact between persons, but are less commonly spread by sharing hats, combs, brushes, towels, and bedding.

Diagnostic Testing

- Examine the hair under a bright light.
- A magnifying glass and fine-toothed comb may be helpful in finding the lice.

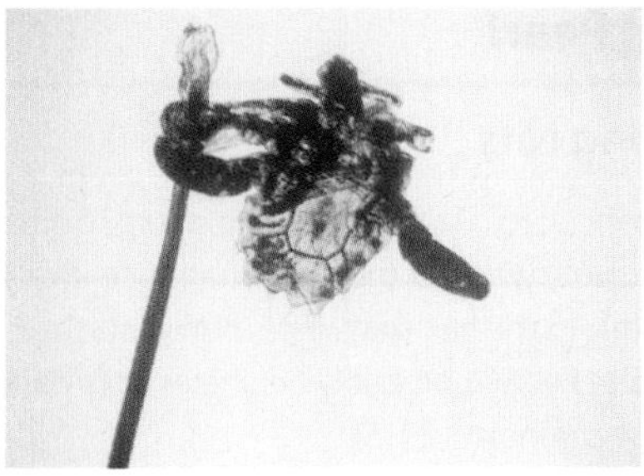

FIGURE 21–10 Nits and lice in hair.

- It is helpful to divide the hair into sections and examine one section or strand at a time.
- Nits are usually found within 1/4 inch of the base of the hair shaft.

Caregiver Education

- Apply a pediculicide shampoo to hair that has been shampooed and towel-dried. Recommended pediculicides for children include permethrin 1% (Nix) and pyrethrin (RID, Clear Lice, Pronto). Leave medication on hair for 10 minutes and then rinse off. Repeat treatment in 7 to 10 days.
- Ivermectin lotion is a prescription medication for children 6 months and older that has been found to eliminate and reduce parasite re-infestations.
- A fine-toothed comb may be used to remove nits from wet hair.
- Soak combs and brushes in hot water with one of the pediculicide shampoos for 15 minutes.
- Wash clothing and bedding in hot, soapy water and dry on hot cycle. Alternately, dry-clean items that cannot be washed.
- Vacuum the floor, mattresses, and soft/stuffed furniture.
- Toys, personal items, and other objects that cannot be laundered can be tied up in a plastic bag for more than 2 weeks.
- Examine the scalps of close contacts and family members.
- Do not spray the floor or other surfaces of the house and furniture with pesticides. These chemicals are toxic and may cause serious adverse effects.

Complementary and Alternative Therapies

- Application of mayonnaise, olive oil, or petroleum jelly has been recommended to suffocate the lice. Parents are instructed to cover the child's hair with the oil-based product, cover with a shower cap overnight, and shampoo the next morning.
- Essential oils from plants or Dimethicone have been explored to treat head lice.
- Hot air with removal of existing nits additionally has shown some promise in studies.
- These treatments have not been proven effective but are widely used (Feldmeier, 2014).

SAFE AND EFFECTIVE NURSING CARE: Clinical Pearl

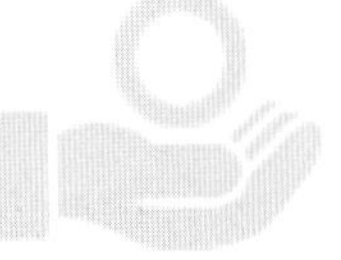

Identifying Nits

It may be difficult to distinguish nits (lice eggs) from dandruff or flaking skin. Note whether the white, translucent, or yellow spot adheres firmly to the hair shaft. If it is firmly attached, it is likely a nit. If it moves freely, it probably originates from dandruff or dry skin (Devore & Schutze, 2015).

CRITICAL COMPONENT

Contraindications for Pediculicide Shampoos

Assess for history of asthma or allergies before recommending pediculicide shampoos. Permethrin or pyrethrin is contraindicated for children with ragweed allergies. These products may cause an allergic reaction or an exacerbation of asthma.

Scabies (Mite Infestation)

Scabies is a skin infestation with a mite called *Sarcoptes scabiei*. This mite lives on human and human-exposed surfaces and causes a significantly pruritic rash. Scabies can occur anywhere on the body but commonly affects the webs of hands and feet and groin folds. In addition to the rash, burrows under the skin may be evident. Scabies often occurs in crowded living conditions resulting in outbreaks. Nurses should be aware of this infestation and how to educate families on elimination and prevention of scabies.

Clinical Presentation

- Mites burrow under the skin, leaving tracks or lines of macules, vesicles, and pustules.
- Itching is severe, especially at night.
- Children younger than 2 years are most likely to be affected on the head and neck, or on the palms and soles of the feet (Fig. 21–11). Older children are most likely to be affected on skin folds between the fingers and toes, wrists, elbows, armpits, waist line, thighs, buttocks, and abdomen (Barry, 2017).

Caregiver Education

- Wash clothing and bedding with hot water and dry on the hot cycle.
- Tie items that cannot be laundered in a plastic bag for more than 5 days.
- Apply permethrin 5% or Ivermectin cream to the entire body from the neck down. Apply at bedtime and leave for 8 to 14 hours. Bathe the child the next morning. The treatment may be repeated in 7 days.
- Over-the-counter creams to relieve itching may be applied to the skin. Examples include Sama and Prax lotion.
- Close contacts of the child also need to be treated.

SAFE AND EFFECTIVE NURSING CARE: Clinical Pearl

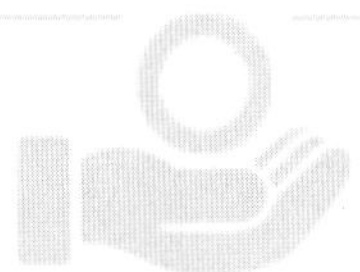

Preventing Secondary Infection

Patients with scabies can experience secondary bacterial infections from skin breakdown secondary to intense pruritus associated with scabies. All patients should be assessed for signs of infection and treated appropriately if present.

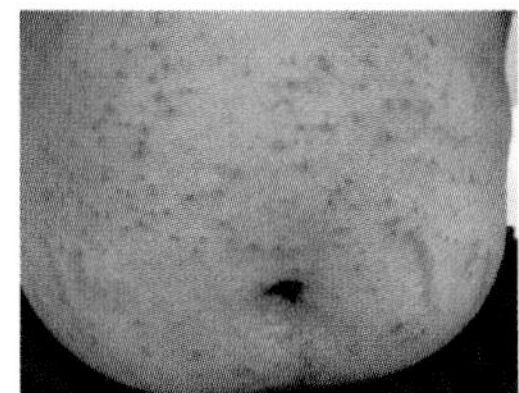

FIGURE 21–11 Child with scabies.

Insect Bites and Stings

These include bites and stings from bees, wasps, hornets, fire ants, and the brown recluse spider.

Clinical Presentation

- Local presentation of stings includes redness, swelling, and pain.
- Systemic presentation caused by an allergic reaction to the insect sting may include emesis, headache, syncope, hives, wheezing, and anaphylactic shock.
- Delayed reactions to stings may occur as long as 1 week later and include hives, fever, joint pain, and vasculitis.
- A brown recluse spider bite may range from mild to severe. In severe bites, the area becomes reddened and painful with a central vesicle or pustule that drains after 3 to 4 days, leaving an ulcer or a necrotic area. There may be systemic responses such as fever, chills, weakness, nausea, and vomiting approximately 12 hours after the bite. Systemic responses do not always occur.

Nursing Interventions

Nursing interventions focus on emergency care for anaphylaxis.

- Assess the skin at the local site and check for hives in other parts of the body.
- Assess for stridor or wheezing, indicating laryngeal edema or bronchospasm.
- Assess for hypotension and tachycardia, indicating anaphylactic shock. Assess level of consciousness.
- Administer epinephrine 0.01 mg/kg subcutaneously or IV as ordered. Repeat every 15 to 20 minutes as needed. Maximum dose is 0.5 mg.
- Give 100% oxygen via nasal cannula or mask.
- Gain IV access; start IV fluids as ordered.
- Administer albuterol nebulizer treatments as ordered for wheezing.
- Give methylprednisolone (corticosteroid) or diphenhydramine (Benadryl) IV as ordered to counteract the allergic reaction.

Caregiver Education

Caregivers should receive education on the following measures related to insect stings and bites.

Emergency Care

- If a child is known to be allergic to an insect sting, caregivers must keep an EpiPen available at all times and be able to inject it intramuscularly (IM) according to directions. Refer to the Safe and Effective Nursing Care: EpiPen Use feature for EpiPen dosages.
- Give oral antihistamine if the child is alert and able to swallow.
- Seek follow-up medical care immediately for any systemic reactions to stings or bites, including spider bites.

Home Care

- Wash the wound, apply ice to the sting or bite, and elevate the extremity. Use ice for 8 to 12 hours as needed to reduce pain and swelling.
- Do not squeeze the stinger. Use tweezers or a scraper to remove the stinger without crushing it.
- Give an antihistamine such as Benadryl orally, dosing according to child's weight and age, or apply it topically as a cream.
- If the child is allergic to insect stings, carry an EpiPen kit with the child; keep one at home and one in the car. Use a medical alert bracelet.
- Wounds that are draining or have a necrotic center must always be assessed and not assumed to be a spider bite. Many "spider bites" diagnosed by caregivers turn out to be staphylococcal infections.
- If a spider bite is confirmed, check on whether tetanus immunizations are up to date.

Complementary and Alternative Therapies

- A baking soda paste made by mixing baking soda with cold water may be soothing to a sting site.

SAFE AND EFFECTIVE NURSING CARE: Understanding Medication

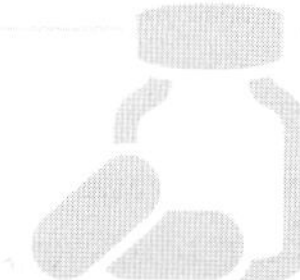

Administration of Epinephrine

Epinephrine 0.01 mg/kg may be given subcutaneously with 0.01 mL/kg of 1:1,000 solution or IV with 0.1 mL/kg of 1:10,000 solution (Czosnowski & Peterson, 2017). Always check the concentration of epinephrine when calculating the volume of medication to administer. For example, to receive a dose of 0.01 mg/kg, a 10-kg child would receive 0.1 mL of 1:1,000 solution or 1 mL of 1:10,000 solution.

Lyme Disease

Lyme disease is caused by the bite of a deer tick that transmits an infective spirochete. Signs and symptoms may appear 3 to 32 days after the tick bite.

Clinical Presentation

- Characteristic skin rash: large, circular rash with central clearing (erythema migrans) (Fig. 21–12)
- Signs and symptoms include fever, headache, aching, and satellite rash

SAFE AND EFFECTIVE NURSING CARE: Clinical Pearl

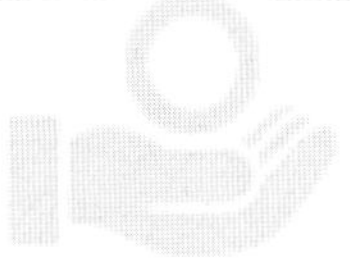

EpiPen Use

Use an EpiPen for children who weight more than 30 kg and an EpiPen Jr for children less than 30 kg. The EpiPen delivers 0.3 mg in 2 mL of 1:1,000 solution IM. The EpiPen Jr delivers 0.15 mg in 2 mL of 1:2,000 solution (Sicherer, Sampson, Eichernfield, & Rotrosen, 2017). Check the expiration date on the EpiPen carefully. Most expire in 2 years. Instructions for EpiPen auto-injector use:

- Remove pen from plastic carrying tube.
- Remove gray cap from wider end of pen. This "arms" the pen for use.
- Grasp the pen in the fist. Do not touch either end.
- The active end of the pen is narrower and black. No needle will be visible. Press the black end at a 90-degree angle into the thigh. Press the black end harder into the thigh until a click or "pop" is heard. This activates the pen and starts the injection of epinephrine.
- Count for 10 to 15 seconds while the epinephrine is being injected.
- Remove the pen at a 90-degree angle. Massage the area.
- There will be a visible needle at this time. Dispose of equipment safely. Place pen back in plastic carrying tube.
- Seek medical help.

(Sicherer et al., 2017)

- Serious clinical manifestations include arthritis, neurological symptoms, meningitis, radiculopathy, and myopericarditis (Sanchez, Vannier, Wormser, & Hu, 2016; Shapiro, 2014)

Diagnostic Testing

- Increased erythrocyte sedimentation rate
- Increased WBC

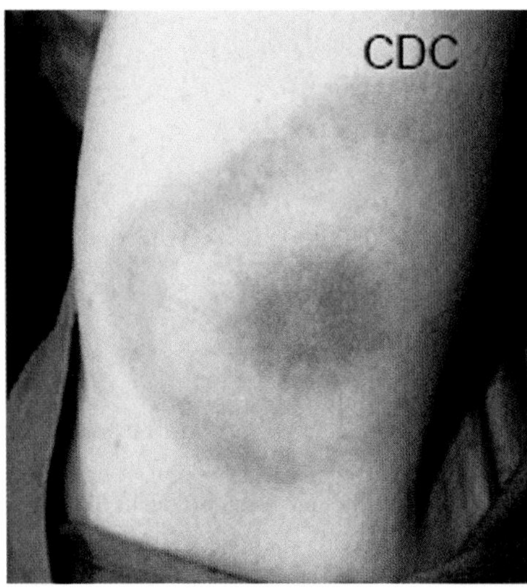

FIGURE 21–12 Lyme disease rash.

- Positive IgM cryoglobulins, rising IgG titers, positive enzyme immunoassay (enzyme-linked immunosorbent assay) or Western blot test

Caregiver Education

Parents and caregivers should receive nurse education on the following topics related to Lyme disease: prevention, home care, and complementary and alternative therapies.

Prevention

- When walking outdoors, avoid areas with tall grass or bushes. Wear light-colored clothing with long sleeves and long pants in the woods. Wear closed shoes and tuck pant legs into socks.
- Spray permethrin on clothing before walking outdoors in wooded areas.
- Use DEET to spray on skin.

Home Care

- First aid for tick removal
- Teach caregivers to be aware of signs and symptoms of Lyme disease after tick bites
- Administration of antibiotics such as amoxicillin or cefuroxime for younger children or doxycycline for children older than 8 years (Shapiro, 2014)

Complementary and Alternative Therapies

- Citronella or lavender oils may be used to prevent tick and other insect bites in children older than 2 years. The effectiveness of these oils is unknown.

CRITICAL COMPONENT

Patients With Neurological Symptoms With Lyme Disease

Facial nerve paralysis and other neurological symptoms are a potentially serious complication of Lyme disease. In patients who present with these symptoms, a lumbar puncture should be performed with evaluation of the cerebrospinal fluid for presence of Lyme disease. In the hospitalized child with Lyme disease, ceftriaxone IM or cefotaxime are effective treatments in children (Sanchez et al., 2016; Shapiro, 2014).

SAFE AND EFFECTIVE NURSING CARE: Clinical Pearl

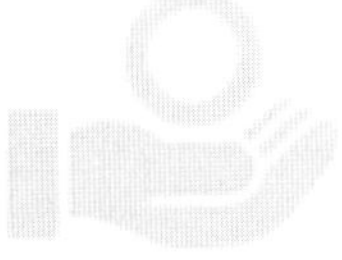

How to Remove Ticks

- Use tweezers to remove the tick directly from the skin.
- Do not squeeze or handle the tick or pull it with bare fingers because tick feces carry disease organisms.
- Use gloves or tissues if gloves are unavailable, and wash hands afterward.
- If part of the tick remains in the skin, soak the skin to soften it and then remove any tick parts in the same way that a splinter would be removed.

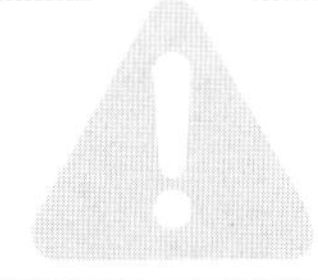

SAFE AND EFFECTIVE NURSING CARE: Promoting Safety

Parents and caregivers should be instructed on using DEET safely as an insect repellant (Alpern, Dunlop, Dolan, Stauffer, & Boulware, 2016; Karwowski et al., 2016).

- Avoid spraying DEET onto a child's skin. Apply the DEET to your hand first and then rub it on the child's skin.
- Do not apply DEET to young children's hands, because they may rub their eyes or place their hands in their mouths.
- Do not use DEET for infants younger than 2 months.
- Do not apply DEET over broken places in the skin.
- Do not spray DEET near food.
- DEET protection: 10% DEET offers protection for 2 hours, and 30% DEET offers protection for 5 hours. These concentrations may be used safely in children. Choose the strength of DEET based on the length of time the child will spend outdoors.
- Use DEET once daily. Do not use DEET products that are combined with sunscreen because frequent application may lead to toxicity.
- Wash skin to remove DEET following time outdoors, and wash clothing that may have been exposed to DEET.

DISORDERS RELATED TO INJURIES

Injury is one of the most common causes of childhood morbidity and mortality across all age groups. Nurses provide care for children with minor and significant injuries. Multiple skin wounds can result from intentional and nonintentional injuries. Wound care is a key part of caring for most injuries. Nurses need to be able to identify and manage injuries appropriately.

Lacerations

A laceration is a tear or cut in the skin, created either surgically or unintentionally through an injury. Based on the depth, size, and location of the laceration, wound management protocol varies significantly. Most lacerations require some type of wound care.

Clinical Presentation

- Assess the size and location of the laceration, determine what type of material broke the skin and whether there are foreign objects remaining in the skin, determine whether the injury took place indoors or outdoors, determine how long ago the injury occurred, and determine whether any first aid was given when the injury occurred.
- Assess for bleeding.
- Assess the neurovascular status of any extremity involved. Determine whether there is limitation in movement. Check color, warmth, capillary refill, and pulses of the extremities involved (Navanandan, Renna-Rodriguez, & DiStefano, 2017).

Nursing Interventions

- Use sterile gauze to apply pressure to the wound if bleeding is present.
- When bleeding is under control, irrigate the wound with normal saline and a syringe.
- Check whether the child's tetanus immunizations are up to date.
- Assist with application of wound closure adhesive strips or suturing as required.
- Apply sterile dressing and antibiotic ointment such as bacitracin or Polysporin as ordered over suture site.
- Cyanoacrylate tissue adhesives may be used to close lacerations that are clean and straight. The adhesive seals the edges of the laceration and forms its own dressing.
- Wounds with a high risk for infection are not sutured initially or may be left open to heal via secondary intention. These include wounds contaminated with dirt or saliva from a bite, wounds that demonstrate a large amount of tissue damage, or wounds that were not sutured within 24 hours of injury.

Caregiver Education

- Give instructions for application of bacitracin or Polysporin ointments and sterile dressings as needed over suture sites. Dressings may range from an adhesive bandage to gauze and tape. For sutured lacerations, keep sterile dressings over the wound for 24 to 48 hours. Keep the wound clean and dry.
- Wound closure adhesive strips are left in place until they fall off naturally or after 7 to 10 days. Keep the area clean and dry.
- If a tissue adhesive is used, an additional dressing is optional. Do not apply ointments over the adhesive. Gentle bathing is permissible, but swimming and scrubbing and pulling at the site are contraindicated.
- Perform hand hygiene carefully before and after caring for wounds.
- Teach caregivers signs of infection in the wound: erythema, tenderness, swelling, drainage, fever. Seek medical help if any of these signs are present.
- Give instructions on when to return for suture removal if applicable. The time needed for healing before sutures are removed depends on the site of the wound, but average length of time varies from 7 to 14 days.
- Pain management is essential during suturing.

Bites (Animal, Human)

Bite wounds from animals or humans may involve punctures, lacerations, and crushed tissue. Cat bites are more likely to inflict puncture wounds that are difficult to clean, and large dogs or other large mammals are more likely to crush tissue or tear the skin.

Clinical Presentation

- Signs of infection may follow the bite incident by a few hours. These include redness, pain, swelling, and subsequent purulent drainage.
- Bites on the hands and feet are most likely to develop infections. Infections are especially severe if the bite involves tendons or joints.

SAFE AND EFFECTIVE NURSING CARE: Clinical Pearl

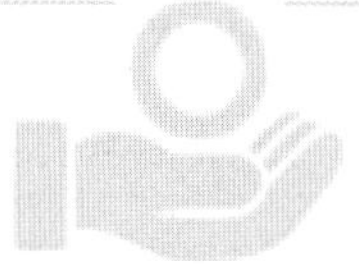

Wound Dressings for the Hospitalized Child

Tips for wound dressings for the hospitalized child include the following:

- Foam dressings come in many shapes and sizes, and may be useful in padding bony prominences or absorbing wound exudates.
- Transparent dressings are useful for securing tubes and IV catheters. They are also effective for covering incisions or dry, shallow wounds.
- Hydrogel sheet dressings are soothing and may be used for covering superficial abrasions or first- and second-degree burns.
- Hydrocolloid dressings are effective for wounds that are in the regeneration or maturation phase of healing.
- Alginate dressings are used to absorb for wounds with moderate-to-heavy drainage.
- Any dressing can contain chemicals that are bactericidal or bacteriostatic. These are referred to as antimicrobial dressings and are used to reduce bacterial load in the wound.

(Black, Cico, & Caglar, 2015; Navanandan et al., 2017; Ubbink, Brolmann, Go, & Vermeulen, 2015)

CRITICAL COMPONENT

Process of Wound Healing

Injured tissue must progress through three stages to complete healing:

- Inflammation or reaction phase: Damage to cells is brought under control, and damaged cellular fragments are removed. Bleeding is controlled and barriers are formed to seal off bacteria.
- Proliferative phase: New tissue is regenerated. The wound is filled with new connective tissue and new epithelium covers the wound.
- Maturation phase: The area is remodeled and restructured, and made stronger. This phase may take weeks or months (Gonzalez, Costa, Andrade, & Medrado, 2016).

- Cat bites are the most likely to become infected. Human bites and other animal bites also transmit bacteria and a risk for infection.
- Muscles, tendons, blood vessels, and nerves may be damaged along with skin and subcutaneous tissue.

Diagnostic Testing

- The most common organism involved in dog and cat bites is *Pasteurella multocida*. However, a variety of organisms can be cultured from bite wounds. *Staphylococcus* and various strains of *Streptococcus* may cause infections.
- Rabies may be transmitted from bites by carnivorous wild animals. The disease is occasionally transmitted by pets that have not been immunized.

Nursing Interventions

- Give immediate wound care. Wounds may be irrigated under pressure with large amounts of sterile saline.
- The wound may be left open and not sutured initially to allow drainage and reduce the chance of infection. Hand bites are not sutured because of the high risk for infection. Bites that are deep, involve puncture wounds, or are more than 8 hours old are not sutured.
- Tissue adhesive dressings are not used for closing bite wounds because of reduced drainage and increased chance of infection.
- Check the child's immunization record to determine whether tetanus immunizations are up to date.
- Dress the wound with antibiotic ointment and a sterile dressing.
- Administer antibiotics as ordered.
- Bites and animal attacks may be very frightening. Provide emotional support for the child and family.

Caregiver Education

Caregivers should be educated on the following measures related to bite injuries: home care and prevention.

Home Care

- Teach caregivers to watch for signs of cellulitis or localized infection: erythema, warmth, red streaking, edema, purulent drainage, fever, and increased pain.
- Teach hand hygiene and wound care with antibiotic ointment and gauze dressing.
- Teach importance of keeping tetanus immunizations up to date.
- Complete the course of oral antibiotics as ordered after bites.

Prevention

- Keep rabies vaccinations up to date for pets.
- Teach children to treat pets with respect and kindness.
- Do not tease animals or annoy them when they are eating or sleeping.
- Do not leave young children alone with a pet.
- Keep dogs on leashes in public.
- Do not handle stray animals, especially if they are sick.
- Prevent aggressive or defensive biting on the part of children.

Sunburns

Sunburns are a result of prolonged or intense exposure to the sun's ultraviolet (UV) rays. Sunburns can vary from mild redness and inflammation to more severe forms including blisters and peeling. Many sunburns can be prevented, and all individuals should be encouraged to wear daily sunscreen to prevent the risk for long-term sun damage and skin cancer.

CRITICAL COMPONENT

Rabies

Rabies can occur after bites from nonimmunized domestic animals, but is most likely to occur after bites from wild animals such as bats, skunks, raccoons, coyotes, foxes, and bobcats. Individuals who are bitten by these animals must receive rabies prophylaxis, and the incident must be reported to the Health Department. A domestic animal that is immunized but is suspected of having rabies is confined for 10 days. If the animal develops signs of rabies, it is killed and the brain is examined. If the examination is positive, the individual who was bitten must receive rabies prophylaxis if not previously treated. Rabies prophylaxis includes passive immunization (rabies immune globulin) that is given initially into the wound and IM. It also includes active immunization (rabies vaccine) that is given as a series of five IM injections over 28 days (Ellis & Ellis, 2014).

Clinical Presentation

- Erythema, tenderness, edema, blistering, itching
- First-degree sunburn: skin redness
- Second-degree sunburn: blistering

Nursing Interventions

- Assess skin for the presence of pediatric melanomas in children who have been exposed to the sun.

Caregiver Education

Caregivers should receive nurse education on the following sunburn-related topics: prevention and home care.

Prevention

- Infants younger than 6 months should not be exposed to direct sunlight.
- Infants older than 6 months and older children should not be exposed to direct sunlight between 10 a.m. and 4 p.m. When children do play outdoors, indirect sunlight is recommended.
- Wearing broad-brimmed hats that protect the face should effectively prevent sunburn.
- Shirts should be worn outdoors.
- Clothing items that contain SPF protection against UV rays are available.
- Apply sunscreen SPF 30 or higher 30 minutes before a child is exposed to the sun and every hour while outdoors. Apply the sunscreen all over the skin.
- Use water-resistant sunscreens for children who are swimming or playing in water.
- Remember that sunlight reflecting off water or snow can damage the skin.
- Children with light complexions sunburn more easily, but children with darker complexions are also vulnerable to sunburn.

Home Care

- Cool baths and cool compresses
- Additional fluids to prevent dehydration
- Skin moisturizers
- Local anesthetic sprays and creams
- Acetaminophen or ibuprofen as needed for pain

CRITICAL COMPONENT

Damaging Ultraviolet Rays

Three types of UV rays are damaging to the skin. UVA rays penetrate the deepest and cause premature aging of the skin. UVB rays have a shorter wavelength but are damaging to outer layers of the skin, causing sunburn and skin cancer. UVC rays are potent, but are filtered by the ozone layer. SPF numbers refer to the protection that sunscreen has against UVB rays. Advise parents to use a sunscreen with an SPF of 30 or greater.

Minor and Major Burns

Minor and major burns can occur as a result of exposure to a heat source or flame. Many burns are preventable, and families must be educated about these preventive measures at well-child visits. Patients with minor burns, such as first-degree or small second-degree burns, can often be managed with outpatient treatment. More significant burns involving larger areas or more extensive skin damage can be life-threatening and require specialized burn care in an intensive care unit or burn unit. Burns often result in significant emotional and physical disability for families. Nurses must understand how to assist families in managing and recovering from these types of injuries.

Clinical Presentation

- Superficial epidermis: red, painful, no blistering
- Superficial partial-thickness epidermis: red, painful, blisters, moist and weeping, blanches with pressure
- Deep partial-thickness epidermis: dry and white, red with blisters if the burn was caused by scalding, less pain experienced than with superficial partial thickness, can feel pressure applied
- Full-thickness burn to epidermis and dermis: no blanching, no pain; white or charred appearance with contact burns
- Electrical burns are deep and may cause more damage internally than is apparent on the skin surface; electrical burns may also trigger cardiac dysrhythmias up to 72 hours after the burn (Fabia, 2016)

Diagnostic Testing

- Arterial blood gases for severe burns or respiratory involvement
- Carboxyhemoglobin levels as indicated for carbon monoxide poisoning if child was in a confined space
- Electrocardiogram and cardiac monitoring as indicated for severe burns or electrical burns
- Wound cultures as needed
- Laboratory assessment may include CBC, basic metabolic panel, phosphorus, magnesium, albumin, serum myoglobin, zinc, prothrombin time, and partial thromboplastin time

Nursing Interventions

Required nursing interventions for burns may include the following measures: emergency care, acute hospital care, chronic hospital care, and chronic home care.

Emergency Care

- Give 100% oxygen if the individual has been burned severely or if the fire was in a confined space. Use a pulse oximeter to monitor oxygen saturation levels. Assist with endotracheal intubation as needed.
- Assess for signs of airway edema or pulmonary insufficiency.
- Place on a cardiac monitor if burns are severe or if the burn is electrical in origin.
- Obtain IV access for fluid replacement. Central venous access is required if burns are severe.
- Remove clothing that is burned, hot in temperature, or contaminated with chemicals. If necessary, cut the clothing away.
- Apply cool, sterile, normal saline compresses to cool and protect the skin.
- Monitor temperature; watch for hypothermia.
- Administer tetanus immunization if needed.
- Provide pain medication as needed.
- Provide emotional support to the child and family.
- Avoid the use of ice on burned skin because it will cause further burns from freezing.

Acute Hospital Care

- Assess for signs of respiratory distress: dyspnea, wheezing, stridor, tachypnea, decreased breath sounds, and retractions.
- Use a pulse oximeter to monitor oxygen saturation levels.
- Administer oxygen or assist with endotracheal intubation as needed.
- Keep head of bed elevated.
- Assess for changes in behavior or level of consciousness.
- Assess for signs of infection: fever; increased redness, swelling, pain; purulent drainage or foul odor.
- Maintain IV access.
- Monitor intake and output. Place Foley catheter to monitor hourly output with severe burns.
- Neurovascular checks every 1 to 4 hours as ordered: color, warmth, capillary refill of extremities, pulse or Doppler signals, ability to move fingers and toes, and sensation. Report decreased movement, decreased Doppler signals, and increased pain in any extremity.
- Assess color of urine, monitoring for presence of myoglobinuria from damaged muscle.
- Assess pain levels frequently, and administer pain medication as ordered before dressing changes and as needed.
- Use sterile technique to assist with dressing changes and application of topical creams or ointments.
- Partial- and full-thickness burns are covered with sterile, nonadherent dressings. Tubular net dressings may be used to anchor dressings onto extremities without tape.
- Insert feeding tube and administer tube feedings as ordered if the child cannot be fed orally or cannot maintain increased caloric requirement because of change in metabolic state.
- Maintain temperature between 37°F and 38.5°F. It is very important to maintain a normal body temperature. Monitor for hypothermia during dressing changes.

Chronic Hospital Care

- Obtain referrals as needed for the child and family: pastoral care according to cultural and spiritual beliefs, child life specialist, occupational therapy, physical therapy, social work, and nutrition.
- Assist with manual debridement of necrotic tissue or whirlpool debridement as indicated. Escharotomy may be required to remove burned areas (eschar).
- Skin grafting is required for children with full-thickness burns.
- Carry out dressing changes and wound care as ordered. Monitor for hypertrophic scarring. Silicone gel sheeting or treatment with allograft skin may reduce hypertrophic scars (Vloemans, Hermans, Van Der Wal, Liebregts, & Middelkoop, 2014).
- Monitor for scar contractures. These contractures may be treated with silicone inserts, pressure, splinting, or surgery as needed.

Chronic Home Care

- Dressing changes are no longer required after new tissue grows over the wound (epithelialization).
- Continue to monitor for hypertrophic scarring and scar contractures (Fig. 21–13).
- Counseling therapy may be needed for the child and family to prevent post-traumatic stress disorder (PTSD) or to help the child and family cope with anxiety, guilt, and depression.

Caregiver Education

Parents and caregivers should receive nurse education on the following topics related to burns: emergency care, acute hospital care, chronic hospital care, and complementary and alternative therapies.

Emergency Care

- First-aid measures for minor burns

Evidence-Based Practice: Dressings for Burn Wound Healing

Vloemans, A., Hermans, M., Van Der Wal, M., Liebregts, J., & Middelkoop, E. (2014). Optimal treatment of partial thickness burns in children: A systematic review. *Burns, 40,* 177–190. doi: 10.1016/j.burns.2013.09.016

Vloemans et al. (2014) examined and analyzed 51 articles to identify optimal wound management in partial- and full-thickness burns. The analysis found that cream under gauze dressings and membranous dressings such as biological dressings or amnion with or without growth factors infused create a moist environment that promotes favorable wound healing. In addition, dressings that contain silver appear to reduce pain, shorten epithelization time, and reduce length of stay, but these are not as extensively studied in pediatrics. The authors note that most studies used tulle gauze dressings with creams such as petroleum jelly and bacitracin as a standard of care even though these measures performed worse in trials when compared to biological dressings.

Nurses should identify and use dressings that promote wound healing, reduce pain, and reduce length of stay for burned children.

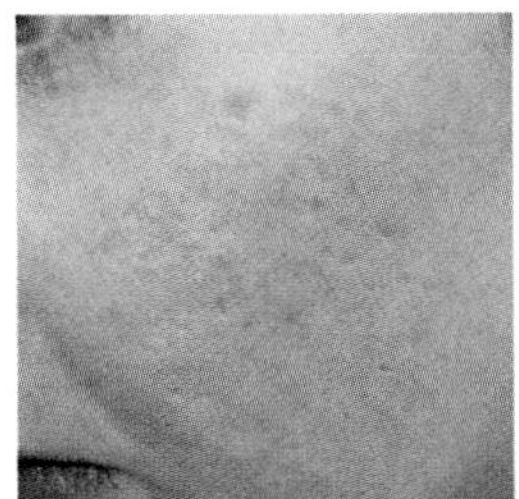

FIGURE 21–13 Child with hypertrophic scarring.

Hospital Care

- Teach the family infection-control measures: hand hygiene, no stuffed toys, no live plants or flowers, and visitor guidelines to prevent exposure to infection.
- Teach the family the plan for therapeutic management. Listen to concerns and answer questions. Include education on dressing changes and debridement, skin grafts, and any surgery required.
- Teach the family the plan for pain management and how often pain medication may be given.

Chronic Home Care

- Teach the family about complications such as infection, scar contractures, hypertrophic scarring, and PTSD.
- Refer to home-based occupational or physical therapy as needed.
- Refer to counseling or therapy as needed.
- Teach family to plan and provide a nutritious, high-protein diet for the child.
- Care for the healing skin: Use moisturizing creams such as cocoa butter, Eucerin, Nivea, Neutrogena, or Vaseline Intensive Care lotion.
- Management of itching while the skin is healing includes use of antihistamines, loose cotton clothing, and baking soda baths.
- Use sunscreen greater than SPF 30 to prevent additional damage to the skin and hyperpigmentation of the healing skin.
- Teach about prevention of burn injuries in the future.

Complementary and Alternative Therapies

- Aloe vera, honey, sugar paste, and papaya are effective topical treatments for superficial and partial-thickness burns when other modalities are not readily available or as adjunct therapy. Use commercial aloe vera products, not live plants.
- Products such as Burnaid that contain tea tree oil may be used as first aid for burns (Bitter & Erickson, 2016).

CRITICAL COMPONENT

Assessing Degree of Burn

- "Rule of nines" estimates body surface area (BSA) burned: head = 9%, anterior trunk = 18%, posterior trunk = 18%, each upper extremity = 9%, each lower extremity = 18%, genitalia = 1% (Fig. 21–14)
- Additional guidelines for assessing burns:
  - First- and second-degree burns covering less than 10% of body are considered minor burns.
  - Burns involving the face, eyes, ears, hands, feet, and genitalia are considered major burns.
  - Burns involving more than 30% of the body are considered major burns (Chemical Hazards Emergency Medical Management, 2017).

SAFE AND EFFECTIVE NURSING CARE: Clinical Pearl

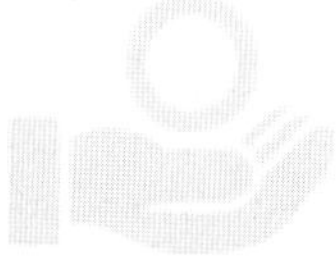

Hospitalization for Burns

Children will require hospitalization if more than 10% total BSA is burned, for full-thickness burns larger than 2% of total BSA, if the burn was electrical or chemical in origin, if there is evidence of smoke inhalation or carbon monoxide poisoning, if there is evidence of abuse or an unsafe environment, or if there are burns to the face, hands, feet, perineum, or joints (Fabia, 2016).

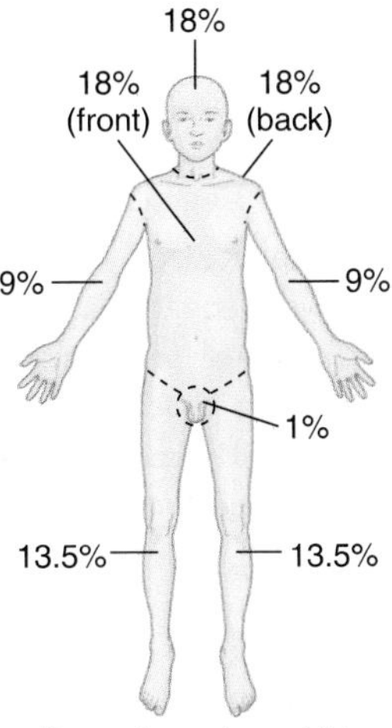

FIGURE 21–14 The rule of nines.

Evidence-Based Practice: Burn Injuries and Post-traumatic Stress

Stoddard, F., Sorrentino, E., Drake, J., Murphy, J., Kim, A., Romo, S., . . . Sheridan, R. (2017). Posttraumatic stress disorder diagnosis in young children with burns. *Journal of Burn Care & Research, 38*(1), e343–e351. doi: 10.1097/BCR.0000000000000386

Hiller, R., Meiser-Stedman, R., Fearon, P., Lobo, S., McKinnon, A., Fraser, A., & Halligan, S. (2016). Research review: Changes in prevalence and symptom severity of child post-traumatic stress disorder in the year following trauma: A meta-analytic study. *Journal of Child Psychology and Psychiatry, 57*(8), 884–898. doi: 10.1111/jcpp.12566

Wurzer, P., Forbes, A., Hundeshagen, G., Andersen, C., Epperson, K., Meyer, W., . . . Finnerty, C. (2017). Two-year follow-up of outcomes related to scarring and distress in children with severe burns. *Journal of Disability and Rehabilitation, 39*(16), 1639–1643. doi: 10.1080/09638288.2016.1209579

Children and families who have suffered from burn injuries may experience anxiety, guilt, depression, and PTSD. PTSD in children appears to be at worst immediately after the injury, with gradual decrease over the first year (Hiller et al., 2016). Improved pain management and support of the family and child decreases symptoms and likelihood of long-term PTSD. However, patients still often have psychological stress and body image disturbances 2 years after burn injury (Wurzer et al., 2017). It is important for nurses to offer emotional support to children and their families after burn injuries and to refer both children and families to therapy or to support groups as part of their discharge planning.

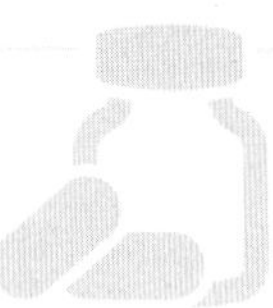

SAFE AND EFFECTIVE NURSING CARE: Understanding Medication

Medications for Treatment of Burns

Bacitracin ointment is effective in the topical treatment of burns. Silver sulfadiazine (Silvadene) may still be used for topical treatment of burns but must never be used in pregnant women, infants younger than 2 months, or children who are allergic to sulfonamides. Bismuth-impregnated petroleum gauze and Biobrane dressings are effective for children with superficial or partial-thickness burns. Other novel approaches supported in the literature are biological membranes, keratinocyte-fibrin sealant sprays, cell suspensions, and substances that contain growth factors (Fabia, 2016; Jeschke & Herndon, 2014).

CRITICAL COMPONENT

Pain Management

Pain management is required when children need debridement and dressing changes with burn injuries. Superficial and partial-thickness burns are very painful. Opiates are effective analgesics for severe or extensive injuries. As healing takes place and the pain becomes less severe, acetaminophen or ibuprofen may offer adequate analgesia. Distraction techniques such as videos, therapeutic play, and virtual reality imaging may also help the child or adolescent to cope with the pain. Parental (family) presence and soothing techniques are important components of pain management in children (Baartmans et al., 2016; De Jong et al., 2014).

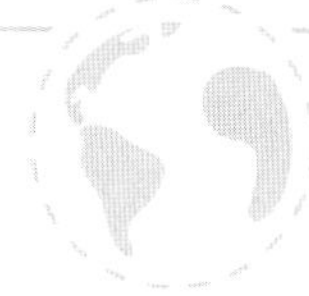

SAFE AND EFFECTIVE NURSING CARE: Cultural Competence

Culture and Risk for Burns

The World Health Organization (2017) reports that approximately 300,000 people die every year from fires, and that risk for burn injuries is higher in low- and middle-income countries. Using open fires for cooking and heating, cooking with pots on ground level, wearing loose-fitting clothing while cooking, and using kerosene appliances account for many burn injuries. Flammable materials used for buildings in developing countries and substandard wiring also lead to fires. The incidence of burns in developed countries has been decreased through smoke detectors, regulation of temperature settings in hot water heaters, and flame-retardant materials in children's clothing. Individuals in low-income countries may not have access to these burn-prevention strategies.

CRITICAL COMPONENT

First Aid for Burns

- Do not use butter, oils, or ice on the burn. These may cause additional injury.
- Perform hand hygiene before caring for burns.
- Superficial burns: Soak the burn in cool water. Apply antibiotic ointment or aloe vera cream.
- Partial-thickness burns with blistering: Soak the burn in cool water. Do not break blisters. Apply antibiotic ointment and non-stick dressing. Change the dressing daily.
- Watch for signs of infection: Signs include increased redness, swelling, pain, or drainage. Seek medical help if there are signs of infection.
- Make sure tetanus immunization is up to date.
- Chemical burns: Wash with large amounts of water. Consult physician or poison control center.
- Electrical burns: Seek medical help. The injury may be worse under the surface of the skin.

SAFE AND EFFECTIVE NURSING CARE: Promoting Safety

Intentional Burn Injury

Some burn injuries in children are intentional. Consider whether the history or the story given is compatible with the severity or pattern of the injury. Also consider whether the injury is compatible with the child's age and development. Refer to child protection services if there is a concern.

CRITICAL COMPONENT

Airway Obstruction and Respiratory Distress With Burn Injury

Be aware of the possibility of airway obstruction if the child was exposed to smoke or to fire within a confined space, or if the child inhaled toxic chemicals. Airway obstruction may be immediate or may progress over 24 to 48 hours. If there is a burn on the face or neck, singed hair on the face, or the presence of carbon particles in the nose or mouth, the individual is at high risk for airway obstruction. Watch for coughing, wheezing, and dyspnea.

If the burn was severe or occurred in a confined space, assume that there may be carbon monoxide poisoning. These burn victims must always be given 100% humidified oxygen (Jeschke & Herndon, 2014).

SAFE AND EFFECTIVE NURSING CARE: Promoting Safety

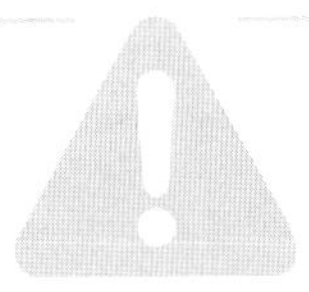

Burn Prevention

Nurses must educate parents on burn prevention strategies.

- Be aware that burns may be chemical, electrical, or thermal.
- Install smoke detectors in homes and check expiration dates on batteries.
- Keep a fire extinguisher in the home.
- Young children and infants are vulnerable to burns from scalding, direct contact with hot objects, and sunburn (Stewart et al., 2016).
- Do not hold infants when cooking or heating bottles.
- Keep curling irons and other hot objects out of infant reach.
- Be aware of infant seat buckles that become hot in the sun.
- Buy fire-retardant clothing for children.
- Cover electrical outlets.
- Keep matches and chemicals locked up.
- Keep pot handles turned inward. Supervise children around burners, hot plates, grills, and griddles. Keep hot objects pushed back on countertops.
- Protect children from stoves and heaters; keep guardrails in front of fireplaces.
- Check bathwater temperature before bathing children. Keep the hot water heater thermostat at 120 degrees.
- Educate children on fire safety and what to do in the event of a fire.
- Educate school-age children on playing safely with fireworks, cooking indoors and outdoors, and playing outdoors where electrical lines are present.
- Prevent sunburn. Refer to earlier Sunburns section.

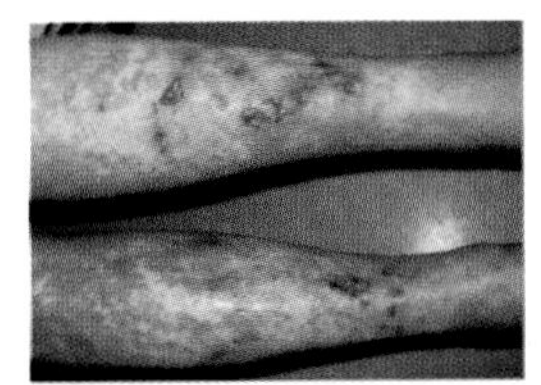

FIGURE 21–15 Child after skin grafting (graft versus host).

CRITICAL COMPONENT

Skin Grafts

When skin grafting is required for burn treatment:

- Burned skin is removed by excision or debridement before skin grafting takes place.
- Autografts: The child's or adolescent's own skin is used for grafting onto the burned area (Fig. 21–15).
- The donor skin may be split partial thickness or full thickness. A power dermatome is used to shave off the skin that will be used for the graft.
- If the area to be grafted is large, the donor skin will be made into a mesh to cover a larger area.
- Allograft: Skin from organ donors is kept preserved or frozen in a skin bank. This skin can be used as a temporary graft only because the body will reject it. It is useful to prevent infection or fluid loss and to allow time for autografting to take place.
- Cultured epithelial autograft: Cells from the patient are used to grow thin sheets of tissue that may be grafted.
- Synthetic products such as the Integra dermal regeneration template may be used to cover the burn temporarily (Fabia, 2016).

Case Study

Impaired Skin Integrity

Meticulous skin care is critical when caring for infants and children in the hospital. These children are at high risk for impaired skin integrity. The nurse is caring for a 1-year-old infant who is confined to the crib. She is not able to take oral feedings, and is receiving IV fluids and IV antibiotics. She has a tracheostomy with oxygen tubing overlying her chest and left shoulder. Additionally, she has a pulse oximeter on her right foot that is covered with tape and attached to her right big toe with a sock covering it.

1. What are risk factors for impaired skin integrity for this infant?
2. How can the nurse prevent skin breakdown in hospitalized children?
3. In areas where skin is not intact, how can healing be promoted?
4. What are potential lesions that may develop?
5. What is appropriate treatment of these lesions?

REFERENCES

Alpern, J. D., Dunlop, S. J, Dolan, B. J., Stauffer, W. M., & Boulware, D. R. (2016). Personal protection measures against mosquitoes, ticks, and other arthropods. *Medical Clinics of North America, 100,* 303–316. doi: 10.1016/j.mcna.2015.08.019

American Academy of Pediatrics. (2015). Tinea capitis. In Kimberlin, D. W., Bardy, M. T., Jackson, M. A., & Long, S. S. (Eds.), *Red Book: 2015 Report of the Committee of Infectious Diseases* (30th ed., pp. 778–781). Elk Grove Village, IL: American Academy of Pediatrics.

Arcangelo, V. P. (2017). Contact dermatitis. In V. P. Arcangelo, A. M. Peterson, J. A. Reinhold, & V. Wilbur (Eds.), *Pharmacotherapeutics for advanced practice: A practical approach (*93-109). Philadelphia: Wolters Kluwer.

Baartmans, M., de Jong, A., van Baar, M., Beerthuizen, G., van Loey, N., Tibboel, D., & Neuwenhuis, M. (2016). Early management in children with burns: Cooling, wound care and pain management. *Burns, 42,* 777–782. doi: 10.1016/j.burns.2016.03.003

Barry, M. (2017). Scabies clinical presentation. *Medscape*. Retrieved from http://emedicine.medscape.com/article/1109204-clinical

Berlowitz, D. (2017). Clinical staging and management of pressure-induced skin and soft tissue injury. *UpToDate,* 1–11. Retrieved from www.uptodate.com/contents/clinical-staging-and-management-pressure-induced-skin-and-soft-tissue-injury

Bitter, C., & Erickson, T. (2016). Management of burn injuries in the wilderness: Lessons from low-resource settings. *Wilderness & Environmental Medicine, 27*(4), 519–525. doi: 10.1016/j.wem.2016.09.001

Black, K., Cico, S., & Caglar, D. (2015). Wound management. *Pediatrics in Review, 36*(5), 207–216. doi: 10.1542/pir.36-5-207

Centers for Disease Control and Prevention. (2014). *Latex allergy: A prevention guide*. Retrieved from https://www.cdc.gov/niosh/docs/98-113/

Chemical Hazards Emergency Medical Management. (2017). Burn triage and treatment-thermal injuries. Retrieve from http://chemm.nlm.nih.gov/burns.htm

Chiocca, E.M. (2015). *Advanced pediatric assessment.* New York: Springer Publishing Company.

Clark, G., Pope, S., & Jaboori, K. (2015). Diagnosis and treatment of seborrheic dermatitis. *American Academy of Family Physicians, 81*(3), 185–190. Retrieved from https://pdfs.semanticscholar.org/87c1/cc0f97f729dde45c98d3d8338fc1e51d6ea7.pdf

Curley, M. A., Razmus, I. S., Robrets, K. E., & Wypij, D. (2003). Predicting pressure ulcer risk in pediatric patients: The Braden Q scale. *Nursing Research, 52*(1), 22–33.

Czosnowski, L., & Peterson, A. (2017). Allergies and allergic reaction. In V. P. Arcangelo, A. M. Peterson, J. A. Reinhold, & V. Wilbur (Eds.), *Pharmacotherapeutics for advanced practice: A practical approach* (pp. 827–842). Philadelphia: Wolters Kluwer.

De Jong, A., Bremer, M., Van Komen, R., Vanbrabant, L., Schuurmans, M., Middelkoop, E., & Va Loey, N. (2014). *Burns, 40,* 38–47. doi: 10.1016/j.burns.2013.09.017

Devore, C.D., & Schutze, G. E. (2015). Head lice. *Pediatrics, 135*(5), e1355–e1365. doi: 10.1542/peds.2015-0746

Du Toit, G., Roberts, G., Sayre, P. H., Bahnson, H. T., Radulovic, S., Santos, A. F., … LEAP Study Team. (2015). Randomized trial of peanut consumption in infants at risk for peanut allergy. *New England Journal of Medicine, 372*(9), 803–813. doi: 10.1056/NEJMoa1414850

Eichenfield, L. F., Bogunewicz, M., Simpson, E. L., Russell, J. J., Block, J. K., Feldman, S. R., & … Paller, A. S. (2015). Translating atopic dermatitis management guidelines into practice for primary care providers. *Pediatrics, 136*(3), 554–565. doi: 10.1542/peds.2014-3678

Ellis, R., & Ellis, C. (2014). Dog and cat bites. *American Academy of Family Physicians, 90*(4), 239–243. Retrieved from http://www.aafp.org/afp/2014/0815/p239.html

Fabia, R. (2016). Surgical treatment of burns in children. *Medscape.* Retrieved from http://reference.medscape.com/article/934173-overview

Feldmeier, H. (2014). Treatment of pediculosis capitis: A critical appraisal of the current literature. *American Journal of Clinical Dermatology, 15,* 401–412. doi: 10.1007/s40257-014-0094-4

Fleisher, D., Sicherer, S., Greenhawt, M., Campbell, D., Chan, E., Muraro, A., … Rosenwasser, L. (2015). Consensus communication on early peanut introduction and the prevention of peanut allergy in high-risk infants. *Pediatrics, 136*(3), 600–604. doi: 10.1542/peds.2015-2394

Gehris, R. P. (2018). Dermatology. In B. J. Zitelli, S. C. McIntire, & A. J. Nowalk (Eds.), *Atlas of pediatric physical diagnosis* (7th ed., pp. 275–340). Philadelphia, PA: Elsevier.

Gonzalez, A., Cost, T., Andrade, Z., & Medrado, A. (2016). Wound healing: A literature review. *Anais Brasileiros DeDermatologia,* 9(15), 614–620. doi: 10.159/abd1806-4841.20164741

Hartman-Adams, H., Banvard, C., & Juckett, G. (2014). Impetigo: Diagnosis and treatment. *American Academy of Family Physicians, 90*(4), 229–235. Retrieved from http://www.aafp.org/afp/2014/0815/p229.html

Hiller, R., Meiser-Stedman, R., Fearon, P., Lobo, S., McKinnon, A., Fraser, A., & Halligan, S. (2016). Research review: Changes in prevalence and symptom severity of child post-traumatic stress disorder in the year following trauma: A meta-analytic study. *Journal of Child Psychology and Psychiatry, 57*(8), 884–898. doi: 10.1111/jcpp.12566

Jeschke, M., & Herndon, D. (2014). Burns in children: Standard and new treatments. *Lancet, 383,* 1168–1178. doi: 10.1016/SO140-6736 (13)61093-4

Karwowski, M., Nelson, J., Stables, J., Feisher, M., Fleming-Dutra, K., Villaueva, J., … Ramussen, S. (2016). Zika virus disease: A CDC update for pediatric health care providers. *Pediatrics, 137*(5), 1–12. doi: 10.1542/peds.2016-0621

Kiss, E., & Heiler, M. (2014). Pediatric skin integrity practice guideline for institutional use: A quality improvement project. *Journal of Pediatric Nursing, 29,* 362–367. doi: 10.1016/j.pedn.2014.01.012

Klunk, C., Domingues, E., & Wiss, K. (2014). An update on diaper dermatitis. *Clinics in Dermatology, 32,* 477–487. doi: 10.1016/j.clindermatol.2014.02.003

Manning, M., Gauvreau, K., & Curley, M. (2015). Factors associated with occipital pressure ulcers in hospitalized infants and children. *American Journal of Critical Care, 24*(4), 342–348. doi: 10.4037/ajcc2015349

National Pressure Ulcer Advisory Panel. (2017). *NPUAP pressure injury stages.* Retrieved from http://www.npuap.org/resources/educational-and-clinical-resources/npuap-pressure-injury-stages/

Navanandan, N., Renna-Rodriguez, M., & DiStefano, M. (2017). Pearls in pediatric wound management. *Clinical Pediatric Emergency Medicine, 18*(1), 53–61. doi: 10.16/j.cpem.2017.01.006

Otsuka, A., Nomura, T., Reknimtr, P., Seidel, J., Honda, T., & Kabashima, K. (2017). The interplay between genetic and environmental factors in the pathogenesis of atopic dermatitis. *Immunological Reviews, 278*(1), 246–262. doi: 10.1111/imr.12545

Pollack, L., Van Santen, K., Weiner, L., Dudeck, M., Edwards, J., & Srinivasan, A. (2016). Antibiotic stewardship programs in U.S. acute care hospitals: Findings from the 2014 national healthcare safety network annual hospital survey. *Clinical Infectious Disease, 63*(4), 443–449. doi: 10.1093/cid/ciw323

Rodriguez, M. (2016). Appropriate treatment of pediatric pressure ulcers among the special needs population in the outpatient clinic: An introduction. *Today's Wound Clinic, 10*(5), 1–4. Retrieved from http://www.todayswoundclinic.com/articles/appropriate-treatment-pediatric-pressure-ulcers-among-special-needs-population-outpatient

Saeki, H., Nakahara, T., Tanaka, A., Kabashima, K., Sugaya, M., Murota, H., … Katoh, N. (2016). Clinical practice guidelines for the management of atopic dermatitis 2016. *Journal of Dermatology, 43*(10), 1117–1145. doi: 10.1111/1346-8138.13392

Salge, T., Vera, A., Antons, D., & Cimiotti, J. (2016). Fighting MRSA infections in hospital care: How organizational factors matter. *Health Services Review,* 53(3), 959–983. doi: 10.1111/1475-6773.12521

Sanchez, E., Vannier, E., Wormser, G., & Hu, L. (2016). Diagnosis, treatment, and prevention of lyme disease, human granulocytic anaplasmosis, and babesiosis. *Journal of American Medical Association, 315*(16), 1767–1777. doi: 10.1001/jama.2016.2884

Schluer, A., Schols, J., & Halfens, R. (2014). Risk and associated factors of pressure ulcers in hospitalized children over 1 year of age. *Journal for Specialists in Pediatric Nursing, 19*(1), 80–89. doi: 10.1111/jspn.12055

Shapiro, E. (2014). Borrelia burgdorferi (Lyme disease). *Pediatrics in Review, 35,* 500–509. doi: 10.1542/pir.35-12-500

Sicherer, S., Sampson, H., Eichenfield, L., & Rotrosen, D. (2017). The benefits of new guidelines to prevent peanut allergy. *Pediatrics, 139*(6), 1–9. doi: 10.1542/peds.2016-4293

Stewart, J., Benford, P., Wynn, P., Watson, M., Coupland, C., Deave, T., ... Kendirck, D. (2016). Modifiable risk factors for scald injury in children under 5 years of age: A multi-centre case-control study. *Burns, 42*(8), 1831–1843. doi: 10.1016/j.burns.2016.06.027

Stoddard, F., Sorrentino, E., Drake, J., Murphy, J., Kim, A., Romo, S., ... Sheridan, R. (2017). Posttraumatic stress disorder diagnosis in young children with burns. *Journal of Burn Care & Research, 38*(1), e343–e351. doi: 10.1097/BCR.0000000000000386

Tume, L., Siner, S., Scott, E., & Lane, S. (2014). The prognostic ability of early Braden Q scores in critically ill children. *Nursing in Critical Care, 19*(2), 98–103. doi: 10.1111/nicc.12035

Ubbink, D. T., Brolmann, F., Go, P., & Vermeulen, H. (2015). Evidence-based care of acute wounds: A perspective. *Advanced Wound Care, 4*(5), 286–294. doi: 10.1089/wound.2014.0592

Vloemans, A., Hermans, M., Van Der Wal, M., Liebregts, J., & Middelkoop, E. (2014). Optimal treatment of partial thickness burns in children: A systematic review. *Burns, 40*, 177–190. doi: 10.1016/j.burns.2013.09.016

World Health Organization. (2017). *WHO launces new document on burn prevention and care.* Retrieved from http://www.who.int/violence_injury_prevention/media/news/13_03_2008/cn/

Wurzer, P., Forbes, A., Hundeshagen, G., Andersen, C., Epperson, K., Meyer, W., ... Finnerty, C. (2017). Two-year follow-up of outcomes related to scarring and distress in children with severe burns. *Journal of Disability and Rehabilitation, 39*(16), 1639–1643. doi: 10.1080/09638288.2016.1209579

Zaenglein, A. L., Pathy, A. L., Schlosser, B. J., Alikhan, A., Baldwin, H. E., Berson, D. S., ... Bhushan, R. (2016). Guidelines of care for the management of acne vulgaris. *Journal of the American Academy of Dermatology, 74*(5), 945–973.e33. doi: 10.1016/j.jaad.2015.12.037

Zampella, J., Kwatra, S., Blanck, J., & Cohen, B. (2016). Tinea in tots: Cases and literature review of oral antifungal treatment of tinea capitis in children under 2 years of age. *Journal of Pediatrics, 183*, 12–18. doi: 10.1016/j.jpeds.2016.12.042

22

Communicable Diseases

Teresa Whited, DNP, APRN, CPNP-PC

LEARNING OUTCOMES

Upon completion of this chapter, the student will be able to:

1. Describe the source and transmission of various communicable diseases.
2. Outline critical components of a history for a child or adolescent with a communicable disease.
3. Describe the clinical presentation of major communicable diseases.
4. Explain diagnostic and laboratory studies used with communicable diseases.
5. Outline recommended immunizations for infants, children, and adolescents.
6. Describe care in the hospital for an infant, child, or adolescent with communicable disease.
7. Plan appropriate isolation techniques to prevent the spread of communicable disease in the hospital.
8. Provide emergency nursing care of children with complications of communicable disease.
9. Develop a home-based plan of care for a child or adolescent with communicable disease.
10. Discuss alternative and complementary therapies used with communicable diseases.
11. Develop a teaching plan for caregivers of children and adolescents with communicable diseases.

IMMUNIZATIONS

Nurses should be aware of the following considerations when it comes to administering immunizations.

- Some immunizations may cause mild fever, or soreness and redness at the injection site. Teach parents how to calculate appropriate doses of acetaminophen to relieve pain or fever after the immunization. Discuss with parents that acetaminophen (Tylenol) or ibuprofen is not needed unless the child is uncomfortable from the fever or pain. These medications are no longer recommended because of potential to decrease immune reaction to vaccine (Wysocki et al., 2017). Warm compresses may also be applied to the injection site.
- Children with mild cold symptoms may receive immunizations. However, if they are moderately to severely ill with or without fever, it is better to hold the immunization until later (CDC, 2017b).
- Legal caregivers must receive a vaccine information statement (VIS) that explains the purpose of the vaccine, possible side effects, and how to care for the child. This statement also informs and questions the caregiver about possible contraindications and allergies to the vaccine. Caregivers must sign a permission form before the child receives the immunization.
- VIS forms can be obtained in many languages.
- All adverse effects of immunizations must be reported. The physician or nurse practitioner may file a Vaccine Adverse Event Report with the Centers for Disease Control and Prevention (CDC, 2017d).
- Documentation must include the lot number of the vaccine. The lot number is recorded on the vaccine label. Documentation also includes the route and site of vaccine administration and the date that the vaccine was given. Copies of permission forms must be kept on file (CDC, 2015a), as well as the manufacturer and source of the vaccine and the date of the VIS form.

Immunizations From Birth to Age 18 Years

Immunizations for children from birth to age 18 years are described by the CDC (2017a) as detailed in Fig. 22–1.

A mild illness is not considered a contraindication to receiving vaccines. Contraindications for each vaccine include a previous severe allergic reaction to any component of the vaccine.

Hepatitis B

- The hepatitis B vaccine is administered to all newborns. If the mother is positive for hepatitis B surface antigen (HBsAg), 0.5 mL of hepatitis B immune globulin (HBIG) is also given.
- Three doses of hepatitis B are given before age 2 years: at birth, at 1 to 2 months of age, and at 9 to 12 months of age.
- If a dose is missed, the series does not have to be restarted. It should be continued.
- A specific contraindication to hepatitis B is a hypersensitivity to yeast (CDC, 2017b).

Hepatitis A

- The hepatitis A vaccine is given to all children 12 months and older.
- This vaccine is especially important in children who are traveling or who are otherwise at risk for the disease.
- The hepatitis A vaccine is not given before 12 months of age.
- Two doses are given, at least 6 to 18 months apart.

Diphtheria, Tetanus, Pertussis/DT

- Four doses are given for infants and toddlers: at 2, 4, 6, and 15 to 18 months.
- A final dose in the series is given between age 4 and 6 years.
- The diphtheria, tetanus, pertussis (DTaP) vaccine may cause irritability, loss of appetite, and localized swelling and tenderness at the injection site. Seizures are a rare side effect of the DTaP due to the pertussis component of the vaccine. However, this vaccine is much safer now because only acellular components are used to manufacture the vaccine.
- DT is for children younger than 7 years who cannot have the pertussis component of the DTaP vaccine.

Haemophilus influenzae Type B

- *Haemophilus influenzae* type B (Hib) is a bacterium that causes infection in various parts of the body.
- This organism was at one time a leading cause of meningitis in young children, and is a significant cause of conjunctivitis, otitis media, and sinusitis.
- The Hib vaccine is given in a series of four doses: at 2, 4, 6, and 12 to 15 months. No additional doses are given after this series.

Rotavirus

Rotavirus is a live attenuated vaccine.

- Rotavirus causes severe diarrhea and dehydration.
- Two vaccinations are available for rotavirus. Based on vaccine use, dosing schedules vary.
- The first immunization is given between 6 and 14 weeks. The series is not started if the infant is more than 14 weeks and 6 days.
- Three doses of RotaTeq vaccination are given orally at 2, 4, and 6 months.
- If Rotarix is given at 2 and 4 months, no additional doses are given.
- Avoid immunization if the child has a history of intussusception, other gastrointestinal disorder, or severe combined immunodeficiency.

Pneumococcal (PCV13 and PPSV23)

- The pneumococcal conjugate vaccine (PCV13) is recommended for children younger than 5 years to protect against *Streptococcus pneumoniae* (pneumococcus).
- PCV13 replaces PCV7. A single additional dose of PCV13 is recommended for all children 14 to 59 months who have received an age-appropriate series of PCV7 and for all children 60 to 71 months with underlying specific medical conditions who have received an age-appropriate series of PCV7.
- Four doses of PCV13 are given in the series: at 2, 4, 6, and 12 to 15 months.
- The pneumococcal polysaccharide vaccine (PPSV23) is used for older children and adults, but may be used in children older than 2 years who have special medical conditions such as a cochlear implant or are asplenic from sickle cell anemia.
- The pneumococcal vaccine protects children from meningitis, otitis media, and other infections.

Inactivated Poliovirus

- Inactivated poliovirus vaccine (IPV) has replaced the live, oral vaccine (OPV) in the United States. IPV is safer to use because OPV contains live viruses and may cause paralysis in immunodeficient children or in close contacts who are immunodeficient.
- IPV is given in a series of four doses: at 2, 4, and 6 to 18 months, and 4 to 6 years.

Influenza

- Children aged 6 months to 18 years should receive an influenza immunization annually.
- Children through 8 years of age who are receiving their first influenza immunization need two doses, at least 4 weeks apart.
- Children older than 2 years have the option of receiving a live, attenuated influenza virus through a nasal spray as an alternative to the injection. However, after recent studies have shown it was less effective during the flu seasons from 2013 to 2016, the CDC did not recommend it for the 2016 to 2017 influenza season (Grohskopf et al., 2016). It is unclear whether this recommendation will persist.
- If used, the nasal spray vaccine is contraindicated for children with asthma and should not be given to children aged 2 to 4 years who have been wheezing within the past 12 months.
- The influenza nasal spray may cause symptoms of mild flu because it is manufactured from a weakened form of the live virus.

(Text continued on page 520)

Recommended Immunization Schedule for Children and Adolescents Aged 18 Years or Younger— United States, 2018.

FOR THOSE WHO FALL BEHIND OR START LATE, SEE THE CATCH-UP SCHEDULE.

These recommendations must be read with the footnotes that follow. For those who fall behind or start late, provide catch-up vaccination at the earliest opportunity as indicated by the green bars. To determine minimum intervals between doses, see the catch-up schedule. School entry and adolescent vaccine age groups are shaded in gray.

Vaccine	Birth	1 mo	2 mos	4 mos	6 mos	9 mos	12 mos	15 mos	18 mos	19-23 mos	2-3 yrs	4-6 yrs	7-10 yrs	11-12 yrs	13-15 yrs	16 yrs	17-18 yrs
Hepatitis B[1] (HepB)	1st dose	←2nd dose→			←3rd dose→												
Rotavirus[2] (RV) RV1 (2-dose series); RV5 (3-dose series)			1st dose	2nd dose	See footnote 2												
Diphtheria, tetanus, & acellular pertussis[3] (DTaP: <7 yrs)			1st dose	2nd dose	3rd dose			←4th dose→				5th dose					
Haemophilus influenzae type b[4] (Hib)			1st dose	2nd dose	See footnote 4		←3rd or 4th dose, See footnote 4→										
Pneumococcal conjugate[5] (PCV13)			1st dose	2nd dose	3rd dose		←4th dose→										
Inactivated poliovirus[6] (IPV: <18 yrs)			1st dose	2nd dose	←3rd dose→							4th dose					
Influenza[7] (IIV)					Annual vaccination (IIV) 1 or 2 doses									Annual vaccination (IIV) 1 dose only			
Measles, mumps, rubella[8] (MMR)					See footnote 8		←1st dose→					2nd dose					
Varicella[9] (VAR)							←1st dose→					2nd dose					
Hepatitis A[10] (HepA)							←2-dose series, See footnote 10→										
Meningococcal[11] (MenACWY-D ≥9 mos; MenACWY-CRM ≥2 mos)			See footnote 11											1st dose		2nd dose	
Tetanus, diphtheria, & acellular pertussis[13] (Tdap: ≥7 yrs)														Tdap			
Human papillomavirus[14] (HPV)														See footnote 14			
Meningococcal B[12]																See footnote 12	
Pneumococcal polysaccharide[5] (PPSV23)											See footnote 5						

Range of recommended ages for all children | Range of recommended ages for catch-up immunization | Range of recommended ages for certain high-risk groups | Range of recommended ages for non-high-risk groups that may receive vaccine, subject to individual clinical decision making | No recommendation

NOTE: The above recommendations must be read along with the footnotes of this schedule.

FIGURE 22–1 Immunization schedule for children from birth through age 18 years of age. *(From Center for Disease Control [CDC]. (2017).* Birth-18 years Recommended Immunization Schedule. *Retrieved from https://www.cdc.gov/vaccines/schedules/hcp/imz/child-adolescent.html)*

Continued

Footnotes — Recommended Immunization Schedule for Children and Adolescents Aged 18 Years or Younger, UNITED STATES, 2018

For further guidance on the use of the vaccines mentioned below, see: www.cdc.gov/vaccines/hcp/acip-recs/index.html.
For vaccine recommendations for persons 19 years of age and older, see the Adult Immunization Schedule.

Additional information

- For information on contraindications and precautions for the use of a vaccine, consult the *General Best Practice Guidelines for Immunization* and relevant ACIP statements, at www.cdc.gov/vaccines/hcp/acip-recs/index.html.
- For calculating intervals between doses, 4 weeks = 28 days. Intervals of ≥4 months are determined by calendar months.
- Within a number range (e.g., 12–18), a dash (–) should be read as "through."
- Vaccine doses administered ≤4 days before the minimum age or interval are considered valid. Doses of any vaccine administered ≥5 days earlier than the minimum interval or minimum age should not be counted as valid and should be repeated as age-appropriate. The repeat dose should be spaced after the invalid dose by the recommended minimum interval. For further details, see Table 3-1, *Recommended and minimum ages and intervals between vaccine doses,* in *General Best Practice Guidelines for Immunization* at www.cdc.gov/vaccines/hcp/acip-recs/general-recs/timing.html.
- Information on travel vaccine requirements and recommendations is available at wwwnc.cdc.gov/travel/.
- For vaccination of persons with immunodeficiencies, see Table 8-1, *Vaccination of persons with primary and secondary immunodeficiencies,* in *General Best Practice Guidelines for Immunization,* at www.cdc.gov/vaccines/hcp/acip-recs/general-recs/immunocompetence.html; and Immunization in Special Clinical Circumstances. (In: Kimberlin DW, Brady MT, Jackson MA, Long SS, eds. *Red Book: 2015 report of the Committee on Infectious Diseases. 30th ed.* Elk Grove Village, IL: American Academy of Pediatrics, 2015:68-107).
- The National Vaccine Injury Compensation Program (VICP) is a no-fault alternative to the traditional legal system for resolving vaccine injury claims. All routine child and adolescent vaccines are covered by VICP except for pneumococcal polysaccharide vaccine (PPSV23). For more information; see www.hrsa.gov/vaccinecompensation/index.html.

1. Hepatitis B (HepB) vaccine. (minimum age: birth)

Birth Dose (Monovalent HepB vaccine only):

- **Mother is HBsAg-Negative:** 1 dose within 24 hours of birth for medically stable infants ≥2,000 grams. Infants <2,000 grams administer 1 dose at chronological age 1 month or hospital discharge.
- **Mother is HBsAg-Positive:**
  - o Give **HepB vaccine** and **0.5 mL of HBIG** (at separate anatomic sites) within 12 hours of birth, regardless of birth weight.
  - o Test for HBsAg and anti-HBs at age 9–12 months. If HepB series is delayed, test 1–2 months after final dose.
- **Mother's HBsAg status is unknown:**
  - o Give **HepB vaccine** within 12 hours of birth, regardless of birth weight.
  - o For infants <2,000 grams, give **0.5 mL of HBIG** in addition to HepB vaccine within 12 hours of birth.
  - o Determine mother's HBsAg status as soon as possible. If mother is HBsAg-positive, give **0.5 mL of HBIG** to infants ≥2,000 grams as soon as possible, but no later than 7 days of age.

Routine Series:

- A complete series is 3 doses at 0, 1–2, and 6–18 months. (Monovalent HepB vaccine should be used for doses given before age 6 weeks.)
- Infants who did not receive a birth dose should begin the series as soon as feasible (see Figure 2).
- Administration of **4 doses** is permitted when a combination vaccine containing HepB is used after the birth dose.
- **Minimum age** for the final (3rd or 4th) dose: 24 weeks.
- **Minimum Intervals:** Dose 1 to Dose 2: 4 weeks / Dose 2 to Dose 3: 8 weeks / Dose 1 to Dose 3: 16 weeks. (When 4 doses are given, substitute "Dose 4" for "Dose 3" in these calculations.)

Catch-up vaccination:

- Unvaccinated persons should complete a 3-dose series at 0, 1–2, and 6 months.
- Adolescents 11–15 years of age may use an alternative 2-dose schedule, with at least 4 months between doses (adult formulation **Recombivax HB** only).
- For other catch-up guidance, see Figure 2.

2. Rotavirus vaccines. (minimum age: 6 weeks)

Routine vaccination:

Rotarix: 2-dose series at 2 and 4 months.

RotaTeq: 3-dose series at 2, 4, and 6 months.

If any dose in the series is either RotaTeq or unknown, default to 3-dose series.

Catch-up vaccination:

- Do not start the series on or after age 15 weeks, 0 days.
- The maximum age for the final dose is 8 months, 0 days.
- For other catch-up guidance, see Figure 2.

3. Diphtheria, tetanus, and acellular pertussis (DTaP) vaccine. (minimum age: 6 weeks [4 years for Kinrix or Quadracel])

Routine vaccination:

- 5-dose series at 2, 4, 6, and 15–18 months, and 4–6 years.
  - o **Prospectively:** A 4th dose may be given as early as age 12 months if at least 6 months have elapsed since the 3rd dose.
  - o **Retrospectively:** A 4th dose that was inadvertently given as early as 12 months may be counted if at least 4 months have elapsed since the 3rd dose.

Catch-up vaccination:

- The 5th dose is not necessary if the 4th dose was administered at 4 years or older.
- For other catch-up guidance, see Figure 2.

FIGURE 22-1—cont'd

For further guidance on the use of the vaccines mentioned below, see: www.cdc.gov/vaccines/hcp/acip-recs/index.html.

4. ***Haemophilus influenzae* type b (Hib) vaccine. (minimum age: 6 weeks)**

Routine vaccination:
- **ActHIB, Hiberix, or Pentacel:** 4-dose series at 2, 4, 6, and 12–15 months.
- **PedvaxHIB:** 3-dose series at 2, 4, and 12–15 months.

Catch-up vaccination:
- **1st dose at 7–11 months:** Give 2nd dose at least 4 weeks later and 3rd (final) dose at 12–15 months or 8 weeks after 2nd dose (whichever is later).
- **1st dose at 12–14 months:** Give 2nd (final) dose at least 8 weeks after 1st dose.
- **1st dose before 12 months and 2nd dose before 15 months:** Give 3rd (final) dose 8 weeks after 2nd dose.
- **2 doses of PedvaxHIB before 12 months:** Give 3rd (final) dose at 12–59 months and at least 8 weeks after 2nd dose.
- **Unvaccinated at 15–59 months:** 1 dose.
- For other catch-up guidance, see Figure 2.

Special Situations:
- **Chemotherapy or radiation treatment**
  12–59 months
  - o Unvaccinated or only 1 dose before 12 months: Give 2 doses, 8 weeks apart
  - o 2 or more doses before 12 months: Give 1 dose, at least 8 weeks after previous dose.

  Doses given within 14 days of starting therapy or during therapy should be repeated at least 3 months after therapy completion.
- **Hematopoietic stem cell transplant (HSCT)**
- 3-dose series with doses 4 weeks apart starting 6 to 12 months after successful transplant (regardless of Hib vaccination history).
- **Anatomic or functional asplenia (including sickle cell disease)**
  12–59 months
  - o Unvaccinated or only 1 dose before 12 months: Give 2 doses, 8 weeks apart.
  - o 2 or more doses before 12 months: Give 1 dose, at least 8 weeks after previous dose.

  Unimmunized persons 5 years or older*
  - o Give 1 dose
- **Elective splenectomy**
  Unimmunized* persons 15 months or older
  - o Give 1 dose (preferably at least 14 days before procedure).
- **HIV infection**
  12–59 months
  - o Unvaccinated or only 1 dose before 12 months: Give 2 doses 8 weeks apart.
  - o 2 or more doses before 12 months: Give 1 dose, at least 8 weeks after previous dose.

  Unimmunized persons 5–18 years*
  - o Give 1 dose
- **Immunoglobulin deficiency, early component complement deficiency**
  12–59 months
  - o Unvaccinated or only 1 dose before 12 months: Give 2 doses, 8 weeks apart.
  - o 2 or more doses before 12 months: Give 1 dose, at least 8 weeks after previous dose.

**Unimmunized* = Less than routine series (through 14 months) OR no doses (14 months or older)

5. **Pneumococcal vaccines. (minimum age: 6 weeks [PCV13], 2 years [PPSV23])**

Routine vaccination with PCV13:
- 4-dose series at 2, 4, 6, and 12–15 months.

Catch-up vaccination with PCV13:
- 1 dose for healthy children aged 24–59 months with any incomplete* PCV13 schedule
- For other catch-up guidance, see Figure 2.

Special situations: High-risk conditions: Administer PCV13 doses before PPSV23 if possible.

Chronic heart disease (particularly cyanotic congenital heart disease and cardiac failure); chronic lung disease (including asthma treated with high-dose, oral, corticosteroids); diabetes mellitus:

Age 2–5 years:
- Any incomplete* schedules with:
  - o 3 PCV13 doses: 1 dose of PCV13 (at least 8 weeks after any prior PCV13 dose).
  - o <3 PCV13 doses: 2 doses of PCV13, 8 weeks after the most recent dose and given 8 weeks apart.
- No history of PPSV23: 1 dose of PPSV23 (at least 8 weeks after any prior PCV13 dose).

Age 6-18 years:
- No history of PPSV23: 1 dose of PPSV23 (at least 8 weeks after any prior PCV13 dose).

Cerebrospinal fluid leak; cochlear implant:

Age 2–5 years:
- Any incomplete* schedules with:
  - o 3 PCV13 doses: 1 dose of PCV13 (at least 8 weeks after any prior PCV13 dose).
  - o <3 PCV13 doses: 2 doses of PCV13, 8 weeks after the most recent dose and given 8 weeks apart.
- No history of PPSV23: 1 dose of PPSV23 (at least 8 weeks after any prior PCV13 dose).

Age 6–18 years:
- No history of either PCV13 or PPSV23: 1 dose of PCV13, 1 dose of PPSV23 at least 8 weeks later.
- Any PCV13 but no PPSV23: 1 dose of PPSV23 at least 8 weeks after the most recent dose of PCV13
- PPSV23 but no PCV13: 1 dose of PCV13 at least 8 weeks after the most recent dose of PPSV23.

Sickle cell disease and other hemoglobinopathies; anatomic or functional asplenia; congenital or acquired immunodeficiency; HIV infection; chronic renal failure; nephrotic syndrome; malignant neoplasms, leukemias, lymphomas, Hodgkin disease, and other diseases associated with treatment with immunosuppressive drugs or radiation therapy; solid organ transplantation; multiple myeloma:

Age 2–5 years:
- Any incomplete* schedules with:
  - o 3 PCV13 doses: 1 dose of PCV13 (at least 8 weeks after any prior PCV13 dose).
  - o <3 PCV13 doses: 2 doses of PCV13, 8 weeks after the most recent dose and given 8 weeks apart.
- No history of PPSV23: 1 dose of PPSV23 (at least 8 weeks after any prior PCV13 dose) and a 2nd dose of PPSV23 5 years later.

Age 6–18 years:
- No history of either PCV13 or PPSV23: 1 dose of PCV13, 2 doses of PPSV23 (1st dose of PPSV23 administered 8 weeks after PCV13 and 2nd dose of PPSV23 administered at least 5 years after the 1st dose of PPSV23).
- Any PCV13 but no PPSV23: 2 doses of PPSV23 (1st dose of PPSV23 to be given 8 weeks after the most recent dose of PCV13 and 2nd dose of PPSV23 administered at least 5 years after the 1st dose of PPSV23).

FIGURE 22-1—cont'd

Continued

For further guidance on the use of the vaccines mentioned below, see: www.cdc.gov/vaccines/hcp/acip-recs/index.html.

- PPSV23 but no PCV13: 1 dose of PCV13 at least 8 weeks after the most recent PPSV23 dose and a 2nd dose of PPSV23 to be given 5 years after the 1st dose of PPSV23 and at least 8 weeks after a dose of PCV13.

Chronic liver disease, alcoholism:

Age 6–18 years:

- No history of PPSV23: 1 dose of PPSV23 (at least 8 weeks after any prior PCV13 dose).

*Incomplete schedules are any schedules where PCV13 doses have not been completed according to ACIP recommended catch-up schedules. The total number and timing of doses for complete PCV13 series are dictated by the age at first vaccination. See Tables 8 and 9 in the ACIP pneumococcal vaccine recommendations (www.cdc.gov/mmwr/pdf/rr/rr5911.pdf) for complete schedule details.

6. **Inactivated poliovirus vaccine (IPV). (minimum age: 6 weeks)**

Routine vaccination:

- 4-dose series at ages 2, 4, 6–18 months, and 4–6 years. Administer the final dose on or after the 4th birthday and at least 6 months after the previous dose.

Catch-up vaccination:

- In the first 6 months of life, use minimum ages and intervals only for travel to a polio-endemic region or during an outbreak.
- If 4 or more doses were given before the 4th birthday, give 1 more dose at age 4–6 years and at least 6 months after the previous dose.
- A 4th dose is not necessary if the 3rd dose was given on or after the 4th birthday and at least 6 months after the previous dose.
- IPV is not routinely recommended for U.S. residents 18 years and older.

Series Containing Oral Polio Vaccine (OPV), *either mixed OPV-IPV or OPV-only series*:

- Total number of doses needed to complete the series is the same as that recommended for the U.S. IPV schedule. See www.cdc.gov/mmwr/volumes/66/wr/mm6601a6.htm?s_cid=mm6601a6_w.
- Only trivalent OPV (tOPV) counts toward the U.S. vaccination requirements. For guidance to assess doses documented as "OPV" see www.cdc.gov/mmwr/volumes/66/wr/mm6606a7.htm?s_cid=mm6606a7_w.
- For other catch-up guidance, see Figure 2.

7. **Influenza vaccines. (minimum age: 6 months)**

Routine vaccination:

- Administer an age-appropriate formulation and dose of influenza vaccine annually.
  - o **Children 6 months–8 years** who did not receive at least 2 doses of influenza vaccine before July 1, 2017 should receive 2 doses separated by at least 4 weeks.
  - o **Persons 9 years and older** 1 dose
- Live attenuated influenza vaccine (LAIV) not recommended for the 2017–18 season.
- For additional guidance, see the 2017–18 ACIP influenza vaccine recommendations (*MMWR* August 25, 2017;66(2):1-20: www.cdc.gov/mmwr/volumes/66/rr/pdfs/rr6602.pdf).

(For the 2018–19 season, see the 2018–19 ACIP influenza vaccine recommendations.)

8. **Measles, mumps, and rubella (MMR) vaccine. (minimum age: 12 months for routine vaccination)**

Routine vaccination:

- 2-dose series at 12–15 months and 4–6 years.
- The 2nd dose may be given as early as 4 weeks after the 1st dose.

Catch-up vaccination:

- Unvaccinated children and adolescents: 2 doses at least 4 weeks apart.

International travel:

- **Infants 6–11 months:** 1 dose before departure. Revaccinate with 2 doses at 12–15 months (12 months for children in high-risk areas) and 2nd dose as early as 4 weeks later.
- **Unvaccinated children 12 months and older:** 2 doses at least 4 weeks apart before departure.

Mumps outbreak:

- Persons ≥12 months who previously received ≤2 doses of mumps-containing vaccine and are identified by public health authorities to be at increased risk during a mumps outbreak should receive a dose of mumps-virus containing vaccine.

9. **Varicella (VAR) vaccine. (minimum age: 12 months)**

Routine vaccination:

- 2-dose series: 12–15 months and 4–6 years.
- The 2nd dose may be given as early as 3 months after the 1st dose (a dose given after a 4-week interval may be counted).

Catch-up vaccination:

- Ensure persons 7–18 years without evidence of immunity (see *MMWR* 2007;56[No. RR-4], at www.cdc.gov/mmwr/pdf/rr/rr5604.pdf) have 2 doses of varicella vaccine:
  - o **Ages 7–12:** routine interval 3 months (minimum interval: 4 weeks).
  - o **Ages 13 and older:** minimum interval 4 weeks.

10. **Hepatitis A (HepA) vaccine. (minimum age: 12 months)**

Routine vaccination:

- 2 doses, separated by 6-18 months, between the 1st and 2nd birthdays. (A series begun before the 2nd birthday should be completed even if the child turns 2 before the second dose is given.)

Catch-up vaccination:

- Anyone 2 years of age or older may receive HepA vaccine if desired. Minimum interval between doses is 6 months.

Special populations:

Previously unvaccinated persons who should be vaccinated:

- Persons traveling to or working in countries with high or intermediate endemicity
- Men who have sex with men
- Users of injection and non-injection drugs
- Persons who work with hepatitis A virus in a research laboratory or with non-human primates
- Persons with clotting-factor disorders
- Persons with chronic liver disease
- Persons who anticipate close, personal contact (e.g., household or regular babysitting) with an international adoptee during the first 60 days after arrival in the United States from a country with high or intermediate endemicity (administer the 1st dose as soon as the adoption is planned—ideally at least 2 weeks before the adoptee's arrival).

11. **Serogroup A, C, W, Y meningococcal vaccines. (Minimum age: 2 months [Menveo], 9 months [Menactra].**

Routine:

- 2-dose series: 11-12 years and 16 years.

Catch-Up:

- Age 13-15 years: 1 dose now and booster at age 16-18 years. Minimum interval 8 weeks.
- Age 16-18 years: 1 dose.

FIGURE 22-1—cont'd

For further guidance on the use of the vaccines mentioned below, see: www.cdc.gov/vaccines/hcp/acip-recs/index.html.

Special populations and situations:
Anatomic or functional asplenia, sickle cell disease, HIV infection, persistent complement component deficiency (including eculizumab use):

- **Menveo**
  - o 1st dose at 8 weeks: 4-dose series at 2, 4, 6, and 12 months.
  - o 1st dose at 7–23 months: 2 doses (2nd dose at least 12 weeks after the 1st dose and after the 1st birthday).
  - o 1st dose at 24 months or older: 2 doses at least 8 weeks apart.
- **Menactra**
  - o Persistent complement component deficiency:
    - — 9–23 months: 2 doses at least 12 weeks apart
    - — 24 months or older: 2 doses at least 8 weeks apart
  - o Anatomic or functional asplenia, sickle cell disease, or HIV infection:
    - — 24 months or older: 2 doses at least 8 weeks apart.
    - — **Menactra** must be administered at least 4 weeks after completion of PCV13 series.

Children who travel to or live in countries where meningococcal disease is hyperendemic or epidemic, including countries in the African meningitis belt or during the Hajj, or exposure to an outbreak attributable to a vaccine serogroup:

- Children <24 months of age:
  - o **Menveo (2-23 months):**
    - — 1st dose at 8 weeks: 4-dose series at 2, 4, 6, and 12 months.
    - — 1st dose at 7-23 months: 2 doses (2nd dose at least 12 weeks after the 1st dose and after the 1st birthday).
  - o **Menactra (9-23 months):**
    - — 2 doses (2nd dose at least 12 weeks after the 1st dose. 2nd dose may be administered as early as 8 weeks after the 1st dose in travelers).
- Children 2 years or older: 1 dose of **Menveo** or **Menactra**.

Note: Menactra should be given either before or at the same time as DTaP. For MenACWY booster dose recommendations for groups listed under "Special populations and situations" above, and additional meningococcal vaccination information, see meningococcal *MMWR* publications at: www.cdc.gov/vaccines/hcp/acip-recs/vacc-specific/mening.html.

12. Serogroup B meningococcal vaccines (minimum age: 10 years [Bexsero, Trumenba].

Clinical discretion: Adolescents not at increased risk for meningococcal B infection who want MenB vaccine.

MenB vaccines may be given at clinical discretion to adolescents 16–23 years (preferred age 16–18 years) who are not at increased risk.

- **Bexsero**: 2 doses at least 1 month apart.
- **Trumenba**: 2 doses at least 6 months apart. If the 2nd dose is given earlier than 6 months, give a 3rd dose at least 4 months after the 2nd.

Special populations and situations:
Anatomic or functional asplenia, sickle cell disease, persistent complement component deficiency (including eculizumab use), serogroup B meningococcal disease outbreak

- **Bexsero**: 2-dose series at least 1 month apart.
- **Trumenba**: 3-dose series at 0, 1-2, and 6 months.

Note: **Bexsero** and **Trumenba** are not interchangeable.
For additional meningococcal vaccination information, see meningococcal *MMWR* publications at: www.cdc.gov/vaccines/hcp/acip-recs/vacc-specific/mening.html.

13. Tetanus, diphtheria, and acellular pertussis (Tdap) vaccine. (minimum age: 11 years for routine vaccinations, 7 years for catch-up vaccination)

Routine vaccination:

- **Adolescents 11–12 years of age:** 1 dose.
- **Pregnant adolescents:** 1 dose during each pregnancy (preferably during the early part of gestational weeks 27–36).
- Tdap may be administered regardless of the interval since the last tetanus- and diphtheria-toxoid-containing vaccine.

Catch-up vaccination:

- **Adolescents 13–18 who have not received Tdap**: 1 dose, followed by a Td booster every 10 years.
- **Persons aged 7–18 years not fully immunized with DTaP**: 1 dose of Tdap as part of the catch-up series (preferably the first dose). If additional doses are needed, use Td.
- **Children 7–10 years** who receive Tdap inadvertently or as part of the catch-up series may receive the routine Tdap dose at 11–12 years.
- **DTaP inadvertently given after the 7th birthday**:
  - o **Child 7–10**: DTaP may count as part of catch-up series. Routine Tdap dose at 11-12 may be given.
  - o **Adolescent 11–18**: Count dose of DTaP as the adolescent Tdap booster.
- For other catch-up guidance, see Figure 2.

14. Human papillomavirus (HPV) vaccine (minimum age: 9 years)

Routine and catch-up vaccination:

- Routine vaccination for all adolescents at 11–12 years (can start at age 9) and through age 18 if not previously adequately vaccinated. Number of doses dependent on age at initial vaccination:
  - o **Age 9–14 years at initiation:** 2-dose series at 0 and 6–12 months. Minimum interval: 5 months (repeat a dose given too soon at least 12 weeks after the invalid dose and at least 5 months after the 1st dose).
  - o **Age 15 years or older at initiation:** 3-dose series at 0, 1–2 months, and 6 months. Minimum intervals: 4 weeks between 1st and 2nd dose; 12 weeks between 2nd and 3rd dose; 5 months between 1st and 3rd dose (repeat dose(s) given too soon at or after the minimum interval since the most recent dose).
- Persons who have completed a valid series with any HPV vaccine do not need any additional doses.

Special situations:

- **History of sexual abuse or assault**: Begin series at age 9 years.
- **Immunocompromised* (including HIV)** aged 9–26 years: 3-dose series at 0, 1–2 months, and 6 months.
- **Pregnancy:** Vaccination not recommended, but there is no evidence the vaccine is harmful. No intervention is needed for women who inadvertently received a dose of HPV vaccine while pregnant. Delay remaining doses until after pregnancy. Pregnancy testing not needed before vaccination.

*See MMWR, December 16, 2016;65(49):1405–1408, at www.cdc.gov/mmwr/volumes/65/wr/pdfs/mm6549a5.pdf.

CS270457-M

FIGURE 22-1—cont'd

- The influenza immunization is contraindicated for individuals who are allergic to previous doses of influenza. Caution should be used in those allergic to eggs or egg products, or those who have moderate to severe acute illness. Hives secondary to egg allergy are not considered a contraindication.

Measles, Mumps, Rubella

Measles, mumps, rubella (MMR) is a live attenuated virus vaccine.

- The minimum age for receiving this immunization is 12 months. Do not give before the first birthday unless traveling outside the United States, in which case the child will need to still receive two doses of vaccine per regular schedule.
- The second dose is generally given at 4 to 6 years of age but may be given before age 4 years if at least 4 weeks have elapsed since the first dose.
- Children may experience maculopapular rash, fever, swollen cheeks, and mild joint pain after receiving the MMR vaccine.
- MMR is contraindicated for persons who are allergic to vaccine components, are pregnant, have immunodeficiency, or have a family history of altered immunocompetence. Caution should be used if the patient is a recent recipient of antibody-containing blood products, intravenous gamma globulin, has a history of thrombocytopenia, has the need for tuberculosis (TB) skin test or IGRA (interferon-gamma release assay) testing, and those with moderate-to-severe acute illness. The TB test may be given before or at the same time as the MMR vaccine or 28 days later.
- The MMR vaccine may be given to a child who is HIV positive as long as he or she is not severely immunocompromised.

Varicella (Varivax)

Varicella is a live attenuated virus vaccine.

- The minimum age for receiving this immunization is 12 months. Do not give before the first birthday.
- The second dose is generally given at 4 to 6 years of age but may be given before age 4 years if at least 3 months have lapsed since the first dose.
- Negative side effects include erythema and soreness at the injection site. A few people may experience a varicella-type rash at the injection site.
- Varicella vaccine is contraindicated for persons who are allergic to components of vaccines or have had previous severe allergic reaction to the vaccines, those with severe immunodeficiency, those who are pregnant, or those with a family history of altered immunocompetence. Caution should be used in those with recent antibody-containing blood products or with moderate-to-severe acute illness.
- The vaccine should not be given if antiviral drugs have been given in the previous 24 hours, and antiviral drugs should be avoided 14 days after the varicella immunization (CDC, 2017b).
- If a child is taking aspirin for another condition such as Kawasaki disease, then the parents/caregivers should be educated about the signs and symptoms of Reye syndrome.

Meningococcal (Menactra or Menveo)

- The meningococcal vaccine is given at 11 to 12 years of age with a booster at 16 years of age. Meningococcal conjugate ACWY is given to children who are 2 to 18 years of age and are at high risk due to asplenia, immunodeficiency disorders, or HIV, or who live in or travel to a country where meningococcal disease is an epidemic (CDC, 2017b).
- Avoid the immunization if the child was allergic to a previous dose or component of vaccine. Use caution in children who have moderate-to-severe acute illness.

Meningococcal Serogroup B Vaccine (MenB-FHbp or MenB-4C)

The meningococcal serogroup B vaccine is recommended for individuals at age 10 and at age 25 years who are at risk for meningitis serogroup B. Increased risks include persistent complement component deficiencies, those with functional or anatomic asplenia, or routine exposure to these diseases. The vaccine can also be given to healthy individuals 16 to 23 years of age for short-term protection against the most common strains of meningococcal disease.

- Two vaccines are licensed in the United States and the vaccines are not interchangeable. When a person starts a dosing series with one type of vaccine, all doses must be completed with the same vaccine type.
- Persons who are at high risk should receive the vaccine in a three-dose series with vaccine spacing of 1 to 2 months following initial vaccine for second vaccine and 6 months for the third dose of the vaccine.
- Persons who are healthy should receive the vaccine in a two-dose series with 6 months spacing between initial and second dose of vaccine.
- It is contraindicated in pregnant/lactating women or in those who have had a severe allergic reaction to the vaccine or any part of the vaccine including latex (Patton, Stephens, Moore, & McNeil, 2017).

Tetanus, Diphtheria, and Acellular Pertussis

- Due to waning immunity to pertussis, it is now recommended that all children 11 to 12 years of age receive one dose of tetanus, diphtheria, and acellular pertussis (Tdap) in place of previous Td.
- All pregnant adolescents/women should receive a dose of Tdap during each pregnancy (ideally 27 to 36 weeks' gestation) regardless of time since previous vaccine (CDC, 2017a).
- Tdap is contraindicated in patients who have had a severe allergic reaction to the vaccine or its components, or who had encephalopathy within 7 days of previous vaccine. Caution should be used in those who have unstable neurological conditions, history of Arthus-type hypersensitivity reactions after previous dose, or moderate-to-severe acute illness (CDC, 2017b).

Human Papillomavirus (HPV-Gardasil)

- The human papillomavirus (HPV) vaccine prevents the most common causes of genital warts and helps prevent cervical, anal, oral, and penile cancers.
- It is recommended to be given at 11 to 12 years of age (minimum age is 9 years) in a two-dose series with a minimum of 6 months between dosing.

- If vaccination is not begun by age 15 years, the patient requires a three-dose series at 0, 1 to 2 months, and 6 months.
- The most common side effect of immunization is syncope. Patients should be encouraged to sit for a few minutes after the dose is given and should be warned of this side effect (CDC, 2017a).
- HPV is contraindicated in those with a severe allergic reaction to the vaccine or its components, and caution should be used in those who are pregnant or have moderate-to-severe acute illness (CDC, 2017b).

CRITICAL COMPONENT

Immunization Success

Vaccines have significantly reduced the incidence of many communicable diseases. For example, diphtheria is now a rare disease in the United States, but was a major health problem in years past. Respiratory diphtheria causes severe illness and death as a result of airway obstruction from a membrane that covers the pharynx or nasal passages. Diphtheria remains a problem is some developing countries, and continued vigilance is needed. However, since widespread vaccination in the United States, only two cases of diphtheria have been reported since 2004. Similarly, polio affected thousands of children until the 1950s, when vaccinations became widespread. Today, the disease has been eliminated from most of the world but is still endemic in several countries worldwide. With the anti-vaccine movement, previously vaccine-preventable diseases such as measles have recurred. Significant outbreaks are reported in areas of poor vaccination, including more than 1,100 cases in 2017. Continued vaccination is essential to prevent the loss of individual and herd immunity required to prevent these communicable diseases (CDC, 2017e, 2017h).

CRITICAL COMPONENT

Types of Immunity

When a person carries antibodies to a disease, he or she has immunity to that disease. There are two types of immunity:

- Active immunity is when a person is exposed to the disease organism and makes his or her own antibodies. Active immunity is permanent or long-lasting.
  - Natural active immunity: a person actually has the infection and is then immune to the disease
  - Vaccine-induced immunity: active immunity to a disease that comes from being immunized with a killed or weakened form of that disease
- Passive immunity is when a person is given antibodies to a disease. This immunity is temporary and lasts for only a few weeks or months.
  - Natural passive immunity: antibodies are passed from mother to fetus by way of the placenta
  - Passive immunity: given through immune globulins to provide immediate protection against a disease (CDC, 2015a)

CRITICAL COMPONENT

Types of Vaccines

Types of vaccines (antigens that stimulate an immune response):

- Inactivated or killed organism (example: inactivated polio virus): The virus is disabled and unable to replicate itself, but it still contains enough of the original characteristics that it can stimulate an immune response.
- Live attenuated or weakened virus (examples: MMR and the varicella vaccine)
- Acellular vaccine (examples: pertussis and Hib): The vaccine contains fragments of cells that stimulate an immune response but does not contain the whole cell.
- Toxoids (examples: tetanus and diphtheria): Toxins produced by the bacteria are inactivated so that they cannot cause harm but can still stimulate an immune response.
- Subunit of virus (example: hepatitis B): Small fragments of viral protein are used.

(CDC, 2015a)

Evidence-Based Practice: Vaccination and Autism

Maglione, M., Das, L., Raaen, L., Smith, A., Chari, R., Newberry, S., . . . Gidengil, C. (2014). Safety of vaccines used for routine immunization of US children: A systematic review. *Pediatrics, 134*(2), 325–337. doi: 10.1542/peds.2014-1079

Jain, A., Marshall, J., Buikema, A., Bancroft, T., Kelly, J. P., & Newschaffer, C. J. (2015). Autism occurrence by MMR vaccine status among US children with older siblings with and without autism. *Journal of the American Medical Association, 313*(15), 1534–1540. doi: 10.1001/jama.2015.3077

Concern regarding vaccine safety has been highly publicized in the media, leading to an anti-vaccine movement and lower vaccination rates. One of the largest controversies is the MMR vaccine's reported link to autism. Despite this report, multiple studies have shown no link to autism related to vaccines or their components. In a systematic review by Maglione et al. (2014), they found strong evidence after review of the literature including more than 66 studies that MMR is not associated with autism. Further, Jain et al. (2015) did a study to identify those with and without older siblings with autism and their rates of autism in association to MMR vaccinations. After searching almost 100,000 charts, they found no association between increased risk for autism with the MMR vaccine even if the older sibling had autism.

To promote adequate vaccination rates, it is important to educate parents and the public regarding the magnitude of evidence of no link between autism and MMR vaccination.

ASSESSMENT

Communicable diseases can affect most body systems and have distinct patterns of presentation. The diagnosis and management of the disease will be based on the subjective and objective findings present in the patient. Nurses should complete a thorough history and physical examination to understand the diagnosis and extent of disease process.

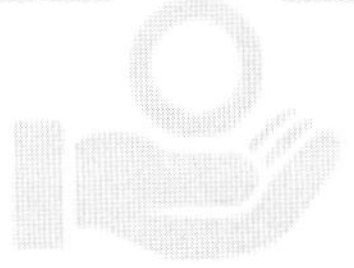

SAFE AND EFFECTIVE NURSING CARE: Clinical Pearl

Routes of Vaccines

- Intramuscular vaccines
  - Diphtheria, tetanus, pertussis (DTaP, DT, Tdap, Td)
  - Hib
  - Hepatitis A
  - Hepatitis B
  - HPV
  - Influenza, trivalent inactivated
  - Meningococcal—conjugate
  - PCV
- Intramuscular or subcutaneous
  - PPSV
  - IPV
- Subcutaneous
  - MMR
  - Varicella
  - Meningococcal—polysaccharide
- Oral
  - Rotavirus

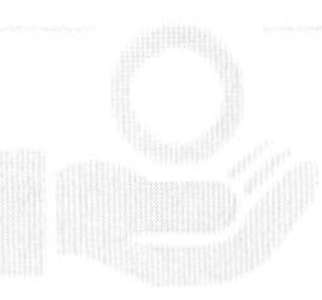

SAFE AND EFFECTIVE NURSING CARE: Clinical Pearl

Reducing Fear of Immunizations by Developmental Stage

Vaccines and needlestick procedures are a source of significant distress for children and families. It is important for clinicians to understand ways to manage vaccine anxiety. Discuss previous vaccine experiences and educate patients and families on what to expect from the vaccinations. Parental coaching on supportive, honest cues assists in managing their child's anxiety.

Based on the child's developmental stage, different comfort measures are more effective:

Infant comfort measures: swaddling, being held by parents with legs exposed, pacifier, feeding, the use of sugary substances to suck on, and distraction objects in older infants

Toddler comfort measures: simple explanations of what to expect, comfort holds by parents or assistant, distraction measures, managing parental anxiety, positive instructions, and positive rewards

School-age comfort measures: more complex preparatory discussions; use of distractions like deep breathing, guided imagery, interactive toys, coaching activities such as counting to the end of procedure, and talking about other things like pets (Stevens & Marvicsin, 2016)

General History

History is essential to assessment of the child who may be experiencing a communicable disease. It is important to ask about the following issues:

- Exposure to the disease: Has the child been around other children who have the communicable disease? Is the child in close contact with other children at daycare or schools? Have family members been exposed to a communicable disease?
- Consider the incubation period of a disease and the length of time it takes for symptoms to appear from the time the child was exposed.
- Has the child had any communicable diseases in the past?
- What immunizations has the child had? Are immunizations up to date with recommended schedule?
- Any child 2 months or younger with a fever of 101°F or higher should be seen by a health-care professional to evaluate for subtle signs of sepsis or other concerning infections. The very young infant does not yet have a fully functioning immune status, and presentations of communicable diseases may be subtle.

Physical Examination

Physical assessment of a child with communicable disease includes assessing prodromal signs and symptoms that may appear before a rash or the main illness appears. The prodromal period is often associated with increased communicability of the disease. Prodromal signs and symptoms may include:

- Coryza (runny nose)
- Cough
- Fever
- Malaise

General signs and symptoms experienced by a child with communicable disease include:

- Changes in behavior—lethargy or irritability
- Skin rashes that may itch and may include macules, papules, pustules, and vesicles
- Enlarged lymph nodes that may vary in location based on the disease but are predominately located in the anterior cervical, posterior cervical, and tonsillar areas
- Fever
- Vomiting and diarrhea
- Pain in any part of the body, including headache, abdominal pain, throat pain, or muscle aches

See Table 22–1 for a list of common communicable diseases.

VIRAL COMMUNICABLE DISEASES

Viral communicable diseases are some of the most common diseases acquired by humans. Thousands of viruses can result in minor illnesses such as the common cold, as well as more significant diseases such as meningitis. This section highlights common and serious viral diseases in childhood.

TABLE 22–1 Summary of Common Communicable Diseases

DISEASE	AGENT	TRANSMISSION	INCUBATION	COMMUNICABILITY
Erythema infectiosum (fifth disease)	Human parvovirus B19 (HPV)	Respiratory secretions	4–21 days	Contagious until rash appears
Hand, foot, mouth disease	Coxsackie or enterovirus	Direct contact	3–6 days	Virus may be shed for several weeks
Hepatitis A	Hepatitis A viral infection	Fecal–oral route Contaminated food	Approximately 30 days	2 weeks before symptoms until 1 week after symptoms
Hepatitis B	HBV viral infection	Blood or blood products Sexual contact	Average 90 days	Can be spread as long as virus is in the blood
Influenza	Influenza type A or B virus	Coughing, sneezing Oral and nasal secretions	1–4 days	1 day before symptoms and 7 days after symptoms
Mononucleosis	Epstein-Barr virus	Saliva Person-to-person sharing of personal objects	30–50 days	Virus may be excreted for months after infection
Mumps (parotitis)	Paramyxovirus	Contact with oral and nasal secretions	16–18 days	2–3 days before swelling of glands to 5 days after swelling starts
Pertussis (whooping cough)	*Bordetella pertussis* bacteria	Oral and nasal secretions	6–21 days	Onset of symptoms for about 2 weeks Nonimmunized infants 6 weeks
RSV bronchiolitis	Respiratory syncytial virus	Hands Oral and nasal secretions Lives on surfaces for hours	4–6 days	Viral shedding 3–4 weeks in infants, 3–8 days in older persons
Roseola (*Exanthem subitum*)	Human herpesvirus 6	Saliva of persons who have the disease or who are carrying virus	9–10 days	Unknown
Rubella (German measles)	Rubella virus	Airborne through respiratory droplets Direct contact with respiratory secretions Found in blood, urine, stool	16–18 days	7 days before rash to 14 days after rash Most children contagious 3–4 days before rash to 7 days after rash
Rubeola (measles)	Rubeola virus	Airborne through respiratory droplets Direct contact with respiratory secretions	8–12 days	1–2 days before prodromal symptoms, 3–5 days before rash, 4 days after rash
Strep throat, Scarlet fever	Group A beta-hemolytic streptococcus	Respiratory droplets Direct contact with secretions	2–5 days	Approximately 10 days 24 hours after antibiotics started
Chickenpox (Varicella zoster)	Varicella zoster virus	Fluid from vesicles Oral, nasal, eye secretions Coughing and sneezing	10–21 days	1 day before rash, while rash is spreading, until all vesicles have crusted

SAFE AND EFFECTIVE NURSING CARE: Promoting Safety

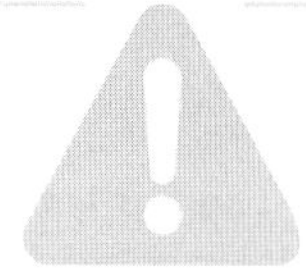

Universal and Standard Precautions

Universal precautions prevent the transmission of HIV, hepatitis B and C, and other blood-borne pathogens. Universal precautions apply to blood, any body fluids that contain blood, semen, and vaginal discharge. Universal precautions provide guidelines for using protective barriers such as gloves, gowns, masks, and eyewear as needed to protect the health-care worker. Guidelines also prevent injuries from needlesticks and other sharp instruments (CDC, 2016).

Standard precautions are more comprehensive than universal precautions and apply to all patients in any setting. Major components of standard precautions include careful hand hygiene, safe injection practices, safe handling of contaminated equipment, and appropriate isolation techniques based on possible exposure to pathogens. Isolation techniques may involve gloves only or may call for gowns, masks (droplet precaution), or eye protection (invasive procedures). Standard precautions also protect the patient by preventing spread of pathogens from health-care providers or equipment to the patient (CDC, 2017g). See Table 22–2 for isolation guidelines in addition to standard precautions.

CRITICAL COMPONENT

Caregiver Education

Situations with an ill child that require emergency medical services include the following (Randolph & McCulloh, 2014):

- Difficulty breathing
- Refusal to lie down
- Blue, gray, or purple tinge on lips or skin
- Fever associated with difficulty breathing or abnormal skin color (pallor, bluish tinge, exceptionally pink)
- Fever with headache or stiff neck
- Behavior changes such as lethargy, acting withdrawn, or becoming more unresponsive
- Seizure activity in a child not known to have seizures and without a plan for managing seizures
- Purple or red rash that is spreading quickly, rash that does not blanch (petechiae)
- Dehydration accompanied by lethargy, sunken eyes, no tears in an infant older than 2 months, decreased urine output
- Vomiting blood, or blood in the stool

Erythema Infectiosum (Fifth Disease)

Erythema infectiosum is commonly referred to as "fifth disease" because it was historically classified as the fifth common red rash in children. Erythema infectiosum commonly affects school-age children 5 to 15 years of age. This rash is a self-limited viral infection but can have persistent lacy rash for several weeks after initial infection.

Disease Process

- Agent: human parvovirus B19 (HPV)
- Transmission: contact with respiratory secretions
- Incubation period: 4 to 21 days
- Communicability: contagious until the rash appears
- Precautions: droplet

Clinical Presentation

- Prodromal: fever, upper respiratory symptoms, headache
- Rash distribution: erythema of the cheeks, giving the appearance of "slapped cheeks." The rash appears after the red cheeks appear and is characterized by a lacy pattern on the trunk and extremities. The rash may disappear and then reappear if the child becomes hot for weeks after the infection (Fig. 22–2).
- Systemic signs and symptoms: no signs or symptoms after the rash has appeared. In adults, there may be pain and swelling of joints (American Academy of Pediatrics [AAP], 2015a).

Diagnostic Testing

Blood testing will reveal the presence of immunoglobulin M (IgM) antibody that indicates immunity to parvovirus B19.

Nursing Interventions

Nursing interventions for patients with fifth disease include emergency care and acute hospital care.

Emergency Care

- Sickle cell crisis may occur with HPV in susceptible persons.

Acute Hospital Care

- Fifth disease may be severe in individuals with immune deficiency disorders.
- A child with HPV who is hospitalized with aplastic crisis or because of immunodeficiency must be placed on droplet precautions.
- A child in aplastic crisis may not have the typical rash, but complain of fever, nausea and vomiting, abdominal pain, malaise, and lethargy.

Caregiver Education

Caregiver education should include the following topics related to Fifth disease.

Emergency Care

- The disease may trigger a crisis in persons with sickle cell disease. It may also trigger aplastic crisis in children who are immunodeficient.

Home Care

- Acetaminophen or ibuprofen for fever or discomfort; adequate hydration

TABLE 22-2 Isolation Guidelines and Standard Precautions

TYPE OF ISOLATION	CONTACT PRECAUTIONS	DROPLET PRECAUTIONS	AIRBORNE PRECAUTIONS
Definition	Prevents disease spread by direct or indirect contact with the patient or patient's environment	Prevents disease spread by close respiratory contact or respiratory secretions	Prevent diseases that remain infectious over long distances, organisms remain suspended in the air
Special equipment	Gown and gloves for contact with patient or contaminated objects and areas in the room Patient-care equipment must be disposable or disinfected after use.	Health-care providers must wear a mask The patient must wear a mask when being transported outside of the room Teach patients to cover mouth with tissue when coughing, dispose of tissue in designated container, wash hands	Health-care providers must wear a mask or respirator depending on specific disease guidelines (refer to Appendix A of CDC isolation guidelines) Airborne infection isolation rooms provide negative pressure, regular air exchanges, and air exhaustion to the outside or to HEPA filters
Considerations	Includes any patient condition with excess wound drainage, body discharges, or fecal incontinence	Pathogens do not remain infectious over long distances; therefore, special ventilation and air handling are not required	Nonimmune health-care providers should not care for these patients
Sample diseases	Bronchiolitis, rotavirus, type A hepatitis in diapered or incontinent patients, impetigo, lice, scabies, poliomyelitis, staphylococcal and streptococcal skin infections Note: smallpox and varicella (chickenpox) require contact and airborne isolation	Influenza, pertussis (whooping cough), *Haemophilus influenzae* type B, epiglottitis or meningitis, meningococcal meningitis, mumps, parvovirus (erythema infectiosum), rubella (German measles), streptococcal group A infections for the first 24 hours, scarlet fever	Measles (rubeola), pulmonary tuberculosis Note: respirators required when caring for patients with tuberculosis Note: smallpox and varicella (chickenpox) require contact and airborne isolation

HEPA, high-efficiency particulate air.

From the Centers for Disease Control and Prevention. (2015). Isolation precautions—Summary of recommendations. *Retrieved from https://www.cdc.gov/infectioncontrol/guidelines/isolation/index.html.*

CRITICAL COMPONENT

Transmission of Fifth Disease to the Fetus

Erythema infectiosum (fifth disease) in pregnant women may be passed on to the fetus and cause severe anemia in the fetus or possible complications such as miscarriage.

- Approximately 50% of pregnant women have had fifth disease in the past and are already immune to parvovirus B19. These women and their fetuses are not affected if exposed. However, all pregnant women should consult their health-care provider if exposure to fifth disease is suspected.
- Less than 5% of pregnant women who are exposed to parvovirus B19 may experience complications, and these usually occur during the first half of the pregnancy.
- To prevent complications from Fifth disease, pregnant women who are in contact with children should practice careful hand hygiene.
- Women of childbearing age can have a blood test to determine whether they have had fifth disease and are therefore immune to this disease (AAP, 2015a; CDC, 2015c).

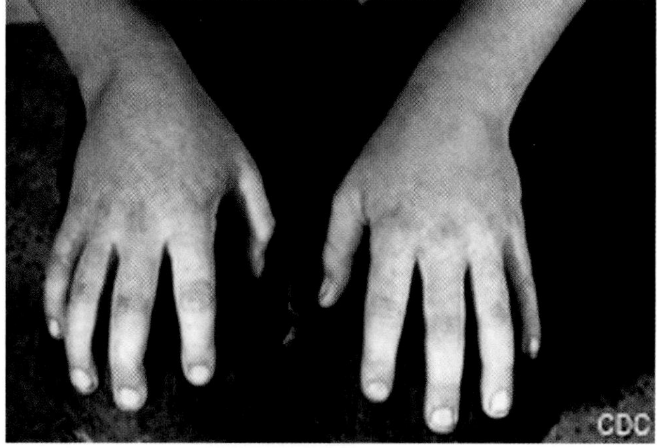

FIGURE 22-2 Child with Fifth disease.

Hand, Foot, and Mouth Disease

Hand, foot, and mouth disease (HFMD) is common among infants and children younger than 10 years. HFMD is a self-limited condition and usually resolves within 10 days without complications. However, the child may have significant difficulty with eating and playing because of the painful lesions to the hands, feet, and mouth. Because multiple strains cause HFMD, children can contract this virus more than once.

Disease Process

- Agent: Coxsackie virus or enterovirus
- Transmission: direct contact, droplet, fecal–oral
- Incubation period: 3 to 6 days
- Communicability: the virus may be shed for several weeks

Clinical Presentation

- Signs and symptoms: cold symptoms, coryza, fever, sore throat
- Small vesicles appear in the mouth and on the palms of the hands and soles of the feet, and may also appear on the genitalia and buttocks (Fig. 22–3)

Diagnostic Testing

- Stool samples and throat swabs can be tested for presence of a virus, but the disease is usually diagnosed clinically.

Caregiver Education

- Careful hand hygiene and disposal of tissues
- Clean surfaces and toys with soap and water, and disinfect with a solution of 1 tablespoon of bleach to 4 cups of water
- Give bland foods and drinks because the mouth may be sore; make sure the child is well hydrated
- Acetaminophen or ibuprofen for pain and fever
- Over-the-counter sprays and mouthwashes that contain local anesthetic to relieve pain in the mouth (CDC, 2017c)

Hepatitis A

Hepatitis A virus (HAV) is a disease process that causes inflammation and decreased liver function. The most common source of HAV is contaminated food or water. Most patients have a mild illness and recover without permanent liver damage within 2 weeks. Longer and more severe disease processes are more common in older children and adults or those with underlying liver issues.

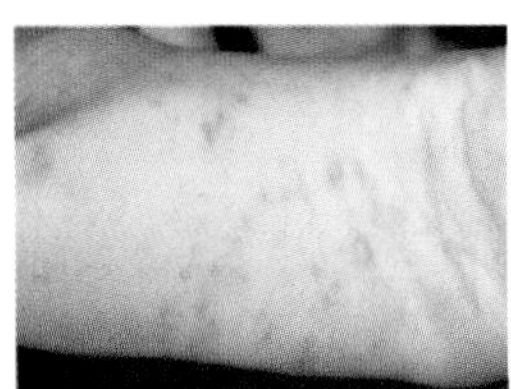

FIGURE 22–3 Blisters in hand, foot, and mouth disease.

Disease Process

- Agent: HAV viral infection
- Transmission: fecal–oral route, contaminated food
- Incubation period: approximately 30 days
- Communicability: most contagious for 2 weeks before onset of symptoms and for 1 week after onset of jaundice

Clinical Presentation

- Fever, malaise, poor appetite, nausea, jaundice, abdominal pain, dark urine
- Children younger than 6 years may have mild or no symptoms; therefore, they may play a significant role in the transmission of HAV

Diagnostic Testing

- Blood test for presence of anti-HAV IgM in the serum
- Other abnormal laboratory work: presence of bilirubin in urine, elevated serum bilirubin, elevated liver enzymes (aspartate transaminase and alanine transaminase)

Nursing Interventions

- Contact isolation if the child is incontinent with feces
- Immune globulin can be given after exposure to prevent or reduce the severity of the disease
- Report incidence to the local health department

Caregiver Education

- Strict hand hygiene and sanitizing of surfaces
- Appropriate rest and activity
- Nutritious, well-balanced diet (Quiros-Tejeira, 2016)

Hepatitis B

Hepatitis B virus (HBV) is a virus that can cause short-term and long-term liver dysfunction. HBV is commonly transmitted through blood or body fluids. Some children younger than 5 years will show no symptoms of HBV; however, 50% of individuals older than 5 will experience signs and symptoms of liver dysfunction and inflammation including jaundice, vomiting, and abdominal pain. The disease process can last from weeks to months; at longer than 6 months, HBV is considered chronic and puts the individual at long-term risk for cirrhosis and liver cancer (CDC, 2015b).

Disease Process

- Agent: HBV viral infection
- Transmission: blood or blood products, sexual contact
- Incubation period: average of 90 days
- Communicability: can be spread as long as the virus is in the blood of an individual; some people are chronic carriers and carry the disease for life

Clinical Presentation

- Symptoms include aching, malaise, joint pain, jaundice, dark urine, loss of appetite, and mild right upper quadrant abdominal pain.
- Children with chronic hepatitis B may be asymptomatic.
- Children with chronic hepatitis B are at risk for development of hepatocellular carcinoma later in life.
- Newborns may acquire HBV perinatally. The CDC (2017f) reports that 40% of infants who do not receive postexposure prophylaxis will experience development of chronic hepatitis B. It is important to administer HBIG in addition to the hepatitis B vaccine if the mother is HBsAg positive.
- High-risk groups among children and adolescents include those living in institutions, those involved in IV drug use, those infected by sexual partners, and children who are hemophiliacs or receive frequent blood transfusions. Individuals who have traveled to Africa or Asia are also at higher risk.

Diagnostic Testing

- Blood tests reveal the HBsAg and the IgM anti-HBc core antibody.
- In chronic hepatitis B, the positive HBsAg persists. Chronic carriers are those who have a positive HBsAg for more than 6 months. HBV DNA markers will also be present.

Nursing Interventions

- Blood-borne precautions (universal precautions)

Caregiver Education

- Teach family members not to share toothbrushes or razors.
- Lifestyle counseling is necessary if risky behaviors such as drug use or sexual activity are present.
- Teach importance of treatment and follow-up.

SAFE AND EFFECTIVE NURSING CARE: Understanding Medication

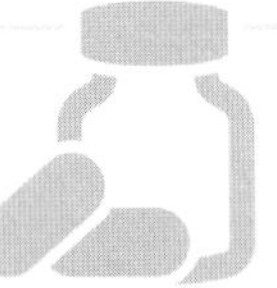

Treatment for Hepatitis B Virus

Two medications may be used for children with chronic HBV:

- Interferon-alpha reduces replication of the HBV virus. It may be given as subcutaneous injection at 6 months. Side effects include fever, aching, joint pain, anorexia, and weight loss.
- Lamivudine inhibits replication of the HBV virus. This drug is given orally, and treatment may last for 1 year. There are fewer side effects than with interferon, but lamivudine may develop resistance (AAP, 2015b; Jonas et al., 2015).

SAFE AND EFFECTIVE NURSING CARE: Cultural Competence

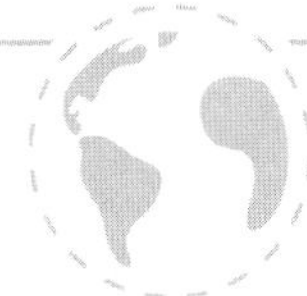

Hepatitis B Among Adoptive Immigrant Children

HBV remains a significant health problem, especially in countries such as Asia and Africa. Approximately 257 million people around the world have HBV. Therefore, nurses and families must be aware that immigrant children and international children who are adopted into families in the United States may have been exposed to this disease. The health history is very important because children may be asymptomatic (WHO, 2017a).

Influenza

Influenza, commonly called the flu, is a very contagious disease process that occurs worldwide annually and is often epidemic. The influenza virus constantly mutates, resulting in new strains annually. The most common months for influenza in the United States are October through May. Most patients have a self-limited disease with common symptoms such as cough, fever, and body aches. However, infants, very young children, those with chronic diseases, and older adults are at increased risk for complications related to the flu, such as pneumonia, encephalitis, myocarditis, pericarditis, and many others. It is important to prevent influenza in all patients, especially individuals in high-risk categories.

Disease Process

- Agent: influenza viruses; influenza may be type A or type B, with type A being much more prevalent
- Transmission: coughing and sneezing; contact with objects contaminated with oral or nasal secretions
- Incubation period: 1 to 4 days
- Communicability: 1 day before symptoms until approximately 7 days after child becomes ill

Clinical Presentation

- Fever, chills, headache, sneezing, cough, malaise, conjunctivitis, and myalgia (aching)

Diagnostic Testing

- Rapid screening for flu virus antigens in nasal secretions

Nursing Interventions

Nursing interventions for influenza among pediatric patients include emergency care and acute hospital care measures.

Emergency Care

- Influenza may trigger croup in infants.

Acute Hospital Care

- Pneumonia is a complication of influenza and may require hospitalization.
- Other complications include ear infections, sinus infections, dehydration, myocarditis, pericarditis, and increased severity of existing medical conditions such as diabetes and asthma.
- Droplet isolation is necessary.

Caregiver Education

- Tylenol or ibuprofen for fever (no aspirin because of risk for Reye syndrome)
- Careful hand washing and disposal of tissues
- Encourage fluids
- Administration of medications within 48 hours of symptoms (see Safe and Effective Nursing Care: Treating Influenza feature)
- Importance of annual influenza immunizations

Complementary and Alternative Therapies

- Multiple herbs, minerals, vitamins, and other treatments may be effective in reducing replication, reducing inflammation, and decreasing length of symptoms for those affected by influenza and other upper respiratory infections. Additional research is needed to identify the safety and efficacy of these therapies (Mousa, 2016).

SAFE AND EFFECTIVE NURSING CARE: Understanding Medication

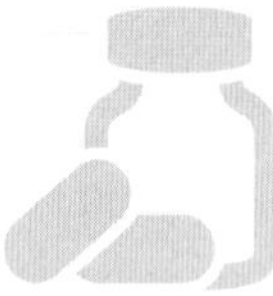

Treating Influenza

Medications for influenza must be given within 48 hours of the onset of symptoms. Two antiviral medications for influenza approved by the U.S. Food and Drug Administration were recommended for the 2016 to 2017 influenza season: oseltamivir (Tamiflu) and zanamivir (Relenza). These medications are effective for both influenza type A and type B. Oseltamivir (Tamiflu) may be given to children older than 1 year and should be given on weight-based dosing. Zanamivir (Relenza) is recommended for children older than 7 years. It is administered as a 10-mg once-daily inhalation medication and is not recommended for children with airway disease such as asthma (AAP Committee on Infectious Diseases, 2016).

Mononucleosis

Mononucleosis is sometimes called mono or the "kissing disease" because it is commonly transmitted through saliva. Mononucleosis is a viral infection caused by the Epstein-Barr virus (EBV); it is most common among adolescent patients but can affect individuals of all ages. This infection results in an increase in white blood cells with a single nucleus, called monocytes or mononuclear lymphocytes. Most patients have a self-limited disease that lasts a few weeks, but rare cases will lead to long-term chronic fatigue syndrome (Cunha, 2017).

Disease Process

- Agent: EBV
- Transmission: person-to-person contact, sharing personal objects such as cups or toothbrushes, through saliva
- Incubation period: 30 to 50 days
- Communicability: virus may be excreted for months after infection

Clinical Presentation

- Fever, sore throat, malaise, pharyngitis, enlarged posterior cervical lymph nodes, with symptoms lasting 1 to 4 weeks (Fig. 22–4)
- May develop splenomegaly or hepatomegaly
- Disease primarily affects adolescents and young adults; children often have very mild symptoms, and adults are usually immune due to previous exposure

Diagnostic Testing

- Positive mono spot test, positive Paul-Bunnell heterophile antibody test, increased lymphocytes, greater than 10% atypical lymphocytes
- EBV antibody titers

Nursing Interventions

- Hospitalization may be needed if the child experiences respiratory distress, abdominal pain with splenomegaly, or dehydration due to inability to swallow adequate fluids.

Caregiver Education

- To prevent injury to spleen, no contact sports for 6 to 8 weeks if spleen is enlarged. Examples of contact sports include basketball, football, soccer, rugby, baseball, boxing, ice hockey, rodeo, wrestling, martial arts, lacrosse, and water polo

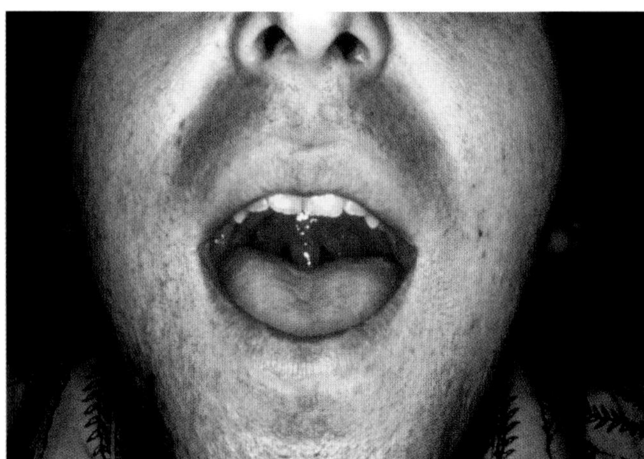

FIGURE 22–4 Pharyngitis in adolescent with mononucleosis.

- Rest, with appropriate quiet activities and play
- Fever management with acetaminophen or ibuprofen
- Hydration and nutrition
- Counseling and emotional support for adolescents who must be on bedrest (Cunha, 2017)

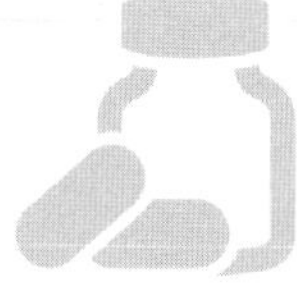

SAFE AND EFFECTIVE NURSING CARE: Understanding Medication

Differentiating Between Mononucleosis and Streptococcal Disease

It may be difficult to distinguish mononucleosis from streptococcal sore throat or pharyngitis. However, health-care providers need to distinguish between the two infections. If ampicillin or amoxicillin is given to an individual with mononucleosis, a maculopapular rash will result.

(Onodi-Nagy et al., 2015)

Mumps (Parotitis)

Mumps is a virus that causes a disease resulting in inflammation primarily of the salivary glands below and in front of the ears. This inflammation can also affect other areas of the body, leading to complications such as sterility in males from orchiditis, hearing loss, encephalitis, and pancreatitis. While the incidence of mumps has significantly declined with immunization, outbreaks continue worldwide, including a significant one in the United States in 2016. Mumps can have systemic symptoms but most commonly present with significant parotid swelling.

Disease Process

- Agent: paramyxovirus
- Transmission: Contact with oral and nasal secretions (droplet spread)
- Incubation period: 16 to 18 days
- Communicability: 2 to 3 days before swelling of salivary glands to 5 days after swelling starts

Clinical Presentation

- Location:
  - Swelling of parotid salivary glands in front of the ear, below the ear, under jaw (Fig. 22–5)
  - Boys may have painful swelling of the testicles (orchitis)
  - Girls may have ovarian involvement with abdominal pain (oophoritis) and breast inflammation (mastitis)
- Systemic signs and symptoms: headache, fever, earache, muscle aches, malaise, loss of appetite

Diagnostic Testing

- IgM enzyme immunoassay is used to detect the mumps virus.

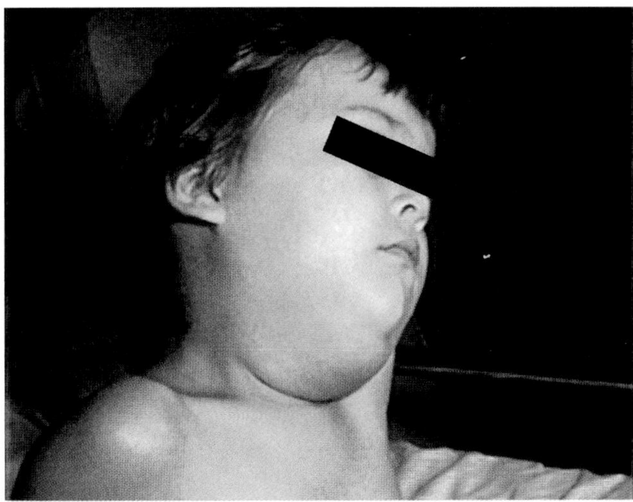

FIGURE 22–5 Child with mumps.

Nursing Interventions

Nursing interventions for patients with the mumps virus include emergency care and acute hospital care.

Emergency Care

- Complications may include meningitis, encephalitis, glomerulonephritis, permanent deafness, sterility, myocarditis, and joint inflammation. Infection during pregnancy may result in fetal death.
- Seek medical care immediately for complications.

Acute Hospital Care

- Droplet spread isolation is required.

Caregiver Education

- Acetaminophen or ibuprofen for fever and pain
- Bland, soft foods
- Bland liquids; avoid citrus juices; keep well hydrated.
- Ice packs or warm compresses to neck for comfort and pain relief
- Snug-fitting underwear and warmth may provide comfort and pain relief for orchitis (CDC, 2015a)

Respiratory Syncytial Virus Bronchiolitis

Respiratory syncytial virus (RSV) is a viral respiratory infection that can affect all ages. RSV is usually well tolerated with symptoms of the common cold in older children, but is the most common cause of bronchiolitis and pneumonia in infants and toddlers. In infants, toddlers, those born prematurely, and those with chronic lung or heart disease, RSV can result in a life-threatening illness. In these individuals, significant respiratory distress, wheezing, and in some cases, respiratory failure can result from RSV. The usual disease process is self-limited to approximately 1 week, with the worst symptoms occurring on days three through five. However, cough and wheezing can persist for up to 3 to 6 weeks after the illness.

Disease Process

- Agent: RSV
- Transmission: contact with saliva and nasal secretions. The virus can live on surfaces for several hours and is readily transmitted by hands.
- Incubation period: This period is usually 4 to 6 days
- Communicability: Viral shedding may last as long as 3 to 4 weeks in infants. In older persons, it is shed for 3 to 8 days.

Clinical Presentation

- Symptoms of a cold in older children: cough, coryza (nasal congestion), fever
- As the disease progresses in infants and young children, there may be respiratory distress with tachypnea, wheezing, retractions, severe coughing, and poor air exchange
- Refer to Chapter 11 for additional information on bronchiolitis.

Diagnostic Testing

- RSV screening

Nursing Interventions

Nursing interventions for RSV include the following measures.

Emergency Care

- The virus may cause respiratory distress in infants and toddlers.
- Emergency treatment may be needed.
- Infants who were born prematurely or who have medical problems such as congenital heart defects are especially vulnerable to the effects of RSV.

Acute Hospital Care

- Hospitalization may be needed for infants with bronchiolitis and pneumonia.
- Contact isolation with gowns and gloves; mask if close to the infant's face
- Frequent assessments of respiratory status
- Schedule activities to allow rest time for infant
- Cool humidified air at bedside
- Administer oxygen as needed
- Hydration with IV fluids if needed

Refer to Chapter 11 for additional information on care of the infant or child with bronchiolitis.

Caregiver Education

- Careful hand hygiene and disposal of tissues
- Cool mist humidifier, hydration
- Do not administer over-the-counter cough/cold products to children younger than 4 years
- Teach parents signs of respiratory distress in an infant and when to seek medical care
- Immunization: infants who are at risk and more vulnerable to RSV due to medical problems may require the palivizumab (Synagis) vaccine to prevent RSV (Ralston et al., 2014)

SAFE AND EFFECTIVE NURSING CARE: Understanding Medication

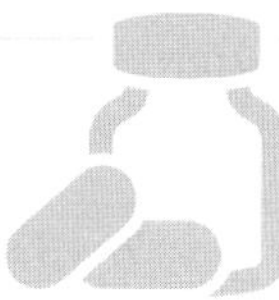

Administration of Palivizumab (Synagis)

The palivizumab (Synagis) vaccine has significantly reduced the incidence of RSV bronchiolitis in infants. This immunization is needed for preterm infants who were born at less than 29 weeks' gestation without chronic lung disease, preterm infants born at 32 weeks' gestation who have chronic lung disease, or children with hemodynamically significant congenital heart disease. The AAP (2015) has given specific guidelines based on gestational ages of infants and risk factors. The dose is given intramuscularly and repeated monthly (every 28 to 30 days) for three to five doses during RSV season. Specific RSV season varies from state to state, but it generally starts in the fall and ends in the spring (AAP, 2015c).

CRITICAL COMPONENT

Signs of Respiratory Distress

Teach parents the signs of respiratory distress for seeking medical care:

- Restlessness, anxiety
- Respiratory rate over 60 in an infant, over 40 in a toddler
- Retractions
- Wheezing
- Distress that increases when lying down
- Breathlessness, gasping, continuous coughing
- Nasal flaring
- Color changes—duskiness around mouth, pallor
- Crowing sound when taking a breath
- Hoarse cry or barking cough

Roseola (Exanthem Subitum, Human Herpes Virus 6)

Roseola is defined as a rose-colored rash and is also called roseola infantum because it is most common among infants and toddlers. Many patients are asymptomatic when they have the virus, but classic presentation of this disease is a high fever that resolves after about 3 to 7 days, after which the rose-colored rash emerges throughout the body. The disease process is usually benign and self-limited, but rarely causes febrile seizures in infants with very high fevers.

Disease Process

- Agent: human herpes virus 6
- Transmission: saliva of persons who have the disease or are carrying the virus; 75% of adults carry the virus in their saliva without symptoms; most people have had roseola by age 4 years

- Incubation period: 9 or 10 days
- Communicability: unknown

Clinical Presentation

- Prodromal: high (potentially as high as 103°F or greater) for 3 to 7 days; the high fever may trigger febrile seizures
- Rash distribution: papular pink or red rash that appears on the day that the fever returns to normal (Fig. 22–6)

Diagnostic Testing

- Typically diagnosed based on the rash. A blood test may look for antibodies.

Nursing Interventions

- Emergency care may be needed for febrile seizures.

Caregiver Education

- Home care includes fever management, sponging with tepid water, and administration of acetaminophen or ibuprofen (Stone, Micali, & Schwartz, 2014).

Rubella (German Measles)

Rubella, sometimes called German measles or 3-day measles, is a contagious viral infection resulting in no symptoms or a mild febrile illness with a rash that lasts approximately 3 days. Rubella infection in infants and children rarely causes significant complications. However, if a pregnant woman is affected, her unborn fetus can develop multiple congenital anomalies such as hearing and vision loss, heart defects, and mental retardation, referred to as congenital rubella syndrome. Given the devastating lifelong consequences to the unborn fetus, it is important that we prevent rubella through adequate immunization.

Disease Process

- Agent: Rubella virus
- Transmission: respiratory droplets or direct contact with respiratory secretions; virus is also found in blood, urine, and stool
- Incubation period: 16 to 18 days
- Communicability: 7 days before rash until 14 days after rash; most children are contagious 3 to 4 days before rash to 7 days after rash

Clinical Presentation

- Prodromal: Children do not have prodromal symptoms. Adolescents may experience mild fever, malaise, sore throat, and headache.
- Rash distribution: Fine red or pink rash that appears on the face first and then spreads downward. The rash lasts approximately 3 days and disappears in the same order that it appeared.
- Systemic signs and symptoms include fever, aching, and posterior cervical lymph nodes tender and swollen (Fig. 22–7).

Caregiver Education

- Home care includes fever management as needed.
- Teach the importance of getting the MMR vaccine before the childbearing years.

CRITICAL COMPONENT

Rubella Infection During Pregnancy

Rubella infection during pregnancy may result in an infant born with congenital rubella syndrome. Problems associated with congenital rubella syndrome are congenital heart defects, congenital cataracts, deafness, mental retardation, miscarriage, and fetal death. These infants may shed the virus and be contagious for 1 year.

(CDC, 2015a)

Rubeola (Measles)

Rubeola is a viral syndrome resulting in a rash for 7 days, often referred to as measles. The disease process is usually a self-limiting moderate illness in most children, presenting with the rash and fever. However, complications such as encephalitis, pneumonia, and death can occur in children younger than 5 years and adults.

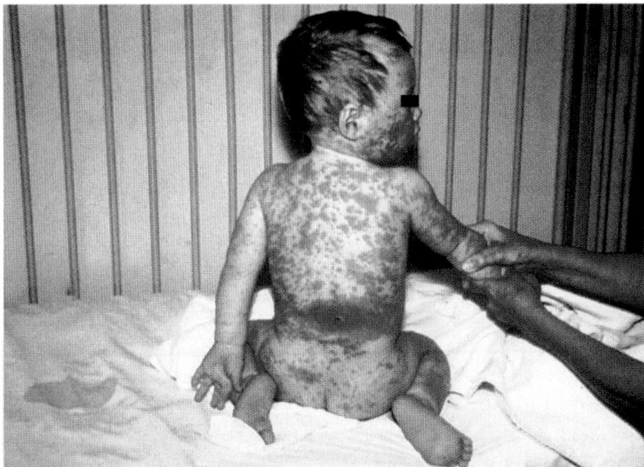

FIGURE 22–6 Child with roseola.

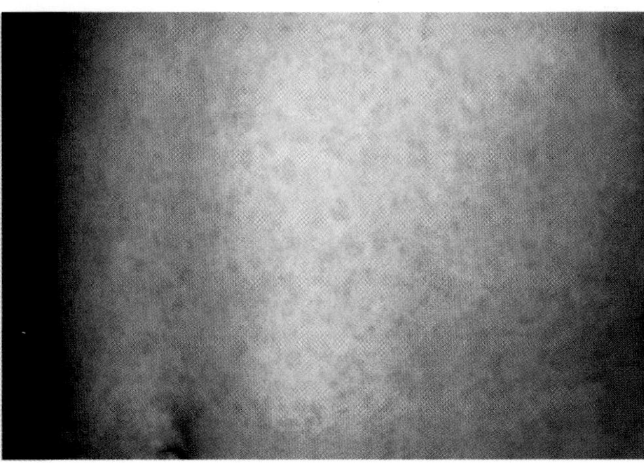

FIGURE 22–7 Child with rubella (German measles).

Prior to immunizations, many children and adults died of complications related to rubeola. Rubeola is still present worldwide and has intermittent outbreaks, most recently in multiple states in the United States in 2017. It is essential to prevent this disease through adequate immunizations to avoid the complications associated with rubeola.

Disease Process

- Agent: measles virus
- Transmission: airborne through respiratory droplets or direct contact with respiratory secretions
- Incubation period: 8 to 12 days
- Communicability: 1 or 2 days before prodromal symptoms, 3 to 5 days before rash, 4 days after rash appears

Clinical Presentation

- Prodromal: coryza, cough, conjunctivitis, fever, malaise; small red spots in the mouth with a bluish white center (Koplik spots; Fig. 22–8)
- Rash distribution: brownish-red macular rash starts at hairline and spreads downward over body
- Systemic signs and symptoms: fever, cough, red, watery eyes, coryza (Fig. 22–9)

Diagnostic Testing

- Blood test to detect antibodies

Nursing Interventions

Nursing interventions for measles include the following measures.

Emergency Care

- Complications include ear infections, diarrhea, encephalitis, pneumonia, seizures, deafness, mental retardation, and death. Seek medical care immediately for complications.

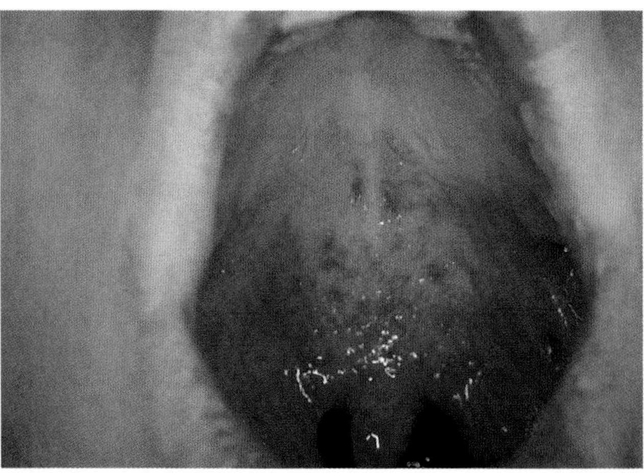

FIGURE 22–8 Koplik spots.

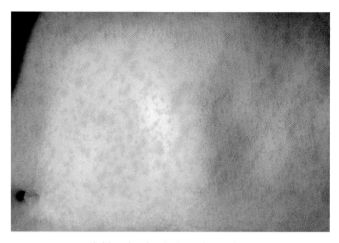

FIGURE 22–9 Child with rubeola (measles) rash.

Acute Hospital Care

- Airborne isolation is required.

Chronic Home Care

- Long-term care, including ventilator care, may be needed for children with brain damage resulting from measles encephalitis.

Caregiver Education

- Manage fever with acetaminophen or ibuprofen.
- Keep child isolated for 5 days after rash appears.
- Dim lights if photophobia exists. Use warm compresses to remove crusting from eyes as needed.
- Give soft, bland foods.
- Keep child well hydrated with plenty of fluids.
- Use cool mist humidifier.

SAFE AND EFFECTIVE NURSING CARE: Cultural Competence

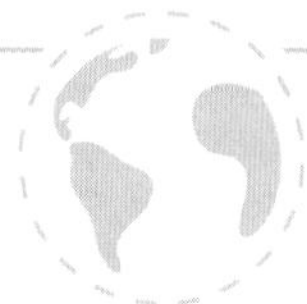

Incidence of Measles Worldwide

Measles is one of the leading causes of death among young children worldwide with an estimated 135,000 people dying of measles in 2015, and it is estimated that measles vaccination prevented 20 million deaths from 2000 to 2015 (WHO, 2017b). Outbreaks of measles in the United States occur in regions with under-vaccination and when travelers or immigrants who have not been immunized in their home countries enter the United States (CDC, 2017e). In recent years, multiple outbreaks have occurred in the United States, the largest occurring in 2014 with 667 cases of measles in multiple states linked to an amusement park in California (CDC, 2017e). It is always important to check immunization records and promote adequate immunization domestically and worldwide.

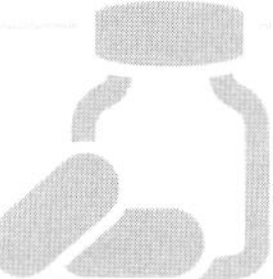

SAFE AND EFFECTIVE NURSING CARE: Understanding Medication

Use of Immune Globulin After Exposure to Measles

- Immune globulin may prevent measles or lessen the severity of the case in unimmunized individuals if given within 6 days of exposure.
- This is especially helpful for infants younger than 6 months, pregnant women, and those who are immunocompromised (CDC, 2015a).

Evidence-Based Practice: Measles and Vitamin A

Bester, J. (2016). Measles and measles vaccination. *JAMA Pediatrics, 170*(12), 1209–1215. doi: 10.1001/jamapediatrics.2016.1787

The World Health Organization has recommended two doses of vitamin A to reduce complications and death from measles in areas of the world where vitamin A deficiency may be present. The recommended dose is 100,000 IU daily for 2 days in infants and 200,000 IU daily for 2 days in older children. A systematic review and meta-analysis by the Cochrane Database of Systematic Reviews found that vitamin A therapy reduced the risk for complications, pneumonia, and death in children younger than 2 years.

Varicella Zoster (Chickenpox)

Varicella zoster virus (VZV) most commonly causes chickenpox in children and rarely may cause shingles. VZV infection most commonly presents in children with the classic rash of maculopapular lesions that begins on the head or trunk, progressing quickly to vesicles with eventual crusting and resolution. The key finding in VZV infection is lesions in all different stages of formation and healing. The most distressing symptom for patients is often the severe pruritus, which can result in scarring or secondary bacterial infections. After initial infection with VZV, the virus lays dormant in the nervous system, often for years. But in some cases, during periods of weakened immune system such as stress, the VZV will result in a secondary infection of shingles in older children and adults. Given the burden of the disease and potential complications, it is essential to prevent this disease process through adequate immunization.

Disease Process

- Agent: VZV
- Transmission: fluid from vesicles of an infected person; secretions from nose, mouth, and eyes; airborne from coughing and sneezing
- Incubation period: 10 to 21 days
- Communicability: 1 day before rash appears, while rash is spreading, and until all vesicles have crusted over

Clinical Presentation

- Prodromal: fever, malaise, coryza
- Rash distribution: The rash first appears on the trunk and face, then spreads to other parts of the body. The rash goes through the stages of macule, papule, vesicle, and scab (crust). All stages are present at the same time. Severe itching may be present (Fig. 22–10).
- Systemic signs and symptoms: fever, headache, dehydration

Diagnostic Testing

- Typically diagnosed by visualizing rash

Nursing Interventions

Nursing interventions for chickenpox include emergency care and acute hospital care.

Emergency Care

- Complications may include bacterial infections of the skin, pneumonia, septicemia, encephalitis, and bleeding problems. Urgent medical care is needed for any complications.

Acute Hospital Care

- Children with chickenpox are not generally hospitalized unless the child is immunocompromised or experiencing complications; IV acyclovir may be given to children in these situations

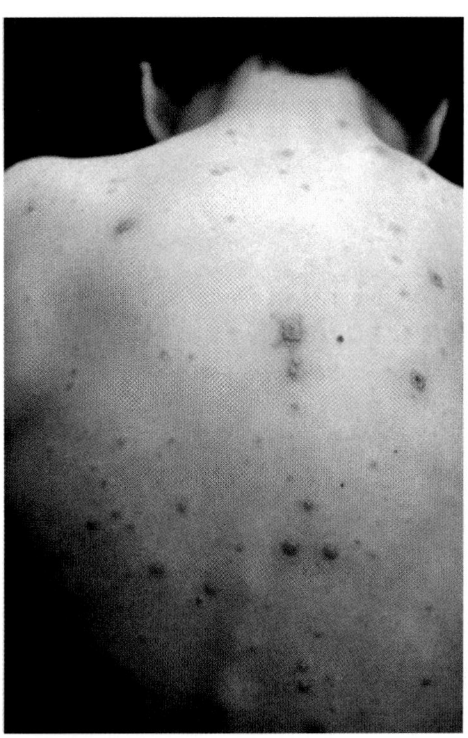

FIGURE 22–10 Child with chickenpox.

- Strict isolation for the hospitalized child, including contact and airborne isolation

Special Considerations

- It is possible to get chickenpox twice. The second case is usually mild, with less fever and few vesicles. Care is the same as for the first case of chickenpox.
- A small percentage of people who receive the chickenpox vaccine get chickenpox, but the disease is mild with fewer lesions. Risk of breakthrough is higher if varicella vaccine is given less than 30 days after the MMR vaccine. Varicella vaccination should be given simultaneously with MMR or longer than 30 days from MMR.
- It is possible to have a mild rash with a few vesicles around the injection site after varicella immunization. These vesicles must be covered with clothing or a nonporous bandage to prevent spread to others. Isolation may be needed if the rash is more widespread.

Caregiver Education

- Use acetaminophen to relieve fever. Aspirin or any medication that contains salicylates should never be used because of the risk for Reye syndrome. The caregiver should receive education on the signs and symptoms of this syndrome.
- Keep child isolated until all vesicles have crusted over.
- Keep the child well hydrated. Offer cool, bland liquids because the inside of the mouth may be affected.
- To help prevent itching, keep child cool, dressed in light cotton, and distracted with play activities. Apply gloves or mittens if necessary; keep fingernails clean and cut short.
- Aveeno (oatmeal powder) or baking soda baths may bring relief.
- Apply calamine or Cetaphil lotion to lesions.

Complementary and Alternative Therapies

- Capsaicin may be used to relieve the pain of shingles (herpes zoster) (CDC, 2015a).

SAFE AND EFFECTIVE NURSING CARE: Promoting Safety

Reye Syndrome

Reye syndrome is a life-threatening disease that primarily affects the brain and liver. It typically follows a viral infection such as chickenpox, influenza, or an upper respiratory infection. The ingestion of aspirin or other medication that contains salicylates during a viral illness greatly increases the probability of development of Reye syndrome. It is important to teach caregivers not to give aspirin or salicylate products to any child or adolescent during a febrile illness.

SAFE AND EFFECTIVE NURSING CARE: Understanding Medication

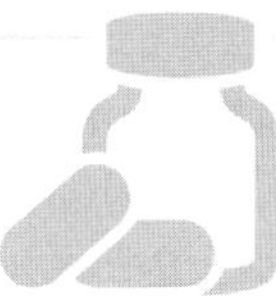

Ibuprofen Administration

Ibuprofen should never be given to infants younger than 6 months secondary to immature renal function that takes 6 to 12 months to reach adult activity. Use of ibuprofen can cause reduction of kidney function (Ziesenitz, Zutter, Erb, & van den Anker, 2017).

CRITICAL COMPONENT

Shingles (Herpes Zoster)

Shingles (herpes zoster) occurs when the VZV that causes chickenpox becomes reactivated in the nervous system, causing a painful, blistering rash in the portion of skin supplied by a particular nerve fiber (dermatome). The person has already completely recovered from chickenpox and the virus that was inactive (latent) becomes active, often years after having chickenpox. Educate caregivers that a child cannot get shingles from someone with chickenpox. However, a child may contract chickenpox from an individual with shingles if there is direct contact with uncovered lesions. Shingles lesions must be covered to prevent spread. It is contagious until all lesions are crusted over (CDC, 2015a).

SAFE AND EFFECTIVE NURSING CARE: Promoting Safety

The Role of Hand Hygiene

The key to preventing the spread of communicable disease is careful hand hygiene. Hands must always be washed before and after caring for infants and children. Caregivers and children must be taught to wash hands before eating and handling food, after using the bathroom or changing diapers, after handling animals, after playing in water or in the sand, and after using tissues to wipe eyes or noses.

BACTERIAL COMMUNICABLE DISEASES

Bacterial communicable diseases are highly contagious, resulting in outbreaks throughout the year, especially in schools, daycare centers, and crowded living conditions. These diseases can often be treated with antibiotics, good hygiene practices, and

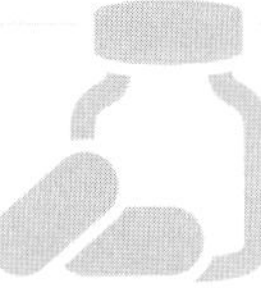

SAFE AND EFFECTIVE NURSING CARE: Understanding Medication

Over-the-Counter Drugs

The AAP urges health-care providers and caregivers to use caution in administering over-the-counter cough and cold medications to young children. Serious side effects have been observed, and studies indicate that cold medications are not effective for children younger than 6 years. In addition, use of these medications may delay important care needed by children. The AAP recommends the use of home remedies such as cool mist humidifiers, saline nose drops, and suctioning bulbs to clear the nares (Lowry & Leeder, 2015).

symptomatic care. Many of these diseases are common in the community but must be treated appropriately to prevent complications in children and adolescents.

Conjunctivitis (Pinkeye)

Conjunctivitis is a disease process that results in erythema and edema of the conjunctiva of the eye, as well as thick, purulent drainage in the case of bacterial infection. Multiple bacteria can result in conjunctivitis, but the most common causes in children are respiratory and skin bacteria such as staphylococcal and streptococcal bacteria. In neonates, sexually transmitted diseases such as herpes simplex virus, gonorrhea, or chlamydia can result in conjunctivitis, which can lead to more serious infections. Most conjunctivitis infections resolve with appropriate treatment. Complications such as vision loss, eye infection, and periorbital cellulitis are rare but significant. It is important for nurses to educate families on conjunctivitis prevention and prompt treatment of eye symptoms.

Disease Process

- Agent: virus or bacteria
- Transmission: contact with discharge from an infected eye, either direct contact or by touching contaminated surfaces
- Communicability: varies depending on organism

Clinical Presentation

- Viral infection: pink or red conjunctiva, edema, watery discharge (Fig. 22–11); may affect only one eye
- Bacterial infection: pink or red conjunctiva, edema, purulent discharge, crusted eyelids in the morning, complaints of itching or pain

Nursing Interventions

- Teach administration of eyedrops as ordered for bacterial infections.

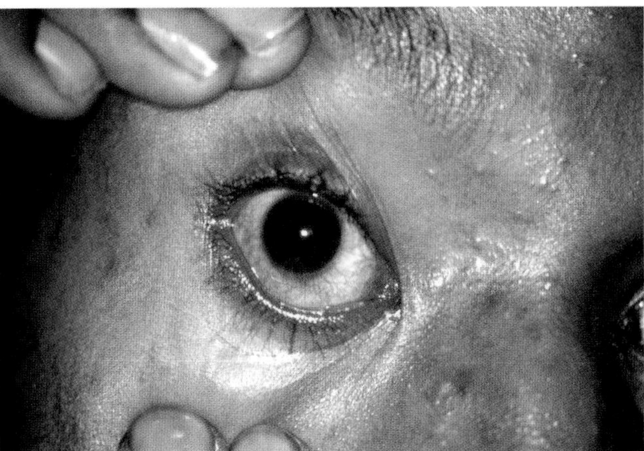

FIGURE 22–11 Child with conjunctivitis.

- If conjunctivitis develops in two or more children in the same setting (home or school), the cause may be adenovirus. This may cause epidemics in school or group settings.

Caregiver Education

- Avoid touching eyes, wash hands carefully after touching eyes, sanitize objects that have been touched by eyes or hands, discard tissues that are used to wipe eyes, and administer eyedrops as ordered.

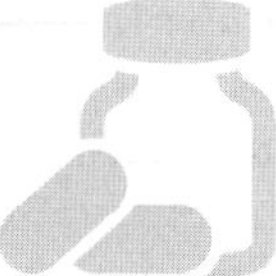

SAFE AND EFFECTIVE NURSING CARE: Understanding Medication

Administering Eyedrops

- Perform hand hygiene.
- Draw the correct amount of medication into the dropper. Do not touch the dropper to the eye or any other surface. The dropper must remain sterile.
- Tilt the child's head back and pull down the lower eyelid. The child can be instructed to look up at the ceiling.
- Squeeze the correct number of medication drops into the pouch formed by pulling down the lower eyelid.
- Allow the child to close the eye. Gently press the tear duct situated in the inner corner of the eye.
- Gently wipe off excess solution with a clean cotton ball or gauze pad.
- Perform hand hygiene.

Pertussis (Whooping Cough)

Pertussis is also known as whooping cough because it causes a characteristic "whoop" sound after paroxysmal coughing fits. In older children and adults, pertussis is usually well tolerated. In infants and very young children, however, this virus often results in a severe respiratory illness that can cause respiratory failure and death. This disease mainly affects babies or children who are not immunized or not fully immunized. Pertussis begins with similar symptoms to a common upper respiratory infection, followed by an increase in symptoms that include the classic paroxysmal coughing fits with posttussive inspiratory whoop and vomiting. Pertussis can cause persistent symptoms for several weeks. Given the consequences to the very young, recent recommendations from the CDC promote a vaccine net of protection around these at-risk infants.

Disease Process

- Agent: *Bordetella pertussis*
- Transmission: oral and nasal secretions
- Incubation period: 6 to 21 days
- Communicability: contagious from the onset of symptoms and for about 2 weeks; infants who have not been immunized may be contagious for at least 6 weeks
- The disease is most dangerous to young infants

Clinical Presentation

- Catarrhal phase that lasts 1 to 2 weeks: cold symptoms, including coryza, mild cough, and fever
- Paroxysmal phase that lasts 1 to 6 weeks or longer: cough ends with crowing (whooping) and may be severe enough to cause vomiting and cyanosis; the classic whoop may not occur in an infant; respiratory distress may be severe
- Recovery phase when cough gradually becomes less severe
- In some children, adolescents, and adults, pertussis may present as a chronic cough that lasts for weeks; the crowing or whooping may not always be present
- Pertussis is becoming more common among adolescents and adults

Diagnostic Testing

- The polymerase chain reaction test identifies genetic material of the *B. pertussis* bacteria in nasal secretions.

Nursing Interventions

- Infants have more severe cases of pertussis and may require hospitalization to manage respiratory distress and dehydration.

Caregiver Education

- Give small amounts of fluid frequently to keep the child hydrated, especially during bouts of vomiting. Refeed or give small amounts of fluid after episodes of coughing and vomiting.
- Teach signs of respiratory distress and dehydration, and urge parents to seek medical care as needed.
- Provide for rest and quiet activities, and avoid stimuli that trigger coughing.
- Use a cool mist humidifier.

CRITICAL COMPONENT

Signs of Dehydration

Teach parents the signs of dehydration for seeking medical care:

- Lethargy
- No tears when crying if older than 2 months
- For young infant, less than five or six wet diapers in 24 hours
- Eyes sunken
- Skin not elastic (poor skin turgor)
- Fontanel sunken

SAFE AND EFFECTIVE NURSING CARE: Understanding Medication

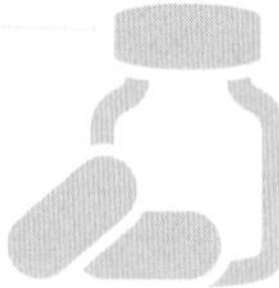

Antibiotic Therapy

Pertussis must be treated with azithromycin (Zithromax), erythromycin, or clarithromycin. Treatment should be started before 21 days into the illness.

SAFE AND EFFECTIVE NURSING CARE: Clinical Pearl

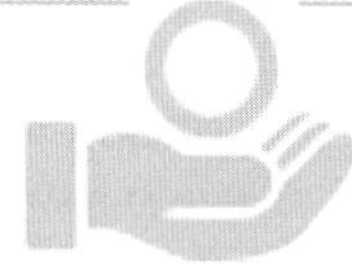

Increased Incidence of Pertussis

In recent years, there has been a significant increase in pertussis incidence in infants, adolescents, and adults. It is now recommended that adolescents 11 to 18 years of age who have completed the recommended DTaP series and adults who have close contact with children receive a single dose of Tdap vaccine. In addition, it is now recommended that pregnant women receive a single dose of Tdap between 27 and 36 weeks' gestation to maximize passive antibody transfer to the infant (CDC, 2015a).

Strep Throat/Scarlet Fever

Strep throat, also known as strep pharyngitis, group A beta-hemolytic streptococcus, or Scarlet fever, is a bacterial infection resulting from group A beta-hemolytic streptococcus. The disease affects all ages but is more common in children older than 2 years, especially school-age children. Strep throat has an abrupt onset of symptoms including a severe sore throat, headache, stomachache, and possible rash called a sandpaper rash (fine, maculopapular, rough rash that occurs especially in the groin, axilla, and neck folds). In some children, the symptoms of strep are subtle, so a good history and physical examination are essential for these children. Prevention and treatment are essential to prevent complications such as rheumatic fever.

Disease Process

- Agent: group A beta-hemolytic streptococcus; causes Group A Streptococcus (GAS) pharyngitis (Fig. 22–12) and may also cause impetigo
- Complications of group A beta-hemolytic streptococcus include rheumatic fever and poststreptococcal glomerulonephritis; please refer to Chapters 12 and 16 for additional information on these diseases
- Transmission: droplet spread, direct contact with secretions
- Incubation period: 2 to 5 days
- Communicability: approximately 10 days without treatment; no longer contagious after 24 hours on antibiotics

Clinical Presentation

- Presentation includes sore throat, fever, headache, enlarged and tender anterior cervical and tonsillar lymph nodes, abdominal pain, and decreased appetite.
- Cough and coryza are not major signs of strep throat. If a child has nasal congestion, the sore throat is likely caused by another organism.
- Children younger than 3 years may have a streptococcal infection without complaining of a sore throat. Symptoms may include fever, irritability, and nasal discharge.
- Scarlet fever is strep throat with a fine, red rash (Fig. 22–13) that has the texture of sandpaper. The rash is more pronounced in the armpits and groin, in the creases of the elbows, and behind the knees. After the rash fades, the skin of the fingers and toes may peel. There may be pallor around the mouth and a white tongue with swollen, red papillae (strawberry tongue; Fig. 22–14).

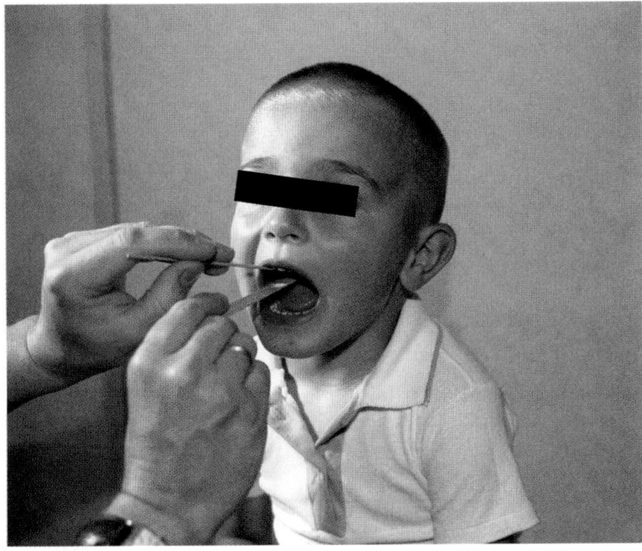

FIGURE 22–12 Child with streptococcal pharyngitis.

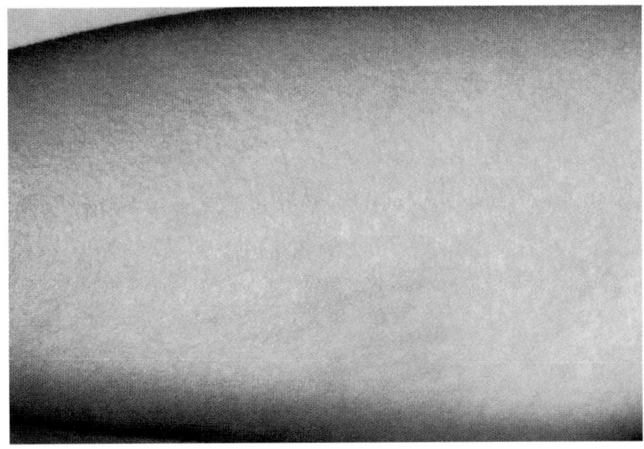

FIGURE 22–13 Child with rash from scarlet fever.

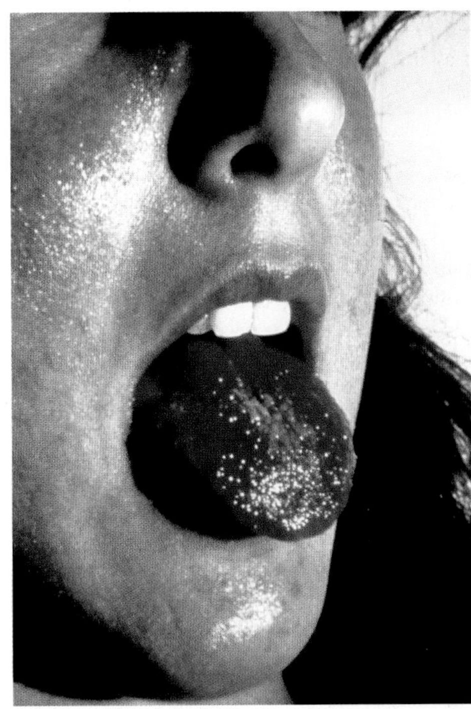

FIGURE 22–14 Child with strawberry tongue.

Diagnostic Testing

- Rapid strep test, throat culture

Nursing Interventions

- Complications of untreated strep throat include glomerulonephritis and rheumatic fever.

Caregiver Education

- Administration of penicillin or amoxicillin as ordered
- Fluids to keep the child hydrated—soups, popsicles, milkshakes

- Cool mist humidifier
- Acetaminophen or ibuprofen for pain and fever
- Replace toothbrush
- Throat lozenges

Complementary and Alternative Therapies

- Saltwater gargles (Bochner, Gangar, & Belamarich, 2017)

See Table 22–1 or refer to Chapter 21 for information on communicable diseases of the skin, refer to Chapter 11 for additional information on bronchiolitis and TB, and refer to Chapter 18 for information on sexually transmitted infections.

Case Study

Keeping Immunizations Current

Immunizations have significantly decreased the incidence of communicable diseases and have helped to keep children well. However, keeping immunization schedules up to date is an ongoing challenge for nurses. The nurse sees multiple children in her pediatric clinic who are not caught up on their immunizations. She is asked by one of the other providers to identify ways to improve immunizations for individual patients and for the community as a whole.

1. What are some creative ways nurses could promote immunizations among children and adolescents?
2. What are some barriers to keeping children immunized?
3. Could combination vaccines be one answer to keeping immunization schedules up to date?
4. How do you overcome vaccine hesitancy in parents who do not wish to immunize their children?

REFERENCES

American Academy of Pediatrics (AAP). (2015a). Parvovirus B19. In D. Kimberlin, M. Brady, M. Jackson, & S. Long (Eds.), *Red Book: 2015 Report of the Committee of Infectious Diseases* (30th ed., pp. 593–596). Elk Grove Village, IL: American Academy of Pediatrics.

American Academy of Pediatrics (AAP). (2015b). Hepatitis B. In D. Kimberlin, M. Brady, M. Jackson, & S. Long (Eds.), *Red Book: 2015 Report of the Committee of Infectious Diseases* (30th ed., pp. 400–423). Elk Grove Village, IL: American Academy of Pediatrics.

American Academy of Pediatrics (AAP). (2015c). Respiratory syncytial virus. In D. Kimberlin, M., Brady, M., Jackson, & S. Long (Eds.), *Red Book: 2015 Report of the Committee of Infectious Diseases* (30th ed., pp. 667–676). Elk Grove Village, IL: American Academy of Pediatrics.

American Academy of Pediatrics (AAP) Committee on Infectious Diseases. (2016). Recommendations for prevention and control of influenza in children, 2016-2017. *Pediatrics, 138*(4), 1–18. doi: 10.1542/peds.2016-2527

Bester, J. (2016). Measles and measles vaccination. *JAMA Pediatrics, 170*(12), 1209–1215. doi: 10.1001/jamapediatrics.2016.1787

Bochner, R., Gangar, M., & Belamarich, P. (2017). A clinical approach to tonsillitis, tonsillar hypertrophy, and peritonsillar and retropharyngeal abscesses. *Pediatrics in Review, 38*(2), 81–92. doi: 10.1542/pir.2016-0072

Centers for Disease Control and Prevention (CDC). (2015a). *Epidemiology and prevention of vaccine-preventable diseases* (13th ed.). Washington DC: Public Health Foundation.

Centers for Disease Control and Prevention (CDC). (2015b). *Isolation precautions.* Retrieved from https://www.cdc.gov/infectioncontrol/guidelines/isolation/index.html

Centers for Disease Control and Prevention (CDC). (2015c). *Parvovirus B19 and fifth disease.* Retrieved from https://www.cdc.gov/parvovirusb19/index.html

Centers for Disease Control and Prevention (CDC). (2016). *Bloodborne infectious diseases: HIV/AIDS, hepatitis B, hepatitis C.* Retrieved from http://www.cdc.gov/niosh/topics/bbp/universal.html

Centers for Disease Control and Prevention (CDC). (2017a). *Child and adolescent schedule.* Retrieved from https://www.cdc.gov/vaccines/schedules/hcp/imz/child-adolescent.html

Centers for Disease Control and Prevention (CDC). (2017b). *Contraindications and precautions.* Retrieved from https://www.cdc.gov/vaccines/hcp/acip-recs/contraindications.html

Centers for Disease Control and Prevention (CDC). (2017c). *Hand, foot, and mouth disease (HFMD).* Retrieved from https://www.cdc.gov/hand-foot-mouth/index.html

Centers for Disease Control and Prevention (CDC). (2017d). *Manual for the surveillance of vaccine-preventable diseases.* Atlanta, GA: Centers for Disease Control and Prevention. Retrieved from https://www.cdc.gov/vaccines/pubs/surv-manual/index.html

Centers for Disease Control and Prevention (CDC). (2017e). *Measles cases and outbreaks.* Retrieved from https://www.cdc.gov/measles/cases-outbreaks.html

Centers for Disease Control and Prevention (CDC). (2017f). *Perinatal transmission.* Retrieved from https://www.cdc.gov/hepatitis/hbv/perinatalxmtn.htm

Centers for Disease Control and Prevention (CDC). (2017g). *Standard precautions for all patient care.* Retrieved from https://www.cdc.gov/infectioncontrol/basics/standard-precautions.html

Centers for Disease Control and Prevention (CDC). (2017h). *What would happen if we stopped vaccinations?* Retrieved from https://www.cdc.gov/vaccines/vac-gen/whatifstop.htm

Cunha, B. (2017). Epstein-Barr virus: Infectious mononucleosis. *Medscape,* 1–18. Retrieved from http://emedicine.medscape.com/article/222040-overview

Grohskopf, L, Sokolow, L., Broder, K., Olsen, S., Karron, R., Jernigan, D., & Bresee, J. (2016). Prevention and control of seasonal influenza with vaccine recommendations of the advisory committee on immunization practices—United States, 2016-2017 influenza season. *Morbidity and Mortality Weekly Report, 65*(5), 1–54. Retrieved from https://www.cdc.gov/mmwr/volumes/65/rr/rr6505a1.htm

Jain, A., Marshall, J., Buikema, A., Bancroft, T., Kelly, J. P., & Newschaffer, C. J. (2015). Autism occurrence by MMR vaccine status among US children with older siblings with and without autism. *Journal of the American Medical Association, 313*(15), 1534–1540. doi: 10.1001/jama.2015.3077

Jonas, M., Lok, A., McMahon, B., Brown, R., Wong, J., Ahmed, A., ... Mohammed, K. (2015). Antiviral therapy in management of chronic hepatitis B viral infection in children: A systematic review and meta-analysis. *Hepatology, 63*(1), 307–318. doi: 10.1002/hep.28278

Lowry, J., & Leeder, S. (2015). Over-the-counter medications: Update on cough and cold preparations. *Pediatrics in Review, 36*(7), 286–298. doi: 10.1542/pir.36-7-286

Maglione, M., Das, L., Raaen, L., Smith, A., Chari, R., Newberry, S., ... Gidengil, C. (2014). Safety of vaccines used for routine immunization of US children: A systematic review. *Pediatrics, 134*(2), 325–337. doi: 10.1542/peds.2014-1079

Mousa, H. (2016). Prevention and treatment of influenza, influenza-like illness, and common cold by herbal, complementary, and natural therapies. *Journal of Evidence-Based Complementary and Alternative Medicine, 22*(1), 166–174. doi: 10.1177/2156587216641831

Onodi-Nagy, K., Kinyo, A., Meszes, A., Garaczi, E., Kemeny, L., & Bata-Csorgo, Z. (2015). Amoxicillin rash in patients with infectious mononucleosis: Evidence of true drug sensitization. *Allergy, Asthma & Clinical Immunology, 11*(1), 1–4. doi: 10.1186/1710-1492-11-1

Patton, M. E., Stephens, D., Moore, K., & MacNeil, J. R. (2017). Updated recommendations for use of MenB-FHbp Serogroup B meningococcal vaccine—Advisory committee on immunization practices, 2016. *MMWR Morbidity and Mortality Weekly Report, 66,* 509–513. doi: 10.15585/mmwr.mm6619a6

Quiros-Tejeira, R. (2016). Hepatitis A—A virus infection in children. *UpToDate.* Retrieved from http://www.uptodate.com/contents/overview-of-hepatitis-a-virus-infection-in-children

Ralston, S., Lieberthal, A., Meissner, H., Alverson, B., Baley, J., Gadornski, A., … Hernandez-Cancio, S. (2014). Clinical practice guideline: The diagnosis, management, and prevention of bronchiolitis. *Pediatrics, 134*(5), e1474–e1502. doi: 10.1542/peds.2014-2742

Randolph, A., & McCulloh, R. (2014). Pediatric sepsis. *Virulence, 5*(1), 179–189. doi: 10.416/viru.27045

Stevens, K., & Marvicsin, D. (2016). Evidence-based recommendations for reducing pediatric distress during vaccination. *Pediatric Nursing, 42*(6), 267–276. Retrieved from http://bd4uz2kj6y.search.serialssolutions.com/?rft.title=Pediatric+nursing&SS_issnh=0097-9805&issn=0097-9805&url_ver=Z39.88-2004&l=BD4UZ2KJ6Y&SS_LibHash=BD4UZ2KJ6Y&SS_ReferentFormat=JournalFormat&rft.genre=article&rft.issn=0097-9805&rft_val_fmt=info%3Aofi%2Ffmt%3Akev%3Amtx%3Ajournal&rft.atitle=evidence-based+recommendations+for+reducing+pediatric+distress+during+vaccination

Stone, R., Micali, G., & Schwartz, R. (2014). Roseola infantum and is causal human herpesvirus. *International Journal of Dermatology, 53*(4), 397–403. doi: 10.1111/ijd.12310

World Health Organization (WHO). (2017a). *Hepatitis.* Retrieved from http://www.who.int/mediacentre/factsheets/fs204/en/

World Health Organization (WHO). (2017b). *Measles.* Retrieved from http://www.who.int/mediacentre/factsheets/fs286/en/

Wysocki, J., Center, K., Brzostek, J., Majda-Stanislwska, E., Szymanski, H., Szenborn, L., … Gurtman, A. (2017). A randomized study of fever prophylaxis and the immunogenicity of routine pediatric vaccinations. *Vaccine, 35*, 1926–1935. doi: 10.1016/j.vaccine.2017.02.035

Ziesenitz, V., Zutter, A., Erb, T., & van den Anker, J. (2017). Efficacy and safety of ibuprofen in infants aged between 3 and 6 months. *Pediatrica Drugs, 19*, 277–290. doi: 10.1007/s40272-017-0235-3

APPENDIX

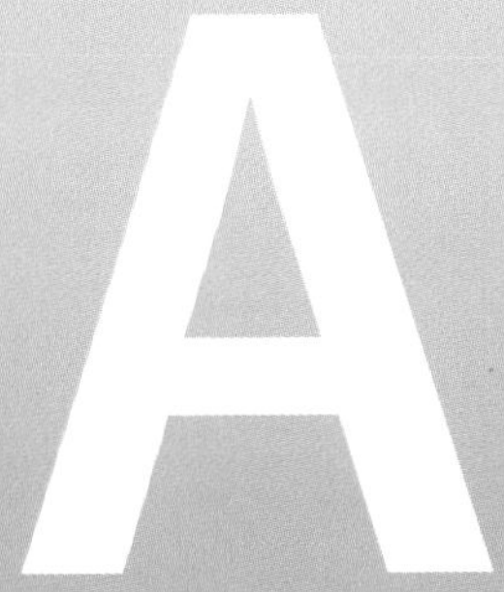

Asthma Action Plan

Asthma Action Plan

For: ______ Doctor: ______ Date: ______

Doctor's Phone Number ______ Hospital/Emergency Department Phone Number ______

GREEN ZONE

Doing Well

- No cough, wheeze, chest tightness, or shortness of breath during the day or night
- Can do usual activities

And, if a peak flow meter is used,

Peak flow: more than ______
(80 percent or more of my best peak flow)

My best peak flow is: ______

Take these long-term control medicines each day (include an anti-inflammatory).

Medicine	**How much to take**	**When to take it**

Before exercise	❒ ______	❒ 2 or ❒ 4 puffs ______	5 minutes before exercise

YELLOW ZONE

Asthma Is Getting Worse

- Cough, wheeze, chest tightness, or shortness of breath, or
- Waking at night due to asthma, or
- Can do some, but not all, usual activities

-Or-

Peak flow: ______ to ______
(50 to 79 percent of my best peak flow)

First

Add: quick-relief medicine—and keep taking your GREEN ZONE medicine.

______ (short-acting beta$_2$-agonist) ❒ 2 or ❒ 4 puffs, every 20 minutes for up to 1 hour
❒ Nebulizer, once

Second

If your symptoms (and peak flow, if used) return to GREEN ZONE after 1 hour of above treatment:
❒ Continue monitoring to be sure you stay in the green zone.

-Or-

If your symptoms (and peak flow, if used) do not return to GREEN ZONE after 1 hour of above treatment:
❒ Take: ______ (short-acting beta$_2$-agonist) ❒ 2 or ❒ 4 puffs or ❒ Nebulizer
❒ Add: ______ (oral steroid) mg per day For ______(3–10) days
❒ Call the doctor ❒ before/ ❒ within ______ hours after taking the oral steroid.

RED ZONE

Medical Alert!

- Very short of breath, or
- Quick-relief medicines have not helped, or
- Cannot do usual activities, or
- Symptoms are same or get worse after 24 hours in Yellow Zone

-Or-

Peak flow: less than ______
(50 percent of my best peak flow)

Take this medicine:

❒ ______ (short-acting beta$_2$-agonist) ❒ 4 or ❒ 6 puffs or ❒ Nebulizer

❒ ______ (oral steroid) mg

Then call your doctor NOW. Go to the hospital or call an ambulance if:
- You are still in the red zone after 15 minutes AND
- You have not reached your doctor.

DANGER SIGNS
- **Trouble walking and talking due to shortness of breath**
- **Lips or fingernails are blue**

- **Take ❒ 4 or ❒ 6 puffs of your quick-relief medicine AND**
- **Go to the hospital or call for an ambulance** ______ (phone) **NOW!**

See the reverse side for things you can do to avoid your asthma triggers.

How To Control Things That Make Your Asthma Worse

This guide suggests things you can do to avoid your asthma triggers. Put a check next to the triggers that you know make your asthma worse and ask your doctor to help you find out if you have other triggers as well. Then decide with your doctor what steps you will take.

Allergens

❐ **Animal Dander**

Some people are allergic to the flakes of skin or dried saliva from animals with fur or feathers.

The best thing to do:

- Keep furred or feathered pets out of your home.

If you can't keep the pet outdoors, then:

- Keep the pet out of your bedroom and other sleeping areas at all times, and keep the door closed.
- Remove carpets and furniture covered with cloth from your home. If that is not possible, keep the pet away from fabric-covered furniture and carpets.

❐ **Dust Mites**

Many people with asthma are allergic to dust mites. Dust mites are tiny bugs that are found in every home—in mattresses, pillows, carpets, upholstered furniture, bedcovers, clothes, stuffed toys, and fabric or other fabric-covered items.

Things that can help:

- Encase your mattress in a special dust-proof cover.
- Encase your pillow in a special dust-proof cover or wash the pillow each week in hot water. Water must be hotter than 130° F to kill the mites. Cold or warm water used with detergent and bleach can also be effective.
- Wash the sheets and blankets on your bed each week in hot water.
- Reduce indoor humidity to below 60 percent (ideally between 30—50 percent). Dehumidifiers or central air conditioners can do this.
- Try not to sleep or lie on cloth-covered cushions.
- Remove carpets from your bedroom and those laid on concrete, if you can.
- Keep stuffed toys out of the bed or wash the toys weekly in hot water or cooler water with detergent and bleach.

❐ **Cockroaches**

Many people with asthma are allergic to the dried droppings and remains of cockroaches.

The best thing to do:

- Keep food and garbage in closed containers. Never leave food out.
- Use poison baits, powders, gels, or paste (for example, boric acid). You can also use traps.
- If a spray is used to kill roaches, stay out of the room until the odor goes away.

❐ **Indoor Mold**

- Fix leaky faucets, pipes, or other sources of water that have mold around them.
- Clean moldy surfaces with a cleaner that has bleach in it.

❐ **Pollen and Outdoor Mold**

What to do during your allergy season (when pollen or mold spore counts are high):

- Try to keep your windows closed.
- Stay indoors with windows closed from late morning to afternoon, if you can. Pollen and some mold spore counts are highest at that time.
- Ask your doctor whether you need to take or increase anti-inflammatory medicine before your allergy season starts.

Irritants

❐ **Tobacco Smoke**

- If you smoke, ask your doctor for ways to help you quit. Ask family members to quit smoking, too.
- Do not allow smoking in your home or car.

❐ **Smoke, Strong Odors, and Sprays**

- If possible, do not use a wood-burning stove, kerosene heater, or fireplace.
- Try to stay away from strong odors and sprays, such as perfume, talcum powder, hair spray, and paints.

Other things that bring on asthma symptoms in some people include:

❐ **Vacuum Cleaning**

- Try to get someone else to vacuum for you once or twice a week, if you can. Stay out of rooms while they are being vacuumed and for a short while afterward.
- If you vacuum, use a dust mask (from a hardware store), a double-layered or microfilter vacuum cleaner bag, or a vacuum cleaner with a HEPA filter.

❐ **Other Things That Can Make Asthma Worse**

- Sulfites in foods and beverages: Do not drink beer or wine or eat dried fruit, processed potatoes, or shrimp if they cause asthma symptoms.
- Cold air: Cover your nose and mouth with a scarf on cold or windy days.
- Other medicines: Tell your doctor about all the medicines you take. Include cold medicines, aspirin, vitamins and other supplements, and nonselective beta-blockers (including those in eye drops).

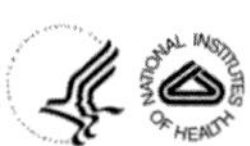

U.S. Department of Health and Human Services
National Institutes of Health

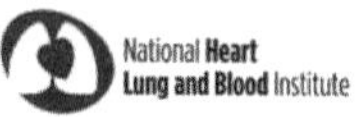

For More Information, go to: www.nhlbi.nih.gov

NIH Publication No. 07-5251
April 2007

APPENDIX

B

Recommended Immunization Schedules for Children and Adolescents Aged 18 Years or Younger

FIGURE 2. Catch-up immunization schedule for persons aged 4 months–18 years who start late or who are more than 1 month behind—United States, 2018.

The figure below provides catch-up schedules and minimum intervals between doses for children whose vaccinations have been delayed. A vaccine series does not need to be restarted, regardless of the time that has elapsed between doses. Use the section appropriate for the child's age. Always use this table in conjunction with Figure 1 and the footnotes that follow.

Vaccine	Minimum Age for Dose 1	Minimum Interval Between Doses			
		Dose 1 to Dose 2	Dose 2 to Dose 3	Dose 3 to Dose 4	Dose 4 to Dose 5
Children age 4 months through 6 years					
Hepatitis B[1]	Birth	4 weeks	8 weeks ***and*** at least 16 weeks after first dose. Minimum age for the final dose is 24 weeks.		
Rotavirus[2]	6 weeks Maximum age for first dose is 14 weeks, 6 days	4 weeks	4 weeks[2] Maximum age for final dose is 8 months, 0 days.		
Diphtheria, tetanus, and acellular pertussis[3]	6 weeks	4 weeks	4 weeks	6 months	6 months[3]
Haemophilus influenzae type b[4]	6 weeks	4 weeks if first dose was administered before the 1st birthday. 8 weeks (as final dose) if first dose was administered at age 12 through 14 months. No further doses needed if first dose was administered at age 15 months or older.	4 weeks[4] if current age is younger than 12 months **and** first dose was administered at younger than age 7 months, **and** at least 1 previous dose was PRP-T (ActHib, Pentacel, Hiberix) or unknown. 8 weeks ***and*** age 12 through 59 months (as final dose)[4] • if current age is younger than 12 months **and** first dose was administered at age 7 through 11 months; OR • if current age is 12 through 59 months **and** first dose was administered before the 1st birthday, **and** second dose administered at younger than 15 months; OR • if both doses were PRP-OMP (PedvaxHIB; Comvax) **and** were administered before the 1st birthday. No further doses needed if previous dose was administered at age 15 months or older.	8 weeks (as final dose) This dose only necessary for children age 12 through 59 months who received 3 doses before the 1st birthday.	
Pneumococcal conjugate[5]	6 weeks	4 weeks if first dose administered before the 1st birthday. 8 weeks (as final dose for healthy children) if first dose was administered at the 1st birthday or after. No further doses needed for healthy children if first dose was administered at age 24 months or older.	4 weeks if current age is younger than 12 months and previous dose given at <7 months old. 8 weeks (as final dose for healthy children) if previous dose given between 7-11 months (wait until at least 12 months old); OR if current age is 12 months or older and at least 1 dose was given before age 12 months. No further doses needed for healthy children if previous dose administered at age 24 months or older.	8 weeks (as final dose) This dose only necessary for children aged 12 through 59 months who received 3 doses before age 12 months or for children at high risk who received 3 doses at any age.	
Inactivated poliovirus[6]	6 weeks	4 weeks[6]	4 weeks[6] if current age is < 4 years 6 months (as final dose) if current age is 4 years or older	6 months[6] (minimum age 4 years for final dose).	
Measles, mumps, rubella[8]	12 months	4 weeks			
Varicella[9]	12 months	3 months			
Hepatitis A[10]	12 months	6 months			
Meningococcal[11] (MenACWY-D ≥9 mos; MenACWY-CRM ≥2 mos)	6 weeks	8 weeks[11]	See footnote 11	See footnote 11	
Children and adolescents age 7 through 18 years					
Meningococcal[11] (MenACWY-D ≥9 mos; MenACWY-CRM ≥2 mos)	Not Applicable (N/A)	8 weeks[11]			
Tetanus, diphtheria; tetanus, diphtheria, and acellular pertussis[13]	7 years[13]	4 weeks	4 weeks if first dose of DTaP/DT was administered before the 1st birthday. 6 months (as final dose) if first dose of DTaP/DT or Tdap/Td was administered at or after the 1st birthday.	6 months if first dose of DTaP/DT was administered before the 1st birthday.	
Human papillomavirus[14]	9 years	Routine dosing intervals are recommended.[14]			
Hepatitis A[10]	N/A	6 months			
Hepatitis B[1]	N/A	4 weeks	8 weeks **and** at least 16 weeks after first dose.		
Inactivated poliovirus[6]	N/A	4 weeks	6 months[6] A fourth dose is not necessary if the third dose was administered at age 4 years or older and at least 6 months after the previous dose.	A fourth dose of IPV is indicated if all previous doses were administered at <4 years or if the third dose was administered <6 months after the second dose.	
Measles, mumps, rubella[8]	N/A	4 weeks			
Varicella[9]	N/A	3 months if younger than age 13 years. 4 weeks if age 13 years or older.			

NOTE: The above recommendations must be read along with the footnotes of this schedule.

Figure 3. Vaccines that might be indicated for children and adolescents aged 18 years or younger based on medical indications

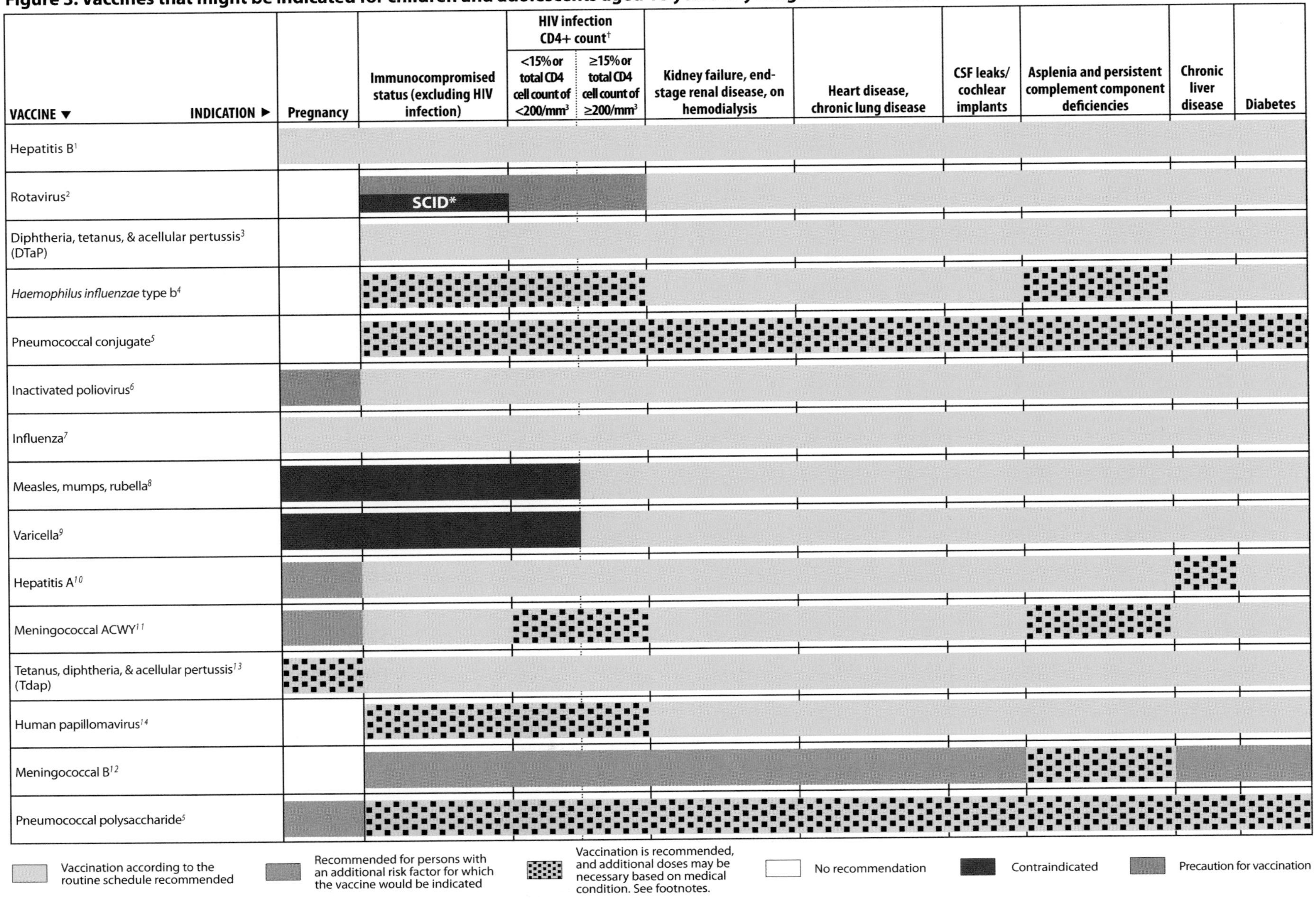

VACCINE ▼ INDICATION ▶	Pregnancy	Immunocompromised status (excluding HIV infection)	HIV infection CD4+ count[†] <15% or total CD4 cell count of <200/mm³	HIV infection CD4+ count[†] ≥15% or total CD4 cell count of ≥200/mm³	Kidney failure, end-stage renal disease, on hemodialysis	Heart disease, chronic lung disease	CSF leaks/ cochlear implants	Asplenia and persistent complement component deficiencies	Chronic liver disease	Diabetes
Hepatitis B[1]										
Rotavirus[2]		SCID*								
Diphtheria, tetanus, & acellular pertussis[3] (DTaP)										
Haemophilus influenzae type b[4]										
Pneumococcal conjugate[5]										
Inactivated poliovirus[6]										
Influenza[7]										
Measles, mumps, rubella[8]										
Varicella[9]										
Hepatitis A[10]										
Meningococcal ACWY[11]										
Tetanus, diphtheria, & acellular pertussis[13] (Tdap)										
Human papillomavirus[14]										
Meningococcal B[12]										
Pneumococcal polysaccharide[5]										

Vaccination according to the routine schedule recommended

Recommended for persons with an additional risk factor for which the vaccine would be indicated

Vaccination is recommended, and additional doses may be necessary based on medical condition. See footnotes.

No recommendation

Contraindicated

Precaution for vaccination

*Severe Combined Immunodeficiency

[†]For additional information regarding HIV laboratory parameters and use of live vaccines; see the General Best Practice Guidelines for Immunization "Altered Immunocompetence" at: www.cdc.gov/vaccines/hcp/acip-recs/general-recs/immunocompetence.html; and Table 4-1 (footnote D) at: www.cdc.gov/vaccines/hcp/acip-recs/general-recs/contraindications.html.

NOTE: The above recommendations must be read along with the footnotes of this schedule.

Footnotes — Recommended Immunization Schedule for Children and Adolescents Aged 18 Years or Younger, UNITED STATES, 2018

For further guidance on the use of the vaccines mentioned below, see: www.cdc.gov/vaccines/hcp/acip-recs/index.html.
For vaccine recommendations for persons 19 years of age and older, see the Adult Immunization Schedule.

Additional information

- For information on contraindications and precautions for the use of a vaccine, consult the *General Best Practice Guidelines for Immunization* and relevant ACIP statements, at www.cdc.gov/vaccines/hcp/acip-recs/index.html.
- For calculating intervals between doses, 4 weeks = 28 days. Intervals of $\geq$4 months are determined by calendar months.
- Within a number range (e.g., 12–18), a dash (–) should be read as "through."
- Vaccine doses administered ≤4 days before the minimum age or interval are considered valid. Doses of any vaccine administered ≥5 days earlier than the minimum interval or minimum age should not be counted as valid and should be repeated as age-appropriate. The repeat dose should be spaced after the invalid dose by the recommended minimum interval. For further details, see Table 3-1, *Recommended and minimum ages and intervals between vaccine doses,* in *General Best Practice Guidelines for Immunization* at www.cdc.gov/vaccines/hcp/acip-recs/general-recs/timing.html.
- Information on travel vaccine requirements and recommendations is available at wwwnc.cdc.gov/travel/.
- For vaccination of persons with immunodeficiencies, see Table 8-1, *Vaccination of persons with primary and secondary immunodeficiencies,* in *General Best Practice Guidelines for Immunization,* at www.cdc.gov/vaccines/hcp/acip-recs/general-recs/immunocompetence.html; and Immunization in Special Clinical Circumstances. (In: Kimberlin DW, Brady MT, Jackson MA, Long SS, eds. *Red Book: 2015 report of the Committee on Infectious Diseases. 30th ed.* Elk Grove Village, IL: American Academy of Pediatrics, 2015:68-107).
- The National Vaccine Injury Compensation Program (VICP) is a no-fault alternative to the traditional legal system for resolving vaccine injury claims. All routine child and adolescent vaccines are covered by VICP except for pneumococcal polysaccharide vaccine (PPSV23). For more information; see www.hrsa.gov/vaccinecompensation/index.html.

1. Hepatitis B (HepB) vaccine. (minimum age: birth)

Birth Dose (Monovalent HepB vaccine only):

- **Mother is HBsAg-Negative:** 1 dose within 24 hours of birth for medically stable infants $\geq$2,000 grams. Infants <2,000 grams administer 1 dose at chronological age 1 month or hospital discharge.
- **Mother is HBsAg-Positive:**
  - o Give **HepB vaccine** and **0.5 mL of HBIG** (at separate anatomic sites) within 12 hours of birth, regardless of birth weight.
  - o Test for HBsAg and anti-HBs at age 9–12 months. If HepB series is delayed, test 1–2 months after final dose.
- **Mother's HBsAg status is unknown:**
  - o Give **HepB vaccine** within 12 hours of birth, regardless of birth weight.
  - o For infants <2,000 grams, give **0.5 mL of HBIG** in addition to HepB vaccine within 12 hours of birth.
  - o Determine mother's HBsAg status as soon as possible. If mother is HBsAg-positive, give **0.5 mL of HBIG** to infants $\geq$2,000 grams as soon as possible, but no later than 7 days of age.

Routine Series:

- A complete series is 3 doses at 0, 1–2, and 6–18 months. (Monovalent HepB vaccine should be used for doses given before age 6 weeks.)
- Infants who did not receive a birth dose should begin the series as soon as feasible (see Figure 2).
- Administration of **4 doses** is permitted when a combination vaccine containing HepB is used after the birth dose.
- **Minimum age** for the final (3rd or 4th) dose: 24 weeks.
- **Minimum Intervals:** Dose 1 to Dose 2: 4 weeks / Dose 2 to Dose 3: 8 weeks / Dose 1 to Dose 3: 16 weeks. (When 4 doses are given, substitute "Dose 4" for "Dose 3" in these calculations.)

Catch-up vaccination:

- Unvaccinated persons should complete a 3-dose series at 0, 1–2, and 6 months.
- Adolescents 11–15 years of age may use an alternative 2-dose schedule, with at least 4 months between doses (adult formulation **Recombivax HB** only).
- For other catch-up guidance, see Figure 2.

2. Rotavirus vaccines. (minimum age: 6 weeks)

Routine vaccination:

Rotarix: 2-dose series at 2 and 4 months.

RotaTeq: 3-dose series at 2, 4, and 6 months.

If any dose in the series is either RotaTeq or unknown, default to 3-dose series.

Catch-up vaccination:

- Do not start the series on or after age 15 weeks, 0 days.
- The maximum age for the final dose is 8 months, 0 days.
- For other catch-up guidance, see Figure 2.

3. Diphtheria, tetanus, and acellular pertussis (DTaP) vaccine. (minimum age: 6 weeks [4 years for Kinrix or Quadracel])

Routine vaccination:

- 5-dose series at 2, 4, 6, and 15–18 months, and 4–6 years.
  - o **Prospectively:** A 4th dose may be given as early as age 12 months if at least 6 months have elapsed since the 3rd dose.
  - o **Retrospectively:** A 4th dose that was inadvertently given as early as 12 months may be counted if at least 4 months have elapsed since the 3rd dose.

Catch-up vaccination:

- The 5th dose is not necessary if the 4th dose was administered at 4 years or older.
- For other catch-up guidance, see Figure 2.

For further guidance on the use of the vaccines mentioned below, see: www.cdc.gov/vaccines/hcp/acip-recs/index.html.

4. ***Haemophilus influenzae* type b (Hib) vaccine. (minimum age: 6 weeks)**

Routine vaccination:
- **ActHIB, Hiberix, or Pentacel:** 4-dose series at 2, 4, 6, and 12–15 months.
- **PedvaxHIB:** 3-dose series at 2, 4, and 12–15 months.

Catch-up vaccination:
- **1st dose at 7–11 months:** Give 2nd dose at least 4 weeks later and 3rd (final) dose at 12–15 months or 8 weeks after 2nd dose (whichever is later).
- **1st dose at 12–14 months:** Give 2nd (final) dose at least 8 weeks after 1st dose.
- **1st dose before 12 months and 2nd dose before 15 months:** Give 3rd (final) dose 8 weeks after 2nd dose.
- **2 doses of PedvaxHIB before 12 months:** Give 3rd (final) dose at 12–59 months and at least 8 weeks after 2nd dose.
- **Unvaccinated at 15–59 months:** 1 dose.
- For other catch-up guidance, see Figure 2.

Special Situations:
- **Chemotherapy or radiation treatment**
  12–59 months
  - o Unvaccinated or only 1 dose before 12 months: Give 2 doses, 8 weeks apart
  - o 2 or more doses before 12 months: Give 1 dose, at least 8 weeks after previous dose.

  Doses given within 14 days of starting therapy or during therapy should be repeated at least 3 months after therapy completion.
- **Hematopoietic stem cell transplant (HSCT)**
- 3-dose series with doses 4 weeks apart starting 6 to 12 months after successful transplant (regardless of Hib vaccination history).
- **Anatomic or functional asplenia (including sickle cell disease)**
  12–59 months
  - o Unvaccinated or only 1 dose before 12 months: Give 2 doses, 8 weeks apart.
  - o 2 or more doses before 12 months: Give 1 dose, at least 8 weeks after previous dose.

  Unimmunized persons 5 years or older*
  - o Give 1 dose
- **Elective splenectomy**
  Unimmunized* persons 15 months or older
  - o Give 1 dose (preferably at least 14 days before procedure).
- **HIV infection**
  12–59 months
  - o Unvaccinated or only 1 dose before 12 months: Give 2 doses 8 weeks apart.
  - o 2 or more doses before 12 months: Give 1 dose, at least 8 weeks after previous dose.

  Unimmunized persons 5–18 years*
  - o Give 1 dose
- **Immunoglobulin deficiency, early component complement deficiency**
  12–59 months
  - o Unvaccinated or only 1 dose before 12 months: Give 2 doses, 8 weeks apart.
  - o 2 or more doses before 12 months: Give 1 dose, at least 8 weeks after previous dose.

**Unimmunized* = Less than routine series (through 14 months) OR no doses (14 months or older)

5. **Pneumococcal vaccines. (minimum age: 6 weeks [PCV13], 2 years [PPSV23])**

Routine vaccination with PCV13:
- 4-dose series at 2, 4, 6, and 12–15 months.

Catch-up vaccination with PCV13:
- 1 dose for healthy children aged 24–59 months with any incomplete* PCV13 schedule
- For other catch-up guidance, see Figure 2.

Special situations: High-risk conditions: Administer PCV13 doses before PPSV23 if possible.

Chronic heart disease (particularly cyanotic congenital heart disease and cardiac failure); chronic lung disease (including asthma treated with high-dose, oral, corticosteroids); diabetes mellitus:

Age 2–5 years:
- Any incomplete* schedules with:
  - o 3 PCV13 doses: 1 dose of PCV13 (at least 8 weeks after any prior PCV13 dose).
  - o <3 PCV13 doses: 2 doses of PCV13, 8 weeks after the most recent dose and given 8 weeks apart.
- No history of PPSV23: 1 dose of PPSV23 (at least 8 weeks after any prior PCV13 dose).

Age 6-18 years:
- No history of PPSV23: 1 dose of PPSV23 (at least 8 weeks after any prior PCV13 dose).

Cerebrospinal fluid leak; cochlear implant:

Age 2–5 years:
- Any incomplete* schedules with:
  - o 3 PCV13 doses: 1 dose of PCV13 (at least 8 weeks after any prior PCV13 dose).
  - o <3 PCV13 doses: 2 doses of PCV13, 8 weeks after the most recent dose and given 8 weeks apart.
- No history of PPSV23: 1 dose of PPSV23 (at least 8 weeks after any prior PCV13 dose).

Age 6–18 years:
- No history of either PCV13 or PPSV23: 1 dose of PCV13, 1 dose of PPSV23 at least 8 weeks later.
- Any PCV13 but no PPSV23: 1 dose of PPSV23 at least 8 weeks after the most recent dose of PCV13
- PPSV23 but no PCV13: 1 dose of PCV13 at least 8 weeks after the most recent dose of PPSV23.

Sickle cell disease and other hemoglobinopathies; anatomic or functional asplenia; congenital or acquired immunodeficiency; HIV infection; chronic renal failure; nephrotic syndrome; malignant neoplasms, leukemias, lymphomas, Hodgkin disease, and other diseases associated with treatment with immunosuppressive drugs or radiation therapy; solid organ transplantation; multiple myeloma:

Age 2–5 years:
- Any incomplete* schedules with:
  - o 3 PCV13 doses: 1 dose of PCV13 (at least 8 weeks after any prior PCV13 dose).
  - o <3 PCV13 doses: 2 doses of PCV13, 8 weeks after the most recent dose and given 8 weeks apart.
- No history of PPSV23: 1 dose of PPSV23 (at least 8 weeks after any prior PCV13 dose) and a 2nd dose of PPSV23 5 years later.

Age 6–18 years:
- No history of either PCV13 or PPSV23: 1 dose of PCV13, 2 doses of PPSV23 (1st dose of PPSV23 administered 8 weeks after PCV13 and 2nd dose of PPSV23 administered at least 5 years after the 1st dose of PPSV23).
- Any PCV13 but no PPSV23: 2 doses of PPSV23 (1st dose of PPSV23 to be given 8 weeks after the most recent dose of PCV13 and 2nd dose of PPSV23 administered at least 5 years after the 1st dose of PPSV23).

For further guidance on the use of the vaccines mentioned below, see: www.cdc.gov/vaccines/hcp/acip-recs/index.html.

- PPSV23 but no PCV13: 1 dose of PCV13 at least 8 weeks after the most recent PPSV23 dose and a 2nd dose of PPSV23 to be given 5 years after the 1st dose of PPSV23 and at least 8 weeks after a dose of PCV13.

Chronic liver disease, alcoholism:

Age 6–18 years:

- No history of PPSV23: 1 dose of PPSV23 (at least 8 weeks after any prior PCV13 dose).

*Incomplete schedules are any schedules where PCV13 doses have not been completed according to ACIP recommended catch-up schedules. The total number and timing of doses for complete PCV13 series are dictated by the age at first vaccination. See Tables 8 and 9 in the ACIP pneumococcal vaccine recommendations (www.cdc.gov/mmwr/pdf/rr/rr5911.pdf) for complete schedule details.

6. **Inactivated poliovirus vaccine (IPV). (minimum age: 6 weeks)**

Routine vaccination:

- 4-dose series at ages 2, 4, 6–18 months, and 4–6 years. Administer the final dose on or after the 4th birthday and at least 6 months after the previous dose.

Catch-up vaccination:

- In the first 6 months of life, use minimum ages and intervals only for travel to a polio-endemic region or during an outbreak.
- If 4 or more doses were given before the 4th birthday, give 1 more dose at age 4–6 years and at least 6 months after the previous dose.
- A 4th dose is not necessary if the 3rd dose was given on or after the 4th birthday and at least 6 months after the previous dose.
- IPV is not routinely recommended for U.S. residents 18 years and older.

Series Containing Oral Polio Vaccine (OPV), *either mixed OPV-IPV or OPV-only series*:

- Total number of doses needed to complete the series is the same as that recommended for the U.S. IPV schedule. See www.cdc.gov/mmwr/volumes/66/wr/mm6601a6.htm?s_cid=mm6601a6_w.
- Only trivalent OPV (tOPV) counts toward the U.S. vaccination requirements. For guidance to assess doses documented as "OPV" see www.cdc.gov/mmwr/volumes/66/wr/mm6606a7.htm?s_cid=mm6606a7_w.
- For other catch-up guidance, see Figure 2.

7. **Influenza vaccines. (minimum age: 6 months)**

Routine vaccination:

- Administer an age-appropriate formulation and dose of influenza vaccine annually.
  - o **Children 6 months–8 years** who did not receive at least 2 doses of influenza vaccine before July 1, 2017 should receive 2 doses separated by at least 4 weeks.
  - o **Persons 9 years and older** 1 dose
- Live attenuated influenza vaccine (LAIV) not recommended for the 2017–18 season.
- For additional guidance, see the 2017–18 ACIP influenza vaccine recommendations (*MMWR* August 25, 2017;66(2):1-20: www.cdc.gov/mmwr/volumes/66/rr/pdfs/rr6602.pdf).

(For the 2018–19 season, see the 2018–19 ACIP influenza vaccine recommendations.)

8. **Measles, mumps, and rubella (MMR) vaccine. (minimum age: 12 months for routine vaccination)**

Routine vaccination:

- 2-dose series at 12–15 months and 4–6 years.
- The 2nd dose may be given as early as 4 weeks after the 1st dose.

Catch-up vaccination:

- Unvaccinated children and adolescents: 2 doses at least 4 weeks apart.

International travel:

- **Infants 6–11 months:** 1 dose before departure. Revaccinate with 2 doses at 12–15 months (12 months for children in high-risk areas) and 2nd dose as early as 4 weeks later.
- **Unvaccinated children 12 months and older:** 2 doses at least 4 weeks apart before departure.

Mumps outbreak:

- Persons ≥12 months who previously received ≤2 doses of mumps-containing vaccine and are identified by public health authorities to be at increased risk during a mumps outbreak should receive a dose of mumps-virus containing vaccine.

9. **Varicella (VAR) vaccine. (minimum age: 12 months)**

Routine vaccination:

- 2-dose series: 12–15 months and 4–6 years.
- The 2nd dose may be given as early as 3 months after the 1st dose (a dose given after a 4-week interval may be counted).

Catch-up vaccination:

- Ensure persons 7–18 years without evidence of immunity (see *MMWR* 2007;56[No. RR-4], at www.cdc.gov/mmwr/pdf/rr/rr5604.pdf) have 2 doses of varicella vaccine:
  - o **Ages 7–12:** routine interval 3 months (minimum interval: 4 weeks).
  - o **Ages 13 and older:** minimum interval 4 weeks.

10. **Hepatitis A (HepA) vaccine. (minimum age: 12 months)**

Routine vaccination:

- 2 doses, separated by 6-18 months, between the 1st and 2nd birthdays. (A series begun before the 2nd birthday should be completed even if the child turns 2 before the second dose is given.)

Catch-up vaccination:

- Anyone 2 years of age or older may receive HepA vaccine if desired. Minimum interval between doses is 6 months.

Special populations:

Previously unvaccinated persons who should be vaccinated:

- Persons traveling to or working in countries with high or intermediate endemicity
- Men who have sex with men
- Users of injection and non-injection drugs
- Persons who work with hepatitis A virus in a research laboratory or with non-human primates
- Persons with clotting-factor disorders
- Persons with chronic liver disease
- Persons who anticipate close, personal contact (e.g., household or regular babysitting) with an international adoptee during the first 60 days after arrival in the United States from a country with high or intermediate endemicity (administer the 1st dose as soon as the adoption is planned—ideally at least 2 weeks before the adoptee's arrival).

11. **Serogroup A, C, W, Y meningococcal vaccines. (Minimum age: 2 months [Menveo], 9 months [Menactra].**

Routine:

- 2-dose series: 11-12 years and 16 years.

Catch-Up:

- Age 13-15 years: 1 dose now and booster at age 16-18 years. Minimum interval 8 weeks.
- Age 16-18 years: 1 dose.

For further guidance on the use of the vaccines mentioned below, see: www.cdc.gov/vaccines/hcp/acip-recs/index.html.

Special populations and situations:
Anatomic or functional asplenia, sickle cell disease, HIV infection, persistent complement component deficiency (including eculizumab use):

- **Menveo**
  - o 1st dose at 8 weeks: 4-dose series at 2, 4, 6, and 12 months.
  - o 1st dose at 7–23 months: 2 doses (2nd dose at least 12 weeks after the 1st dose and after the 1st birthday).
  - o 1st dose at 24 months or older: 2 doses at least 8 weeks apart.
- **Menactra**
  - o Persistent complement component deficiency:
    - — 9–23 months: 2 doses at least 12 weeks apart
    - — 24 months or older: 2 doses at least 8 weeks apart
  - o Anatomic or functional asplenia, sickle cell disease, or HIV infection:
    - — 24 months or older: 2 doses at least 8 weeks apart.
    - — **Menactra** must be administered at least 4 weeks after completion of PCV13 series.

Children who travel to or live in countries where meningococcal disease is hyperendemic or epidemic, including countries in the African meningitis belt or during the Hajj, or exposure to an outbreak attributable to a vaccine serogroup:

- Children <24 months of age:
  - o **Menveo (2-23 months):**
    - — 1st dose at 8 weeks: 4-dose series at 2, 4, 6, and 12 months.
    - — 1st dose at 7-23 months: 2 doses (2nd dose at least 12 weeks after the 1st dose and after the 1st birthday).
  - o **Menactra (9-23 months):**
    - — 2 doses (2nd dose at least 12 weeks after the 1st dose. 2nd dose may be administered as early as 8 weeks after the 1st dose in travelers).
- Children 2 years or older: 1 dose of **Menveo** or **Menactra**.

Note: Menactra should be given either before or at the same time as DTaP. For MenACWY booster dose recommendations for groups listed under "Special populations and situations" above, and additional meningococcal vaccination information, see meningococcal *MMWR* publications at: www.cdc.gov/vaccines/hcp/acip-recs/vacc-specific/mening.html.

12. Serogroup B meningococcal vaccines (minimum age: 10 years [Bexsero, Trumenba].

Clinical discretion: Adolescents not at increased risk for meningococcal B infection who want MenB vaccine.

MenB vaccines may be given at clinical discretion to adolescents 16–23 years (preferred age 16–18 years) who are not at increased risk.

- **Bexsero**: 2 doses at least 1 month apart.
- **Trumenba**: 2 doses at least 6 months apart. If the 2nd dose is given earlier than 6 months, give a 3rd dose at least 4 months after the 2nd.

Special populations and situations:
Anatomic or functional asplenia, sickle cell disease, persistent complement component deficiency (including eculizumab use), serogroup B meningococcal disease outbreak

- **Bexsero**: 2-dose series at least 1 month apart.
- **Trumenba**: 3-dose series at 0, 1-2, and 6 months.

Note: **Bexsero** and **Trumenba** are not interchangeable.

For additional meningococcal vaccination information, see meningococcal *MMWR* publications at: www.cdc.gov/vaccines/hcp/acip-recs/vacc-specific/mening.html.

13. Tetanus, diphtheria, and acellular pertussis (Tdap) vaccine. (minimum age: 11 years for routine vaccinations, 7 years for catch-up vaccination)

Routine vaccination:

- **Adolescents 11–12 years of age:** 1 dose.
- **Pregnant adolescents:** 1 dose during each pregnancy (preferably during the early part of gestational weeks 27–36).
- Tdap may be administered regardless of the interval since the last tetanus- and diphtheria-toxoid-containing vaccine.

Catch-up vaccination:

- **Adolescents 13–18 who have not received Tdap**: 1 dose, followed by a Td booster every 10 years.
- **Persons aged 7–18 years not fully immunized with DTaP**: 1 dose of Tdap as part of the catch-up series (preferably the first dose). If additional doses are needed, use Td.
- **Children 7–10 years** who receive Tdap inadvertently or as part of the catch-up series may receive the routine Tdap dose at 11–12 years.
- **DTaP inadvertently given after the 7th birthday**:
  - o **Child 7–10**: DTaP may count as part of catch-up series. Routine Tdap dose at 11-12 may be given.
  - o **Adolescent 11–18**: Count dose of DTaP as the adolescent Tdap booster.
- For other catch-up guidance, see Figure 2.

14. Human papillomavirus (HPV) vaccine (minimum age: 9 years)

Routine and catch-up vaccination:

- Routine vaccination for all adolescents at 11–12 years (can start at age 9) and through age 18 if not previously adequately vaccinated. Number of doses dependent on age at initial vaccination:
  - o **Age 9–14 years at initiation:** 2-dose series at 0 and 6–12 months. Minimum interval: 5 months (repeat a dose given too soon at least 12 weeks after the invalid dose and at least 5 months after the 1st dose).
  - o **Age 15 years or older at initiation:** 3-dose series at 0, 1–2 months, and 6 months. Minimum intervals: 4 weeks between 1st and 2nd dose; 12 weeks between 2nd and 3rd dose; 5 months between 1st and 3rd dose (repeat dose(s) given too soon at or after the minimum interval since the most recent dose).
- Persons who have completed a valid series with any HPV vaccine do not need any additional doses.

Special situations:

- **History of sexual abuse or assault**: Begin series at age 9 years.
- **Immunocompromised* (including HIV)** aged 9–26 years: 3-dose series at 0, 1–2 months, and 6 months.
- **Pregnancy:** Vaccination not recommended, but there is no evidence the vaccine is harmful. No intervention is needed for women who inadvertently received a dose of HPV vaccine while pregnant. Delay remaining doses until after pregnancy. Pregnancy testing not needed before vaccination.

*See MMWR, December 16, 2016;65(49):1405–1408, at www.cdc.gov/mmwr/volumes/65/wr/pdfs/mm6549a5.pdf.

CS270457-M

APPENDIX

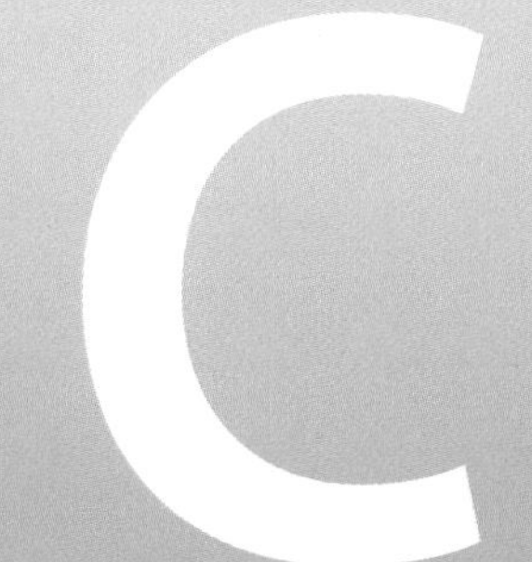

Car Seat Safety

Using the correct car seat or booster seat can be a lifesaver: make sure your child is always buckled in an age- and size-appropriate car seat or booster seat.

Birth 1 2 3 4 5 6 7 8 9 10 11 12+

Age by Years*

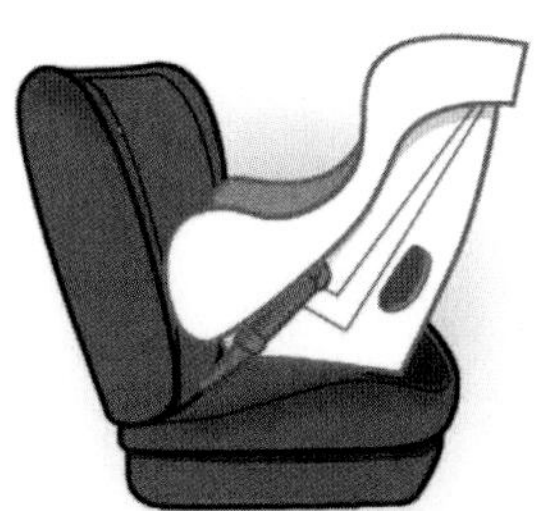

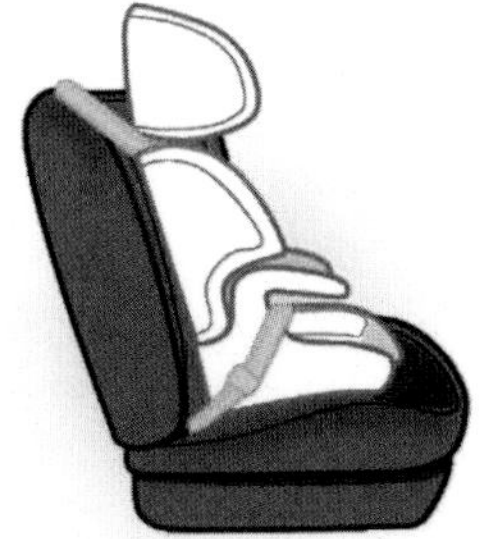

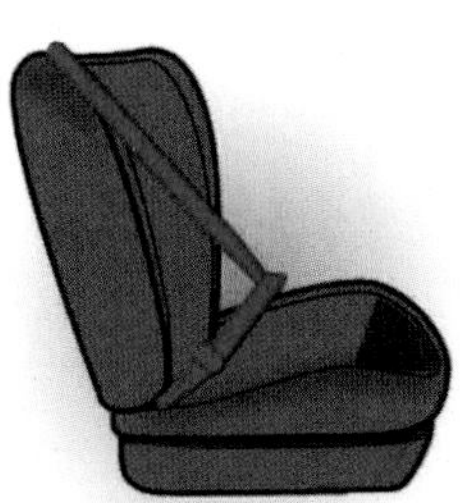

REAR-FACING CAR SEAT

Birth up to Age 2*
Buckle children in a rear-facing seat until age 2 or when they reach the upper weight or height limit of that seat.

FORWARD-FACING CAR SEAT

Age 2 up to at least age 5*
When children outgrow their rear-facing seat, they should be buckled in a forward-facing car seat until at least age 5 or when they reach the upper weight or height limit of that seat.

BOOSTER SEAT

Age 5 up until seat belts fit properly*
Once children outgrow their forward-facing seat, they should be buckled in a booster seat until seat belts fit properly. The recommended height for proper seat belt fit is 57 inches tall.

SEAT BELT

Once seat belts fit properly without a booster seat
Children no longer need to use a booster seat once seat belts fit them properly. Seat belts fit properly when the lap belt lays across the upper thighs (not the stomach) and the shoulder belt lays across the chest (not the neck).

Keep children ages 12 and under in the back seat. Never place a rear-facing car seat in front of an active air bag.

**Recommended age ranges for each seat type vary to account for differences in child growth and height/weight limits of car seats and booster seats. Use the car seat or booster seat owner's manual to check installation and the seat height/weight limits, and proper seat use.*

Child safety seat recommendations: American Academy of Pediatrics.
Graphic design: adapted from National Highway Traffic Safety Administration.

APPENDIX

D

Growth Charts

2 to 20 years: Boys
Stature-for-age and Weight-for-age percentiles

NAME ______________________

RECORD # ______________

Mother's Stature ______________ Father's Stature ______________

Date	Age	Weight	Stature	BMI*

***To Calculate BMI**: Weight (kg) ÷ Stature (cm) ÷ Stature (cm) x 10,000
or Weight (lb) ÷ Stature (in) ÷ Stature (in) x 703

AGE (YEARS)

12 13 14 15 16 17 18 19 20

STATURE

in: 76 74 72 70 68 66 64 62 60

cm: 190 185 180 175 170 165 160 155 150

Stature percentiles: 97 90 75 50 25 10 3

in: 62 60 58 56 54 52 50 48 46 44 42 40 38 36 34 32 30

cm: 160 155 150 145 140 135 130 125 120 115 110 105 100 95 90 85 80

3 4 5 6 7 8 9 10 11

WEIGHT

kg: 105 100 95 90 85 80 75 70 65 60 55 50 45 40 35 30 25 20 15 10

lb: 230 220 210 200 190 180 170 160 150 140 130 120 110 100 90 80 70 60 50 40 30

Weight percentiles: 97 90 75 50 25 10 3

lb: 80 70 60 50 40 30

kg: 35 30 25 20 15 10

AGE (YEARS)

2 3 4 5 6 7 8 9 10 11 12 13 14 15 16 17 18 19 20

Published May 30, 2000 (modified 11/21/00).
SOURCE: Developed by the National Center for Health Statistics in collaboration with the National Center for Chronic Disease Prevention and Health Promotion (2000).
http://www.cdc.gov/growthcharts

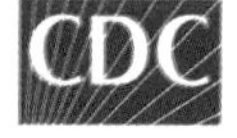

SAFER • HEALTHIER • PEOPLE™

2 to 20 years: Girls
Stature-for-age and Weight-for-age percentiles

NAME ______________________

RECORD # ______________

Mother's Stature ____________ Father's Stature ____________

Date	Age	Weight	Stature	BMI*

***To Calculate BMI**: Weight (kg) ÷ Stature (cm) ÷ Stature (cm) x 10,000
or Weight (lb) ÷ Stature (in) ÷ Stature (in) x 703

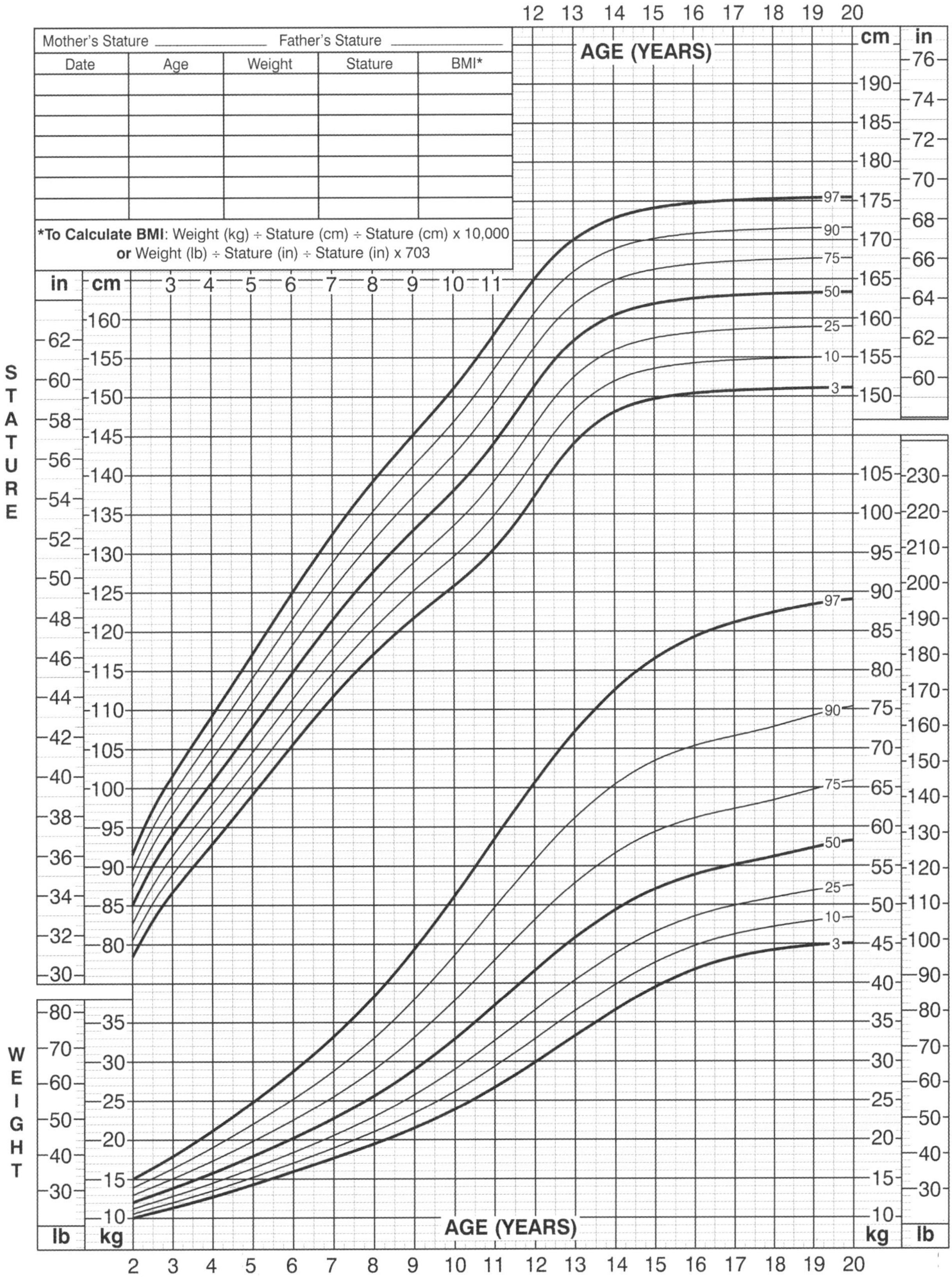

AGE (YEARS)

12 13 14 15 16 17 18 19 20

cm in

STATURE

in cm 3 4 5 6 7 8 9 10 11

Stature percentiles: 97, 90, 75, 50, 25, 10, 3

cm: 80 85 90 95 100 105 110 115 120 125 130 135 140 145 150 155 160 165 170 175 180 185 190

in: 30 32 34 36 38 40 42 44 46 48 50 52 54 56 58 60 62 64 66 68 70 72 74 76

WEIGHT

Weight percentiles: 97, 90, 75, 50, 25, 10, 3

kg: 10 15 20 25 30 35 40 45 50 55 60 65 70 75 80 85 90 95 100 105

lb: 30 40 50 60 70 80 90 100 110 120 130 140 150 160 170 180 190 200 210 220 230

lb kg AGE (YEARS) kg lb

2 3 4 5 6 7 8 9 10 11 12 13 14 15 16 17 18 19 20

Published May 30, 2000 (modified 11/21/00).
SOURCE: Developed by the National Center for Health Statistics in collaboration with
the National Center for Chronic Disease Prevention and Health Promotion (2000).
http://www.cdc.gov/growthcharts

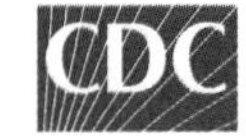

SAFER • HEALTHIER • PEOPLE™

Birth to 36 months: Boys
Length-for-age and Weight-for-age percentiles

NAME ______________________

RECORD # ______________

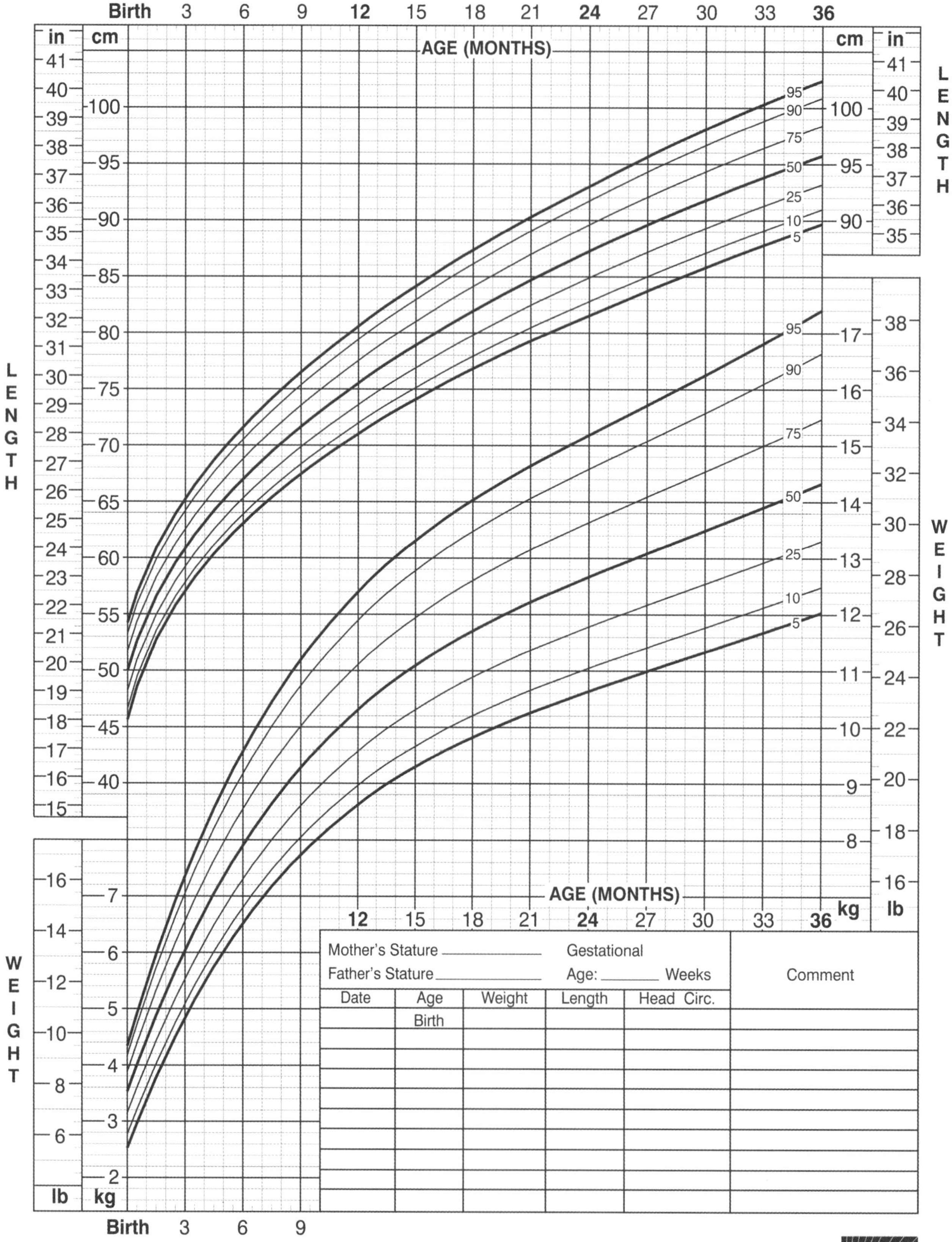

Mother's Stature ____________ Gestational
Father's Stature ____________ Age: ________ Weeks

Date	Age	Weight	Length	Head Circ.	Comment
	Birth				

Published May 30, 2000 (modified 4/20/01).
SOURCE: Developed by the National Center for Health Statistics in collaboration with the National Center for Chronic Disease Prevention and Health Promotion (2000).
http://www.cdc.gov/growthcharts

CDC
SAFER • HEALTHIER • PEOPLE™

Birth to 36 months: Girls
Length-for-age and Weight-for-age percentiles

NAME ______________________

RECORD # ______________

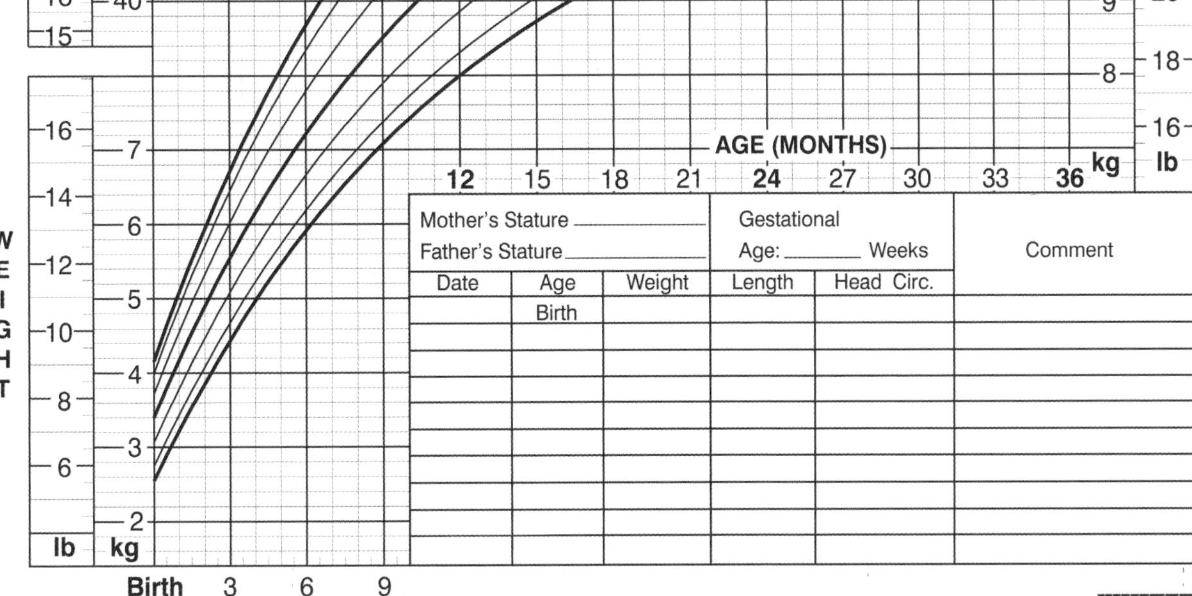

Mother's Stature ______			Gestational		Comment
Father's Stature ______			Age: ______ Weeks		
Date	Age	Weight	Length	Head Circ.	
	Birth				

Published May 30, 2000 (modified 4/20/01).
SOURCE: Developed by the National Center for Health Statistics in collaboration with the National Center for Chronic Disease Prevention and Health Promotion (2000).
http://www.cdc.gov/growthcharts

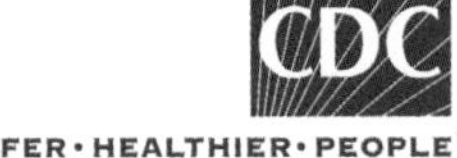

APPENDIX E

Pediatric Fluid and Electrolyte Requirements

How to Calculate Maintenance Fluid Requirements in Children

1. Body surface area (BSA) method (commonly used in children >10 kg):
   1,500–2,000 mL/m²/day ÷ 24 = fluid rate in mL/hr

   Example: Calculate maintenance fluids in mL/hr for a child with a BSA of 0.8 m².

   Answer: 1,500 mL/m²/day × 0.8 m² = 1,200 mL/day ÷ 24 hr = 50 mL/hr

   2,000 mL/m²/day × 0.8 m² = 1600 mL/day ÷ 24 hr = 66.6 mL/hr

   Range: 50–66.6 mL/hr
2. Body weight method (100/50/20 rule or Holliday–Segar [1957] formula):

<10 kg	100 mL/kg/day
11–20 kg	1,000 mL + 50 mL/kg for each kg >10
>20 kg	1,500 mL + 20 mL/kg for each kg >20

   Example: Calculate maintenance fluids in mL/hr for a child weighing 25 kg.

   Answer: 1,500 mL + 20 mL/kg × 5 kg = 1,500 mL + 100 mL = 1,600 mL

   1,600 mL ÷ 24 hr = 66.6 mL/hr

Caloric Requirements (Approximate)

Preterm infants	120 Kcal/kg/day
Infants	100 Kcal/kg/day
Young child	80 Kcal/kg/day
Older child	60 Kcal/kg/day

Minimum Urine Output

Infants	2 mL/kg/hr
Children 1–12 years	1 mL/kg/hr
Adolescents >12 years	0.5 mL/kg/hr

Calculating Body Mass Index

Take the child's weight in pounds divided by the height in inches multiplied by the height in inches, then multiply the results by 703. The results are dependent on the child's age.

$$\frac{\text{weight (lbs)}}{\text{height (in.)} \times \text{height (in.)}} \times 703 = \text{BMI (body mass index)}$$

REFERENCE

Holliday, M. A., & Segar, W. E. (1957). The maintenance need for water in parenteral fluid therapy. *Pediatrics, 19*, 823–832.

Photo and Illustration Credits

Chapter 1

Figure 1–1. Courtesy of the National Institutes of Health, www.nih.gov.

Figure 1–4. PediaSIM pediatric simulation photo courtesy of CAE Healthcare. © 2011 CAE Healthcare.

Chapter 3

Figure 3–1. Copyright fotosearch.com.

Figure 3–10. From Ward, S. L., & Hisley, S. M. (2016). *Maternal-child nursing care: Optimizing outcomes for mothers, children, and families* (2nd ed., p. 67). Philadelphia: F.A. Davis. Courtesy of Family Ties Project, Washington, DC: Life Planning for Families Affected by HIV/AIDS.

Chapter 4

Figure 4–2. Courtesy of Craig Froehle, PhD.

Figure 4–3. Copyright 2017 LanguageLine Solutions.

Chapter 5

Figure 5–1. Courtesy of the Back to Sleep campaign, Eunice Kennedy Shriver National Institute of Child Health and Human Development, National Institutes of Health and Human Services, http://www.nichd.nih.gov/sids.

Figure 5–2. **A,** From the Scottish Government. Copyright Crown Copyright. Contains public sector information licensed under the Open Government License v3.0. Retrieved from https://news.gov.scot/news/baby-boxes-begin. **B,** Courtesy of Rebecca Leutke.

Figures 5–3. From Ward, S. L., & Hisley, S. M. (2016). *Maternal-child nursing care: Optimizing outcomes for mothers, children, and families* (2nd ed., p. 1398). Philadelphia: F.A. Davis.

Figure 5–5. From Ward, S. L., & Hisley, S. M. (2016). *Maternal-child nursing care: Optimizing outcomes for mothers, children, and families* (2nd ed., p. 1402). Philadelphia: F.A. Davis.

Figure 5–6. From the National Institute of Child Health and Human Development. Retrieved from http://www.nichd.nih.gov/sids.

Chapter 7

Figure 7–1. From Chapman, L., & Durham, R. (2014). *Maternal-newborn nursing: The critical components of nursing care* (2nd ed., p. 428). Philadelphia: F.A. Davis.

Figure 7–2. From Ward, S. L., & Hisley, S. M. (2016). *Maternal-child nursing care: Optimizing outcomes for mothers, children, and families* (2nd ed., p. 640). Philadelphia: F.A. Davis.

Figure 7–3. From Ward, S. L., & Hisley, S. M. (2016). *Maternal-child nursing care: Optimizing outcomes for mothers, children, and families* (2nd ed., p. 643). Philadelphia: F.A. Davis.

Figure 7–4. From Ward, S. L., & Hisley, S. M. (2009). *Maternal-child nursing care: Optimizing outcomes for mothers, children, and families* (Enhanced, revised revision, p. 174). Philadelphia: F.A. Davis.

Figure 7–5. From Chapman, L., & Durham, R. (2014). *Maternal-newborn nursing: The critical components of nursing care* (2nd ed., p. 434). Philadelphia: F.A. Davis.

Figure 7–6. From Ward, S. L., & Hisley, S. M. (2016). *Maternal-child nursing care: Optimizing outcomes for mothers, children, and families* (2nd ed., p. 646). Philadelphia: F.A. Davis.

Figure 7–7. From Chapman, L., & Durham, R. (2010). *Maternal-newborn nursing: The critical components of nursing care* (p. 284). Philadelphia: F.A. Davis.

Figure 7–8. From Ward, S. L., & Hisley, S. M. (2016). *Maternal-child nursing care: Optimizing outcomes for mothers, children, and families* (2nd ed., p. 721). Philadelphia: F.A. Davis. Courtesy of St. Luke's Hospital, Bethlehem, PA.

Figure 7–9. From Ward, S. L., & Hisley, S. M. (2016). *Maternal-child nursing care: Optimizing outcomes for mothers, children, and families* (2nd ed., p. 651). Philadelphia: F.A. Davis.

Figure 7–10. From Chapman, L., & Durham, R. (2014). *Maternal-newborn nursing: The critical components of nursing care* (2nd ed., p. 461). Philadelphia: F.A. Davis.

Figure 7–11. From Ward, S. L., & Hisley, S. M. (2016). *Maternal-child nursing care: Optimizing outcomes for mothers, children, and families* (2nd ed., p. 676). Philadelphia: F.A. Davis.

Figure 7–12. From Ward, S. L., & Hisley, S. M. (2016). *Maternal-child nursing care: Optimizing outcomes for mothers, children, and families* (2nd ed., p. 677). Philadelphia: F.A. Davis.

Figure 7–13. From Ward, S. L., & Hisley, S. M. (2016). *Maternal-child nursing care: Optimizing outcomes for mothers, children, and families* (2nd ed., p. 679). Philadelphia: F.A. Davis.

Figure 7–15. From Ward, S. L., & Hisley, S. M. (2016). *Maternal-child nursing care: Optimizing outcomes for mothers, children, and families* (2nd ed., p. 657). Philadelphia: F.A. Davis.

Figure 7–19. From Durham, R. & Chapman, L. (2014). *Maternal-newborn nursing: The critical components of nursing care* (2nd ed., p. 404). Philadelphia: F.A. Davis.

Figure 7–20. From Scanlon, V., and Sanders, T. (2015). *Essentials of anatomy and physiology* (7th ed., p. 512). Philadelphia: F.A. Davis.

Figures 7–21 and 7–22. Copyright 2011, Medela Corporation, McHenry, Illinois.

Figure 7–23. From Ward, S. L., & Hisley, S. M. (2016). *Maternal-child nursing care: Optimizing outcomes for mothers, children, and families* (2nd ed., p. 699). Philadelphia: F.A. Davis.

Figure 7–24. From Ward, S. L., & Hisley, S. M. (2016). *Maternal-child nursing care: Optimizing outcomes for mothers, children, and families* (2nd ed., p. 699). Philadelphia: F.A. Davis.

Figure 7–25. From Durham, R. & Chapman, L. (2014). *Maternal-newborn nursing: The critical components of nursing care* (2nd ed., p. 405). Philadelphia: F.A. Davis.

Acrocyanosis. From Dillon, P. M. (2007). *Nursing health assessment: A critical thinking case studies approach* (2nd ed., pp. 855–867). Philadelphia: F.A. Davis.

Milia. From Dillon, P. M. (2007). *Nursing health assessment: A critical thinking case studies approach* (2nd ed., pp. 855–867). Philadelphia: F.A. Davis.

Lanugo. From Dillon, P. M. (2007). *Nursing health assessment: A critical thinking case studies approach* (2nd ed., pp. 855–867). Philadelphia: F.A. Davis.

Vernix caseosa. From Dillon, P. M. (2007). *Nursing health assessment: A critical thinking case studies approach* (2nd ed., pp. 855–867). Philadelphia: F.A. Davis.

Jaundice. From Dillon, P. M. (2007). *Nursing health assessment: A critical thinking case studies approach* (2nd ed., pp. 855–867). Philadelphia: F.A. Davis.

Epstein's pearls. From Dillon, P. M. (2016). *Nursing health assessment: The foundation of clinical practice* (3rd ed., p. 414). Philadelphia: F.A. Davis.

Natal teeth. From Dillon, P. M. (2016). *Nursing health assessment: The foundation of clinical practice* (3rd ed., p. 414). Philadelphia: F.A. Davis.

Ballard Gestational Age Assessment Tool. From Ballard J. L., et al. (1991). New Ballard score, expanded to include extremely premature infants. *Journal of Pediatrics, 119*, 418. Reprinted with permission.

Chapter 8

Figure 8–1. From Dillon, P. M. (2007). *Nursing health assessment: A critical thinking case studies approach* (2nd ed., p. 893). Philadelphia: F.A. Davis.

Figure 8–2. From the Centers for Disease Control and Prevention (CDC) (2011). https://phil.cdc.gov/ImageidSearch.aspx, ID 14040 Photo Credit: Amanda Mills.

Figure 8–3. **A,** From Merkel, S., et al. (1997). The FLACC: A behavioral scale for scoring postoperative pain in young children. *Pediatric Nurse, 23*(3), 293–297. Copyright 1997 by Jannetti Co., University of Michigan Medical Center. Reprinted with permission. **B,** From Wong-Baker FACES™ Pain Scale, Copyright 1983, Wong-Baker FACES™ Foundation. http://www.WongBakerFACES.org. Reprinted with permission.

Figure 8–5. From Dillon, P.M. (2007). *Nursing health assessment: A critical thinking case studies approach* (2nd ed., p. 895). Philadelphia: F.A. Davis.

Chapter 9

Figures 9–1 and 9–5. Courtesy of Daniel C. Rausch, BSN, RN.

Figure 9–2. From the Centers for Disease Control and Prevention, Joseph Strycharz, Ph.D.; Kyong Sup Yoon, Ph.D.; Frank Collins, Ph.D (2006). https://phil.cdc.gov/ImageidSearch.aspx, ID 10854

Figures 9–3 and 9–4. From the National Highway Traffic Safety Administration Image Library. https://icsw.nhtsa.gov/nhtsa/ImageLibrary/

Chapter 10

Figure 10–1. From the Office of Disease Prevention and Health Promotion. *Healthy People 2020.* http://www.healthypeople.gov

Figure 10–2. From Dillon, P. M. (2007). *Nursing health assessment: A critical thinking case studies approach* (2nd ed., p. 99). Philadelphia: F.A. Davis.

Figure 10–3. From Dillon, P. M. (2016). *Nursing health assessment: The foundation of clinical practice* (3rd ed., p. 227). Philadelphia: F.A. Davis.

Figure 10–4. From Dillon, P. M. (2016). *Nursing health assessment: The foundation of clinical practice* (3rd ed., p. 369). Philadelphia: F.A. Davis.

Figure 10–5. From Dillon, P. M. (2007). *Nursing health assessment: A critical thinking case studies approach* (2nd ed., p. 708). Philadelphia: F.A. Davis.

Stage 1 male sexual development. From Dillon, P. M. (2016). *Nursing health assessment: The foundation of clinical practice* (3rd ed., p. 298). Philadelphia: F.A. Davis.

Stage 2 male sexual development. From Dillon, P. M. (2016). *Nursing health assessment: The foundation of clinical practice* (3rd ed., p. 298). Philadelphia: F.A. Davis.

Stage 3 male sexual development. From Dillon, P. M. (2016). *Nursing health assessment: The foundation of clinical practice* (3rd ed., p. 298). Philadelphia: F.A. Davis.

Stage 4 male sexual development. From Dillon, P. M. (2016). *Nursing health assessment: The foundation of clinical practice* (3rd ed., p. 298). Philadelphia: F.A. Davis.

Stage 5 male sexual development. From Dillon, P. M. (2016). *Nursing health assessment: The foundation of clinical practice* (3rd ed., p. 298). Philadelphia: F.A. Davis.

Stage 1 female maturation. From Dillon, P. M. (2016). *Nursing health assessment: The foundation of clinical practice* (3rd ed., p. 276). Philadelphia: F.A. Davis.

Stage 2 female maturation. From Dillon, P. M. (2016). *Nursing health assessment: The foundation of clinical practice* (3rd ed., p. 276). Philadelphia: F.A. Davis.

Stage 3 female maturation. From Dillon, P. M. (2016). *Nursing health assessment: The foundation of clinical practice* (3rd ed., p. 276). Philadelphia: F.A. Davis.

Stage 4 female maturation. From Dillon, P. M. (2016). *Nursing health assessment: The foundation of clinical practice* (3rd ed., p. 276). Philadelphia: F.A. Davis.

Stage 5 female maturation. From Dillon, P. M. (2016). *Nursing health assessment: The foundation of clinical practice* (3rd ed., p. 276). Philadelphia: F.A. Davis.

Chapter 11

Figure 11–1. From Dillon, P.M. (2007). *Nursing health assessment: A critical thinking case studies approach* (2nd ed., p. 394). Philadelphia: F.A. Davis.

Figure 11–2. From Centers for Disease Control and Prevention (1995), https://phil.cdc.gov/ImageidSearch.aspx, ID 6379.

Figure 11–3. From Dillon, P. M. (2007). *Nursing health assessment: A critical thinking case studies approach* (2nd ed., p. 369). Philadelphia: F.A. Davis.

Figures 11–4, 11–5, and 11–7. From Centers for Disease Control and Prevention, Antibiotic Prescribing and Use in Doctor's Offices, https://www.cdc.gov/antibiotic-use/community/index.html.

Figure 11–6. From Dillon, P. (2016). *Nursing health assessment: The foundation of clinical practice* (3rd ed., p. 99). Philadelphia: F.A. Davis.

Figure 11–9. Images provided by Allergan and Michael Juderka. AeroChamber®, AeroChamber Plus®, Flow-Vu®, AeroChamber Plus Flow-Vu®, ComfortSeal®, and AeroBear® are registered trademarks of Trudell Medical International.

Chapter 12

Figures 12–1, 12–2, and 12–3. From Ward, S. L., & Hisley, S. M. (2016). *Maternal-child nursing care: Optimizing outcomes for mothers, children, and families* (2nd ed., p. 1020). Philadelphia: F.A. Davis.

Figures 12–4 and 12–5. From Ward, S. L., & Hisley, S. M. (2016). *Maternal-child nursing care: Optimizing outcomes for mothers, children, and families* (2nd ed., p. 1021). Philadelphia: F.A. Davis.

Figure 12–6. From Ward, S. L., & Hisley, S. M. (2009). *Maternal-child nursing care: Optimizing outcomes for mothers, children, and families* (Enhanced, revised revision, p. 872). Philadelphia: F.A. Davis.

Figure 12–7. From Ward, S. L., & Hisley, S. M. (2016). *Maternal-child nursing care: Optimizing outcomes for mothers, children, and families* (2nd ed., p. 200). Philadelphia: F.A. Davis.

Figure 12–9. From Ward, S. L., & Hisley, S. M. (2009). *Maternal-child nursing care: Optimizing outcomes for mothers, children, and families* (Enhanced, revised revision, p. 679). Philadelphia: F.A. Davis.

Figure 12–10. From Ward, S. L., & Hisley, S. M. (2016). *Maternal-child nursing care: Optimizing outcomes for mothers, children, and families* (2nd ed., p. 1027). Philadelphia: F.A. Davis.

Figure 12–11. From Ward, S. L., & Hisley, S. M. (2016). *Maternal-child nursing care: Optimizing outcomes for mothers, children, and families* (2nd ed., p. 1025). Philadelphia: F.A. Davis.

Figure 12–12. From Ward, S. L., & Hisley, S. M. (2016). *Maternal-child nursing care: Optimizing outcomes for mothers, children, and families* (2nd ed., p. 1026). Philadelphia: F.A. Davis.

Figures 12–13 and 12–21. From Ward, S. L., & Hisley, S. M. (2016). *Maternal-child nursing care: Optimizing outcomes for mothers, children, and families* (2nd ed., p. 1037). Philadelphia: F.A. Davis.

Figure 12–14. From Centers for Disease Control and Prevention. Congenital heart defects: Tricuspid atresia. https://www.cdc.gov/ncbddd/heartdefects/tricuspid-atresia.html.

Figure 12–16. From Ward, S. L., & Hisley, S. M. (2016). *Maternal-child nursing care: Optimizing outcomes for mothers, children, and families* (2nd ed., p. 1030). Philadelphia: F.A. Davis.

Figures 12–17 and 12–18. From Ward, S. L., & Hisley, S. M. (2016). *Maternal-child nursing care: Optimizing outcomes for mothers, children, and families* (2nd ed., p. 1029). Philadelphia: F.A. Davis.

Figure 12–19. From Ward, S. L., & Hisley, S. M. (2016). *Maternal-child nursing care: Optimizing outcomes for mothers, children, and families* (2nd ed., p. 1031). Philadelphia: F.A. Davis.

Figures 12–20 and 12–22. From Ward, S. L., & Hisley, S. M. (2016). *Maternal-child nursing care: Optimizing outcomes for mothers, children, and families* (2nd ed., p. 1035). Philadelphia: F.A. Davis.

Figure 12–23. From Ward, S. L., & Hisley, S. M. (2016). *Maternal-child nursing care: Optimizing outcomes for mothers, children, and families* (2nd ed., p. 1038). Philadelphia: F.A. Davis.

Figure 12–24. From Ward, S. L., & Hisley, S. M. (2016). *Maternal-child nursing care: Optimizing outcomes for mothers, children, and families* (2nd ed., p. 1034). Philadelphia: F.A. Davis.

Chapter 13

Figures 13–1, 13–3, 13–7, and 13–9. From Gilman, S., & Newman, S. W. (2003). *Manter and Gatz's essentials of clinical neuroanatomy and neurophysiology* (10th ed.) Philadelphia: F.A. Davis.

Figure 13–2. From Scanlon, V., & Sanders, T. (2015). *Essentials of anatomy and physiology* (7th ed., p. 195). Philadelphia: F.A. Davis.

Figure 13-6. Courtesy of the Epilepsy Foundation of America, Washington, D.C. Reprinted with permission.

Tonic neck reflex. From Dillon, P. M. (2016). *Nursing health assessment: The foundation of clinical practice* (3rd ed., p. 421). Philadelphia: F.A. Davis.

Palmar grasp reflex. From Dillon, P. M. (2016). *Nursing health assessment: The foundation of clinical practice* (3rd ed., p. 421). Philadelphia: F.A. Davis.

Moro flex or startle reflex. From Dillon, P. M. (2016). *Nursing health assessment: The foundation of clinical practice* (3rd ed., p. 421). Philadelphia: F.A. Davis.

Blinking (glabellar). From Dillon, P. M. (2016). *Nursing health assessment: The foundation of clinical practice* (3rd ed., p. 424). Philadelphia: F.A. Davis.

Babinski reflex. From Dillon, P. M. (2016). *Nursing health assessment: The foundation of clinical practice* (3rd ed., p. 422). Philadelphia: F.A. Davis.

Rooting reflex. From Dillon, P. M. (2016). *Nursing health assessment: The foundation of clinical practice* (3rd ed., p. 423). Philadelphia: F.A. Davis.

Stepping reflex. From Dillon, P. M. (2016). *Nursing health assessment: The foundation of clinical practice* (3rd ed., p. 422). Philadelphia: F.A. Davis.

Sucking reflex. From Dillon, P. M. (2016). *Nursing health assessment: The foundation of clinical practice* (3rd ed., p. 423). Philadelphia: F.A. Davis.

Traction (pull to sit). From Dillon, P. M. (2016). *Nursing health assessment: The foundation of clinical practice* (3rd ed., p. 425). Philadelphia: F.A. Davis.

Chapter 14

Figure 14–1. From the National Institute on Drug Abuse, "Drugs, Brains, and Behavior: The Science of Addiction," August 2010. Retrieved October 10, 2012, from http://www.drugabuse.gov/publications/science-addiction/drugs-brain.

Figure 14–2. From "Sniffing Markers Destroys Your Brain," reproduced with permission from the National Inhalant Prevention Coalition, 1991.

Chapter 15

Figures 15–1. From Scanlon, V., & Sanders, T. (2011). *Essentials of anatomy and physiology* (6th ed., p. 399). Philadelphia: F.A. Davis.

Chapter 16

Grade 1. From Custer, J., and R. Rau (2009). The Harriet Lane Handbook: A Manual for Pediatric House Officers, 17th Edition. Reprinted with permission from Elsevier Mosby.

Grade 2. From Custer, J., and R. Rau (2009). The Harriet Lane Handbook: A Manual for Pediatric House Officers, 17th Edition. Reprinted with permission from Elsevier Mosby.

Grade 3. From Custer, J., and R. Rau (2009). The Harriet Lane Handbook: A Manual for Pediatric House Officers, 17th Edition. Reprinted with permission from Elsevier Mosby.

Grade 4. From Custer, J., and R. Rau (2009). The Harriet Lane Handbook: A Manual for Pediatric House Officers, 17th Edition. Reprinted with permission from Elsevier Mosby.

Grade 5. From Custer, J., and R. Rau (2009). The Harriet Lane Handbook: A Manual for Pediatric House Officers, 17th Edition. Reprinted with permission from Elsevier Mosby.

Chapter 17

Figure 17–3. From Ward, S. L., & Hisley, S. M. (2016). *Maternal-child nursing care: Optimizing outcomes for mothers, children, and families* (2nd ed., p. 1097). Philadelphia: F.A. Davis.

Figure 17–4. From Ward, S. L., & Hisley, S. M. (2016). *Maternal-child nursing care: Optimizing outcomes for mothers, children, and families* (2nd ed., p. 1100). Philadelphia: F.A. Davis.

Teaching Parents How to Inject Insulin. From Ward, S. L., & Hisley, S. M. (2016). *Maternal-child nursing care: Optimizing outcomes for mothers, children, and families* (2nd ed., p. 1099). Philadelphia: F.A. Davis.

Chapter 18

Figure 18–1. From Ward, S. L., & Hisley, S. M. (2016). *Maternal-child nursing care: Optimizing outcomes for mothers, children, and families* (2nd ed., p. 138). Philadelphia: F.A. Davis.

Figure 18–2. From Dillon, P. M. (2007). *Nursing health assessment: A critical thinking case studies approach* (2nd ed., p. 612). Philadelphia: F.A. Davis.

Figure 18–3. From the Centers for Disease Control and Prevention, Department of Health and Human Services. (1979). Retrieved from https://phil.cdc.gov/ImageidSearch.aspx, ID 4819.

Figure 18–4. From the Centers for Disease Control and Prevention, Department of Health and Human Services. (1978). Retrieved from https://phil.cdc.gov/ImageidSearch.aspx, ID 3719.

Figure 18–5. From Dillon, P. M. (2007). *Nursing health assessment: A critical thinking case studies approach* (2nd ed., p. 613). Philadelphia: F.A. Davis.

Figure 18–6. From Scanlon, V., & Sanders, T. (2015). *Essentials of anatomy and physiology* (7th ed., p. 503). Philadelphia: F.A. Davis.

Figure 18–7. From Ward, S. L., & Hisley, S. M. (2016). *Maternal-child nursing care: Optimizing outcomes for mothers, children, and families* (2nd ed., p. 699). Philadelphia: F.A. Davis.

Figure 18–8. From Dillon, P. M. (2016). *Nursing health assessment: The foundation of clinical practice* (3rd ed., p. 309). Philadelphia: F.A. Davis.

Figure 18–9. From Centers for Disease Control and Prevention, Department of Health and Human Services. (1986). Retrieved from https://phil.cdc.gov/ImageidSearch.aspx, ID 5237

Figure 18–10. From Centers for Disease Control and Prevention, Department of Health and Human Services. (1963). Retrieved from https://phil.cdc.gov/ImageidSearch.aspx, ID 2246

Figure 18–11. From the National Cancer Institute, U.S. National Institutes of Health. (1988). Retrieved from http://visualsonline.cancer.gov/details.cfm?imageid=2323

Figure 18–12. **A,** From Centers for Disease Control and Prevention, Department of Health and Human Services, and Dr. Godfrey P. Oakley. (1974). Retrieved from https://phil.cdc.gov/ImageidSearch.aspx, ID 2634. **B,** Courtesy of D.M. Kocisko.

Figure 18–13. From Dillon, P. M. (2016). *Nursing health assessment: The foundation of clinical practice* (3rd ed., p. 142). Philadelphia: F.A. Davis.

Figure 18–15. Copyright www.genetic-diseases.net. Reprinted with permission.

Figure 18–16. From Centers for Disease Control and Prevention, Department of Health and Human Services. Retrieved from https://phil.cdc.gov/ImageidSearch.aspx, ID 2567

Chapter 19

Figure 19–1. From the Centers for Disease Control and Prevention/Sickle Cell Foundation of Georgia, Jackie George, Beverly Sinclair. (2009). Photograph by Janice Haney Carr. Retrieved from https://phil.cdc.gov/ImageidSearch.aspx, ID 11690.

Figure 19–2. From the Centers for Disease Control and Prevention, Aaron L. Sussell. (1999). Retrieved from https://phil.cdc.gov/ImageidSearch.aspx, ID 73333.

Figure 19–3. From the Centers for Disease Control and Prevention, Cynthia Goldsmith. Retrieved from https://phil.cdc.gov/ImageidSearch.aspx, ID 8241.

Figure 19–6. From Ward, S. L., & Hisley, S. M. (2009). *Maternal-child nursing care: Optimizing outcomes for mothers, children, and families* (Enhanced, revised revision, p. 1357). Philadelphia: F.A. Davis.

Figure 19–7. From Ward, S. L., & Hisley, S. M. (2009). *Maternal-child nursing care: Optimizing outcomes for mothers, children, and families* (Enhanced, revised revision, p. 1374). Philadelphia: F.A. Davis.

Figure 19–8. From the Centers for Disease Control and Prevention, Robert S. Craig. (1967). Retrieved from https://phil.cdc.gov/ImageidSearch.aspx, ID 6050.

Figures 19–9 and 19–11. From the National Cancer Institute.

Figure 19–10. From the Centers for Disease Control and Prevention, James Gathany. (2005). Retrieved from https://phil.cdc.gov/ImageidSearch.aspx, ID 8277.

Chapter 20

Figure 20–1. From Dillon, P. M. (2007). *Nursing health assessment: A critical thinking case studies approach* (2nd ed., p. 687). Philadelphia: F.A. Davis.

Figure 20–2. From Ward, S. L., & Hisley, S. M. (2016). *Maternal-child nursing care: Optimizing outcomes for mothers, children, and families* (2nd ed., p. 1173). Philadelphia: F.A. Davis.

Figure 20–3. From Ward, S. L., & Hisley, S. M. (2016). *Maternal-child nursing care: Optimizing outcomes for mothers, children, and families* (2nd ed., p. 1197). Philadelphia: F.A. Davis.

Figure 20–17. From Ward, S. L., & Hisley, S. M. (2016). *Maternal-child nursing care: Optimizing outcomes for mothers, children, and families* (2nd ed., p. 1185). Philadelphia: F.A. Davis.

Figure 20–18. From Wise, C. (2015). *Orthopaedic manual therapy: From art to evidence* (5th ed.). Philadelphia: F.A. Davis.

Figure 20–19. From Legangie, P., & Norkin, C. (2011). *Joint structure and function* (5th ed.). Philadelphia: F.A. Davis.

Figure 20–20. From May, B., & Lockard, M. (2011). *Prosthetics & orthotics in clinical practice*. Philadelphia: F.A. Davis.

Chapter 21

Figure 21–1. From Curley, M. A. Q., Razmus, I. S., Roberts, K. E., & Wypij, D. (2003 January/February). Predicting pressure ulcer risk in pediatric patients: The Braden Q Scale. *Nursing Research, 52*(1), 22–23. Reprinted with permission.

Figure 21–3. From Dillon, P. M. (2016). *Nursing health assessment: The foundation of clinical practice* (3rd ed., p. 72). Philadelphia: F.A. Davis.

Figure 21–4. From Dillon, P. M. (2007). *Nursing health assessment: A critical thinking case studies approach* (2nd ed., p. 258). Philadelphia: F.A. Davis.

Figures 21–5 and 21–6. From Freiman, A., & Barankin, B. (2006). *Derm notes: Dermatology clinical pocket guide* (p. 53). Philadelphia: F.A. Davis.

Figure 21–7. From Freiman, A., & Barankin, B. (2006). *Derm notes: Dermatology clinical pocket guide* (p. 104). Philadelphia: F.A. Davis.

Figure 21–8. From Dillon, P. M. (2016). *Nursing health assessment: The foundation of clinical practice* (3rd ed., p. 63). Philadelphia: F.A. Davis.

Figure 21–9. From Dillon, P. M. (2016). *Nursing health assessment: The foundation of clinical practice* (3rd ed., p. 55). Philadelphia: F.A. Davis.

Figure 21–10. From Dillon, P. M. (2016). *Nursing health assessment: The foundation of clinical practice* (3rd ed., p. 121). Philadelphia: F.A. Davis.

Figure 21–11. From Freiman, A., & Barankin, B. (2006). *Derm notes: Dermatology clinical pocket guide* (p. 142). Philadelphia: F.A. Davis.

Figure 21–12. From the Centers for Disease Control and Prevention, Department of Health and Human Services, 2007. Retrieved from https://phil.cdc.gov/ImageidSearch.aspx, ID 9875.

Figure 21–13. From Freiman, A., & Barankin, B. (2006). *Derm notes: Dermatology clinical pocket guide* (p. 144). Philadelphia: F.A. Davis.

Figure 21–14. From Taber's Cyclopedic Medical Dictionary Index (22nd ed.). (2016). Philadelphia: F.A. Davis.

Figure 21–15. From Freiman, A., & Barankin, B. (2006). *Derm notes: Dermatology clinical pocket guide* (p. 194). Philadelphia: F.A. Davis.

Chapter 22

Figure 22–1. From the Centers for Disease Control and Prevention. (2018). Birth-18 years Recommended Immunization Schedule. Retrieved from https://www.cdc.gov/vaccines/schedules/hcp/imz/child-adolescent.html.

Figure 22–2. From the Centers for Disease Control and Prevention, Department of Health and Human Services. Retrieved from http://www.nlm.nih.gov/medlineplus/fifthdisease.html.

Figure 22–3. From Freiman, A., & Barankin, B. (2006). *Derm Notes: Dermatology Clinical Pocket Guide* (p. 95). Philadelphia: F.A. Davis.

Figure 22–4. From the Centers for Disease Control and Prevention, Department of Health and Human Services, Dr. N. J. Flumara, Dr. Gavin Hart (1976). Retrieved from https://phil.cdc.gov/ImageidSearch.aspx, ID 3805

Figure 22–5. From the Centers for Disease Control and Prevention, Department of Health and Human Services, NIP/Barbara Rice (1976). Retrieved from http://phil.cdc.gov/phil/details.asp?pid=130

Figure 22–6. From the Centers for Disease Control and Prevention, Department of Health and Human Services, Arthur E. Kaye (1969). Retrieved from https://phil.cdc.gov/ImageidSearch.aspx, ID 3318.

Figure 22–7. From the Centers for Disease Control and Prevention, Department of Health and Human Services (1975). Retrieved from https://phil.cdc.gov/ImageidSearch.aspx, ID 4514.

Figure 22–8. From the Centers for Disease Control and Prevention, Department of Health and Human Services, Dr. Heinz F. Eichenwald. (1958). Retrieved from https://phil.cdc.gov/ImageidSearch.aspx, ID 3187.

Figure 22–9. From the Centers for Disease Control and Prevention, Department of Health and Human Services, Dr. Heinz F. Eichenwald. (1958). Retrieved from https://phil.cdc.gov/ImageidSearch.aspx, ID 3168.

Figure 22–10. From the Centers for Disease Control and Prevention, Department of Health and Human Services (1995). Retrieved from https://phil.cdc.gov/ImageidSearch.aspx, ID 6121.

Figure 22–11. From the Centers for Disease Control and Prevention, Department of Health and Human Services, Joe Miller, V.D. (1976). Retrieved from https://phil.cdc.gov/ImageidSearch.aspx, ID 6784.

Figure 22–12. From the Centers for Disease Control and Prevention, Department of Health and Human Services, Dr. M. Moody (n.d.). Retrieved from https://phil.cdc.gov/ImageidSearch.aspx, ID 10190.

Figure 22–13. From the Centers for Disease Control and Prevention, Department of Health and Human Services (1975). Retrieved from https://phil.cdc.gov/ImageidSearch.aspx, ID 5163.

Figure 22–14. From the Centers for Disease Control and Prevention, Department of Health and Human Services (1984). Retrieved from https://phil.cdc.gov/ImageidSearch.aspx, ID 5120.

INDEX

Note: A *b* indicates content appears in a boxed feature on the page. An *f* indicates a figure. A *t* indicates a table.

B

C

F

J

K

L

M

Q

R

S

T

U

V

W

X

Z